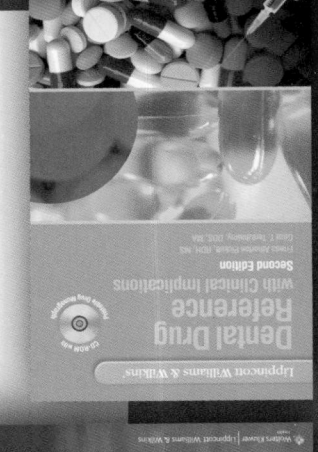
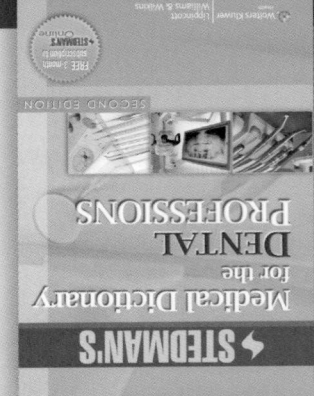
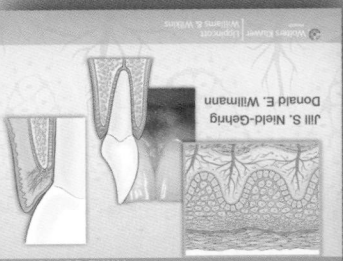
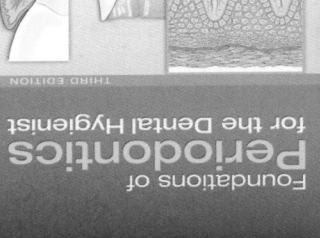
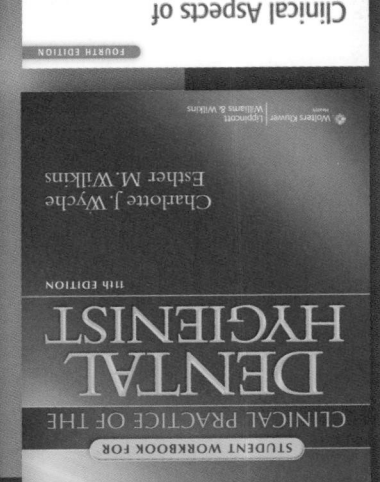

CONTENTS

CLINICAL PRACTICE OF THE
DENTAL HYGIENIST

11th EDITION

Esther M. Wilkins, BS, RDH, DMD

Department of Periodontology
Tufts University, School of Dental Medicine
Boston, Massachusetts
and
Forsyth School of Dental Hygiene
Massachusetts College of Pharmacy and Health Sciences
Boston, Massachusetts

Contributing Editor

Charlotte J. Wyche, RDH, MS

Department of Periodontics and Oral Medicine
University of Michigan School of Dentistry
Ann Arbor, Michigan

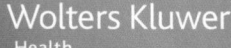
Wolters Kluwer | Lippincott Williams & Wilkins
Health
Philadelphia · Baltimore · New York · London
Buenos Aires · Hong Kong · Sydney · Tokyo

Acquisitions Editor: Julie Stegman
Managing Editor: Meredith L. Brittain
Marketing Manager: Shauna Kelley
Designer: Doug Smock
Production Service: Aptara, Inc.

Eleventh Edition

© 2013 by LIPPINCOTT WILLIAMS & WILKINS, a WOLTERS KLUWER business
Two Commerce Square
2001 Market Street
Philadelphia, PA 19103 USA
LWW.com

Printed in China

Library of Congress Cataloging-in-Publication Data

Wilkins, Esther M.
  Clinical practice of the dental hygienist / Esther M. Wilkins;
contributing editor, Charlotte J. Wyche. – 11th ed.
  p. ; cm.
  Includes bibliographical references and index.
  ISBN 978-1-60831-718-9
  I. Wyche, Charlotte J. II. Title.
  [DNLM: 1. Dental Prophylaxis–Outlines. 2. Dental
Hygienists–Outlines. WU 18.2]
  617.6′01–dc23

                    2011042671

Care has been taken to confirm the accuracy of the information presented and to describe generally accepted practices. However, the authors, editors, and publisher are not responsible for errors or omissions or for any consequences from application of the information in this book and make no warranty, expressed or implied, with respect to the currency, completeness, or accuracy of the contents of the publication. Application of the information in a particular situation remains the professional responsibility of the practitioner.

The authors, editors, and publisher have exerted every effort to ensure that drug selection and dosage set forth in this text are in accordance with current recommendations and practice at the time of publication. However, in view of ongoing research, changes in government regulations, and the constant flow of information relating to drug therapy and drug reactions, the reader is urged to check the package insert for each drug for any change in indications and dosage and for added warnings and precautions. This is particularly important when the recommended agent is a new or infrequently employed drug.

Some drugs and medical devices presented in the publication have Food and Drug Administration (FDA) clearance for limited use in restricted research settings. It is the responsibility of the health care provider to ascertain the FDA status of each drug or device planned for use in their clinical practice.

To purchase additional copies of this book, call our customer service department at (800) 638-3030 or fax orders to (301) 223-2320. International customers should call (301) 223-2300.

Visit Lippincott Williams & Wilkins on the Internet: at LWW.com. Lippincott Williams & Wilkins customer service representatives are available from 8:30 am to 6 pm, EST.

                                        10 9 8 7 6 5 4 3

CCS0614

DEDICATION

The eleventh edition of *Clinical Practice of the Dental Hygienist* is dedicated to all past and present students who have studied from the ten preceding editions. Gratitude is expressed to their teachers in the many different dental hygiene programs around the world, for their leadership in, and devotion to, dental hygiene education.

A very special recognition goes to the students of the first ten classes in dental hygiene at the University of Washington in Seattle for whom the original "mimeographed" syllabus was created. They are remembered with much appreciation because their need for text study material made this book possible in the first place.

Esther M. Wilkins

CONTRIBUTORS

Caren M. Barnes, RDH, BS, MS
Department of Dental Hygiene
University of Nebraska Medical Center, College of
    Dentistry
Lincoln, Nebraska

Barbara L. Bennett, CDA, RDH, MS
Department of Dental Hygiene, Allied Health Division
Texas State Technical College
Harlingen, Texas

Elain Benton, RDH, BS, CTTS
Department of Public Health Sciences
Texas A&M HSC Baylor College of Dentistry
Dallas, Texas

Sara L. Beres, RDH, BA, MS
Department of Dental Hygiene
Sheridan College
Sheridan, Wyoming

Tessie Lamadrid Black, RDH, BS
Consultant
Braintree, Massachusetts

Patricia A. Cohen, RDH, BS, MS
Department of Periodontology
School of Dental Medicine
Tufts University
Boston, Massachusetts

Marilyn Cortell, RDH, MS
Department of Dental Hygiene
New York City College of Technology
Brooklyn, New York

Jane Carolyn Cotter, RDH, MS
Department of Dental Hygiene
Texas A&M HSC Baylor College of Dentistry
Dallas, Texas

Ernestine R. Daniels, RDH, BS
Department of Dental Hygiene
Florida State College at Jacksonville
Jacksonville, Florida

Kathryn Ragalis Davis, RDH, MS, DMD
Department of General Dentistry
Tufts University School of Dental Medicine
Boston, Massachusetts

Barbara Dawidjan, RDH, MEd
Quinsigamond Community College
Worcester, Massachusetts

Teresa Butler Duncan, RDH, BS
Department of Dental Hygiene
School of Health Related Professions
University of Mississippi Medical Center
Jackson, Mississippi

Janet M. Gruber, RDH, MPA
Department of Dental Hygiene
Farmingdale State College of New York
Farmingdale, New York

Donna F. Homenko, RDH, MEd, PhD
Department of Dental Hygiene and Bioethics
Cuyahoga Community College
Cleveland, Ohio

Janis G. Keating, RDH, MA
Dental Professional Sales
Philips Sonicare
Stamford, Connecticut

Pamela S. Kennard, BSN, RDH, MA
Department of Dental Hygiene
State College of Florida
Bradenton, Florida

Cynthia Biron Leiseca, RDH, EMT, MA
DH Methods of Education, Inc.
Fernandina Beach
Amelia Island, Florida

Judi S. Luxmore, RDH, BAS, MS
(Retired) Department of Periodontology and
    Dental Hygiene
University of Detroit Mercy School of Dentistry
Detroit, Michigan

Deborah M. Lyle, RDH, BS, MS
Department of Marketing
Water Pik, Inc.
Morris Plains, New Jersey

Deborah S. Manne, RDH, RN, MSN, OCN
Department of Otolaryngology—Head and Neck Surgery
St. Louis University School of Medicine
St. Louis, Missouri

Stacy A. Matsuda, RDH, BS, MS
Department of Periodontology
School of Dentistry
Oregon Health and Science University
Portland, Oregon

Durinda J. Mattana, RDH, MS
Department of Periodontology and Dental Hygiene
School of Dentistry
University of Detroit-Mercy
Detroit, Michigan

Laura Mueller-Joseph, RDH, MS, EdD
Department of Dental Hygiene
Farmingdale State College
Farmingdale, New York

Luisa Nappo-Dattoma, RDH, RD, EdD
Department of Dental Hygiene
Farmingdale State College
Farmingdale, New York

Karen A. Raposa, RDH, MBA
Clinical Education Manager
Hu-Friedy Manufacturing Co., LLC
Chicago, Illinois

Pamela S. Ridilla, RDH, MS
School of Dental Sciences
Daytona State College
Daytona Beach, Florida

Janet B. Selwitz-Segal, RDH, CDA, MS
(Retired) Massachusetts College of Pharmacy and
    Health Sciences
Boston, Massachusetts

Donna J. Stach, RDH, MEd
Department of Surgical Dentistry, Division of
    Periodontics
School of Dental Medicine
University of Colorado
Aurora, Colorado

Tammy K. Swecker, BSDH, MEd
Division of Dental Hygiene
Virginia Commonwealth University
Richmond, Virginia

Terri S. I. Tilliss, RDH, MS, MA, PhD
Department of Graduate Orthodontics
School of Dental Medicine
University of Colorado
Aurora, Colorado

Esther M. Wilkins, BS, RDH, DMD
Department of Periodontology
School of Dental Medicine
Tufts University
Boston, Massachusetts

Lane Wilson-Foreman, CDA, RDH, BS
Department of Dental Health Programs
Tallahassee Community College
Tallahassee, Florida

Charlotte J. Wyche, RDH, MS
Department of Periodontics and Oral Medicine
University of Michigan School of Dentistry
Ann Arbor, Michigan

Dental hygienists are oral healthcare specialists with professional goals centered on the prevention and/or control of oral disease and the maintenance of oral and general health. As primary health care professionals, dental hygienists can apply their knowledge and skills in a wide variety of areas related to clinical practice, education, research, public health, and advocacy for health promotion and disease prevention. Dental hygienists collaborate with dentists and members of other health professions to provide oral health care that links with total body health care. New emphasis on the effect of oral health on systemic health challenges dental hygienists to widen their scope of practice.

OBJECTIVES

Objectives of the 11th edition include:

- To help prepare the beginning dental hygiene student to recognize the requirements of evidence-based dental hygiene practice.
- To develop skills and knowledge for entry into the profession.
- To help when studying for Licensure Board examinations; the condensed outline form aids to make review easier.
- To update professional hygienists already in practice, and assist long-term practitioners to recognize the new responsibility to apply evidence-based scientific approaches to patient care.

THE TEXTBOOK PLAN

Highlights

Highlights of *Clinical Practice of the Dental Hygienist*, 11th edition include

- New chapters for orientation to clinical practice describe Evidence-based Dental Hygiene Practice (Chapter 2) and Effective Health Communication (Chapter 3).
- Emphasis on professional ethics starts in the opening chapter and threaded throughout the text.
- Essential to preparation for practice is the application all-necessary attention to infection control for practitioners and patients during all clinical procedures.

- Three chapters (Chapters 4, 6, and 7) include infection control and ergonomic health for the clinical practitioner and patient.
- The final chapter in Section I, Orientation to Clinical Dental Hygiene Practice, is Chapter 8, Introduction to Documentation. Documentation is the newest addition to the Dental Hygiene Process of Care, which is illustrated Figure I-1.

Organization of the Textbook

As in past editions, sections of *Clinical Practice of the Dental Hygienist* are sequenced to conform to the Dental Hygiene Process of Care. There are eight sections in the 11th edition, five of which are specifically identified by name with the recognized components of the Process of Care. They are: *assessment, dental hygiene diagnosis, care planning, implementation,* and *evaluation.*

The textbook opens with chapters devoted to an introduction to the profession of dental hygiene and chapters related to preparation for practice. They include infection control and ergonomic health for the clinical practitioner and patient. The final large section, Section VIII, applies the process of care to patients with special needs.

The eight major sections are:

    I. Orientation to Clinical Dental Hygiene Practice
   II. Preparation for Dental Hygiene Practice
  III. The Process of Care: Assessment
  IV. The Process of Care: Dental Hygiene Diagnosis and Care Planning
   V. The Process of Care: Implementation: Prevention
  VI. The Process of Care: Implementation: Clinical Treatment
 VII. The Process of Care: Evaluation of Dental Hygiene Care Outcomes
VIII. Patients With Special Needs

Supplementary information is available in Appendices:

    I. American Dental Hygienists' Association Code of Ethics for Dental Hygienists
   II. Canadian Dental Hygienists' Association Code of Ethics
  III. International Federation of Dental Hygienists Code of Ethics

IV. Guidelines for Infection Control in Dental Health-Care Settings—2003
V. Average Measurements of Human Teeth
VI. Prefixes, Suffixes, and Combining Forms
VII. Charting Symbols and Standardized Abbreviations Useful for Documenting Dental Hygiene Care

FEATURES OF THE NEW EDITION

All chapters have been updated, and many have been extensively revised. Each chapter includes the following features:

- Detailed **outline format** for the text makes it easier to study and locate information quickly. In this era of information growth related to new research and products available for professional clinical practice as well as teaching patients self-care, the condensation of printed material into outline form can provide busy, overloaded students with a new efficiency for learning.
- **Chapter outlines** at the opening of each chapter provide a preliminary review for readers before they start to concentrate on the meat of the chapter; the outline can help readers locate material within the chapter at any time.
- **Key Words boxes** near the beginning of each chapter identify spelling and definition for the new vocabulary of the particular chapter. Each key word is listed in the index, so a quick reference to definitions in other chapters is possible.
- **Everyday Ethics boxes** ("EEs") provide students with the opportunity to become aware of and discuss clinical problems from real-life practice. Principles of ethical dental hygiene practice need to be brought into the curriculum at an early stage if students are to develop into ethical practitioners. This feature has been continued from previous editions because of expressed appreciation of teachers and students. Previously used "EEs" have been revised and many new ones created.
- **Factors to Teach the Patient boxes** have been an appreciated feature for many editions. They help students to select topics from the chapter that need special emphasis while teaching patients self-care and responsibility for oral health for their own lifetime as well as that of their family and community.
- **Emphasis on the new sixth section of the Process of Care, Documentation,** brings to full cycle the clinical care of a patient. Having sample Progress notes for the varieties of patients illustrated in this textbook can increase students' awareness of the significance of such notes in the permanent record of each patient.
- New to this edition, **a video camera icon** appears next to those sections for which video clips are available on the companion website. See the

"Additional Resources" section of this preface for more information.

STUDENT WORKBOOK

A unique study guide, *Student Workbook for Clinical Practice of the Dental Hygienist,* prepared by Charlotte J. Wyche for the 9th and 10th editions, has been recognized as a major contribution to student learning. The 11th edition workbook, revised to highlight new chapters and updated information from the textbook, also contains revised crossword and word search puzzles.

Everyday Ethics boxes in the workbook include new individual learning, cooperative learning, or discovery activities designed to help the student reflect on or apply ethical theory-related "Questions for Consideration" found in the textbook. Activities and questions related to patient case scenarios, patient assessment summaries, and documentation of patient care provide an emphasis on case-based application of knowledge.

ADDITIONAL RESOURCES

Clinical Practice of the Dental Hygienist, 11th edition includes additional resources for both instructors and students that are available on the book's companion Web site at http://thepoint.lww.com/Wilkins11e.

Instructors

Approved adopting instructors will be given access to the following additional resources:

- Brownstone test generator
- PowerPoint presentations
- Lesson plans
- Image bank of all the images and tables in the book
- WebCT and Blackboard ready cartridge
- Answers to the exercises found in *Student Workbook to Accompany Clinical Practice of the Dental Hygienist,* by Charlotte J. Wyche and Esther M. Wilkins (book available for separate purchase)

Students

Students who have purchased *Clinical Practice of the Dental Hygienist,* 11th edition have access to the following additional resources:

- 20 videos that show techniques and procedures
- Quiz bank
- Stedman's audio pronunciation guide for select clinical terms, customized to the text

In addition, purchasers of the text can access the searchable full text online by going to the *Clinical Practice of the Dental Hygienist,* 11th edition Web site at http://thePoint.lww.com/Wilkins11e. See the inside front cover of this text for more details, including the passcode you will need to gain access to the Web site.

ACKNOWLEDGMENTS

A textbook of the size and scope of *Clinical Practice of the Dental Hygienist* shows the work of many contributors. Comments and suggestions come from teachers, students, and practitioners from around the world, as the book has been translated into a variety of languages. Any suggestion, whether for one word or whole chapters, is welcomed and considered. It is hoped that this new edition will bring comments and requests as in the past.

Recognition for Our Contributors

We start with expressed recognition and appreciation to our listed contributors (pages iv to v) for their new or revised chapters or other assigned responsibility. Each has spent much time for selective revision and to survey the literature for new material and references.

Other Appreciation

Appreciation is expressed to the following:

K. Vendrell Rankin, DDS. This professor, associate chair, and certified tobacco treatment specialist in the Department of Public Health Science at Texas A&M Health Science Center Baylor College of Dentistry is recognized for providing information and guidance for Chapter 33, The Patient Who Uses Tobacco.

Marcia Williams of Newton, Massachusetts. Many illustrations for this and previous editions have been the work of our talented artist. Her personal interest and patience in preparing new, revising previous, and adding color to enhance the line drawings, is acknowledged with sincere gratitude.

Pamela Breitschneider, BA, MEd, PhD. For her help with many chapters for computer searches for the new research provided over the entire 2 to 3 years while revision was in action, generous assistance is greatly appreciated.

Marie V. Gillis, RDH, MS. Marie is recognized for contributions in the revision of Chapter 30, The Patient with Orthodontic Appliances, and for her work on the videos available on the book's companion website (see the "Additional Resources" section earlier in this preface for details).

Gail Schoonmaker. Gail was instrumental in restyling many of the references to conform with the National Library of Medicine style, formatting many of the tables, and seeking the permissions for the book.

The Community College of Philadelphia. This school, its students, and its faculty hosted and appear in the videos found on this book's companion Web site (see the "Additional Resources" section earlier in this preface for details). Special thanks go to Theresa Grady, RDH, MEd, Dental Hygiene Program Director, for coordinating the location, props, and models for the videos.

Our Readers. And, finally, an expression of appreciation goes to our readers over the years: students, teachers, and practicing dental hygienists. Send us your comments and suggestions. As stated in the first edition: It is hoped that through greater understanding of each patient's oral and general health needs, more complete and effective dental hygiene services can be rendered.

Esther M. Wilkins

REVIEWERS

Barbara Adams, RDH, BS, MA
Dental Hygiene
Wallace State Community College
Hanceville, Alabama

Sandra Nagel Beebe, RDH, PhD
Southern Illinois University Carbondale
Carbondale, Illinois

LynnAnn B. Bryan, BSDH, MEd
Marquette University School of Dentistry
Milwaukee, Wisconsin

Mychelle Vedder-Burton
CUNY Hostos
Bronx, New York

Dianne Chadbourne, RDH, BS, MDH
MCPHS/Forsyth School of Dental Hygiene
Boston, Massachusetts

Kimberlee Clark, RDH, BS, MEd
Dental Hygiene
Western Career College-San Jose
San Jose, California

Charles Crosby, DDS, JD
Dental Health Professions
York Technical College
Rock Hill, South Carolina

Barbara R. Ellis, RDH, MA
Monroe Community College
Rochester, New York

Marie Varley Gillis, RDH, MS
(Retired) Education Affiliates
Washington, DC

Jane Gray, RDH, MEd
University of Oklahoma College of Dentistry
Oklahoma City, Oklahoma

Sheila Gross, CDA, RDH, BA, MS
Health Sciences
Northeast Wisconsin Technical College
Green Bay, Wisconsin

Stephanie Harrison, BS, MA
Dental Hygiene
Community College of Denver
Denver, Colorado

Sherry Heaney, RDHAP, MEd
Dental Hygiene
Western Career College
San Jose, California

Suzette Jestin, CDA, PID, BEd
Dental
Vancouver Community College and University of British
    Columbia
Vancouver, British Columbia

Heather Nelson
Columbia College
Calgary, Alberta

Carolyn Ray, RDH, MEd
Dental Hygiene
University of Oklahoma
Oklahoma City, Oklahoma

Salim Rayman
Hostos Community College
Bronx, New York

David Reff, BS, DDS
Dental Assisting and Dental Hygiene Programs
Apollo College
Boise, Idaho

Amanda Richardson, RDH, BS
Department of Dental Hygiene
University of Louisiana at Monroe
Caldwell Hall Monroe, Louisiana

Judy Romano, AS, BS, MA
Dental Hygiene/Dental Assisting
Hudson Valley Community College
Troy, New York

Natalie Vanoli, RDH, BS, RDHAP
Dental Hygiene
Western Career College
San Jose, California

Lucille Ann Zarbo
School of Dental Hygiene
Erie Community College
Williamsville, New York

CONTENTS

CHAPTER 5

EXPOSURE CONTROL: BARRIERS FOR PATIENT AND CLINICIAN   60

CHAPTER 6

INFECTION CONTROL: CLINICAL PROCEDURES   72

CHAPTER 7

PATIENT RECEPTION AND ERGONOMIC PRACTICE   88

CHAPTER 8

INTRODUCTION TO DOCUMENTATION   100

SECTION III

ASSESSMENT   113

CHAPTER 9

PERSONAL, DENTAL, AND MEDICAL HISTORIES   115

CHAPTER 26

PROTOCOLS FOR PREVENTION AND CONTROL OF DENTAL CARIES 377

CHAPTER 27

ORAL INFECTION CONTROL: TOOTHBRUSHES AND TOOTHBRUSHING 386

CHAPTER 28

INTERDENTAL CARE AND IRRIGATION 408

CHAPTER 29

DENTIFRICES AND MOUTHRINSES 423

CHAPTER 30

THE PATIENT WITH ORTHODONTIC APPLIANCES 436

Orientation to Clinical Dental Hygiene Practice

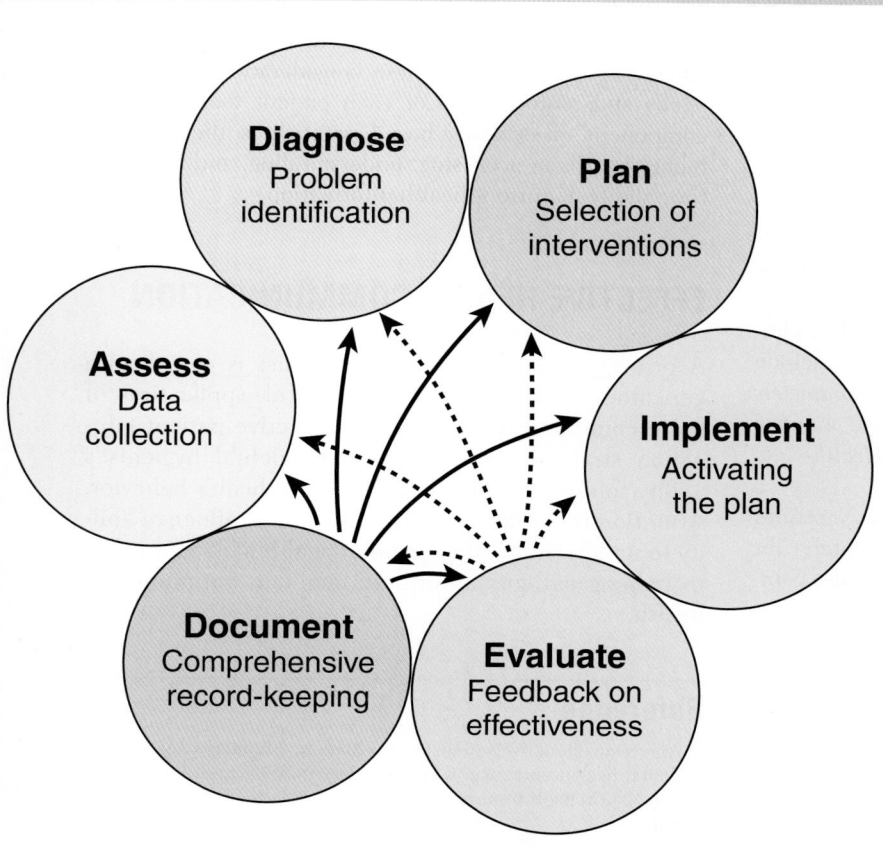

FIGURE I-1 **The Dental Hygiene Process of Care.**

INTRODUCTION

Professional dental hygiene practice is not defined only by the clinical duties that are traditionally associated with private practice dental care settings. The dental hygienist is an educated and licensed primary healthcare provider who fills numerous roles that contribute to better oral health. In addition, the dental hygienist is concerned with the general health and well-being of both individual patients and population groups. The chapters in this section of the book outline the professional roles and responsibilities of the dental hygienist as they apply in all practice settings.

THE PROFESSIONAL DENTAL HYGIENIST

The professional status of dental hygiene practice is dedicated to the following:

- Application of a dental hygiene process of care that meets standards for clinical dental hygiene practice
- Application of ethical standards and core values outlined in professional Codes of Ethics to dental hygiene practice in every setting
- Application of evidence-based, best-practice dental hygiene interventions
- Ability to communicate and build rapport with individuals and groups of all ages and across cultures, using patient education strategies that motivate positive health behavior changes

STANDARD OF CARE IN DENTISTRY AND DENTAL HYGIENE

Many health profession and government organizations develop and disseminate documents that outline practice parameters or provide clinical guidelines for providing clinical care. Examples of these types of documents include the American Academy of Periodontology *Parameters of Care* (page xx) and the Center for Disease Control *Guidelines for Infection Control in Dental Health-Care Settings* (Appendix IV, page 1096).

The American Dental Hygienists' Association *Standards for Clinical Dental Hygiene Practice*[1] outlines criteria for competency in dental hygiene care illustrated by the components of the Dental Hygiene Process of Care.

THE DENTAL HYGIENE PROCESS OF CARE

The dental hygiene process of care is the basis for providing preventive, educational, and therapeutic dental hygiene services that meet accepted standards of patient care. The process, illustrated by **Figure I-1**, as well as similar figures that are repeated on each section heading page, explains the series of interrelated steps that the dental hygienist follows to provide clinical patient care. The process of care makes a full cycle.

The overall process is explained in Chapter 1. Each step in the process is described more completely throughout the sections of the textbook.

ETHICAL APPLICATIONS

Basic ethical concepts are described in the introduction to each section of the textbook. Reference charts are included to summarize important ethical information. In each chapter, ethical decision making is illustrated in an Everyday Ethics scenario with questions that can be used to guide class discussions or individual reflection.

EVIDENCE-BASED DENTAL HYGIENE PRACTICE

The evidence-based practice of dental hygiene is about selecting healthcare interventions that are supported by current research and take into consideration the unique needs and requirements of each patient too. A critical component of evidence-based practice is the development of skills in accessing, understanding, and analyzing the validity of current health information.

EFFECTIVE HEALTH COMMUNICATION

A primary role of the dental hygienist is as a health educator. Understanding and skillful application of basic communication skills and effective patient education strategies can enhance the dental hygienist's ability to motivate positive changes in health behavior. Attention to patient characteristics that influence ability to understand and respond to health messages is key to helping patients attain and maintain optimum oral health.

Reference

1. American Dental Hygienists' Association. Standards for clinical dental hygiene practice. Chicago: ADHA; 2008. p. 3. [cited 2011 Feb 12]. Available from: www.adha.org/downloads/adha_standards08.pdf

The Professional Dental Hygienist

ESTHER M. WILKINS, BS, RDH, DMD
LAURA MUELLER-JOSEPH, RDH, MS, EDD
CHARLOTTE J. WYCHE, RDH, MS
DONNA F. HOMENKO, RDH, MED, PHD

Chapter Outline

The dental hygienist is a licensed primary healthcare professional, oral health educator, and clinician who provides preventive, educational, and therapeutic services supporting total health for the control of oral diseases and the promotion of oral health. Dental hygiene services are provided in general and specialty dental practices, programs for research, professional education, community health, hospital and institutional care of disabled persons, as well as for federal programs, the armed services, and dental product promotion in the corporate industry. Key words relating to dental hygienists and their practice are defined in **Box 1-1**.

ROLES OF DENTAL HYGIENE

- Within the wide span of dental hygiene practice areas, dental hygienists may serve in a variety of capacities.
- With the challenges brought about by advances in scientific research and changes in healthcare systems, the scope of practice has widened.
- Dental hygienists serve in several interrelated roles, including that of clinician, educator, researcher, administrator/manager, and advocate.
- All roles are interconnected through their common application to public health.

| **BOX 1-1** | **Key Words and Abbreviations** |

Professional Dental Hygienist

ADHA: American Dental Hygienists' Association.

ADHP: Advanced Dental Hygiene Practitioner

CDHA: Canadian Dental Hygienists' Association.

CEU: continuing education unit; 1 unit commonly refers to 1 clock hour of instruction.

Collaborative Practice of Dental Hygiene: the science of the prevention and treatment of oral disease through the provision of educational, assessment, preventive, clinical, and other therapeutic services in a collaborative working relationship with a consulting dentist, but without general supervision.

Competency: the skills, understanding, and professional values of an individual ready for beginning dental hygiene practice.

Continuing education: postlicensure short-term educational experiences for refresher, updating, and renewal; continuing education units may be required for relicensure.

Cotherapist: term used to describe the relationships between patient, dentist, and dental hygienist when coordinating the efforts to attain and maintain the oral health of the patient.

Dental hygiene care plan: the services within the framework of the total treatment plan to be carried out by the dental hygienist, patient, and caregiver.

Dental hygiene care: the science and practice of the prevention of oral diseases; the integrated preventive and treatment services administered for a patient by a dental hygienist.

Dental hygiene diagnosis: identification of an existing or potential oral health problem that a dental hygienist is qualified and licensed to treat.

Dental hygiene process of care: an organized systematic group of activities that provides the framework for delivering quality dental hygiene care.

Dental hygienist: dental health specialist whose primary concern is the maintenance of oral health and the prevention of oral disease (see also opening paragraph, page 3).

Dentistry: the evaluation, diagnosis, prevention, and/or treatment (nonsurgical, surgical, or related procedures) of diseases, disorders, and/or conditions of the oral cavity, maxillofacial area, and/or the adjacent and associated structures and their impact on the human body, provided by a dentist, within the scope of his/ or her education, training, and experience, in accordance with the ethics of the profession and applicable law (American Dental Association).

Direct supervision: the dentist has diagnosed and authorized the condition to be treated, remains on the premises while the procedure is performed, and approves the work performed before dismissal of the patient.

General supervision: the dentist has authorized the procedure for a patient of record but need not be present when the authorized procedure is carried out by a licensed dental hygienist. The procedure is carried out in accordance with the dentist's diagnosis and treatment plan.

Health promotion: the process of enabling people to increase control and improve their health through self-care, mutual aid, and the creation of healthy environments.

Health: state of physical, mental, and social well-being, not only the absence of disease.

Hygiene: the science of health and its preservation; a condition or practice, such as cleanliness, that is conducive to the preservation of health.

IFDH: International Federation of Dental Hygienists

Intervention: an action taken by a dental hygienist to maintain or restore a patient's optimal oral health.

License by credential: acceptance for licensure by a regulatory body (state, province) on the evidence from a license obtained in another state where equivalent standards and requirements are required; also called reciprocity, a mutual or cooperative exchange.

Oral hygiene: procedures for preservation of health of the oral cavity; personal maintenance of cleanliness and other measures recommended by dental professionals.

Personal supervision: while the dentist is personally treating a patient, the dental hygienist is authorized to aid in the treatment by concurrently performing a supportive procedure.

Primary healthcare: employs the techniques and agents to abort the onset of disease, to reverse the progress of the initial stages of disease, or to arrest the disease process before treatment becomes necessary.

Profession: occupation or calling that requires specialized knowledge, methods, and skills, as well as preparation, from an institution of higher learning, in the scholarly, scientific, and historic principles underlying such methods and skills; a profession continuously enlarges its body of knowledge, functions autonomously in formulation of policy, and maintains high standards of achievement and conduct; members of a profession are committed to continuing study, place service above personal gain, and are committed to providing practical services vital to human and social welfare.

Prognosis: a forecast of the probable course and outcome of the treatment of a condition or disease.

Supervision: term applied to a legal relationship between dentist and dental team members in practice. Each practice act defines the type of supervision required.

BOX 1-2	The ADHA Roles of Dental Hygienists

CLINICIAN
Assesses, diagnoses, plans, implements, and evaluates treatment for prevention, intervention, and control of oral diseases while practicing in collaboration with other professionals.

EDUCATOR
Uses educational theory and methodology to analyze health needs, develops health promotion strategies, and delivers and evaluates the results of attaining or maintaining oral health for individuals or groups.

PUBLIC HEALTH
All roles of the dental hygienist are considered to be **interrelated** within the context of improving the public's health by promoting oral health.

RESEARCHER
Applies the scientific method to select appropriate therapies, educational methods, or content; interprets and applies findings and solves problems.

ADMINISTRATOR/MANAGER
Applies organizational skills, communicates objectives, identifies and manages resources, and evaluates and modifies programs of health, education, or healthcare.

ADVOCATE
Influences legislators, health agencies, and other organizations to bring existing health problems and available resources together to resolve problems and improve access to care. Analyzes barriers to change; develops mechanisms to effect change; implements processes and evaluates the success of programs that promote health for individuals, families, or communities; and promotes lifestyle changes for individual patients.

- Areas of responsibility in this variety of roles are defined in **Box 1-2** and illustrated in **Figure 1-1**.

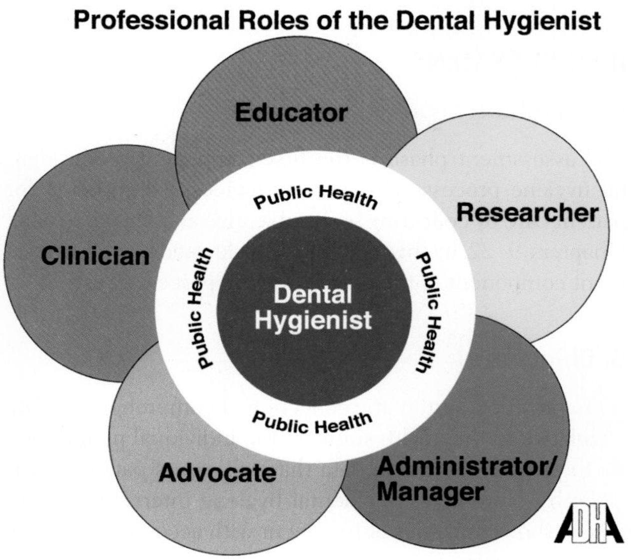

Professional Roles of the Dental Hygienist

FIGURE 1-1 **American Dental Hygienists' Association Professional Roles of the Dental Hygienist.** This graphic represents the six interconnected roles of the dental hygienist and positions the role of public health as an integral component of the other roles of clinician, educator, researcher, administrator/manager, and advocate. (Used with permission from the American Dental Hygienists' Association, Chicago, IL.)

DENTAL HYGIENE CARE

The term "dental hygiene care" is used to denote all integrated preventive and treatment services administered for a patient by a dental hygienist. This term is parallel to the commonly used term "dental care," which refers to the services provided by the dentist.

- Clinical services, both dental and dental hygiene, have limited long-range probability of success if the patient does not understand the need for cooperation in daily procedures of personal care and diet and for regular appointments for professional care.
- Educational and clinical services, therefore, are mutually dependent and inseparable in the total dental hygiene care of the patient.

Dr. Alfred C. Fones, the "father of dental hygiene," emphasized the important role of education. In the first textbook for dental hygienists, he wrote:

"It is primarily to this important work of public education that the dental hygienist is called. She must regard herself as the channel through which dentistry's knowledge of mouth hygiene is to be disseminated. The greatest service she can perform is the persistent education of the public in mouth hygiene and the allied branches of general hygiene."[1]

- Dental hygiene has changed and the scope of practice has developed from Dr. Fones's original concept.
- Scientific information about the prevention of oral diseases has been advancing steadily.
- The public has become increasingly aware of the need for dental hygiene care and the importance of oral health instruction.
- The clinical practice of the dental hygienist integrates specific care with instructional services required by the individual patient.

TYPES OF SERVICES

The clinical and educational responsibilities of the dental hygienist are divided into preventive and therapeutic services. Clinical and educational activities are inseparable and overlap as patient care is planned and accomplished.

I. PREVENTIVE SERVICES

Preventive services are the methods employed by the clinician and/or patient to promote and maintain oral health. Preventive services fall into three groups: primary, secondary, and tertiary.

- *Primary prevention* refers to measures carried out so that disease does not occur and is truly prevented.
  Example: An example of primary prevention is the fluoridation of water supplies.
- *Secondary prevention* involves the treatment of early disease to prevent further progression of potentially irreversible conditions that, if not arrested, can lead eventually to extensive rehabilitative treatment or even loss of teeth.
  Example: Removal of all calculus and dental biofilm while debriding a root surface in a relatively shallow periodontal pocket is an example of secondary prevention in that the treatment contributes to the prevention of continued attachment loss and the formation of a deep pocket.
- *Tertiary prevention* uses methods to replace lost tissues and to rehabilitate the oral cavity to a level where function is as near normal as possible after secondary prevention has not been successful.
  Example: An example of tertiary prevention is the replacement of a missing tooth using a fixed partial denture or implant and therefore restoring function.

II. EDUCATIONAL SERVICES

- Educational services are the strategies developed for an individual or a group to elicit behaviors directed toward health.
- Educational aspects of dental hygiene service permeate the entire patient care system.
- The preparation for clinical treatment, the outcomes of treatment, and the long-term success of both preventive and therapeutic services depend on the patient's understanding of each procedure and on the daily care of the oral cavity.

III. THERAPEUTIC SERVICES

- Therapeutic services are clinical treatments designed to arrest or control disease and maintain oral tissues in health.
- Dental hygiene treatment services are an integral part of the overall treatment plan.
- All scaling and root debridement along with the steps in posttreatment care are parts of the therapeutic phase in the treatment of periodontal infections.
- Placement of a pit and fissure sealant is an example of both a preventive and a therapeutic service.

DENTAL HYGIENE PROCESS OF CARE

The dental hygiene process of care includes assessment, dental hygiene diagnosis, planning, implementation, evaluation, and documentation.[2] As a process, the procedures performed are continual in nature and may overlap or occur simultaneously.

I. PURPOSES OF THE DENTAL HYGIENE PROCESS OF CARE

- To provide a framework within which individualized needs of the patient can be met.
- To identify the causative and risk factors of a condition that can be reduced, eliminated, or prevented by the services of a dental hygienist.

II. ASSESSMENT[3]

A. Definition

The assessment phase is the first component of the dental hygiene process. This phase provides a foundation for patient care by collecting both subjective and objective data. Chapters 9–22 in this textbook are devoted to the assessment component of the dental hygiene process of care.

B. Objectives

- To provide a systematic collection of comprehensive data relative to the health status of the individual patient.
- To provide evaluation data that will assess patient status both before and after dental hygiene interventions and will show outcomes of treatment with accomplishment of patient goals.

C. Subjective Data

- Obtained by observation and interaction with the patient

■ Includes chief complaint, perception of health, personal care, and the value placed on oral health.

D. Objective Data

■ Includes physical and oral assessment.
■ Records clinical and radiographic findings that show evidence of changes/disease in extra- and intraoral soft tissues, teeth, and periodontal tissues.

III. DENTAL HYGIENE DIAGNOSIS[4]

A. Definition

The dental hygiene diagnosis identifies the health behaviors of an individual patient as well as the actual or potential oral health problems that dental hygienists are educated and licensed to treat. The diagnosis provides the basis on which the dental hygiene care plan is designed, implemented, and evaluated. For preparation of the dental hygiene diagnosis, the data from the assessment phase are analyzed critically and interpreted. Chapter 23 (page 340) provides more information about the dental hygiene diagnosis.

B. Objectives

■ To identify the health behaviors of each patient as well as the actual or potential oral health problems that dental hygienists are licensed to treat.
■ To provide the basis on which the dental hygiene care plan is designed, implemented, and evaluated.
■ To justify the treatment proposed to the patient.
■ To challenge the dental hygienist to assume responsibility for patient care and to move beyond a rote system of clinical practice.

C. Data Processing

■ Use critical thinking skills to collect and interpret information.
■ Include the classification, interpretation, and validation of information collected during the assessment phase.
  A. *Classification.* Classification of data involves the sorting of information into specific categories such as general systemic, oral soft tissue, periodontal, dental, and oral hygiene. As information is organized, pertinent data are interpreted according to the patients' needs.
  B. *Interpretation.* Data interpretation relies upon critical thinking to identify significance. The cognitive processes of analysis, synthesis, inductive reasoning, and deductive reasoning are the basis for determining a diagnosis.
  C. *Validation.* Validation is an attempt to verify the accuracy of data interpretation. Validation can assist in recognizing errors, isolating discrepancies, and identifying the need for additional information.

TABLE 1-1	EXAMPLES OF DENTAL HYGIENE DIAGNOSTIC STATEMENTS	
PROBLEM		**CAUSE (RISK FACTORS AND ETIOLOGY)**
Halitosis	*Related to*	Dental biofilm accumulation on the tongue
Cervical abrasion	*Related to*	Incorrect toothbrushing
Potential for dental caries	*Related to*	Deep occlusal pits and fissures
Bleeding on probing	*Related to*	Marginal dental biofilm
Anxiety	*Related to*	Dental phobia

■ Compare findings with standards or norms.
■ Recognize deviations or abnormalities.
■ Analyze abnormalities with respect to significance.
■ Direct interaction with the patient.
■ Consultation with other healthcare professionals.
■ Comparison of data with an authoritative reference.

D. Formulate the Dental Hygiene Diagnosis

■ Focus on a patient's individual needs.
■ Determine potential or actual problems that can be prevented, minimized, or resolved by independent or interdependent interventions.
■ Identify the patient's condition or potential for risk.
■ Specify the causative and contributing factors, such as environmental, psychological, sociocultural, and physiological factors believed to be related to the health condition.
■ Provide safe and effective care. Dental hygienists diagnose within the scope of dental hygiene.
■ Express the problem and cause, for example, "Generalized brown tooth stains related to the use of cigars."
■ Sample diagnostic statements are provided in **Table 1-1**.

IV. THE DENTAL HYGIENE CARE PLAN[5]

A. Definition

Dental hygiene care planning is the selection of interventions to be performed by the patient, the dental hygienist, or others to meet the needs of the patient in attaining oral health. Chapters 23 and 24 describe care planning and provide a template for development of a written dental hygiene care plan.

B. Objectives

■ To develop strategies to meet the individual needs of the patient as identified by the dental hygiene diagnosis.
■ To incorporate priorities, goals, interventions, and expected outcomes.

C. Establish Priorities

- Priorities are determined by the immediacy of the condition, the severity of the problems, and available resources.
- Patients are active participants in the identification of priorities.

D. Set Goals

- Each problem is accompanied by a goal.
- Goals are directly related to the problem and represent the anticipated level of achievement.

E. Determine Interventions

- Interventions are dental hygiene therapies or patient educational activities that reduce, eliminate, or prevent the cause and risk factors related to the problem.
  Example: For the prevention of halitosis, dental hygiene interventions may include tongue cleaning and patient instruction about the papillae on the tongue that trap biofilm.

F. Identify Expected Outcomes (Prognosis)

- Expected outcomes represent measurable criteria for each intervention.
- Selected according to the anticipated effectiveness of the interventions.
- Provide a way to evaluate the results of the intervention.
  Example: An expected outcome following a patient education intervention about tongue anatomy might be that the patient is now able to perform a self-evaluation of tongue cleanliness.

G. Present the Dental Hygiene Care Plan

- To the dentist for integration with the comprehensive care plan.
- To the patient for complete understanding of the interventions needed and the appointment requirements.

H. Obtain Informed Consent (Page 359)

- Demonstrates that the care plan has been thoroughly explained to the patient.
- Determines the willingness of the patient to participate.

V. IMPLEMENTATION

A. Definition

The implementation phase is the activation of the care plan. Here the dental hygiene services are performed and personal daily oral care instructions are given. The concepts and procedures associated with implementation of dental hygiene care are presented in Chapters 25–45.

B. Objectives

- To put the care plan into action.
- To perform identified dental hygiene interventions to be fulfilled by the dental hygienist, the patient during self-care, and other caregivers.

VI. EVALUATION

A. Definition

At this point, the process of care comes full circle. The evaluation phase is used to determine if the patient needs to be retreated, referred, or placed on maintenance. Evaluation of dental hygiene care is detailed in Chapter 46 (page 725).

B. Objectives

- To compare current health status with baseline data.
- To assess progress or lack thereof toward the stated goal.
- To determine change or modification of the care plan.
- To determine maintenance interval according to the patient's health status and adherence to personal oral hygiene protocols.

C. Maintenance Phase

- The maintenance phase of care has also been termed "continuing care" or "supportive therapy."
- It may be scheduled at intervals of 3, 4, or 6 months depending on the patient's health status and adherence to personal daily care.
- All patients need to be placed on a maintenance program to prevent progression or recurrence of disease and to maintain an optimum level of health. Maintenance is described further in Chapter 47 (page 733).

VII. DOCUMENTATION

A. Definition

The process of detailing all assessment data, diagnosis, care plan, treatments, teaching, and evaluation in a condensed consistent format for the patient's permanent record. It represents a chronologic history of the patient's total care. Details for documentation are described in Chapter 8.

B. Objectives

- To document all components of the dental hygiene process of care (assessment, diagnosis, planning, implementation, and evaluation).
- To record legible, concise and accurate information.
- To recognize ethical and legal responsibilities of record keeping including guidelines outlined in state and province regulations and statutes.

- To ensure compliance with the Health Information Portability and Accountability Act (HIPAA).
- To respect and protect the confidentiality of patient information.

C. Documentation of Assessment Findings

- Subjective and objective data is documented using appropriate medical/dental terminology and abbreviations.
- Recordings of objective data follow protocols for periodontal charting, restorative, and other dental charting on standard clinic or computer forms.

D. Documentation of the Dental Hygiene Diagnosis

- Provides clearly written statements that link assessment findings with possible causes that can be prevented, minimized, or resolved by dental hygiene interventions.

E. Documentation of the Dental Hygiene Care Plan

- A step-by-step sequential plan is outlined for dental hygiene care that addresses the dental hygiene diagnosis in appropriate medical/dental terminology.
- All components of the care plan are stated to include the estimated time needed for each appointment.

F. Documentation of Dental Hygiene Interventions

- Dental hygiene interventions are recorded on a treatment-rendered form with appropriate date of service.

- The signature of the provider of care accompanies each entry.
- As part of a legal dental hygiene record, handwritten documents and signatures are required to be legibly written in black or blue permanent ink.

G. Documentation of Dental Hygiene Care Evaluation

- Evaluation of each intervention is recorded to show it as a completed or a continuing procedure.
- Reference to the next step for patient care will include reference to the need for continued dental hygiene treatment, maintenance dental hygiene therapy, or referral for dental care.

VIII. APPLICATIONS FOR THE PROCESS OF CARE

The six components of the dental hygiene process of care serve as the foundation for clinical practice of the dental hygienist. In Chapter 24 (page 351), the Dental Hygiene Care Plan is illustrated by the utilization of the *Patient-Specific Dental Hygiene Care Plan* (Figure 24-1). The plan provides a framework for completing and recording the details of the various components of the process.

DENTAL HYGIENE ETHICS

The ethics of a profession provide the general standards of right and wrong that guide the behavior of the members in that profession. Key words relating to ethics and ethical principles are defined in **Box 1-3**.

BOX 1-3	Key Words

Ethics

Autonomy: the act of self-determination by persons with the ability to make a choice or decision. Autonomy exists for both the dental hygienist and the patient.

Beneficence: the act of doing good.

Confidentiality: involves the rights of patients to privacy; a duty of dental hygienists is to protect privileged communication.

Core values: basic values of a profession; guide to choices or actions by implying a preference for what is deemed to be acceptable in the profession.

Ethical dilemma: a problem that involves two morally correct choices or courses of action. There may not be a single answer and, depending on the choice, the outcomes can differ.

Ethical issue: a common problem wherein a solution is readily grounded in the governing practice act, recognized laws, or acceptable standards of care. Decisions involving ethical issues are generally more clearly defined than are dilemmas.

Ethics: a sense of moral obligation; a system of moral principles that governs the conduct of a professional group, planned by them for the common good of people; principles of morality.

Justice/fairness: fair treatment according to an equitable distribution of benefits and burdens; impartiality; a core value.

Moral: a principle or habit with respect to right or wrong behavior.

Nonmaleficence: avoidance of harm to others; a core value.

Rights: expectations by the patient that correlate with the duties of a professional person when providing care.

Societal trust: maintaining a bond of trust in the relationships between the dental hygienist and patients, other professional persons, and the public.

Veracity: a duty to tell the truth when information is disclosed to patients about treatment.

Virtue: character trait; one must intend to act virtuously as a professional. Examples include honesty, compassion, care, and wisdom.

The members of a profession

- Have extensive specialized education
- Possess an intellectual body of knowledge from study and research
- Provide services important for the common good of society, for example, dental hygienists provide preventive, educational, and therapeutic services that protect and enhance the overall health of the public
- Maintain an organization of members that sets professional standards
- Exercise autonomy and judgment
- Adhere to their own code of ethics.

THE CODE OF ETHICS

- Describes professional conduct.
- Outlines responsibilities and duties of each member toward patients, colleagues, and society in general.

I. PURPOSES OF THE CODE OF ETHICS

- To increase the awareness of, and sensitivity to, ethical situations in practice.
- To define a standard of conduct that will give each individual a strong sense of ethical consciousness in professional practice as well as in all phases of life.

II. DENTAL HYGIENE CODES

- The Codes of the American Dental Hygienists' Association, the Canadian Dental Hygienists' Association, and the International Federation of Dental Hygienists can be read in Appendices I, II, and III (pages 1085–1095).
- Each dental hygienist is responsible for the study and application of the code of the particular association in which membership is held.

CORE VALUES

"Core Values" are selected principles of ethical behavior that can be considered the heart of the code of a profession.

I. CORE VALUES IN DENTAL HYGIENE

- Individual autonomy and respect for human beings
- Confidentiality
- Societal trust
- Beneficence
- Nonmaleficence
- Justice and fairness
- Veracity

II. PERSONAL VALUES

- Value development begins at an early age and is influenced by familial, social, and economic factors.

- Life experiences, grounded in previous successes and failures, serve as a foundation for professional virtues.
- Members of a health profession can benefit from periodic self-assessment of individual values, attitudes, and responsibilities.

III. THE PATIENT FIRST

- The responsibility to put the patient first is foremost.
- Dental hygienists are ethically, morally, and legally responsible to provide oral care for all patients without discrimination.
- Ethical decision making and professional behavior are reflected in every aspect of dental hygiene practice.

IV. LIFELONG LEARNING: AN ETHICAL DUTY

- To ensure optimal care for each patient.
- To maintain competency.
- To learn scientific advances from new research.
- To provide evidence-based patient care.
- To apply consistent ethical reasoning.
- To ensure fulfillment of each patient's rights.

ETHICAL APPLICATIONS

A dental hygienist may be involved in a variety of moral, ethical, and legal situations as part of the daily routine. In ethics, a problem situation is considered either an *ethical issue* or an *ethical dilemma*.

I. ETHICAL ISSUE

- More clearly defined than a dilemma.
- A common problem wherein a solution is grounded in the governing practice act, recognized laws, or accepted standards of care based on the standard rules of practice.

II. ETHICAL DILEMMA

- A problem that may involve two morally correct choices or courses of action.
- May not have a single answer and, depending on the choice, the outcomes can differ.
- To resolve a dilemma, the facts are gathered, ethical principles and theories are applied, and options are explored.

III. STEPS IN THE RESOLUTION OF AN ISSUE OR A DILEMMA

- STEP 1 Dental Hygiene Situation
  A. Is this situation an ethical issue or a dilemma?
  B. What is the chief concern/problem?
  C. Summarize the history of the situation.
  D. List all the facts from all the people involved.

- STEP 2 Individual Preferences
  A. What are the rights of the individuals involved?
  B. In a clinical case: has informed consent been obtained?
- STEP 3 Choices *versus* Alternatives
  A. Which core values apply to this case?
  B. Describe the realistic alternatives that exist.
  C. Explain the benefits and disadvantages of all possible outcomes.
- STEP 4 Case Parameters
  A. Does the "scope of practice" apply to the situation? If so, explain.
  B. What financial, legal, or cultural factors need consideration?
  C. Compare the anticipated action with acceptable professional standards.
  D. Is there a conflict of interest between the patient, dental providers, or other individuals?
  E. Is there a need for an outside source to be consulted?

IV. SUMMARY: THE FINAL DECISION

- Many factors can be used to solve a dilemma.
- All dental healthcare providers involved in the decision process can participate in a follow-up evaluation of the action taken.
- Once a decision has been made, the concluding assessment should be: Is the decision/action that is selected morally defensible? In essence, can the choice to solve the dilemma be defended?
- A professional dental hygienist may need to defend it to the patient, the dentist, members of the dental team, a state board, or even a court of law.
- Most importantly, the decision must be defensible based on standards of practice established for the dental hygiene profession.

V. APPLICATIONS: EVERYDAY ETHICS

Various ethical issues and dilemmas are presented throughout this book for discussion and consideration. The examples are found in special boxes called "Everyday Ethics" and usually appear at the end of the chapter where the problem may apply.

LEGAL FACTORS IN PRACTICE

- The law must be studied and respected by each dental hygienist practicing within the state, province, or country.
- Although the various practice acts have certain basic similarities, differences in scope and definition exist.
- Terminology varies, but each practice act regulates the patient services that may be practiced by the licensed dental hygienist. Changes may be made from time to time.

- A frequent review of the practice acts and/or regulations will keep the dental health professional up to date.

PERSONAL FACTORS IN PRACTICE

- Each dental hygienist represents the entire profession to the patient being served.
- The dental hygienist's expressed or demonstrated attitudes toward dentistry, dental hygiene, and other health professions, as well as toward health services and preventive measures, will affect the subsequent attitude of the patient toward other dental hygienists and dental hygiene care in general.
- Members of health professions who exemplify the traits they hold as objectives for others enhance probability of positive response and cooperation from their patients.

Many personal factors of general physical health, oral health, cleanliness, appearance, and mental health are to be considered. A few of these are included here:

- *General Physical Health.* Optimum physical health depends to a great extent on a well-planned diet, sufficient amount of sleep, and adequate amount of exercise.

  Because of the occupational hazards of dental personnel, routine examinations at least annually need to include tests for hearing, sight, urinary mercury, and certain communicable diseases. Immunizations are described on page 61.

- *Oral Health.* The maintenance of a clean, healthy mouth demonstrates by example that the dental hygienist follows the teachings of the dental and dental hygiene professions relative to prevention and control of oral disease.
- *Mental Health.* The mental health of the dental hygienist is reflected in interpersonal relationships and the ability to inspire confidence through a display of professional and emotional maturity. Adequate physical health, recreation, and participation in professional and community activities contribute to optimum mental health.

SPECIAL PRACTICE AREAS

A wide range of settings is available for the practice of a dental hygienist. Likewise, a wide range of patient problems requires specialized knowledge and skills.

I. DENTAL SPECIALTIES

A dentist may conduct an ethical limited practice in the following nine areas of dentistry:[6]

- Dental Public Health
- Endodontics
- Oral and Maxillofacial Pathology
- Oral and Maxillofacial Surgery
- Orthodontics and Dentofacial Orthopedics

- Pediatric Dentistry
- Periodontics
- Prosthodontics
- Oral and Maxillofacial Radiology

Education and training for certification in the dental specialties require a minimum of 2 or 3 years of graduate or postdoctoral study and the successful completion of written and practical examinations. Masters and postdoctoral specialty degrees require three or more years beyond basic dental education.

II. DENTAL HYGIENE SPECIALTIES

Although licensure is not required universally for dental hygienists to practice within a specialty, educational curricula exist for certain areas.

- Advanced degrees for dental hygiene education and public health have been available for many years.
- Other dental hygienists with masters or doctoral degrees have majored in nutrition and dietetics, business and administration, and law, as well as a variety of sciences.
- In other special areas, short-term courses have been developed, such as for instruction in the care of patients with disabilities.
- In-service training may be available in long-term care institutions, hospitals, and skilled nursing facilities.
- Other dental hygienists have learned to practice in a specialty through private study, special conferences, and personal experience.
- In 1999 the state of Minnesota[7] approved the development of master-level degree programs to prepare dental hygienists as Oral Health Providers (OHP) who will be licensed in that state to provide preventive and basic restorative dental services directly to underserved populations.
- A 2009 PEW Report[8] recognized that creating new mid-level oral health care providers, such as the Advanced Dental Hygiene Practitioner (ADHP) proposed by the American Dental Hygienists' Association could enhance access to oral health services for underserved populations.

The clinical practice of the dental hygienist can include many specialty areas.

- Private practice orthodontics, pediatric dentistry, and periodontics clinics particularly value dental hygienists as partners in prevention.
- Many states have enacted collaborative practice legislative initiatives[9] and adopted practice rules that allow dental hygienists to provide care autonomously for underserved populations in specifically designated public health settings.
- Other dental hygienists are involved in special clinics with a variety of health specialists, where patients with dental deformities such as cleft lip and/or palate or with oral cancer are under care.
- In other facilities, dental hygienists serve with a combined medical and dental team in the treatment of patients with severe systemic diseases; patients with physical, mental, or emotional handicapping conditions; or patients with combinations of any of the problems mentioned.

OBJECTIVES FOR PROFESSIONAL PRACTICE

I. OVERALL GOALS

- A dental hygienist's self-assessment is essential in attaining goals of perfection for service to each patient and in collaboration with the dentist in a total dental and dental hygiene care program.
- Personal objectives are outlined and reviewed frequently in a plan for continued self-improvement.
- The overall professional goals of the dental hygiene profession relate to health promotion and disease prevention.
- The goal of each dental hygienist with respect to patient care is *to aid individuals and groups in attaining and maintaining optimum oral health*. Other personal objectives are related to this primary one.

II. PERSONAL GOALS

The professional dental hygienist will:

- Exemplify the highest degree of professional ethics and conduct.
- Plan and carry out effectively the dental hygiene services essential to the total care program for each individual patient.
- Apply evidenced-based knowledge and understanding of the basic and clinical sciences in the recognition of oral conditions and the prevention of oral diseases.
- Apply evidenced-based scientific knowledge and skill to all clinical and instructional procedures.
- Recognize each patient as an individual and adapt care planning and interventions accordingly.
- Identify and care for the needs of patients who have unusual general health problems that affect dental hygiene procedures.
- Demonstrate interpersonal relationships that permit attending the patient with assurance and presenting dental health information effectively.
- Provide a complete and personalized instructional service to help each patient become motivated toward changes in oral health behavioral practices.
- Practice safe and efficient clinical routines for the application of standard precautions for infection control.
- Apply a continuing process of self-evaluation in clinical practice throughout professional life.
- Recognize the need for lifelong learning to acquire updated knowledge through reading professional literature and enrolling in continuing education programs.
- Maintain membership and participate actively in the local, national, and international dental hygiene professional associations.

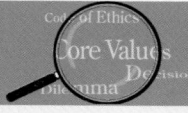
Everyday Ethics

The first term of the dental hygiene curriculum has just finished. The instructor asks for student volunteers to help at the college's health fair to provide basic routine brushing and flossing directions to people who stop at the dental hygiene information table. Three students, Alice, Annette, and Josephine, sign up to volunteer for this community service. The day before the health fair, which takes place on a Saturday, Annette is asked to work in the dental office where she is employed part-time. Since she really needs the money, she decides not to attend the health fair and instead goes to work without telling anyone.

Questions for Consideration
1. In general, would this situation be described as a professional issue or an ethical dilemma? Why?
2. Discuss Annette's actions in terms of the core ethical values.
3. What aspects of the Dental Hygiene Code of Ethics can you use to support your choice of action?

DOCUMENTATION

The professional dental hygienist carefully documents all aspects of patient care in the patient's permanent record to provide:

- A comprehensive, accurate, and ongoing record of all aspects of the dental hygiene process of care.
- Documentation that adheres to ethical and legal standards.
- Objective, factual (rather than judgmental or subjective) statements that respect the integrity of the patient, the practitioner, and the practice.

Factors To Teach The Patient

- The role of the dental hygienist as a cotherapist with each patient and with members of the dental profession.
- The moral and ethical nature of becoming a dental hygiene professional.
- The scope of service of the dental hygienist as defined by various practice acts.
- The interrelationship of instructional and clinical services in dental hygiene patient care.
- The patient's potential state of oral health and how it can be improved and maintained.

References

1. Fones AC, editor. Mouth hygiene. 4th ed. Philadelphia: Lea & Febiger; 1934. 248 p.
2. American Dental Hygienists' Association. Standards for clinical dental hygiene practice. Chicago: American Dental Hygienists' Association; 2008. [cited 2010 Feb 18] Available from: www.adha.org/downloads/adha_standards08.pdf
3. Mueller-Joseph L, Petersen M. Dental hygiene process: diagnosis and care planning. Albany: Delmar; 1995. 9–14 pp.
4. Ibid. pp. 20–5.
5. Ibid. pp. 46–55.
6. American Dental Association. Principles of ethics and code of professional conduct. Chicago: American Dental Association; 2009. [cited 2010 Feb 18] 13 p. Available from: http://www.ada.org/prof/prac/law/code/index.asp
7. American Dental Hygienists' Association. The history of introducing a new provider in Minnesota. Chicago: American Dental Hygienists' Association; 2009 [cited 2010 Feb 23]. 2 p. Available from: www.adha.org/downloads/MN_Mid-Level_History_and_Timeline.pdf
8. The PEW Center on the States, National Academy for State Health Policy, WK Kellogg Foundation. Help wanted: a policy maker's guide to new dental providers. Washington DC: The PEW Center on the States; 2009 May. pp. 18, 23–5.
9. American Dental Hygienists' Association [Internet]. Chicago: American Dental Hygienists' Association; © 2010. Stateline: the latest legislative news in oral health from coast to coast; update February 2010 [cited 2010 Feb 23]; about 20 screens. Available from: http://www.adha.org/governmental_affairs/stateline.htm

Evidence-Based Dental Hygiene Practice

JUDI S. LUXMORE, RDH, BAS, MS
CHARLOTTE J. WYCHE, RDH, MS

Chapter Outline

The main goal of clinical dental hygiene practice is to improve and maintain the oral health of the patient. Clinical questions and/or problems that arise on a daily basis require current and reliable information to identify best-practice treatment interventions and oral self-care recommendations that will improve the patient's health.

■ The concepts of evidence-based practice will assist dental hygienists in formulating a plan for objective, effective, and scientifically sound interventions that meet patient needs and assure positive health outcomes.

■ Key words related to evidence-based practice and research are found in **Box 2-1**.

EVIDENCE-BASED PRACTICE

I. DEFINITION

■ A formalized approach to clinical care in which the clinician, in consultation with the patient, uses the best scientific evidence available to make decisions about clinical treatment options and techniques/equipment patients will need to optimize daily personal oral care.

■ Evidence-based practice involves two fundamental principles:
1. Evidence alone is never sufficient to make a clinical decision.
2. A hierarchy of evidence, discussed more completely later in the chapter, exists to guide clinical decision making.

BOX 2-1	Key Words

Evidence-Based Dental Hygiene Practice

Best practice: approach or intervention that has been deter-mined to be efficient and effective in producing good health outcomes based on repeatable research evidence collected over time on large, diverse groups of people.

Biomedical databases: organized collection of medically related journal articles, research reports, theses, and /or dissertations typically in digital form.

Case Control Series (retrospective): study design in which persons with a disease of interest (cases) are compared with those without the disease (controls); researchers look back to identify possible causes.

Case reports: professional article that describes the diagnos-tic, preventive, and therapeutic services rendered to one patient with an unusual or complex condition.

Case studies: in-depth analysis and description of a series of cases of an unusual or complex condition.

Clinical significance: practical difference noted by research-ers that can be applied to patient care.

Cohort studies (follow-up or prospective): study where the same subjects are followed over a period to observe the occurrence of a particular event.

Comparison group: group of individuals in a study that do not receive the treatment when nonrandom methods are used for sample selection.

Descriptive statistics: research that provides an accurate interpretation of characteristics of a particular person, event, or group in real-life situations; research that is conducted to discover new meaning, describe what exits, determine the frequency with which something occurs, and categorize information.

Editorial: article in a newspaper or magazine that expresses the opinion of its editor or publisher.

Evidence: everything that is used to determine or demon-strate the truth of an assertion.

Evidence-based dental hygiene (EBDH) practice: refers to a scientific, research-supported approach to decide dental hygiene interventions for each patient.

Inferential statistics: numerical data designed to allow gen-eralization from a sample to a population.

In vitro ("test tube") research: manipulation of organs, tissues, cells, and biomolecules in a controlled, artificial environment.

Intervention: treatment that is manipulated during the conduct of a study to produce an effect on the dependent variable.

Levels of evidence: hierarchy for making clinical judgments related to patient care based on types of research studies.

Meta-analysis: statistical process used during a systematic review to combine data from various studies into one analysis.

Opinion: belief or conclusion held with confidence but not substantiated by positive knowledge or proof.

Outcome: end result that follows from an action.

Randomized controlled double-blind studies (RCT): the most rigorous type of clinical experiment; most commonly used in testing the efficacy or effectiveness of health care ser-vices or health technologies.

Reference citation: a number or other notation contained in the text of a manuscript that refers to the published or unpub-lished source of the information listed in a reference list.

Scientific evidence: Evidence that has been repeatedly tested through research with valid and reliable methods.

Search engine: a computer program that uses key words or terms to locate documents or data from the World Wide Web or other Internet databases.

Statistical significance: identifies the extent to which the results are not due to chance. Statistical significance is indicated in research by the "p-value" notation.

Systematic reviews: critical evaluation of all published studies that investigate a specific question by a group of experts using preestablished criteria to produce a sum-mary of results.

Tutorial: a method of transferring knowledge or instructions needed to complete a specific task, using an individual or small group interactive-type learning setting that seeks to teach by example; online tutorials are available on a variety of topics.

Validity: ability to measure what was intended.

Variable: factors in a research study that can be manipulated and measured.

II. PURPOSE

- To answer clinical questions quickly and efficiently.
- To identify research-supported, best-practice interven-tions that contribute to positive patient outcomes.
- To ensure application of the most up-to-date practice interventions in the delivery of patient care.

III. NEED FOR EVIDENCE-BASED PRACTICE[1]

- Patients are becoming more sophisticated about searching the Internet for health information.

- Patients expect the clinician to know the latest developments in health care and will value a prac-titioner who can discuss and help them evaluate information obtained elsewhere.
- Dental hygienists who are up-to-date with evidence-based dental hygiene (EBDH) practice can help determine the relevance, validity, and reliability of information that patients are accessing on their own.
- Differences in practice procedures
  - Clinicians are not consistently knowledgeable about new therapies.

- There may be inconsistencies between dental hygiene schools' teachings and procedures tested by regional examination for licensure.
- Gap between current research knowledge and application into practice
  - A practitioner's limited personal journal collection, rather than an extensive range of scientific publications, may remain the dominant source for making treatment decisions.
  - Ability to access, or an individual's selection of, continuing education courses can affect the clinical practitioner's knowledge of current therapies.
  - Gap in knowledge of up-to-date care widens the longer time that clinicians have been out of school.
  - Evidence-based decision-making behaviors and research analysis skills may not be well understood by every dental professional.
- Information explosion management[2]
  - The rate of published research increases yearly.
  - Effective strategies to disseminate new evidence are limited by large number of publications and by lag time between research completion and publication.
  - Clinicians' time to access a growing number of publications with new information is limited.
- Changing educational requirements
  - Curriculum reform reports the need for more complete integration of basic science with clinical coursework.
  - Knowledge of research methods and electronic biomedical database searching are critical for finding clinical answers quickly.
  - Practice that applies to higher-level thinking and problem-solving skills is needed to assure comprehensive management of dental hygiene care.

IV. EVIDENCE-BASED DECISION-MAKING PROCESS[3]

The evidence-based decision-making process for dental hygiene care is based on an interaction between four components as illustrated in **Figure 2-1**.

- *Scientific evidence.* Review of relevant and current clinical research of high quality identifies best-practice treatment choices.
- *Patient preferences or values.* The patient's needs, wants, and expectations are considered, respected, and weighted (i.e., cultural, religious, capabilities).
- *Clinical/patient circumstances.* The unique and specific particulars of each individual patient are considered (i.e., age, health concerns, disease state).
- *Clinician's experience and judgment.* The clinical skill and experiences of the clinician enhance the ability to identify quickly the patient's health, risks, needs, and potential for various interventions.

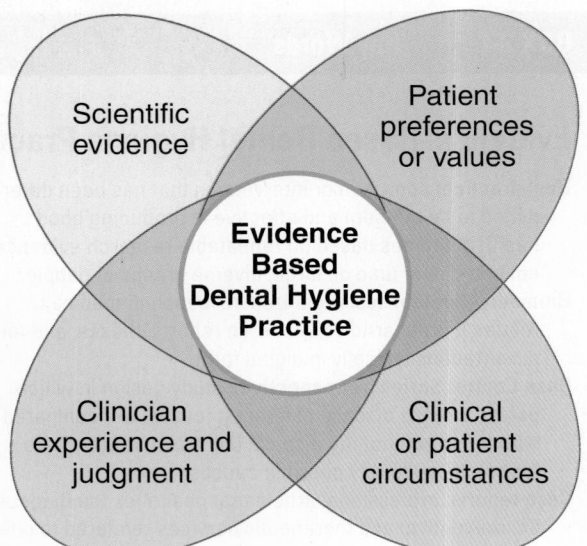

FIGURE 2-1 **An Evidence-Based Decision-Making Model for Dental Hygiene Practice.**

V. SKILLS NEEDED FOR EVIDENCE-BASED DENTAL HYGIENE PRACTICE

A variety of skills are needed to implement EBDH into everyday clinical practice. Finding evidence to support treatment and preventive interventions and recommendations requires the dental hygienist to:

- *Understand EBDH practice.* A variety of tutorials, listed in **Box 2-2**, that inform about the evidence-based decision-making process are available on the Internet by typing the term "evidence-based" into an Internet search engine.
- *Follow a systematic approach.* As described below, a step-by step approach to asking questions related to clinical practice will ensure success.
- *Read and understand research.* Practice will help the dental hygienist recognize reliable *versus* unreliable information through an understanding of the types of

BOX 2-2	Evidence-Based Tutorials

- **University of North Carolina at Chapel Hill Health Sciences Library:** http://www.hsl.unc.edu/Services/Tutorials/EBM/welcome.htm
- **Information Services Department of the Library of the Health Sciences-Chicago at the University of Illinois at Chicago:** http://ebp.lib.uic.edu/
- **University of Rochester Medical Center:** http://www.urmc.rochester.edu/hslt/miner/resources/evidence_based/
- **SUNY Downstate Medical Center:** http://library.downstate.edu/EBM2/contents.htm

publications and articles, research methods, and statistical analysis.

■ *Be computer literate.* Development of critical thinking skills is necessary to evaluate Web-based information or efficiently and effectively search the scientific literature via databases of biomedical references.

■ *Embrace self-directed learning.* Development of a plan for continuing education and reading of professional literature will help to maintain up-to-date knowledge.

A SYSTEMATIC APPROACH

A systematic method is required to identify and select research findings and other science-based information related to a particular patient's oral and systemic health. **Figure 2-2** illustrates a step-by-step procedure, explained later in the chapter, that will aid the practitioner in the development of these crucial skills.[3]

I. DETERMINE CLINICAL ISSUE

■ Asking the right question is fundamental, and critical, to the evidence-based decision-making process.

■ Include important characteristics of the patient (i.e., age, gender).

II. DEVELOP RESEARCHABLE QUESTION

A good, researchable question includes four parts, referred to as PICO.[3] Examples of PICO questions related to dental hygiene practice can be found in **Table 2-1**.

■ *Patient problem or population (P):* What are the most important characteristics of the patient or population of interest?

■ *Intervention (I):* Which main intervention, prognostic factor, or exposure is being considered?

■ *Comparison (C):* What is the main alternative to compare with the intervention? The clinical question does not always need a specific comparison.

■ *Outcome (O):* What is the desired outcome, accomplishment, measure, improvement, or effect?

III. SEARCH FOR EVIDENCE: CONDUCT REVIEW OF LITERATURE

Select appropriate resources and conduct a search for science-based information. Scientific articles can still be accessed in a traditional library, but more often, searches are accomplished on a computer using an appropriate search engine or database.[3]

■ An Internet search engine is designed to search for information on the World Wide Web.

■ The search results are generally presented in a list of results (websites or articles related to the topic) and are often called "hits."

■ Use of popular general search engines, such as Google or the Wikipedia, may lead to some results, but accuracy and unbiased sources of information can rarely be assured. Only a fraction of all of the resources available will be displayed.

■ Web search engines can also provide access to government agencies and independent organizations that offer a variety of statistical data and other information regarding medicine and health.

■ Dedicated search engines (such as PubMed) that are devoted to specific professional literature databases provide access to information from scholarly articles in biomedical and other health-related journals.

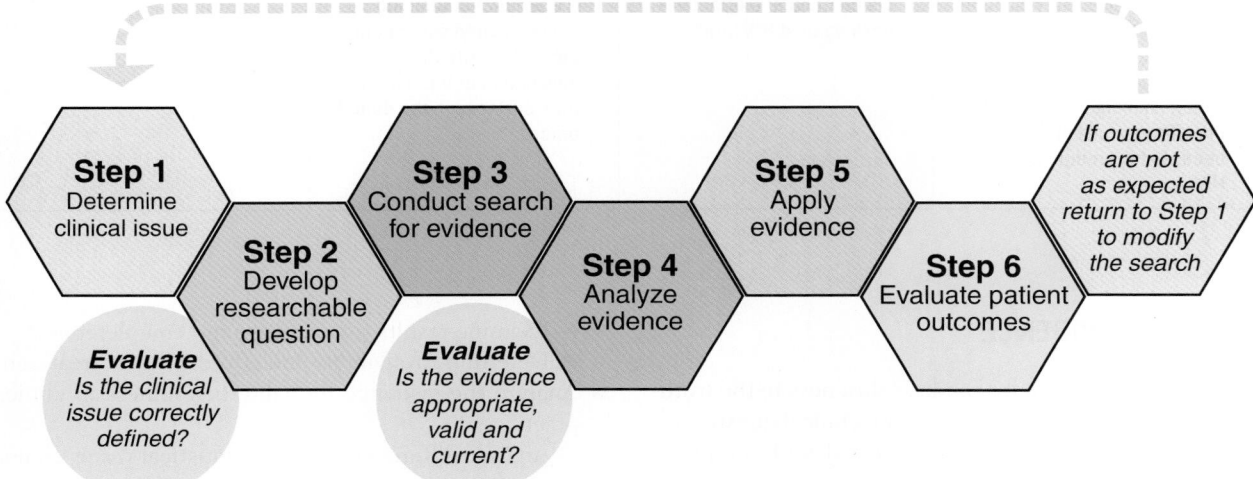

FIGURE 2-2 **Steps for a Systematic Approach to Evidence-Based Dental Hygiene Practice.** Evaluation is an ongoing and important component of the process.

TABLE 2-1	EXAMPLE OF PICO QUESTIONS AND LITERATURE SEARCH RESULTS

Scenario	PICO	PICO Question	Relevant Articles from PubMed Literature Search
Mrs. Winnie: Is a 79-year-old African-American woman who presents for a routine maintenance appointment. Her health history identifies that she has arthritis. She states that because of limited wrist and hand mobility, she has been having trouble maneuvering a toothbrush to reach all surfaces of her teeth. Her friend told her about a new kind of toothbrush that has curved bristles that are able to brush both inner and outer surfaces of the teeth at the same time.	**Patient/Problem:** Limited hand mobility **Intervention:** Regular tooth-brush **Comparison:** Curved-bristle toothbrush **Outcome:** Effective biofilm removal/healthy gingiva	For a patient with limited hand/wrist movement, will a curved-bristle toothbrush be as effective at removing biofilm from all surfaces of the teeth as a regular tooth-brush is?	Selected results from about 5 related journal articles: ■ Chava VK. An evaluation of the efficacy of a curved bristle and conventional tooth-brush. A comparative clinical study. *J Periodontol.* 2000 May;71(5):785–9. ■ Arici S, Alkan A, Arici N. Comparison of different tooth-brushing protocols in poor-toothbrushing orthodontic patients. *Eur J Orthod.* 2007 Oct;29(5):488–92.
Mrs. Arthur: Is an attractive 48-year-old mother of two who has come into the clinic for her regular check-up. She is very interested in whitening her teeth because her thirtieth high school reunion is coming up in 1 month. She has heard about various bleaching methods and is wondering which method would be right for her. She is on a limited budget, but is willing to pay the extra expense if an in-office treatment will get her teeth whiter.	**Patient/Problem:** Wants teeth whitened **Intervention:** In-office profes-sional bleaching procedure **Comparison:** At-home or over-the-counter bleaching system **Outcome:** Lighter tooth color *NOTE: Research about compara-tive cost is done in addition to the literature search.	For a patient who is dissatis-fied with her tooth color, will using an over-the-counter bleaching system be as effective as in-office bleaching?	Selected results from more than 100 related journal articles: ■ da Costa JB, McPharlin R, Paravina RD, Ferracane JL. Comparison of at-home and in-office tooth whitening using a novel shade guide. *Oper Dent.* 2010 Jul–Aug;35(4):381–8. ■ Zekonis R, Matis BA, Cochran MA, Al Shetri SE, Eckert GJ, Carlson TJ. Clinical evalua-tion of in-office and at-home bleaching treatments. *Oper Dent.* 2003 Mar–Apr;28(2):114–21.
Rick Snyder: Is a new dental rep and your office is in his territory. Rick is excited and anxious to tell you about a new product his company has recently developed for surface disinfection. The new product contains sodium lauryl sulfate and alcohol. Rick claims his product is better than the product containing dimethyl-benzyl ammonium chloride that the office is currently using because his product kills the HIV virus.	**Problem:** New disinfection products **Intervention:** Dimethylbenzyl ammonium chloride **Comparison:** Sodium lauryl sulfate and alcohol **Outcome:** Adequate surface disinfection and effective-ness against HIV virus.	Will a product containing sodium lauryl sulfate and alcohol be as effective as a product containing dimeth-ylbenzyl ammonium chlo-ride to disinfect surfaces in the dental office? Will a product containing sodium Lauryl sulfate and alcohol be effective in elimination of the HIV virus from surfaces in the dental office?	■ An intensive PubMed search did not find any usable research article that might guide decision making about these questions. *NOTE: An option is to ask Rick to pro-vide any unpublished or "in press" studies he is aware of that support his claim.

IV. ANALYZE EVIDENCE

■ Analyze the evidence for validity (closeness to the truth and how well the studies answer the clinical question).[4]

   ■ Determine if report follows logical and complete steps of research process.

   ■ Determine if focus of study is similar to patient's concerns.

   ■ Examine results for accuracy and completeness.

   ■ Determine availability and affordability of treatment.

■ Analyze the evidence for value (usefulness in clinical practice).[5,6]

   ■ Analyze difference between statistical *versus* clinical significance.

   ■ Determine if treatment outcomes are large enough to justify treatment.

■ Determine if researchers have provided a critical argument for using results in clinical practice.

V. APPLY EVIDENCE

■ Return to the patient and apply the evidence, guided by clinical expertise/experience and the patient's preferences.
■ Consider potential results in association with the patient's needs and the clinician's ability to obtain results.

VI. EVALUATE RESULTS

■ Determine if the evidence-based decision-making process was successfully carried out.
■ Decide if additional search strategies and information are needed.
■ Determine whether a modification of original outcome goal is needed.
■ Begin the process again if patient outcome is not successful.

READING AND UNDERSTANDING RESEARCH

The sources for obtaining scientific information are growing daily. Knowing how to determine the validity and reliability of information is paramount for selecting successful patient care strategies and interventions. A checklist of questions to ask when considering the validity of a publication is found in **Box 2-3**.

I. PUBLICATION TYPES

■ Textbooks. Good as background resources but, because of a drawn-out publication process, can become outdated quickly.

BOX 2-3	Questions to Ask When Considering the Validity of a Publication

■ Who is sponsoring?
■ Is there an editorial review board? Are the articles peer reviewed?
■ What are the credentials of the contributors?
■ Are there advertisements? How many?
■ Are there good-quality production standards?
■ Is manuscript preparation information included?
■ What type of articles are included? (i.e., Informational? Opinion/editorial? Case reports? Scientific study?)

■ Commercial-based journals/magazines.
  ■ Often free, which means that they are based on product sponsorship.
  ■ Articles may be written by in-house staff member without professional credentials.
  ■ Most carry informational articles; however, some have articles summarizing recent research that contain reference citations, but may not include all available scientific studies.
■ Professional journals
  ■ Produced by professional organizations. Membership dues payment is required or publications are a benefit of being a member.
  ■ Part or all of the publication is devoted to scientific studies. Most contain articles with supporting reference citations.
■ Peer-reviewed (refereed) publications
  ■ Before publication of any scholarly article or research report in these journals, one or more dental hygiene experts or statisticians have critically examined all components of the manuscript. Peer-reviewed journals usually list all review board members and their credentials in each issue of the journal.
  ■ After receiving feedback from the reviewers, the article is not published until the author revises the manuscript to address significant concerns or answer questions expressed by the reviewers.
  ■ The purpose of this process is to help assure the validity and unbiased nature of the supporting review of the literature, the research results, and the conclusions or recommendations put forth by the author.

II. RESEARCH APPROACHES

■ Qualitative
  ■ Results are reported using a narrative; often uses quotations.
  ■ Systematic; subjective approach.
  ■ Uses numbers only to report demographic information.
■ Quantitative
  ■ Results reported in numbers.
  ■ Data can be counted and analyzed by descriptive or inferential statistics.

III. RESEARCH TYPES

■ Descriptive
  ■ Often, a first step in classifying and organizing information.
  ■ Asks "how often" or "to what extent" something occurs.
  ■ Helps identify relationships that can be further explored in subsequent studies.
■ Correlational
  ■ Looks at the relationship between two or more variables.

■ Determines the strength and type of relationships.
■ Variables are not manipulated; no cause and effect is determined.
■ Experimental
 ■ Intervention variables are manipulated to discover the effect of one variable on another (i.e., Does A cause B?)
 ■ Contains a control group and randomly assigned subjects; provides an intervention to only the experimental group.
■ Quasi-experimental
 ■ Designed to examine cause-and-effect relationships.
 ■ Has less control by researcher than true experimental designs.
 ■ No control group; or subjects may not be randomly assigned.

IV. LEVELS OF EVIDENCE

The concept of "levels of evidence" is used to evaluate the strength (scientific rigor and quality) of scientific evidence and to provide a hierarchy for making clinical judgments related to patient care. Six levels shown in **Figure 2-3** are organized based on types of research.

■ The three highest levels of evidence provide the strongest basis for making clinical decisions; the less relevant research method types follow in descending order.
■ The levels are often visualized as a pyramid because there are a smaller number of studies in the more clinically valuable top levels compared with the number of studies in the lower levels.

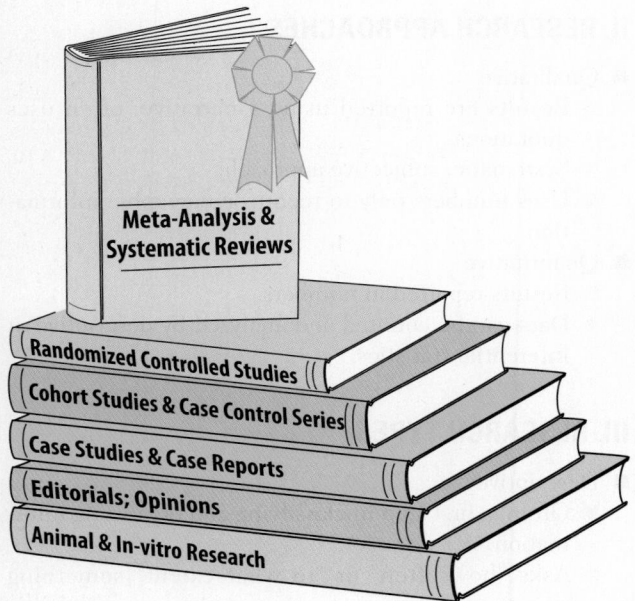

FIGURE 2-3 **Levels of Evidence Pyramid.** Source: SUNY Health Sciences. Guide to research methods: The evidence pyramid [Internet]. New York; SUNY (State University of New York) Downstate Medical Center; c 2009. Evidence Based Medicine Course; 2004 Jan 6 [cited 2010 Oct 21]. [about 1 screen] Available from: http://library. downstate.edu/EBM2/2100.htm

■ Systematic reviews and meta-analysis: the highest level of evidence.
 ■ A systematic review is a critical evaluation of all published studies that investigate a specific question by a group of experts using preestablished criteria to produce a summary of results.
 ■ Meta-analysis is the statistical process used during a systematic review to combine data from various studies into one analysis.
■ Randomized controlled double-blind studies (RCT): the most rigorous clinical studies
 ■ RCT is a type of scientific experiment most commonly used in testing the efficacy or effectiveness of health care services or health technologies.
 ■ It eliminates selection bias, balancing both known and unknown factors, in the assignment of treatments.
■ Cohort studies and case–control series
 ■ Cohort (follow-up or prospective): study where the same subjects are followed over a period of time to observe the occurrence of a particular event.
 ■ Case–control (retrospective): study design in which persons with a disease of interest (cases) are compared with those without the disease (controls); researchers look back to identify possible causes.
■ Case studies and case reports
 ■ Case report: a professional article that describes the diagnostic, preventive, and therapeutic services rendered to one patient with an unusual or complex condition.
 ■ Case study: an in-depth analysis and description of a series of cases of an unusual or complex condition.
■ Editorials and opinions
 ■ Editorial: an article in a newspaper or magazine that expresses the opinion of its editor or publisher.
 ■ Opinion: a belief or conclusion held with confidence but not substantiated by positive knowledge or proof.
■ Animal and in vitro research.

INTERNET-BASED HEALTH INFORMATION

I. COMPUTER/INTERNET LITERACY

■ The amount of online information is overwhelming.
■ Finding valid and reliable information from an appropriate website takes an understanding of both location and content.
■ Skills using Internet search engines to find health information and analyze the content are enhanced by practice.

II. CONTENT ANALYSIS[7–10]

A. Choose the correct online source for reliable information.
 ■ Many popular search engines lead to newspaper and magazine articles or websites that may not

<table>
<tr><td>**BOX 2-4**</td><td>**Databases for Locating Biomedical Information**</td></tr>
</table>

- **MEDLINE (PubMed), http://www.ncbi.nlm.nih.gov/pubmed/:** A service of the U.S. National Library of Medicine that includes over 16 million citations from MEDLINE and other life science journals for biomedical articles back to the 1950s; includes links to full-text articles and related resources.
- **CINAHL (Cumulative Index to Nursing and Allied Health Literature), http://www.cinahl.com/:** A bibliographic database that includes abstracts of nursing and allied health articles.
- **Cochrane Library (The Cochrane Collaboration), http://www.cochrane.org/:** An international nonprofit and independent organization; produces and disseminates systematic reviews of health care interventions and promotes the search for evidence in the form of clinical trials and other studies of interventions.
- **ADA's EBD website (The American Dental Association's Evidence-Based Dentistry), http://ebd.ada.org:** A dental informatics resource; provides practitioners with access to current scientific information that is easy to comprehend and that can be quickly reviewed at the point of care.
- **National Institutes of Health, http://health.nih.gov:** A searchable encyclopedia of health topics.

provide science-based, research-supported information.

- Reliable biomedical information can be found by using:
  - search engines such as EviDents (http://medinformatics.uthscsa.edu/) or the American Dental Association Center for Evidence-Based Dentistry (http://ebd.ada.org/Default.aspx)
  - databases such as those listed in **Box 2-4**
- Other online resources include e-published professional journals or newsletters, professional association- or government-published guidelines, and association, government, or education websites.

B. Determine the purpose of the site (e.g., to educate, entertain, or market products?). Be familiar with domain names and what they mean.
  - .edu and .gov are considered reliable sites for educational and governmental information.
  - .org indicates nonprofit organizations. An understanding of the mission and purpose of the organization is important.
  - .com, .biz, and .net tend to be from special-interest groups or advertising (possibly for profit).

C. Analyze the information to make sure it is relevant.
  - Topic covered in-depth?
  - Bibliography present?

  - References to other websites included?
  - All points of view covered?

D. Determine who is responsible for the information (i.e., author and publisher).
  - Author – credentials and contact information given?
  - Publisher of the site? To locate the publisher, look at the site address (URL), the website's home page, under links such as "About Us" or "Our Mission," or at the bottom of the page.

E. Determine the accuracy and objectivity of the site.
  - Accuracy
    - Information similar to other sources (textbooks/journal articles)?
    - Reference citations provided?
  - Objectivity
    - Conflicts of interest and/or bias apparent?
    - All points of view discussed?
    - Credentials of the author and publisher (to determine the underlying connection) provided?

F. Note how well the site is maintained.
  - Up-to-date
    - Last update indicated?
    - Publication date for specific information?
  - Quality control
    - Easy to navigate and find what is needed?
    - Links current and working?
    - Grammar and spelling errors?

G. Put it all together (strengths and weaknesses of website).
  - Weigh the appropriateness of all the aforementioned factors to determine if the website is worthwhile in relation to the topic and the clinical situation.
  - In addition, organizations such as the Health on the Net Foundation[11] and the URAC Health Website Accreditation Program[12] provide certification that is aimed at assuring accurate and objective health information on the Internet. Sites that display a symbol of accreditation from these organizations have met specific guidelines intended to assure the quality of health information they provide.

ETHICS IN RESEARCH[13]

- Ethics in research is about the responsibility of researchers to conduct nonbiased research, report accurate results, and protect the rights of individuals who participate as research subjects.
- Many dental hygienists will never actively fulfill the role of dental hygiene researcher. However, each can look for evidence that ethical principles were followed when reading the report of a research study.
- Basic ethical principles and decision-making guidelines are discussed on page 9 and also in Section Introductions throughout this textbook.

I. ETHICAL STANDARDS

The same ethical theories and ethical principles that guide professional interactions of the dental hygienist with patients, dental colleagues, other health care providers, and community members can also be applied to conducting research. Some examples are:

■ Honesty
■ Concepts of right and wrong or fairness
■ **Norms for conduct** that distinguish between acceptable and unacceptable behavior and treatment
■ Reliance on a professional Code of Ethics or other guidelines to make decisions for addressing ethical issues and dilemmas

II. ETHICAL RESEARCH INVOLVING HUMAN SUBJECTS

Ethical standards in research are designed to protect individuals who participate as research subjects, with regard to their rights to:

■ Self-determination
■ Privacy
■ Anonymity and confidentiality
■ Fair treatment
■ Protection from discomfort and harm
■ Understand the risks and benefits of participating in the study
■ Informed consent

III. INFORMED CONSENT FOR RESEARCH

■ Is a written consent form, signed by each individual who participates in a study subjects.
■ Is a standardized form provided for all study participants and is included within the research proposal.
■ Includes complete and advanced information about the nature of a study and what the study participant can expect.
■ Contains a statement of possible benefits and/or risks of the study.
■ Contains a confidentiality statement assuring the participant of anonymity.

IV. INSTITUTIONAL REVIEW BOARD

■ Before conducting any research study, a federal mandate requires the institution in which the project is being implemented to evaluate the research proposal.
■ The institutional review board (IRB) is a group of individuals within the institution who review research proposals submitted by researchers. The group can require modifications before approving research or disapprove research based on its review.
■ Purpose of IRB review is to protect the rights and welfare of human subject volunteers in research.
■ Published research articles often include a statement that IRB approval was received before conducting the study.

DOCUMENTATION

If current research findings from a journal article or other source are used to plan dental hygiene recommendations/interventions, the following factors are included in the patient's record:

■ The PICO question used to search for information
■ Citations for references that support the recommendation/intervention
■ Patient factors that may influence the recommendation/intervention
■ Timeline for evaluation of patient response to the recommendation/intervention
■ An example patient progress note is found in **Box 2-5**.

| **BOX 2-5** | **Example Progress Note for Documenting an EBDH Intervention** |

Patient presents for routine maintenance appointment with history of arthritis and limited hand/wrist movement. She asks about using a new kind of curved bristle toothbrush that her friend has told her about. Review of the literature (P = limited hand mobility, I = regular toothbrush, C = curved-bristle toothbrush, O = effective biofilm removal, healthy gingiva) found evidence that this kind of toothbrush can have successful clinical outcomes [Chava VK. An evaluation of the efficacy of a curved bristle and conventional toothbrush: a comparative clinical study. *J Periodontol.* 2000 May; 71(5):785–9.]

Patient states that she knows where she can purchase this kind of brush. Instruction provided on basic technique for using the curved bristle toothbrush. Patient will bring the toothbrush at her next scheduled maintenance appointment in 3 months and her success in biofilm removal with this brush will be assessed.

Signed: _____, RDH Date: _____

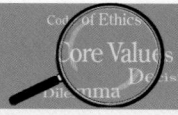

Everyday Ethics

After discussing a new surface disinfection product with Rick, a dental product representative, and conducting a review of the literature related to the efficacy and safety of the primary ingredient, Sondra, the dental hygienist, reports to the office manager that there is no scientific evidence that supports the claim that this product is as good as what they are already using for surface disinfection in their clinic. The office manager, who has been dating Rick for the last few months, is in charge of ordering all office supplies, orders the product anyway and tells Sondra that she selected it because the product is considerably less expensive than what they have been using. She supports her decision by restating the claims in the company's brochure related to the efficacy of the product.

Questions for Consideration

1. Explain why this situation is an ethical issue as well as an ethical dilemma for Sondra?
2. What is the chief concern/problem related to this situation? What are the long-term implications if Sondra is not able to resolve the situation?
3. What core values apply as Sondra considers alternatives for resolving this situation? What personal values might Sondra review as she considers alternative actions to pursue?

Factors To Teach The Patient

■ A result from one study does not necessarily provide the best answer. The type of study, patient parameters, and other factors are taken into consideration before a decision is made about best-practice interventions.

■ Research method, study design, source of information, and many other factors can affect the validity, reliability, and usefulness of health-related information.

■ A statistical significance cited in a study does not mean that clinically it is the best decision for a patient.

References

1. Forrest JL, Miller SA, Overman PO, Newman MG. Evidence-based decision making: a translational guide for dental professionals. Philadelphia: Lippincott, Williams & Wilkins; 2009. pp. 1–3.
2. Aravamudhan K, Frantsve-Hawley J. American Dental Association's resources to support evidence-based dentistry. *J Evid Based Dent Pract.* 2009 Sep;9(3):139–44.
3. Forrest J, Miller S. Evidence-based decision making in action: Part 1–finding the best clinical evidence. *J Contemp Dent Pract.* 2002 Aug;3(3):10–26.
4. Sutherland SE. Evidence-based dentistry: Part V. Critical appraisal of the dental literature: papers about therapy. *J Can Dent Assoc.* 2001 Sept;67(8):442–5.
5. Forrest JL, Miller SA, Overman PO, Newman MG. op. cit., pp. 128–32.
6. Forrest J, Miller S. Evidence-based decision making in action: Part 2–evaluating and applying the clinical evidence. *J Contemp Dent Pract.* 2003 Feb15;4(1):42–52.
7. Cornell University Library. Five Criteria for Evaluating Web Pages [Internet]. Ithaca (NY): Cornell University; 2010 June 28 [cited 2010 Nov 15]; [1 screen]. Available from: http://olinuris.library.cornell.edu/ref/research/webcrit.html
8. Northern Virginia Community College. Research Tools: Website Evaluation: a brief guide to evaluating websites [Internet]. Northern Virginia Community College, copyright 2010 [cited 2010 Nov 15]; [1 screen]. Available from: http://www.nvcc.edu/library/research-tools.htm
9. University of California at Berkley. Evaluating Web Pages: Techniques to Apply & Questions to Ask [Internet]. Berkley: University of California at Berkley; 2010 March 23 [cited 2010 Nov 15]; [1 screen]. Available from: http://www.lib.berkeley.edu/TeachingLib/Guides/Internet/Evaluate.html
10. University Of Michigan Library. Criteria for Website Evaluation [Internet]. Ann Arbor (MI): University of Michigan; 2010 August 10 [cited 2010 Nov 15]; [1 screen]. Available from: http://guides.lib.umich.edu/content.php?pid=30524
11. Health on the Net Foundation. HONCode Certification: What is it? [Internet]. Geneva, Switzerland: Health on the Net Foundation; 2010 March 1 [cited 2010 Nov 15]; [about 7 screens]. Available from: http://www.hon.ch/HONcode/Pro/Visitor/visitor.html
12. URAC. Health Website and Health Content Vendor Accreditation Program [Internet]. Washington DC: URAC; copyright 2003–2010 [cited 2010 Nov 15]; [1]. Available from: http://www.urac.org/programs/prog_accred_HWS_po.aspx
13. Aita M, Richer M. Essentials of research ethics for healthcare professionals. *Nurs Health Sci.* 2005 Jun;7(2):119–25.

Effective Health Communication

CHARLOTTE J. WYCHE, RDH, MS

Chapter Outline

Health communication is the use of communication strategies that enhance ability to provide patient-centered health information, motivate positive changes in health behaviors, and achieve improved health outcomes. In the context of dental hygiene care, good communication skills help patients embrace healthy behaviors of all types that allow them to attain and maintain oral health. Key words related to health communication are found in **Box 3-1**.

HEALTH COMMUNICATION

I. OBJECTIVES OF HEALTH COMMUNICATION

Healthy People 2020 health communication objectives[1] related to direct patient care include:

- Shared decision-making between patients and providers
- Personalized, targeted, accurate, accessible, and actionable information, self-management tools, and resources
- Increase of health literacy skills

II. SKILLS AND ATTRIBUTES OF EFFECTIVE HEALTH COMMUNICATORS

Healthcare providers who most effectively deliver preventive interventions demonstrate the following during patient interactions:[2]

- Expertise and knowledge in health and prevention
- Understanding of learning/behavior change theories and principles of good communication
- Relationship building skills

BOX 3-1	Key Words

Health Communication

Affect: as used by mental health professionals, refers to an expressed or observed emotional response or lack of expression of emotional response (flat or restricted affect).

Communication: a process of defining the meaning of a message shared between a sender and one or more intended recipients.

- **Mass Communication:** communication from one source intended to reach a large group of individuals.
- **Nonverbal Communication:** sending and receiving wordless messages; usually refers to body language, gestures, facial expressions, eye contact, and verbal elements such as rhythm and intonation.
- **Verbal Communication:** sending and receiving messages using words; usually defined as spoken or written communication.

Culture: refers to a learned set of beliefs, values, attitudes, convictions, and behaviors that are common to a group (especially an ethnic group) of people and usually passed down from generation to generation.

Cultural competence: a set of congruent attitudes, skills, behaviors, and policies that enable effective cross-cultural communication for delivery of oral health services.

Cultural sensitivity: refers to making an effort to understand the language, culture, and behaviors of diverse individuals and groups.

Culturally effective oral healthcare: refers to a dynamic relationship between provider and patient that results in culturally relevant and culturally specific oral healthcare recommendations; delivery of oral healthcare services in a way that is respectful of and responsive to the cultural norms and linguistic needs of individual patients.

Decoding: the reverse process of encoding; the receiver takes the words, gestures, or other signs to recreate the thought.

Diadic: refers to one-on-one communication between two people; in contrast to communication among a group or from one person toward a group of individuals.

Encode: refers to the translation of a thought into words, gestures, or other linguistic signs that will allow thoughts to be expressed in some understandable way to another; encoding can be verbal or nonverbal, oral, visual, or tactile.

Feedback: the receiver's direct response to a communicated message.

Haptics: touch as a form or component of communication.

Kinesics: body language or physical movement.

Linguistic competence: refers to providing culturally appropriate oral and written health information for persons with limited proficiency in English (or other dominant local language).

Mass Media: methods of communication that uses technology (such as print, television, or Internet) to reach a large, diverse audience.

Neurolinguistics: the study of the causes and effects of language disorders and how to communicate with individuals with language disorders (such as aphasia).

Occulesics: eye behavior, such as direct or indirect eye contact, during communication.

Oral health disparities: significant differences in oral health status and/or access to oral health services between one population and another; populations affected by disparities include racial and ethnic minorities, the elderly, and persons with disabilities.

Plain language publication: written health information that uses simplified terminology, pictures, or any other method that can enhance understanding for patients with limited language proficiency.

Pragmatics: study of the impact of language and how people use language.

Proxemics: refers to the component or dimension of physical space or distance in the context of human communication.

Semantics: study of the meaning of language.

Stereotype: an attitude or judgment (either positive or negative) made about people that is usually not based on personal experience but rather on what has been learned from other sources; seeing individuals from a population group as having no individuality as though all have the same characteristics.

Vocalics: cues, such accent, loudness, tempo, pitch, cadence, and tone, that occur during verbal communication.

- Interview and role modeling skills
- Assessment for readiness to change behaviors
- Attention to the patient's attitudes and beliefs
- Personal attributes of confidence and flexibility

III. ATTRIBUTES OF EFFECTIVE HEALTH INFORMATION[3]

Recommendations made by a health educator are more likely to be effective if the patient perceives that the information is:

- Evidence-based, accurate, balanced, and reliable
- Consistent with information from other sources
- Culturally and linguistically appropriate

- Delivered in an easily understood and accessible way
- Provided when the patient is most ready to receive it
- Repeated and reinforced over time

 ## TYPES OF COMMUNICATION

- Communication is a process that involves at least two, and sometimes multiple, individuals.
- The source, who has a desire to communicate some specific concept, encodes and then transmits a message to at least one receiver who decodes the message.
- This process can then reverse itself and the receiver becomes the sender of a return message that may or

may not provide direct feedback to the original message that was sent.

- The effectiveness of the communication depends on how closely the encoding and the decoding match. Barriers to effective communication are discussed later in the chapter.
- All communication is either verbal or nonverbal. Each can be subdivided into vocal and nonvocal.

I. VERBAL

- A form of communication based on language or words.
- Vocal communication is spoken language.
- Nonvocal communication is based on signs or signals that express language concepts, and include writing, Braille, and sign language.

II. NONVERBAL

Messages expressed by body language or affective (expressive) display can influence or interfere with a healthcare provider's ability to communicate, perhaps even more than the verbal method used. Some nonverbal, nonvocal factors include:

- Body position (posture or use of social space)
- Movement of body parts such as hands or arms
- Eye movements and facial expression.
- Appearance (grooming and dress)

Nonverbal, vocal factors include:

- Vocal qualifiers (volume, pitch, tempo and cadence)
- Vocal characterizers (crying, laughing).

III. MEDIA COMMUNICATION

- Media communication refers to the use of tools or technology to convey information.
- Media communication can be directed to an individual recipient (written care plan provided for an individual patient) or to a wider, more diverse target audience (patient education brochures developed by a professional association or health information on the Internet).

BARRIERS TO EFFECTIVE COMMUNICATION

It is rare that every message coded and transmitted by a sender is decoded and understood with complete accuracy by the receiver. Multiple factors that can affect the way health messages are understood are described in **Table 3-1**.

- Many of the factors listed in the table overlap in their description; more than one barrier may exist and have an effect on an attempt at communication.

TABLE 3-1	BARRIERS TO EFFECTIVE HEALTH COMMUNICATION
BARRIER	**DESCRIPTION**
Cultural	Differences in social norms or perceptions related to differences in gender, age, language, economic, or ethnic background
Interpersonal	Discomfort related to perceptions about the individual; appearance causes distraction; individuals don't see "eye-to-eye" or relate well to each other
Attitudinal	Lack of sensitivity or respect; over or under-confidence displayed by either patient or clinician
Physical	Distractions related to the physical environment; noise levels; face-to-face positioning not used.
Physiological	Inability to hear, see, touch or vocalize as required to communicate
Physocological	Emotional factors such as fear or pain cause distraction
Insufficient knowledge	Either the clinician is not well informed and cannot provide sufficient information or the patient has low health literacy and cannot understand the information provided
Lack of access to knowledge	Inability to access media or use technology to find information
Lack of interest	Patient is not ready to engage in health behavior change; clinician is experiencing "burn out" or disinterest in patient education
Information overload	Too much information on too many topics is provided at one time; no written reinforcement is provided
Poor communication skills	Either the patient or the clinician is not able to respond or provide feedback to messages received; clinician uses "jargon" or professional terminology that the patient does not understand

- All of the factors listed can provide a barrier to communication in either direction between the clinician and the patient.
- Dental hygienists who strive to develop good listening skills, enhance their ability to assess a patient's needs, and approach each individual with empathy and respect can go far toward overcoming the barriers to effective health communication.

HEALTH LITERACY

Health literacy is a set of cognitive and social skills that determine the ability of a patient to obtain, understand, or respond to health messages and be motivated to make health decisions that promote and maintain good health.[4] A large part of even an educated population may have low health literacy and often these are the patients with the highest treatment needs and the greatest barriers to receiving health information.

I. HEALTH LEARNING CAPACITY[5]

The level of a patient's health literacy depends on not only the reading level but also the complex interaction of cognitive and psychosocial skills. Skills that support health-learning capacity are listed in **Table 3-2**.

II. ASSESS AND ADDRESS HEALTH LITERACY[4]

To enhance communication with all patients regardless of health literacy level:

- Assess health literacy level and provide an individualized approach for every patient.
- Ensure a clinic environment that is helpful and user friendly by providing clear directions, visible and clearly written signs or universal symbols, and color-coded maps where necessary.

TABLE 3-2	SKILLS NECESSARY FOR HEALTH LEARNING TO INCREASE HEALTH LITERACY CAPACITY
DOMAINE	**SKILL SET**
Cognitive	Information processing ability Attention Short and long-term memory capacity Reasoning ability
Combined Cognitive/Psychosocial	Numeracy (ability with numbers) Verbal ability Reading
Psychosocial	Self-efficacy Communication ability Previous health-related experience

Source: Wolf MS, Wilson EA, Rapp DN, Waite KR, Bocchini MV, Davis TC, Rudd RE. *Pediatrics*. 2009 Nov;124 Suppl 3: S275–S281.

- Encourage patients to write down and bring questions about their oral health to each appointment.
- Provide health history, informed consent forms that are written in plain language. Provide help if required in completing forms.
- Build on the patient's current knowledge base to encourage healthy decision making.
- Provide written patient education materials that use plain, easily understandable language rather than materials that use professional jargon or provide complex explanation of patient conditions.
- Use visual aids for education materials when appropriate.
- Monitor to determine understanding of all forms and education materials. The "teach-back" method of asking patients to explain following instructions is a helpful approach.

COMMUNICATION THEORIES

Effective health communication is grounded in basic communication theory. The ultimate goal of health communication is to persuade behavior change that will support optimum health. Communication and persuasion theories most often associated with oral health research are discussed briefly in the following sections.[6]

I. HEALTH BELIEF MODEL

- Basic premise is that if people are informed, they will make good health-related decisions.
- Steps in this staged model are listed in **Table 3-3**. Each step is dependent on the previous step.

Limitations of this model are that information alone is not usually sufficient to change behaviors and that most behavior change does not follow a logical series of stepwise changes.

II. THEORY OF REASONED ACTION

- Based on the premise that individuals form an intention to make health-related changes on the basis of knowledge, personal values, and two different kinds of belief.
- *Behavioral beliefs* are attitudes held by the individual, formed on their understanding of relative risks, benefits, and possible outcomes. Knowledge and perception of personal health influence behaviors.
- *Normative beliefs*, based on community or social norms and expectations held by others who influence the individual, also can exert a powerful influence on intentions, attitudes, and behaviors.
- This theory is most useful in predicting health behavior change in situations in which both the behavioral beliefs and normative beliefs are stable and consistent and when there are no extraneous factors that affect the individual's intention to change behavior.

TABLE 3-3	HEALTH BELIEF MODEL—BEHAVIOR CHANGE STEPS

TO MAKE A BEHAVIOR CHANGE, INDIVIDUALS MUST BELIEVE THAT	EXAMPLE RELATED TO ORAL DISEASE
They are **susceptible** to the condition.	The patient smokes cigars and research indicates that tobacco use increases the risk for oral cancer.
The condition is a **serious threat** to their health.	Statistics show that oral cancer can lead to disfigurement and even death.
The condition **can be prevented** or changed.	Research demonstrates that quitting smoking can significantly lower the risk of oral cancer.
They are **capable of actions** that can make the change happen.	The dental hygienist can provide help and support for individuals who want to quit using tobacco (see Chapter 33 for more information).

III. SELF-EFFICACY

- Based on the individual's belief that actions will affect outcome.
- Increased self-efficacy can be gained by experiencing success, learning from the success of others, and through verbal persuasion.
- While high self-efficacy regarding a specific area (such as oral self-care) can be a predictor of successful behavioral change, use of this theory for comprehensive health behavior change can be limited if the patient has low self-efficacy in another area (such as ability to limit carbohydrates in the diet).

IV. LOCUS OF CONTROL

- Based on the perception of personal control over issues related to health.

- Those with an internal locus of control believe that their personal actions determine their health status.
- Those with an external locus of control believe that health and illness are determined by external factors and that changing behaviors will not really have a positive effect overall.

V. TRANSTHEORETICAL MODEL AND STAGES OF CHANGE

- This theory states that individuals move along a continuum of predictable steps to change health-related behaviors.
- Healthcare providers can assess where the patient is on the continuum and provide individualized interventions and recommendations based on the patient's readiness to change.
- The six stages of change in the continuum are described in **Table 3-4**.

TABLE 3-4	COMPONENTS OF THE TRANSTHEORETICAL MODEL AND STAGES OF CHANGE

STEPS AND DESCRIPTION	IMPLICATIONS FOR DENTAL HYGIENE CARE
Precontemplation No intention of behavior change	Provide information and initiate discussion regarding risks.
Contemplation Considering behavior change (within 6 months)	Assist patient in examining pros and cons of proposed behavior change.
Preparation Ready and actively planning to make the change	Provide information, support, encouragement, and follow-up to be sure the behavior change has been initiated.
Action The behavior change has been adopted	Provide support, encouragement, and follow-up to make sure the behavior change continues.
Maintenance The change has been continuous for at least 6 months.	Provide encouragement and continued follow-up to support during potential relapse.
Termination Not often reached—as if the previous behavior did not even exist; return to old behavior is highly unlikely	Celebrate: recognize success and continue to reinforce reduced risk for oral disease.

Courtesy of Terri Tilliss, RDH, MS, MA, PhD.

- Motivational interviewing, a patient education approach described in the next section, is based on the Transtheoretical Model or the Stages of Change theory.

MOTIVATIONAL INTERVIEWING

(Contributed by Terri Tilliss, RDH, MS, MA, PhD)

- Health education strategies that provide new knowledge, make recommendations, and demonstrate products and procedures may not result in the necessary changes in patient behavior.
- Attempts by oral healthcare providers to encourage oral self-care behaviors using traditional methods may involve negative concepts such as confrontation, guilt, defensiveness, and resistance.
- Motivational interviewing is a well-accepted, patient-centered communication alternative that can help increase a patient's engagement in their own oral care and strengthen commitment to health-related behavior changes.[7–10]
- Differences between the motivational interviewing and traditional patient education approaches are listed in **Table 3-5**.

I. BACKGROUND

- First utilized in the early 80s for client-centered psychotherapy.
- Derived from the supportive and empathic counseling style of Carl Rogers.[11]
- Supported by the Stages of Change theory, also known as the Transtheoretical Model.[12]

- Was applied to health-related behavior change in the late 90s by Miller and Rollnick[13] and others.

II. KEY COMPONENTS

The motivational interviewing approach changes the relationship between the patient and the healthcare provider, putting the patient in charge. Key components of the motivational interviewing approach include:[9]

- Expressing empathy, acceptance, and respect for the patient
- Recognizing inconsistencies between current actions/behaviors and the patient's own health-related goals
- Recognizing, understanding, and exploring resistance to change
- Eliciting self-motivation discussion
- Supporting self-efficacy

III. CHARACTERISTICS OF EFFECTIVE TECHNIQUE[7,14]

- Establish rapport. Raise the patient's awareness and ask for permission to discuss the topic.
- Acknowledge the patient's concerns, priorities, and arguments against change; express empathy and acceptance rather than scold.
- Avoid confrontation when dealing with resistance.
- Assess readiness for change and tailor interventions to facilitate movement along the continuum.
- Provide feedback. Incorporate active listening skills that are attentive to what the patient is saying and convey interest and concern.

TABLE 3-5	**DIFFERENCES BETWEEN TRADITIONAL PATIENT EDUCATION AND MOTIVATIONAL INTERVIEWING**
TRADITIONAL	**MOTIVATIONAL INTERVIEWING**
Persuasive	Supportive
Similar motivational approach for all patients	Patient-directed counseling or coaching approach
Clinicians decide/select behaviors to be changed	Patients make the decisions and are considered the "expert" in directing their own life
Clinician assumes the "power role" and patient is subordinate	Respects patient autonomy
Patient's ambivalence and resistance are not directly addressed	Ambivalence is explored and resistance is resolved
Assumes all patients are ready for behavior change	Recognizes that readiness for change occurs in stages
Clinician does most of the talking, creating a monolog	Patient and clinician engage in a dialogue
Clinician instills knowledge, insight, and motivation	Seeks to evoke intrinsic motivation for behavior change
Motivation often based on guilt, intimidation, or scare tactics	Builds trust within patient–clinician relationship that supports change

Courtesy of Terri Tilliss, RDH, MS, MA, PhD.

- Listen more than talk, especially at the beginning of a conversation.
- Practice attentive listening rather than multitasking during conversations.
- Sit eye-to-eye with the patient rather than with the patient in a reclined position or standing/sitting taller than the patient does.
- Convey a nonjudgmental attitude, reinforce an atmosphere of respect and valuing of the individual, even if the behavior is not acceptable.
- Maintain a calm, unhurried demeanor.
- Use a normal tone of voice and vocabulary that is appropriate, but does not talk down, to the patient.
- Look for clues, share your thoughts and observations, and ask questions.
- Do not jump to conclusions.
- Link information to activities of daily living to help provide context for recommendations.

- Employ reflective listening skills and paraphrase patient statements to evaluate accuracy.
- Ask open-ended questions that help patient identify and word through concerns or ambivalence to change.
- Support self-efficacy and allow patient to explore their health goals, desires, and potential for successful behavior change.
- Shift the responsibility for goal achievement to the patients, but let them know that support is available.

COMMUNICATION ACROSS THE LIFESPAN

Irrespective of the patient's age, building rapport is the key to effective health communication. Tips for establishing rapport with patients of all ages are found in **Box 3-2**. Key points related to specific age groups are discussed in the subsequent sections.

I. CHILDREN AND ADOLESCENTS[15]

The oral health needs of young children are more specifically discussed in Chapter 49 on pages 754 to 773. Information about oral health issues during adolescence is found on pages 787 to 793.

A. Infants (Birth to 12 Months)

Infants communicate primarily through their senses of touch, sight, and hearing. Techniques the clinician can use to communicate with an infant during a dental hygiene examination include:

- Interact playfully with a receptive infant by mimicking facial expressions, rocking, and talking softly or singing.

- Encourage an adult who is familiar with the infant to distract and comfort the child.
- Wait until the infant is calm to approach closely.

B. Toddlers and Preschoolers (Ages 1 to 2 and 3 to 5)

- Although dependent on adults for their care, most children appreciate and respond to being approached directly.
- Development of a sense of self enhances the need to assert independence and maintain control over any situation.
- Offer encouragement and gentle hints or engage in "parallel" actions to demonstrate, rather than directly assisting, to promote success in age appropriate self-care tasks.
- Calmly distract or direct toward an alternative behavior to counter defiance or inappropriate behavior.
- State specifically what the child is expected to do rather than criticize to effectively control unwanted behavior.
- Ask simple, specifically focused questions to help the child remember past experiences.
- To overcome the limited ability to process auditory information and short attention span, provide brief, truthful, and simple instructions and responses to questions.
- Toddlers are beginning to converse in short sentences, but if the adult becomes impatient or abrupt, the child may feel frustrated or ashamed and become unresponsive.
- Children this age understand more than they are given credit for but often misinterpret language that is not familiar to them; therefore, serious discussions or use of certain words may distress them.

C. School-Age Children (6 through 12)

- The ability is developing to understand serious events logically and comprehend impact on themselves.
- More aware of the needs of others but may be reluctant to state their own needs. Third-person statements such as "I know a child who was afraid and this is what he did." may help overcome anxieties.
- The ability and desire to respond to simple questions can allow the dental hygienist to assess knowledge and misconceptions.

D. Adolescents (13 through 18)

- Marked by intense and often extreme feelings about situations and persons in their world.
- Strongly independent and desire to have their viewpoint considered with respect.
- Tendency to withdraw or become hostile if they feel they are misunderstood.
- A straightforward approach that explains and then solicits input into a discussion on topics that interest the adolescent is most effective to build rapport and establish trust.

■ Confidentiality laws, which vary from state to state, can help determine what behavior-related information the dental hygienist discusses with a parent or guardian. Anything that is an immediate safety issue (such as thoughts of suicide) is related immediately.

To develop a rapport and a trusting relationship with an adolescent patient:

■ Address the adolescent directly even when parent/guardian is present.
■ Ensure that the adolescent has the opportunity to ask and answer questions independently (privately) as well as with parents/guardians.[16]

II. OLDER ADULTS[17]

Oral health issues related to aging are discussed in Chapter 52 on pages 804 to 806. Providing effective health education for aging patients who are experiencing a communication difficulty requires respect for the needs of the individual and response to functional ability or limitations. Suggestions for communicating with older individuals experiencing communication difficulty are listed in **Box 3-3**.

A. Physical and Cognitive Changes

■ Cognitive disabilities are more likely to be present as an individual ages and to interfere with understanding health-related information.
■ Communication disorders such as dysarthria and aphasia are associated with conditions that are more common in an aging population.
■ Sensory loss (particularly hearing loss) can provide challenges in interpersonal communication.
■ Physiologic changes may occur in speech patterns, including voice tremor, pitch, loudness, and speaking rate.

B. Communication Predicament[18,19]

■ Healthcare providers often use an inappropriate over-modification of speech and language when addressing older patients.
■ *Accommodative speech* refers to use of a high-pitched tone of voice, a "sing song" cadence, and relatively simplistic language when addressing an older adult.

BOX 3-3	Suggestions for Communicating With Older Adults Experiencing Communication Difficulty

■ Identify communication barriers and modify communication approach appropriately.
■ Identify and avoid "elderspeak."
■ Practice speech that affirms and respects the patient level of competence and independence.

■ Use of *terms of endearment* (honey, sweetie, dearie) and *diminutive* forms of a patient's name can reflect a lack of respect for the individual as an adult person.
■ Use of plural pronouns ("Are we ready for our appointment?") can imply that the patient cannot act alone or make independent decisions.
■ This "baby talk" or "elderspeak" approach to communication does not enhance comprehension and can be perceived as patronizing or demeaning.

COMMUNICATION WITH CAREGIVERS

■ Many patients with disabling conditions and also young children rely on someone else to help with or provide daily self-care regimens. The dental hygienist then communicates with the caregiver or parent as well as the patient.
■ In a group conversation, keep the primary focus on the patient by maintaining eye contact and directing comments/questions to the patient, if appropriate, as well as the caregiver.
■ Assess patient needs and caregiver relationships carefully to determine the extent of the caregiver's role in daily self-care.
■ Encourage the caregiver to allow the patient to maintain as much independence as possible.

CULTURAL CONSIDERATIONS

Culturally sensitive delivery of dental hygiene services can make a positive difference in oral health outcomes.[20] A cultural awareness checklist is found in **Box 3-4**.

I. CULTURE AND HEALTH

A. Effects of Culture on Oral Health Status

The increasing diversity of ethnic/racial communities and linguistic groups in the United States presents a challenge to the delivery of oral health services.

■ Health disparities related to cultural and ethnic background exist in the healthcare system.[21]
■ Each individual patient presents with learned patterns of health knowledge and behaviors that "must be transcended to achieve equal access and quality health care."[22]
■ Ignoring culture can lead to negative health consequences and/or poor clinical outcomes.[23]

Culture and language can influence:[22]

■ Beliefs and behaviors related to health, healing, and wellness.
■ Perceptions of illness, diseases, and their causes.
■ Attitudes of patients toward accessing health services or attitudes toward healthcare providers.

BOX 3-4	A Checklist to Enhance Cultural Awareness During Patient Care

- Examine and recognize any personal bias that may affect communication when working with patients from a different culture.
- Conduct all patient assessments with cultural sensitivity in mind.
- Assess to determine the patient's cultural identification and, if necessary, research to identify implications for dental hygiene practice.
- Determine language barriers, identify patient's preferred method of communication, and regularly double-check to assure comprehension.
- Identify religious and health-related beliefs, views, or misconceptions that may influence dental hygiene interventions.
- Identify and address cultural dietary considerations.
- Double-check verbal and nonverbal signs routinely to determine the level of the patient's trust of healthcare providers.

Source: Seibert PS, Stridh-Igo P, Zimmerman CG. A checklist to facilitate cultural awareness and sensitivity. J Med Ethics 2002 Jun;28(3):143–146.

- Attitudes and behaviors of providers who may have learned a set of values that are different from those of their patients.

B. Culturally Effective Oral Care

- Meeting each patient's individual oral care needs is the hallmark of dental hygiene practice.
- The ability to provide effective oral health education and dental hygiene services for culturally diverse patients requires the ability to assess, be sensitive to, and respect each patient's cultural differences.
- Culturally effective dental hygiene care respects each patient's health beliefs, practices, values, customs, and traditions in the plan for dental hygiene care.

II. CROSS-CULTURAL COMMUNICATION

Communication with patients from other cultures is enhanced when the dental hygienist develops knowledge about and avoids stereotyping traditional behaviors and values of a patient's cultural group. Knowing some general principles can enhance communication.

A. Nonverbal Communication

Some culturally related differences in nonverbal communication are identified in **Table 3-6**. To communicate successfully the dental hygienist will:

- Follow the patient's lead for touching or personal space.
- Use hand and arm gestures with caution.

- Be careful interpreting facial expressions.
- Follow the patient's lead for making eye contact.

B. Language Proficiency

- Simplify language as much as possible without speaking down to the patient.
- Eliminate professional jargon.
- Use pictures, diagrams, and demonstrations to help increase understanding.
- Provide "plain language" health information publications to reinforce and support compliance with oral health recommendations.

C. Using an Interpreter

When the patient's skills in the dominant language are not sufficient to assure informed consent or compliance with recommendations, a professional interpreter can be used to enhance communication. Family members or friends are not the same as a professional interpreter.

- A professional interpreter will have proficiency in both languages as well as an ability to convey complex information completely and accurately. Informal interpreters are more likely to modify important information or interject their own opinions, beliefs, or prejudices.
- It is particularly inadvisable to ask children to interpret sensitive health information.
- Focus on and direct all communication to the patient, with pauses to allow the interpreter to translate.

D. Family Decision Making

- In many cultures, an individual's health problem is considered to be a family problem.
- Involvement of certain family members in the treatment planning process may be a key factor in assuring compliance with recommendations.
- Sensitivity is needed when family members or children, even older children, are involved in the discussion.

III. ATTAINING CULTURAL COMPETENCE

Cultural and linguistic competence is the ability of healthcare providers and organizations to understand and respond to the needs of culturally diverse populations for whom they provide care. Achieving cultural competence in providing healthcare is a process[24] that requires a commitment to cultural awareness, a motivation to engage in cultural encounters, and an ongoing acquisition of cultural knowledge and communication skills. The dental hygienist who strives to become adept at providing culturally effective care:

- Values (and not simply tolerates) diversity.
- Conducts honest self-assessment to determine how personal health beliefs, traditions, and biases influence ability to relate to culturally different individuals.

TABLE 3-6	NONVERBAL COMMUNICATION AND CROSS-CULTURAL CONSIDERATIONS
ATTRIBUTE	**EXPLANATION**
Facial Expressions	■ Smiling, winking, and blinking may not signify the same intent in all cultures. ■ People from some cultures point at an object by shifting eyes or pursing lips because pointing with a hand or finger is inappropriate. ■ Expressions of pain and discomfort may differ among cultures or according to family experiences. Some cultures value stoicism while others seem to emote effusively.
Gestures	■ Hand signs can be interpreted in many ways among cultures. ■ Some commonly used gestures, such as the "OK" finger-thumb circle shape or the "thumbs-up" gesture have vulgar connotations for members of some cultures.
Head Movements and Physical Postures	■ Head movement signs for "yes" and "no" vary greatly in some cultures. ■ Some cultures nod head (as in "yes") to indicate attention to or respect for the speaker—even if the answer to the question is not yes or if they do not understand what is being said. ■ Standing with hands on hips might indicate a challenge to members of some cultures. ■ Many cultures consider slouching or poor posture as a sign of disrespect. ■ Showing the bottom of the shoe (resting foot on top of knee while sitting) is considered impolite in some cultures.
Personal Space and Touching	■ Individuals from some cultures are accustomed to standing or sitting very close and sometimes touching, even during casual interactions; others may express alarm if the provider stands or sits too close. ■ A light touch, a brief kiss on the cheek, or warm handshake is common in some cultures, even among people who have just met or individuals of the same gender. ■ In some cultures, such physical contact may be extremely inappropriate. ■ In some cultures, touching or accepting an article with the left hand is considered unclean.
Eye Contact	■ In some cultures making direct eye-to-eye contact is a sign of respect; in others, it is a sign of disrespect especially if done by a child or toward an authority figure such as a healthcare provider. ■ The "languid" or half-closed eyes of individuals from some cultures in not necessarily a sign of disrespect or inattention.

Source: Management Sciences for Health (MSH) [Internet]. Cambridge: MSH, US. Department of Health and Human Services, Health Resources and Services Administration, and Bureau of Primary Health Care: c 2010. Non-verbal communication: the provider's guide to quality and culture. [cited 2010, Aug 27]; [about 13 screens]. Available from: http://erc.msh.org/mainpage.cfm?file=4.6.0.htm&module=provider&language=English

■ Actively acquires knowledge about patients' health beliefs, behaviors, and cultural norms.
■ Is nonjudgmental regarding cultural traditions and beliefs.
■ Avoids stereotypes.
■ Routinely adapts delivery of dental hygiene care in a way that reflects understanding of each patient's diversity and unique oral health needs.

IV. CULTURAL COMPETENCE AND THE DENTAL HYGIENE PROCESS OF CARE

Respect for each patient's cultural differences, healthcare practices, health beliefs, and values can be integrated into all areas of the dental hygiene process of care.[25]

A. Assessment

The ability to collect accurate, complete assessment data is the key to providing dental hygiene interventions that meet patient needs.

■ Culturally effective nonverbal communication and listening skills help build trust and patient rapport that can facilitate the transfer of essential personal health information.
■ Skillful, nonjudgmental questioning can help elicit cultural specific data such as health beliefs and values, as well as avoid misunderstandings about a patient's culturally related health practices.
■ Asking permission before touching a patient during the extra- and intraoral examination procedures can avoid problems with cultural differences in personal space.

B. Diagnosis

A dental hygiene diagnosis is predicated on a clear understanding of the patient's history, medical status, symptoms, and current treatment modalities. The culturally competent dental hygienist will prepare diagnostic statements that take into consideration:

■ Culture-specific health risks that are related to oral status
■ Cultural practices that may impact the patient's oral health status

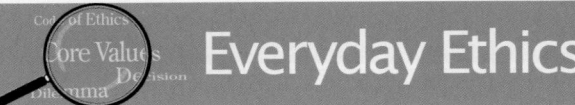

Everyday Ethics

Abelena Flores, a 65-year-old Mexican-American female who presents to the clinic for the first time for her initial assessment appointment. Mrs. Flores speaks English moderately well, but Lisel, the dental hygienist, notices that she is not able to read the health history and seems to be confused during more complex explanations. Lisel offers to obtain a medical translator for the next appointment, but Mrs. Flores insists that her son, who speaks English and her son's new wife who does not speak English, will accompany her to help interpret and make decisions about the treatment plan Lisel will present to her at that visit. Lisel is concerned that the family members will not be knowledgeable enough to be able to explain the needed treatment so that informed consent can be obtained.

Lisel considers arranging for a friend who is a medical translator to be present without telling Mrs. Flores beforehand. Lisel knows that her patient will not be charged for that service because the medical translator is a volunteer who has provided free translation services at the clinic in the past.

Questions for Consideration
1. Is this an ethical issue or an ethical dilemma for Lisel?
2. Explain which Core Values (Table II-1, page 38) Lisel will need to consider as she determines what action to take regarding the use of a translator during Mrs. Flores next appointment.
3. How might personal values related to Lisel's and Mrs. Flores' cultural differences affect Lisel's ethical duty in resolving this situation?

C. Planning

The dental hygiene care plan formulates oral health goals that meet the needs of each individual patient realistically. The goals identified in the plan are based on a synthesis of needs determined by the dental hygienist and those expressed by the patient.

- A culturally sensitive dental hygiene care plan respects and takes into consideration the patient's current health practices and beliefs.
- With the patient's input, the plan may be devised to accept, modify, or eliminate current culturally relevant healthcare practices.
- The plan is sensitive to the practices, products, or substances that the patient's culture prohibits, such as mouthrinses containing alcohol for patients in some cultures.
- A culturally and linguistically sensitive approach to communicating the dental hygiene care plan can facilitate informed consent for dental hygiene interventions.

D. Implementation

Culturally appropriate communication can enhance the patient's cooperation during treatment.

- Knowledge of culturally determined expressions of pain and discomfort during treatment can help the dental hygienist determine appropriate pain control measures during treatment.
- Language appropriate instructions before, during, and after each procedure can enhance patient compliance with treatment.
- "Plain language" oral health materials can enhance patient compliance with recommendations.

E. Evaluation

A dental hygienist who is sensitive to cultural differences evaluates treatment success on the basis of goals determined in a previously prepared culturally relevant care plan.

- Feedback provided for the patient respects culturally diverse beliefs and values related to oral health.
- Self-evaluation regarding the cultural effectiveness of the practitioner's approach can provide insight for planning modifications to the patient's continuing care plan.

DOCUMENTATION

When documenting communication aspects of a patient visit, the following factors are included:

- Patient's age, gender, and ethnicity
- Factors or observations related to health literacy level

BOX 3-5	**Example Progress Note Documenting the Communication Aspects of a Patient Visit**

Sixty-five-year-old African-American male presents for initial data collection appointment. Patient has significant hearing loss and does not use a hearing aid but reads lips during casual conversation. He prefers to ask complex questions and receive answers by writing on a notepad. Patient summarized or restated to demonstrate that he understood what was discussed and stated that all of his questions were answered. Initial data collection completed. Next visit: Presentation of care plan and begin oral hygiene instructions.

Signed: _____, RDH Date: _____

- Cultural characteristics that can affect communication or delivery of dental hygiene care
- Significant factors such as patient hearing loss, need to communicate with caregiver, use of an interpreter, and description of specific modifications made to accommodate those factors
- An example progress note that documents communication aspects of a patient visit is found in **Box 3-5**

Factors To Teach The Patient

- The dental hygienist's ability to provide good dental hygiene care is affected by the willingness and ability of the patient to communicate accurate and complete information about health status, needs, and concerns.
- The patient's motivation to follow oral health recommendations is affected by the rapport established and the trust developed between the patient and the clinician.

References

1. U.S. Department of Health and Human Services. Healthy people 2020: topics and objectives. Health Communication and Information Technology: overview [Internet]. Washington, DC: U.S. Department of Health and Human Services; 2010 Dec [cited 2011 Jan 3] Available from: http://www.healthypeople.gov/2020/topicsobjectives2020/overview.aspx?topicid=18
2. Burke LE, Fair J. Promoting prevention: skill sets and attributes of health care providers who deliver behavioral interventions. *J Cardiovasc Nurs.* 2003 Sep–Oct;18(4):256–66.
3. U.S. Department of Health and Human Services. Healthy people 2010: objectives for improving health. 2nd ed. Washington, DC: U.S. Government Printing Office; 2000 Nov. Volume 1, Part A, Focus Area 11-Health communication;11.3–11.22.
4. Horowitz AM, Kleinman DV. Oral health literacy: the new imperative to better oral health. *Dent Clin North Am.* 2008 Apr;52(2):333–44, vi.
5. Wolf MS, Wilson EA, Rapp DN, Waite KR, Bocchini MV, Davis TC, Rudd RE. Literacy and learning in health care. *Pediatrics* 2009 Nov;124 Suppl 3:S275–S281.
6. Hollister MC, Anema MG. Health behavior models and oral health: a review. *J Dent Hyg.* 2004 Summer;78(3):6.
7. Britt E, Hudson SM, Biampied NM. Motivational interviewing in health settings: a review. *Patient Educ Couns.* 2004 May;53(2):147–55.
8. Harrison R, Benton T, Everson-Stewart S, Weinstein P. Effect of motivational interviewing on rates of early childhood caries: a randomized trial. *Pediatr Dent.* 2007 Jan–Feb;29(1):16–22.
9. Williams KB, Bray KK. Increasing patient engagement in care: motivational interviewing. *Access.* 2009 May–Jun;23(5):36–9.
10. Yevlahova D, Satur J. Models for individual oral health promotion and their effectiveness: a systematic review. *Aust Dent J* 2009 Sep;54(3):190–7.
11. Rogers CR. *On becoming a person: a therapist's view of psychotherapy.* New York: Houghton Mifflin; 1961.
12. Prochaska JO, DiClemente CC. Transtheoretical therapy: toward a more integrative model of change. *Psychother Theor Res Pract.* 1982;19(3):276–88.
13. Miller WR, Rollnick S. Motivational interviewing: preparing people for change. New York: Guilford Press; 2002.
14. Emmons KM, Rollnick S. Motivational interviewing in health care settings. Opportunities and limitations. *Am J Prev Med.* 2001 Jan;20(1):68–74.
15. Deering C, Cody D. Communicating with children and adolescents. *Am J Nurs.* 2002 Mar;102(3):34–41.
16. Mappa P, Baverstock A, Finlay F, Verling W. Current Practice with regard to 'seeing adolescents on their own' during outpatient consultations. *Int J Adolesc Med Health.* 2010 Apr–Jun;22(2): 301–5.
17. Yorkston KM, Bourgeois MS, Baylor CR. Communication and aging. *Phys Med Rehabil Clin N Am.* 2010 May;21(2)309–19.
18. Brown A, Draper P. Accommodative speech and terms of endearment: elements of a language mode often experienced by older adults. *J Adv Nurs.* 2003 Jan;41(1):15–21.
19. Williams K, Kemper S, Hummert ML. Enhancing communication with older adults: overcoming elderspeak. *J Gerontol Nurs.* 2004 Oct;30(10):17–25.
20. Rayman S, Almas K. Transcultural barriers and cultural competence in dental hygiene practice. *J Contemp Dent Pract.* 2007 May 1;8(4):43–51.
21. U.S. Department of Health and Human Services, Agency for Healthcare Research and Quality: 2008 National Healthcare Disparities Report (Publication # 09–0002). Rockville, MD: Agency for Healthcare Research and Quality; 2008 March. p. 2. [cited 2010 Nov 20]. Available from: www.ahrq.gov/qual/nhdr08/nhdr08.pdf
22. U.S. Department of Health and Human Services. Cultural Competency: What is Cultural Competency? [Internet]. Rockville, MD: Office of Minority Health Office of Minority Health; 2009 Oct 19 [modified cited 2010 Nov 20] [1 screen]. Available from: http://minorityhealth.hhs.gov/templates/browse.aspx?lvl=2&lvlID=11
23. Management Sciences for Health Electronic Resource Center, U.S. Department of Health and Human Services, Health Resources and Services Administration, and Bureau of Primary Healthcare. Cambridge, MA; Management Sciences for Health. ©2010: The Provider's Guide to Quality and Culture: Health Disparities: Clinical Outcomes. [cited 2010 Nov 20] [about 9 screens] Available from: http://erc.msh.org/mainpage.cfm?file=7.1.0.htm&module=provider&language=English
24. Campinha-Bacote J. The Process of Cultural Competence in the Delivery of Healthcare Services: a model of care. *J. Transcult. Nurs.* 2002 Jul;13(3):181–4.
25. Fitch P. Cultural competence and dental hygiene care delivery: Integrating Cultural Care into the Dental Hygiene Process of Care. *J Dent Hyg.* 2004 Winter;78(1):11–21.

Preparation for Dental Hygiene Practice

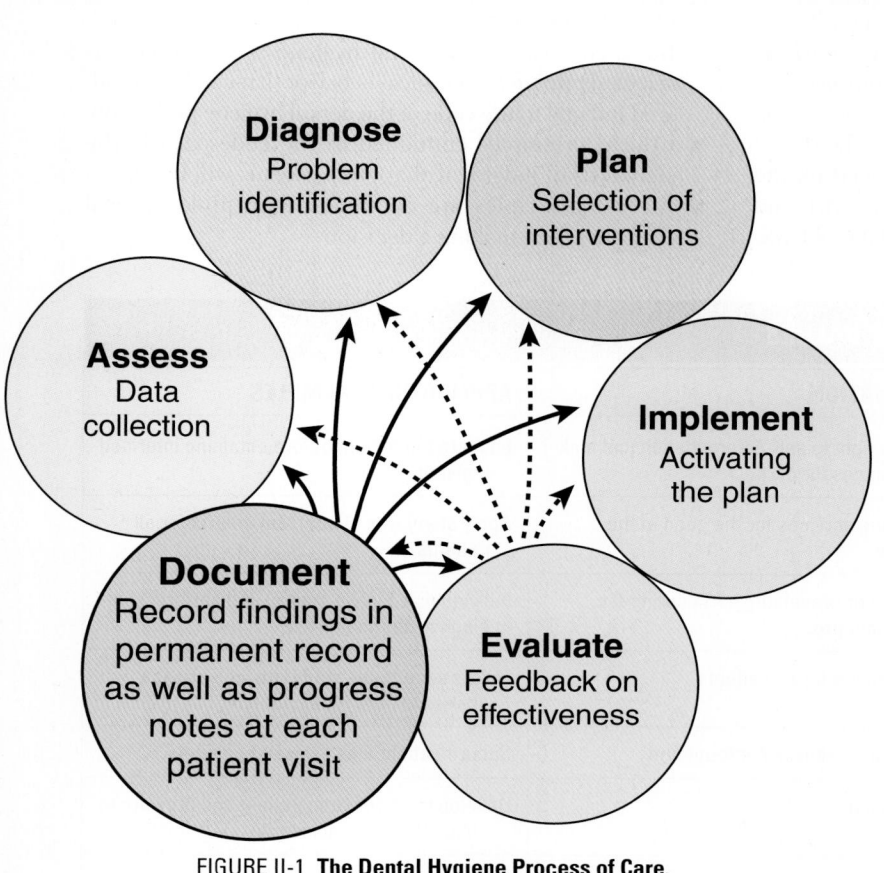

FIGURE II-1 **The Dental Hygiene Process of Care.**

INTRODUCTION

Preparation for dental hygiene care centers on the use of standard precautions for infection control to insure the safety of the patients and the clinician. In oral healthcare practice, an objective is to protect the health and safety of patients, dental personnel, and others who come in contact with the environment of the clinic or office. Health services facilities, including dental facilities, must be places for cure and prevention, not for increasing risk of disease or discomfort following inadequate precautionary measures and habits of the professional personnel.

■ The first responsibility of the entire team is to develop and maintain work practices for all appointments that will prevent direct or indirect cross-infection between dental personnel and patients and from one patient to another.
■ The second responsibility is to document all patient care activities in a comprehensive, ethical, and standardized manner.

Chapters in this section:

■ Provide specific information about the chain of infection and the microorganisms that can be transmitted in the dental setting when standard precautions are not observed.
■ Describe specific materials and procedures necessary for safe clinical practice. Appendix IV on page 1096 is related to these chapters and contains the United States Centers for Disease Control and Prevention *Guidelines for Infection Control in Dental Health-Care Settings.*
■ Outline procedures for reception and seating of the patient. To support the health and welfare of the dental hygiene practitioner, special emphasis is placed on the ergonomic factors of body posture and hand, wrist, and arm positions for prevention of musculoskeletal problems.

■ Describe methods for the systematic documentation of patient assessment data and patient visit activities.

THE DENTAL HYGIENE PROCESS OF CARE

Documentation of each aspect of patient care is an integral component of the Dental Hygiene Process of Care that is linked to every other step, as illustrated in **Figure II-1**. Preparation for clinical practice does not form a specific step; however, practices described in this section protect the patient and the practitioner and are encompassed within all of the components of the process.

ETHICAL APPLICATIONS

A dental hygienist may be involved in a variety of moral, ethical, and legal situations during practice. Principles of ethics are applied to all professional actions related to the process of care. The goal is to increase the awareness of, and sensitivity to, ethical situations during practice. An overview of the core values with definitions and applications is found in **Table II-1**.

■ Basic core values and principles, as outlined in the various *Dental Hygiene Codes of Ethics* found in the Appendices starting on page 1085, are applied in every phase of the dental hygiene appointment.
■ Basic core values in dental hygiene are identified as selected principles of ethical behavior that can be considered integral to the code of the dental hygiene profession.
■ Ethical principles contained in the codes clarify the standards of judgment that professionals will follow.
■ Ethical principles are combined with philosophical theories when making a decision.

TABLE II-1	DENTAL HYGIENE CORE VALUES	
ETHICAL PRINCIPLE/CORE VALUE	**EXPLANATION**	**APPLICATION EXAMPLES**
Autonomy	Patient's right to self-determination and making choices for care	Educate the patient before obtaining informed consent.
Beneficence	Performing services for the good of the patient	Apply standards of infection control for all patients.
Nonmaleficence	Removing or preventing harm during the treatment process	Individualize biofilm control and perform subgingival debridement.
Justice	Fair treatment for all patients	Follow acceptable standards and provide access to care for all patients.
Confidentiality	Protection of sensitive information	Secure patient files in locked cabinets.
Veracity	Truth-telling	Develop trust between patient and provider to obtain the medical history.
Fidelity	Keeping promises	Help a fearful patient be comfortable by using local anesthesia or nitrous oxide.

CHAPTER 4

Infection Control: Transmissible Diseases

BARBARA L. BENNETT, CDA, RDH, MS

Chapter Outline

For dental healthcare personnel (DHCP), infection and communicable disease can lead to illness, disability, and loss of work time. In addition, patients, family members, and community contacts can become exposed, may become ill, and lose productive time or suffer permanent after-effects.

■ In oral healthcare practice, the objective is to protect patients, dental personnel, and others who may become exposed to infectious agents in the environment of the office or clinic.

- Health services facilities, including dental facilities, are places for cure and prevention, not for dissemination of disease due to inadequate precautionary measures and habits of the professional personnel.
- The first responsibility of the entire dental team is to organize and maintain a system for the sterilization, disinfection, and care of instruments and equipment.
- The second step is to develop and maintain work practices for all appointments that will prevent direct or indirect cross-infections between dental personnel and patients and from one patient to another.
- **Box 4-1** lists and defines terms that apply to the transmission of infectious agents.

STANDARD PRECAUTIONS

- Previous infection control recommendations from the United States Centers for Disease Control and Prevention (CDCP) were focused on the risk of transfer of the blood-borne pathogens, and the term **universal precautions** was used.
- With recognition that other body fluids besides blood carry infectious agents, the new concepts have been enclosed within the all-inclusive term **standard precautions**.

I. STANDARD PRECAUTIONS: DEFINITION[1]

A. Integrate and expand the elements of universal precautions.
B. Represent a standard of care that protects DHCP and their patients from pathogens that can be spread by blood or any other body fluid, excretion, or secretion.
C. Apply to contact with the following:
- Blood
- All body fluids, secretions, and excretions (except sweat), regardless of whether they contain blood
- Nonintact skin
- Mucous membranes

II. ADDITIONAL TRANSMISSION-BASED PRECAUTIONS

A. Droplet precautions
- Close respiratory or mucous membrane contact transmitted through airborne droplets (sneezing, coughing).
- Examples: *Mycobacterium tuberculosis*, influenza, chickenpox transmitted through airborne droplets (sneezing, coughing)
B. Contact precautions
- Reduce risk of transmission of organisms and specific diseases by direct skin or indirect contact.
- Examples: Vancomycin-resistant enterococci, Methicillin-resistant *Staphylococcus aureus*
C. Airborne precautions
- Reduce risk of airborne transmission of infectious agents by droplet nuclei.
- Special air handling and ventilation required.
- Examples: *Legionella pneumophila*, *M. tuberculosis*

MICROORGANISMS OF THE ORAL CAVITY

I. ORIGIN

- *In utero* the oral cavity is sterile, but after birth within a few hours to one day a simple oral flora develops.[2]
- The microorganisms are transmitted to the infant from the mother and other family members or caretakers.
- As the infant grows, there is continuing introduction of microorganisms normal for an adult oral cavity. The microbiota of the adult is very complex.[2]
- Many of the salivary bacteria come from the dorsum of the tongue, but some are from mucous membranes and gingival/periodontal tissues.
- High counts of total microorganisms are found in dental biofilm, periodontal pockets, and carious lesions.

II. INFECTION POTENTIAL

- Intact mucous membrane of the oral cavity provides some protection against infection.
  - Pathogenic (disease-producing), potentially pathogenic, or nonpathogenic microorganisms may be present in the oral cavity of each patient.
- Pathogenic organisms may be transient.
- Patients may be carriers of certain diseases. Inadvertent transmission to subsequent susceptible patients or to dental personnel may occur because of inappropriate work practices, such as careless handwashing, unhygienic personal habits, or inadequate sterilization and handling of sterile instruments and materials.

III. CROSS-CONTAMINATION

- Spread of microorganisms from one source to another: person to person, or person to an inanimate object and then to another person.
- Recognition of the many possibilities for the transfer of infection in a dental office or clinic provides a basis for planning the system of sterilization, disinfection, and handling of instruments and equipment.

THE INFECTIOUS PROCESS

I. ESSENTIAL FEATURES FOR DISEASE TRANSMISSION

A chain of events is required for the spread of an infectious agent. The six essential links are shown in **Figure 4-1** and described here:

- An *infectious agent*, the *invading organism* (bacterium, virus, fungus, rickettsia, protozoa). Each organism has its own specific reaction in an infected host.
- *A reservoir* where the invading organisms live and multiply. The infectious agent has its own essential environment,

(*continued on page 43*)

BOX 4-1 **Key Words**

Disease Transmission

Aerosol: an artificially generated collection of particles suspended in air.

Microbial aerosol: suspension of particles in the air that consists partially or wholly of microorganisms; it may be capable of causing an infection.

Anergy: diminished reactivity to specific antigen(s); inability to react to skin-test antigen (even if person is infected with the organism tested) because of immunosuppression.

Antibody: a soluble protein molecule produced and secreted by body cells in response to an antigen; it is capable of binding to that specific antigen.

Antigen: a substance that is capable, under appropriate conditions, of inducing a specific immune response and of reacting with the products of that response, that is, with the specific antibody.

Carrier: a person who harbors a specific infectious agent in the absence of discernible clinical disease and serves as a potential source of infection. The carrier state may be temporary, transient, or chronic.

Asymptomatic carrier: an individual who harbors pathogenic organisms without clinically recognizable symptoms; a carrier may infect those contacted.

CDCP: United States Centers for Disease Control and Prevention, Department of Health and Human Services, Public Health Service, Atlanta, GA 30333.

CFU: colony-forming unit.

Communicable period of a disease: the time during which an infectious agent may be transferred directly or indirectly from an infected person to another person; the communicable period may include or overlap the incubation period.

Droplet: diminutive drop, such as the particles of moisture expelled while coughing, sneezing, or speaking, that may carry infectious agents.

ELISA or EIA: an enzyme-linked immunosorbent assay; a laboratory test to detect antibody in the blood serum.

Western blot (WB): a laboratory test for antibody that is more specific than EIA and is used to validate seropositive reactions to the EIA.

Endemic: the constant presence of a disease or infectious agent within a geographic area.

Epidemic: widespread occurrence of cases of an illness in a community or region; greater than the expected number of cases for the particular population.

Fomite or fomes: an inanimate object or material on which disease-producing agents (microorganisms) may be conveyed.

HCP: healthcare personnel; **DHCP:** dental healthcare personnel.

Healthcare-associated infection: an infection associated with or acquired during a medical or surgical intervention; replaces nosocomial, which is limited to an adverse infectious outcome occurring in a hospital.

Herpes Simplex 1 skin related viruses:

Herpes gladiatorum: infection transmitted by skin contact among wrestlers and other athletes. Incidence as high as 3% has been reported among high school wrestlers.

Herpes barbae: herpes simplex spread over the bearded part of the face due to minor injuries of daily shaving or contamination from razor.

Immunity: the resistance that a person has against disease; it may be natural or acquired.

Passive immunity: short-duration immunity either naturally attained by transplacental transfer from the mother or artificially acquired by inoculation of specific protective antibodies.

Active immunity: immunity either naturally attained by infection, with or without clinical manifestations, or artificially acquired by inoculation of the agent in a killed, modified, or variant form; in response, the body produces its own antibodies; usually lasts for years.

Incubation period: the time interval between the initial contact with an infectious agent and the appearance of the first clinical sign or symptom of the disease.

Infection: a state caused by the invasion, development, or multiplication of an infectious agent into the body.

Primary infection: first time; no preexisting antibodies.

Latent infection: persistent infection following a primary infection in which the causative agent remains inactive within certain cells.

Recurrent infection: symptomatic reactivation of a latent infection.

Infectious agent: organism capable of producing an infection.

Jaundice: yellowness of skin, sclerae, mucous membranes, and excretions due to hyperbilirubinemia and deposition of bile pigments. Also called *icterus*.

Microbiota: the microscopic living organisms of a region.

Pandemic: widespread epidemic usually affecting the population of an extensive region, several countries, or sometimes the entire globe.

Parenteral: injection by a route other than the alimentary tract, such as subcutaneous, intramuscular, or intravenous.

Parotitis: inflammation of the parotid gland.

Pathogen: a virus, microorganism, or other substance that causes disease.

Opportunistic pathogen: capable of causing disease only when the host's resistance is lowered.

Percutaneous: by way of, or through, the skin.

Permucosal: by way of, or through, a mucous membrane.

Prion: abnormal infectious protein particle lacking nucleic acid that has been implicated as the cause of certain neurodegenerative diseases; an example is Creutzfeldt-Jacob disease.

Prodrome: early or premonitory symptom (adj: prodromal).

Replication: process by which viruses reproduce and multiply.

Retrovirus: virus with RNA as its core genetic material; requires the enzyme reverse transcriptase to convert its RNA into proviral DNA.

Risk population: group having an increased prevalence of infection, increased chances or likelihood of infection, and increased prevalence of disease carriers.

(*continued*)

Disease Transmission (*Continued*)

Serologic diagnosis: the identification of a disease by serum markers of that specific condition.

Seroconversion: after exposure to the etiologic agent of a disease, the blood changes from negative ("seronegative") to positive ("seropositive") for the serum marker for that disease; the time interval for conversion is specific for each disease.

Serum marker: a specific finding (such as an antibody or antigen) by laboratory blood analysis that identifies an existing disease state. May be referred to as a "titer."

Shedding (viral): presence of virus in body secretions, in excretions, or in body surface lesions with potential for transmission.

Standard precautions: an approach to infection control to protect DHCP and patients from pathogens that can be spread by blood or any other body fluid, secretion, or excretion (except sweat), regardless of whether they contain blood.

STD: sexually transmitted disease.

Surveillance (of disease): continuing scrutiny of all aspects of occurrence and spread of a disease that are pertinent to effective control.

Susceptible host: host not possessing resistance against an infectious agent.

Transmission (horizontal): passage of an infectious agent from one individual to another.

Vertical transmission: passage of an infectious agent from one generation to another by breast milk or across the placenta.

Universal precautions: an approach to infection control in which all human blood and certain human body fluids are treated as if known to be infectious for HIV, HBV, and other blood-borne pathogens.

Vector: a carrier that transfers an infectious microorganism from one host to another.

Biologic vector: an arthropod, insect, or other living carrier in whose body the infecting organism multiplies before becoming infective to the recipient.

Vehicle: a substance or object that serves as an intermediate means by which an infectious agent is transported and introduced into a susceptible host through a suitable portal of entry.

Virion: complete virus particle made up of the **nucleoid** (the genetic material) **and capsid** (the shell of protein that protects the nucleoid).

Virulence: the degree of pathogenicity or disease-evoking power of an infectious agent.

Virus: a subcellular genetic entity capable of gaining entrance into a limited range of living cells and capable of replication only within such cells; a virus contains either DNA or RNA but not both. (DNA and RNA are defined in Box 4-2, page 55.)

Window period: the time between exposure resulting in infection and the presence of detectable serum antibody; antibody test is negative but infectious agent is transmissible during the window period.

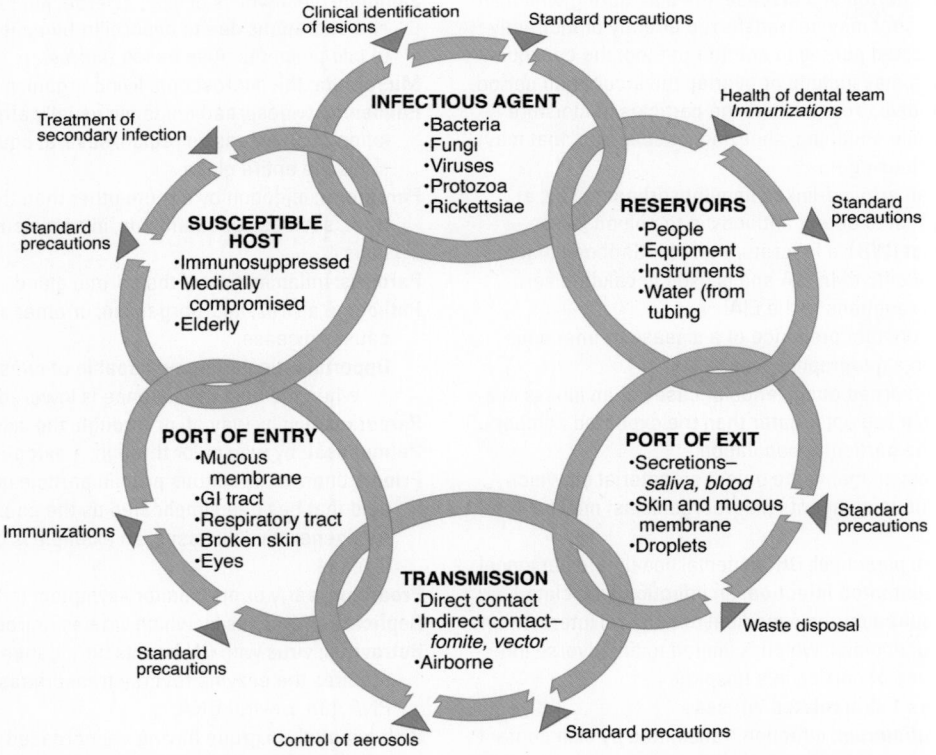

FIGURE 4-1 **Interventions to Break the Chain of Disease Transmission.** A break in the chain of six major links is required for the spread of an infectious agent. Standard precautions are applied to interrupt the chain.

which may be inanimate matter, an insect, or human cells or blood. For example, soil is the reservoir for tetanus, and humans are reservoirs for herpetic infections.

- A *port of exit* or mode of escape from the reservoir. Organisms exit through various body systems, such as the respiratory tract, or through skin lesions. Escape from the blood stream may be through skin abrasions, hypodermic needles, or dental instruments.
- A *mode of transmission*, which may be direct, person to person, or indirect by way of an intermediate vehicle, such as contaminated hands or a hypodermic needle. Transmission by a droplet may be direct from the respiratory tract of one person to the oral cavity of the receiving host. Droplets also may pass indirectly to hands or inanimate objects to be transferred indirectly to the susceptible host.
- A port *of entry* or mode of entry of the infectious agent into the new host. Modes of entry may be similar to modes of escape, such as the respiratory tract, mucous membranes, or a break in the skin.
- A *susceptible host* that does not have immunity to the invading infectious agent.

A heart valve may be defective because of a congenital or acquired condition. Such a valve may be susceptible to infective endocarditis resulting from a bacteremia created during dental or dental hygiene instrumentation.

II. AIRBORNE INFECTION

A. Dust-borne Organisms

- *Clostridium tetani* (tetanus bacillus), and enteric bacteria are among the organisms that may travel in the dust brought in from outside and that moves in and about dental treatment areas.
- When doors are opened and closed and people pass in and out, dust is set into motion that can settle on instruments, other objects, or people.
- Infectious microorganisms also can reach dust from the oral cavities of patients by way of large airborne particles.
- Dust-borne organisms can be sources of contamination for dental instruments and the hands of dental personnel.
- Surface disinfection of all equipment contacted during an appointment contributes to control of dust-borne pathogens.
- Procedures for surface disinfection are described on pages 83–84.

B. Aerosol Production

Airborne particles are usually classified by size as either aerosols or spatter. They are constantly being produced.

1. Aerosols

- A particle of a true aerosol is less than 50 μ in diameter; nearly all are less than 5 μ.[3]

- Aerosols are biologic contaminants that occur in solid or liquid form, are invisible, and may remain suspended in air for long periods.
- Aerosol particles (sometimes called droplet nuclei) that are 5 μ or smaller may be breathed deep into the lungs.
- Larger particles get trapped higher in the respiratory tree.
- The tiny particles may contain respiratory disease–producing organisms or traces of mercury or amalgam that collect in the lung because they are not biodegradable.

2. Spatter

- Heavier, larger particles may remain airborne a relatively short time because of size and weight, then drop or spatter on objects, people, and the floor.
- Spatter is composed of particles greater than 50 μm in diameter that usually fall within 2 feet of origin.[3]
- Spatter may be visible, particularly after it has landed on skin, hair, clothing, or environmental surfaces where gross contamination can result.

3. Origin

- Produced during all intraoral procedures, including examination and treatment.
- When produced by air spray, air–water spray, handpiece activity, or ultrasonic scaling, the number of aerosols increases to tremendous proportions.

4. Contents

- *Microorganisms.* An aerosol may contain a single organism or a clump of microorganisms adhered to a dust or debris particle contained within a liquid droplet.
- *Particles from Cavity Preparation.* Tooth fragments; microorganisms from saliva, biofilm, and/or oropharynx/nasopharynx; oil from a handpiece; and water from the cooling equipment may be in aerosols following cavity preparation.
- *Ultrasonic Scaling.* The many microorganisms found in the aerosols from ultrasonic scalers may include *Staphylococcus aureus, albus,* and *pyogenes; Streptococcus viridans;* lactobacilli; actinomyces; pneumococci; and diphtheroids.[4] Viruses also may be spread by ultrasonic instruments.

5. Concentration

- Bacteria-laden aerosols and spatter are in greater concentration close to the site of instrumentation; the quantity decreases with distance.
- Aerosols travel with air currents and may move from room to room.

III. PREVENTION OF TRANSMISSION

A. Airborne Infection Can Be Controlled By

- Elimination or limitation of the organisms at their source
- Interruption of transmission

■ Protection of the potentially susceptible recipient
■ Carefully monitored procedures for all patients with or without a known serious communicable disease

B. Preprocedural Oral Hygiene Measures

■ Biofilm removal: toothbrushing and flossing by the patient
■ Use of an antiseptic mouthrinse to reduce the numbers of bacteria contained in aerosols

C. Interruption of Transmission

■ As much use of a rubber dam, high-volume evacuation, and manual instrumentation as possible
■ Installation of air-control methods to supply adequate ventilation, filtration, and relative humidity
■ Employing vacuum cleaning to remove dirt and micro-organisms rather than dust-arousing housekeeping methods. The cleaner needs to have a filter to prevent the escape of organisms after they are suctioned.

D. Clean Water

■ Use water that meets EPA regulatory standards for drinking water (less than 500 CFU/ml of heterotrophic water bacteria).
■ Waterlines need to be flushed for at least 20–30 seconds between patients during the day to reduce contamination.[5]
  A. Flushing dental waterlines clears planktonic micro-organisms; however, the effects are transient.
  B. Additional methods to treat biofilm are needed to assure treatment water quality.

E. Protection of the Clinician

■ Use masks, shields, and protective eyewear to prevent direct contact of spatter and aerosols with the faces of the dental team.

F. Protection of the Patient

■ Use protective eyewear to prevent direct spatter and aerosols to the face and eyes.

PATHOGENS TRANSMISSIBLE BY THE ORAL CAVITY

■ Selected pathogens that may be transmitted by way of the oral cavity and their disease manifestations, mode of transfer, and incubation and communicability periods are listed in **Table 4-1**.
■ Pathogens are often present within the oral cavity without producing oral signs or symptoms, a fact of particular importance to the total consideration of prevention of disease transmission.

■ Tuberculosis, viral hepatitis, herpetic infections, and acquired immunodeficiency syndrome (HIV/AIDS) are included in this chapter because of the special problems they create in personal and patient care.

TUBERCULOSIS

Mycobacterium tuberculosis, the etiologic agent in tuberculosis (TB), is a resistant organism that requires special consideration when sterilization and disinfection methods are selected and administered. Clinical procedures are planned to prevent exposure and infection from this serious disease.

■ Drug-resistant TB may occur when patients are non-compliant in their required extended drug therapy or if the medication is not available.
■ Multidrug-resistant TB (MDR-TB) refers to resistance to at least two of the first-line drugs.
■ Extensively drug-resistant TB (XDR-TB) refers to resistance to first-line drugs and at least one of three second-line drugs.[6]

I. TRANSMISSION

A. Inhalation[7]

■ Tuberculosis is contracted when a vulnerable person inhales aerosolized droplet nuclei containing tubercle bacilli from sputum and saliva of an infected individual during coughing, sneezing, speaking, or singing. **(Figure 4-2)**.
■ Use of ultrasonic and other handpieces, and of air–water spray, create aerosols that can carry the tubercle bacilli.

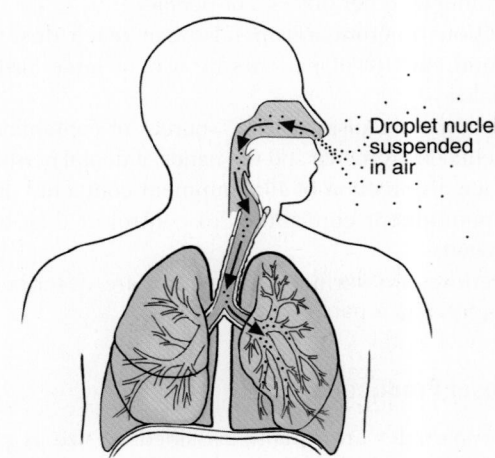

FIGURE 4-2 **Droplet Nuclei.** Many potentially pathogenic microorganisms are disseminated by aerosols and spatter. The primary mode of transmission of tubercle bacilli is by droplet nuclei breathed directly into the lung. (Source: McInnes ME. Essentials of communicable disease. 2nd ed. St. Louis: The C.V. Mosby Co.; 1975).

- Droplet nuclei are small enough to pass through over 95% bacterial filtration efficiency required of standard surgical masks, and may remain suspended in the air for hours. Standard precautions may be insufficient to protect the DHCP from transmission of tuberculosis in the healthcare setting.[7]
- Airborne infection isolation measures are necessary (NIOSH).[7]

B. Factors Affecting Transmission of Tuberculosis

- The degree to which the infected person produces infectious droplets
- The amount and duration of exposure
- The susceptibility of the recipient.
- Some patients are more contagious than are others. Maximum communicability is usually just before the disease is diagnosed, when the person may have a severe cough and other respiratory symptoms.

C. Areas of Infection

- Infection of the lungs is most common.
- Extrapulmonary TB: the tubercle bacillus also infects lymph nodes, meninges (tuberculous meningitis), kidneys, bone, skin, and the oral cavity.
- Figure 65-5 shows a tuberculosis ulcer of the tongue (page 996).

II. CLINICAL MANAGEMENT

Official recommendations from the Centers of Disease Control and Prevention (CDCP)[7] include the following:

1. Risk assessment conducted annually.
2. Dental Health Care Personnel (DHCP). Screen all newly employed DHCP for latent TB infection and TB disease; any DHCP with persistent cough (more than 3 weeks) or other suggestive symptoms are referred promptly for medical evaluation.
3. Medical history. Patients are routinely questioned about TB history and symptoms suggestive of TB infection; history is updated regularly.
4. Referral. Patients with symptoms or history suggestive of tuberculosis are referred immediately for medical evaluation.
5. Deferral of elective dental treatment: Table 65-6 (page 995) provides a patient management guide.
6. Urgent Dental Care. Patients suspected of active TB infection are treated only in a facility with an airborne isolation room. Respiratory protection with a minimum N95 disposable filtration mask is used when caring for a patient with active (or suspected active) TB.
7. Separation of suspected or confirmed tuberculosis patients. Patients are isolated in a separate area until referral to the appropriate facility can be made.

VIRAL HEPATITIS

Hepatitis or inflammation of the liver has multiple causes, which includes the following:[8]

- Viral and bacterial infections
- Toxins and certain medications
- Heavy alcohol use

I. HEPATITIS VIRUSES: CATEGORIES

A. Viruses with oral-fecal route of transmission by unsanitary food handling and water
   - Hepatitis A virus and Hepatitis E virus
   - Not an occupational concern for DHCP
B. Viruses with blood-borne route of transmission by contact with infected body fluids
   - Hepatitis B virus (HBV), hepatitis C virus (HCV), and hepatitis D virus (HDV)
   - Chronic or carrier disease state may occur with HBV, HCV, and HDV
   - Directly impact the practice of dental hygiene and patient care
C. New hepatitis viruses
   - Hepatitis F, Hepatitis G, and transfusion-transmitted viruses identified9
   - Role in disease progression is unclear.
D. **Table 4-2** lists the hepatitis terminology with abbreviations and significance.

HEPATITIS B

- Hepatitis B is a serious, endemic, worldwide disease. It can occur at any age. Immunization is necessary for newborns and at all ages.
- **Figure 4-3** shows a diagram of the hepatitis B virus.
- Among professional personnel, both medical and dental, the use of strict sterilization of equipment and materials, aseptic techniques, and self-protection measures is mandatory.

I. TRANSMISSION

A. Blood and Other Body Fluids

- Almost all body fluids including blood and blood products and saliva contain HBV, although no transmission of HBV infection due to saliva alone has been documented.
- Transmission of HBV can also occur from inanimate objects that have been exposed.

B. Modes of Transmission[10]

Hepatitis B is transmitted through percutaneous and permucosal exposure.

- Percutaneous including intravenous, intramuscular, and subcutaneous

(continued on page 49)

TABLE 4-1	INFECTIOUS DISEASES				
INFECTIOUS AGENT	**DISEASE OR CONDITION**	**ROUTE OR MODE OF TRANSMISSON**	**INCUBATION PERIOD**	**COMMUNICABLE PERIOD**	**VACCINE**
Human immuno-deficiency virus (HIV)	Acquired immunode-ficiency syndrome (AIDS) HIV infection	Blood and blood products (infected IV needles) Sexual contact Transplacental and perinatal	To detectable antibodies: <1 mo To disease diagnosis: <1 y–15 y or more	From asymptomatic through life	Vaccine in progress
Hepatitis A virus (HAV)	Type A hepatitis "Infectious" hepatitis	Fecal–oral Contaminated food, water, shellfish	15–50 d (average 28–30 d)	2–3 wk before onset (jaundice) to 8 d after disease symptoms abate	Yes
Hepatitis B virus (HBV)	Type B hepatitis "Serum" hepatitis	Blood Saliva and all body fluids Sexual contact Perinatal	2–6 mo (average 60–90 d)	Before and during clinical signs Carrier state: indefinite	Yes
Hepatitis C virus (HCV)	Type C hepatitis	Percutaneous Blood Exposure to contaminated needles	2 wk–6 mo (average 6–9 wk)	1 wk before onset **of** symptoms, persists in most persons indefinitely Carrier state: indefinite	No No
Delta hepatitis virus (HDV) Delta agent	Delta hepatitis	Coinfection with HBV Blood Sexual contacts Perinatal	2–8 wk	All phases of active infection	HBV vaccine
Hepatitis E virus (HEV) ET-NANB	Type E hepatitis Enterically transmitted non-A, non-B	Fecal–oral Contaminated water	15–64 d	Not known	No
Herpes simplex virus Type 1 (HSV-1) Type 2 (HSV-2)	Acute herpetic Gingivostomatitis Herpes labialis Ocular herpetic Herpetic whitlow Genital herpes	Saliva Direct contact (lip, hand) Indirect contact (on objects, limited survival) Sexual contact	2–12 d	Labialis: 1 d before lesions are crusted Acute stomatitis: 7 wk after recovery Asymptomatic infection: with viral shedding Reactivation period: with viral shedding	No
Varicella-zoster virus (VZV)	Chicken pox Herpes zoster (shin-gles)	Direct contact Indirect contact Airborne droplet	10–21 d Average 14–16 d	1–5 d prior to onset of rash until all vesicles are crusted of vesicles	Yes
Epstein–Barr virus (EBV)	Infectious Mononucleosis Oral hairy leukoplakia	Direct contact Saliva	4–6 wk	Prolonged Pharyngeal excretion 1 y after infection	No
Cytomegalovirus (CMV)	Neonatal cytomegalo-virus infection Cytomegaloviral disease	Perinatal Direct contact (most body secretions) Blood transfusion Organ transplantation Saliva	3–12 wk postpartum 3–8 wk after transfu-sion or transplant	Months to years	No
Mycobacterium tuberculosis	Tuberculosis	Droplet nuclei Sputum Saliva	2–10 wk	As long as viable bacilli are discharged in sputum	B.C.G. (Bacille Calmette Guérin)
Corynebacterium diphtheriae	Diphtheria	Direct and Indirect	2–5 d	2–4 wk	Yes

TABLE 4-1	INFECTIOUS DISEASES (*Continued*)				
INFECTIOUS AGENT	**DISEASE OR CONDITION**	**ROUTE OR MODE OF TRANSMISSON**	**INCUBATION PERIOD**	**COMMUNICABLE PERIOD**	**VACCINE**
Treponema pallidum	Syphilis Congenital syphilis	Direct contact Transplacental	10 d–3 mo	Variable and indefinite 2–4 y	No
Neisseria gonorrhoeae	Gonorrhea Gonococcal pharyngitis	Direct contact Indirect (short survival of organisms)	1–14 d	May continue for months and years if untreated	No
Bordetella pertussis	Whooping cough Pertussis	Direct contact with discharges	6–20 d	Untreated: from early catarrhal stage to 3 wk after paroxysmal cough	Yes
Mumps virus (paramyxovirus)	Infectious parotitis (mumps)	Direct contact (saliva) Airborne droplet	12–25 d (average 16–18 d)	12–25 d after exposure From 6 to 7 d before symptoms until 9 d after swelling	Yes
Poliovirus types 1, 2, 3	Poliomyelitis	Direct contact (saliva) Droplet Fecal–oral	7–14 d	As long as virus is secreted, most infectious 7–10 d before and after onset of symptoms	Yes
Influenza viruses (A, B, C)	Influenza	Nasal discharge Respiratory droplets	Average 2 d	3–5 d from clinical onset, longer in children and immunocompromised	Yes
Measles virus (Morbillivirus)	Rubeola (measles)	Direct contact Saliva Airborne droplet	7–18 d to fever, 14 d to rash	Few days before fever to 4 d after rash appears	Yes
Rubella virus (togavirus)	Rubella (German measles) Congenital rubella syndrome	Nasopharyngeal Secretions Direct contact Airborne droplets Maternal infection first trimester	14–21 d	From 1 wk before to at least 4 d after rash appears Highly communicable Infants shed virus for months after birth	Yes
Group A streptococci (beta-hemolytic) Streptococcus pyogenes	Streptococcal sore throat Scarlet fever Impetigo Erysipelas	Respiratory droplets Direct contact	1–3 d	10–21 d, untreated Many nasal oropharyngeal carriers	No
Staphylococcus aureus Staphylococcus epidermidis	Abscesses Boils (furuncle) Cellulitis Impetigo Bacterial pneumonia	Saliva Exudates Respiratory droplets Nasal discharge	4–10 d Variable and indefinite	While lesions drain and carrier state persists	No
Candida albicans	Candidiasis	Secretions Excretions (oral, skin, vaginal)	Variable 2–5 d for "thrush" in children	While lesions are present	No
Streptococcus pneumoniae	Pneumonia Pneumococcal pneumonia	Droplet Direct contact Indirect	1–3 d Not well determined	While virulent organisms are discharged	Yes

Source: Heymann DL, ed. Control of communicable diseases manual. 19th ed. Washington: American Public Health Association; 2008.

TABLE 4-2	VIRAL HEPATITIS: ABBREVIATIONS AND THEIR SIGNIFICANCE	
ABBREVIATION	**TERM**	**SIGNIFICANCE**
Hepatitis A		
HAV	Hepatitis A virus	Etiologic agent for hepatitis A
anti-HAV	Antibody to hepatitis A virus	Acute or resolved infection Protective immune response to infection
Hepatitis B		
HBV	Hepatitis B virus (Dane particle)	Etiologic agent for hepatitis B Current HBV infection
HBsAg	Hepatitis B surface antigen	Surface marker in acute disease and carrier state Indicates infectivity
anti-HBs	Antibody to hepatitis Bs antigen	Indicates (1) **Active immunity** to HBV (past infection) (2) **Passive immunity** from HBIG (3) Immune response from HB vaccine
HbeAg	Hepatitis Be antigen	Presence indicated viral replication and high infectivity, found in both acute and chronic carrier states
Anti-Hbe	Antibody to Hepatitis Be antigen	Seroconversion from e antigen to e antibody is a predictor of long-term clearance of HBV in patients
HbcAg	Hepatitis B core antigen	Nucleocapsid core of Hepatitis B virus
anti-HBc	Hepatitis B core antibody	Indicates prior HBV infection
Hepatitis C		
HCV	Hepatitis C virus	Etiologic agent for hepatitis C Indicates acute disease and chronic state
anti-HCV	Antibody to hepatitis C virus	Does not indicate immunity in >50% of persons infected
Hepatitis D		
HDV	Hepatitis delta virus	Etiologic agent for hepatitis D Only infectious in presence of acute or chronic HBV infection
HDV-Ag	Delta antigen	Detectable during early acute HDV infection
anti-HDV	Antibody to hepatitis D virus	Indicates acute, resolved, or chronic infection
Hepatitis E		
HEV	Hepatitis E virus	Etiologic agent for hepatitis E
anti-HEV	Antibody to hepatitis E virus	Indicates acute or resolved infection
Immune globulins		
IG	Immune globulin	Contains antibodies to HAV and low-titer HBV antibodies
HBIG	Hepatitis B immune globulin	Contains high-titer antibodies to HBV

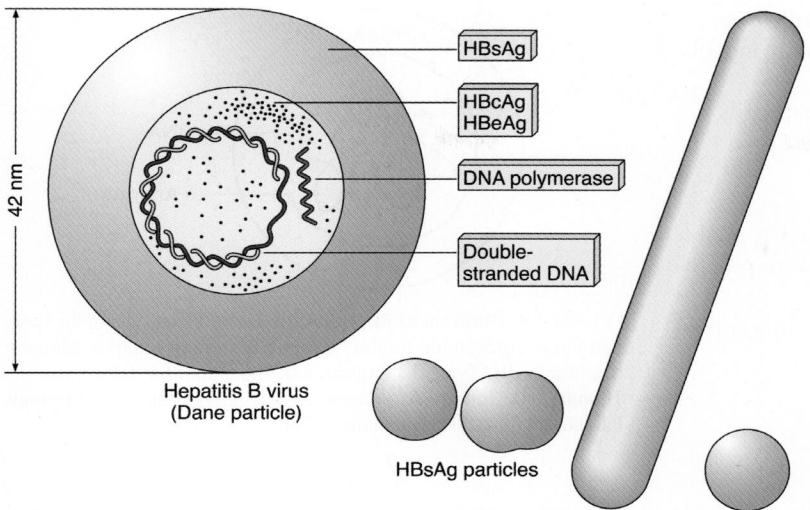

FIGURE 4-3 **Diagram of the Hepatitis B Virus.** Hepatitis B virus is a 42-nanometer DNA virus hepadnavirus, composed of an inner nucleocapsid core (HBcAg) surrounded by a lipoprotein coat containing the surface antigen (HBsAg). Inside the core particle is a single molecule of circular, partially double-stranded DNA, an endogenous DNA polymerase, and HBeAg. Spherical and tubular particles of HBsAg circulate in infected blood in great numbers. (Reprinted with permission from Rubin E, Farber JL. *Pathology.* 3rd ed. Philadelphia: Lippincott Williams & Wilkins; 1999.)

- Accidents with needlestick and other sharp instruments
- Exchanging contaminated needles, syringes, and other intravenous drug paraphernalia.
- Sexual exposure
- Infection from blood transfusion and blood products: rare since donor and blood screening was instituted in 1985.

C. Perinatal Transmission

1. Maternal transmission of HBV to the fetus is efficient and not rare.
    - HBV-infected mothers positive for both HBsAg and HBeAg: high risk for infant to be infected and become chronic carrier.
    - Can lead to chronic liver disease or cancer of the liver later in life.
2. Prevention
    - Screen all pregnant women for presence of HBsAg.
    - Provide Hepatitis B vaccine and Hepatitis B Immune Globulin (HBIG) to infants born to HB-infected mothers within 12 hours of birth to protect them from infection.[11]

D. Carrier State or Chronic Hepatitis B

- All HBsAg-positive persons are potentially infective. Chronically infected individuals vary in infectivity from high (HBeAg-positive, elevated HBV-DNA) to moderate (anti-HBe-positive).
- A chronic carrier of HBV is an individual with the HBsAg-positive serological results in the blood on at least two occasions at least 6 months apart.
- A carrier state may also result following a subclinical undiagnosed exposure and may be unknown to the individual.

E. Immunity

- Protective immunity follows infection if antibodies (anti-HBsAg) develop to the hepatitis B surface antigen.
- The antibody may be present, although unknown, whether immunity was acquired following a subclinical, or otherwise unrecognized case of hepatitis B.

II. PREVENTION

- Hepatitis B viruses cause serious illness, including acute and chronic hepatitis, cirrhosis, and liver cancer, sometimes leading to disability and death.
- Hepatitis B is a critical occupational hazard for dental personnel because of their close association with the potentially infected body fluids of patients.
- Every healthcare individual requires immunization so that the possibilities of disease acquisition and transmission can be minimized.

A. Preventive Methods

- Prenatal testing of all pregnant women for HBsAg to identify household contacts who need to be vaccinated.
- Universal immunization of infants and children to be accomplished during routine healthcare visits when vaccinations are usually administered. Hepatitis vaccine can be combined with other childhood immunizations to reduce the number of injections.
- Immunization of adolescents and adults, particularly those at high risk. Eventually, as the universal vaccination of children continues, adult requirements will be lessened.
- Enforce blood bank control measures.
    - A. Screening of donors; reject individuals with history of viral hepatitis, drug addiction, recent transfusion or tattoo, and travelers from HBV endemic areas.
    - B. Strict testing for all donated blood.

■ Enforce use of disposable syringes and needles.
  A. For acupuncture, skin testing, parenteral inoculations, body piercing
  B. Education of public to expect certain standards

B. Active Immunization: The Vaccines

■ Effective Hepatitis B vaccines have been available since 1982 for pre-exposure and postexposure prophylaxis.
■ All vaccines act to stimulate antibodies and convey immunity.

HEPATITIS C

■ A serologic test for antibody to HCV became available in 1991, and routine blood screening was implemented in 1992.

I. TRANSMISSION[12]

■ Hepatitis C is primarily transmitted parenterally and other modes similar to Hepatitis B.
■ Transmission rarely occurs from mucous membrane exposures to blood, and no transmission has been documented from intact or non-intact skin exposures to blood.
■ Environmental contamination with blood containing HCV is not a significant risk for transmission in the healthcare setting.
■ Sexual partners of HCV-infected persons

II. PREVENTION

■ Education and behavior modification is essential since no vaccine is available for Hepatitis C.
■ Strict attention to standard infection control procedures for all healthcare personnel.
■ Measures recommended for hepatitis B can be applied to hepatitis C.

HEPATITIS D

■ The delta hepatitis virus, also called the delta agent, cannot cause infection except in the presence of HBV infection.
■ The diagram in **Figure 4-4** shows the delta antigen surrounded by HBsAg.

I. TRANSMISSION

■ Delta infection is superimposed on HBsAg carriers.
■ Occurs primarily in persons who have had multiple exposures to HBV: particularly patients with hemophilia and intravenous drug users.

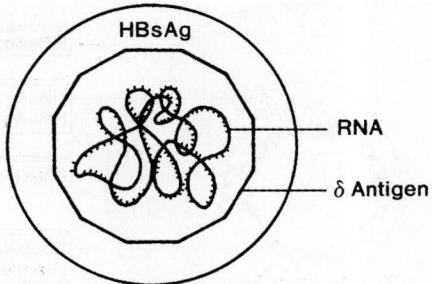

FIGURE 4-4 Diagram of the Hepatitis Delta Virus. The delta agent antigen is surrounded by the hepatitis B surface antigen. (Source: Hoofnagle JH. Type D hepatitis and the hepatitis delta virus. In: Thomas HC, Jones EA, editors. Recent advances in hepatology. Edinburgh: Churchill Livingstone; 1986.)

■ Transmission is similar to that of HBV; by direct exposure to contaminated blood and serous body fluids, contaminated needles and syringes, sexual contacts, and perinatal transfer.[13]

II. PREVENTION

■ All measures to prevent hepatitis B will prevent delta hepatitis because HDV is dependent on the presence of HBV.
■ Immunization with hepatitis B vaccine also protects the recipient from delta hepatitis infection.

HERPESVIRUS DISEASES

■ Herpesviruses are endemic worldwide, and each virus causes a wide variety of disease entities that are highly infectious.
■ Herpesvirus diseases are a significant public health problem because of the lack of effective therapeutics and vaccines.
■ Of the many identified herpesviruses, the eight major types that are known to infect humans are listed in **Table 4-3** with their abbreviations and some of the infections they cause.

I. GENERAL CHARACTERISTICS

■ Herpesviruses produce diseases with latent, recurrent, and sometimes malignant tendencies. For example, herpes simplex type 2 (HSV2) has been implicated in cervical cancer; herpes simplex type 1(HSV1) in oral cancer, and Epstein–Barr virus (EBV; HHV4) has been implicated in various types of cancer.[14]
■ Herpesviruses travel along sensory nerve pathways to specific ganglia where they may remain latent and become reactivated to produce recurrent infection after certain stimuli or when the body's immunity is significantly lowered.
  A. HSV1 travels to the trigeminal ganglion **(Figure 4-5)**.

TABLE 4-3	HERPESVIRUSES	
HERPESVIRUS NUMBER	**NAME OF VIRUS AND ABBREVIATION**	**INFECTIONS**
HHV1	Herpes simplex virus, type 1 **HSV1**	Herpetic gingivostomatitis Herpes labialis Herpetic whitlow Herpetic conjunctivitis
HHV2	Herpes simplex virus, type 2 **HSV2**	Genital herpes
HHV3	Varicella-zoster virus **VZV**	Chicken pox Shingles
HHV4	Epstein–Barr virus **EBV**	Infectious mononucleosis Oral hairy leukoplakia Lymphoepithelial cysts of parotid gland Lymphatic cancers Nasophyarngeal cancers Periapical lesions Periodontal disease severity
HHV5	Human cytomegalovirus **CMV**	Asymptomatic infections Severe Associated with periapical pathosis and increased severity of periodontal diseases along with EBV and HSV Immunosuppressed persons: CMV retinitis, neurologic deficiencies, pneumonia
HHV6	Herpes lymphotropic virus **HLV**	Roseola (*exanthem infantum*) Immune system suppression Seen in HIV-periodontitis with EBV
HHV7	Human herpes virus 7 **HHV7**	Primary infection in childhood Asymptomatic or Roseola-like macular cutaneous eruptions Infection may occur following bone marrow and solid organ transplants
HHV8	Kaposi's sarcoma–related virus **KSRV** or **KS**	Development of Kaposi's sarcoma

Source: Kessler HP. Herpes virus infections: a review for the dental practitioner. *Texas Dent* J. 2005 Feb;122(2):150.

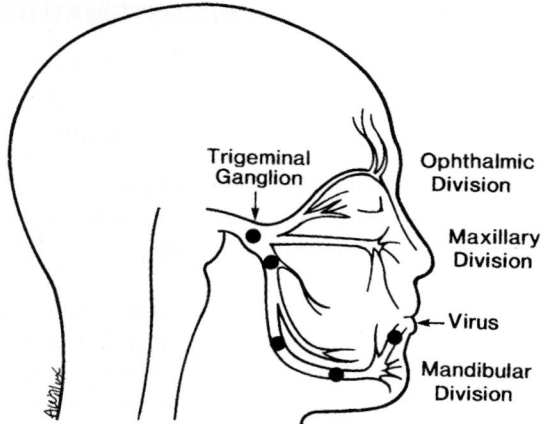

FIGURE 4-5 **Latent Infection of Herpes Simplex Virus.** Path of the virus traced from point of viral penetration on lip to establishment of latent infection in the trigeminal ganglion.

B. HSV2 goes to the thoracic, lumbar, and sacral dorsal root ganglia.
C. Varicella-zoster virus (VZV) travels to the sensory ganglia of the vagal, spinal, or cranial nerves.
◼ Immunosuppressed patients have more frequent and severe herpes infections.
◼ Herpesviruses are among the opportunistic organisms in acquired immunodeficiency syndrome (HIV/AIDS).

II. RELATION TO PERIODONTAL INFECTIONS[15]

◼ Human herpesviruses occur in periodontitis pockets with relatively high prevalence.
◼ Herpesvirus-positive periodontitis lesions involving CMV, EBV, and other herpesviruses have higher levels of periodontopathic bacteria. An apparent association exists between active infection of certain herpesviruses and periodontitis.[16]
◼ Infection with herpesviruses can suppress a patient's immunity. As a result, subgingival overgrowth of opportunistic periodontal pathogens can occur and periodontal disease symptoms can be more severe.

HHV1 HERPES SIMPLEX VIRUS TYPE 1 (HSV1)

Infection with HSV-1 is widespread, and it is estimated that up to 90% of adults have antibodies to the virus. Primary infection usually occurs in children but may occur at any age, and especially in the immunocompromised.[17]

◼ Antibodies (anti-HSV) are produced but do not guarantee immunity to recurrent herpes or to other herpesvirus infections.
◼ Sulcular epithelium can serve as a reservoir for the viruses. Anti-HSV is present in the gingival sulcus fluid. Trauma to the oral area during a dental or dental hygiene appointment may trigger a herpetic recurrence.

I. PRIMARY HERPETIC GINGIVOSTOMATITIS

- Many cases of primary infection with HSV1 are asymptomatic or mild and isolated to marginal and attached gingiva.
- Acute herpetic gingivostomatitis is the most common pattern of symptomatic primary herpetic infection. Full-blown herpetic gingivostomatitis presents with widespread oral ulcers that also may involve the pharyngeal areas.
- When clinical disease is evident, gingivostomatitis and pharyngitis are the most frequent manifestations, with fever, malaise, severe pain often interfering with the ability to eat, and lymphadenopathy for 2 to 7 days.
- Painful oral vesicular lesions may occur on the gingiva, mucosa, tongue, and lips.
- Manifestations may vary from mild to severely dehabilitating.
- A patient may be a subclinical carrier, and reactivation from the trigeminal ganglia **(Figure 4-5)** may be followed by asymptomatic excretion of the viruses in the saliva.
- Reactivation may also lead to herpetic ulcerations of the lip, the typical "cold sore."

II. HERPES LABIALIS (COLD SORE, FEVER BLISTER)

- Both HSV-1 and HSV-2 cause genital and oral–facial infections that cannot be distinguished clinically, although they are antigenically different.
- HSV-1 is spread predominantly through infected lesions in oral and ocular areas, and is found in mucous membranes and skin above the waist.
- Recurrent HSV symptomatic lesions are common and may occur at or near the primary lesion at the vermillion border of the lower lip. Triggers include trauma, stress, sunlight, illness, or any conditions that deplete the patient's immune system.
- Dental and dental hygiene appointments with associated emotional stress and oral trauma involved may be triggers of HSV lesions.
- Six to 24 hours before the lesion appears, pain, burning, slight stinging, or sensations of localized warmth and erythema of the affected epithelium with slight swelling serve as a forewarning. A group of vesicles forms, eventually ruptures, and crusting follows; healing may take up to 10 days.
- Lesions are infectious, shedding the virus. Care must be taken by the patient because autoinfection (to the eye, nose, or genitals, for example) is possible, as is infection of other people.

III. HERPETIC WHITLOW

- Herpetic whitlow is the herpes simplex infection of the fingers that results from the virus entering through minor skin abrasions most frequently around a fingernail.
- Whitlow was common among DHCP before wearing gloves became a requirement; standard precautions have almost eliminated the incidence of whitlow among DHCP.

IV. OCULAR/OPHTHALMIC HERPES

- Herpes simplex lesions in the eye can be a primary or recurrent infection of HSV-1 or HSV-2.
- Transmission can occur from splashing saliva or fluid from a vesicular lesion directly into an unprotected eye.
- Prevent ocular herpetic infection by using standard precautions and the use of proper personal protection including eye covering for both clinician and patient.

HHV2 HERPES SIMPLEX VIRUS TYPE 2 (HSV2)

- HSV2 is commonly known as genital herpes, but it also occurs as an oral and perioral infection.
- **Neonatal herpes** is a serious disease that can cause delayed mental development, blindness, neurological problems and death to the newborn infected during childbirth. Obstetricians may recommend delivery by cesarean section to women with active genital herpes to avoid transmission to the infant.
- Antiviral therapy can suppress HSV2 lesions. The latency of the virus never can be eradicated.

CLINICAL MANAGEMENT FOR HERPES

- Terminology may be a problem, so such terms as "fever blisters" or "cold sores" need to be used to ensure patient understanding.
- Postpone appointment with patient with active lesion
- Explain the contagiousness to the patient: prodromal stage can be the most transmissible to other patients and clinicians.
- Contagiousness, with possible transmission to other patients
- Autoinoculation possible from instrumentation that can splash viruses to the patient's eye or extend the lesion to the nose.
- Irritation to the lesions can prolong the course and increase the severity of the infection.

HHV3 VARICELLA-ZOSTER VIRUS (VZV)

- Chickenpox (varicella) and shingles (herpes zoster) are caused by the same virus, the varicella-zoster virus.
- Chickenpox is the primary infection, with latency occurring.
- Reactivation may occur many years later in the form of herpes zoster or shingles.

I. CHICKEN POX/VARICELLA INFECTION

- Chickenpox is an extremely contagious childhood disease.
- Transmission occurs by respiratory droplets and direct skin contact with articles soiled by discharges from the vesicles and the respiratory tract.
- Chickenpox can be life threatening in children who are immunocompromised, such as those with HIV infection.
- Live attenuated vaccine has been available in the United States since 1995 and has reduced reported infections.
- Primarily a disease of children, chickenpox may occur in adults not previously exposed; adults have a more serious course of illness with more complications.[18]

II. SHINGLES/ZOSTER INFECTION

- Chickenpox leaves a lasting immunity, but the VZV remains latent in the dorsal root ganglia.
- Reactivation in adulthood may result from immunosuppression such as from drug therapy or HIV/AIDS infection, and in people with advanced neoplastic disease.
- Lifetime risk for herpes zoster is highest in the elderly and immunocompromised persons; prevalence increases with age.
- A live attenuated VZV vaccine, Zostavax, approved for use in adults 60 years of age and older, greatly reduces prevalence as well as morbidity and mortality of the disease.[19]

HHV4 EPSTEIN–BARR VIRUS (EBV)

- The Epstein–Barr virus, EBV, is one of the most common human viruses; many cases may be asymptomatic.
- EBV has been associated with a variety of diseases **(Table 4-3)**; it can remain latent and become reactivated, especially if the immune system becomes compromised.
- Infectious mononucleosis (IM)
  A. Mononucleosis is a symptomatic disease caused by infection with the EBV.
  B. Viruses can be excreted through the saliva even when the patient has no symptoms of disease; there may be a long period of communicability or a lasting carrier state.[20]
  C. Prevention: minimize contact with saliva by frequent handwashing, avoiding drinking from a common container; standard precautions by DHCP.
- Oral hairy leukoplakia
  A. EBV replicates within epithelial cells in oral hairy leukoplakia; it is considered a marker for immunosuppression.
  B. Oral hairy leukoplakia can be identified in HIV-infected individuals by the clinical appearance of white linear patches along the lateral border of the tongue.

HHV5 CYTOMEGALOVIRUS (CMV)

- Cytomegalovirus infections are widespread as shown in **Table 4-3**.
- The most severe disease develops in infants infected *in utero* and in immunocompromised patients, including HIV/AIDS. Infection with CMV is a serious complication of AIDS.
- Transmission[21]
  A. Respiratory droplets, especially among children. Children attending day care have a high prevalence of CMV infection.
  B. Blood transfusion: cause of post-transfusion mononucleosis.
  C. Post-transplant infection: for solid organs and bone marrow.
  D. Sexual transmission through semen, vaginal fluid, or saliva.
- Neonatal transmission
  A. Virus from the mother's primary or recurrent infection can infect the infant *in utero,* in the birth canal, or through breast milk.
  B. Cytomegalovirus infection in a fetus may lead to a child that is premature, is anemic, or has mental disabilities, microcephaly, motor disabilities, deafness, or chronic liver disease.
- Prevention
  A. Personal hygiene: handwashing.
  B. Utilization of standard precautions by healthcare personnel.
  C. Seropositivity of donor checked before organ transplant and other surgery.

HHV6 HERPES LYMPHOTROPHIC VIRUS (HLV)

- Widespread distribution among humans; prevalence of close to 90% by age 5 in the United States.[17]
- Commonly isolated from saliva and transmitted by respiratory droplets
- Primary infection is usually asymptomatic; latency in CD4 T lymphocytes HLV6 persists indefinitely.
- Clinical infection presents as childhood infection (6 months to 2 years): *Roseola infantum*; a serious disease that is a major cause of emergency room visits and hospitalizations in this age group: produces high temperature and rash.
- HHV6 can produce a variety of neurologic diseases, including encephalitis and febrile seizures.
- Reactivation depresses the immune system; depletes CD4 lymphocytes; may be a cofactor in HIV/AIDS progression.
- Reactivation can also occur after bone marrow transplantation and solid organ transplants, and may be complicated by rejection of the transplant.

HHV7 HUMAN HERPES VIRUS (HHV)

- Closely related to HHV6, prevalent in the general population; reactivation of latent infection is common in immunocompromised persons.
- Primary infection very common in childhood, is usually asymptomatic.
- Symptomatic disease causes roseola-like macular cutaneous eruption.
- Infection may occur following bone marrow and solid organ transplants.
- Periodontal connection: gingival tissue may serve as a reservoir for HHV7; high prevalence of HHV7 was detected in both periodontally diseased and in healthy gingival tissue.[16]

HHV8 KAPOSI'S SARCOMA–RELATED HERPESVIRUS (KSRV)

- Human herpesvirus-8 (HHV-8) seroprevalence among the general population in the United States is low, and is much greater among men with male sexual partners. In persons with normal immune system, primary infection is usually asymptomatic.
- Kaposi's sarcoma (KS) is considered an AIDS-defining lesion. The overall incidence of KS has dropped dramatically since effective antiretroviral therapy (ART) has become available.
- Virus is also found in saliva; circulating B lymphocytes are the major cell of latency.
- Associated symptoms include transient fever, lymphadenopathy, arthralgias; they occur primarily in the immunocompromised.[22]

HIV/AIDS INFECTION

- Acquired immunodeficiency syndrome (AIDS) is a severe pandemic disease caused by infection with the *human immunodeficiency virus* (HIV). A diagram of HIV-1 virus is shown in **Figure 4-6**.
- HIV was first recognized in 1981 as a cluster of diseases that were characterized by a loss of cellular immunity.[23]
- The major types of HIV are HIV-1 and HIV-2. HIV-1 is more prevalent in the United States and Europe, and has been extensively researched. It will be the primary focus of this chapter.
- HIV-2 was isolated in West Africa and later in Europe and North America and has been shown to have similar characteristics as HIV-1, although pathogenicity and transmission may be slightly lower.
- The HIV diseases are slow, progressive, often lethal diseases with the ability to persist within cells such as macrophages for long periods.

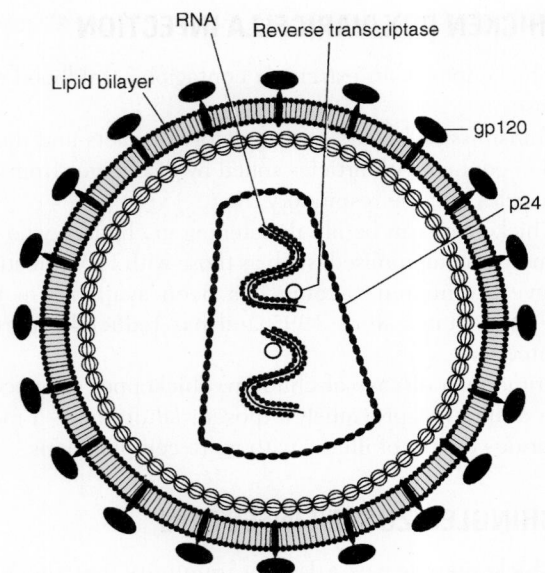

FIGURE 4-6 **Diagram of the Human Immunodeficiency Virus (HIV-1).** The envelope of the virion is composed of the lipid bilayer with glycoproteins (gp120). The core contains two strands of RNA, enzymes, and core proteins.

A. Manifestations of HIV range from mild abnormalities in immune response without apparent signs and symptoms to a variety of life-threatening infections and malignant conditions.

B. **Box 4-2** provides abbreviations and terminology relating to HIV-1 infection and AIDS.

I. TRANSMISSION

- All bodily secretions of a patient with HIV infection contain HIV, however only blood, semen, vaginal secretions, and breast milk contain sufficient amounts of the virion to transmit infection.
- *Blood transfusion* was a source of HIV infection before availability of serological testing (1985). In developing countries where testing is not available, transfusions still may be a significant source of HIV transmission and a problem for travelers.
- Modes of transmission
  A. Sexual contact accounts for the majority of cases of transmission in adults.
  B. Exposure to blood and blood products
  C. Perinatal (vertical transmission)
    1. *In utero*: HIV can be effectively transmitted across the placenta.
    2. *During delivery*: the passage through an infected birth canal.
    3. *Breast-feeding* increases transmission risk.

II. SEROLOGICAL TESTS[23]

- **Serological** tests for antibodies to HIV have been commercially available since 1985.

BOX 4-2	Key Words

HIV and AIDS

AIDS: acquired immunodeficiency syndrome.

AZT (ZDV): zidovudine, retrovir; drug used for the treatment of HIV infection and AIDS; first antiviral drug approved by the United States Food and Drug Administration (FDA).

CD4+: T-helper lymphocyte; primary target cell for HIV infection; CD4+ count decreases with the severity of HIV-related illness.

DNA: deoxyribonucleic acid; a nucleic acid found in a cell nucleus; a carrier of genetic information.

HAART: highly active antiretroviral therapy containing several antiretroviral medications; the combination has been more effective than monotherapy in the treatment of HIV.

HIV: human immunodeficiency virus; causes AIDS.

HIV antibody: antibody to human immunodeficiency virus; antibody can be detected in the blood 6 to 8 weeks after infection.

IDU: injection-drug user.

KS: Kaposi sarcoma; a malignant vascular tumor; an opportunistic neoplasm that may occur in people with HIV infection.

LAV: lymphadenopathy-associated virus; one of the former names for HIV.

MMWR: *Morbidity and Mortality Weekly Report;* publication of the United States Centers for Disease Control and Prevention (CDCP), Atlanta, GA.

OHL: oral hairy leukoplakia.

PCP: pneumocystis pneumonia; caused by *Pneumocystis jiroveci:i* an opportunistic infection that occurs in people with HIV infection.

PGL: persistent generalized lymphadenopathy.

PWA: person with AIDS.

RNA: ribonucleic acid; a nucleic acid found in cytoplasm and in the nuclei of certain cells; RNA directs the synthesis of proteins and replaces DNA as a carrier of genetic codes in some viruses

---

- EIA or ELISA (enzyme-linked immunosorbent assay) are the most commonly used screening tests and are highly sensitive and specific.
- Confirmatory testing includes the Western blot or indirect fluorescent antibody (IFA) test.
- Count of T-helper cells (CD4+) or percentage is the most used marker to evaluate the progression of HIV infection and to help clinicians make treatment decisions.

CLINICAL COURSE OF HIV-1 INFECTION

I. INCUBATION PERIOD

- Detection of the antibody in the blood, or seroconversion, occurs within 6 weeks to 6 months after exposure to the HIV virus. Presence of the antibody indicates HIV infection.
- Viral production is high throughout all stages of the infection.
- Incubation period from establishment of infection to the appearance of symptoms of AIDS may be 15 years or longer.

II. ACUTE SEROCONVERSION SYNDROME (PRIMARY HIV INFECTION)

- CD4+ T lymphocytes more than 500.[24]
- Within 2–3 weeks of infection, flulike symptoms varying from mild to profound may appear: symptoms may be vague so a diagnosis of HIV is not made.

- Detectable HIV antibody (anti-HIV) as a serum marker of the infection may be found.

III. EARLY SYMPTOMATIC HIV DISEASE

- CD4+ T lymphocytes 200–500 cells; continued increase in viremia.[24]
- Systemic symptoms are night sweats, weight loss, diarrhea, fever, malaise, general weakness.
- Opportunistic infections begin to occur.
- Oral lesions become more common; candidiasis may be predictive of the development of full-blown AIDS in untreated patients within two years.

IV. LATE-STAGE DISEASE: AIDS

- CD4+ cell count falls below 200.
- *Pneumocystis jirovecii* pneumonia (PCP) is a presenting feature with other AIDS-defining diseases.[25]
- Presentation of full-blown AIDS is highly variable and is affected by the host's prior exposure to chronic infections and treatment.

V. SYMPTOMS: AIDS INDICATING CONDITIONS[26]

- CD4+ numbers decline.
- Opportunistic infections (OI) become more frequent, extensive, and severe.
- AIDS-dementia complex occurs; often as progressive encephalopathy with significant neurologic dysfunction.

■ Tuberculosis infection: risk for progression from latent to active TB in HIV-infected individual is greater than in the general population.

■ Constitutional disease: HIV wasting syndrome: long-term fever, severe weight loss, anemia, chronic diarrhea, and chronic weakness are all effects of loss of immune response and repeated opportunistic diseases.

■ Neoplasms: several neoplasms, related to the underlying immunodeficiency, are common indicators of HIV-1 infection and AIDS including KS, primary B-cell lymphoma of the brain, non-Hodgkin's lymphoma, and cervical or rectal carcinoma.

■ Untreated, the disease usually progresses to death in 1 to 3 years.

ORAL MANIFESTATIONS OF HIV-1 INFECTION

■ Oral manifestations of HIV infection are significant indicators of HIV infection and markers of disease progression.

■ Integrate with patient history for early recognition and referral for medical evaluation and testing.

■ Early intervention is possible with drugs to slow down the process of the disease, prevent severe complications, and improve long-term quality of life.

■ The advent of highly active antiretroviral therapy (HAART) has greatly changed the overall prevalence and patterns of oral manifestations of HIV disease.

■ **Table 4-4** lists oral lesions according to frequency of the association with HIV infection.

I. EXTRAORAL EXAMINATION

A careful extraoral assessment is essential at each appointment.

A. Lymphadenopathy

■ Palpation for enlarged lymph nodes is a routine part of every extraoral examination.

■ Persistent generalized lymphadenopathy (PGL) is an early sign of HIV infection and a marker for AIDS progression.

B. Skin Lesions

■ Several conditions listed in **Table 4-4** develop in the skin.

■ Examples are KS, VZV, and human papillomavirus lesions.

II. INTRAORAL EXAMINATION[27]

■ Intraoral lesions are shown in **Table 4-4**.

■ Prevalence of oral manifestations has changed since the use of HAART.

TABLE 4-4	ORAL LESIONS ASSOCIATED WITH HIV/AIDS	
GROUP I: LESIONS STRONGLY ASSOCIATED WITH HIV-INFECTION	**GROUP II: LESIONS LESS COMMONLY ASSOCIATED WITH HIV-INFECTION**	**GROUP III: LESIONS SEEN WITH HIV-INFECTION**

Candidiasis
  Erythematous
  Psuedomembranous
Hairy leukoplakia
Kaposi's sarcoma (KS)
Non-Hodgkin's lymphoma
Periodontal infections
  Linear gingival erythema
  Necrotizing (ulcerative) gingivitis
  Necrotizing (ulcerative) periodontitis
	Bacterial infections
	  Mycobacterium avium-intracellulare
	  Mycobacterium tuberculosis
	Melanotic hyperpigmentation
	Necrotizing (ulcerative) stomatitis
	Salivary gland disease
	  Dry mouth due to decreased salivary flow
	  Unilateral or bilateral swelling of major salivary glands
	Viral infections
	  Herpes simplex virus
	  Human papillomavirus (warty-like lesions)
	  Condyloma *acuminatum*
	  Focal epithelial hyperplasia
	  Verruca *vulgaris*
	  Varicella-zoster virus (VZV)
	  Herpes zoster varicella
	Thrombocytopenic purpura
	Ulceration NOS (not otherwise specified)
		Bacterial infections
		  Actinomyces israelii
		  Escherichia coli
		  Klebsiella pneumoniae
		Cat-scratch disease
		Drug reactions:
		  Ulcerative erythema multiforme
		  Lichenoid
		  Toxic epidermolysis
		Viral infections
		  Cytomegalovirus
		  Molluscum *contagiosum*
		Fungal infection other than Candidiasis:
		  Cryptococcus neoformans
		  Geotrichum candidum
		  Histoplasma capsulatum
		  Mucoraceae (mucormycosis/zygomycosis)
		  Aspergillus flavus
		Neurologic disturbances
		  Facial palsy
		  Trigeminal neuralgia
		Epithelioid (bacillary) angiomatosis
		Recurrent apthous stomatitis

Source: EC-Clearinghouse on Oral Problems Related to HIV Infection and WHO Collaborating Centre on Oral Manifestations of the Human Immunodeficiency Virus. Classification and diagnostic criteria for oral lesions in HIV infection. *J Oral Pathol Med.* 1993 Aug;22(7):289–91.

A. Fungal Infections

- Oral candidiasis, the most frequently occurring oral infection; increases as HIV disease progresses.
- Candidiasis may be recognized by clinical examination, or the dentist may request the use of exfoliative cytology for definitive diagnosis.

B. Viral Infections

- Examples: herpes simplex, oral hairy leukoplakia, oral lesions of VZV, human papilloma virus, and cytomegalovirus ulcers.
- Lesions tend to be more widespread, occur in atypical patterns, and may persist for months.

C. Bacterial Infections: Gingival and Periodontal Infections

- Atypical gingival changes may be an initial indicator of undiagnosed HIV infection.
- Patients with HIV infection who maintain a high level of personal and professional oral care may present with healthier periodontal tissues.
- Periodontal infections associated with HIV infection tend to show more severe symptoms and to progress more rapidly.
  A. Linear gingival erythema (LGE)
  1. Presents as unusual of pattern of gingivitis with a distinctive band of erythema at the free gingival margin, extending 2 to 3 mm apically.
  2. LGE occurs independently of oral hygiene status, and does not respond as expected to improved personal biofilm control and periodontal therapy.
  B. Necrotizing ulcerative gingivitis (NUG) and periodontitis (NUP)
  1. Increased incidence of NUG with marked ulceration.
  2. NUG may progress to involve underlying bone and result in NUP, characterized by rapid attachment loss and severe tissue destruction.
  3. Deep pocketing rarely occurs; the extensive gingival and alveolar bone tissue destruction results in bone sequestrum.
  4. Attachment loss of more than 6 mm within a 6-month period is not uncommon.

III. DENTAL HYGIENE MANAGEMENT

- DHCPs may be the first to suspect HIV infection when oral manifestations and symptoms are recognized; referral for appropriate medical care is indicated.
- Dental healthcare professionals are ethically and legally obligated to treat HIV infected patients of record and other patients seeking treatment. The patients are protected by the American with Disabilities Act.
- To assist HIV infected patients in maintaining their oral health can significantly improve their quality of life

by reducing pain and susceptibility to other opportunistic infections.
- Pain and oral manifestations may be caused by the disease or from adverse drug effects of HAART.
- Adverse effects of the primary antiretroviral medication Zidovudine (ZVD/AZT) are nausea and vomiting, which can be severe enough to contribute to dental caries and dental erosion.
- Emphasis on immaculate personal oral care and frequent professional periodontal therapy. Fluoride varnish needs to be included in the preventive oral hygiene program for all ages.

PREVENTION OF HIV INFECTION

- Until a vaccine is available, prevention depends to a large degree on community education for attitudinal and behavioral changes.
- Health education efforts need to be focused on awareness of risk, modes of transmission of the HIV, and the preventive measures necessary to halt its transmission especially in high-risk groups.
- Dental personnel who are well informed with accurate, current information that can provide care for HIV-infected patients give support to community health programs.

I. GOALS

A. Primary Prevention

- The goal of primary prevention (for those not infected) is to lower the rate at which new cases of HIV infection appear.
- Programs for women, particularly of childbearing age; intravenous drug users who share needles; and teenagers are focused to reach the most vulnerable groups.
- HIV testing is required for all pregnant women and all newborns to control the increasing numbers of children with HIV infection.
- Provide routine testing for HIV as with other diseases.

B. Secondary Prevention

- The goals of secondary prevention (for seropositive individuals) are to reduce the rate of transmission and to introduce treatment early.
- Early intervention may postpone severe clinical manifestations of advanced illness.
- A leading part of the program is to counsel the HIV-infected individuals to practice safe sex* and to cooperate with the program to screen and counsel their sexual contacts and families.

---

*"Practice Safe Sex" is meant to include barrier protection and no exchange of body fluids (saliva, semen, vaginal secretions), in accord with recommended guidelines.

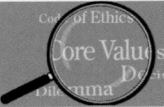

Everyday Ethics

Mr. Sands, a new patient to the dental hygiene clinic, had completed his admission history and basic examination at a previous appointment. He is assigned to Jenny because she needs more credits for patients with heavy calculus. He is scheduled today for his personal instruction for home care, and scaling for the first quadrant.

When Jenny starts to read the record before clinic opened, she learns that Mr. Sands has a history of Hepatitis C. She immediately makes up an excuse and asks Marilyn, her classmate in the clinic unit next to hers, to treat Mr. Sands, while she, Jenny, attends to the two pediatric patients scheduled for sealants with Marilyn. Marilyn has already prepared for the appointment with the children and needs the four credits toward her sealants requirement, although she also needs credits for a patient with heavy calculus.

Questions for Consideration

1. Which of the dental hygiene Core Values (Table II-1, page 38) is Jenny violating by her actions to avoid caring for this patient?
2. Is this an ethical dilemma or an ethical issue for Marilyn? How can Marilyn resolve the problem? What might be the consequences for both if Marilyn reports Jenny's action to the instructor in charge? What if Jenny does a similar thing in the future?
3. Using the "Steps in the Resolution of an Issue or a Dilemma" listed on pages 10–11, determine a course of action that can help Marilyn resolve the problem.

II. ONGOING PROGRAMS

- Strict testing for blood donors and all tissue organ donors, as well as identification and counseling of recipients of blood transfusions before 1985 and their sexual partners. The incubation period has been shown to be much longer than was originally thought.
- With early diagnosis and medical intervention, people with HIV infection can be symptom free and healthy and can live longer than was possible earlier in the epidemic.

BOX 4-3	Example Progress Note

Patient presented with large apthous ulcer during routine maintenance appointment and states that he is getting these lesions fairly frequently. Intraoral examination revealed excellent oral hygiene with small calculus deposits on the lingual of the mandibular anteriors and on proximal of mandibular premolars. Periodontal assessment is stable chronic slight periodontitis. Medical history indicated he is taking Zidovudine (ZVD), saquinavir, and Viramune for treatment of HIV, and has been in treatment for the past two years. He reported that his condition is well-controlled and that his CD4+ count was 700 at his last medical appointment and his viral load was low. RDH demonstrated use of intraoral "brush picks" to better access the premolar and molar proximal areas, and patient was responsive to oral hygiene instructions. Patient was referred to physician for consultation regarding apthous ulcer recurrences.

Signed: _____, RDH Date: _____

DOCUMENTATION

Suggested documentation for the patient with an infectious disease includes the following:

- If the patient is under treatment for an infectious condition, note the patient's medication, its purpose, adverse effects, and effects on oral health.
- Record all consultations with specialists.
- When patient is not being treated, record referral and purpose.
- Record results of specific laboratory tests (CD4+ counts, neutrophil counts, and others) that potentially affect dental hygiene treatment; note those values at each appointment.
- Box 4-3 provides a sample Progress Note.

Factors To Teach The Patient

- Reasons for postponing an appointment when a herpes lesion ("fever blister" or "cold sore") is present on the lip.
- Importance of not touching or scratching the lesion because of self-infection to fingers or eyes, for example.
- How the viruses can survive on objects and transfer infection to other people.
- How to help by keeping the medical history up-to-date by informing of additional exposures and immunizations to communicable diseases for self and family members.
- Importance of oral health to overall systemic health.
- Preparation for a dental or dental hygiene appointment by thorough mouth cleaning with toothbrush and dental floss to lower the bacterial count and thus lessen aerosol contamination in the treatment room.

References

1. Centers for Disease Control and Prevention. Guidelines for infection control in dental health-care settings – 2003. *MMWR*. 2003 Dec 19;52(RR-17):16. Available from: http://www.cdc.gov/mmwr/PDF/rr/rr5217.pdf

2. Socransky SS, Manganiello SD. The oral microbiota of man from birth to senility. *J Periodontol*. 1971 Aug;42(8):485–94.

3. Harrel SK, Molinari J. Aerosols and splatter in dentistry: a brief review of the literature and infection control implications. *J Am Dent Assoc*. 2004 Apr;135(4):429–37.

4. Larato DC, Ruskin PF, Martin A. Effect of an ultrasonic scaler on bacterial counts in air. *J Periodontol*. 1967 Nov–Dec;38(6):550.

5. Molinari JA, Harte JA. *Cottone's practical infection control in dentistry*. 3rd ed. Baltimore: Lippincott Williams & Wilkins; 2009. Chapter 13, How to choose and use environmental surface disinfectants; p. 190.

6. Heymann DL, ed. *Control of communicable diseases manual*. 19th ed. Washington: American Public Health Association; 2008. Tuberculosis; pp. 642–4.

7. Centers for Disease Control and Prevention. Guidelines for preventing the transmission of *Mycobacterium tuberculosis* in health-care settings, 2005. *MMWR*. 2005 Dec 30;54(RR-17):19–20. Available from: http://www.cdc.gov/mmwr/PDF/rr/rr5217.pdf

8. National Prevention Information Network [Internet]. Atlanta: CDC NPIN Resource Center; [updated 2010 Nov 22]. Viral hepatitis; [updated 2010 Oct 15; cited 2010 May 19]; [1 p.]. Available from: http://www.cdcnpin.org/scripts/hepatitis/index.asp

9. Centers for Disease Control and Prevention. *The ABCs of hepatitis*. Atlanta: CDC; 2010 June. Publication No.: 21–1076. Available from: http://www.cdc.gov/hepatitis/Resources/Professionals/PDFs/ABCTable_BW.pdf

10. Heymann. op.cit., p.286.

11. Centers for Disease Control and Prevention. Updated U.S. Public Health Service guidelines for the management of occupational exposures to HBV, HCV, and HIV and recommendations for postexposure prophylaxis. *MMWR*. 2001 June 29;50(RR-11):1–42. Table 3, Recommended postexposure prophylaxis for exposure to hepatitis B virus; [about screen 21]. Available from: http://www.cdc.gov/mmwr/preview/mmwrhtml/rr5011a1.htm#tab3

12. Heymann. op.cit., pp.293–5.

13. Heymann. op.cit., pp.295–7.

14. Heymann. op.cit., pp.300–2.

15. Slots J. Herpesviruses in periodontal diseases. *Periodontol 2000*. 2005 June;38(1):33–62.

16. Cassai E, Galvan M, Trombelli L, Rotola A. HHV-6, HHV-7, HHV-8 in gingival biopsies from chronic adult periodontitis patients. A case-controlled study. *J Clin Periodontol*. 2003 Mar;30(3):184–91.

17. Kessler HP. Herpes virus infections: a review for the dental practitioner. *Tex Dent J*. 2005 Feb;122(2):150–65.

18. Heymann. op.cit., pp.109–12.

19. Centers for Disease Control and Prevention. Prevention of herpes zoster. *MMWR*. 2008 June 6;57(05):1–30. Available from: http://www.cdc.gov/mmwr/preview/mmwrhtm/rr5705al.htm

20. Heymann. op.cit., pp.428–30.

21. Heymann. op.cit., pp.161–4.

22. Heymann. op.cit., pp.398–9.

23. Heymann. op.cit., pp.1–9.

24. Centers for Disease Control and Prevention. Revised surveillance case definitions for HIV infection among adults, adolescents and children aged <18 months and for HIV infection and AIDS among children aged 18 months to <13 years – United States, 2008. *MMWR*. 2008 Dec 5;57(RR-10):1–8. Available from: http://www.cdc.gov/mmwr/preview/mmwrhtml/rr5710a1.htm?s_rr5710a1_e

25. Centers for Disease Control and Prevention. Appendix A: AIDS-defining conditions. *MMWR*. 2008 Dec 5;57(RR-10):9. Available from: http://www.cdc.gov/mmwr/preview/mmwrhtml/rr5710a2.htm

26. Reznik DA, O'Neal C. www.HIVdent.org: the Internet's HIV/AIDS oral health resource [Internet]. [place unknown]: HIVdent; c1996–2007. Oral manifestations of HIV/AIDS in the HAART era; [cited 2010 May 5]; [about 5 screens]. Available from: http://www.hivdent.org/_oralmanifestations_OralManifestations_OMHAHO502.htm

27. Centers for Disease Control and Prevention. Guidelines for the prevention and treatment of opportunistic infections among HIV-exposed and HIV-infected children. *MMWR*. 2009 Sep 4;58(RR-11):1–3. Available from: http://www.cdc.gov/mmwr/preview/mmwrhtml/rr5811a1.htm

CHAPTER

Exposure Control: Barriers for Patient and Clinician

ESTHER M. WILKINS, BS, RDH, DMD

Chapter Outline

PERSONAL PROTECTION FOR THE DENTAL TEAM
I. Immunizations
II. Management Program

CLINICAL ATTIRE
I. Gown or Uniform
II. Hair and Head Covering
III. Outside Wear

USE OF FACE MASK: RESPIRATORY PROTECTION
I. Mask Efficiency
II. Use of a Mask

USE OF PROTECTIVE EYEWEAR
I. Indications for Use of Protective Eyewear
II. Protective Eyewear

III. Suggestions for Clinical Application

HAND CARE
I. Bacteriology of the Skin
II. Hand Care

HANDWASHING PRINCIPLES
I. Rationale
II. Purposes
III. Facilities

METHODS OF HANDWASHING
I. Indications
II. Definitions
III. Routine Handwash
IV. Antiseptic Handwash
V. Antiseptic Hand Rub
VI. Surgical Antisepsis

GLOVES AND GLOVING
I. Criteria for Selection of Treatment/Examination Gloves
II. Types of Gloves
III. Procedures for Use of Gloves
IV. Factors Affecting Glove Integrity

LATEX HYPERSENSITIVITY
I. Clinical Manifestations
II. Individuals at High Risk of Latex Sensitivity
III. Management

DOCUMENTATION

EVERYDAY ETHICS

FACTORS TO TEACH THE PATIENT

REFERENCES

Exposure control refers to all procedures during clinical care necessary to provide top-level protection from exposure to infectious agents for members of the dental team and their patients. Dental healthcare personnel (DHCP) have a professional obligation to serve *all* patients with comprehensive oral care, including patients with known or unknown communicable diseases. The practice of *standard precautions* means that the body fluids of all patients are treated as if they were infectious.

■ An organized system for exposure control is needed.
■ A written exposure control plan is prepared to serve as a guide for the entire team.[1] The written plan can be the basis for training new personnel.

■ Consistency between DHCPs is necessary to maintain standards of asepsis and to prevent cross-contamination.
■ As new research and commercial products become available, the written protocol is revised.
■ Using the protocol and transferring the objectives and overall aims to the clinical setting are the responsibilities of each member of the dental team.
■ Physical barriers and other requirements of the protocol provide safety for both the DHCP and the patients.
■ Refer to Appendix IV (page 1096) to review specific recommendations from the U.S. Department of Health and Human Services.
■ Selected terms for the application of exposure control and immunizations are defined in **Box 5-1**.

BOX 5-1	**Key Words**

Exposure Control

Allergen: substance, protein or nonprotein, capable of inducing allergy or specific hypersensitivity; can enter the body by being inhaled, swallowed, touched, or injected.

Antimicrobial soap: a soap containing an active ingredient against skin microorganisms.

Atopy: clinical hypersensitivity state or allergy with a hereditary predisposition; includes hay fever, eczema, and asthma.

Barrier protection: refers to placing a physical barrier between the patient's body fluids (such as blood and saliva) and the healthcare personnel (HCP) to prevent disease transmission.

Barriers for HCP: include gloves, mask, protective eyewear, and protective clothing (gown).

Barriers for patient: include protective eyewear, head cover during surgeries, and rubber dam during restorative and sealant procedures.

Booster dose: amount of immunogen (vaccine, toxoid, or other antigen preparation), usually smaller than the original amount, injected at an appropriate interval after the primary immunization to sustain the immune response to that immunogen.

Exposure incident: a specific eye, mouth, mucous membrane, nonintact skin, or parenteral contact with blood or other potentially infectious material that results from the performance of one's usual professional duties.

Hypoallergenic: property of a substance that indicates it does not create a hypersensitive reaction; may apply to various chemicals; not specified on manufacturer's' labels.

Immunization: the process of rendering a subject immune to a particular disease by stimulation with a specific antigen to promote antibody formation in the body.

Inoculation: introduction of antigenic material or vaccine; more frequently used to refer to introduction of material into a culture medium.

Latex allergy: an acquired hypersensitivity reaction to the proteins found in natural rubber latex (NRL).

Occupational exposure: reasonably anticipated skin, eye, mucous membrane, or parenteral contact with blood or other potentially infectious materials that may result from the performance of one's usual duties.

PPD: purified protein derivative for tuberculin intracutaneous skin test for tuberculosis; positive reaction means previous infection with *Mycobacterium tuberculosis*.

Rhinitis: inflammation of the mucous membrane of the nose; may result from infection by bacteria or virus, or may be a seasonal (hay fever) or nonseasonal allergic reaction.

Toxoid: toxin treated by heat or chemical agent to destroy its deleterious properties without destroying its ability to combine with, or stimulate the formation of, antitoxin; examples of toxoids used for active immunization are tetanus and diphtheria.

Tuberculin test (Mantoux): a test for the presence of active or inactive tuberculosis; a positive test is denoted by redness and induration at the injection site by 48 to 72 hours after injection.

Vaccination: process of introducing a vaccine into the body to produce immunity to a specific disease.

Vaccine: a suspension of attenuated or killed microorganisms administered for the prevention or treatment of an infectious disease.

PERSONAL PROTECTION FOR THE DENTAL TEAM

The continuing health and productivity of dental health-care personnel depend to a large degree on the individuals' efforts to maintain themselves in a high standard of good health as expressed in Chapter 1, page 11. Resistance to disease, if exposed, is enhanced in a person with top-level health habits.

■ Loss of work time, personal suffering, long-term systemic effects, and even exclusion from continued practice are possible results from communicable disease infection.

■ The only safe procedure is to practice defensively at all times, with specific precautions for personal protection.

■ All clinical staff members need to be well aware of the signs and symptoms of diseases that are occupational hazards for clinical dental and dental hygiene practitioners.

■ All are encouraged to seek early diagnosis and treatment of a seemingly minor condition that could be the initial symptom of a more serious communicable disease.

I. IMMUNIZATIONS

Dental personnel in a hospital setting are subject to the rules and regulations for all hospital employees. Policies often require certain immunizations for new employees if written proof of immunizations is not available and tests for antibodies prove to be negative.

■ In private dental practices, individual initiative is required to maintain standards of safety for all dental team members relative to immunizations.

■ Basic immunizations recommended for healthcare workers include at least the vaccines for hepatitis B, influenza, MMR (measles, mumps, rubella), and varicella-zoster. As research provides more vaccines, health care personnel will seek additional immunizations.

■ General recommendations on immunizations are reviewed annually by the Advisory Committee on Immunization Practices (ACIP).[2]

■ At the time of employment, it is reasonable for a dentist-employer to request a record of current immunizations and the most recent updating from employees, as well as specific tests, such as for tuberculosis. Immunization for rubella is particularly important for female employees of childbearing age.

II. MANAGEMENT PROGRAM

A. Recommended

- Records for personal immunizations are regularly updated.
- The needs differ in different climates, countries, and locations. Persons changing work location, or traveling for participation in dental hygiene programs, need to become aware of specific precautions.

B. Obtaining Tests

Obtain tests promptly when exposed to certain infectious diseases and seek prophylactic immunization as indicated and available.

C. Written Records

- Keep confidential written records of immunizations, boosters, and reimmunizations; plan for regular follow-up.
- When the status of current immunizations is known, time is saved by not needing a susceptibility test before initiating passive immunizations when accidental exposure occurs.

 CLINICAL ATTIRE

The wearing apparel of clinicians and their assistants is vulnerable to contamination from splash, spatter, aerosols, and patient contact. The recommended gown or uniform is designed and cared for in a manner that minimizes cross-contamination.

I. GOWN OR UNIFORM

- Gowns or uniforms are expected to be clean and maintained as free as possible from contamination.
- Wearing clinic coats over street clothes is not recommended because of the exposure of the street clothes to infectious material.

A. Solid, Closed Front

- The garment is closed at the neck and fastened or tied back, preferably.
- The fabric is disposable or can be washed commercially and withstand washing with bleach.

B. Length

- Long garment to cover knees when seated for patient treatment.
- Long sleeves with fitted cuffs permit protective gloves to extend over the cuffs.

C. No Pockets

- Pockets are too readily available for placing contaminated objects, such as writing implements or keys.
- Gloved hands, prepared for patient treatment, are kept from touching objects or being placed in pockets.

D. Protection for Gown or Uniform

- A washable or a disposable apron may be used over the gown when clinical services that involve blood, spatter, or aerosols are performed.

E. Laundering

- Commercial laundry services are preferred.
- When laundered at home, the items from a dental office or clinic need to be kept separate and treated with household bleach for disinfection.

II. HAIR AND HEAD COVERING

- Hair is worn off the shoulders and fastened back away from the face.
    - When longer, it needs to be held within a head cover.
    - Because the hair is exposed to much contamination, an appropriate head cover is advised when using handpieces and ultrasonic or air-powder polishing instruments.
- Facial hair needs to be covered with a face mask and face shield.

III. OUTSIDE WEAR

Clinic uniforms and shoes are not to be worn outside the clinic practice setting.[3] When clinical clothing is worn outside, contamination can be carried from, and brought into, the treatment area.

 USE OF FACE MASK: RESPIRATORY PROTECTION

Basic personal barrier protection is composed of face mask, protective eyewear, and gloves.

- The use of the face mask is described first because it needs to be positioned first when preparing for clinical care procedures.
- The protective eyewear is placed second. After that, the hands can be washed before gloving.
- Dispersion of particles of debris, polishing agents, calculus, and water, all of which are contaminated by the patient's oral flora, occurs regularly during instrumentation.
- The greatest aerosols are created following the use of a handpiece, prophylaxis angle, or power-driven ultrasonic scaler.
- Evidence of the spread of particles appears on the splashed face, protective eyewear, and uniform and on the coverall placed over the patient for protection from the spray.

BOX 5-2	Characteristics of an Ideal Mask

1. No contact with the wearer's nostrils or lips
2. Has a high bacterial filtration efficiency rate
3. Fits snugly around the entire edges of the mask
4. No fogging of eyewear
5. Convenient to put on and remove
6. Made of material that does not irritate skin or induce allergic reaction
7. Does not collapse during wear or when wet

I. MASK EFFICIENCY

A. Criteria: Essential Characteristics (Box 5-2)

- *Filtration* (measured in BFE = bacterial filtration efficiency).
  - Standard masks block filtration of particles as small as 3 μm with a filter efficiency greater than 95%.
  - Particles of 3 μm and smaller can penetrate to the alveoli of the lower respiratory tract, where their infectivity is increased.
  - Droplet nuclei (*Mycobacterium tuberculosis*) range from 0.5 to 1 μm and are a risk in healthcare settings.[4]
- *Fit.* Proper fit over face is vital to protect against inhaling droplet nuclei from aerosols.
- *Moisture absorption.* Soak through is an important factor. Lining needs to be impervious. Mask must be changed for each patient and not worn longer than 1 hour.
- *Comfort.* Degree of comfort encourages compliance in wearing.

B. Materials

- Various materials have been used for masks, including gauze and other cloth, plastic foam, fiberglass, synthetic fiber mat, and paper.
- In research studies, foam, paper, and cloth were found to be the least adequate filters of aerosols, whereas glass fiber and synthetic fiber mat were shown to be the most effective.[5,6]
- Particulate Respirator Mask (PRM)
  - Use for potentially infectious patient (active tuberculosis) when ventilation is poor, and procedure likely to produce droplet spatter or aerosols of oral or respiratory fluids.
  - Heavy-duty mask designed for the essential tight fit.

II. USE OF A MASK

- Adjust the mask and position eyewear before a handwash.
- Use a fresh mask for each patient.
  - Change mask each hour or more frequently when it becomes wet.

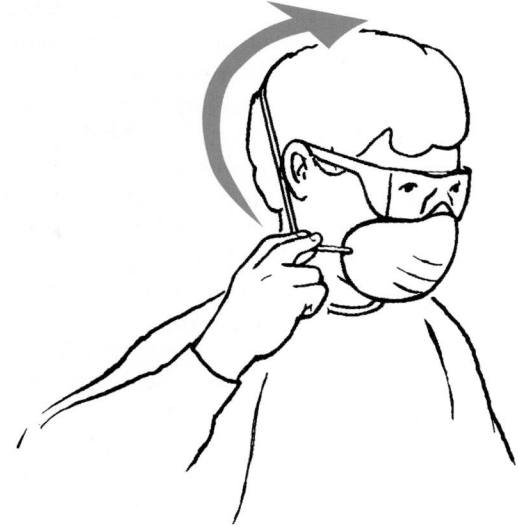

FIGURE 5-1 Removal of Mask. Handle only by the elastic or tie strings, carefully avoiding the contaminated mask.

- Chin-cover face shield needs to be supplemented with a fitted mask.
- Keep the mask on after completing a procedure while still in the presence of aerosols.
  - Particles smaller than 5 μm remain suspended longer (up to 24 hours) than do larger particles and can be inhaled directly into terminal lung alveoli.
  - Removal of a mask in the treatment room immediately following the use of aerosol-producing procedures permits direct exposure to airborne organisms.
- Mask removal
  - Grasp side elastic or tie strings to remove **(Figure 5-1)**.
  - Never handle the outside of a contaminated mask with gloved or bare hands. Never place the mask under the chin.

USE OF PROTECTIVE EYEWEAR

Eye protection for the dental team members and patients is necessary to prevent physical injuries and infections of the eyes.

- Severe and disabling eye accidents and infections have been reported.[7-9]
- Eye involvement may lead to pain, discomfort, loss of work time, and, in certain instances, permanent injury.
- Accidents can occur at any time, and as with most accidents, they occur when least prepared for or expected.
- Eye infections can follow the accidental dropping of an instrument on the face or the splashing of various materials from a patient's oral cavity into the eye.

- Contamination can be introduced from saliva, biofilm, carious material, pieces of old restorative materials during cavity preparation, bacteria-laden calculus during scaling, and any other microorganisms contained in aerosols or spatter.
- An aerosol created by a power-driven scaler can be heavily contaminated with oral microorganisms.
- Careful, deliberate techniques and instrument management, with evacuation and other procedures for the control of oral fluids, contribute to the prevention of accidents and infections of the eyes.
- All measures described for the prevention of airborne disease transmission by aerosols and spatter apply to eye protection.
- The most effective defense is the use of protective eyewear by all involved—dental team members and patients.

I. INDICATIONS FOR USE OF PROTECTIVE EYEWEAR

A. Dental Team Members

- Protective eyewear is worn for all procedures.
- For dental personnel who do not require corrective lens for vision, protective eyewear with clear lens can be a routine part of clinical dress.

B. Patients

- Protective eyewear is essential for each patient at each appointment.
- The patient's medical history will reflect types of eye surgery, implants, or other special concerns.
- Patients with their own prescription lenses may prefer to wear them, but for the safety of the patient's glasses, the use of the protective eyewear provided in the office or clinic may be advisable.

II. PROTECTIVE EYEWEAR

A. General Features of Acceptable Eyewear

- Wide coverage, with side shields, to protect around the eye.
- Shatterproof; made of strong, sturdy plastic.
- Lightweight.
- Flexible and with rounded smooth edges to prevent discomfort if pressed against the nose or ears.
- Easily disinfected.
  - A. Smooth surface areas to prevent accumulation of infectious material.
  - B. Disinfectant used cannot damage or distort the frames or lens.
- A clear or lightly tinted lens, rather than a very dark lens, permits the dental team members to watch the patient's reactions and maintain contact and response.

- Protection against glare. Certain patients may request tinted lenses or prefer to wear their own sunglasses when their eyes are especially sensitive to the dental light.

B. Types of Eyewear

Many styles, including regular eyeglass shapes and those described as follows, have been used.

- *Goggles* **(Figure 5-2A)**. Shielding on all sides of the glasses may give the best protection, provided they fit closely around the edges. Goggle-style coverage is especially necessary for protection during laboratory work.
- *Eyewear With Side Shields* **(Figure 5-2B** and **C)**. A side shield can provide added protection. For the member of the dental team who depends on a prescription lens, separate side shields are available that can be connected to the bows.

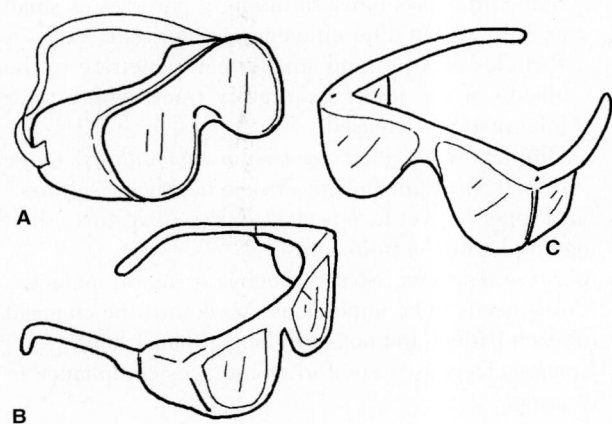

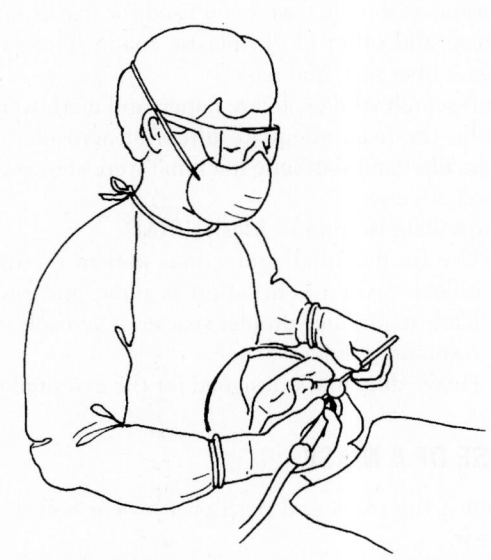

FIGURE 5-2 **Protective Eyewear.** Protective cover for both patient and clinician may be goggles-style (**A**) or glasses with side shields (**B** and **C**).

■ *Eyewear With Curved Frames.* When the sides of the eyewear are curved back, they may provide a protection somewhat similar to that offered by those with the side shield.
■ *Postmydriatic Spectacles Used by Ophthalmologist.* Disposable glasses are available that are made of flexible plastic.
■ *Child-Sized.* Child-sized sunglasses and children's play spectacles have been used.

C. Face Shield

A clinician needs to wear a face shield over a regular mask when aerosol-producing handpiece, power scaler, or power polishing equipment is used.

III. SUGGESTIONS FOR CLINICAL APPLICATION

A. Patient Instruction

A patient who has not been asked to wear protective eyewear at previous appointments will appreciate a simple explanation of the reasons for doing so.

B. Contact Lenses

Dental team members and patients who wear contact lenses always need to wear protective eyewear over them during dental and dental hygiene procedures.

C. Care of Protective Eyewear

■ Run eyewear under water stream to remove abrasive particles. Rubbing an abrasive agent over the plastic lens can create scratches.
■ Materials used for protective lens may be damaged by some disinfectants. Clean with detergent and rinse thoroughly. Air-dry.
■ Check periodically for scratches on the lens, and replace appropriately.

D. Eye Wash Station

■ Do not connect the eye wash station equipment to a sink used by clinicians for patient preparation.
■ It must not be connected to the regular faucets unless the hot water source is turned off permanently.

HAND CARE

In the infectious process of disease transmission, the hands may serve as a *means of transmission* of the blood, saliva, and dental biofilm from a patient, and the hands, especially under the fingernails, may serve as a *reservoir* for microorganisms.

■ *Skin breaks in the hands may serve as a port of entry* for potentially pathogenic microorganisms.

■ By caring properly for the hands, using effective washing procedures, and following the basic rules for gloving, primary cross-contamination can be controlled.
■ A conscious effort is made to keep the gloved hands from touching objects other than the instruments and disinfected parts of the equipment prepared for the immediate patient.

I. BACTERIOLOGY OF THE SKIN

A. Resident Bacteria

■ Many relatively stable bacteria inhabit the surface epithelium or deeper areas in the ducts of skin glands or depths of hair follicles; ultimately, they are shed with the exfoliated surface cells, or with excretions of the skin glands.
■ The flora may be altered by newly introduced pathogens or reduced by washing.
■ Resident bacteria tend to be less susceptible to destruction by disinfection procedures.

B. Transient Bacteria

■ Transient bacteria reflect continuous contamination by routine contacts; some bacteria are pathogens and may act temporarily as residents.
■ They may be washed away or, in the event that a skin break exists, may cause an autogenous infection.
■ Most transients can be removed with soap and water by washing thoroughly.

II. HAND CARE

A. Fingernails

■ Maintain clean, smoothly trimmed, short fingernails with well-cared-for cuticles to prevent breaks where microorganisms can enter.
■ Effects of short nails.
  A. Make handwashing more effective because of fewer microorganisms harbored under the nails.[10]
  B. Prevent cuts from long nail in disposable gloves.
  C. Permit selection of a closer fit of glove; longer glove fingers may be required to protect nails.
  D. Allow greater dexterity during instrumentation.
  E. Decrease chance of patient discomfort.

B. Wristwatch and Jewelry

■ Remove hand and wrist jewelry at the beginning of the day.
■ Microorganisms can become lodged in crevices of rings, watchbands, and watches, where cleaning is impossible.

C. Gloves

- After handwashing, don gloves. Never expose open skin lesions or abrasions to a patient's oral tissues and fluids.
- After glove removal, wash hands to remove microorganisms.

HANDWASHING PRINCIPLES

I. RATIONALE

- Effective and frequent handwashing can reduce the overall bacterial flora of the skin and prevent the organisms acquired from a patient from becoming skin residents.
- It is impossible to sterilize the skin, but every attempt is made to reduce the bacterial flora to a minimum.

II. PURPOSES

The objective of all handwashing is to reduce the bacterial flora of the hands to an absolute minimum. An effective handwash procedure can be expected to accomplish the following:

- Remove surface dirt and transient bacteria
- Dissolve the normal greasy film on the skin
- Rinse and remove all loosened debris and microorganisms

III. FACILITIES

A. Sink

- Use a sink with a foot pedal or electronic control for water-flow control to avoid contamination to/from faucet handles.
- For regular sink, turn on water at the beginning and leave on through the entire procedure. Turn faucets off with the towel after drying hands.
- Clean around brim of sink with disinfectant. The sink must be of sufficient size so that contact with the inside of the wash basin can be avoided easily. A sink cannot be sterilized and can become highly contaminated.
- Prevent contamination of clothing by not leaning against the sink.
- Use a separate area and sink reserved for instrument washing. Contaminated instruments must be removed from the treatment room before preparation for the next patient.

B. Soap

- Use a liquid surgical scrub containing an antimicrobial agent. Povidone–iodine (iodophore) has a broad spectrum of action.
- Apply from a foot- or knee-activated or electronically controlled dispenser to avoid contamination to and from a hand-operated dispenser or cake soap. Rinsing is a necessary part of the handwashing procedure.

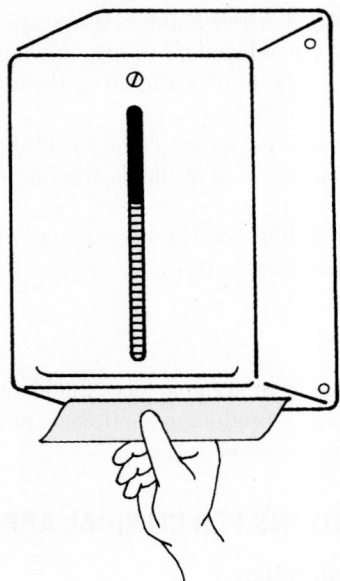

FIGURE 5-3 Towel Dispenser. Correct type of dispenser that requires no contact except with the towel itself, which hangs down from the container.

C. Scrub Brushes

- Avoid overvigorous use of a brush to minimize skin abrasion. Skin irritation and abrasion can leave openings for additional cross-contamination.
- Disposable sponges are available commercially and may be preferred when a scrub brush is traumatic to the skin.

D. Towels

- Obtain disposable towel from a dispenser that requires no contact except with the towel itself, which hangs down **(Figure 5-3)**.
- Cloth towels are not recommended.

 METHODS OF HANDWASHING

Handwashing is considered the most important single procedure for the prevention of cross-contamination.

I. INDICATIONS

- Before and after treating each patient (before glove placement and after glove removal)
- Before regloving after removing gloves that are torn, cut, or punctured
- After barehanded touching inanimate objects that may be contaminated with blood or saliva
- When hands are visibly soiled
- Before leaving the treatment room

II. DEFINITIONS[11]

A. Routine Handwash

- Water and nonantimicrobial soap (plain soap)
- To remove soil and transient microorganisms

B. Antiseptic Handwash

- Water and antimicrobial liquid soap (e.g., chlorhexidine, iodine and iodophors, chloroxylenol [PCMX], triclosan)
- To remove or destroy transient microorganisms and reduce resident flora

C. Antiseptic Hand Rub

- Alcohol-based hand rub (contains 60–95% ethanol or isopropanol)
- To remove or destroy transient microorganisms and reduce resident flora

D. Surgical Antisepsis (Also Called Surgical Scrub)

- Water and antimicrobial liquid soap (e.g., chlorhexidine, iodine and iodophores, chloroxylenol [PCMX], triclosan)
- To remove or destroy transient microorganisms and reduce resident flora with a persistent or prolonged effect that inhibits proliferation or survival of microorganisms

III. ROUTINE HANDWASH

- Wet hands, apply soap; avoid hot water.
- Rub hands together for at least 15 seconds; cover all surfaces of fingers, hands, and wrists.
- Interlace fingers and rub to cover all sides.
- Rinse under running water; dry thoroughly with disposable towels.
- Turn off faucet with the towel.
- Bar soap harbors microorganisms; keep on soap rack where drainage and drying are possible.

IV. ANTISEPTIC HANDWASH

A. Preliminary Steps

- Remove watch and jewelry from hands.
- Fasten hair back securely.
- Don protective eyewear and mask before handwashing to prevent contamination of washed hands ready for gloving.
- Use cool water.

B. Handwashing Procedure

- Lather hands, wrists, and forearms quickly with liquid antimicrobial soap.
- Rub all surfaces vigorously; interlace fingers and rub back and forth with pressure.

- Rinse thoroughly, running the water from fingertips down the hands. Keep water running.
- Repeat two more times. One lathering for 3 minutes is less effective than are three short latherings and three rinses in 30 seconds. The latherings serve to loosen the debris and microorganisms and the rinsings wash them away.
- Use paper towels for drying, taking care not to recontaminate.

V. ANTISEPTIC HAND RUB

- Wash away visible dirt before use.
- Decontaminate hands with an alcohol-based hand rub.
- Apply the product (follow manufacturer's directions for amount to use) to the palm of one hand, and rub hands together.
- Rub hands vigorously, covering all surfaces of fingers and hands, until the hands are dry.

VI. SURGICAL ANTISEPSIS

- Each hospital or oral surgery clinic has rules and regulations for surgical antisepsis. These will be posted over the scrub sinks.
- A surgical antisepsis performed as the first one of a day will be 10 minutes and subsequent ones may be 3–5 minutes. Following treatment of a contagious or isolated patient, the procedure will take at least 5 minutes.

A. Preliminary Steps

1. Remove watch and jewelry. Place hair and beard coverings and make sure hair is completely covered. Don protective eyewear and mask.
2. Open sterile brush package to have ready.
3. Wash hands and arms, using surgical liquid antimicrobial soap to remove gross surface dirt before using the scrub brush. Lather vigorously with strong rubbing motions, 10 on each side of hands, wrists, and arms. Interlace the fingers and thumbs to clean the proximal surfaces.
4. Rinse thoroughly from fingertips across hands and wrists. Hold hands higher than elbows throughout the procedure. Leave water running.
5. Use orangewood stick from the sterile package to clean nails. Rinse.

B. First Hand

1. Lather the hands and arms and leave the lather on to increase the exposure time to the antimicrobial ingredient.
2. Apply surgical liquid antimicrobial soap, and begin the brush procedure. Scrub in an orderly sequence without returning to areas previously scrubbed.
3. First hand and arm.
   - Brush back and forth across nails and fingertips, passing the brush under the nails.

■ Fingers and hand: Use small circular strokes on all sides of the thumb and each finger, overlapping strokes for complete coverage.
■ Continue to wrist. Apply more soap to maintain a good lather.
■ When arm is completed, leave lather on.

C. Second Hand

1. Repeat on the other arm. Some systems require the use of a second sterile brush for the second hand. When this is so, discard the first brush into the proper container and obtain the second brush.
2. At one-half of scrub time, rinse hands and arms thoroughly, first one and then the other, starting at the fingertips and letting water pass down over the arm.
3. Lather and repeat.
4. At the end of time (or counts), rinse thoroughly, each arm separately, from fingertips. Apply towel from fingertips to elbow without reapplying to hand area.
5. Hold hands up and clasped together. Proceed to dressing area for gowning and gloving.

 GLOVES AND GLOVING

Wearing gloves is standard practice to protect both the patient and the clinician from cross-contamination.

I. CRITERIA FOR SELECTION OF TREATMENT/ EXAMINATION GLOVES

A. Safety Factors: Infection Control

■ Effective barrier; evidence from manufacturer of quality control standards.
■ Impermeable to patient's saliva, blood, and bacteria.
■ Strength and durability to resist tears and punctures.
■ Impervious to materials routinely used during clinical procedures.
■ Nonirritating or harmful to skin; use nonlatex gloves when patient or clinician is allergic.
■ Length: glove cuff extends to provide coverage over cuff of long sleeve.

B. Ergonomic Choice Factors

■ Fit hand well; no interference with motion.
■ Tactile sense not decreased.
■ No tight pull over palm or between thumb and index finger.

II. TYPES OF GLOVES

A. Material

■ Latex
■ Nonlatex: neoprene, block copolymer, vinyl, *N*-nitrile

B. For Patient Care

■ *Nonsterile Single-Use Examination/Treatment.* Latex, nonlatex
■ *Presterilized Single-Use Surgical.* Latex, nonlatex

C. Utility Gloves

■ *Heavy Duty.* Latex, nonlatex (puncture resistant for clinic cleanup)
■ *Plastic.* Food handler's glove to wear as overglove

III. PROCEDURES FOR USE OF GLOVES

A. Mask and Eyewear Placement

■ Place mask and protective eyewear before handwashing and gloving.
■ Prevent the need for manipulating the mask around the face and hair after washing the hands.

B. Pregloving Handwash

■ Use an antiseptic handwash before gloving.
■ Hands must be dried thoroughly to control moisture inside glove and thus discourage growth of bacteria.

C. Glove Placement

■ Always glove and deglove in front of the patient; a patient may need assurance that gloves are new and used only for that appointment.
■ Place gloves over the cuff of long-sleeved clinic wear to provide complete protection of arms from exposure to contamination.

D. Avoiding Contamination

■ Keep gloved hands away from face, hair, clothing (pockets), telephone, patient records, clinician's stool, and all parts of the dental equipment that have not been predisinfected and covered with a barrier material.

E. Torn, Cut, or Punctured Glove

■ Remove immediately, wash hands thoroughly, and don new gloves.

F. Removal of Gloves

■ Develop a procedure whereby gloves can be removed without contaminating the hands from the exposed external surfaces of the gloves.
■ **Figure 5-4** illustrates one system for glove removal.
■ Wash hands promptly after glove removal. Organisms on the hands multiply rapidly inside the warm, moist environment of the glove, even when no external contamination has occurred.

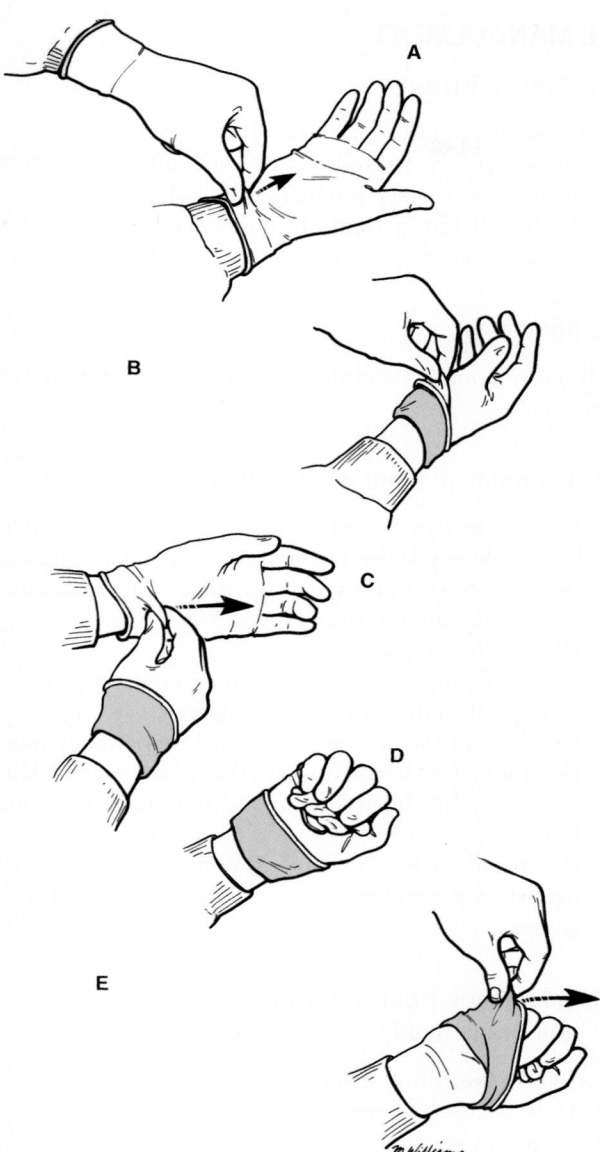

FIGURE 5-4 **Steps for Removal of Gloves.** (**A**) Use left fingers to pinch right glove near edge to fold back. (**B**) Fold edge back without contact with clean inside surface. (**C**) Use right fingers to contact outside of left glove at the wrist to invert and remove. (**D**) Bunch glove into the palm. (**E**) With ungloved left hand, grasp inner noncontaminated portion of the right glove to peel it off, enclosing other glove as it is inverted.

IV. FACTORS AFFECTING GLOVE INTEGRITY

A. Length of Time Worn

New pair for each patient is the basic requirement; total time worn should be no longer than 1 hour; when gloves develop a sticky surface, remove, wash hands, and reglove with a fresh pair.

B. Complexity of the Procedure

Certain procedures are more likely to promote perforations, especially when sharp instruments must be changed frequently.

C. Packaging of the Gloves

Top gloves of a new package are tightly packed and can be torn when removed; must be handled carefully until pressure is relieved.

D. Size of Glove

When too long, the extra material at the fingertips can get caught, torn, or in the way; picking up small objects is difficult, especially sharp instruments.

E. Pressure of Time

Stress; working too fast increases the risk of glove damage.

F. Storage of Gloves

Keep in cool, dark place; exposure to heat, sun, or fluorescent light increases potential for deterioration and perforations.

G. Agents Used

Certain chemicals react with the glove material; for example, petroleum jelly, alcohol, and products made with alcohol tend to break down the glove integrity.

H. Hazards From the Hands

Long fingernails and rings worn inside gloves.

LATEX HYPERSENSITIVITY

Patients and clinicians may have or may develop sensitivity to natural rubber latex. Symptoms of a hypersensitive reaction range from a dermatitis to a life-threatening anaphylactic shock. The only available treatment for latex allergy is avoiding all contact.

- Latex sensitivity is due to the protein allergens and to additives used when the commercial latex is prepared.
- Latex allergens occur in any equipment or product used that contains natural rubber latex (NRL).
- Gloves are the most frequently used item that contains latex.
- When gloves are powdered (cornstarch), the allergen can become airborne and be dispersed throughout the clinical area and on the personnel.
- Equipment listed in **Box 5-3** may contain NRL. However, many of the items also are made of alternative materials. When the label on a product does not list the contents, the manufacturer can be contacted to identify latex-free items.

BOX 5-3	Equipment That May Contain Latex

Bite blocks	O ring (on ultrasonic insert)
Blood pressure cuff	Orthodontic elastics
Gloves	Rubber polishing cup
Goggles	Stethoscope
Lead apron cover	Stopper in anesthesia
Masks (elastic head band)	carpule
Mixing bowl	Suction adapter
Nitrous oxide nosepiece	
and tubing Rubber dam	

I. CLINICAL MANIFESTATIONS

A. Methods of Exposure

- Aeroallergen inhalation (from powdered gloves)
- Donning gloves
- Mucosal contact

B. Type I Hypersensitivity (Immediate Reaction)

- Urticaria: hives
- Dermatitis: rash, itching
- Nasal problems: sneezing, itchy nose, runny nose
- Respiratory reaction: breathing difficulty, asthmalike wheezing, coughing
- Eyes: watery, itchy
- Drop in blood pressure: shock
- Anaphylaxis

C. Type IV Hypersensitivity (Delayed Reaction)

Contact dermatitis develops 6 to 72 hours after contact.

II. INDIVIDUALS AT HIGH RISK OF LATEX SENSITIVITY

A. Have Had Frequent Exposure to Latex Products

- Occupational exposure: healthcare personnel who wear latex gloves regularly for patient care or have worked in a rubber manufacturing plant.
- Multiple medical surgeries or treatments requiring placement of rubber tubes or drains. Examples: genitourinary anomalies, spina bifida.

B. Have Other Documented Allergies

Examples: food allergies (avocado, banana, kiwi fruit, chestnuts, papaya, peanuts).

III. MANAGEMENT

A. Medical History

- Questions in history will reveal all allergies.
- Questions directed to latex may not suffice. Questions about other specific products need to be asked.
- Advise allergic patients to obtain and wear an alert badge (bracelet).

B. Document

All information is carefully recorded for continuing reference.

C. Appointment Planning for Allergic Patient

- *Early in the Day when Powdered Gloves Are Used.* Meet before glove powder contaminates the air throughout the facility or outerwear of clinical attire becomes laden with airborne latex.
- *Clean Clinical Areas*
  - Person preparing room must wear nonlatex gloves.
  - Wipe all surfaces to remove allergen.
- *No Latex in the Treatment Room.* Use nonlatex products for high-risk patients (whether or not specific latex sensitivity has been known and reported in the history).
- *Prepare Latex-Free Carts.*[12] Materials and gloves, for use when seeing high-risk patients, can be readied in advance.

D. Emergency Treatment Equipment and Drugs Ready

1. Inform the entire dental team of appointment.
2. Have a latex-free emergency cart available.[15]
3. Alert for emergency.

DOCUMENTATION

Documentation needs to record the following:

- Irregularities related to personal protection that could have influenced the procedures of a routine appointment.
- How the special needs were taken care of for a patient with an allergy to latex.
- Unexpected need to refer a patient suspected of infection with tuberculosis.
- Information in Medical Alert that patient is sensitive to Latex.

  A sample progress note may be found in **Box 5-4.**

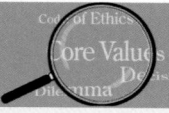

Everyday Ethics

After Mr. Green's dental hygiene treatment is completed, the dentist, Dr. Root, is notified so that the final examination can be made. Dr. Root comes in shortly and sits down next to the patient. He browses through the notations made in the patient's chart and then picks up the mirror and explorer to proceed with a clinical examination. It is apparent that he has not washed his hands and may not even have donned a new pair of gloves since he left the other treatment room. A similar situation has happened occasionally before.

Questions for Consideration

1. Mabel, the dental hygienist, notes that the dentist did not change his gloves or wash his hands. Is Mable faced with an ethical dilemma or an ethical issue? Explain.

2. Read the nine "Standards of Professional Responsibility" in the ADHA Code of Ethics in Appendix I (pages 1085–1086). Explain which of the standards are involved and how each is violated if Mable does not address this issue with Dr. Root.

3. Use the steps for making decisions on page 10 to determine some actions that Mable might take to address this situation both immediately and long term.

BOX 5-4	Example Progress Note

Initial appointment for new patient to our practice. History form and questions completed.

Radiographs taken and clinical charting begun. Interesting new patient who asked many questions about procedures and why we needed to wear mask and glasses and other equipment because she "didn't have a cold or anything I could 'catch.'" Said they didn't do anything like that at her previous dental office. Made appointment in 2 weeks for completion of treatment plan with Dr. Wyman.

Signed: _____, RDH Date: _____

Factors To Teach The Patient

- Need for the patient's complete history for the protection of both the patient and the professional person.
- Purposes for use of barriers (face mask, protective eyewear, and gloves) by the clinician for the benefit of the patient.
- Importance of eye protection.
- Significance of handwashing in the control of disease transmission (everywhere, not only dental office or clinic.

References

1. United States Department of Labor, Occupational Safety and Health Administration. Controlling Occupational Exposure to Bloodborne Pathogens in Dentistry, OSHA 3129, 1992. United States Government Printing Office: 1992–312–410/64790.

2. United States Department of Health and Human Services, Centers for Disease Control and Prevention. General recommendations on immunization. *MMWR.* 2006 Dec 1;55(RR–15):1–48.

3. Federation Dentaire Internationale, Commission on Dental Practice. Technical report: recommendations for hygiene in dental practice. *Int Dent J.* 1979 Mar;29(1):72–9.

4. United States Centers for Disease Control. Guidelines for preventing the transmission of *mycobacterium tuberculosis* in health-care facilities. *MMWR.* 1994 Oct 28;43(RR–13):1–132.

5. Micik RE, Miller RL, Leong AC. Studies on dental aerobiology: III. Efficacy of surgical masks in protecting dental personnel from airborne bacterial particles. *J Dent Res.* 1971 May–Jun;50(3):626–30.

6. Miller RL, Micik RE. Air pollution and its control in the dental office. *Dent Clin North Am.* 1978 Jul;22(3):453–76.

7. Cooley RL, Cottingham AJ, Abrams H, Barkmeier WW. Ocular injuries sustained in the dental office: methods of detection, treatment, and prevention. *J Am Dent Assoc.* 1978 Dec;97(6):985–8.

8. Wesson MD, Thornton JB. Eye protection and ocular complications in the dental office. *Gen Dent.* 1989 Jan–Feb;37:19.

9. Roberts-Harry TJ, Cass AE, Jagger JD. Ocular injury and infection in dental practice: a survey and a review of the literature. *Br Dent J.* 1991 Jan 5;170(1):20–2.

10. Allen AL, Organ RJ. Occult blood accumulation under the fingernails: a mechanism for the spread of blood-borne infection. *J Am Dent Assoc.* 1982 Sep;105(3):455–9.

11. United States Department of Health and Human Services, Centers for Disease Control and Prevention Guidelines for infection control in dental health-care settings–2003. *MMWR.* 2003 Dec 19;52(RR–17):15.

12. Falcone KJ, Powers DO. Latex allergy: implications for oral health care professionals. *J Dent Hyg.* 1998 Summer;72(3):25–32.

Infection Control: Clinical Procedures

ESTHER M. WILKINS, BS, RDH, DMD

Chapter Outline

INFECTION CONTROL

The success of a planned system for control of disease transmission depends on the cooperative effort of each member of the dental health team. The aim is to provide the highest level of infection control possible and practical that will ensure a safe environment for both patients and the clinical team.

The presence of specific disease-producing organisms is rarely known; therefore, application of protective, preventive procedures is needed before, during, and following *all* patient appointments. Definitions and abbreviations related to infection control are provided in **Box 6-1**.

BOX 6-1 **Key Words**

Key Words and Abbreviations: Infection Control

ADA: American Dental Association, 211 E. Chicago Ave., Chicago, IL 60611.

Antimicrobial agent: any agent that kills or suppresses the growth of microorganisms.

Antiseptic: a substance that prevents or arrests the growth or action of microorganisms either by inhibiting their activity or by destroying them; term used especially for preparations applied topically to living tissue.

Asepsis: free from contamination with microorganisms; includes sterile conditions in tissues and on materials, as obtained by exclusion, removing, or killing organisms.

Aseptic technique: procedures carried out in the absence of pathogenic microorganisms.

Bioburden: a microbiologic load, that is, the number of contaminating organisms present on a surface before sterilization or disinfection.

Biofilm: the surface film that contains microorganisms and other biologic substances.

Biohazard: a substance that poses a biologic risk because it is contaminated with biomaterial that has a potential for transmitting infection.

Biologic indicator: a preparation of nonpathogenic microorganisms, usually bacterial spores, carried by an ampule or a specially impregnated paper enclosed within a package during sterilization and subsequently incubated to verify that sterilization has occurred.

Broad spectrum: indicates a range of activity of a drug or chemical substance against a wide variety of microorganisms.

Chain of asepsis: a procedure that avoids transfer of infection. The "chain" implies that each step, related to the previous one, continues to be carried out without contamination.

Chemical indicator: a color change stripe or other mark, often on autoclave tape or bag, used to monitor the process of sterilization; color change indicates that the package has been brought to a specific temperature, but color change is not an indicator of sterilization.

Contamination: introduction of microorganisms, blood, or other potentially infectious material or agent onto a surface or into tissue.

Decontamination: disinfection; use of physical or chemical means to remove, inactivate, or destroy pathogenic microorganisms on a surface or item to the extent that they are no longer capable of transmitting infectious disease; the surface or item is rendered safe for handling, use, or disposal.

Disinfectant: an agent, usually a chemical, but may be a physical agent, such as x-rays or ultraviolet light, that destroys microorganisms but may not kill bacterial spores; refers to substances applied to inanimate objects.

EPA: United States Environmental Protection Agency, Washington, DC.

EPA registered: number on a label indicates that the product has the acceptance of EPA.

FDA: United States Food and Drug Administration, 5600 Fishers Lane, Rockville, MD 20857; regulates food, drugs, biologic products, medical devices, radiologic products.

Infection control: the selection and use of procedures and products to prevent the spread of infectious disease.

Infectious waste: contaminated with blood, saliva, or other substances; potentially or actually infected with pathogenic material; officially called "regulated" waste.

Invasive procedure: entry into tissues during which bleeding occurs or the potential for bleeding exists.

Healthcare-associated infection: an infection associated with or acquired during a medical or surgical intervention; replaces **nosocomial**, which is limited to an adverse infectious outcome occurring in a hospital.

OSAP: Organization for Safety and Asepsis Procedures Research Foundation, P.O. Box 6297, Annapolis, MD 21401.

OSHA: United States Occupational Safety and Health Administration, Department of Labor, Washington, DC 20210.

PEP: postexposure prophylaxis.

PPE: personal protective equipment.

Sanitation: the process by which the number of organisms on inanimate objects is reduced to a safe level. It does not imply freedom from microorganisms and generally refers to a cleaning process.

Shelf life: stability of an item after it has been prepared; length of time a substance or preparation can be kept without changes occurring in its chemical structure or other properties.

Sporicide: substance that kills spores.

Sterilization: process by which all forms of life, including bacterial spores, are destroyed by physical or chemical means.

Synergism: the joint action of agents so that their combined effect is greater than the sum of their individual parts.

Waste:

Contaminated waste: items that have contacted blood or other body secretions.

Hazardous waste: poses a risk to humans or the environment.

Infectious waste: capable of causing an infectious disease.

Regulated waste: liquid blood or saliva, sharps contaminated with blood or saliva, and nonsharp solid waste saturated with or caked with liquid or semisolid blood or saliva or tissue including teeth (OSHA).

Toxic waste: capable of having a poisonous effect.

I. OBJECTIVES

The following are necessary to prevent the transmission of infectious agents and eliminate cross-contamination:

- Reduction of available pathogenic microorganisms to a level at which the normal resistance mechanisms of the body may prevent infection.
- Elimination of cross-contamination by breaking the chain of infection (Figure 4-1, page 42).
- Application of standard precautions by treating each patient as if all human blood and body fluids are known to be infectious for HIV, HBV, HCV, and other bloodborne pathogens.

II. BASIC CONSIDERATIONS FOR SAFE PRACTICE

Basic factors involved in the conduct of safe practice include the following, to be described in this chapter:

- Treatment room features
- Instrument management
- Preparation for appointment
- Unit water lines
- Environmental surfaces
- Care of sterile instruments
- Patient preparation
- Summary of procedures for the prevention of disease transmission
- Disposal of waste

TREATMENT ROOM FEATURES

- The design of many treatment rooms may not be conducive to ideal planning for infection control.
- Changes can be made in routines so that updated, preferred systems can be adapted.
- When renovations or a new dental office or clinic are anticipated, plans can reflect the most advanced knowledge available relative to safety and disease control.
- A partial list of notable features is included here and illustrated in **Figure 6-1**. The objective is to have materials, shapes, and surface textures that facilitate the effective use of infection control measures.

A. Unit

- Designed for easy cleaning and disinfection, with smooth, uncluttered surfaces.
- Removable hoses that can be cleaned, disinfected, and covered.
- Syringes with autoclavable tips or fitted with disposable tips.
- Handpieces with antiretraction valves that can be autoclaved.
- Use of barrier covers where possible.

B. Dental Chair

- Foot-operated controls.
- Surface and seamless finish of easily cleaned plastic material that withstands chemical disinfection without damage or discoloring; cloth upholstery to be avoided.

C. Light

- Removable handle for sterilization or disposable barrier cover.

D. Clinician's Chair

- Smooth, plastic seat cover that is easily disinfected and has a minimum of seams and creases.
- Set (before gloving) at correct height for individual clinician.

E. Floor

- No cloth carpeting.
- Smooth floor covering, easily cleaned, nonabsorbent.

F. Sink

- Smooth material (stainless steel).
- Wide and deep enough for effective handwashing without splashing.
- Automatic water faucets and soap dispensers with electronic, "hand," "knee," or foot-operated controls.
- Separate room or area for contaminated instrument care.

G. Supplies

- All sterilizable or disposable.

H. Waste

- Receptacle with opening large enough to prevent contact with sides when material is dropped in; heavy-duty plastic bag liner to be sealed tightly for disposal.
- Separate sharps disposal.
- Small biohazard receptacle near treatment area to receive contaminated sponges and other waste, for disposal in large waste container clearly marked for contaminated waste.

 INSTRUMENT PROCESSING CENTER

The processing center for care, cleaning, packaging, sterilizing, and storing instruments is located definitely apart from the treatment rooms.

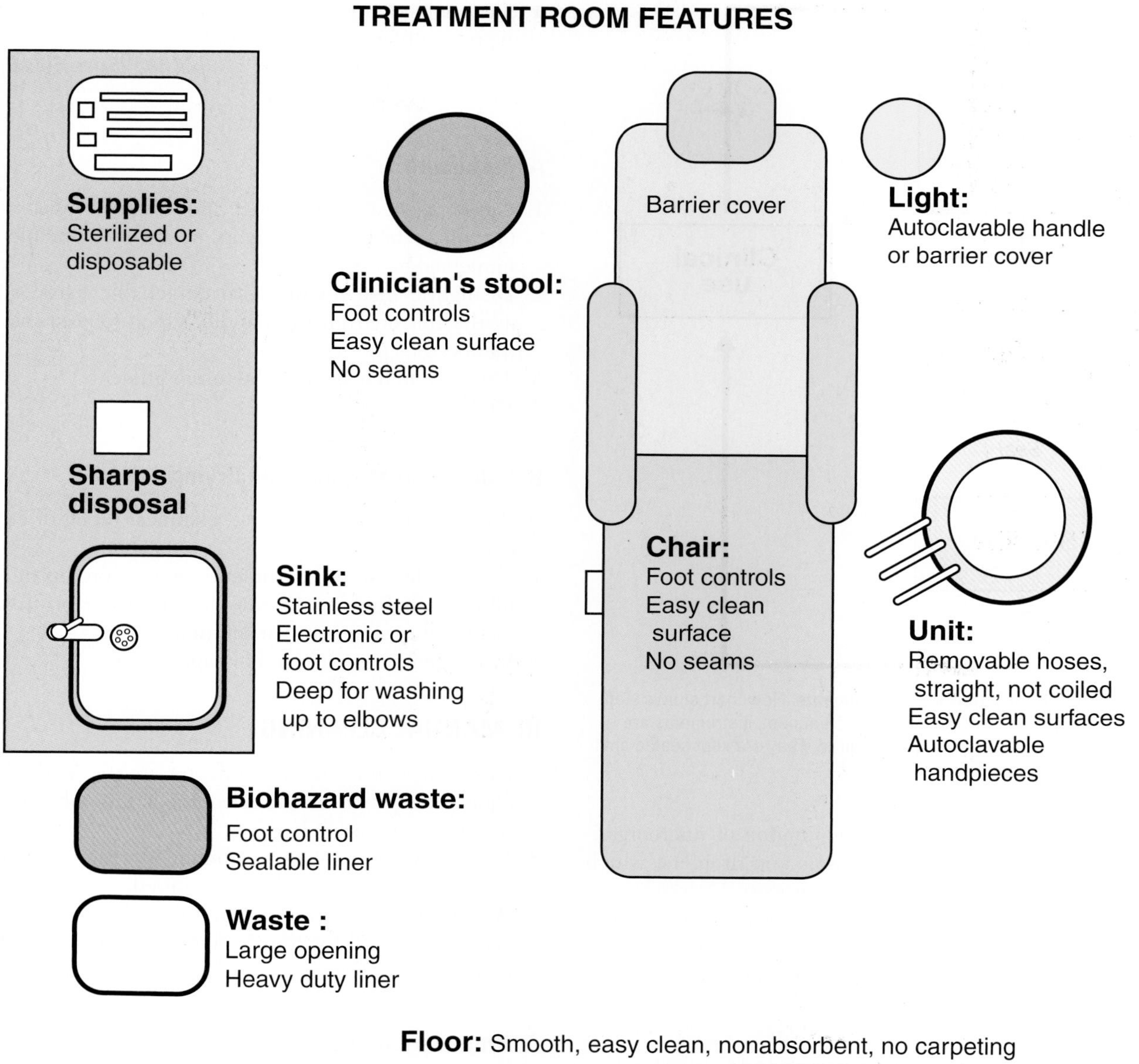

TREATMENT ROOM FEATURES

Supplies:
Sterilized or
disposable

**Sharps
disposal**

Clinician's stool:
Foot controls
Easy clean surface
No seams

Barrier cover

Light:
Autoclavable handle
or barrier cover

Sink:
Stainless steel
Electronic or
 foot controls
Deep for washing
 up to elbows

Chair:
Foot controls
Easy clean
 surface
No seams

Unit:
Removable hoses,
 straight, not coiled
Easy clean surfaces
Autoclavable
 handpieces

Biohazard waste:
Foot control
Sealable liner

Waste :
Large opening
Heavy duty liner

Floor: Smooth, easy clean, nonabsorbent, no carpeting

FIGURE 6-1 **Optimal Treatment Room Features.**

- The successful practice of standard precautions to prevent cross-contamination depends on the development of, and strict adherence to, a planned program for instrument management.
- A good rule is to learn the most effective, safe system and then to follow that method without exception.
- A specific routine is easier for the entire dental team to follow, and peer review is in-built.
- The basic steps in the recirculation of instruments from the time an appointment procedure is completed until the instruments are sterilized and ready for use in a continuing clinical appointment are shown in the flowchart in **Figure 6-2**. Each of the steps is described in the following sections.

CLEANING PROCEDURES[1]

The three basic methods for precleaning instruments before sterilization are using washer/thermal disinfector, ultrasonic processing, or manual scrubbing. Benefits from the use of washer/thermal disinfector and ultrasonic cleaning over manual scrubbing include the following:

- Increased efficiency in obtaining a high degree of cleanliness.
- Reduced danger to clinician from direct contact with potentially pathogenic microorganisms.
- Improved effectiveness for disinfection.

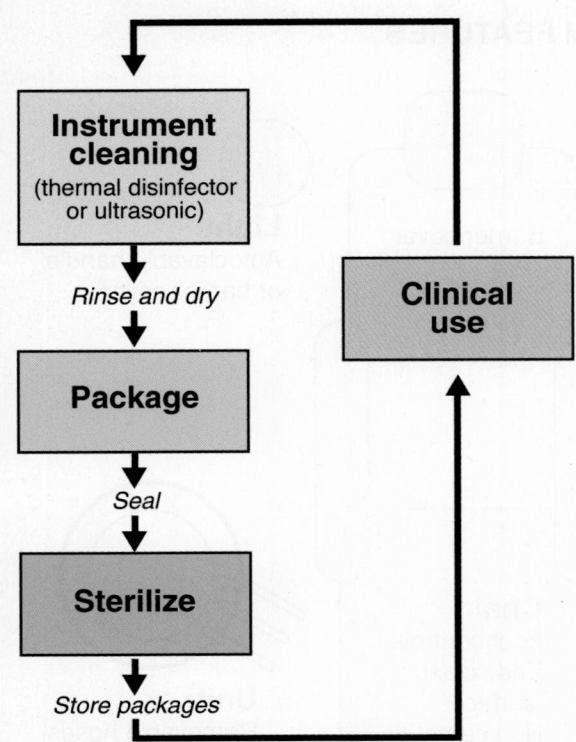

FIGURE 6-2 **Recirculation of Instruments.** Flowchart shows step-by-step process. At the completion of treatment, instruments are cleaned, packaged, sterilized, and stored. They are kept sealed until patient appointment begins.

■ Elimination of possible dissemination of microorganisms through release of aerosols and droplets, which can occur during the scrubbing process.
■ Penetration into areas of the instruments where the bristles of a brush may be unable to contact.
■ Ideally the instruments are contained within a cassette so that little or no handling is required.

I. INSTRUMENT WASHER/THERMAL DISINFECTOR

■ The *instrument washer* uses high-velocity hot water and a detergent to clean instruments. Some models are equipped to dry the instruments. Household dishwashers are different, and not appropriate for dental instruments.
■ The *instrument washer/thermal disinfector* differs from the plain washer by having a higher degree of temperature, so that it disinfects as well as cleans the instruments.
■ Disinfection means that the instruments in cassettes can be handled while packaging.

II. ULTRASONIC PROCESSING

■ Ultrasonic cleaning before sterilization is safer than manual cleaning. Manual cleaning of instruments is a dangerous, difficult, and time-consuming procedure.

■ Ultrasonic equipment is maintained and used according to manufacturer's guidelines.
■ *Ultrasonic processing is not a substitute for sterilization; it is only a cleaning process.*

A. Procedure

1. Guard against overloading; the solution must contact all surfaces. Instruments need to be completely immersed.
2. Dismantle instruments with detachable parts, such as the mirror from the handle. Open jointed instruments.
3. Time accurately by manufacturer's guide.
4. Drain, rinse, and air-dry.

B. Indications for Thorough Drying

■ When sterilizing by dry heat, chemical vapor, or ethylene oxide.
■ Nonstainless steel instruments require predip in rust inhibitor before steam autoclaving; water on instruments dilutes the antirust solution.
■ Instruments are packaged in paper wrap.

III. MANUAL CLEANING

■ Ultrasonics and washer-disinfector are the methods of choice, but when manual cleaning is the only alternative, precautions are heeded.
■ Ideally the instruments are contained within a cassette so that little or no handling is required.
■ When instruments are not in a cassette, transfer forceps are needed for transferring contaminated instruments.

A. Procedure for Manual Scrubbing

1. Wear heavy-duty gloves, protective eyewear, and mask.
2. Dismantle instruments with detachable parts. Open jointed instruments.
3. Use detergent and scrub with a long-handled brush under running water; hold the instruments low in the sink. Scrubbing one instrument at a time minimizes risk of puncture injury.
4. Brush with strokes away from the body; use care not to splash and contaminate the surrounding area.
5. Rinse thoroughly.
6. Dry on paper towels (same reasons as those listed for ultrasonic processing).

B. Care of Brushes

1. Color code brushes to distinguish from handwash brushes.
2. Soak and wash contaminated brushes in detergent; rinse thoroughly and sterilize.

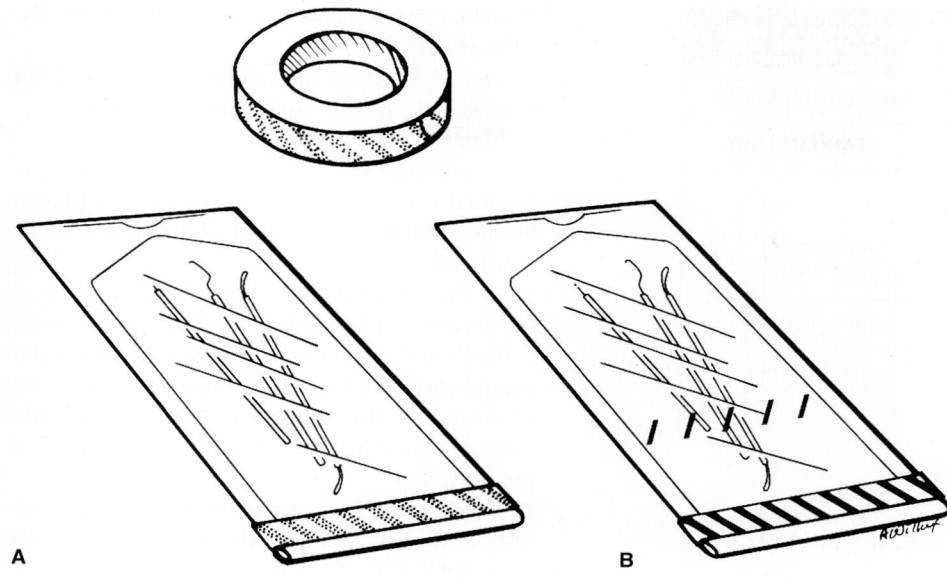

FIGURE 6-3 **Process Indicator Tape (A) Before autoclaving. (B) After autoclaving.** The change of color in the stripes indicates that the package has been subjected to the proper temperature for sterilization but does not show sterilization. A biologic indicator is also needed for periodic monitoring to determine that the autoclave is functioning properly and that sterilization is actually taking place.

A

B

PACKAGING STEP

I. PURPOSES

A. To prevent contamination of newly sterilized instruments as soon as they are removed from the sterilizer.
B. To provide a means of storing instruments to keep them in sets for individual appointment use and sterilized and ready for immediate use on opening.

II. INSTRUMENT ARRANGEMENT

A. Preset cassettes or packages can be preplanned to contain all the items usually needed for a particular appointment.
B. Each package is dated and marked for identification of contents: for examples, *Adult Scaling and Root Planing; Examination.*
C. Clear packages with self-seal permit instrument identification without special labeling. **Figure 6-3** shows clear, "see-through" packages for easy identification of package contents.

III. PREPARATION

A. Materials

- Each method of sterilization has specific requirements, and the manufacturers' recommendations are followed.
- Sturdy wrapping is necessary to prevent punctures or tears that break the chain of asepsis and require a repeat of the process.
- The wrap permits the steam or chemical vapor to pass through the contents.

B. Seal

- Indicator tape is used. Pins, paper clips, or other types of metal fasteners are not used because they provide holes for the entry of microorganisms.
- Chemical indicator tape is used to seal all packages, except when the wrap has built-in indicators. The chemical, usually in the form of a series of stripes, changes color during the sterilization process **(Figure 6-3)**.
- The change of color means that the autoclave reached a designated temperature required for penetration but does not designate sterilization.
- Distinct black stripes will appear. A lighter color change may be a warning signal that the autoclave function needs to be checked.
- The striped indicator tape is left on the sealed package and thereby serves to identify those packages ready for use. Packages are kept completely sealed until unwrapped in front of the patient.

STERILIZATION

I. APPROVED METHODS

Each of the methods listed here is described in the sections following. **Table 6-1** summarizes the operating requirements of each.

A. Steam under pressure (autoclave)
B. Dry heat
C. Chemical vapor

II. SELECTION OF METHOD

- All materials and items cannot be treated by the same system of sterilization.

TABLE 6-1	METHODS FOR STERILIZATION	
METHOD	**STERILIZING REQUIREMENT**	
	TIME	**TEMPERATURE**
Steam under pressure (autoclave) 1) Gravity displacement 2) Prevacuum	15–30 min 3.5–10 min	250°F (121°C) 270°F (132°C)
Dry heat oven	120 min	320°F (160°C)
Unsaturated chemical vapor	20 min	270°F (132°C)

- Supplement with disposable single-use products when sterilization is not possible.
- The method for sterilization selected provides complete destruction of all microorganisms, viruses, and spores and yet must not damage the instruments and other materials.
- Procedures cannot be overly complex, or many errors in processing may occur.
- Careful, specific use of sterilizing equipment in accord with the manufacturer's specifications is necessary.
- Incomplete sterilization frequently results from inadequate preparation of the materials to be sterilized (cleaning, packaging), misuse of the equipment (overloading, timing, temperature selection), or inadequate maintenance.

III. TESTS FOR STERILIZATION

Sterilization is the process by which all forms of life are destroyed. That definition provides the rationale for testing whether a sterilizer is working properly. Three tests are used: an external and an internal chemical indicator and a biologic monitor.

- **External Chemical Indicator:** to seal the package and change color to show the autoclave temperature has been reached (**Figure 6-3**).
- **Internal Chemical Indicator:** color change assesses instrument exposure to temperature and steam for the required time.
- **Biologic Monitor:** tests that the autoclave is functioning properly.
  A. The testing system requires the use of selected test microorganisms that are put through a regular cycle of sterilization and then are cultured. When no growth occurs, the sterilizer has performed with maximum efficiency.
  B. *Microorganisms Used*
     1. Steam Autoclave: *Geobacillus stearothermophilus* (formerly *Bacillus stearothermophilus*) vials, ampules, or strips.

2. Dry Heat Oven: *Bacillus atrophaeus* (formerly *Bacillus subtilis*) strips.
3. Chemical Vapor: *Geobacillus/stearothermophilus* (formerly *Bacillus stearothermophilus*) strips.

C. *Procedures*
  1. The ampule, vial, or strip is placed in the center of a package, which in turn is placed in the middle of the load of packages to be sterilized.
  2. After the cycle has been completed at the customary time and temperature, the ampule or strip is incubated. Ampules and vials show the color change associated with no living microorganisms, whereas the strip organisms are cultured and show no growth if the sterilizer has performed properly.
  3. **Table 6-2** shows indications for performing spore tests in dental settings. Records that are kept show dates and outcomes.

D. *Frequency*
  1. At least weekly testing is recommended; more often when heavy autoclave use.
  2. Equipment can be obtained for performing the testing, or commercial mail-in services are available.

TABLE 6.2	SPORE TESTING
WHEN	**WHY**
Once per week	To verify proper use and functioning
Whenever a new type of packaging material or tray is used	To ensure that the sterilizing agent is getting inside to the surface of the instruments
After training of new sterilization personnel	To verify proper use of the sterilizer
During initial uses of a new sterilizer	To make sure unfamiliar operating instructions are being followed
First run after repair of a sterilizer	To make sure that the sterilizer is functioning properly
With every implantable device and hold device until results of test are known	Extra precaution for sterilization of item to be implanted into tissues
After any other change in the sterilizing procedure	To make sure change does not prevent sterilization

Source: Adapted with permission from Miller CH, Palenik CJ. Sterilization, disinfection, and asepsis in dentistry. In: Block SS. Disinfection, sterilization, and preservation. 4th ed. Philadelphia: Lea & Febiger; 1991. p. 680.

MOIST HEAT: STEAM UNDER PRESSURE

Destruction of microorganisms by heat takes place because of inactivation of essential cellular proteins or enzymes. Moist heat causes coagulation of protein.

I. AUTOCLAVE TYPES

- *Gravity Displacement*: Self-generation of steam forces out the air; steam enters to penetrate through the cassettes or packages
- *High-Speed Prevacuum*: pump removes the air from the chamber and allows faster penetration of the steam for sterilizing.
- A time/temperature comparison of the two autoclave systems is provided in **Table 6-1**.

II. USE

- Moist heat may be used for all materials except oils, waxes, and powders that are impervious to steam or for materials that cannot be subjected to high temperatures.

III. PRINCIPLES OF ACTION

- Sterilization is achieved by action of heat; pressure serves only to attain high temperature.
- Sterilization depends on the penetrating ability of steam.
- Air must be excluded, otherwise steam penetration and heat transfer are prevented.
- Space between objects is essential to ensure access for the steam.
- Materials must be thoroughly cleaned and air-dried; adherent material can provide a barrier to the steam.
- Air discharge occurs in a downward direction; load must be arranged for free passage of steam toward bottom of autoclave.

IV. EVALUATION OF STEAM UNDER PRESSURE

A. Advantages

- All microorganisms, spores, and viruses are destroyed quickly and efficiently.
- Wide variety of materials may be treated; most economical method of sterilization.

B. Disadvantages

- May corrode carbon steel instruments if precautions are not taken.
- Unsuitable for oils or powders that are impervious to heat.

DRY HEAT

The action of dry heat is oxidation.

I. USE

- Primarily for materials that cannot safely be sterilized with steam under pressure.
- For oils and powders when they are thermostabile at the required temperatures.
- For small metal instruments enclosed in special containers or that might be corroded or rusted by moisture.

II. PRINCIPLES OF ACTION

- Sterilization is achieved by heat that is conducted from the exterior surface to the interior of the object; the time required to penetrate varies among materials.
- Sterilization can result when the whole material is treated for a sufficient length of time at the required temperature; therefore, timing for sterilization must start when the entire contents of the sterilizer have reached the peak temperature needed for that load.
- Oil, grease, or organic debris on instruments insulates and protects microorganisms from the sterilizing effect.

III. OPERATION

A. Temperature

A temperature of 160°C (320°F) maintained for 2 hours; 170°C (340°F) for 1 hour. Timing starts after the desired temperature has been reached.

B. Penetration Time

Heat penetration varies with different materials, and the nature and properties of various materials is considered.

C. Care

Care is taken not to overheat because certain materials can be affected. Temperatures over 160°C (320°F) may destroy the sharp edges of cutting instruments.

IV. EVALUATION OF DRY HEAT

A. Advantages

- Useful for materials that cannot be subjected to steam under pressure.
- When maintained at correct temperature, this method is well suited for sharp instruments.
- No corrosion compared with steam under pressure.

B. Disadvantages

- Long exposure time required; penetration slow and uneven.
- High temperature critical to certain materials.

CHEMICAL VAPOR STERILIZER

The unsaturated chemical vapor sterilizer is also called the Chemiclave or Harvey sterilizer.

A combination of alcohols, formaldehyde, ketone, water, and acetone heated under pressure produces a gas that is effective as a sterilizing agent.

I. USE

Chemical vapor sterilization cannot be used for materials or objects that can be altered by the chemicals that make the vapor or that cannot withstand the high temperature. Examples are low-melting plastics, liquids, or heat-sensitive handpieces.

II. PRINCIPLES OF ACTION

Microbial and viral destruction results from the permeation of the heated formaldehyde and alcohol. Heavy, tightly wrapped, or sealed packages would not permit the penetration of the vapors.

III. OPERATION

A. Temperature

From 132°C (270°F) with 20–40 pounds pressure in accord with the manufacturer's directions.

B. Time

Minimum of 20 minutes after the correct temperature and pressure have been attained. Time is extended for a large load or a heavy wrap.

C. Cooling at the Completion of the Cycle

Instruments are dry. Instruments need a short period for cooling.

IV. CARE OF STERILIZER

Depending on the amount of use, refilling is needed by at least every 30 cycles. In accord with manufacturer's instructions, the condensate tray is removed, the exhausted solution emptied, and the tray cleaned.

V. EVALUATION OF CHEMICAL VAPOR STERILIZER

A. Advantages

- Corrosion- and rust-free operation for carbon steel instruments.
- Ability to sterilize in a relatively short total cycle.
- Ease of operation and care of the equipment.

B. Disadvantages

- Adequate ventilation is needed; cannot use in a small room.
- Slight odor, which is rarely objectionable.

CARE OF STERILE INSTRUMENTS

- Instruments stored without sealed wrappers are only momentarily sterile because of airborne contamination.
- Labeled, sterilized, and sealed packages are stored unopened in clean, dry cabinets or drawers. Paper-wrapped packages are handled carefully to prevent tearing. All stored packages are dated and used in rotation.
- Packages wrapped and sealed in paper may not need resterilizing for several months to 1 year.
- Plastic or nylon wrap with a tape or heat seal may be expected to remain sterile longer.
- The expected shelf life before resterilizing depends on the area surrounding the stored packages. A closed, protected area without exposure, such as a cabinet or drawer that can be disinfected routinely, is preferred.

CHEMICAL DISINFECTANTS

Chemical disinfectants are used in several forms, including as surface disinfectants, immersion disinfectants, immersion sterilants, and hand antimicrobials. Each variety has specific chemicals, dilutions, and directions for application.

I. CATEGORIES

Disinfectants are categorized by their biocidal activity as high level, intermediate level, or low level. Biocidal activity refers to the ability of the chemical disinfectant to destroy or inactivate living organisms.

A. High Level

High-level disinfectants inactivate spores and all forms of bacteria, fungi, and viruses. Applied at different time schedules, the high-level chemical is either a disinfectant or a sterilant.

B. Intermediate Level

Intermediate-level disinfectants inactivate all forms of microorganisms but do not destroy spores.

C. Low Level

Low-level disinfectants inactivate vegetative bacteria and certain lipid-type viruses but do not destroy spores, tubercle bacilli, or nonlipid viruses.

II. USES

A. Environmental Surfaces Disinfection

Following each appointment, the treatment area is cleaned and disinfected.

B. Dental Laboratory Impressions and Prostheses

Impressions can be carriers of infectious material to a dental laboratory. Completed prostheses must be disinfected before delivery to a patient.

III. PRINCIPLES OF ACTION

- Disinfection is achieved by coagulation, precipitation, or oxidation of protein of microbial cells or denaturation of the enzymes of the cells.
- Disinfection depends on the contact of the solution at the known effective concentration for the optimum period of time.
- Items are thoroughly cleaned and dried because action of the agent is altered by foreign matter and dilution.
- A solution has a specific shelf life, use life, and reuse life. Some may be altered by changes in pH, or the active ingredient may decrease in potency. Check manufacturer's directions.

IV. CRITERIA FOR SELECTION OF A CHEMICAL AGENT

The objective is to select a product that is effective in the control of microorganisms and practical to use. Properties of an ideal disinfectant are shown in **Box 6-2**.

- EPA approval.
  - Use EPA-registered hospital disinfectant for low-level requirements.
  - Use EPA-registered hospital disinfectant with a tuberculocidal claim for intermediate and high especially when there is visible blood or other potentially infectious material.
- Manufacturer's informational literature and container labels
  - Provide facts about the product that ensure its effectiveness.
  - When the label has insufficient information, the manufacturer is contacted and instructions are obtained.
  - The criteria include at least the following: must be tuberculocidal, bacteriocidal, virucidal, and fungicidal.
  - Label must state:
    1. Effectiveness and stability expressed by
       a. *Shelf life*: the expiration date indicating the termination of effectiveness of the unopened container.
       b. *Use life*: the life expectancy for the solution once it has been activated but not actually put to use with contaminated items.

BOX 6-2	Properties of an Ideal Disinfectant

1. Broad spectrum:
   Has the widest possible antimicrobial spectrum.
2. Fast acting:
   Needs a rapidly lethal action on all vegetative forms and spores of bacteria and fungi, protozoa, and viruses.
3. Not affected by physical factors:
   Active in the presence of organic matter, such as blood, sputum, and feces.
   Be compatible with soaps, detergents, and other chemicals encountered in use.
4. Nontoxic
5. Surface compatibility:
   Not corrode instruments and other metallic surfaces.
   Not cause the disintegration of cloth, rubber, plastics, or other materials.
6. Residual effect on treated surfaces
7. Easy to use
8. Odorless:
   An inoffensive odor would facilitate its routine use.
9. Economical:
   Cost not prohibitively high.

Source: Molinari JA, Harte JA. Cottone's practical infection control in dentistry. 3rd ed. Philadelphia: Lippincott Williams & Wilkins, 2009. Chapter 12, Environmental surface infection control: disposable barriers and chemical disinfection; p. 173.

c. *Reuse life*: the amount of time a solution can be used and reused while being challenged with instruments that are wet or coated with bioburden.
2. Directions for activation (mixing proportions).
3. Type of container for storage and place (conditions such as heat and light).
4. Directions for use
   a. Precleaning and drying of items to be submerged.
   b. Time/temperature ratio.
5. Instructions for disposal of used solution.
6. Warnings
   a. Toxic effects (on eyes, skin).
   b. Specific directions for emergency care in the event of an accident (e.g., splash in eye).
   c. Keep manufacturer's *Materials Safety Data Sheets* for reference.

- After the product has been selected, it is the responsibility of the dental personnel to use it as directed to obtain the best possible infection control.

PREPARATION OF THE TREATMENT ROOM

- The cleanliness and neatness of the treatment room reflect the character and conscientiousness of the dental personnel.
- The patient, with limited knowledge of dental science, may judge the ability of the dental personnel by the appearance of the office or clinic.
- Other patients may inquire about sterilization and infection control.
- The patient's attitude is important, but more important is the relationship of cleanliness to the presence of microorganisms. The need is to provide clinical services in an environment that minimizes cross-contamination.
- The orderliness and immaculate cleanliness of the treatment rooms result from continuing care. An excellent test for the effects of care and any minor oversights is for each dental team member to sit in the dental chair occasionally and look around at what the patient sees from that vantage point.

I. OBJECTIVES

Effective care of instruments and equipment contributes to the following:

- Control of disease transmitted by way of environmental surfaces.
- An increase in the working efficiency of the office personnel.
- An atmosphere of cleanliness and orderliness that contributes to the patient's and the clinician's well-being.
- An increase in the patient's confidence in the ability of the dental personnel.

- The maintenance of the working efficiency of office equipment and instruments.
  A. To prolong their span of usefulness.
  B. To contribute to patient safety.
- A decrease in the occurrence of unpleasant odors in the office.

II. PRELIMINARY PLANNING

Preparation of the treatment room when time between appointments is limited requires an efficient procedural system. The classification of inanimate objects (**Table 6-3**) provides a guide for analysis.

First, all surfaces and items that will be used or contacted during the appointment can be categorized and listed as critical, semicritical, or noncritical. The most logical and scientific sequence for preparation for the appointment can then be outlined.

A. Hand "Touch Contacts"

Only contacts essential to the service to be performed are made. Planning ahead to have materials ready so that cabinet knobs or drawer handles do not have to be contacted is an example.

B. Sterilizable Items

Critical and semicritical items are sterilized or are disposable.

C. Disposable Items

Disposable items are used wherever possible.

TABLE 6-3	CLASSIFICATION OF INANIMATE OBJECTS		
SURFACE CATEGORY	**DEFINITION**	**STERILIZATION/DISINFECTION**	**EXAMPLES**
Critical	Penetrate soft tissue or bone	Sterilize or disposable	Needles Curets Explorers Probes
Semicritical	Touch intact mucous membrane, oral fluids Does not penetrate	Sterilize after each use High-level disinfection when sterilization cannot be used	Radiographic biteblock Ultrasonic handpiece Amalgam condenser Mirror
Noncritical	Do not touch mucous membranes (only contact unbroken epithelium)	Cleaning and tuberculocidal intermediate-level disinfection	Light handles Certain x-ray machine parts Safety eyewear
Environmental	No contact with patient surfaces (or only intact skin)	Cleaning and intermediate to low disinfection	Counter tops Equipment surfaces Housekeeping surface

D. Items That May Be Covered

Barrier coverings prevent contamination from reaching surfaces. Covers for light handles, counter tops, x-ray machine parts, and water faucets are examples. Care is taken when removing the covers not to contaminate the object beneath.

E. Items That Require Chemical Disinfection

Objects and surfaces that cannot be included in one of the preceding categories are treated with a chemical disinfectant. If the material is not compatible with the chemical action of the disinfectant, a substitute item, which is either disposable or coverable, will be needed.

III. CLEAN AND DISINFECT ENVIRONMENTAL SURFACES

A. Agent

- The effectiveness of the disinfection procedure is the result of two actions:
  A. The physical rubbing and removal of contaminated material.
  B. The chemical inactivation of the living microorganisms.
- Do not store gauze sponges in the solution. Use a spray bottle to dispense the disinfectant.

B. Procedure

1. Wear heavy-duty household gloves and mask.
2. Use several large gauze sponges or paper towels. The use of small sponges wastes time. A disinfectant soaked sponge in each hand can decrease the time of cleaning certain objects. Contaminated objects, such as tubings, can be held with one sponge while scrubbing with the other sponge.
3. Spraying of a disinfectant must be followed by vigorous scrubbing for cleaning. When applied only by spray without scrubbing, the agent does not penetrate or remove the film of microorganisms.
4. Scrub the disinfectant over the entire surface, with attention to irregularities where contaminated material can aggregate.
5. Spray and leave the surfaces wet.

IV. UNIT WATER LINES

- A biofilm of microorganisms can form on the inside of the water-line tubings during overnight standing.
- Tests have been conducted on tubings to handpieces, water syringes, and ultrasonic scalers. When the lines were flushed for 2 minutes, the microbial counts were reduced.[1]
- Contaminated water cannot be used for surgical purposes or during the irrigation of pocket areas because infective microorganisms can be introduced.

- If contaminated water is directed forcefully into a pocket, microorganisms can enter the tissue and infection or bacteremia can result.
- Procedure for clinical use:
  A. Flush all water lines at least 2 minutes at the beginning of each day.
  B. Run water through water tubing for 30 seconds before and 30 seconds after each patient appointment.
- Refer to Appendix IV (page 1096) for the recommendations from the U.S. Department of Health and Human Services.

PATIENT PREPARATION

- The use of preprocedural rinsing and toothbrushing has been shown to lower the numbers of oral bacteria and, therefore, to lower the numbers of infected aerosols created during instrumentation.
- Oral procedures that require penetration of tissues, such as giving anesthesia by injection or scaling subgingival pocket surfaces, can introduce bacteria into the tissues and hence into the bloodstream. Organisms injected into the tissue could multiply and create an abscess. Because of natural resistance, the body can handle and destroy invading microorganisms, provided the numbers can be kept to a minimum.
- Practical procedures for the preparation of a patient include preprocedural oral hygiene measures and rinsing with an antimicrobial mouthrinse. These contribute to the prevention of disease transmission.

I. PREPROCEDURAL ORAL HYGIENE MEASURES

A. Toothbrushing

- Toothbrushing disturbs and removes microorganisms. When a patient is being trained in dental biofilm control measures and needs supervision at each appointment, a double purpose can be accomplished.
- Demonstration of biofilm removal from the teeth, tongue, and gingiva contributes to lowering the microbial count before treatment procedures.

B. Rinsing

- The numbers of bacteria on the gingival or mucosal surfaces can be reduced by the use of a preprocedural antiseptic mouthrinse.[2]
- The substantivity of 0.12% chlorhexidine provides a lowered bacterial count for more than 60 minutes. Preprocedural rinsing before injections is advised.

II. APPLICATION OF A SURFACE ANTISEPTIC

A. Before Injection of Anesthetic[3]

■ As a needle is introduced into the mucosa for penetration to deeper tissues, microorganisms on the surface can be carried into the tissue.

■ An antiseptic applied before the injection can decrease the risk of introducing septic material into the soft tissue.

B. Before Scaling and Other Dental Hygiene Instrumentation[4]

■ *Instrumentation* in a sulcus or pocket and around the gingival margin can create breaks in the tissue where bacteria can enter.

■ Subgingival instrumentation in a pocket with broken down sulcular epithelium contributes to the entrance of bacteria into the underlying tissues and bacteremia.

■ *Procedure*. Dry the surface and swab the area before instrumentation. Use an antiseptic solution to irrigate the sulci and pockets carefully.

SUMMARY OF STANDARD PROCEDURES

Basic procedures for clinical management are listed here.

I. PATIENT FACTORS

■ Prepare a comprehensive patient history. Refer patients suspected of carrying infectious disease for medical evaluation.

■ Ask the patient to rinse with an antimicrobial mouthrinse to reduce the numbers of oral microorganisms.

■ Provide protective eyewear.

■ Avoid elective procedures for a patient who is suffering from a communicable condition, such as a respiratory infection, or who has an open lesion on or about the lips or oral tissues, for the benefit of all who would be subjected to exposure.

II. CLINIC PREPARATION

■ Run water through all water lines, including the air–water syringe, handpieces, and ultrasonic unit, for 2 minutes at the start of the day and for at least 30 seconds before and after each use during the day.

■ Disinfect all environmental surfaces that may be "touch surfaces" during the appointment. Make an orderly sequence for surface disinfection. Apply barrier covers as indicated.

■ Sterilize instruments and all other equipment that can be sterilized by one of the methods for complete sterilization. Maintain closed sterilized packages until ready for use.

III. FACTORS FOR THE DENTAL TEAM

■ Have medical examinations; keep immunizations up to date; have appropriate testing on a periodic basis.

■ Always use mask, protective eyewear, gloves, and a clean closed-front gown with fitted wrist cuffs.

■ Utilize thorough hand hygiene and cleansing before donning and after removal of gloves.

■ Develop habits that minimize contacts with switches and other parts of the dental unit, dental chair, light, and clinician's stool, and avoid all environmental contacts unrelated to the procedure at hand.

IV. TREATMENT FACTORS

A. Hypodermic Needles

■ Use a safe recapping method (Figure 37-6, page 571) to prevent accidental penetration or self-inoculation.

■ Place used needles into a puncture-resistant sharps container.

■ Dispose of all partially emptied carpules of anesthetics.

B. Removable Oral Prostheses

■ Routinely, gloves are worn to receive a septic prosthesis from a patient.

■ Place the prosthesis in a disposable cup and cover with a disinfectant. Use a fresh solution of 0.05% iodophor in water, or a 1:5 dilution of 5% sodium hypochlorite. Clean by ultrasonics.

■ When a lathe is used for cleaning the denture, wear goggles and a mask and use a sterile ragwheel and fresh pumice. Pumice is used only once and caught on a disposable paper liner in the dustbin and discarded.

V. POSTTREATMENT

■ Use heavy puncture-resistant gloves to handle used instruments.

■ Follow routines to disinfect, clean, and prepare the instruments for sterilization.

■ Contaminated waste is secured in plastic disposal bags.

■ Disinfect safety eyewear for patient and dental team members.

OCCUPATIONAL POST-EXPOSURE MANAGEMENT

Accidents happen even to the most skillful clinician. Accidental percutaneous (laceration, needle stick) or permucosal (splash to eye or mucosa) exposure to blood or other body fluids requires prompt action.

I. SIGNIFICANT EXPOSURES

- Percutaneous or permucosal stick or wound with needle or sharp instrument contaminated with blood, saliva, or other body fluids.
- Contamination of any obviously open wound, nonintact skin, or mucous membrane with blood, saliva, or a combination.
- Exposure of patient's body fluids to unbroken skin is not considered a significant exposure.

II. PROCEDURE FOLLOWING EXPOSURE

- Immediately wash the wound with soap and water; rinse well.
- Flush nose, mouth, eyes, or skin with clear water, saline, or a sterile irrigant.
- Report to designated official.
- Complete an incident report as required.
- Follow the required predetermined, posted procedures of the clinic, institution, or individual practice setting.

III. FOLLOW-UP

- Report signs and symptoms associated with HIV seroconversion.
- Obtain medical evaluation of any illness involving fever, rash, lymphadenopathy.
- Pursue counseling and further testing.

DISPOSAL OF WASTE

Types of waste are defined in **Box 6-1**. Each type of waste requires special handling.

I. REGULATIONS

- Investigate the regulations of each town or city sanitation division for rules concerning disposal of contaminated waste.

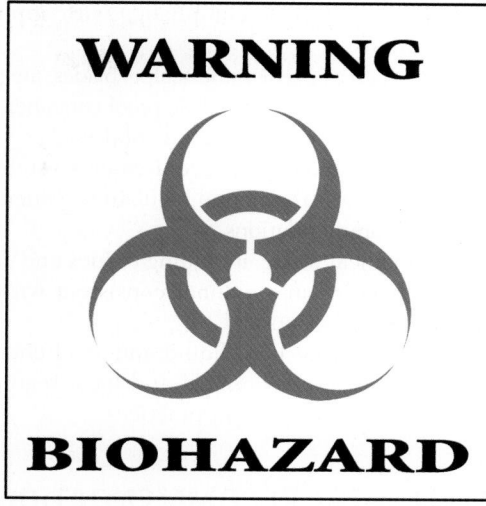

FIGURE 6-4 **Universal Label for Hazardous Material.** A hazard-warning label should be fluorescent orange or orange-red with lettering or a symbol in a contrasting color. The label must be attached to containers used to store or transport waste. A label is not required for regulated waste that has been decontaminated (such as dental waste that has been autoclaved).

- **Figure 6-4** illustrates the universal label required by the United States Occupational Safety and Health Administration (OSHA). The labels must be attached to containers used to store or transport hazardous waste materials.

II. GUIDELINES

- Disposable materials, such as gloves, masks, wipes, paper drapes, or surface covers, that are contaminated with blood or body fluids are carefully handled and discarded in sturdy, impervious plastic bags to minimize human contact.
- Blood, suctioned fluids, or other liquid waste may be carefully poured into a drain that is connected to a

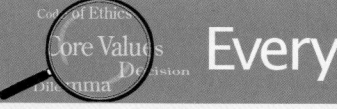 Everyday Ethics

Kimberly, the dental hygienist, is about to begin the patient examination when she notices that the indicator tape on the sterilizing cassette had not changed color. She excuses herself and finds out from the receptionist that a call to the repair service has been made because the autoclave has been shutting down before completion of the cycle. It is after 1:00 PM and patients are scheduled all afternoon.

Questions for Consideration
1. When proper sterile technique is not followed, what ethical principles and core values are involved? Describe Kimberly's duty to her patients.
2. Use the steps to decision making (page 10) to determine possible solutions for this situation. Describe how each could be defended to the patient, the dentist, and other dental team members.
3. Which ADHA professional roles (Box 1-2, page 5) does Kimberly serve in when she plans to make changes that ensure that this kind of situation does not happen again? Explain each role and how it applies for Kimberly.

sanitary sewer system in compliance with applicable local regulations.

- Sharp items, such as needles and scalpel blades, are placed intact into a puncture-resistant, leak-proof container.
- Human tissue and contaminated solid wastes can be disposed of according to the requirements established by local or state environmental regulatory agencies and published recommendations.
- Infectious medical waste, including tissues and culture media, are handled in a manner consistent with local regulations before disposal.
- Disposal methods for both liquid and solid chemicals vary with the type of chemical and local regulations governing waste-management practices.

SUPPLEMENTAL RECOMMENDATIONS

I. CLEANING THE FACE

- Check and clean the exposed parts of the face not covered by mask or protective eyewear, where spatter collects, as an aid to disease control as well as for general sanitation.
- In reality, cleaning the face several times each day and washing before eating is a logical procedure for personal hygiene and safety.

II. SMOKING AND EATING

Smoking and eating are banned in treatment areas.

III. RECEPTION AREA

- Select only toys and other reception area items that can be cleaned and disinfected.
- Provide hand sanitizer gel in the reception area.

IV. STERILIZATION MONITORING

- Keep a written record of dates when processing tests and biologic monitor tests are performed for each sterilizer.
- Indicate advance dates for the next testing clearly on a calendar or other reference point.
- Perform tests made weekly on the same day to simplify remembering.

V. OFFICE POLICY MANUAL

- Include in the clinic or office policy manual outlines of procedures to follow for standard precautions.
- Addresses for sources of various materials can be kept in a special reference section of the manual.
- Emergency procedures to follow when accidentally exposed are defined clearly.

DOCUMENTATION

Documentation for a patient with concerns about infection control procedures would include:

- Name, record number, address, telephone, email
- Medical history for history of hepatitis B, hepatitis C, or HIV; high-risk history associated with these diseases; patient consent to be tested for HBV, HCV, HIV
- HIV-positive patient: current medications and previously taken, if they were ineffective; most recent viral load, current CD4 if known
- A sample Progress Note for a patient with concerns about infection control procedures can be reviewed in **Box 6-3**.

BOX 6-3	Example Progress Note

Patient presents for routine maintenance appointment. Health history update indicates patient has been recently diagnosed as HIV positive. She was concerned about her increased risk for opportunistic infections as well as the fact that her condition might increase risk for other patients seen in the office. Explained that standard precautions and infection control procedures used during all patient treatment are designed to protect all patients from cross-contamination. Discussed importance of her oral health and need for ideal homecare. New appointments planned.

Signed: _____, RDH Date: _____

 **Factors To Teach The Patient**

- The meaning of "standard precautions" and what is included under the term; how these precautions protect the patient and the dental team members.
- The contribution of the accurately completed medical and dental personal history to the provision of the best, safest treatment possible.
- Methods for sterilization of instruments, including handpieces; how the autoclave or other sterilizer is tested daily or weekly.
- Facts about the normal oral flora and the factors that influence an increased number of bacteria on the tongue, mucosa, and in the dental biofilm on the teeth.
- Methods for personal daily control of the oral bacteria through biofilm control and tongue brushing.
- Reasons for preprocedural rinsing.
- Method for thorough rinsing.

References

1. Gross A, Devine MJ, Cutright DE. Microbial contamination of dental units and ultrasonic scalers. *J Periodontol.* 1976 Nov;47(11):670–3.
2. Veksler AE, Kayrouz GA, Newman MG. Reduction of salivary bacteria by pre-procedural rinses with chlorhexidine 0.12%. *J Periodontol.* 1991 Nov;62(11):649–51.
3. Connor JP, Edelson JG. Needle tract infection. A case report. *Oral Surg Oral Med Oral Pathol.* 1988 Apr;65(4):401–3.
4. Fine DH, Korik I, Furgang D, Myers R, Olshan A, Barnett ML, Vincent J. Assessing preprocedural subgingival irrigation and rinsing with an antiseptic mouthrinse to reduce bacteremia. *J Am Dent Assoc.* 1996 May;127(5):641–2.

7 CHAPTER

Patient Reception and Ergonomic Practice

ESTHER M. WILKINS, BS, RDH, DMD

Chapter Outline

The patient's presence in the office or clinic is an expression of confidence in the dentist and the dental hygienist. Confidence is inspired by the reputation for professional knowledge and skill, the appearance of the office, and the actions of the workers in it.

■ The physical arrangement and interpersonal relationships provide the setting for specific services to be performed.
■ The patient's well-being is the all-important consideration throughout the appointment.
■ At the same time, the clinician must function effectively and efficiently in a manner that minimizes stress and fatigue to ensure personal health.
■ Muscular skeletal disorders, repetitive stress injuries, and cumulative trauma disorders are common work-related conditions for dental hygienists that require continuing preventive physical and mental energy on the part of each clinical dental hygienist.

■ The science of ergonomics has provided information for the development of standards for human performance and workplace design that can maximize health, comfort, and efficiency for dental hygienists in clinical practice.
■ Key words related to ergonomics, patient reception and care, and workplace design are defined in **Box 7-1**.

PREPARATION FOR THE PATIENT

I. TREATMENT AREA

The requirements for preparation of the treatment area are *standard precautions* for all patients whether or not the presence of a communicable disease is known.

■ *Environmental surfaces*. All contact areas are thoroughly disinfected or covered to control cross-contamination.

Chair Positioning and Ergonomic Practice

Body language: a set of nonverbal signals, including body movements, postures, gestures, and facial expressions, that gives expression to various physical, mental, and emotional states.

Body mechanics: the field of physiology that studies muscular actions and functions in the maintenance of the posture of the body.

Cumulative trauma: disorders of the musculoskeletal, autonomic, and peripheral nervous system caused by repeated, forceful, and awkward movements of the human body, as well as by exposure to mechanical stress, vibration, and cold temperatures.

Ergonomics: study of human performance and workplace design to maximize health, comfort, and efficiency.

Kyphosis: naturally occurring concave forward curve present in the thoracic region of spine when viewed from the side.

Lordosis: naturally occurring convex forward curve present in the cervical and lumbar regions of the spine when viewed from the side.

Postural hypotension: also called orthostatic hypotension; a fall in blood pressure associated with dizziness, syncope, and blurred vision that occurs upon standing or when standing motionless in a fixed position.

Risk factor: anything that puts the clinician or the patient at risk or increases their risk of exposure to an identified hazard.

Safe work practice: any work practice that improves clinician and patient safety. This includes but is not limited to decreased physical demands, improved layout, environmental factors, and work process organization.

Stress: a physical, chemical, or emotional factor that causes physical or mental tension and may be a factor in disease causation or fatigue.

Supine: flat position with head and feet on the same level.

Trendelenburg: the modified supine position when the head is lower than the heart.

Work-related musculoskeletal disorder, repetitive strain injury, cumulative trauma disorder, bioaccumulated stress: terms used to describe disorders of the musculoskeletal, autonomic, and peripheral nervous system caused by repeated, forceful, and awkward movements, as well as by exposure to mechanical stress, vibration, and cold temperatures. Often work-related.

Work simplification: application to clinical procedure of time and motion studies, analysis of instruments and equipment, and body mechanics to provide the patient with a smooth, systematic, simplified approach for comprehensive dental hygiene therapy.

- *Instruments.* Sterile packaged instruments remain sealed until the start of the appointment.
- *Equipment.* Prepare and make ready other materials that will be used, such as for the determination of blood pressure and patient instruction. Anticipate specific needs for procedures being delivered.
- *Patient's dental chair.* Upright for current patient reception; chair arm up for access.
- *Clinician's chair.* Set at proper height for the entire day when same clinician will be there.

II. RECORDS

- For the patient of record, the patient's medical and dental history for pertinent appointment information, updating, and assessment are reviewed.
- Read previous appointment progress notes to focus the current treatment plan.
- Anticipate examination procedures and new record making for a new patient.

PATIENT RECEPTION

I. INTRODUCTIONS

- The dental assistant or the dentist may introduce the new patient to the dental hygienist, but more frequently, a self-introduction is in order.

- The patient is greeted by name, and the hygienist's name is clearly stated, for example, "Good morning, Mrs. Smith; I am Anna Jones, the dental hygienist."
- Wearing a name tag for the patient's convenient observation is helpful.
- Procedure for introducing the patient to others:
  A. A lady's name always precedes a gentleman's.
  B. An older person's name precedes the younger person's (when of the same sex and when the difference in age is obvious).
  C. In general, the patient's name precedes that of a member of the dental personnel.
  D. An older patient is not called by the first name except at the patient's request.

II. ESCORT PATIENT TO DENTAL CHAIR

- Invite patient to be seated and adjust the chair as needed.
- Assist the elderly, disabled, or very small children; guide into the chair (support the patient's arm when patient requests or accepts it.)
- Assist with wheelchair. Bring wheelchair adjacent to the dental chair. Wheelchair procedures are described in Chapter 56, pages 857–859.
- Suggestions for helping the patient with a vision impairment may be found in Chapter 59, page 910.

A. Place handbag in a safe place, if possible within the patient's view.

B. Provide protective eyewear. When a patient removes personal corrective eyeglasses to substitute those provided, make sure the personal glasses are placed in their case in a safe place.

 POSITION OF THE PATIENT

I. GENERAL POSITIONS

Four body positions for delivery of care are shown in **Figure 7-1**.

A. Upright

This is the initial position for patient reception from which chair adjustments are made.

B. Semi-Upright

Patients with certain types of cardiovascular, respiratory, or vertigo problems may need this position.

C. Supine

■ In a supine or flat position the brain is on the same level as the heart.
■ A patient is ideally situated for support of the circulation; rarely could a patient faint while lying in a supine position.
■ Position used most for treatment procedures.

D. Trendelenburg

■ The patient is in the supine position and tipped back and down 35° to 45° so that the heart is higher than the head.

II. THE DENTAL CHAIR

■ A dental chair provides complete body support for the patient, which increases patient relaxation.
■ A comfortable patient is more compliant and allows the procedure to be completed more efficiently.
■ Seat and leg support moves as a unit; back and headrest move as a unit; both are power controlled.
■ Has a thin back so that the chair may be lowered close to the clinician's elbow height.
■ Chair base permits the chair to be lowered as needed for appropriate treatment position.
■ Chair controls need to be available to both the assistant and clinician.

III. USE OF DENTAL CHAIR

A. Prepositioning for Patient Reception

■ Chair at low level; back upright.
■ Chair arm raised on side of approach.

B. Adjustment Steps

■ Patient is seated with back upright.
■ Chair seat and foot portion are raised first to help the patient settle back.
■ Lower back to the supine position for maxillary instrumentation and to a 20° angle with the floor for mandibular treatment.
■ Request patient to slide up to rest the head at upper edge of the headrest or backrest and turn head to left or right as needed for visibility and access.
■ Adjust chair until patient's mouth is at the clinician's elbow height with shoulder relaxed **(Figure 7-2)**.

C. Conclusion of Appointment

■ Move instrument tray away and turn off light.
■ Slowly raise back of chair and tilt chair forward.

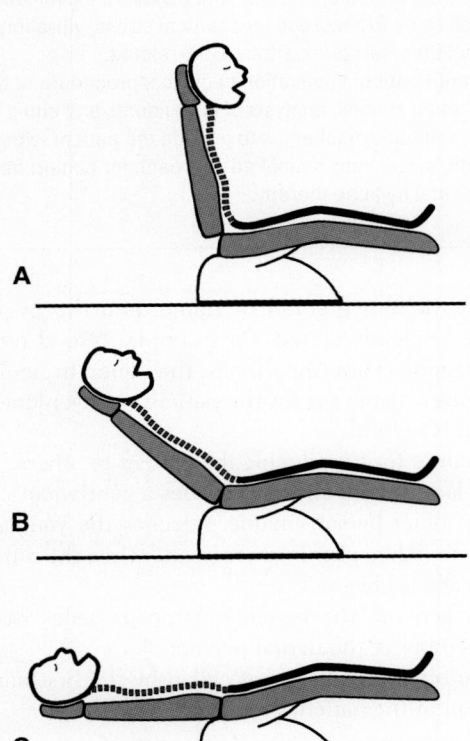
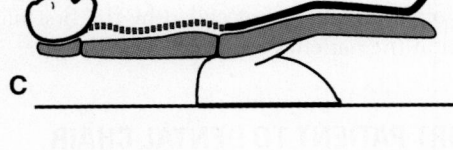
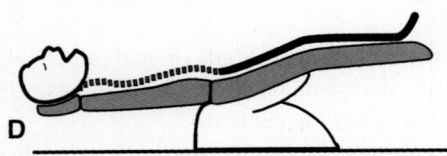

FIGURE 7-1 **Basic Patient Positions. (A)** Upright. **(B)** Semi-upright. **(C)** Supine or horizontal with the brain on the same level as the heart. **(D)** Trendelenburg, with the brain lower than the heart and the feet slightly elevated.

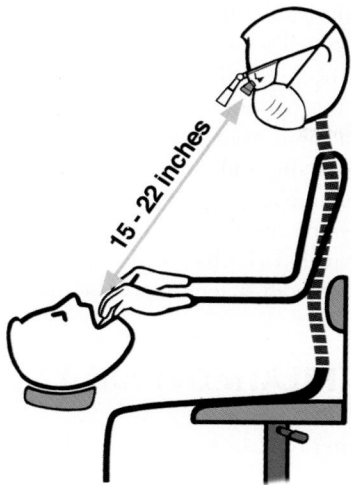

FIGURE 7-2 Clinician's Working Distance. Acceptable positioning shows the patient at the clinician's elbow level and the oral cavity of the patient between 15 and 22 inches from the clinician's eyes.

▪ Request patient to remain seated in upright position briefly to avoid postural hypotension.

D. Contraindications for Supine Position

▪ Review patient history for indications of need for adaptation.
▪ Patient may request a position variation.
▪ Conditions that may contraindicate the supine position include congestive heart disease, vertigo, and a breathing difficulty such as emphysema, severe asthma, or sinusitis.
▪ During the third trimester of pregnancy, some women may be uncomfortable. Chair positioning for the pregnant patient is described on page 748 and illustrated in Figure 48-2, page 749.

 ## POSITION OF THE CLINICIAN

▪ The clinician is in neutral working position, with good access, light, and visibility, which in turn contribute to an efficient procedure.
▪ The patient is positioned so that a thorough, biologically oriented service may be performed conveniently and efficiently within a reasonable length of time.
▪ The positions of the patient and the clinician are interdependent.
▪ When clinician and patient positioning is considered, it is realistic to remember that the patient's position will be assumed for a relatively short time compared with that of the clinician.

NEUTRAL WORKING POSITION

I. OBJECTIVES

Objectives concern the health of the clinician, the service to be performed, and the effect on the patient.

The preferred neutral position attempts to accomplish the following:

▪ Contribute to and preserve rather than detract from clinician's health and wellness.
▪ Contribute to ease and efficacy of performance that encourages patient cooperation.
▪ Allow endurance for prolonged periods of peak efficiency.
▪ Reduce potential for overexertion and injury from mental and physical stress and fatigue.
▪ Give the patient a sense of well-being, security, and confidence.
▪ Accommodate a patient with special needs.

II. THE EFFECTS OF NEUTRAL WORKING POSITION

▪ Neutral working position (NWP) needs to be developed, practiced daily, and made habitual.
▪ Habitual neutral position will translate to all activities, outside of work as well. An internal environment can be created for on-going physical ease, comfort, safety, and activity.
▪ Without practicing the principles of neutral position on a regular daily basis, a clinician can experience discomfort, pain, and work-related stress disorders. The long-term result can be shortened or compromised career longevity with changes in daily life activities.

Analysis and assessment of posture can give direction to corrections for treatment. A posture assessment instrument is available.[1]

III. DESCRIPTION OF NEUTRAL SEATED POSITION

▪ *Back:* in neutral alignment with natural spinal curves, including cervical lordosis, thoracic kyphosis, and lumbar lordosis
▪ *Head:* on top of neutral spine with forward neck flexion between 15 and 20 degrees or less.
▪ *Eyes:* directed downward to prevent neck and eye strain.
▪ *Shoulders:* relaxed and parallel with the hips and floor.
▪ *Elbows:* close to the body.
▪ *Forearms:* parallel with the floor.
▪ *Wrist:* forearm and wrist are in a straight line.
▪ *Thighs:* full body weight distributed evenly on seat; comfortable space (about 3 inches) between edge of seat and back of knee.
▪ *Knees:* slightly apart.
▪ *Feet:* flat on the floor.

IV. CLINICIAN/PATIENT POSITIONING

A. Distance

▪ Patient's oral cavity is adjusted to clinician's elbow height.

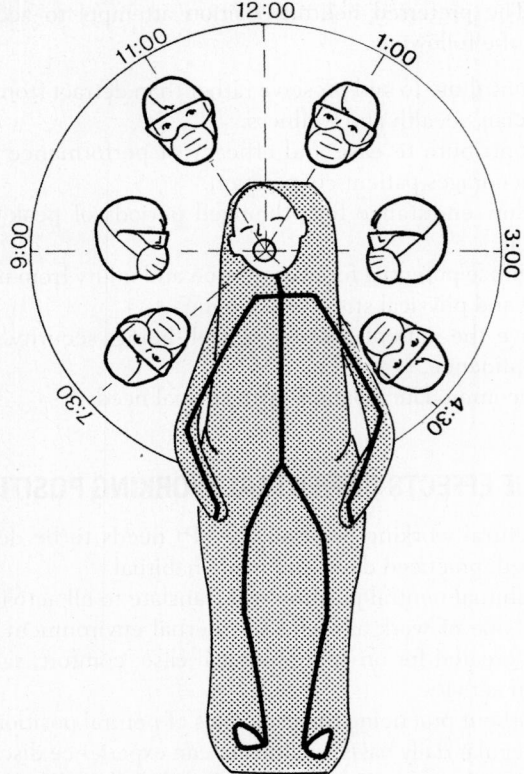

FIGURE 7-3 **Range of Positions for Clinician.** The patient's head is placed at the upper edge of the backrest or headrest for convenient access by the clinician during treatment. The range of positions is compared with the numbers on a clock.

- Distance from clinician's eyes to the patient's oral cavity when the clinician is seated in neutral position will be within the range of 15 to 22 inches **(Figure 7-2)**.
- The distance is defined as the "working distance," which is a significant measurement when fitting loupes for an individual clinician.

B. Selection

- Neutral working position is combined with effective access to the patient for treatment procedures.
- Orientation of position of the clinician to patient can be compared to the hours of a clock around the patient's head with 12:00 noon at the top of the patient's head as shown in **Figure 7-3**.
- Clock hours correspond with clinician/patient relation associated with instrumentation in different areas of the patient's oral cavity.

C. Flexibility

Orientation for the right-handed clinician is associated with 8:00 AM to 2:00 to 3:00 PM; and for the left-handed clinician orientation is associated with 10:00 to 11:00 AM to 4:00 PM.

- Access and visual adjustment determines which side the clinician will select for a given procedure.
- Movement of the clinician's chair freely on wheels and turning of the patient's head facilitate positioning and patient treatment from either side.
- Crossing over the midline improves access and visibility in certain areas.
- In treatment rooms with limited space, the dental chair may be swiveled to change the angle of the chair to allow the clinician space to move across the midline.

 # THE TREATMENT AREA

- The treatment area centers around the patient's oral cavity.
- The entire "work area" refers to the dental chair with patient, the unit, and the instrument tray as they are positioned for the convenience and accessibility of the clinician and assistant for 4-handed dental hygiene.
- For the clinician, the essentials for access and visibility for patient care are provided by the flexibility of movement of the clinician's chair and appropriate lighting, supplemented by the clinician's own visibility enhanced by wearing magnification loupes with head light.

I. THE CLINICIAN'S CHAIR

- The chair is a significant adjunct to implement ergonomic practice.
- Optimal design provides adequate support and the opportunity and means to change body posture frequently during the workday as clinicians, patients, and procedures change.
- The clinician adjusts the chair to personal specifications.
- Many clinicians own their own chair to accommodate or prevent a personal health problem.

A. Characteristics of an Acceptable Chair

- *Base:* broad and heavy with no fewer than four casters; a chair with five casters provides greater stability.
- *Seat:* seamless upholstery, padded firmly; accommodates requirements for neutral seated position.
- *Height:* adjustable for wide personal variability.
- *Back:* adjustable lumbar support to accommodate different positions, procedures, and clinicians.
- *Mobility:* completely mobile; built with free-rolling casters; not connected to other dental equipment; free movement around the patient's head for instrumentation from either side.
- *Adjustment:* multiple adjustments for different positions, procedures, and clinicians; mechanisms easy to learn and use.
- *Infection control friendly:* all surfaces able to withstand standard precautions regimen.

II. VISION: LIGHTING

- During treatment, visibility in the oral cavity is prerequisite to thoroughness without undue trauma to the tissues.
- With adequate light, efficiency increases, treatment time is decreased, and patient cooperation increases.
- Many lighting options are available. All need to be directed properly to the oral cavity for adequate visualization, optimal patient care, and clinician comfort and safety.

A. Dental Light: Suggested Features

- Is readily adjustable both vertically and horizontally.
- Beam of light is capable of being focused.
- Set within a comfortable arm's reach.
- Does not require awkward or forceful movement to position it for visualization.

B. Dental Light: Location

Attachment

- Unit attachment.
- Ceiling-mounted light on a track is most versatile.

Dual Lighting

- Advantages of the use of two clinic lights have been demonstrated with a supine patient position in a contoured chair.
- One light directed from the front of the patient may be attached to the dental unit; the other light is mounted on a ceiling track.

C. Dental Light: Adjustment Principles

- Light allows clear illumination of entire treatment area.
- **Figure 7-4** shows position of light for maxillary and mandibular treatment.

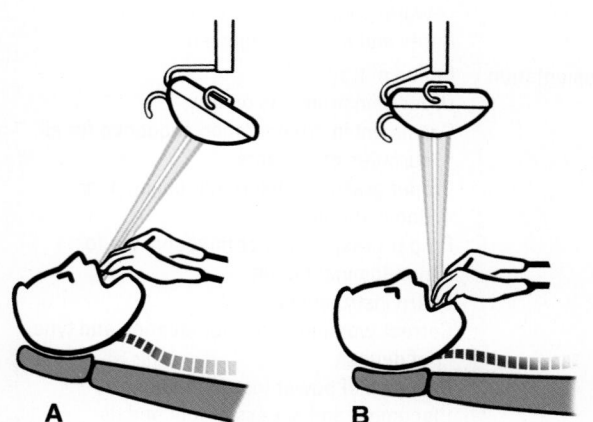

FIGURE 7-4 **Lighting.** Light does not obstruct clinician, allows clear illumination of the treatment area. **(A)** Maxillary arch; chin up position; beam of light often between 60°→ 45° angle to floor. **(B)** Mandibular arch; chin down position; beam of light nearly perpendicular to floor.

III. VISION: MAGNIFICATION[2]

Magnification is needed to improve visualization, support neutral working position, and enhance treatment procedures.

A. Choice of Loupe Systems

- Through-the-lens: adjusted with the clinician's prescription as needed.
- Flip-up for magnification only.
- Loupes with head light: for added improvement in visualization.

B. Features

- Proper fit is essential to successful incorporation of magnification into the clinician's treatment environment.
- Proper fit is dependent on the clinician's working distance and neutral position.
- Clinicians need to research the differences to select best option.

IV. HANDPIECES

- Technology has provided handpieces that are ergonomically compatible with procedures clinicians provide.
- Designs are smaller, lighter, and better fitted to dental hygienists' hands.

A. Ergonomically Designed Handpieces

- Are lightweight, decreasing stress on hand and wrist.
- Fit in the contours of the clinician's hand and allow functional light grasp.
- Reduce fatigue and strain.
- Allow maneuverability.
- Provide power assist without strain.
- Produce less heat buildup.
- Are available in a cordless option.

V. CORDS

A. Management

- Managing cords is a significant aspect of ergonomic practice.
- Cords are part of dental units and are an integral part of delivery of care for every patient.
- Ultrasonics, air/water syringes, slow-speed handpieces and all power-driven equipment requires cords connected to a power source.
- Improper management and inefficient design of the cords can increase drag on hand, wrist, and arm increasing risk of repetitive injury.
- Care is needed that cords can be sanitized, and are not dragging on the floor of the clinic.

B. Curly Cords

- Can cause excessive stretching and pulling by clinician.
- Associated with bending, reaching, and awkward postures to position for treatment.
- Increase the strain on hand, wrist, arm, and shoulder of clinician.
- Provide an ergonomic risk by increasing fatigue level and creating muscle imbalances.
- Straight cords may be generally easier to manage.

 ERGONOMIC PRACTICE

I. SCOPE OF ERGONOMIC DENTAL HYGIENE

- Includes all practices that make work safe, decrease strain and fatigue, eliminate hazards, and improve work process affecting health and well-being of clinician and patient.
- Terminology related to ergonomics is included in **Box 7-1**.
- **Box 7-2** lists items of the equipment, work layout, and work process organization that need attention during practice if physical occupational disorders are to be prevented.

II. RELATED OCCUPATIONAL PROBLEMS

- The physical challenges inherent in dental hygiene practice place the clinicians at risk for developing work-related musculoskeletal disorders.
- **Table 7-1** describes a variety of disorders that can occur among clinicians.
- Prevention of the slow developing conditions is a daily responsibility.

III. ERGONOMIC RISK FACTORS

- Prevention begins with the recognition of the risk factors that can point to potential body injury and more serious permanent musculoskeletal disorders.[3,4]
- **Table 7-2** lists and defines significant risk factors and provides examples of various practices that can lead to musculoskeletal disorders.

 SELF-CARE FOR THE DENTAL HYGIENIST

- Responsible self-care and attention to the risk factors of musculoskeletal disorders are central to ergonomic practice.
- Self-care is built on but not limited to all safe work practices that incorporate ergonomic principles for health and well-being. Self-care includes but is not limited to:

BOX 7-2	Ergonomic Practice		
Equipment	Personal protective equipment Lighting (**Figure 7-4**) Magnification Properly fitted gloves Instruments balanced, sharp, of varied diameters, with knurling on handles Power instruments Handpiece lightweight and ergonomically designed Cords and cord maintenance Foot pedals Suction Air/water syringe	**Work Process Organization**	Clinician neutral working posture (NWP) Use of magnification system supporting NWP Clinician/patient positioning (CPP) Light within easy arm's reach with clear illumination of treatment area Access and management of suction and air/water syringe Cords and cord management
Work Layout	Uncluttered, easy access to patient, patient records, computer, radiographs Counters clear with designated area for documentation Instrument tray within easy reach Light fixture easy to move and adjust Orderly tray set-up with complete armamentarium for services to be delivered Convenient treatment room set-up and design for patient chair, air/water syringe, suction, cords, foot pedals	**Instrumentation**	Reach of tray Order of instruments on tray Consistent instrumentation sequence for all surfaces of sextants Proper grasp and fulcrum technique for dominant hand Proper grasp and fulcrum technique for nondominant hand Sharp instruments Correct working stroke for location and type of deposit Inclusion of power instrumentation Placement and access of foot pedals Selective polishing Placement and access to overgloves Documentation procedure

TABLE 7-1	MUSCULOSKELETAL DISORDERS AFFECTING DENTAL HYGIENISTS

With any symptoms or any ongoing discomfort, take action to find the source of the problem and how to relieve the symptom. Prevention is the best course of action. Early intervention will decrease the risk of a more involved condition or a more costly injury. If not addressed in a timely manner any of these conditions could lead to a limited ability to practice or total disability.

CONDITION	CAUSES	SYMPTOMS
Carpal Tunnel Syndrome A symptomatic compression of the median nerve within the carpal tunnel **(Figure 7-5)**.	Deviations of wrist from neutral. Pinch grasp with insufficient rest.	Numbness; tingling in the thumb, index, and middle fingers.
Thoracic Outlet Syndrome Painful disorder of the fingers, hand, and/or wrist from compression of the brachial nerve plexus and vessels between the neck and shoulder.	Tilting head forward. Hunched and/or rounded forward shoulders. Continuously reaching overhead.	Numbness, tingling, and/or pain in the hand or wrist.
Bursitis Inflammation of the bursa.	Areas of friction or impingement anywhere in the body, usually the shoulder.	Decreased range of motion. Aching.
Tendonitis Painful inflammation of the wrist resulting in strain.	Repeated wrist extension or palmar flexion.	Pain in the wrist, especially along the outer edges of the hand rather than through the center of the wrist.
Disc Herniation Displacement of the nucleus of the disc with resultant pressure on the spinal cord or peripheral nerves.	Prolonged, static postures of forward flexion, hyperextension, lateral bending, or rotation of the spine. Can present on cervical, thoracic, or lumbar areas of the spine.	Pain, numbness, tingling of the arm, fingers, lower back, hip, or leg.

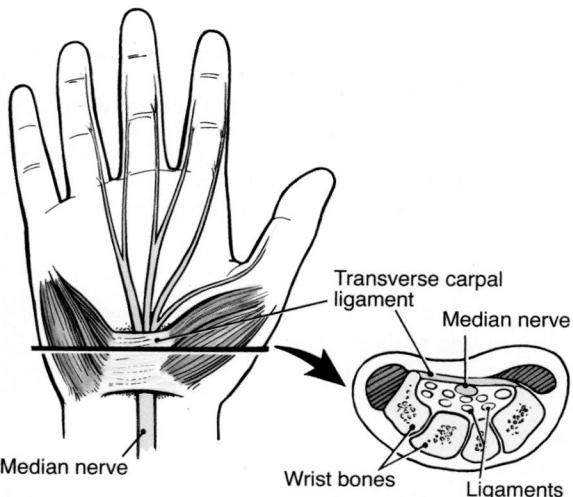

FIGURE 7-5 **Anatomy of the Wrist.** Left, the median nerve passes through the transverse carpal tunnel of the wrist and branches to innervate the thumb, the index and middle fingers, and the medial aspect of the ring finger. Right, cross section of wrist shows the median nerve passing through the carpal tunnel. The tunnel is formed by the concave arch of the carpal (wrist) bones and roofed over by the transverse carpal ligament.

- *Physical fitness:* Immunizations, healthy diet, adequate sleep, exercise.
- *Standard precautions:* Personal protective equipment (PPE).
- *Clinical practice:* Clinician/patient positioning (CPP), instrument selection and use, prevention of sharps injuries.
- *Neutral working position:* In all activities, not only clinical practice.
- *Stress management:* Reasonable patient scheduling, adequate breaks.

I. DAILY FUNCTIONAL MOVEMENT EXERCISES

- In dental hygiene practice, it is necessary to give constant attention to maintaining a healthy spine.
  A. Achieving neutral work posture throughout the work day.
  B. Performing effective clinician/patient positioning, and practicing daily functional movement exercises will protect and encourage a healthy spine.[5]

TABLE 7-2	ERGONOMIC RISK FACTORS

Intensity (strength or concentration of exposure), frequency (how often is the exposure), and duration (length of time of exposure) are related to the detrimental effects of the risk factor. A combination of risk factors intensifies risk and increases potential for injury.

RISK FACTOR	DEFINITION	EXAMPLE
Prolonged Awkward Position	Body postures that deviate from the normal resting or neutral positions.	Twisting the torso during instrumentation. Arm raised when scaling.
Static Positions Long-Term Static Load	Assuming and holding any position for a long period; stresses the body, accelerates fatigue and discomfort.	Bending neck for long periods. Retracting cheek with nondominant hand without stable fulcrum. Prolonged seated posture.
Repetition	Performing the same motion or series of motions continually or frequently.	Scaling and root planing. Probing. Exposing radiographs.
Force/Grasp	Physical effort needed to lift, push, pull, grasp, and pinch items in the work environment. Often required to handle and control equipment and tools. Force increases as contact area decreases.	Manual instrumentation. Exposing radiographs.
Environmental	Can directly influence comfort and risk of injury.	Cold. Heat. Poor lighting. Noise.
Vibration	The physical exposure to rapidly oscillating tools or machinery.	Tools such as jackhammers. Additional research is needed to demonstrate effect power scaling and handpieces have on dental personnel.
Insufficient Rest	Performing the same motion or series of motions continually or frequently without sufficient recovery time for muscles.	Scaling procedures. Probing. Exposing radiographs. Unreasonable patient scheduling. Insufficient breaks.
Stress	A physical, chemical, or emotional factor that causes bodily or mental tension and may be a factor in disease causation or fatigue. Involves clinician perception of control of work environment and psychosocial factors.	Having no control over scheduling. Delivering care when patient arrives late. Poor team communication. Insufficient input concerning workload at work.
Poor Physical Fitness	Decreased capacity for body to resist the negative consequences of physical demands of dental hygiene practice.	Demands of long periods of sitting. Demands of repeated instrumentation.

- A healthy spine requires that it be flexible. To accomplish a flexible spine, encourage movement in all directions so that no one area of the spine becomes overused, limiting its movement potential and affecting other areas of the spine.
- With impingement of an area of the spine for any length of time, blood flow and oxygenation to the area is affected.
- Chronic poor postural habits can lead to nerve impingement resulting in chronic pain and possible injury.
- Practicing daily functional movement exercises for the spine and other joints in the practice setting and at home is a preventive strategy for all dental personnel.

A. Objectives of Exercises

With consistent practice, the following can be accomplished:

- Stretch, lengthen, and maintain the health of muscles.
- Support the structure of the natural curves of the spine.
- Stabilize range of motion of the joints.
- Maintain balance of musculoskeletal system.
- Maintain flexibility and comfort.
- Decrease stress of physical challenges on internal systems.
- Aid in development and maintenance of good postural work habits.

Box 7-3	Example Progress Note

Josie came in crutches with the surprise of having a broken hip but trying to be her usual cheerful self. It was an auto accident, so there were many sore places all over she said. Said she was tired of her "dirty mouth" and figured she must have a lot of tartar because they didn't help her keep her mouth clean in the hospital or Rehab and she has had trouble holding her arms up to clean her teeth right. One of her grandchildren (18 years old) brought her and helped her into the dental chair. She asked not to be tipped way back, and didn't like being tipped even a little. I did most of the exam standing up. Examination showed limited opening of mouth, posterior teeth areas of biofilm, some calculus; probing mostly within 3 mm range with a few bleeding spots; sensitivity to cold facial 20, 21. Recommended changing to desensitizing dentifrice. She called off the appointment before scaling and said she'd make another appointment in a couple of weeks.

She was obviously exhausted but seemed proud that she had done that much.

Signed: _____, RDH Date: _____

- Improve awareness to develop skill in creating necessary adjustments to maintain dynamic postural integrity.
- Foster ideal upright posture that translates to all functional movement.
- Retrain muscles and develop neuromuscular patterns for good postural habits that will transfer to all life activities.
- Develop a safe internal environment for injury prevention.

- Provide a structurally organized base upon which to build strength and conditioning.

B. Functional Movement Exercises

- Sequence designed specifically for dental personnel to:
  - Create functional movement patterns.
  - Gently stretch and lengthen muscles that have occupational demands.
  - Encourage full range of motion for healthy joints.
  - Support the natural curves of the spine.
  - Exercises can be performed during clinical practice hours, at chairside between patients, in nonpatient areas of the office, and/or at home.[6]
  - Do movement exercises slowly and with awareness. **Figure 7-6** describes and illustrates a series of functional movement exercises.
  - Other exercises for use during dental hygiene practice are shown in Figure 38-20, page 597.

DOCUMENTATION

Documentation for a patient with requirements for a personalized dental chair positioning during instrumentation would include:

- Medical history notations indicating health history and current problem causing breathing difficulties.
- Potential emergency that could occur if patient is over-stressed; need for preparation at future appointments.
- Notation for reference to length of appointment and time of day if needed.
- A sample progress note can be reviewed in **Box 7-3**.

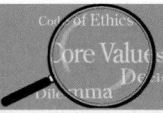 Everyday Ethics

After practicing for a few years as a dental hygienist, Delia has developed chronic pain in her neck, back, and hands. As a result, she knows that her instrumentation is affected and patients are not receiving definitive scaling at their appointments.

Questions for Consideration

1. What is Delia's ethical responsibility to herself in this situation? (Note the ADHA Code of Ethics for Dental Hygienists, Section 7, Standards of Professional Responsibility, page 1086 in Appendix I.)
2. Explain which Core Values (page 38, Table II-1) apply to Delia's ethical responsibility to her patients if her ability to perform dental hygiene treatment is compromised?
3. Explain which of the questions included in the steps for making ethical decisions (page 10) might help direct Delia in determining actions she can take now to assure that her patients continue to receive the best possible dental hygiene care.

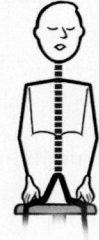

A. Sitting in neutral position, close eyes, do full diaphragm breathing. Allow abdomen to be full as lungs become full. Exhale with lips slightly parted.

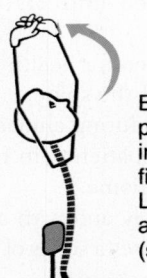

B. Standing or sitting in neutral position, stretch both arms up, interlace fingers, turn interlaced fingers so that palms are up. Look at hands and follow with eyes as you pull hands backward (spinal extension). Return to neutral.

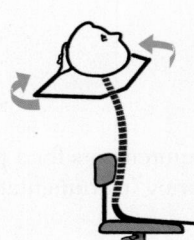

C. Standing or sitting in neutral position, interlace fingers and place on back of head; push elbows backward while slowly looking upward then slowly return to neutral. Chin moves up towards ceiling. Inhale as you look up and exhale as you return to neutral (thoracic extension).

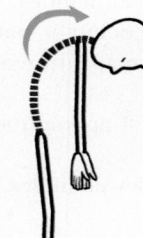

D. Standing in neutral position, slowly bend forward, rounding the back, gently bring the chin in the direction of the chest, letting the arms and hands hang down freely (spinal flexion).

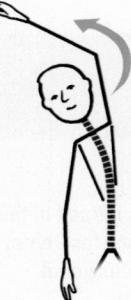

E. Standing in neutral position, raise left arm, palm facing toward midline; right arm hangs by side, palm facing hip. Bend trunk to the right and return to neutral. Right ribs flex and come closer together. Left ribs extend and move away from each other.
Repeat on opposite side.

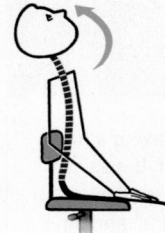

F. As chest moves forward and upward allow the head to move back (thoracic extension); chin moves in an upward direction. Inhale fully, count to five; exhale as you slowly return to neutral. Jaw remains relaxed.

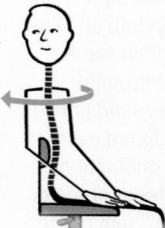

G. Sitting in neutral position, palms resting on thighs. Very gently look over right shoulder and allow right shoulder to move back as left shoulder moves forward (spinal rotation). Right palm will move along thigh back toward hip. Left palm will move forward along thigh toward knee.
Repeat on opposite side.

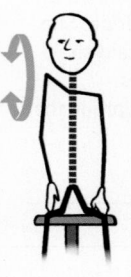

H. Shoulders relaxed in neutral position. Move right shoulder up toward right ear, backward and down. Do this movement in a clockwise direction 10 times and in a counter-clockwise direction 10 times. This movement should be done slowly and with awareness of movement of shoulder in all directions. Repeat on opposite side.

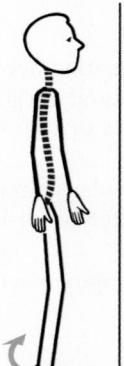

I. Standing, roll onto balls of feet, roll back onto heels of feet. Stand near wall for support.

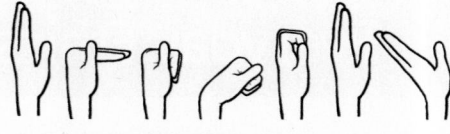

J. Tendon gliding exercise for fingers, hand and wrist. This is a fluid movement involving movement of wrist as you perform the sequence, left to right.

FIGURE 7-6 **Functional Movement Exercises.** Movements for each exercise are repeated in 10 unit cycles, seated or standing with weight supported evenly by both feet flat on the floor. The ideal plan is to perform some segments after each patient.

Factors To Teach The Patient

- How certain positions of the clinician are necessary for safe ergonomic practice and patient care.
- How patient cooperation makes it possible for the dental hygienist to practice with less stress and strain to prevent musculoskeletal discomfort and pain, and deliver better patient care.

References

1. Simmer-Beck M, Branson B. Posture perfect. *Dimens Dent Hyg.* 2005 May;3(5):14–19.
2. Branson B, Simmer-Beck M. Visual acuity without injury. *Dimens Dent Hyg.* 2009 Sep;7(9):46–9.
3. Michalak-Turcotte C, Sanders M. A problem solving approach. *Dimens Dent Hyg.* 2005 Sep;3(9):18–21.
4. Michalak-Turcotte C, Sanders M. Developing a plan of action. *Dimens Dent Hyg.* 2005 Nov;3(11):20–2.
5. Valachi B, Valachi K. Preventing musculoskeletal disorders in clinical dentistry. Strategies to address the mechanisms leading to musculoskeletal disorders. *J Am Dent Assoc.* 2003 Dec;134(12):1604–12.
6. Valachi B. Improving your musculoskeletal health. *Dimens Dent Hyg.* 2003 Jun–Jul;1(3):20–6.

Introduction to Documentation

CHARLOTTE J. WYCHE, RDH, MS

Chapter Outline

Complete, accurate examinations and patient information maintained in comprehensive records and chartings are basic requirements of providing patient care. Accurate documentation is essential to a safe, thorough, and caring dental hygiene practice. **Box 8-1** defines key terms related to patient records and charting.

THE PATIENT RECORD

I. PURPOSES AND CHARACTERISTICS

■ Patient health records provide a means of communication between the members of the health team themselves, as well as with their patients.

■ Coordinated planning and continuity of care can be facilitated.

■ Patient records serve as a basis for the evaluation of the quality of care and aid when a review is made of the effectiveness of patient care practices.

■ Data from health records are utilized in research and education.

■ Documentation in the patient's record is considered legal evidence in any legal or forensic situation.[1]

■ Patient record entries are:
   ■ recorded promptly during or following treatment
   ■ recorded using clear, concise, subjective statements
   ■ dated
   ■ signed by the clinician

BOX 8-1	Key Words

Records and Charting

Chart: a form or graphic used as a component of a patient's permanent health record.

Charting: the process of tabulating clinical information on a graphic form.

Encryption: translation of computerized data into a secret code; the most effective way to achieve data security; in order to read an encrypted file, the reader needs access to a secret key or password that enables changing the "cipher text" into plain text.

Forensic: pertaining to or used in legal proceedings.

Forensic dentistry: refers to the use of dental records or oral health data to identify individuals for legal proceedings.

Malpractice: professional negligence; an act or an omission by a health care provider that causes injury to a patient; a deviation from acceptable standards of care.

Patient record: a written document that contains information identifying an individual patient, such as a patient's name, address, and phone number, as well as information related to that particular patient's care, such as health history information, dental charting items, treatment dates, and treatment codes.

Electronic record: in a computerized database management system, a record is a complete set of information. Records are composed of electronic fields, each of which contains space for one item of information.

Sign: objective, observable evidence of an illness or disorder; a physical manifestation of a disorder that is apparent to a trained healthcare provider and sometimes to the patient.

Symptom: any change in the body or its function that is perceived by the patient; the subjective experience of a disease or disorder.

Triage: screening and classification of individuals in order to make optimal use of treatment resources; sorting and allocating relative priority for patient treatment needs.

Unique identifier: secret name and/or password used by an individual to access computerized information that is not available to others who do not have permission to access the information.

II. COMPONENTS OF A PATIENT RECORD[2]

The format of the patient record will vary among practices and clinics. All information collected during the initial examination and during continuing patient appointments is an official part of the permanent records.

- All components of the dental hygiene process of care are included.[3]
- Comprehensive, regularly updated health histories and vital signs are documented.
- All findings from the comprehensive initial patient assessment are recorded.
- The comprehensive dental treatment plan and the dental hygiene care plan are included.
- Additional assessment and treatment information from each patient visit is documented and dated.
- Additional components of the patient record include:
  - informed consent forms
  - radiographs
  - study casts
  - photographs
  - copies of correspondence with dental specialists or medical practitioners.
- Each component of the patient record is marked with patient identification and/or demographic information.

III. THE HANDWRITTEN RECORD

- Historically, dental healthcare personnel have maintained the individual patient's records by longhand on paper.
- Handwritten records are recorded legibly and written in ink.
- Records have also been dictated into a machine to be typewritten into the permanent record later.
- Mistakes are corrected by placing a single line through the error, writing the correct information immediately after, and signing the entry.
- If a late entry is necessary, the new information:
  - follows the most recent entry in the patient record
  - is noted as a late entry
  - includes the date and time that the late entry was made.
- Systems may involve the completion of forms with topics and spaces to check off and spaces for writing descriptive information and/or prose-style summary.
- Strict infection control protocols are required to prevent contamination of paper records during patient care.

IV. THE ELECTRONIC RECORD[4]

A. Characteristics

- Computerized records have provided a faster, more convenient, and better organized mode of information gathering and preserving.

- A variety of custom software programs are available.
- Systems may provide methods for documenting dental and periodontal assessments with automated, voice-activated recordings.
- Other systems include printing off hard copies for the patient when indicated.
- Computerized systems have advantages for integration of the records into the total practice.
  - Complete patient information, appointment schedules, medical alerts, and financial aspects can be included.
  - Data can be accessed from anywhere within the system by authorized personnel.
- Infection control protocols include providing plastic barriers for computer keyboard and mouse disinfection of chairside monitors.

B. Features

The electronic clinical record is not only a repository of information but has additional potential for providing increased functionality in clinical decision making and evaluation of patient care outcomes.[5] Previous professional liability court actions in the United States have established the validity of electronic healthcare records.[5] Specially designed software and record storage systems can:

- Standardize terminology used for data entry
- Improve efficiency and accountability[6]; speed up entry of information and encourage entry of more comprehensive information
- Increase the legibility of information
- Provide easier, faster access to clinical information
- Enhance communication[6] with patients and with consulting dental specialists or other multidisciplinary team members who may not be together at one clinical site
- Provide new ways of analyzing clinical information and outcomes of various clinical treatment approaches or treatment procedures
- Maintain digital radiographs and photographs within the patient record.

V. ABBREVIATIONS AND SYMBOLS

The use of unique abbreviations that are not easily understood by others can cause clinical or legal problems. A selected list of standard abbreviations and symbols developed by the American Dental Association[7] is found in Appendix VII on page 1122.

PRIVACY OF PATIENT RECORDS

Given the global nature of computerized systems for storing and retrieving health information, healthcare workers have addressed the concept of privacy of computerized information. Legislation is in place in the United States, Canada, and some European countries to protect the privacy of patient information.[5]

- The Health Information Portability and Accountability Act of 1996 (HIPAA) took effect for dental practices in the United States on April 14, 2003. The law provides federal privacy standards that protect patient records and other health related information in an emerging electronic information environment.[8]
- Some states may have stricter laws that take precedence over the federal standards.
- The HIPAA is basically comprises three key sets of rules concerning privacy, confidentiality, and security of patient information.[8]

I. PRIVACY

Refers to a patient's right to keep health information private and control who can access it. Patients have the right to:[9]

- Receive a copy of personal health records.
- Ask to change incorrect or incomplete information.
- Receive a report on when, why, and with whom their health information is shared.
  - Free once a year.
  - Within 60 days of request.
- Decide, in some cases (such as marketing), whether health information can be shared.
- Ask to be contacted regarding health information in a specific location or by a specific method such as telephone or mail.
- File a complaint with the provider, health insurer, or United States government regarding concerns about use of their health information.

II. CONFIDENTIALITY

Refers to the responsibility that healthcare providers have to protect patients' confidential health information.

1. Healthcare providers are responsible for:[9]
   - Complying with protocols that protect patient information to avoid inappropriate disclosure.
   - Providing patients with a "notice of privacy practices" document at the beginning of their care.
2. Employers are responsible for:[8,9]
   - Educating employees about confidentiality of patient information.
   - Implementing security measures, policies, and formal protocols that protect patient information.
   - Conducting analysis of security risks and vulnerabilities.
   - Establishing sanctions for workforce members who fail to comply with policies.

III. SECURITY

- Refers to policies, procedures, and tools used to keep individually identifiable patient information private.
- The rule provides for a uniform level of protection for health information that is electronically stored or transmitted.
- Required components[9] include the use of:
  - Technology that protects against unauthorized access to stored patient data that uses unique patient identifier and treatment code sets when transmitting patient health information[10]
  - Encryption technology so patient information cannot be understood if it is intercepted.
  - Technology that verifies information has not been changed during electronic transmission.

IV. STORAGE SYSTEMS

- In all systems, the privacy of personal patient information must be respected.
- For written records, a filing system is needed that provides accessibility to the health records by authorized personnel only.
- Computerized records require several computer terminals at desks or in treatment rooms where authorized personnel can access required information.

DOCUMENTING THE INTRA- & EXTRAORAL EXAMINATION

- A specific objective of the intra- and extraoral examination as a part of the total patient assessment is the recognition of deviations from normal that may be signs and symptoms of disease.

- Signs and symptoms of disease are the deviations from normal that are recorded in the patient's record. Additional information about signs and symptoms is found in Chapter 11, on page 147.
- The need for careful, thorough examination cannot be overemphasized. Concentration and attention to detail are necessary in order that each slight deviation from normal may be entered on the record.

TOOTH NUMBERING SYSTEMS

Different systems are used in different dental offices and clinics worldwide. The three most commonly used tooth designation systems[11] are described here:

I. CONTINUOUS NUMBERS 1 THROUGH 32

This tooth numbering method is referred to as the *Universal* or *ADA*[12] system. **Figure 8-1** shows the crowns of the teeth with the corresponding numbers.

A. Permanent Teeth

- Start with the right maxillary third molar (number 1).
- Follow around the arch to the left maxillary third molar (16).
- Descend to the left mandibular third molar (17).
- Follow around to the right mandibular third molar (32).

B. Primary or Deciduous Teeth

- Use continuous upper case letters A through T in the same order as described for the permanent teeth.
- Right maxillary second molar (A) around to left maxillary second molar (J).

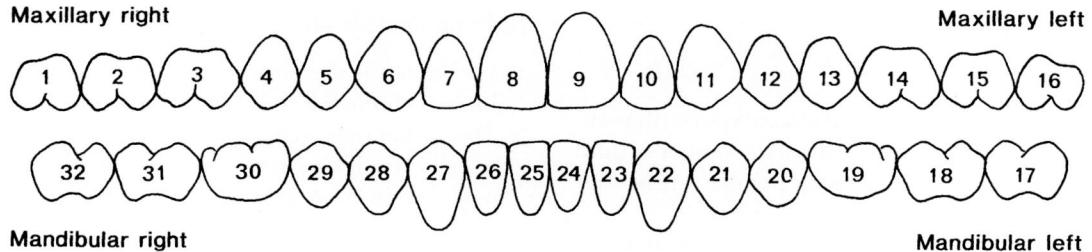

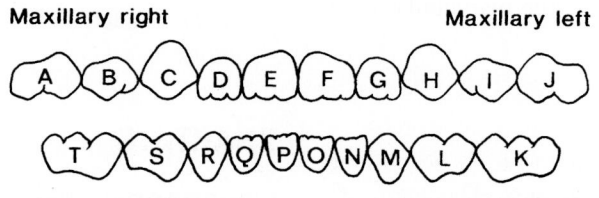

FIGURE 8-1 **Universal Tooth Numbering (American Dental Association).** *Above,* permanent dentition designated by numbers 1 through 32, starting at the maxillary right with 1 and following around to the maxillary left third molar (number 16) to the left mandibular third molar (number 17) and around to the right mandibular third molar (number 32). *Below,* primary teeth are designated by letters in the same sequence.

PERMANENT TEETH

Q-1															Q-2
Maxillary right															Maxillary left
18	17	16	15	14	13	12	11	21	22	23	24	25	26	27	28
48	47	46	45	44	43	42	41	31	32	33	34	35	36	37	38
Mandibular right															Mandibular left
Q-4															Q-3

PRIMARY TEETH

Q-5										Q-6
Maxillary right										Maxillary left
55	54	53	52	51	61	62	63	64	65
85	84	83	82	81	71	72	73	74	75
Mandibular right										Mandibular left
Q-8										Q-7

FIGURE 8-2 **International Tooth Numbering (Fédération Dentaire Internationale).** Each quadrant is numbered 1 through 4, with number 1 on the maxillary right, number 2 on the maxillary left, number 3 on the mandibular left, and number 4 on the mandibular right. Each tooth in a quadrant is numbered 1 through 8 from the central incisor. Quadrants of the primary dentition are numbered from 5 through 8. It is a 2-digit system.

■ Descend to left mandibular second molar (K) and around to the right mandibular second molar (T).

II. F.D.I. TWO-DIGIT

The F.D.I. system is also called the *International* system.[13,14]

A. Permanent Teeth

Each tooth is numbered by the quadrant (1 to 4) and by the tooth within the quadrant (1 to 8).

■ *Quadrant Numbers*
  1 = Maxillary right
  2 = Maxillary left
  3 = Mandibular left
  4 = Mandibular right
■ *Tooth Numbers Within Each Quadrant.* Start with number 1 at the midline (central incisor) to number 8, third molar. **Figure 8-2** shows each tooth number in the four quadrants.
■ *Designation.* The digits are pronounced separately. For example, "two-five" (25) is the maxillary left second premolar, and "four-two" (42) is the mandibular right lateral incisor.

B. Primary or Deciduous Teeth

Each tooth is numbered by quadrant (5 to 8) to continue with the permanent quadrant numbers. The teeth are numbered within each quadrant (1 to 5).

■ *Quadrant Numbers*
  5 = Maxillary right
  6 = Maxillary left
  7 = Mandibular left
  8 = Mandibular right
■ *Tooth Numbers Within Each Quadrant.* Number 1 is the central incisor, and number 5 is the second primary molar.
■ *Designation.* The digits are pronounced separately. For example, "eight-three" (83) is the mandibular right primary canine, and "six-five" (65) is the maxillary left second primary molar.

III. QUADRANT NUMBERS 1 THROUGH 8

Names to identify this method are the *Palmer System* or *Set-square.*[15]

A. Permanent Teeth

■ Each tooth is designated using the numbers 1 (central incisor) through 8 (third molar) in each quadrant.
■ The appropriate quadrant for each tooth is designated using a specific pattern of vertical and horizontal lines as shown in **Figure 8-3**.

B. Primary or Deciduous Teeth

■ Upper case letters A through E are used instead of the numbers.

CHARTING

I. PURPOSE

The purpose of each type of charting is defined by its title:

■ *Dental chart.* Includes diagrammatic representation of existing conditions of the teeth.

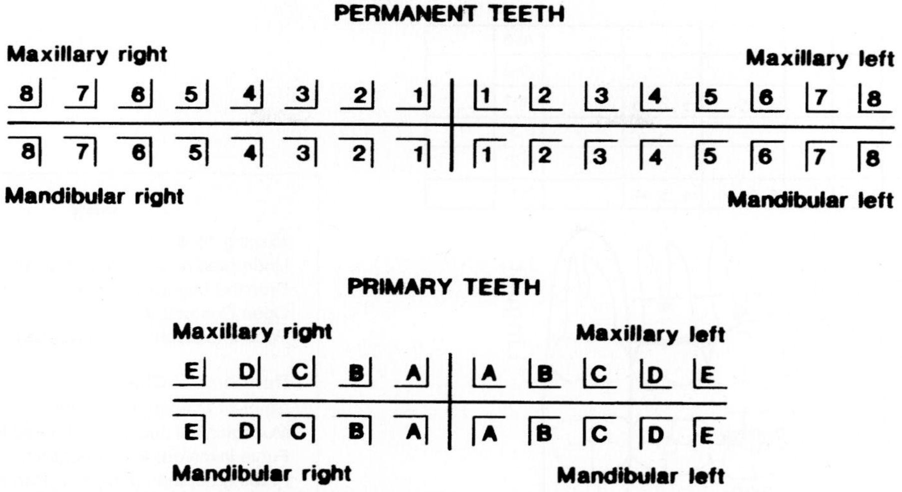

PERMANENT TEETH

Maxillary right   Maxillary left

8 | 7 | 6 | 5 | 4 | 3 | 2 | 1 | 1 | 2 | 3 | 4 | 5 | 6 | 7 | 8

8 | 7 | 6 | 5 | 4 | 3 | 2 | 1 | 1 | 2 | 3 | 4 | 5 | 6 | 7 | 8

Mandibular right   Mandibular left

PRIMARY TEETH

Maxillary right   Maxillary left

E | D | C | B | A | A | B | C | D | E

E | D | C | B | A | A | B | C | D | E

Mandibular right   Mandibular left

FIGURE 8-3 **Palmer System Tooth Numbering.** Each permanent tooth is designated by number 1 through 8, starting at the central incisor of each quadrant. Quadrants are designated by horizontal and vertical lines. Primary teeth are identified by the letters A through E, starting at the central incisor.

■ *Periodontal chart.* Indicates clinical features of the periodontium.

■ The use of separate chart forms to record the special features of periodontal and dental finding is preferable, but the two may be combined on one chart.

■ Dental and periodontal charts are updated routinely to record changes in the patient's oral features over time.

■ Neatness in the markings of symbols, drawings, and labels goes hand in hand with the accuracy of the examination itself.

An accurate, detailed, and carefully recorded charting is used as follows:

A. For Care Planning

The charting is a graphic representation of the existing condition of the patient's teeth and periodontium from which needed treatment procedures can be organized into a treatment plan.

B. For Treatment

During dental and dental hygiene appointments, the charting is useful for guiding specific procedures.

C. For Evaluation

The outcome and degree of lasting effects of treatment are determined by comparing the findings of the initially recorded examination with periodic follow-up examinations.

D. For Protection

In the event of misunderstanding by a patient, or if legal questions should arise, the records and chartings are realistic evidence.

E. For Identification

In the event of emergency, accident, or disaster, a patient may be identified by the teeth for which a record has been maintained.

II. FORMS USED FOR CHARTING

■ Many variations of chart forms are in current use, some available commercially, some designed by the individual practitioner to meet particular needs.

■ Specifications for an adequate form include ample space to chart neatly, accurately, and completely; to label as needed for clarity; and to record in a manner that can be interpreted by all who use it.

■ *Anatomic Drawings of the Complete Teeth.* Figure 8-4 provides a typical example of a form that may be used for periodontal and/or dental charting.

■ *Geometric.* A diagrammatic representation that provides space to record findings for each tooth. Examples of geometric charting forms used to record a patient's disclosed biofilm for teaching personal disease control are shown in Figures 22-1 and 22-2 (pages 316 and 317).

III. SEQUENCE FOR CHARTING

A. Basic Entries

■ *Name, Birth Date.*
■ *Date of Examination.* Every entry must be dated.
■ *Missing Teeth.* When radiographs are available in advance, missing teeth can be charted before the clinic appointment. Whether dental or periodontal charting

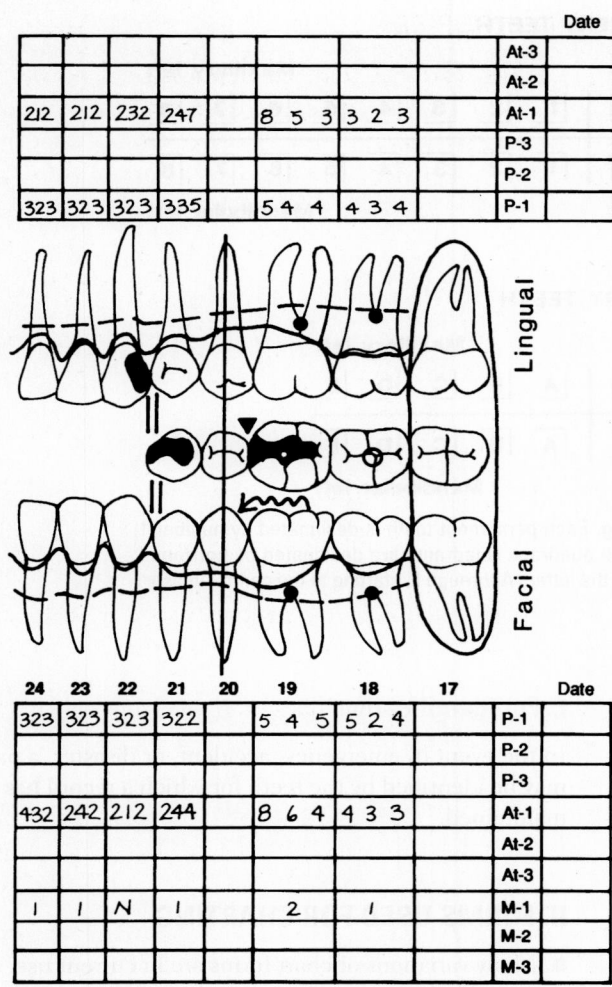

FIGURE 8-4 Periodontal and Dental Charting. Section of a charting (mandibular left quadrant) shows combined dental and periodontal charting. Dental caries and restorations are usually marked with colored pencils, such as blue for restorations and red for dental caries, on the anatomic crowns or roots. The gingival margin is clearly drawn to show areas of recession. Boxes at the apices of each tooth provide spaces for probing depths and clinical attachment level recordings, as well as for mobility notations.

Key

Missing Tooth: | or X
Unerupted or impacted: Encircle tooth
Drift and Migration: ⌇⌇⌇
Open Contact: ||
Food Impaction: ↓ (at occlusal)

Periodontal Chart
Gingival Margin: Black line
Mucogingival Junction: Dashed line
Furca involved: ● (in furcation)
Probing depths: (mm) P-1, P-2, P-3
Clinical attachment level: (mm) At-1, At-2, At-3

Dental Chart
Dental Caries: red
Restorations: blue
Defective Restoration: circle with red
Overhang: ▼ (at occlusal)
Mobility: (+, N, 1, 2, 3) M-1, M-2, M-3
Fremitus: F-1 (recorded on maxillary only)

is completed first, marking the missing teeth will be necessary.

B. Systematic Procedure

1. The use of a set routine is prerequisite to accomplishing a complete and accurate charting, not only for the tooth surface-to-surface pattern but also for the parts of the charting itself.
2. Charting of all of one kind of item for the entire mouth, rather than complete chartings of one tooth, helps to obtain accuracy because only one train of thought is required at a time.
   - For example, in the dental charting, record all the restorations first.
   - Then start again at the first tooth and chart all the deviations from normal.
   - Charting all restorations and deviations for each tooth separately is a less efficient method.

C. Before Patient Appointment

Radiographs and study casts prepared at an initial appointment before clinical examination for charting help to conserve patient chair time.

D. Radiographic Charting

- The following may be charted from radiographs without the presence of the patient: missing, unerupted, impacted teeth; endodontic restorations; overhanging margins of existing restorations; proximal surface carious lesions; and any other deviation from normal evident from the radiographs.
- Supplemental and confirmational observations and checks are made during the clinical examination with the patient. For example, when an overhanging restoration is noted and a carious lesion is suspected but not visible on the radiograph because the

restoration superimposes, examination by exploration is required.

E. Study Casts

Record the classification of occlusion (page 275 in Chapter 18).

PERIODONTAL RECORDS

- The patient's permanent records include the itemized findings of all the clinical and radiographic examinations.
- Prepare entries that are clear and easily understood by all who read them and use them in continuing treatment.
- Additions to the records are made to show the progress of treatment and comparative observations throughout the series of treatment appointments.
- After the periodontium has been brought to a state of health, a maintenance plan is outlined.
- At each succeeding appointment, new and comparative records and chartings are made.

I. CLINICAL OBSERVATIONS OF THE GINGIVA

Clinical observations are recorded either on the chart form or in the patient progress notes during each patient visit. Examine gingiva and record findings before disclosing agent is used for plaque-score.

A. Describe Gingiva

- Color, size, position, shape, consistency, and surface texture; extent of bleeding when probed; and areas where there is minimal attached gingiva (in Chapter 14, page 219, and Table 14-1, page 217).

B. Describe Distribution of Gingival Changes

Localized or generalized; specify the areas of severest disease involvement. Use tooth numbers to identify adjacent gingival tissue.

II. ITEMS TO BE CHARTED

- Missing teeth
- Location of bridges, pontics, and implants
- Gingival line (margin) and mucogingival lines (junctions)
- Probing depths
- Areas of suspected mucogingival involvement
- Furcation involvement
- Abnormal frenal attachments
- Mobility and fremitus of teeth

III. DEPOSITS

Deposits can be recorded on forms such as the one illustrated in **Figure 8-4** or on dental index forms, which are illustrated on page 316.

A. Stains

- *Extrinsic*. Record type of stain, color, distribution; specific location by tooth number; whether slight, moderate, or heavy.
- *Intrinsic*. Record separately from extrinsic and identify by type when known.

B. Soft Deposits

- *Food Debris*. Distribution and amount. Record location by teeth when the biofilm control instruction requires special emphasis on a particular area.
- *Dental Biofilm*.
  A. Record direct observations with or without disclosing agent; include distribution and degree or amount.
  B. Record biofilm film index or score (Chapter 22, pages 315–321).

C. Calculus

- Record distribution and amount of supragingival and subgingival calculus separately for treatment planning purposes.
- Record subgingival calculus in periodontal pockets on the probing chart illustrated in **Figure 8-4**.

IV. FACTORS RELATED TO OCCLUSION

Clinical signs of trauma from occlusion are described on page 279. The following list is for consideration with other records for the treatment planning.

A. Mobility of Teeth

Record degree of mobility for each tooth (in Chapter 15, page 245). In **Figure 8-4**, an example of a method for recording mobility is shown.

B. Fremitus (page 239)

- Fremitus determination is described in Chapter 15 (page 239).
- Record the significance in relation to mobility.

C. Possible Food Impaction Areas

- Inquire of patient where fibrous foods usually catch between the teeth.
- Use dental floss to identify inadequate contact areas that may contribute to food impaction. An example of one method for recording an open contact is shown by

the vertical parallel lines between teeth numbered 21 and 22 in **Figure 8-4**.

D. Occlusion-Related Habits

■ Observe for evidence of, and question patient concerning, such parafunctional habits as bruxism or clenching.
■ Note wear patterns and facets on study cast.
■ Note attrition.

V. RADIOGRAPHIC FINDINGS

Specific notes are made to correlate the radiographic findings with the clinical observations just listed. Details of radiographic findings in periodontal disease are described on page 240. The following are recorded in relation to the specific teeth involved:

■ Height of bone as related to the cementoenamel junction.
■ Horizontal or angular shape of remaining bone.
■ Intact, broken, or missing crestal lamina dura.
■ Furcation involvement.
■ Widening of periodontal ligament space.
■ Overhanging fillings, large carious lesions, and other dental biofilm–retention factors.

VI. SEVERITY OF PERIODONTAL DISEASE

■ Determination of the severity of periodontal disease is based on analysis of gingival changes, periodontal probing recordings, sites of bleeding on probing, clinical attachment level, tooth mobility and fremitus, and the radiographic findings.
■ A dental or dental hygiene diagnosis statement can be developed using the disease classifications outlined in Table 16-1 as a reference.

DENTAL RECORDS

The patient's permanent records include the itemized clinical and radiographic findings related to the teeth along with subjective symptoms reported by the patient. Information about conditions related to the teeth is included in Chapter 17. Occlusion and mobility of teeth have been included with the periodontal examination because the causes of mobility are related to the patient's periodontal status.

■ After initial entries are recorded, additions are made to show the progress of treatment. At each periodic maintenance visit, new and comparative records and chartings are prepared.
■ The need for meticulous examination and recording cannot be overemphasized. Finding and recording a carious lesion may mean saving a tooth for the

patient's lifetime; inadvertent neglect of a tooth may lead eventually to a need for endodontic therapy or even extraction.

I. THE ANATOMIC TOOTH CHART FORM

Figure 8-4 is an example of a quadrant of dental charting using anatomic tooth drawings. When charting, clinical and radiographic findings are coordinated.

II. ITEMS TO BE CHARTED

A list of basic items to be charted includes:

■ Missing teeth.
■ Existing restorations. Note restorative materials so that the care plan can designate selective polishing agents that will not harm the surfaces of restorations.
■ Fixed and removable prostheses.
■ Dental sealants.
■ Overhangs, open contacts, open margins, and other irregularities.
■ Cavitated carious lesions and questionable demineralized noncavitated lesions.
■ Inadequate contact areas and observed proximal surface roughness. Use dental floss. Fraying of dental floss as it is passed over a rough proximal surface may mean the defective margin of a restoration, a sharp cavity margin, or dental calculus.
■ Pulp vitality. Record numbers in the permanent record. Chart forms sometimes include a specific place for the recording of such data.
■ Tooth sensitivity. The patient may report hypersensitive areas. Record the tooth number and surface for reference during the treatment phase.

CARE PLAN RECORDS

■ Along with a comprehensive dental treatment plan, a formal dental hygiene care plan that includes dental hygiene diagnostic statements and addresses the patient's risk factors is included in the patient's record.
■ Chapter 24, starting on page 352, provides more information about developing a dental hygiene care plan.
■ The initial care plan developed during an initial examination, as well as copies of updated plans are included as part of the comprehensive, permanent patient record.

INFORMED CONSENT

Documentation of informed consent obtained before initiating treatment is an essential component of each patient's record. Information about obtaining and documenting informed consent is found in Chapter 24 on page 358.

BOX 8-2	Essential Components of a Patient Progress Note

- Purpose of the visit
- History review
- Assessment findings
- Description of treatment provided
- Drugs (including topical or local anesthetic) administered during treatment or prescribed by the dentist.
- Self care and other instructions provided
- Referrals, consultations with physician or dental specialist
- Laboratory tests ordered; results of laboratory tests
- Next visit appointments scheduled or recommended; appointment cancellations.
- Details related to patient conversations, including telephone and e-mail.
- Signature of clinician and date

BOX 8-3	Example of a Progress Note Using the SOAP Format

Patient presents for reassessment of self-oral care 2 weeks following oral hygiene instruction.

S = Patient states that he notices a reduction in biofilm following oral self-care instructions provided at the previous appointment.

O = Today's "Plaque-Free Score" = 89%; SBI score = 2.

A = "Plaque-Free Score" compared with previous score of 22%; SBI score compared with previous score of 5. Significant improvement in biofilm control noted in all areas except facial surfaces of maxillary molars.

P = Patient congratulated on areas of success. Additional instruction provided specifically related to biofilm removal on posterior facial and proximal tooth surfaces. Patient observed while brushing and flossing maxillary molar areas using a mirror. Next visit: 3 months re-evaluation.

Signed: _____, RDH Date: _____.

PATIENT VISIT AND TREATMENT RECORDS

I. PURPOSE

Documentation completed during or immediately following a patient visit, sometimes referred to as a progress note, is a chronological history of treatment received by the patient during each appointment.[16] Dental hygiene progress notes document all aspects of the dental hygiene process of care and records all interactions between the patient and the practice.[3]

II. ESSENTIALS OF GOOD PROGRESS NOTES[1,16]

Each entry in the patient record is dated and signed by the clinician. In addition to documentation about treatment rendered, essential components of the patient progress note are listed in **Box 8-2**.

Information that is **never** included in the patient record includes:

- The clinician's personal opinion
- Speculation
- Derogatory statements
- Information about financial matters, professional disputes, legal actions, or risk-management protocol

III. SYSTEMATIC DOCUMENTATION

- A systematic, standardized approach to writing patient progress notes assures that no details are missing from the patient's record.

- Many clinicians develop their own systematic approach to make sure documentation is comprehensive.
- Several more formalized documentation systems have been developed. One approach, which uses the acronym SOAP as a guide, is well accepted for use in the medical, and dental professions.[17–19]
- **Table 8-1** defines the components of the SOAP acronym and provides examples of factors that are included in patient progress notes.
- **Box 8-3** provides an example of a patient progress note written using the SOAP format.

IV. RISK REDUCTION AND LEGAL CONSIDERATIONS[1]

- Malpractice allegations can, unfortunately, occur against even a dental hygienist who routinely meets every standard when providing dental hygiene care.
- Because litigation can occur years after the patient visit when the details and even the patient may have been forgotten, excellent comprehensive documentation in each patient record entry is the best protection for the clinician against allegations of wrongdoing.

V. EXAMPLE PROGRESS NOTES

An example progress note, related to a clinical situation, can be reviewed in each chapter of this book.

	DESCRIPTION	EXAMPLES
TABLE 8-1	**COMPONENTS OF SOAP DOCUMENTATION AND EXAMPLES OF FACTORS TO INCLUDE IN PROGRESS NOTES**	

	DESCRIPTION	EXAMPLES
S	**Subjective** Characteristics perceived by the patient or clinician	■ Patient's age ■ Patient's gender ■ Type of appointment scheduled ■ Medical history findings ■ Patient's chief complaint ■ Patient's self-care regimen ■ Social history
O	**Objective** Characteristics observed during examination	■ Head and neck exam findings ■ Periodontal exam findings; bleeding; soft tissue condition ■ Hard tissue exam findings; current cavitated carious lesions and demineralized noncavitated lesions ■ Radiographic findings ■ Comparison of current findings with previous findings
A	**Assessment/Analysis** Identification of problems or patient needs	■ Risk factors for oral disease ■ Caries risk level ■ Calculus level ■ Current periodontal diagnosis/case type and status ■ Periodontal disease risk level
P	**Procedures** Interventions performed or planned	■ Dental hygiene interventions performed ■ Medicaments or local anesthesia applied and to which teeth ■ Consults with dentist or other health providers ■ Self-care instructions ■ Goals for patient improvement ■ Pending/planned dental hygiene interventions

Source: Jacks ME, Blue C, Murphy D. Short- and long-term effects of training on dental hygiene faculty members' capacity to write SOAP notes. *J Dent Educ.* 2008 Jun;72(6):719–24.

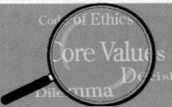 # Everyday Ethics

Mrs. Belvedere, the office manager in Dr. Grain's office, has online access to all electronic patient records from her computer at home. With Dr. Grain's permission, she often uses her home email to contact patients and insurance companies regarding treatment plans, insurance coverage, or financial records. Patients receive HIPAA information about confidentiality and security of their information, but are not told that Mrs. Belvedere has access to their records at her home. Hanna, who is a new dental hygienist in the office, inadvertently finds out that sensitive patient information is being sent out from the same home email account that is used by both Mrs. Belvedere's husband and her adult son. When Hanna approaches Dr. Grain about the potential breach in security of patient information, he seems unconcerned.

Questions for Consideration

1. What dental hygiene core values are being compromised if Hanna decides not to follow through to try to change the situation?
2. What standards of professional responsibility, identified in the ADHA code of ethics, apply in this situation?
3. Which ethical theories, as described in Table III-1 on page 114, can support Hanna as she decides how to approach Mrs. Belvedere and Dr. Grain to make changes in the way patient records and information are handled?

Factors To Teach The Patient

- Interpretation of all recordings; meaning of all numbers used, such as for probing depths.
- The importance of making a complete study of the patient's oral problems before beginning treatment.
- Advantages of cooperation and patience in furnishing information that will help dental personnel to interpret observations accurately so that the correct diagnosis and appropriate treatment plan can be made.
- Assurance that all information received is completely confidential.
  - Patient records are locked when the office is closed.
  - Access to patient records and computers that contain patient information is limited to only certain personnel.
  - Electronic transfer of patient information is secure.

References

1. Dym H. Risk management techniques for the general dentist and specialist. *Dent Clin North Am.* 2008 Jul;52(3):563–77, ix.
2. American Association of Dental Boards. Guidelines on the dental patient record. Chicago: American Association of Dental Boards; 2009. pp. 4–12.
3. American Dental Hygienists Association. Standards for clinical dental hygiene practice. Chicago: American Dental Hygienists' Association; 2008. p. 9.
4. Emmott L. Electronic dental records in dentistry. *J Am Coll Dent.* 2010 Winter;77(1):10–12.
5. Rhodes PR. The electronic patient record In: Rose LF, Mealey B, Genco RJ, Cohen DW, eds. *Periodontics, medicine, surgery, and implants.* St. Louis: Elsevier; 2004. pp. 163–71.
6. Hudis S. Converting to electronic dental records. *J Am Coll Dent.* 2010 Winter;77(1):13–15.
7. American Dental Association. Dental abbreviations, symbols and acronyms. 2nd ed. Chicago: American Dental Association; 2008. pp. 5–20.
8. Chasteen J, Murphy G, Forrey A, Heid D. The health insurance portability accountability act and the practice of dentistry in the United States: System security. *J Contemp Dent Pract.* 2004 Aug 15;5(3):158–67.
9. Chasteen J, Murphy G, Forrey A, Heid D. The Health Insurance Portability and Accountability Act: practice of dentistry in the United States: privacy and confidentiality. *J Contemp Dent Pract.* 2003 Feb 15;4(1):59–70.
10. Chasteen J, Murphy G, Forrey A, Heid D. The health insurance portability and accountability act and the practice of dentistry in the United States: electronic transactions. *J Contemp Dent Pract.* 2003 Nov 15;4(4):108–20.
11. Peck S, Peck L. A time for change of tooth numbering systems. *J Dent Educ.* 1993 Aug;57(8):643–7.
12. American Dental Association. System of Tooth Numbering and Radiograph Mounting. Chicago: American Dental Association; 1968, October.
13. Fédération Dentaire Internationale. Two-digit system of designating teeth. *Int Dent J.* 1971 March;21(1):104.
14. Türp JC, Alt KW. Designating teeth: The advantages of the FDI's two-digit system. *Quintessence Int.* 1995 Jul;26(7):501–4.
15. Palmer C. Palmer's dental notation. *Dent Cosmos.* 1891;33:194.
16. American Association of Dental Boards. op.cit. pp. 9–10.
17. Nunn PJ, Chaney SC. The SOAP system. *RDH.* 1994 Jun;14(6):22–24, 54.
18. Rethman J. Clean up your records with SOAP. S (subjective findings), O (objective findings), A (assessment), P (plan). *Dent Today.* 1995 Aug;14(8):80.
19. Sleszynski SL, Glonek T, Kuchera WA. Standardized medical record: a new outpatient osteopathic SOAP note form: validation of a standardized office form against physician's progress notes. *J Am Osteopath Assoc.* 1999 Oct;99(10):516–29.

Assessment

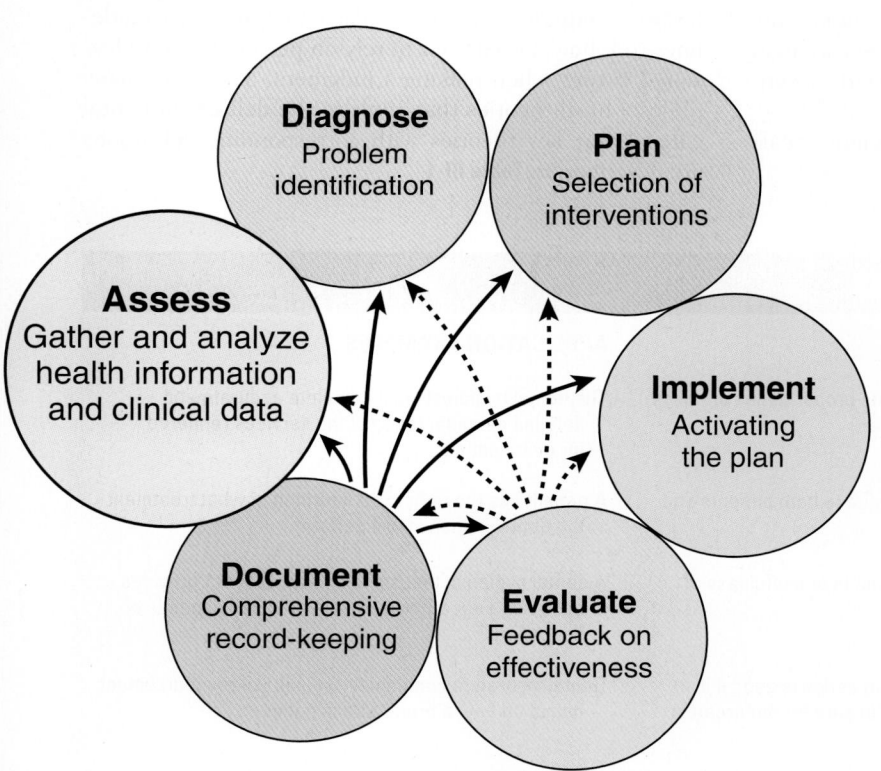

FIGURE III.1 **The Dental Hygiene Process of Care.**

Diagnose
Problem
identification

Plan
Selection of
interventions

Assess
Gather and analyze
health information
and clinical data

Implement
Activating
the plan

Document
Comprehensive
record-keeping

Evaluate
Feedback on
effectiveness

INTRODUCTION

The chapters in this section include descriptions for the preparation and assembling of materials and information that will be analyzed to develop an individualized care plan. Basic procedures for collecting data are outlined in the chapters in this section. Critical analysis of the data identifies patient problems that will be used to formulate the dental hygiene diagnosis.

THE DENTAL HYGIENE PROCESS OF CARE

Assessment is the first step in the dental hygiene process of care, as illustrated in **Figure III-1** on the previous page. Basically, the initial assessment is a collection of all pertinent facts and materials to use in planning care and as a guide during all treatment. After care has been provided, recollection of assessment data evaluates the outcomes of dental hygiene interventions.

An efficiently conducted assessment can benefit the patient. The documentation and critical analysis of assessment findings include the following:

- Provide a permanent, continuing, accurate, and complete record of the patient's oral and general health.
- Help formulate dental hygiene diagnostic statements from which a patient-oriented dental hygiene care plan can be formulated that outlines individualized preventive and treatment interventions.
- Guide instrumentation during dental hygiene treatment.

- Provide the basis to correlate dental hygiene care with the comprehensive dental treatment plan.

Built into the sequence of clinical procedures is the initiation of steps for arresting oral disease processes and controlling etiologic factors. The prevention plan is geared to help prevent episodes of recurrence of oral disease. Comprehensive and accruate assessment data aids the dental hygienist in identifying the following:

- Health-related factors that affect the management of dental hygiene care
- Risk factors for oral or systemic disease
- Description of personal and culturally related habits that affect oral status
- Health-related attitudes of the patient and the value placed on maintenance of oral health and the prevention of disease
- Oral hygiene methods and communication strategies that meet the patient's needs

ETHICAL APPLICATIONS

An ethical theory offers a general view or approach to an ethical problem. In healthcare, theories are often based on norms or rules that ask which type of action is morally correct. A dental professional may consider the most favorable outcome of a particular situation, what guidelines to follow, or whether to rely on personal and professional virtues when making a judgment. There are many philosophical theories that apply to the delivery of dental care. A few key theories with corresponding definitions are described in **Table III-1**.

TABLE III-1	SOME ETHICAL THEORIES	
THEORY	**DEFINITION**	**APPLICATION EXAMPLES**
Deontology	A study of rules by following the proper duties or obligations pertaining to one's role.	The dental hygienist must complete accurate and detailed documentation of the services rendered for every patient.
Rights Theory	Focusing on what is rightfully due to both patients and providers.	A patient has the right to be informed of what treatment the dental hygienist will perform.
Teleology	Concerned with the consequences or usefulness of one's actions, goal-driven.	A dental hygienist that stays on schedule but provides chairside education to meet the individual needs of the patient.
Utilitarianism	A form of teleology that says an action is good if it brings about the greatest pleasure for the greatest number of people.	Dental insurance companies set limits of reimbursement based on how a procedure is coded
Virtue Ethics	A moral theory that is concerned with the virtuous qualities of a professional's character (compassion, empathy, honesty, respect, wisdom, patience).	Always being honest and offering the best care to every patient.

CHAPTER 9

Personal, Dental, and Medical Histories

CHARLOTTE J. WYCHE, RDH, MS
ESTHER M. WILKINS, BS, RDH, DMD

Chapter Outline

INTRODUCTION

For safe, scientific dental and dental hygiene care, a meaningful, complete patient health history is an essential part of the complete assessment. With successive appointments, the history is carefully reviewed and considered along with new findings. Key words relating to the preparation and use of the histories are defined in **Box 9-1**.

The history directs and guides steps to be taken in preparation for, during, and following appointments. Some important points about the patient history are listed here.

■ The history is needed before oral examination procedures with periodontal probe and explorer are carried out.

■ The use of instruments that would manipulate the soft tissue around the teeth is contraindicated until after it has been determined whether antibiotic premedication is required.

■ When a question exists about the medical history as described by the patient, or when an unusual or abnormal condition is observed, consultation with the patient's physician or referral for examination of the patient who does not have a physician is mandatory.

■ Even emergency treatment, such as for the relief of pain, is postponed tentatively or kept to a minimum until the patient's status is determined.

BOX 9-1 **Key Words**

Personal, Medical, and Dental Histories

Allergy: state of abnormal and individual hypersensitivity acquired through exposure to a particular allergen.

Antibiotic premedication: provision of an effective antibiotic before invasive clinical procedures that can create a transient bacteremia, which, in turn, can cause infective endocarditis or other serious infection.

Bacteremia: presence of microorganisms in the bloodstream.

Drug interaction: a change in the effect of one drug when a second drug is introduced concomitantly; the change may be desirable, adverse, or inconsequential.

Forensic: pertaining to or applied in legal proceedings.

Forensic dentistry: dentolegal science; the relation and application of dental facts to legal problems, as in using the teeth for identifying the dead.

Hematogenous: produced or derived from blood; disseminated through the bloodstream.

Immunocompromised: when the immune response is attenuated by administration of immunosuppressive drugs, by irradiation, by malnutrition, or by certain disease processes.

Informed consent: a medicolegal document that holds providers responsible for ensuring that patients understand the risks and benefits of a procedure or medication before it is administered.

OTC: over the counter; nonprescription drug; pertains to distribution of drugs directly to the public without prescription.

PDR: *Physicians' Desk Reference*; contains current information about the actions, side effects, and interactions of drugs; a new edition is published annually.

Premedication: preliminary medication; may be for the purpose of allaying apprehension, preventing bacteremia, or otherwise facilitating the clinical procedure.

SBE: subacute bacterial endocarditis, now called infective endocarditis.

I. SIGNIFICANCE

The significance of taking a complete and accurate patient history cannot be overestimated because:

- Oral conditions reflect the general health of the patient; dental procedures may complicate or be complicated by existing pathologic or physiologic conditions elsewhere in the body.
- General health factors influence response to treatment, such as tissue healing, and thereby influence the outcomes that may be expected from oral care.
- The state of the patient's health is constantly changing. Therefore, the history represents only the period in the patient's life during which the history was made.

II. PURPOSES OF THE HISTORY

Carefully prepared personal, medical, and dental histories are used in comprehensive patient care to:

- Provide information pertinent to the etiology and diagnosis of oral conditions and the total patient care plan.
- Reveal conditions that necessitate precautions, modifications, or adaptations during appointments to ensure that dental and dental hygiene procedures will not harm the patient and that emergency situations will be prevented.
- Aid in the identification of possible unrecognized conditions for which the patient will be referred for further diagnosis and treatment.
- Permit appraisal of the general health and nutritional status, which, in turn, contributes to the prognosis of success in patient care and instruction.

- Give insight into emotional and psychological factors, attitudes, and prejudices that may affect present appointments as well as continuing care.
- Document records for reference and comparison over a series of appointments for periodic follow-up.
- Furnish evidence in legal matters if questions arise.[1]
- Identify cultural beliefs and practices that affect risk for oral disease.
- Determine ethnic/racial influences on risk factors for oral disease.

HISTORY PREPARATION

The general methods in current use for obtaining a health history are the *interview*, the *questionnaire*, or a combination of the two. There are several systems for obtaining the history.

I. SYSTEMS

A. Preappointment Information

- Basic information obtained before the initial assessment appointment can save time and facilitate the process.
- A brief telephone screening interview can help determine potential medical problems and need for premedication, and it can identify medically compromised or physically challenged patients for whom modifications in routine care may be needed.

B. Self-History

- Because a self-history can be prepared at home, the history form can be mailed to the patient in advance of the first appointment.

■ This kind of form might include some items that can be checked or circled, as in a questionnaire, and some space to allow the patient to provide additional information.

C. Brief History

■ A brief history of vital items is obtained during an initial emergency visit; a more complete history is obtained at a succeeding appointment.

■ Purposes of brief history are to prepare for emergency care and to learn of any condition that may contraindicate instrumentation.

■ Brief history may be in the form of a questionnaire; an interview for follow-up provides opportunity for individual evaluation.

D. Complete History

■ A complete patient history is made at the initial visit and is a combination of interview and questionnaire.

■ At successive appointments, the complete history is reviewed with the patient and changes are considered when planning patient care.

II. RECORD FORMS

A. Basic History Forms

■ Many varying forms are in current use.

■ Forms are available commercially or from the American Dental Association (ADA),[2] but many dentists and dental hygienists prefer to develop their own and have a form printed to their specifications.

■ ADA and other organizations have basic history forms that have been translated into a variety of languages. Many are available on the Internet.

B. Characteristics of an Adequate Form

The number of items or questions included is not necessarily indicative of the value of the form. The extensive and involved form may be as practical or impractical as the brief checklist that permits no detailed description. Success in use depends on function and a clear common understanding of the meaning of the recorded information to all who refer to it.

An adequate basic history form will:

■ Provide for conventional notation of important details in a logical sequence.

■ Permit quick identification of special needs of a patient when the history is reviewed before each appointment.

■ Allow ample space to record the patient's own words whenever possible in the interview method, or for self-expression by the patient on a questionnaire.

■ Have space for notes concerning attitudes and knowledge as stated or displayed by the patient during the history-taking or other later appointments.

■ Be of a size consistent with the complete patient record forms for filing and ready availability.

■ Be provided, whenever possible, in a version that has been translated to the patient's primary or dominant language.

C. Supplementary Forms

■ A secondary, more detailed questionnaire can be used to determine additional information for specialized topics.

■ The basic questionnaire reveals whether the topic applies to the individual, and if the answer is positive, additional information is requested.

Example. Simple questions on the basic questionnaire indicate the use of tobacco products. Completion of another questionnaire provides details about the type of tobacco used and frequency of use. Figure 34-4 (page 506) illustrates a tobacco use assessment form.

III. INTRODUCTION TO THE PATIENT

■ Educate the patient about why the information requested in the history is essential before treatment can be undertaken.

■ Convey the idea that oral health and general health are interrelated, without creating undue alarm concerning potential ill effects or harmful sequelae from required treatment.

■ To build rapport, allow children to participate in their history preparation, but most of the information will need to be supplied by a parent or legal guardian. The signature of the responsible adult is required on the record.

IV. LIMITATIONS OF A HISTORY

Many patients cannot or will not provide complete or, in certain cases, correct information when answering medical or dental history questions. Reasons for inaccuracy or incompleteness of information can include:

■ Problems related to the method of obtaining the histories, how the questions are worded, or an inadvertent lack of neutrality in the attitude of the person preparing the history.

■ Difficulty in comprehending a self-administered test because the patient cannot read, or has a language barrier.

■ The location in which the questionnaire is completed. A crowded reception area where other patients can see the form and the checks made does not provide sufficient privacy.

■ The patient's limited knowledge and inability to understand the relationship between certain diseases or conditions and dental treatment. Information may seem irrelevant, so it is withheld.

■ Reticence to discuss a health condition that may be embarrassing, such as history of infectious or communicable disease. The patient may fear refusal of treatment, particularly if such had been a previous experience in other dental practices.

THE QUESTIONNAIRE

Positive findings on a questionnaire are explained further in a personal interview. A questionnaire by itself cannot be expected to satisfy the overall purposes of the history, but it can be adapted best to phases of the personal history, some aspects of the dental history, and factual information in the medical history.

I. TYPES OF QUESTIONS

The health questionnaires available from the American Dental Association (adult questionnaire in **Figure 9-1** and child questionnaire in **Figure 9-2**) provide useful examples of questions essential to patient evaluation.[2]

A. System Oriented

- Direct questions or topics that check whether the patient has had a disease of, for example, the digestive system, respiratory system, or urinary system may be used.
- The questions may contain references to body parts, for example, the stomach, lungs, kidneys.
- Questions can then be directed to the specific disease state and the dates and duration.

B. Disease Oriented

- A typical set of questions for the patient to check may start with "Do you have, or have you had, any of the following diseases or problems?"
- A listing under that question contains such items as diabetes, asthma, or rheumatic fever arranged alphabetically or grouped by systems or body organs.
- Follow-up questions can determine dates of illness, severity, and outcome.

C. Symptom Oriented

- In the absence of previous or current disease states, questions may lead to a suspicion of a condition, which, in turn, can provide an opportunity to recommend and encourage the patient to schedule an examination by a physician.
- Examples of the symptom-oriented questions are "Are you thirsty much of the time?" "Does your mouth frequently become dry?" or "Do you have to urinate (pass water) more than six times a day?"
- Positive answers could lead to tests for diabetes detection.

D. Culture Oriented

Questions related to the patient's cultural background can help to:

- Identify ethnic or gender-related increase in risk for systematic or oral disease.
- Determine traditional culturally related health/illness behaviors that may influence dental hygiene interventions or recommendations.
- Identify herbal preparations or other traditional medications used by the patient that may affect oral care or risk for disease.

II. ADVANTAGES OF A QUESTIONNAIRE

- Broad in scope; useful during the interview to identify positive areas that need additional clarification.
- Time-saving.
- Consistent; all selected questions are included, and none is omitted because of time or other factors.
- Patient has time to think over the answers; not under pressure, nor under the eyes of the interviewer.
- Patient may write information that might not be expressed directly in an interview.
- Legal aspects of a written record with patient's signature.

III. DISADVANTAGES OF A QUESTIONNAIRE (IF USED ALONE WITHOUT A FOLLOW-UP INTERVIEW)

- Impersonal; no opportunity to develop rapport.
- Inflexible; no provision for additional questioning in areas of specific importance to an individual patient.

THE INTERVIEW

In long-range planning for the patient's health, much more is involved than asking questions and receiving answers. The rapport established at the time of the interview contributes to the continued cooperation of the patient.

I. PARTICIPANTS

- The interviewer is alone with the patient or parent of the child patient and, if necessary, a qualified professional translator/interpreter.
- The history is never to be taken in a reception area when other patients are present.

II. SETTING

- A consultation room or office is preferred; move the patient away from the atmosphere of the treatment room, where thoughts may be on the techniques to be performed.
- The treatment room may be the only available place with privacy. If the treatment room is used for a patient interview:
  A. Seat patient comfortably in upright position.
  B. Turn off running water and dental light, and close the door.
  C. Sit on clinician's stool to be at eye level with the patient.

Health History Form

ADA.
American Dental Association
www.ada.org

E-mail: _____ Today's Date: _____

As required by law, our office adheres to written policies and procedures to protect the privacy of information about you that we create, receive or maintain. Your answers are for our records only and will be kept confidential subject to applicable laws. Please note that you will be asked some questions about your responses to this questionnaire and there may be additional questions concerning your health. This information is vital to allow us to provide appropriate care for you. This office does not use this information to discriminate.

Name: _____
    Last   First   Middle

Home Phone: *Include area code* ( )

Business/Cell Phone: *Include area code* ( )

Address: _____
    Mailing address

City: _____ State: _____ Zip: _____

Occupation: _____

Height: _____ Weight: _____ Date of birth: _____ Sex: M F

SS# or Patient ID: _____ Emergency Contact: _____ Relationship: _____ Home Phone: ( ) Cell Phone: ( )
    Include area codes

If you are completing this form for another person, what is your relationship to that person?

Your Name _____ Relationship _____

Do you have any of the following diseases or problems:
    (Check DK if you Don't Know the answer to the question)

	Yes	No	DK
Active Tuberculosis	☐	☐	☐
Persistent cough greater than a 3 week duration	☐	☐	☐
Cough that produces blood	☐	☐	☐
Been exposed to anyone with tuberculosis	☐	☐	☐

If you answer yes to any of the 4 items above, please stop and return this form to the receptionist.

Dental Information *For the following questions, please mark (X) your responses to the following questions.*

	Yes	No	DK
Do your gums bleed when you brush or floss?	☐	☐	☐
Are your teeth sensitive to cold, hot, sweets or pressure?	☐	☐	☐
Does food or floss catch between your teeth?	☐	☐	☐
Is your mouth dry?	☐	☐	☐
Have you had any periodontal (gum) treatments?	☐	☐	☐
Have you ever had orthodontic (braces) treatment?	☐	☐	☐
Have you had any problems associated with previous dental treatment?	☐	☐	☐
Is your home water supply fluoridated?	☐	☐	☐
Do you drink bottled or filtered water?	☐	☐	☐
If yes, how often? Circle one: DAILY / WEEKLY / OCCASIONALLY			
Are you currently experiencing dental pain or discomfort?	☐	☐	☐

	Yes	No	DK
Do you have earaches or neck pains?	☐	☐	☐
Do you have any clicking, popping or discomfort in the jaw?	☐	☐	☐
Do you brux or grind your teeth?	☐	☐	☐
Do you have sores or ulcers in your mouth?	☐	☐	☐
Do you wear dentures or partials?	☐	☐	☐
Do you participate in active recreational activities?	☐	☐	☐
Have you ever had a serious injury to your head or mouth?	☐	☐	☐

Date of your last dental exam: _____
What was done at that time? _____

Date of last dental x-rays: _____

What is the reason for your dental visit today? _____

How do you feel about your smile? _____

Medical Information *Please mark (X) your response to indicate if you have or have not had any of the following diseases or problems.*

	Yes	No	DK
Are you now under the care of a physician?	☐	☐	☐

Physician Name: _____ Phone: *Include area code* ( )

Address/City/State/Zip: _____

	Yes	No	DK
Are you in good health?	☐	☐	☐
Has there been any change in your general health within the past year?	☐	☐	☐

If yes, what condition is being treated? _____

Date of last physical exam: _____

	Yes	No	DK
Have you had a serious illness, operation or been hospitalized in the past 5 years?	☐	☐	☐

If yes, what was the illness or problem? _____

	Yes	No	DK
Are you taking or have you recently taken any prescription or over the counter medicine(s)?	☐	☐	☐

If so, please list all, including vitamins, natural or herbal preparations and/or diet supplements:

_____
_____
_____
_____

FIGURE 9-1 Adult Health History Form. (Copyright © 2010 American Dental Association. All rights reserved. Reprinted by permission). (*continued*)

Medical Information *Please mark (X) your response to indicate if you have or have not had any of the following diseases or problems.*

(Check DK if you Don't Know the answer to the question)	Yes	No	DK
Do you wear contact lenses?	☐	☐	☐

Joint Replacement. Have you had an orthopedic total joint (hip, knee, elbow, finger) replacement? ☐ ☐ ☐
Date: _____ If yes, have you had any complications?_____

Are you taking or scheduled to begin taking either of the medications, alendronate (Fosamax®) or risedronate (Actonel®) for osteoporosis or Paget's disease? ☐ ☐ ☐

Since 2001, were you treated or are you presently scheduled to begin treatment with the intravenous bisphosphonates (Aredia® or Zometa®) for bone pain, hypercalcemia or skeletal complications resulting from Paget's disease, multiple myeloma or metastatic cancer? ☐ ☐ ☐
Date Treatment began: _____

	Yes	No	DK
Do you use controlled substances (drugs)?	☐	☐	☐
Do you use tobacco (smoking, snuff, chew, bidis)?	☐	☐	☐

If so, how interested are you in stopping?
(Circle one) VERY / SOMEWHAT / NOT INTERESTED

Do you drink alcoholic beverages? ☐ ☐ ☐
If yes, how much alcohol did you drink in the last 24 hours? _____
If yes, how much do you typically drink In a week? _____

WOMEN ONLY Are you:
	Yes	No	DK
Pregnant?	☐	☐	☐
Number of weeks: _____			
Taking birth control pills or hormonal replacement?	☐	☐	☐
Nursing?	☐	☐	☐

Allergies - Are you allergic to or have you had a reaction to: To all **yes** responses, specify type of reaction.

	Yes	No	DK
Local anesthetics_____	☐	☐	☐
Aspirin _____	☐	☐	☐
Penicillin or other antibiotics_____	☐	☐	☐
Barbiturates, sedatives, or sleeping pills _____	☐	☐	☐
Sulfa drugs _____	☐	☐	☐
Codeine or other narcotics_____	☐	☐	☐

	Yes	No	DK
Metals_____	☐	☐	☐
Latex (rubber) _____	☐	☐	☐
Iodine _____	☐	☐	☐
Hay fever/seasonal _____	☐	☐	☐
Animals_____	☐	☐	☐
Food _____	☐	☐	☐
Other _____	☐	☐	☐

Please mark (X) your response to indicate if you have or have not had any of the following diseases or problems.

	Yes	No	DK
Artificial (prosthetic) heart valve	☐	☐	☐
Previous infective endocarditis	☐	☐	☐
Damaged valves in transplanted heart	☐	☐	☐
Congenital heart disease (CHD)			
Unrepaired, cyanotic CHD	☐	☐	☐
Repaired (completely) in last 6 months	☐	☐	☐
Repaired CHD with residual defects	☐	☐	☐

Except for the conditions listed above, antibiotic prophylaxis is no longer recommended for any other form of CHD.

	Yes	No	DK		Yes	No	DK
Cardiovascular disease.	☐	☐	☐	Mitral valve prolapse	☐	☐	☐
Angina	☐	☐	☐	Pacemaker	☐	☐	☐
Arteriosclerosis	☐	☐	☐	Rheumatic fever	☐	☐	☐
Congestive heart failure	☐	☐	☐	Rheumatic heart disease	☐	☐	☐
Damaged heart valves	☐	☐	☐	Abnormal bleeding	☐	☐	☐
Heart attack	☐	☐	☐	Anemia	☐	☐	☐
Heart murmur	☐	☐	☐	Blood transfusion	☐	☐	☐
Low blood pressure	☐	☐	☐	If yes, date:_____			
High blood pressure	☐	☐	☐	Hemophilia	☐	☐	☐
Other congenital heart				AIDS or HIV infection	☐	☐	☐
defects	☐	☐	☐	Arthritis	☐	☐	☐

	Yes	No	DK
Autoimmune disease	☐	☐	☐
Rheumatoid arthritis	☐	☐	☐
Systemic lupus erythematosus	☐	☐	☐
Asthma	☐	☐	☐
Bronchitis	☐	☐	☐
Emphysema	☐	☐	☐
Sinus trouble	☐	☐	☐
Tuberculosis	☐	☐	☐
Cancer/Chemotherapy/ Radiation Treatment	☐	☐	☐
Chest pain upon exertion	☐	☐	☐
Chronic pain	☐	☐	☐
Diabetes Type I or II	☐	☐	☐
Eating disorder	☐	☐	☐
Malnutrition	☐	☐	☐
Gastrointestinal disease	☐	☐	☐
G.E. Reflux/persistent heartburn	☐	☐	☐
Ulcers	☐	☐	☐
Thyroid problems	☐	☐	☐
Stroke	☐	☐	☐
Glaucoma	☐	☐	☐

	Yes	No	DK
Hepatitis, jaundice or liver disease	☐	☐	☐
Epilepsy	☐	☐	☐
Fainting spells or seizures	☐	☐	☐
Neurological disorders	☐	☐	☐
If yes, specify:_____			
Sleep disorder	☐	☐	☐
Mental health disorders	☐	☐	☐
Specify:_____			
Recurrent Infections	☐	☐	☐
Type of infection:_____			
Kidney problems	☐	☐	☐
Night sweats	☐	☐	☐
Osteoporosis	☐	☐	☐
Persistent swollen glands in neck	☐	☐	☐
Severe headaches/ migraines	☐	☐	☐
Severe or rapid weight loss	☐	☐	☐
Sexually transmitted disease	☐	☐	☐
Excessive urination	☐	☐	☐

Has a physician or previous dentist recommended that you take antibiotics prior to your dental treatment? ☐ ☐ ☐

Name of physician or dentist making recommendation:	Phone:

Do you have any disease, condition, or problem not listed above that you think I should know about? ☐ ☐ ☐
Please explain:

NOTE: Both Doctor and patient are encouraged to discuss any and all relevant patient health issues prior to treatment.
I certify that I have read and understand the above and that the information given on this form is accurate. I understand the importance of a truthful health history and that my dentist and his/her staff will rely on this information for treating me. I acknowledge that my questions, if any, about inquiries set forth above have been answered to my satisfaction. I will not hold my dentist, or any other member of his/her staff, responsible for any action they take or do not take because of errors or omissions that I may have made in the completion of this form.

Signature of Patient/Legal Guardian:	Date:

FOR COMPLETION BY DENTIST

Comments:_____

FIGURE 9-1 (*continued*)

Child Health/Dental History Form

ADA
American Dental Association
www.ada.org

Patient's Name			Nickname	Date of Birth
LAST	FIRST	INITIAL		

Parent's/Guardian's Name	Relationship to Patient

Address			
PO OR MAILING ADDRESS	CITY	STATE	ZIP CODE

Phone		Sex M ❑ F ❑
Home	Work	

Have you (the parent/guardian) or the patient had any of the following diseases or problems?... ❑ Yes ❑ No
1. Active Tuberculosis, 2. Persistent cough greater than a three-week duration, 3.Cough that produces blood?
If you answer yes to any of the three items above, please stop and return this form to the receptionist.

Has the child had any history of, or conditions related to, any of the following:

❑ Anemia	❑ Cancer	❑ Epilepsy	❑ HIV +/AIDS	❑ Mononucleosis	❑ Thyroid
❑ Arthritis	❑ Cerebral Palsy	❑ Fainting	❑ Immunizations	❑ Mumps	❑ Tobacco/Drug Use
❑ Asthma	❑ Chicken Pox	❑ Growth Problems	❑ Kidney	❑ Pregnancy (teens)	❑ Tuberculosis
❑ Bladder	❑ Chronic Sinusitis	❑ Hearing	❑ Latex allergy	❑ Rheumatic fever	❑ Venereal Disease
❑ Bleeding disorders	❑ Diabetes	❑ Heart	❑ Liver	❑ Seizures	❑ Other_____
❑ Bones/Joints	❑ Ear Aches	❑ Hepatitis	❑ Measles	❑ Sickle cell	

Please list the name and phone number of the child's physician:

Name of Physician _____Phone _____

Child's History

                                            Yes No

1. Is the child taking any prescription and/or over the counter medications or vitamin supplements at this time? .... 1. ❑ ❑
   If yes, please list: _____
2. Is the child allergic to any medications, i.e. penicillin, antibiotics, or other drugs? If yes, please explain: _____ 2. ❑ ❑
3. Is the child allergic to anything else, such as certain foods? If yes, please explain: _____ 3. ❑ ❑
4. How would you describe the child's eating habits?_____
5. Has the child ever had a serious illness? If yes, when: _____ Please describe: _____ 5. ❑ ❑
6. Has the child ever been hospitalized? .... 6. ❑ ❑
7. Does the child have a history of any other illnesses? If yes, please list: _____ 7. ❑ ❑
8. Has the child ever received a general anesthetic? .... 8. ❑ ❑
9. Does the child have any inherited problems?... 9. ❑ ❑
10. Does the child have any speech difficulties?.. 10. ❑ ❑
11. Has the child ever had a blood transfusion?.. 11. ❑ ❑
12. Is the child physically, mentally, or emotionally impaired? .... 12. ❑ ❑
13. Does the child experience excessive bleeding when cut? .... 13. ❑ ❑
14. Is the child currently being treated for any illnesses? .... 14. ❑ ❑
15. Is this the child's first visit to a dentist? If not the first visit, what was the date of the last dentist visit? Date: _____ 15. ❑ ❑
16. Has the child had any problem with dental treatment in the past? .... 16. ❑ ❑
17. Has the child ever had dental radiographs (x-rays) exposed? .... 17. ❑ ❑
18. Has the child ever suffered any injuries to the mouth, head or teeth? .... 18. ❑ ❑
19. Has the child had any problems with the eruption or shedding of teeth? .... 19. ❑ ❑
20. Has the child had any orthodontic treatment? .... 20. ❑ ❑
21. **What type of water does your child drink?** ❑ City water ❑ Well water ❑ Bottled water ❑ Filtered water
22. **Does the child take fluoride supplements?** .... 22. ❑ ❑
23. **Is fluoride toothpaste used?** .... 23. ❑ ❑
24. How many times are the child's teeth brushed per day? _____ When are the teeth brushed?_____ 24. ❑ ❑
25. Does the child suck his/her thumb, fingers or pacifier?.. 25. ❑ ❑
26. At what age did the child stop bottle feeding? Age _____ Breast feeding? Age _____
27. Does child participate in active recreational activities? .... 27. ❑ ❑

NOTE: Both doctor and patient are encouraged to discuss any and all relevant patient health issues prior to treatment.
I certify that I have read and understand the above. I acknowledge that my questions, if any, about inquiries set forth above have been answered to my satisfaction. I will not hold my dentist, or any other member of his/her staff, responsible for any action they take or do not take because of errors or omissions that I may have made in the completion of this form.

Parent's/Guardian's Signature _____Date _____

For completion by dentist
Comments _____
_____
_____
_____

For Office Use Only: ❑ Medical Alert ❑ Premedication ❑ Allergies ❑ Anesthesia Reviewed by_____
Date _____

FIGURE 9-2 Child Health History Form. (Copyright © 2010 American Dental Association. All rights reserved. Reprinted by permission).

III. POINTERS FOR THE INTERVIEW

Interviewing involves communication between individuals. Communication implies the transmission or interchange of facts, attitudes, opinions, or thoughts, through words, gestures, or other means.

■ Through tactful but direct questioning, communication can be successful, and the patient will give all known information. Frequently, the patient is unaware of a health problem.

■ The most effective attitude for the clinician to portray is one of friendly understanding, reassurance, and acceptance.

■ Genuine interest and willingness to listen when a patient wishes to describe symptoms, complaints, or current health practices not only aids in establishing the rapport needed but frequently provides insight into the patient's real attitudes and prejudices.

■ By asking simple questions at first and more personal questions later after rapport has developed, the patient will be more relaxed and frank in answering.

■ Self-confidence and gentle efficiency on the part of the interviewer help give the patient a feeling of confidence.

■ Skill is required because tact, ingenuity, judgment, and cultural sensitivity are taxed to the fullest in the attempt to obtain accurate and complete information from the patient.

■ The culturally sensitive dental hygienist will be aware of nonverbal communication issues when interviewing a patient from a different culture (see Table 3-6, page 33).

IV. INTERVIEW FORM

■ The interviewer may use a structured form with places to check and fill in.

■ Another method is to record on blank sheets from questions created from a guide list of essential topics.

■ Either type of form can involve reference to the positive or negative answers on a previously completed questionnaire.

■ Familiarity with the items on the history permits the interviewer to be direct and informal without reading from a fixed list of topics, a method that may lack the personal touch necessary to gain the patient's confidence.

■ When appropriate, the patient's own words are recorded.

V. ADVANTAGES OF THE INTERVIEW

■ Personal contact contributes to development of rapport for future appointments.

■ Flexibility for individual needs; details obtained can be adapted for supplementary questioning.

VI. DISADVANTAGES OF THE INTERVIEW

■ Time consuming when not prefaced with questionnaire.

■ Unless a list is consulted, items of importance may be omitted.

■ Patient may be embarrassed to talk about personal conditions and may hold back significant information.

ITEMS INCLUDED IN THE HISTORY

Information obtained by means of the history is directly related to how the goals for patient care are established and will be accomplished. In **Tables 9-1–9-3**, items are listed with possible medications and other treatments the patient may have or has had, along with suggested considerations for appointment procedures.

■ In specialized practices, objectives may require increased emphasis on certain aspects.

■ The age group most frequently served would influence the material needed. *Example.* Parental history and prenatal and postnatal information may take on particular significance for the treatment of a small child; in a pediatric dentistry practice, a special form could be devised to include all essential items.

■ Insight and awareness shown while preparing the patient history depend on background knowledge of the manifestations of systemic diseases and the medications for various conditions.

■ Objectives for the items to include in the various parts of the history are listed here.

I. PERSONAL HISTORY (TABLE 9-1)

The basic objectives in gathering personal information about the patient are to:

■ Collect data essential for appointment planning and business aspects.

■ Identify need for approval for care of a minor patient and/or other legal requirements.

■ Determine the need for consultation with the patient's physician.

■ Determine culturally appropriate communication measures.

II. DENTAL HISTORY (TABLE 9-2)

The dental history contributes to the care provider's knowledge of:

■ The immediate problem, chief complaint, cause of present pain, or discomfort of any kind in the oral cavity.

■ Risk assessment forms, such as the American Association of Pediatric Dentistry Caries Risk

TABLE 9-1	ITEMS FOR THE PERSONAL HISTORY	

ITEMS TO RECORD IN PATIENT HISTORY	RECORD NOTES	CONSIDERATIONS FOR APPOINTMENT PROCEDURES
1. Name Addresses: residence and business Telephone numbers Gender Ethnic/racial category Marital status For child: name of parent or guardian For parent: age and sex of children	Accurate recording necessary for business aspects of dental practice	Aids in establishing rapport Instruction applicable to entire family Advice concerning fluorides for children Determine need for interpreter
2. Birth date	Whether of age or a minor Oral conditions related to age changes; diseases, healing, and other possible characteristics	Informed consent of parent or guardian necessary for care of minor or person with a mental handicap; signature is obtained Approach to patient instruction
3. Birthplace and residence in early years	Presence of fluoride in drinking water Food and eating patterns Conditions endemic to certain areas	Effects of fluoride on teeth Instruction in dietary needs adapted to cultural practices
4. Occupation: present and former Spouse's occupation For child: parent's occupation	May be a factor in etiology of certain diseases, dental stains, occlusal wear May affect diet, oral habits, general health	Instruction applied to specific needs Dexterity in use of self-care devices related to dexterity gained from occupation Influence on oral care of entire family For child: which parent will supervise and assist child in oral care
5. Physician	Name, address, and telephone number For consultation	Consultation indicated: (1) when disease symptoms are suspected but patient does not state (2) in an emergency (3) Medication/premedication
6. Referred by and address	To whom to send referral acknowledgment and appreciation	Contribution to rapport with patient Patient referred by another patient may have concept of the office procedures

Assessment Tool (CAT)[3] and the American Dental Association Caries Risk Assessment forms[4,5] provide essential information for planning individualized dental hygiene interventions based on the patient's needs.

- The previous dental hygiene and dental care as described by the patient, including preventive care, periodontal treatments, and the extent of restorative and prosthetic replacement, as well as any adverse effects.
- The attitude of the patient toward oral health and care of the mouth as may be indicated by previous periodic dental and dental hygiene treatments and family history of oral care.
- The personal daily care exercised by the patient as evidence of knowledge of the purposes of continuing care and of the value placed on the teeth and their supporting structures.

- The patient's current beliefs and attitudes about health, illness, and oral health.
- Culturally related health practices that may impact the patient's oral health.

III. MEDICAL HISTORY (TABLE 9-3)

Objectives of the medical history are to determine whether the patient has or has had any conditions in the following categories:

A. Conditions That May Complicate Certain Kinds of Dental and Dental Hygiene Treatment

Examples. Lowered resistance to infection; uncontrolled hypertension; or systemic disease that requires treatment before stressful dental procedures, particularly surgery, can be carried out.

TABLE 9-2	ITEMS FOR THE DENTAL HISTORY	

ITEMS TO RECORD IN THE HISTORY	RECORD NOTES	CONSIDERATIONS FOR APPOINTMENT PROCEDURES
1. Reason for present appointment	Chief complaint in patient's own words Pain or discomfort Onset, symptoms, duration of an acute condition	Need for immediate treatment Attitude toward dentistry and preventive care
2. Previous dental appointments	Date of last treatment Services performed Regularity	Patient knowledge concerning regular dental care Cooperation anticipated
3. Anesthetics used	Local, general Adverse reactions	Choice of anesthetic
4. Radiation history	Type, number, dates of dental and medical radiographs Therapeutic radiation Availability of dental radiographs from previous dentist Amount of exposure considered with exposure for medical purposes	Amount of exposure; limitations Patient's appreciation for need and use of radiographs
5. Family dental history	Parental tooth loss or maintenance	Attitude toward saving teeth and preventive dentistry Culturally related oral health beliefs and practices
6. Previous treatment	Type of treatment; frequency of maintenance appointments Whether referred to specialist	Attitude toward specialized care Previous familiarity with role of dental hygienist
a. periodontal	History of acute infection (necrotizing ulcerative gingivitis) Surgery; posttreatment healing	Attitude toward self-care and disease control
b. orthodontic	Age during treatment; completion date Previous problem Habit correction	For current treatment, consultation with orthodontist needed to determine instructions
c. endodontic	Dates, etiology	Periodic recheck
d. prosthodontic	Types of prostheses	Care of prostheses and abutment teeth
e. other	Extent of restorations Tooth loss Implants	Understanding prevention
7. Injuries to face or teeth	Causes and extent Fractured teeth or jaws	Limitation of opening Special care during healing
8. Temporomandibular joint	History of injury, discomfort, disease, dislocation Previous treatment	Effect on opening; accessibility during instrumentation
9. Habits	Clenching, bruxism Mouth breathing Biting objects; fingernails, pipe stem, thread, other Cheek or lip biting Patient awareness of habits	Tension of patient Instruction relative to effects of habits
10. Tobacco use	Form of tobacco, amount used Frequency Knowledge of effects on oral tissues	Instruction concerning oral effects Tobacco cessation program Periodontal risk Dental stains; dentifrice selection

TABLE 9-2	ITEMS FOR THE DENTAL HISTORY (*Continued*)	
ITEMS TO RECORD IN THE HISTORY	**RECORD NOTES**	**CONSIDERATIONS FOR APPOINTMENT PROCEDURES**
11. Fluorides	Systemic, topical, dates Residence during tooth development years Amount of fluoride in drinking water	Current preventive procedures and need for reevaluation

12. Biofilm control procedures	Toothbrushing: current procedures
	   type of brush (manual or powered)
	   texture of filaments
	   frequency of use
	   age of brush; frequency of having a new brush
	Dentifrice
	   name
	   how selected; reason
	Additional cleansing devices and frequency of use
	   dental floss
	   water irrigation
	   implants care
	Mouthrinse or other agents:
	   frequency, purpose
	Source of instruction in care of oral cavity
		Present practice and previous instruction
		New instruction needed; reception by patient
		Relation of techniques to prevention of dental caries and periodontal infections
		Supervision of child by parent: current practices
		Problems of habit change

B. Conditions or Diseases That Require Special Precautions or Premedication Before Treatment

Examples. Increased osteonecrosis risk related to previous treatment with bisphosphonates; or antibiotic coverage for the patient at risk for infective endocarditis (IE).

C. Conditions Under Treatment by a Physician That Require Medicating Drugs That May Influence or Contraindicate Certain Procedures

Examples. Anticoagulant therapy requires consultation with physician; antihypertensive drugs may alter the choice of local anesthetic used.

D. Gender or Ethnic/Racial Influences That Increase Risk for Systemic and Oral Disease

Example. American Indians and African Americans have increased risk for diabetes and a related increased risk for periodontal disease.

E. Allergic or Untoward Reactions

Examples. Latex hypersensitivity; medication or material for which there was a previous adverse reaction.

F. Diseases and Drugs With Manifestations in the Mouth

Examples. Hematologic disorders; phenytoin-induced gingival overgrowth; infectious diseases such as herpesvirus.

G. Communicable Diseases That Endanger the Dental Personnel

Examples. Active tuberculosis; viral hepatitis; herpes; syphilis.

H. Physiologic State of the Patient

Examples. Pregnancy; puberty; menopause; birth control pills.

IMMEDIATE APPLICATIONS OF PATIENT HISTORIES

- Information from the histories influences all aspects of total patient care and dental hygiene care planning.
- Immediate evaluation of the histories is necessary before proceeding to complete the assessment.
- Together with information from all other parts of the diagnostic work-up, the patient histories are essential for the preparation of the dental hygiene care plan.

I. MEDICAL CONSULTATION

Dentist and physician need to consult relative to the patient's current therapy and medications or to elements of the patient's past health status that could influence present dental treatment needs.[6]

(continued page 130)

TABLE 9-3	ITEMS FOR THE MEDICAL HISTORY		
ITEM TO RECORD IN HISTORY	**RECORD NOTES**	**MEDICATIONS AND TREATMENT MODALITIES**	**CONSIDERATIONS FOR APPOINTMENT PROCEDURES**
1. **General health and appearance**	Disabilities Overall impression of well-being Patient's appraisal of own health		Response, cooperation, and attitude to expect during appointments
2. **Medical examination**	Date of most recent examination Reason for the examination Tests performed; results Anticipated surgery	New prescriptions received Previous prescriptions continued	Verification with physician for added information Need for superior state of oral health in advance of surgery 1. When long recovery is expected and patient may miss maintenance appointments 2. Before transplant, heart surgery, or prosthesis
3. **Major illnesses, hospitalizations, surgeries**	Causes of illness Type and duration of treatment Anesthetics used Convalescence Course of healing: normal, not normal	Medications, treatments	Influence of illnesses on health and care of the oral cavity Anesthetic choice Expected outcome from gingival treatment
4. **Age factors**	Problems of health in different age groups Elderly: multiple disease entities; patient may need to bring the containers for identification of medications	See individual medical problem Update drug regimen at each appointment	Effects on dental and dental hygiene procedures and personal care
5. **Height and weight**	Weight changes over past years or months Obesity Undernourishment Child growth pattern	Diet pills Substance abuse	Marked weight change may be a symptom of undiagnosed disease; suggest referral for medical examination Influence on dietary instructions for oral health
6. **Medications prescribed by physician**	Reasons: relation to dental care Frequency Patient's regularity of taking Sugar content of liquid medicines, effect on dental caries (also true of over-the-counter [OTC] items) Previous history of bisphosphonate use	List all drugs by name Ask patient for drugs, medicine, injections, tonics, vitamins, patches, pills, capsules, to get a complete answer Dosage; route of administration	Consultation with physician concerning adjustments in dosage for dental or dental hygiene appointments Indications for premedication Side effects of drugs (e.g., increased risk of osteonecrosis with history of bisphosphonate use).
7. **Self-medication**	Type, frequency OTC preparations Substance abuse	Pain relievers Sleeping tablets Cough syrup Antacids Cathartics Vitamins Diet pills	Information not revealed by patient could complicate treatment Lack of interest in oral health, only pain relief Drug side effects
8. **Family medical history**	Predisposition to certain diseases (e.g., diabetes) History of diseases that occur in the family	Cultural beliefs about medications	May help patient seek medical examination when symptom suggests possible disease
9. **Daily diet**	Recommendations of patient's physicians, past and present Vitamin supplements Appetite Regularity of meals Food likes and dislikes	Vitamin supplements	Instructions to be given relative to oral health Prognosis for healing after treatment Need for dietary review and analysis

TABLE 9-3	ITEMS FOR THE MEDICAL HISTORY (*Continued*)		
ITEM TO RECORD IN HISTORY	**RECORD NOTES**	**MEDICATIONS AND TREATMENT MODALITIES**	**CONSIDERATIONS FOR APPOINTMENT PROCEDURES**

10. Alcohol consumption	Frequency
	Amount
	Substance abuse
		Recovering alcoholic:
		  May be taking disulfiram,
		  Avoid all alcohol-containing preparations including commercial mouthrinses
			Excessive use: effect on anesthesia; increased healing time
			Poor nutritional state is common; lack of oral care
			Avoid alcohol-containing mouthrinse
			May result in poor patient cooperation

11. Allergies	Determine substances to which the patient is allergic
	  Latex
	  Anesthetics
	  Penicillin
	  Medicaments
	  Foods
	  Iodine
		Antihistamines
		Inhalers
		Decongestants
		Steroids
			Preparation for emergency
			Xerostomia
			Avoid use of substances to which the patient is allergic

12. Arthritis	Joint pain Immobility Temporomandibular joint involvement	Aspirin Nonsteroidal anti-inflammatory drugs Corticosteroids Total joint replacements	Antibiotic premedication: consult physician if treated with chemotherapeutic agent Dental chair adjustment
13. Blood disorder	Type and duration of disease Leukemia: remission, thrombocytopenia	Vitamins Minerals: iron (iron-deficiency anemia) Folic acid supplement (sickle cell anemia) Antineoplastic drugs	Consultation with physician Need for high level of oral health Antibiotic premedication Immunosuppression Increased bleeding Oral lesions
14. Bleeding	Bleeding associated with previous dental appointments History of disorder with coagulation problem History of transfusions or other blood products Check use of aspirin (relation to bleeding tendency) Laboratory tests for bleeding time, coagulation may be needed	Anticoagulant medication Hemophilia factor replacement	Emergency prevention through preappointment precautions May need to apply direct pressure or hemostatic agent after scaling Special measures for hemophilia
15. Cancer	Head and neck radiation effects on oral cavity, salivary glands Dental and dental hygiene therapy updated before start of surgery, radiation therapy, or immunosuppression Blood count before dental and dental hygiene therapy Previous history of bisphosphonate prescription.	Radiation therapy Fluoride therapy: daily topical application Antineoplastic drugs, alkylating agents, antimetabolites, antibiotics, plant alkaloids, steroids	Bleeding; infection; poor healing response Avoid trauma to tissues Effect on oral radiographic survey: prevention of overexposure Dental caries: preventive measures Xerostomia: substitute saliva Increased risk of osteonecrosis with history of bisphosphonate use.
16. Cardiovascular diseases	Consultation with physician Refer for examination when patient seems unsure of problem	Cardiac glycosides Antiarrhythmics Antianginals Antihypertensives Anticoagulants	Minimize stress Premedication for stress Ascertain that medications have been taken Monitor vital signs

(continued)

TABLE 9-3		ITEMS FOR THE MEDICAL HISTORY (*Continued*)	
ITEM TO RECORD IN HISTORY	**RECORD NOTES**	**MEDICATIONS AND TREATMENT MODALITIES**	**CONSIDERATIONS FOR APPOINTMENT PROCEDURES**
a. Congenital heart disease	Susceptibility to infective endo- carditis Type of problem; date of rheu- matic fever		Antibiotic premedication may be required
b. Previous history of infective endo- carditis	Susceptibility to recurrence of infective endocarditis Type of problem; date		Antibiotic premedication may be required
c. Hypertension	Symptom of other disease state Monitoring blood pressure for each appointment Anesthesia: limit epinephrine or omit as recommended by physician	Diuretics Antiadrenergic agents Vasodilators Angiotensin-converting enzyme inhibitors Calcium channel-blocking agent	Postural hypotension (raise dental chair slowly) Xerostomia: saliva substitute and fluoride rinse may be needed Gingival enlargement (drug side effect)
d. Angina pectoris	Prepare for symptoms; have ready amyl nitrite inhalant or nitroglycerin tablets or spray	Amyl nitrite, nitroglycerin, or other antianginal drugs	Allay fears and prevent stress Morning appointment
e. Heart diseases	History of disease symptoms of fatigue, shortness of breath, or cough Consult with physician	Glycosides (digitalis) Anticoagulants Antiarrhythmic drugs Pacemaker	Monitor vital signs Short, more frequent appoint- ments Change dental chair slowly Patient with breathing problem (sleeps with two or more pil- lows) may need semi-upright position Bleeding tendency associated with anticoagulant Check use of ultrasonic (pace- maker)
f. Surgically cor- rected cardiovas- cular lesions	Type, date of surgery Consultation with physician Before surgical procedure, when possible: the patient needs complete oral evaluation and corrective dental work done, with motivation to high level of oral personal care daily	No tobacco use Anticoagulants Cyclosporine Nifedipine	Antibiotic premedication vital for synthetic valves or other replacements, indefinitely Gingival bleeding can be expected Gingival enlargement
g. Cerebrovascular accident (stroke)	Date of onset; residual disabilities Speech, vision, mental function	No tobacco; low-salt diet Anticoagulants Antihypertensives Vasodilator Steroid Anticonvulsant	Gingival bleeding likely when anti- coagulants are used Adapt procedures for physical disability
17. **Communicable diseases**	History of diseases; immuniza- tions Present disease; communicability Residence or extended trips in countries with high endemic incidence of certain diseases Risk group factor	Immunizations Drug therapy for current infection	Appointment postponement
a. Hepatitis B	Jaundice history Clarification of type of hepatitis Laboratory clearance	Vaccine of HBV	Precautions against percutane- ous injury

TABLE 9-3	ITEMS FOR THE MEDICAL HISTORY (*Continued*)		
ITEM TO RECORD IN HISTORY	**RECORD NOTES**	**MEDICATIONS AND TREATMENT MODALITIES**	**CONSIDERATIONS FOR APPOINTMENT PROCEDURES**
b. Tuberculosis	Active or passive Cough Duration of disease	Isoniazid Rifampin Pyrazinamide	Length of treatment; infectivity diminished after few months of treatment
c. Sexually transmitted infections (STIs)	May not obtain history of STIs Oral and pharyngeal lesions may be indicators of disease	Antibiotics	Infectiousness diminishes with antibiotic therapy for gonorrhea and syphilis Refer to physician and postpone treatment when lesions or other signs suggest infection Caution for risk from previously treated diseases
d. Herpes	Lesions can be transmitted readily	Nondefinitive; symptomatic and palliative treatment Acyclovir	Postpone routine care when oral lesions are present
e. HIV infection AIDS	Risk group identification Oral manifestations	Wide variety of opportunistic infections and complications require variety of drugs	Oral lesions Complete sterilization and barrier procedures as for all patients
18. Diabetes mellitus	Uncontrolled: requires antibiotic premedication Undiagnosed: excess thirst, appetite, and urination Family incidence: help in finding susceptible undiagnosed Severe advanced diabetes: complications (vision, kidney, cardiovascular, nervous system)	Insulin Diet control Hypoglycemics	Prepare for emergency; insulin; apple juice; frosting Appointment time related to insulin therapy and mealtime Need frequent maintenance appointments Periodontal disease accelerated Referral for tests for suspected undiagnosed
19. Ears	Deafness or degree of hearing impairment Infections, ringing, dizziness, balance	Treatment for infection Hearing aid	Adaptations for communication and biofilm control instruction
20. Endocrine	Age-group relations to certain conditions Growth, development Menstruation, menopause	Thyroid hormone supplement Antithyroid Estrogen/progestin Oral contraceptives Corticosteroids	Emphasis on high level of biofilm control Any patient taking steroids may need antibiotic premedication for appointments Monitor blood pressure
21. Epilepsy	Type, frequency of seizures precipitating factors Preparation for emergency seizure	Anticonvulsant Sedative	Minimize stress Medications make patient drowsy, less alert Valproic acid requires bleeding time before treatment
22. Eyes	Disturbance of vision Purpose for corrective eyeglasses or contact lenses Manifestations of systemic disease	Eyedrops (e.g., glaucoma)	Avoid epinephrine if glaucoma Protective eyewear during appointment Adaptations for communication with limited sight
23. Gastrointestinal	Nature and treatment of the disease Diet restriction prescribed by physician	Antacids Antidiarrheals Laxatives Antispasmodics	Patient instruction in accord with prescribed diet and medication Xerostomia

(*continued*)

TABLE 9-3	ITEMS FOR THE MEDICAL HISTORY *(Continued)*		
ITEM TO RECORD IN HISTORY	**RECORD NOTES**	**MEDICATIONS AND TREATMENT MODALITIES**	**CONSIDERATIONS FOR APPOINTMENT PROCEDURES**
24. **Kidney**	Renal disease; kidney stones Hemodialysis: hypertension, anemia, hepatitis carrier Transplant: hypertension, hepatitis	Salt restriction Many drugs are nephrotoxic Immunosuppressive drugs (cyclosporine)	Monitor blood pressure Bleeding tendency Poor healing Susceptibility to infection Limited stress tolerance
25. **Liver**	History of jaundice, hepatitis Impaired drug metabolism Cirrhosis: history of alcoholism	Nutritional emphasis Abstinence from alcohol	Laboratory test for hepatitis Bleeding problems
26. **Mental, psychiatric**	Emotional problems hinder oral care	Antipsychotic drugs Antianxiety drugs Tranquilizers Antidepressants Antiparkinsonism drugs	Limited stress tolerance Xerostomia (side effect) Avoid mouthrinse containing alcohol
27. **Physical activity**	Overall health consciousness	Good health habits Regular exercise	Contribute to cooperative attitude in maintaining oral health
28. **Physical disabilities**	Extent, cause, duration Type of treatment related to individual condition Consultation with physician or medical specialist	Pain reliever Muscle relaxant Anticonvulsant	Adjustment of physical arrangements Wheelchair accessibility and transfer Adaptations of techniques and instruction Consult for antibiotic premedication for certain conditions: for example: prosthetic joint replacement, shunt
29. **Pregnancy**	Month, parturition date Possible oral manifestations History of previous pregnancies Iron deficiency anemia	Iron Folic acid Multivitamins	Adjust physical position for comfort Frequent appointments for maintaining high level of oral hygiene
30. **Respiration**	Breathing problems Persistent cough Cough up blood Chest pain Precipitation of asthmatic attack	Codeine cough syrup Antihistamine Bronchial dilator Expectorant Decongestant Steroid	Dental chair position Ultrasonic and air-powder polisher contraindicated Anesthesia choice: nitrous oxide contraindicated No aerosol agents

A. Telephone or Personal Contact

- Immediate consultation may be needed so that urgent treatment may proceed.
- Follow-up in writing is essential because without legal record of the advice or decision, a misunderstanding could result.

B. Written Request

- A letter of formal request is the preferred procedure for medical consultation.
- A prepared form can be developed with spaces for filling in the specific questions and with space in the lower half for the physician to complete confidential information from the patient's medical record or to provide the necessary recommendations.

C. Referrals

- The patient is referred for medical examination when signs of a possible disease condition are apparent.
- The patient is referred for laboratory tests when recent test results are not available or follow-up tests are needed.

II. RADIATION

- When a patient is receiving radiation therapy or has had recent radiation for other purposes, a conference with the physician or oncologist involved is recommended to discuss the quantity of radiation to be received from any necessary dental radiographs.
- No apparent rationale exists for precluding a properly justified dental radiographic examination because of a history of radiation therapy.[7]

III. PROPHYLACTIC PREMEDICATION

■ Selected patients at risk for IE receive antibiotic premedication before any oral tissue manipulation that could create a bacteremia.

■ The patient history and the information in **Box 9-2A** are reviewed to identify a patient needing premedication in accordance with the recommendations of the American Heart Association Guidelines.

■ Routine use of antibiotic premedication is never indicated. The patient may be at less risk from the dental procedure than from the potential side effects of an antibiotic. Overuse of antibiotics can induce microbial resistance and, rarely, allergy or toxicity to the drug used.[8]

■ The subgingival use of instruments (for example, probe, explorer, or curet) is withheld until the risk has been determined, the condition has been discussed with the patient's physician, the prescription has been obtained, and taken as directed.

■ The oral antibiotic prescription is required one hour before instrumentation begins to assure the adequate concentration in the blood during and immediately following the actual instrumentation.

■ At-risk patients already taking an antibiotic for other health conditions may require additional antibiotic prophylaxis before dental and dental hygiene instrumentation. A different class of antibiotic is prescribed rather than to increase the dose of the current drug being taken.[8]

BOX 9-2A	Medical Conditions That Require Antibiotic Premedication Before Dental and Dental Hygiene Treatment

Antibiotic prophylaxis with dental procedures is recommended only for patients with cardiac conditions associated with the highest risk of adverse outcomes from endocarditis, including:

■ Prosthetic cardiac valve
■ Previous endocarditis
■ Congenital heart disease only in the following categories:
   A. Unrepaired cyanotic congenital heart disease, including those with palliative shunts and conduits
   B. Completely repaired congenital heart disease with prosthetic material or device, whether placed by surgery or catheter intervention, during the first six months after the procedure. *(Prophylaxis is recommended because endothelialization of prosthetic material occurs within 6 months of the procedure.)*
   C. Repaired congenital heart disease with residual defects at the site or adjacent to the site of a prosthetic patch or prosthetic device (which inhibit endothelialization)
■ Cardiac transplantation recipients with cardiac valvular disease

Source: American Heart Association: Endocarditis Prophylaxis Information. [Internet] Dallas: American Heart Association; c2011 [cited 2011 Jan 20]. Available at: http://www.americanheart.org/presenter.jhtml?identifier=11086

PRETREATMENT ANTIBIOTIC PROPHYLAXIS

I. AMERICAN HEART ASSOCIATION (AHA) GUIDELINES

A. Brief Historical Review[8]

■ The AHA has made recommendations for the prevention of IE for many years. The first document was published in 1955. There have been nine revisions since then including the latest one in 2007.

■ The 1960 report described the possible emergence of penicillin-resistant oral microorganisms as a result of prolonged therapy for prevention of IE. Prevention for child patients was also described.

■ The revised recommendations published in 1972 were endorsed for the first time by the American Dental Association (ADA). At that time, the maintenance of good oral hygiene was emphasized as a strong influence on the prevention of IE.

■ The 1997 revised document characterized high-, moderate-, and low-risk cardiac conditions with prophylaxis not recommended for low-risk patients. Also in 1997, it was clarified that most cases of IE are not the result of an invasive treatment procedure but are from bacteremias that result from daily activities, for examples, bacteremias created by toothbrushing, flossing, oral irrigation, toothpicks, and chewing.

B. Rationale for 2007 Revision[9]

■ Former guidelines were based more on expert opinion or individual case studies; current guidelines attempt to be more supported by scientific evidence.

■ Frequent exposure to random bacteremias that result from daily activities are more likely to cause IE than treatment procedures performed at spaced dental and dental hygiene appointments.

■ Antibiotic prophylaxis may prevent a very small number of cases of IE, if any, in patients receiving a dental or dental hygiene treatment procedure.

■ There are risks of antibiotic-associated adverse events that may exceed the benefit, if any, of antibiotic therapy.

■ Maintenance of optimal oral health with daily biofilm removal may reduce the incidence of IE due to bacteremias caused by daily activities. Such prevention can be more significant than prophylactic antibiotics given occasionally for a dental or dental hygiene invasive treatment procedure.

■ Literature reviews found no evidence-based method to decide exactly which procedures require prophylactic antibiotic premedication and which do not need it.

■ Other factors that limit conducting controlled research are:
   A. the low incidence of IE.
   B. the wide variety of types of cardiac diseases.
   C. the wide variety of invasive dental procedures.
   D. antibiotic premedication does not always prevent IE following a dental invasive procedure.

II. RECOMMENDATIONS BASED ON THE FOLLOWING FOUR PRINCIPLES:[9]

■ Only an extremely small number of cases of IE might be prevented by antibiotic prophylaxis for dental procedures even if such prophylactic therapy were 100% effective.
■ IE prophylaxis for dental procedures is recommended only for patients with underlying cardiac conditions associated with the highest risk of adverse outcomes from IE.
■ For patients with these underlying cardiac conditions, prophylaxis is recommended for all dental procedures that involve manipulation of gingival tissue, the periapical region of teeth, or perforation of the oral mucosa.
■ Prophylaxis is not recommended based solely on an increased lifetime risk of acquisition of IE.

III. MEDICAL CONDITIONS THAT REQUIRE ANTIBIOTIC PREMEDICATION BEFORE INVASIVE DENTAL AND DENTAL HYGIENE PROCEDURES

■ **Box 9-2A** lists the cardiac conditions for which antibiotic prophylaxis is recommended.
■ **Box 9-2B** lists the following:
   A. Dental and dental hygiene procedures for which endocarditis prophylaxis is recommended.
   B. Procedures for which prophylaxis is NOT needed.
■ The American Academy of Orthopedic Surgeons (AAOS)[11] recommends that "clinicians consider antibiotic prophylaxis for all total joint replacement patients before any invasive procedure that may cause bacteremia."

IV. RECOMMENDED ANTIBIOTIC PROTOCOL

■ **Table 9-4** provides the recommended antibiotic prescriptions for prevention of cardiac endocarditis.

ASA DETERMINATION

With the completion of the patient histories, an overall estimate of medical risk of a patient can be

---

BOX 9-2B	Dental and Dental Hygiene Procedures for Which Endocarditis Prophylaxis Is Recommended for Patients in BOX 9-2A

All dental and dental hygiene procedures that involve:

■ Manipulation of gingival tissue
■ The periapical region of teeth
■ Perforation of the oral mucosa

need antibiotic premedication (**Table 9-4**)

The following procedures and events do NOT need prophylaxis:

■ Routine anesthetic injections through noninfected tissue
■ Taking dental radiographs
■ Placement of removable prosthodontic or orthodontic appliances
■ Adjustment of orthodontic appliances
■ Placement of orthodontic brackets
■ Shedding of primary teeth
■ Bleeding from trauma to the lips or oral mucosa.

Source: American Heart Association. Endocarditis Prophylaxis Information. [Internet] Dallas: American Heart Association; c2011 [cited 2011 Jan 20]. Available at: http://www.americanheart.org/presenter.jhtml?identifier=11086

---

made. American Society of Anesthesiologists (**ASA**) **Physical Status Classification System**[11,12] (Table 23-1, page 342) describes six categories of physical status provides examples of adaptations necessary for providing dental hygiene care for a patient in each category.

■ **ASA I:** A patient without apparent systemic disease: a normal healthy patient.
■ **ASA II:** A patient with mild systemic disease.
■ **ASA III:** A patient with severe systemic disease that limits activity but is not incapacitating.
■ **ASA IV:** A patient with an incapacitating systemic disease that is a constant threat to life.
■ **ASA V:** A moribund patient not expected to survive 24 hours with or without care.

REVIEW AND UPDATE OF HISTORY

■ Updating the patient's health history at each appointment is essential.
■ Changes in health status revealed by interim medical examinations or evidenced by reported illness or hospitalizations are recorded and considered during continuing treatment.

TABLE 9-4	PROPHYLACTIC REGIMENS FOR DENTAL, ORAL, RESPIRATORY TRACT, OR ESOPHAGEAL PROCEDURES		
		REGIMEN—SINGLE DOSE 30–60 MIN BEFORE PROCEDURE	
SITUATION	**AGENT**	**ADULT**	**CHILD***
Standard general prophylaxis	Amoxicillin	2.0 g orally	50 mg/kg orally
Unable to take oral medications	Ampicillin **or** Cefazolin or celtriaxone	2.0 g IM or IV[†] 1.0 g IM or IV	50 mg/kg IM or IV 50 mg/kg IM or IV
Allergic to penicillins or ampicillin—oral	Cephalexin[‡] **or** Clindamycin **or** Azithromycin or Clarithromycin	2.0 g orally 600 mg orally 500 mg orally	50 mg/kg orally 20 mg/kg orally 15 mg/kg orally
Allergic to penicillins and unable to take oral medications	Cefazolin or ceftriaxone[†] **or** Clindamycin	1.0 g IM or IV 600 mg IM or IV	50 mg/kg IM or IV 25 mg/kg IM or IV

*Total child dose never exceeds adult dose
[†]IM = intramuscularly; IV = intravenously.
[‡]Cephalosporins are not prescribed for individuals with immediate-type hypersensitivity reaction (urticaria, angioedema, or anaphylaxis) to penicillins or ampicillin.
Source: American Heart Association. Endocarditis Prophylaxis Information. [Internet] Dallas: American Heart Association; c2011 [cited 2011 Jan 20]. Available at: http://www.americanheart.org/presenter.jhtml?identifier=11086

■ Post a wall plaque that states *"Please Advise Us of Any Change in Your Medical History Since Your Last Visit"* in an appropriate place in a dental office or clinic to remind patients about the importance of updating information at each appointment.

Following a review of the previously recorded history, questions can be directed to the patient to compare the present condition with the previous one and to determine at least the following:

■ Interim illnesses; changes in health
■ Visits to physician; reasons and results
■ Laboratory tests performed and the results; blood, urine, or other analyses
■ Current medications
■ Changes in the oral soft tissues and the teeth observed by the patient

DOCUMENTATION

■ Date all records.
■ Keep handwritten permanent records, such as signed health history forms in ink.
■ Provide a specific line on a health history form for the signature of the patient.[1,2] The completed history for a minor is signed by a parent or guardian. A signature is also needed on the informed consent form.
■ Maintain all information obtained for a patient history in strictest privacy.

■ For patients with special health problems that require premedication, use some type of coded tab to alert all dental personnel to check the medical history before each appointment.
■ Analyze the usefulness of items on the patient history form periodically, and plan for revision as scientific evidence reveals new information.
■ Progress notes document regular update of forms completed and changes in personal, dental, or health history since last appointment.
■ Box 9-3 provides an example of a progress note related to completion of personal, dental, and medical histories.

BOX 9-3	Example Progress Note: Related to Updating a Patient's Medical History

Forty-five-year-old patient presents for routine 6-month maintenance appointment. Update of health history: interview and new health history form completed and signed. Changes from last appointment: recent diagnosis of hypertension and physician prescription for Lisinopril ACE inhibitor, 10 mg. Patient began taking medication 2 weeks ago. No additional changes noted.

Signed: _____, RDH Date: _____

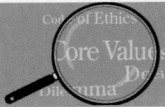

Everyday Ethics

Chris, the dental hygienist, was waiting for her new patient at 1:00 pm. All she knew was that Irana was 70 years old, from Russia, and could speak and understand English fairly well. Chris heard the front door to the office open and went out to greet her patient. The little lady was on the arm of a teenage boy who quickly helped Irana to a chair and turned to leave after saying to Chris (pointing to the patient) "Just back from hospital. They fixed her heart and told her to get her teeth cleaned to keep her healthy. Car not parked." Then to his grandmother "Back in an hour," before he rushed out.

Chris ushered Irana into the treatment room and helped her into the chair, then started the history questions with "What were you in the hospital for?" Irina grabs Chris' arm and firmly requests, "Want teeth cleaned." Chris attempts to explain why she is asking the questions about her health. Then she asks for her physician's name, and permission to call the physician to obtain the information. Irina points to her heart, but just becomes more agitated and keeps repeating

"Want teeth cleaned" and refuses to give approval to call her doctor. Chris is alarmed at the thought of providing care for this patient without complete information about her health history, but hates to waste the scheduled appointment time, given her well-filled schedule and the number of patients clamoring for appointments.

Questions for Consideration

1. Professionally and ethically, what are a dental hygienist's responsibilities to take time to help a patient understand the seriousness of an illness and the need for a complete personal, dental, and medical history before receiving dental treatment?
2. Provide an example of how each of the ethical theories (Table III-1, page 114) might apply as Chris determines how to resolve this issue?
3. Which of the dental hygiene core values apply as Chris determines what action to take?

Factors To Teach The Patient

- The need for obtaining the personal, medical, and dental history before performance of dental and dental hygiene procedures, and the need for keeping the histories up to date.
- The assurance that recorded histories are kept in strict professional confidence.
- The relationship between oral health and general physical health.
- The interrelationship of medical and dental care.
- All patients who require antibiotic premedication need special attention paid to (1) the importance of preventive dentistry, (2) the imperative need for regular dental care, and (3) the necessity for taking the prescribed prescription 1 hour before the appointment starts.

References

1. Robbins KS. Medicolegal considerations. In: Malamed SF, editor. *Medical emergencies in the dental office*. 6th ed. St Louis: Mosby; 2002. pp. 93–103.
2. American Dental Association. Medical history form (5500). Chicago: ADA Department of Salable Materials; copyright 2007 [cited 2010 Dec 10]. 2 pages. Available from: https://siebel.ada.org/ecustomer_enu/start.swe?SWECmd=Start&SWEHo=siebel.ada.org
3. American Academy of Pediatric Dentistry, Council on Clinical Affairs. Policy on use of a caries-risk assessment tool (CAT) for infants, children, and adolescents. *Pediatr Dent*. 2008–2009;30 (7 Suppl):29–33.
4. American Dental Association. Caries risk assessment form (age >6). Chicago: ADA; ©2008 [cited 2010 Dec 10]. 2 pages. Available from: www.ada.org/sections/professionalResources/docs/topics_caries_over6.doc
5. American Dental Association. Caries risk assessment form (age 0–6). Chicago: ADA; ©2008 [cited 2010 Dec 10]. 2 pages. Available from: www.ada.org/sections/professionalResources/docs/topics_caries_under6.doc
6. Chiodo GT, Rosenstein DI. Consultation between dentists and physicians. *Gen Dent*. 1984 Jan–Feb;32(1):19–22.
7. Department of Health and Human Services (US), Food and Drug Administration, Center for Devices and Radiological Health. *Selection of patients for x-ray examinations: dental radiographic examinations*. Washington: Superintendent of Documents; 1988. p. 10. HHS Publication FDA 88–8274.
8. Pallasch TJ, Slots J. Antibiotic prophylaxis and the medically compromised patient. *Periodontol 2000*. 1996 Feb;10:107–38.
9. Wilson W, Taubert KA, Gewitz M, Lockhart PB, Baddour LM, Levison M, Bolger A, Cabell CH, Takahashi M, Baltimore RS, Newburger JW, Strom BL, Tani LY, Gerber M, Bonow RO, Pallasch T, Shulman ST, Rowley AH, Burns JC, Ferrieri P, Gardner T, Goff D, Durack DT. Prevention of infective endocarditis: guidelines from the American Heart Association: a guideline from the American Heart Association Rheumatic Fever, Endocarditis, and Kawasaki Disease Committee, Council on Cardiovascular Disease in the Young, and the Council on Clinical Cardiology, Council on Cardiovascular Surgery and Anesthesia, and the Quality Care and Outcomes Research Interdisciplinary Working Group. *Circulation*. 2007 Oct 9;116(15):1736–54.
10. American Academy of Orthopaedic Surgeons (AAOS). Information Statement Antibiotic Prophylaxis for Patients With Joint Replacements [Internet]. Washington, DC:AAOS; ©2009 Feb [updated 2010 Jun; cited 2011 Jan 20]; [1 screen]. Available from: http://www.aaos.org/about/papers/advistmt/1033.asp
11. American Society of Anesthesiologists. New classification of physical status. *Anesthesiology*. 1963 Jan–Feb;24(1)111.
12. ASA Physical Status Classification System [Internet]. Park Ridge, IL: American Society of Anesthesiologists; c2005–10 [updated 2008; cited 2010 Mar 4]. Available from: http://www.asahq.org/clinical/physicalstatus.htm

CHAPTER 10

Vital Signs

ESTHER M. WILKINS, RDH, DMD

Chapter Outline

INTRODUCTION

Determination of four vital signs—*body temperature, pulse and respiratory rates,* and *blood pressure*—is considered standard procedure in patient care. **Table 10-1** summarizes the normal values of the four basic vital signs for adolescents and adults.

Adding a fifth new vital sign—*smoking status*—gives the opportunity to introduce early in the encounter with the patient the significance of smoking to general and oral health. The fact that smoking is the number one preventable cause of illness and death more than justifies including smoking status as a vital sign.[1] **Figure 10-1** illustrates a vital signs stamp to use for convenient recording of all five signs.

I. PATIENT PREPARATION AND INSTRUCTION

- Seat patient in upright position, at eye level for instruction.
- Explain the vital signs and obtain consent.

- Explain how vital signs can affect dental hygiene and dental treatment.
- During the process, explain each step as needed by the individual patient.

II. DENTAL HYGIENE CARE PLANNING

- Recording vital signs contributes to the proper systemic evaluation of a patient in conjunction with the complete medical history.
- Dental hygiene care planning and appointment sequencing are directly influenced by the findings.
- When vital signs are not within normal, advise the patient to check with the physician.
- Referral for medical evaluation and treatment is indicated.
- Key words related to the vital signs are defined in Box 10-1.

TABLE 10-1	ADULT VITAL SIGNS	
Vital Sign	**Values of Significance in Dental and Dental Vital Sign Hygiene Appointments**	
Body Temperature (Oral)	Normal 37.0°C (98.6°F) Normal range 35.5–37.5°C (96–99.5°F)	
Pulse Rate	Normal range 60–100/min	
Respiration	Normal range 14–20/min	
Blood Pressure Category	**Systolic mmHg**	**Diastolic mmHg**
Normal	<120	<80
Prehypertension	120–139	80–89
Hypertension **Stage 1** **Stage 2**	140–159 >160	90–99 >100

Source: Data from The seventh report of the joint national committee on prevention, detection, evaluation, and treatment of high blood pressure. Bethesda (MD): National Heart, Lung, and Blood Institute Health Information Center; 2003 May. 52 p. N.I.H. Publication No. 03-5233.

BODY TEMPERATURE

While preparing the patient history and making the extraoral and intraoral examinations, the need for taking the tempera-

```
                VITAL SIGNS

NAME_____ DATE_____
Blood Pressure _____
Pulse _____
Temperature _____
Respiratory Rate _____
Smoking Status  Current  Former  Never
(please circle)
```

FIGURE 10-1 **Vital Signs Stamp for a Patient's Record.** (Source: Fiore MC. The new vital sign. Assessing and documenting smoking status. *JAMA.* 1991 Dec;266(22):3183–4).

ture may become apparent, or the dentist may have requested the procedure in conjunction with current oral disease.

I. INDICATIONS FOR TAKING THE TEMPERATURE

- For the new patient's initial permanent record along with all vital signs.
- For complete examination during a maintenance appointment.
- When oral infection is known to be present.
  - Necrotizing ulcerative gingivitis or periodontitis.
  - Apical or periodontal abscess.
  - Acute pericoronitis.
- With other vital signs, prior to administration of local anesthetic.
- At any appointment when the patient reports illness or there is a suspected infection.

BOX 10-1	Key Words

Vital Signs

Anoxia: oxygen deficiency; a reduction of oxygen in the tissues can lead to deep respirations, cyanosis, increased pulse rate, and impairment of coordination.

Apnea: temporary cessation of breathing; absence of spontaneous respirations.

Auscultation: listening for sounds produced within the body; may be performed directly or with a stethoscope.

Bradycardia: unusually slow heartbeat evidenced by slowing of the pulse rate.

Core temperature: the temperature of the deep tissues of the body; remains relatively constant; contrasts with body surface temperature, which rises and falls in response to environment.

Diastole: the phase of the cardiac cycle in which the heart relaxes between contractions and the two ventricles are dilated by the blood flowing into them; diastolic pressure is the lowest blood pressure.

Diurnal: pertaining to or occurring during the daytime or period of light.

Hypertension: systolic blood pressure of 140 mmHg or greater and diastolic blood pressure of 90 mmHg or greater.

Hyperthermia: higher-than-normal body temperature.

Hypothermia: lower-than-normal body temperature.

Korotkoff sounds: the sounds heard during the determination of blood pressure; sounds originating within the blood passing through the vessel or produced by vibratory motion of the arterial wall.

Normotensive: normal tension or tone; of or pertaining to having normal blood pressure.

Pulse pressure: the difference between systolic and diastolic blood pressure; normally 40 mmHg.

Pyrexia: an abnormal elevation of the body temperature above 37.0°C (98.6°F).

Stethoscope: instrument used to hear and amplify the sounds produced by the heart, lungs, and other internal organs.

Systole: the contraction, or period of contraction, of the heart, especially the ventricles, during which blood is forced into the aorta and the pulmonary artery; systolic pressure is the highest, or greatest, pressure.

Tachycardia: unusually fast heartbeat; at a rate greater than 100 beats per minute.

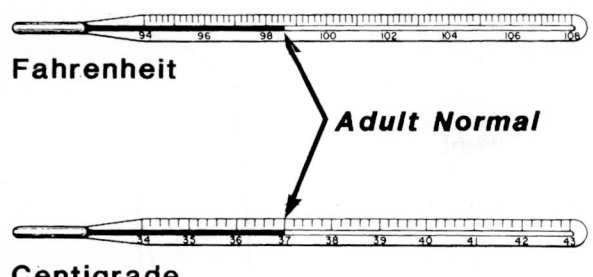

Fahrenheit

Adult Normal

Centigrade

FIGURE 10-2 **Thermometers.** Centigrade and Fahrenheit thermometers compared. Adult normal temperature is shown at 37.0°C and 98.6°F.

- Protection of the health of the healthcare personnel and patients or families who may be exposed secondarily.
- Special significance during epidemics when community exposures are at risk.
- For patient's referral for medical care when indicated.

II. MAINTENANCE OF BODY TEMPERATURE

A. Normal

- *Adults.* The normal average temperature is 37°C (98.6°F), as illustrated in **Figure 10-2**. The normal range is from 35.5° to 37.5°C (96° to 99.5°F).
- *Older adults.* Over 70 years of age, the average temperature is slightly lower (36.0°C, 96.8°F).
- *Children.* There is no appreciable difference between boys and girls. Average temperatures are as follows:
  - First year—37.3°C (99.1°F).
  - Fourth year—37.5°C (99.4°F).
  - Fifth year—37°C (98.6°F).
  - Twelfth year—36.7°C (98.0°F).

B. Temperature Variations

1. *Fever (pyrexia).* Values over 37.5°C (99.5°F).
2. *Hyperthermia.* Values over 41.0°C (105.8°F).
3. *Hypothermia.* Values below 35.5°C (96.0°F).

C. Factors that Alter Body Temperature

1. *Time of day.* Highest in late afternoon and early evening; lowest during sleep and early morning.
2. *Temporary increase.* Exercise, hot drinks, smoking, or application of external heat.
3. *Pathologic states.* Infection, dehydration, hyperthyroidism, myocardial infarction, or tissue injury from trauma.
4. *Decrease.* Starvation, hemorrhage, or physiologic shock.

III. METHODS OF DETERMINING TEMPERATURE

A. Locations for Measurement

- *Oral:* patient needs to be able to breathe through the nose and hold lips closed; must not have sore mouth, very dry mouth, or recent oral surgery.

- *Forehead:* for disposable thermometer.
- *Ear:* with a tympanic device.
- *Medical/hospital applications:* also use axilla or rectum for assessment.

B. Types of Thermometers

Electronic With Digital Readout

- Cover with disposable protective sheath.
- Place under tongue; short time required.
- Read on the digital display.

Tympanic

- Cover with protective sheath.
- Insert gently into ear canal.
- Short exposure (2–5 seconds) before record appears on digital unit.

Mercury in Glass: Oral, Blue Tip; Rectal, Red Tip

- Used less because of danger for breakage with mercury spill that must be cleaned up using specified procedures.
- Sheath cover used for infection protection.
- Takes longer time before reading than other types.
- More difficult to see and read mercury column.

Disposable Single-Use Chemical Strip

- Apply to appropriate skin area, usually the forehead.
- Color changes denote temperature.

IV. CARE OF PATIENT WITH TEMPERATURE ELEVATION

A. Temperature Over 41°C (105.8°F)

- Treat as a medical emergency.
- Transport to a hospital for medical care.

B. Temperature 37.6° to 41°C (99.6°C to 105.8°F)

- Check possible temporary or factitious cause, such as hot beverage or smoking, and observe patient while repeating the determination.
- Review the dental and medical history.
- Postpone elective oral care when there are signs of respiratory infection or other possible communicable disease.

 PULSE

- The pulse is the intermittent throbbing sensation felt when the fingers are pressed against an artery.
- It is the result of the alternate expansion and contraction of an artery as a wave of blood is forced out from the heart.
- The pulse rate or heart rate is the count of the heartbeats.

■ Irregularities of strength, rhythm, and quality of the pulse are noted while counting the pulse rate.

I. MAINTENANCE OF NORMAL PULSE

A. Normal Pulse Rates

■ *Adults.* There is no absolute normal. The adult range is 60 to 100 beats per minute, slightly higher for women than for men.
■ *Children.* The pulse or heart rate falls steadily during childhood.
  ■ *In utero*—150 beats per minute (bpm).
  ■ At birth—130 bpm.
  ■ Second year—105 bpm.
  ■ Fourth year—90 bpm.
  ■ Tenth year—70 bpm.

B. Factors that Influence Pulse Rate

An unusually fast heartbeat (over 100 beats per minute in an adult) is called *tachycardia;* an unusually slow heartbeat (below 50) is *bradycardia.*

■ *Increased pulse.* Caused by exercise, stimulants, eating, strong emotions, extremes of heat and cold, and some forms of heart disease.
■ *Decreased pulse.* Caused by sleep, depressants, fasting, quiet emotions, and low vitality from prolonged illness.
■ *Emergency situations.* Listed in Tables 69-4 and 69-5 (pages 1076 and 1080).

II. PROCEDURE FOR DETERMINING PULSE RATE

A. Sequence

The pulse rate is obtained following the body temperature. When the mercury in a glass thermometer is used, the pulse can be counted while the thermometer is in the mouth.

B. Sites

The pulse may be felt at several points over the body.

■ *Radial pulse*: at the wrist **(Figure 10-3).**
■ Other sites convenient for use in a dental office or clinic are the *temporal* artery on the side of the head in front of the ear, or the *facial* artery at the border of the mandible.
■ *Carotid pulse*: used during cardiopulmonary resuscitation (Figure 69-6, page 1069) for an adult.
■ *Brachial pulse*: used for an infant **(Figure 10-3).**

C. Prepare the Patient

1. Tell the patient what is to be done.
2. Have the patient in a comfortable position with arm and hand supported, palm down.

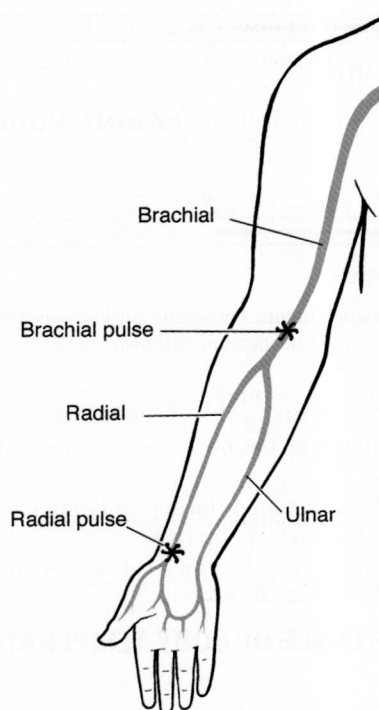

FIGURE 10-3 **Arteries of the Arm.** Note the location of the radial pulse. The brachial pulse may be felt just before the brachial artery branches into the radial and ulnar arteries.

3. Locate the radial pulse on the thumb side of the wrist with the tips of the first three fingers **(Figure 10-4).** Do not use the thumb because it contains a pulse that may be confused with the patient's pulse.

D. Count and Record

■ When the pulse is felt, exert light pressure and count for 1 clocked minute. Use the second hand of a watch or clock. Check with a repeat count when question rate or quality.

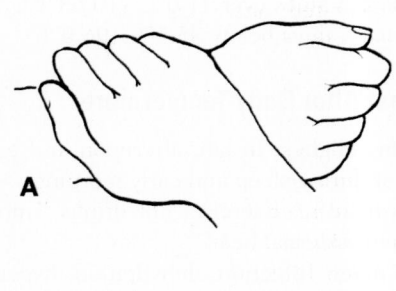

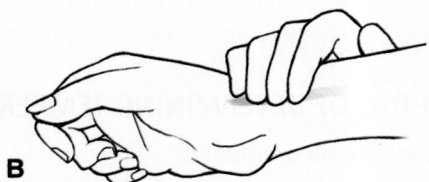

FIGURE 10-4 **Determination of Pulse Rate. (A)** Correct position of hands. **(B)** The tips of the clinician's first three fingers are placed over the radial pulse located on the thumb side of the ventral surface of the wrist.

- While taking the pulse, observe the following:
  A. Rhythm: regular, regularly irregular, irregularly irregular.
  B. Volume and strength: full, strong, poor, weak, thready.
- Record the date, pulse rate, other characteristics in patient's record.
- A pulse rate over 100 is considered abnormal for an adult.

 # RESPIRATION

- The function of respiration is to supply oxygen to the tissues and to eliminate carbon dioxide.
- Variations in normal respirations may be shown by such characteristics as the rate, rhythm, depth, and quality and may be symptomatic of disease or emergency states.

I. MAINTENANCE OF NORMAL RESPIRATIONS

A respiration is one breath taken in and let out.

A. Normal Respiratory Rate

- *Adults.* The adult range is from 14 to 20 per minute, slightly higher for women.
- *Children.* The respiratory rate decreases steadily during childhood. Averages are as follows:
  - First year—30 per minute.
  - Second year—25 per minute.
  - Eighth year—20 per minute.
  - Fifteenth year—18 per minute.

B. Factors that Influence Respirations

Many of the same factors that influence pulse rate also influence the number of respirations. A rate of 12 per minute or fewer is considered subnormal for an adult; over 28 is accelerated; and rates over 60 are extremely rapid and dangerous.

1. *Increased respiration.* Caused by work and exercise, excitement, nervousness, strong emotions, pain, hemorrhage, shock.
2. *Decreased respiration.* Caused by sleep, certain drugs, pulmonary insufficiency.
3. *Emergency situations.* Listed in Tables 69-4 and 69-5 (pages 1076 and 1080).

II. PROCEDURES FOR OBSERVING RESPIRATIONS

A. Determine Rate

1. Make the count of respirations immediately after counting the pulse.
2. Maintain the fingers over the radial pulse.
3. Respirations must be counted so that the patient is not aware, as the rate may be voluntarily altered.

4. Count the number of times the chest rises in 1 clocked minute. It is not necessary to count both inspirations and expirations.

B. Factors to Observe

1. *Depth.* Describe as shallow, normal, or deep.
2. *Rhythm.* Describe as regular (evenly spaced) or irregular (with pauses of irregular lengths between).
3. *Quality.* Describe as strong, easy, weak, or labored (noisy). Poor quality may have an effect on body color; for example, a bluish tinge of the face or nail beds may mean an insufficiency of oxygen.
4. *Sounds.* Describe deviant sounds made during inspiration, expiration, or both.
5. *Position of patient.* When the patient assumes an unusual position to secure comfort during breathing or prefers to remain seated upright, mark records accordingly.

C. Record

Record all findings in the patient's record.

 # BLOOD PRESSURE

- Information about the patient's blood pressure is essential during dental and dental hygiene appointments because special adaptations may be needed.
- Blood pressure readings most usually are recorded with the medical history and other assessment data.
- Readings taken at the start of an appointment can be significantly higher than at the end of treatment.[2]
- To establish a baseline reading and determine the need for patient referral for medical attention, more than one reading is advised. A comparison of the reading at the beginning of the appointment with one at the close of appointment when the patient is relaxed may be helpful.
- Screening for blood pressure in dental practices has been shown to be an effective health service for all ages since many patients are unaware that they have hypertension.
- Growing evidence indicates that primary hypertension is detectable and occurs commonly in young children and adolescents.[3]
- Cardiovascular diseases are described starting page 1078. That information can be a helpful introduction and is recommended for reading in conjunction with this section on the techniques for obtaining blood pressure.

I. COMPONENTS OF BLOOD PRESSURE

- Blood pressure is the force exerted by the blood on the blood vessel walls.
- When the left ventricle of the heart contracts, blood is forced out into the aorta and travels through the large arteries to the smaller arteries, arterioles, and capillaries. The vessels of the heart are shown in Figure 66-1 on page 1008.

- The pulsations extend from the heart through the arteries and disappear in the arterioles.
- During the course of the cardiac cycle, the blood pressure is changing constantly.

A. Systolic Pressure

Systolic pressure is the peak or the highest pressure. It is caused by ventricular contraction. The normal systolic pressure is less than 120 mmHg.

B. Diastolic Pressure

Diastolic pressure is the lowest pressure. It is the effect of ventricular relaxation. The normal diastolic pressure is less than 80 mmHg.

C. Pulse Pressure

The pulse pressure is the difference between the systolic and diastolic pressures.

II. FACTORS THAT INFLUENCE BLOOD PRESSURE

A. Maintenance of Blood Pressure

Blood pressure depends on the following:

1. Force of the heartbeat (energy of the heart).
2. Peripheral resistance; condition of the arteries; changes in elasticity of vessels, which may occur with age and disease.
3. Volume of blood in the circulatory system.

B. Factors that Increase Blood Pressure

1. Exercise, eating, stimulants, and emotional disturbance.
2. Use of oral contraceptives; blood pressure increases with age and length of use.

C. Factors that Decrease Blood Pressure

1. Fasting, rest, depressants, and quiet emotions.
2. Such emergencies as fainting, blood loss, shock (Tables 69-4 and 69-5, pages 1076 and 1080).

III. EQUIPMENT FOR DETERMINING BLOOD PRESSURE

A sphygmomanometer is made up of a pressure measuring device (manometer) and an inflatable cuff to wrap around the arm or under certain circumstances, the leg.

A. Mercury Sphygmomanometer (Analog)

- Traditional system, but mercury is a potential health hazard because of mercury spillage.
- Has shown to be more accurate and consistent than other types.

B. Aneroid Sphygmomanometer (Analog)

- Compact, portable glass-enclosed gauge with needle for registration of blood pressure.
- Requires regular calibration to keep accurate.

C. Electronic Sphygmomanometer (Digital)

- Automatic determination of blood pressure without use of stethoscope.

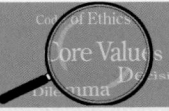 Everyday Ethics

Gracie was having a very busy day and at 10:15 A.M. was already late for the 10:00 A.M. patient, Mr. McElroy, who had arrived early and was waiting in the reception area. While completing his history, to save time, she copied over the blood pressure recording from his previous appointment just two weeks ago. It had been 130/83, only slightly into the pre-hypertension level.

The appointment was planned for the maxillary left quadrant with anesthesia. After the scaling was complete and Mr. McElroy was climbing out of the dental chair, looking a bit unsteady as he stood up, he casually remarked: "I just remembered while you were working that my Doc gave me a new prescription—I suppose I should have told you before. But it is only one pill a day—for keeping the blood pressure down. I don't have any trouble anyway, he just wanted to be sure."

Questions for Consideration
1. Explain how the principles of beneficence and maleficence apply to Gracie's actions with Mr. McElroy's examination and charting procedures.
2. Has Gracie placed the office at risk for a possible medical emergency given Mr. McElroy's physical status? Answer by describing the rights and duties of both the hygienist and the patient.
3. Who is responsible for ensuring that accurate documentation has been completed on all patients—from an ethical and a quality assurance perspective?

D. Wrist or finger devices are considered to be less accurate and are not considered for professional use.

E. Stethoscope

- Consists of a diaphragm or cupped endpiece that transmits and sends sound through tubes to the earpieces
- Used with mercury or aneroid-type analog sphygmomanometers

IV. PROCEDURE FOR DETERMINING BLOOD PRESSURE

A. Prepare Patient

1. Tell patient briefly what is to be done. Detailed explanations should be avoided because they may excite the patient and change the blood pressure.
2. Seat patient comfortably, with the arm slightly flexed, with palm up, and with the whole forearm supported on a level surface at the level of the heart.
3. Use either arm unless otherwise indicated, for example, by a handicap. Repeat blood pressure determinations should be made on the same arm, because a variation in pressure may exist between arms.
4. Take pressure on bare arm, not over clothing. Loosen a tight sleeve.
5. Select cuff size as described in **Figure 10-5**.

B. Apply Cuff

1. Apply the completely deflated cuff to the patient's arm, supported at the level of the heart. If the arm rests on

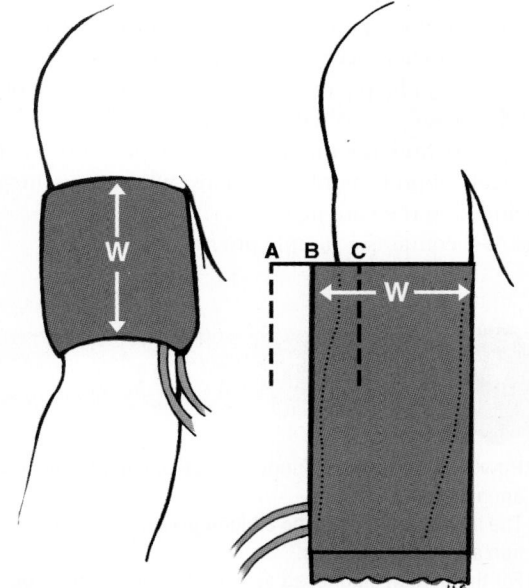

FIGURE 10-5 **Selection of Cuff Size.** The correct width (W) is 20% greater than the diameter of the arm where applied. (A) Too wide. (B) Correct width. (C) Too narrow.

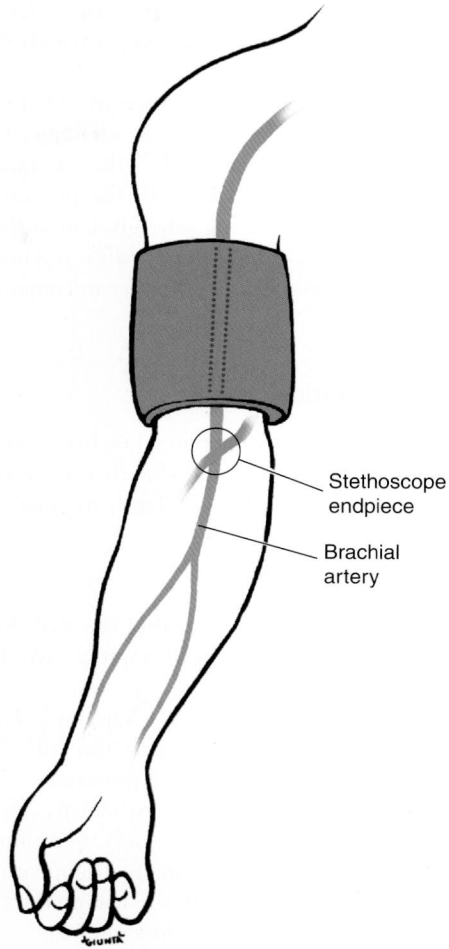

FIGURE 10-6 **Blood Pressure Cuff in Position.** The lower edge of the cuff is placed approximately 1 inch above the antecubital fossa. The stethoscope endpiece is placed over the palpated brachial artery pulse point approximately 1 inch below the antecubital fossa and slightly toward the inner side of the arm.

the arm of a dental chair, higher than the heart, the diastolic pressure may show a small but significant increase.[4]
2. Place the portion of the cuff that contains the inflatable bladder directly over the brachial artery. The cuff may have an arrow to show the point that is placed over the artery. The lower edge of the cuff is placed 1 inch above the antecubital fossa **(Figure 10-6)**. Fasten the cuff evenly and snugly.
3. Adjust the position of the gauge for convenient reading.

C. Locate the Radial Pulse (Figures 10-3 and 10-4)

1. Palpate 1 inch below the antecubital fossa to locate the brachial artery pulse **(Figure 10-3)**.
2. Hold the fingers on the pulse.

D. Determine Maximum Inflation Level (MIL)

1. Close the needle valve (air lock) attached to the hand control bulb firmly but so it may be released readily.

2. Pump to inflate the cuff until the radial pulse stops. Monitor the gauge to note the level at which the pulse disappears.

3. Continue to pump until the gauge reads 20 or 30 points beyond where the radial pulse was no longer felt. This is the maximum inflation level (MIL). It means that the brachial artery is collapsed by the pressure of the cuff and no blood is flowing through. *Unless the MIL is determined, the level to which the cuff is inflated will be arbitrary. Excess pressure can be very uncomfortable for the patient.*

E. Position the Stethoscope

Place the endpiece over the palpated brachial artery, 1 inch below the antecubital fossa, and slightly toward the inner side of the arm **(Figure 10-6)**. Hold lightly in place.

F. Deflate the Cuff Gradually

1. Release the air lock slowly so that the dial drops very gradually and steadily, approximately two to three lines per second.

2. Listen for the first sound: *systole* ("tap tap"). This is the beginning of the flow of blood past the cuff. Note the number on the dial as the *systolic pressure*.

3. Continue to release the pressure slowly. The sound will continue, first becoming louder, then diminishing and becoming muffled, until finally disappearing. Note the number on the dial where the last distinct tap was heard. That number is the *diastolic pressure*.

4. Release further (about 10 points) until all sounds cease. That is the second diastolic point. In some clinics and hospitals, the last sound is taken as the diastolic pressure.

5. Let the rest of the air out rapidly.

G. Repeat for Confirmation

■ Wait 30 seconds before inflating the cuff again.

■ More than one reading is needed within a few minutes to determine an average and ensure a correct reading.

H. Record

■ Write date and arm used.

■ Record blood pressure as a fraction, for example, 120/80.

V. BLOOD PRESSURE FOLLOW-UP CRITERIA

■ Dental personnel have an obligation to advise and *refer for further evaluation.*

■ Diagnosis of hypertension would never be made or treatment started on the basis of an isolated reading.

■ When the blood pressure is routinely within the normal range (120/80), it needs to be rechecked within 2 years.

BOX 10-2	Example Progress Note

Patient postponed regular maintenance appointment over a month; blood pressure seems to stay in the same range within a few mm though still in the prehypertension level (140/82). I explained how much more calculus had accumulated and what that meant to the attachment level. He said he would try harder; he had noticed more bleeding. Uses his hand brush more than his electric one because he is "on the road so much." I suggested a travel type electric to keep in his suitcase; he caught on and said "which kind"?

Signed: _____, RDH Date: _____

■ Rechecking within 1 year is recommended for persons at increased risk for hypertension, such as family history, weight gain, obesity, African American, use of oral contraceptives, smoking, and excessive alcohol consumption.

■ Lifestyle modifications are indicated for all levels of blood pressure classification.[5] Consultation with a patient's physician is indicated prior to dental or dental hygiene treatment when either reading is ≥180/110. **(Table 10-1)**.

DOCUMENTATION

Documentation in the permanent record of a patient with a high blood pressure would include the following:

■ Carefully documented medical history with regular updates at each maintenance appointment.

■ Reminder to help patient realize the importance of regularly taking prescribed medication.

■ Prepared and documented blood pressure reading at each appointment especially when anesthesia is included in the care plan.

■ **Box 10-2** contains a sample progress note.

Factors To Teach The Patient

■ How vital signs can influence dental and dental hygiene appointments.

■ The importance of having a blood pressure determination at regular intervals.

■ For the patient diagnosed as hypertensive, encourage regular continuing use of prescription drugs for control of high blood pressure.

References

1. Fiore MC. The new vital sign. Assessing and documenting smoking status. *JAMA*. 1991 Dec;266(22):3183–4.
2. Nichols C. Dentistry and hypertension. *J Am Dent Assoc*. 1997 Nov;128(11):1557–62.
3. U.S. Department of Health and Human Services. The fourth report on the diagnosis, evaluation, and treatment of high blood pressure in children and adolescents. Washington, DC: US Department of Health and Human Services, National Institutes of Health, National Heart, Lung, and Blood Institute; 2005:1.
4. Beck FM, Weaver JM, Blozis GG, Unverferth DV. Effect of arm position and arm support on indirect blood pressure measurements made in a dental chair. *J Am Dent Assoc*. 1983 May;106(5):645–7.
5. Chobanian AV, Bakris GL, Black HR, Cushman WC, Green LA, Izzo JL Jr, Jones DW, Materson BJ, Oparil S, Wright JT Jr, Roccella EJ; Joint National Committee on Prevention, Detection, Evaluation, and Treatment of High Blood Pressure. National Heart, Lung, and Blood Institute; National High Blood Pressure Education Program Coordinating Committee. *The seventh report of the joint national committee on prevention, detection, evaluation, and treatment of high blood pressure*. Bethesda (MD): National Heart, Lung, and Blood Institute Health Information Center; 2003 May. 52 p. N.I.H. Publication No. 03-5233.

Extraoral and Intraoral Examination

ESTHER M. WILKINS, BS, RDH, DMD

Chapter Outline

A careful overall observation of each patient and a thorough examination of the oral cavity and adjacent structures are essential to total assessment before care planning. A variety of lesions may be observed for which the patient may or may not report subjective symptoms. Recognition, treatment, and follow-up of specific lesions may be of definite significance to the present and future general and oral health of the patient.

Despite the occurrence of many seemingly minor lesions, the danger of oral malignancies remains a definite possibility. Every effort must be made to detect potentially cancerous lesions early.

■ Each area of the mucous membrane is examined, and minor deviations from normal are given prompt attention.

■ A life may depend on an oral examination. Routine examination for each new patient and at each maintenance appointment provides a realistic approach to the control of oral disease.

■ The oral tissues are sensitive indicators of the general health of the individual. Changes in these structures may be the first indication of subclinical disease processes in other parts of the body.

■ Prerequisite to the recognition of deviations from the normal appearance of the oral cavity is knowledge and understanding of the normal morphology, anatomy, and physiology of the oral cavity and the surrounding area.

■ Box 11-1 defines terms used for extraoral and intraoral examination.

BOX 11-1	Key Words

Extraoral/Intraoral Examination

Aphtha: a little white or reddish ulcer.

Crust: outer scablike layer of solid matter formed by drying of a body exudate or secretion.

Cyst: a closed, epithelial-lined sac, normal or pathologic, that contains fluid or other material.

Dorsal: back surface; opposite of ventral.

Epidermis: outermost and nonvascular layers of the skin composed of basal layer, spinous layer, granular layer, and horny layer.

    Corium: the dermis or true skin just beneath the epidermis; well supplied with nerves and blood vessels.

Erosion: soft tissue slightly depressed lesion in which the epithelium above the basal layer is denuded.

Erythema: red area of variable size and shape; reaction to irritation, radiation, or injury.

Exophytic: growing outward.

Exostosis: a benign bony growth projecting from the surface of bone.

Fissure: a narrow slit or cleft in the epidermis where infected ulceration, inflammation, and pain can result.

Forensic: pertaining to or used in legal proceedings.

Idiopathic: of unknown etiology.

Indurated: hardened; abnormally hard.

Lymphadenopathy: disease of the lymph nodes; regional lymph node enlargement.

Morphology: science that deals with form and structure.

Palpation: perceiving by sense of touch.

Papilla: small, nipple-shaped projection or elevation (papillary: adjective).

Patch: circumscribed flat lesion larger than a macule; differentiated from surrounding epidermis by color and/or texture.

Pedunculated: elevated lesion attached by a thin stalk.

Petechia: hemorrhagic nonraised spot of pinpoint to pinhead size.

Polyp: any growth or mass protruding from a mucous membrane.

Pseudomembrane: a loose membranous layer of exudate that contains microorganisms, precipitated fibrin, necrotic cells, and inflammatory cells produced during an inflammatory reaction on the surface of a tissue.

Punctate: marked with points or punctures differentiated from the surrounding surface by color, elevation, or texture.

Purulent: containing, forming, or discharging pus.

Rubefacient: reddening of the skin.

Scar: cicatrix; mark remaining after healing of a wound or healing following a surgical intervention.

Sclerosis: induration or hardening.

Sessile: elevated lesion with a broad base.

Temporomandibular disorder (TMD): a collective term that includes a wide range of disorders of the masticatory system characterized by one or more of the following: pain in the preauricular area, temporomandibular joint (TMJ), and muscles of mastication, with limitation or deviation in mandibular motion and TMJ sounds during mandibular function.

Torus: bony elevation or prominence usually located on the midline of the hard palate (torus palatinus) and the lingual surface of the mandible in the premolar area (torus mandibularis).

Trismus: motor disturbance of the trigeminal nerve, especially spasm of the masticatory muscles with difficulty in opening the mouth.

Ventral: inferior surface; opposite of dorsal.

Verruca: a wartlike growth.

OBJECTIVES

A thorough examination is essential to the total care of the patient. The dental hygienist will:

■ Observe the patient overall, as well as in all areas in and about the oral cavity, and record those areas that appear to deviate from normal and that may be evidence of disease.

■ Screen each patient at each appointment to detect lesions that may be pathologic, particularly those that may be cancerous.

■ Recognize a need for postponement of the current appointment because of evidence of communicable disease or in deference to the need for urgent medical consultation and/or treatment.

■ Prevent the development of advanced, irreversible, or untreatable oral disease by early recognition of initial lesions.

■ Identify suspected conditions that require additional testing and referral for medical evaluation.

■ Identify extraoral and intraoral deviations from normal for which dental hygiene care and instruction may need special adaptations.

■ Provide a means of comparison of individual oral examinations over a series of maintenance appointments, and thus determine the effects of dental and dental hygiene care and the success of patient instruction.

■ Provide information for continuing records of the patient's dental hygiene diagnosis and care plan for legal purposes.

COMPONENTS OF EXAMINATION

■ The current concept of patient care is that the total patient is being treated, not only the oral cavity, and particularly not only the teeth and their immediate surrounding tissues.

- The examination is, therefore, all-inclusive to detect possible physical, mental, or psychological influences of the whole patient on the oral health.
- Thorough examination becomes a routine part of each patient appointment so that treatment for the control and prevention of oral diseases will be effective.

I. TYPES OF EXAMINATIONS

A. Complete

- A complete examination includes a thorough summary of all the components of the assessment. The extraoral and intraoral examination is a component of a patient's complete assessment.
- The complete examination prior to comprehensive treatment is essential for each new patient. When a dental or periodontal treatment emergency is apparent, a limited examination may be a necessary at the start.
- The complete examination is required for the routine maintenance of a treated patient.

B. Screening

- Screening implies a brief, preliminary examination, usually for a particular purpose.
- A screening may be for initial patient assessment and triage to determine priorities for treatment.
- *Community Screening*: a survey of a group of individuals to identify the prevalence of a particular disease or condition within that population.

C. Limited

A type of screening made for an emergency situation. It may be used in the management of an acute condition.

D. Follow-up

- Limited follow-up examination to check the healing following a treatment. Example: after initial therapy for necrotizing ulcerative gingivitis (in Chapter 41, page 652).
- To remove a dressing and/or sutures.

E. Maintenance/Reevaluation

- Maintenance after a specific period of time following the completion of the Care Plan and the anticipated restoration to health.
- A maintenance examination is a complete reassessment from which a new dental hygiene diagnosis and care plan are derived.

II. METHODS FOR EXAMINATION

- The extraoral and intraoral examination is accomplished by various visual and tactile, manual and Instrumental methods.

- Patient position, optimum lighting, and effective retraction for accessibility and visibility contribute to the accuracy and completeness of the examination.

A. Visual Examination

- *Direct Observation.* Visual observation is carried out in a systematic order to note surface appearance (color, contour, size) and to observe movement and other evidence of function.
- *Radiographic Examination.* The use of radiographs can reveal deviations from the normal not noticeable by direct vision.
- *Transillumination.* A strong light directed through a soft tissue or a tooth to enhance examination is useful for detecting irregularities of the teeth and locating calculus. Hold the mouth mirror to view from the lingual to see the translucency.

B. Palpation

- Palpation is examination using the sense of touch through tissue manipulation or pressure on an area with the fingers of one hand or both.
- *Digital.* Use of a single finger. Example: Index finger applied to the lingual side of the mandible beneath the canine and premolar area to determine presence of a torus mandibularis.
- *Bidigital.* Use of finger and thumb of same hand. Example: palpation of the lips (**Figure 11-1**).
- *Bimanual.* Use of finger or fingers and thumb from each hand applied simultaneously in coordination. Example: index finger of one hand palpates on the floor of the mouth inside, while a finger or fingers from the other hand press on the same area from under the chin externally (**Figure 11-2**).
- *Bilateral.* The two hands are used at the same time to examine corresponding structures on opposite sides of the body. Comparisons can be made. Example: fingers place beneath the chin to palpate the submandibular lymph nodes (**Figure 11-3**).

C. Instrumentation

- Examination instruments, such as a periodontal probe and an explorer are used for specific examination of the teeth and periodontal tissues.

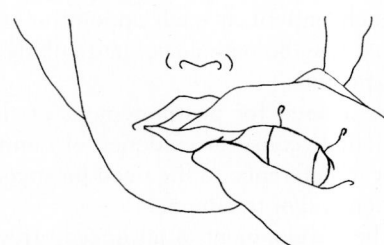

FIGURE 11-1 **Bidigital Palpation.** Palpation of the lip to illustrate the use of a finger and thumb of the same hand.

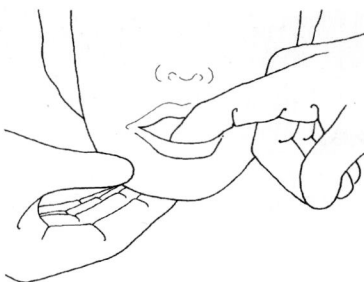

FIGURE 11-2 **Bimanual Palpation.** Examination of the floor of the mouth by simultaneous palpation with fingers of each hand in apposition.

■ Probe and explorer are described in Chapter 15, pages 226–238.

D. Percussion

■ Percussion is the act of tapping a surface or tooth with the fingers or an instrument.
■ Information about the status of health of the part is determined either by the response of the patient or by the sound. When a tooth is known to be sensitive in any way, percussion needs to be avoided.

E. Electrical Test

■ An electric pulp tester may be used to detect the presence or absence of vital pulp tissue.
■ Methods for use of a pulp tester are described in Chapter 17, page 268.

F. Auscultation

■ Auscultation is the use of sound.
■ Example: The sound of clicking of the temporomandibular joint when the jaw is opened and closed. **Figure 11-5** shows examination of the temporomandibular joint.

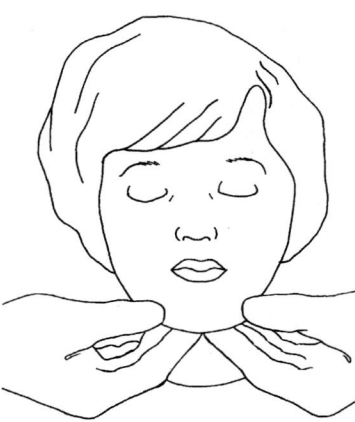

FIGURE 11-3 **Bilateral Palpation.** Bilateral palpation is used to examine corresponding structures on opposite sides of the body.

III. SIGNS AND SYMPTOMS

■ A specific objective for patient examination as a part of the complete assessment is the recognition of deviations from normal that may be signs or symptoms of disease.
■ The need for careful, thorough examination cannot be overemphasized. Concentration and attention to detail are necessary if the signs and symptoms of early disease are to be recognized and documented.
■ General signs and symptoms may occur in various disease conditions. Example: fever, or increase in body temperature accompanies most infections.
■ A *pathognomonic* sign or symptom is unique to a particular disease and may be used to distinguish that condition from other diseases or conditions.

A. Signs

■ A sign is any abnormality that can be identified by a healthcare professional while examining a patient.
■ A sign is an *objective symptom*.
■ Examples of signs: observable changes such as color, shape or consistency or abnormal findings revealed by the use of a probe, explorer, radiograph, or other instrument for disease detection.

B. Symptoms

■ A symptom is also any departure from normal that may be indicative of disease.
■ A symptom is a subjective abnormality that can be observed by the patient.
■ Examples are pain, tenderness, and bleeding when toothbrushing as described by the patient.

IV. PREPARATION FOR EXAMINATION

■ Review the patient's health histories and other parts of the records.
■ Examine radiographs on view box or in the computer.
■ Explain the procedures to be performed.
■ Help the patient decide about allowing the clinician to have access for a complete head and neck examination. When a patient is wearing a scarf or other head/neck covering for cultural or religious purposes, the dental hygienist uses culturally sensitive communication skills (Chapter 3, page 8).

SEQUENCE OF EXAMINATION

A recommended sequence for examination is outlined in **Table 11-1**, in which factors to consider during appointments are related to the actual observations made and recorded. The sequence presented in **Table 11-1** is adapted from *Detecting Oral Cancer*, available from the National Institutes of Health.[1]

TABLE 11-1	EXTRAORAL AND INTRAORAL EXAMINATION	

ORDER OF EXAMINATION	TO OBSERVE	INDICATION AND INFLUENCES ON APPOINTMENTS
1. Overall Appraisal of Patient	Posture, gait General health status; size Hair; scalp Breathing; state of fatigue Voice, cough, hoarseness	Response, cooperation, attitude toward treatment Length of appointment
2. Face	Expression: evidence of fear or apprehension Shape: twitching; paralysis Jaw movements during speech Injuries; signs of abuse	Need for alleviation of fears Evidence of upper respiratory or other infections Enlarged masseter muscle (related to bruxism)
3. Skin	Color, texture, blemishes Traumatic lesions Eruptions, swellings Growths	Relation to possible systemic conditions Need for supplementary history Biopsy or other treatment to recommend Influences on instruction in diet
4. Eyes	Size of pupils Color of sclera Eyeglasses (corrective) Protruding eyeballs	Dilated pupils or pinpoint may result from drugs, emergency state Eyeglasses essential during instruction Hyperthyroidism
5. Nodes (Palpate) (Figure 11-4) a. Pre- and postauricular b. Occipital c. Submental; submandibular d. Cervical chain e. Supraclavicular	Adenopathy; lymphadenopathy Induration	Need for referral Medical consultation Coordinate with intraoral examination
6. Temporomandibular Joint (Palpate) (Figure 11-5)	Limitations or deviations of movement Tenderness; sensitivity Noises: clicking, popping, grating	Disorder of joint; limitation of opening Discomfort during appointment and during personal biofilm control
7. Lips a. Observe closed, then open b. Palpate (Figure 11-1)	Color, texture, size Cracks, angular cheilosis Blisters, ulcers Traumatic lesions Irritation from lip-biting Limitation of opening; muscle elasticity; muscle tone Evidences of mouthbreathing Induration	Need for further examination: referral Immediate need for postponement of appointment when a lesion may be communicable or could interfere with procedures Care during retraction Accessibility during intraoral procedures Patient instruction: dietary, special biofilm control for mouthbreather
8. Breath Odor	Severity Relation to oral hygiene, gingival health	Possible relation to systemic condition Alcohol use history; special needs
9. Labial and Buccal Mucosa, Left and Right Examined Systematically a. Vestibule b. Mucobuccal folds c. Frena d. Opening of Stensen's duct e. Palpate cheeks	Color, size, texture, contour Abrasions, traumatic lesions, cheekbite Effects of tobacco use Ulcers, growths Moistness of surfaces Relation of frena to free gingiva Induration	Need for referral, biopsy, cytology Frena and other anatomic parts that need special adaptation for radiography or impression tray Avoid sensitive areas during retraction
10. Tongue a. Vestibule b. Lateral borders c. Base of tongue (retract) (Figure 11-6) d. Deviation on extension	Shape: normal asymmetric Color, size, texture, consistency Fissures; papillae Coating Lesions: elevated, depressed, flat Induration	Need for referral, biopsy, cytology Need for instruction in tongue cleaning

(continued)

TABLE 11-1	EXTRAORAL AND INTRAORAL EXAMINATION (*Continued*)	
ORDER OF EXAMINATION	**TO OBSERVE**	**INDICATION AND INFLUENCES ON APPOINTMENTS**
11. Floor of Mouth a. Ventral surface of tongue b. Palpate (Figure 11-2) c. Duct openings d. Mucosa, frena e. Tongue action	Varicosities Lesions: elevated, flat, depressed, traumatic Induration Limitation or freedom of movement of tongue Frena; tongue-tie	Large muscular tongue influences retraction, gag reflex, accessibility for instrumentation Film placement problems
12. Saliva	Quantity; quality (thick, ropy) Evidence of dry mouth; lip wetting Tongue coating	Reduced in certain diseases, by certain drugs Special dental caries control program Influence on instrumentation Need for saliva substitute
13. Hard Palate	Height, contour, color Appearance of rugae Tori, growths, ulcers	Need for referral, biopsy, cytology Signs of tongue thrust, deviate swallow Influence on radiographic film placement
14. Soft Palate, Uvula	Color, size, shape Petechiae Ulcers, growths	Referral, biopsy, cytology Large uvula influences gag reflex
15. Tonsillar Region, Throat	Tonsils: size and shape Color, size, surface characteristics Lesions, trauma	Referral, biopsy, cytology Enlarged tonsils encourage gag reflex Throat infection, a sign for appointment postponement

I. SYSTEMATIC SEQUENCE FOR EXAMINATION

The advantages of following a routine order for examination include the following:

- Minimal possibility of overlooking an area and missing details of importance.
- Increased efficiency and conservation of time.
- Maintenance of a professional atmosphere, which inspires the patient's confidence.

II. STEPS FOR THOROUGH EXAMINATION (TABLE 11-1)

A. Extraoral

1. Observe patient during reception and seating to note physical characteristics and abnormalities, and make an overall appraisal.
2. Observe head, face, eyes, and neck, and evaluate the skin of the face and neck.
3. Palpate the salivary glands and lymph nodes. **Figure 11-4** shows the location of the major lymph nodes of the face, oral regions, and neck.
4. Observe mandibular movement and palpate the temporomandibular joint **(Figure 11-5)**. Relate to items from questions in the medical/dental history.[2,3]

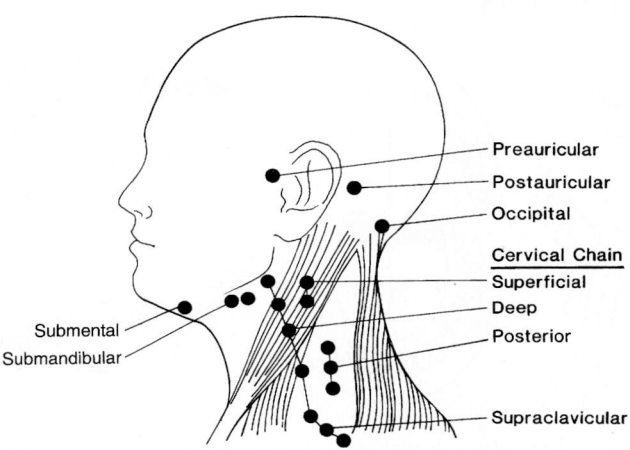

FIGURE 11-4 **Lymph Nodes.** The locations of the major lymph nodes into which the vessels of the facial and oral regions drain.

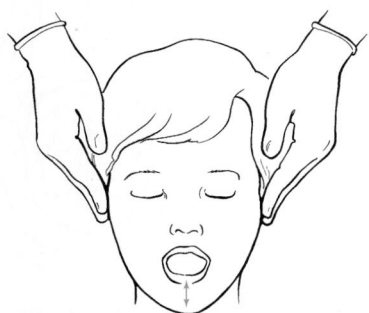

FIGURE 11-5 **Assessment of the Temporomandibular Joint.** The joint is palpated as the patient opens and closes the mouth.

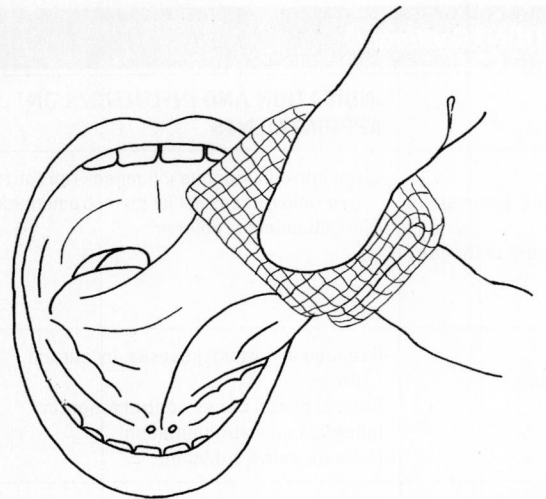

FIGURE 11-6 **Examination of the Tongue.** To observe the posterior third of the tongue and the attachment to the floor of the mouth, hold the tongue with a gauze sponge, retract the cheek, and move the tongue out, first to one side and then the other, as each section of the mucosa is carefully examined.

B. Intraoral

1. Make a preliminary examination of the lips and intraoral mucosa by using a mouth mirror or a tongue depressor.
2. View and palpate lips, labial and buccal mucosa, and mucobuccal folds.
3. Examine and palpate the tongue, including the dorsal and ventral surfaces, lateral borders, and base. Retract to observe posterior third, first to one side then the other **(Figure 11-6)**. The papillae of the tongue are shown in Figure 14-2 (page 210).
4. Observe mucosa of the floor of the mouth. Palpate the floor of the mouth **(Figure 11-2)**.
5. Examine the hard and soft palates, tonsillar areas, and pharynx. Use a mirror to observe the oropharynx, naso-pharynx, and larynx.

6. Note amount and consistency of the saliva and evidence of dry mouth.

DOCUMENTATION OF FINDINGS

I. RECORDS

A. Record Form (Paper or Computer)

1. Contains adequate space for complete descriptions of lesions observed; not merely a check sheet.
2. Contains spaces for successive examinations at follow-up and maintenance appointments.

B. Information to Record

A complete description of each finding includes the location, extent, size, color, surface texture or configurations, consistency, morphology, and history.

II. HISTORY

Questions directed to the patient provide necessary information in the management of an oral lesion. Because alarming the patient must be avoided, judgment is needed for selecting the appropriate time to obtain the history of a lesion.

- Whether the lesion is known or not known to the patient; previous evaluation.
- If known, when first noticed; if recurrence, previous date.
- Duration; changes in size and appearance.
- Symptoms.

III. LOCATION AND EXTENT

When a lesion is first seen, its location is noted in relation to adjacent structures. A printed diagram of parts of the oral cavity drawn into the record form can be a valuable aid for marking the location **(Figure 11-7)**. Descriptive

Draw outlines of abnormalities in proper locations
MUCOSAL ABNORMALITIES

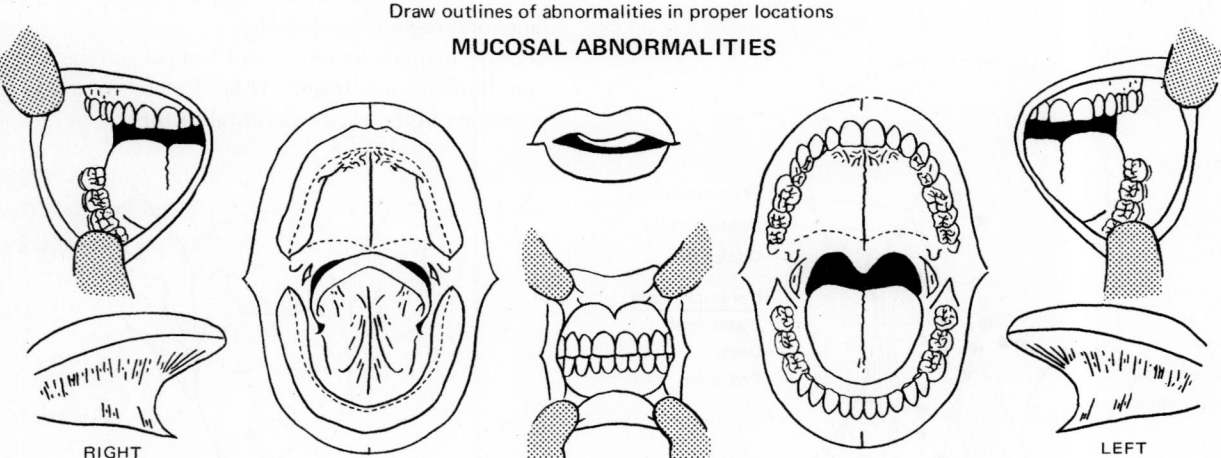

RIGHT   LEFT

FIGURE 11-7 **Record Form for Clinical Findings.** As part of a clinical examination record form, deviations from normal can be drawn to show the location and relative size. (Courtesy of the University of Southern California School of Dentistry.)

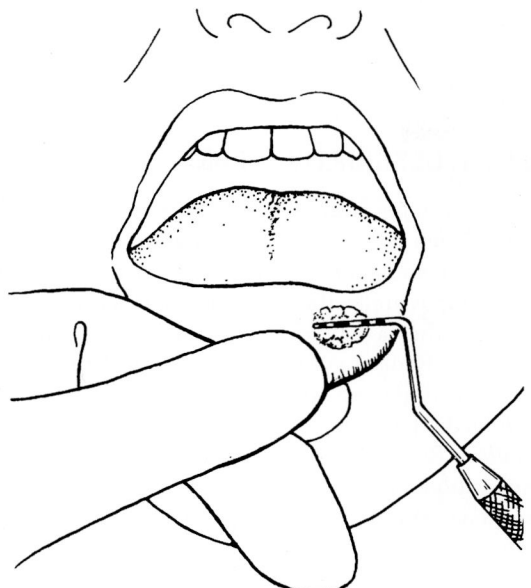

FIGURE 11-8 Use of a Probe to Measure a Lesion. In addition to the exact location, the width and length of a lesion is recorded. Using the probe provides a convenient method.

words to define the location and extent include the following:

- *Localized.* Lesion limited to a small focal area.
- *Generalized.* Involves most of an area or segment.
- *Single lesion.* One lesion of a particular type with a distinct margin.
- *Multiple lesions.* More than one lesion of a particular type. Lesions may be
  - Separate. Discrete, not running together; may be arranged in clusters.
  - Coalescing. Close to each other with margins that merge.

IV. PHYSICAL CHARACTERISTICS

A. Size and Shape

- Record length and width in millimeters.
- The height of an elevated lesion may be significant.
- Use a probe to measure, as shown in **Figure 11-8**.

B. Color

- Red, pink, white, and red and white are the most commonly seen.
- Other more rare lesions may be blue, purple, gray, yellow, black, or brown.

C. Surface Texture

- A lesion may have a smooth or an irregular surface.
- The texture may be papillary, verrucous or wartlike, fissured, corrugated, or crusted.
- Other descriptive terms are defined in **Box 11-1** with the key words.

D. Consistency

- Lesions may be soft, spongy, resilient, hard, or indurated.

MORPHOLOGIC CATEGORIES[4]

- Most lesions can be classified readily as *elevated, depressed,* or *flat* as they relate to the normal level of the skin or mucosa.
- Flowcharts **Figures 11-9A** Elevated Lesions, **11-9B** Depressed Lesions, and **11-9C** Flat Lesions break down the terms used for describing lesions in each category.

I. ELEVATED LESIONS (FIGURE 11-9A)

An elevated lesion is above the plane of the skin or mucosa. Elevated lesions are considered *blisterform* or *nonblisterform*.

A. Blisterform

Blisterform lesions contain fluid and are usually soft and translucent. They may be vesicles, pustules, or bullae.

1. *Vesicle.* A vesicle is a small (1 cm or less in diameter), circumscribed lesion with a thin surface covering. It may contain serum or mucin and appear white.
2. *Pustule.* A pustule may be more or less than 5 mm in diameter. It contains pus. Pus gives the pustule a yellowish color.
3. *Bulla.* A bulla is large (more than 1 cm). It is filled with fluid, usually mucin or serum, but may contain blood. The color depends on the fluid content.

B. Nonblisterform

Nonblisterform lesions are solid and do not contain fluid. They may be papules, nodules, tumors, or plaques. Papules, nodules, and tumors are also characterized by the base or attachment. As shown in **Figure 11-10**, the *pedunculated* lesion is attached by a narrow stalk or pedicle, whereas the *sessile* lesion has a base as wide as the lesion itself.

1. *Papule.* A papule is a small (pinhead to 5 mm in diameter), solid lesion that may be pointed, rounded, or flat-topped.
2. *Nodule.* A nodule is larger than a papule (greater than 5 mm but less than 1 cm).
3. *Tumor.* A tumor is 2 cm or greater in width. In this context, "tumor" means a general swelling or enlargement and does not refer to neoplasm, either benign or malignant.
4. *Plaque.* A plaque is a slightly raised lesion with a broad, flat top. It is usually larger than 5 mm in diameter, with a "pasted on" appearance.

II. DEPRESSED LESIONS (FIGURE 11-9B)

A depressed lesion is below the level of the skin or mucosa. The outline may be regular or irregular, and there may be a flat or raised border around the depression. The depth is usually described as superficial or deep. A deep lesion is greater than 3 mm deep.

A. Ulcer

Most depressed lesions are ulcers and represent a loss of continuity of the epithelium. The center is often gray to yellow, surrounded by a red border. An ulcer may result from the rupture of an elevated lesion (vesicle, pustule, or bulla).

B. Erosion

An erosion is a shallow, depressed lesion that does not extend through the epithelium to the underlying tissue.

III. FLAT LESIONS (FIGURE 11-9C)

A flat lesion is on the same level as the normal skin or oral mucosa. Flat lesions may occur as single or multiple lesions and have a regular or irregular form.

A *macule* is a circumscribed area not elevated above the surrounding skin or mucosa. It may be identified by its color, which contrasts with the surrounding normal tissues.

IV. OTHER DESCRIPTIVE TERMS

- *Crust.* An outer layer, covering, or scab that may have formed from coagulation or drying of blood, serum, or pus, or a combination. A crust may form after a vesicle breaks; for example, the skin lesion of chicken pox is first a macule, then a papule, then a vesicle, and then a crust.
- *Erythema.* Red area of variable size and shape.
- *Exophytic.* Growing outward.
- *Indurated.* Hardened.
- *Papillary.* Resembling a small, nipple-shaped projection or elevation.
- *Petechiae.* Minute hemorrhagic spots of pinhead to pinpoint size.

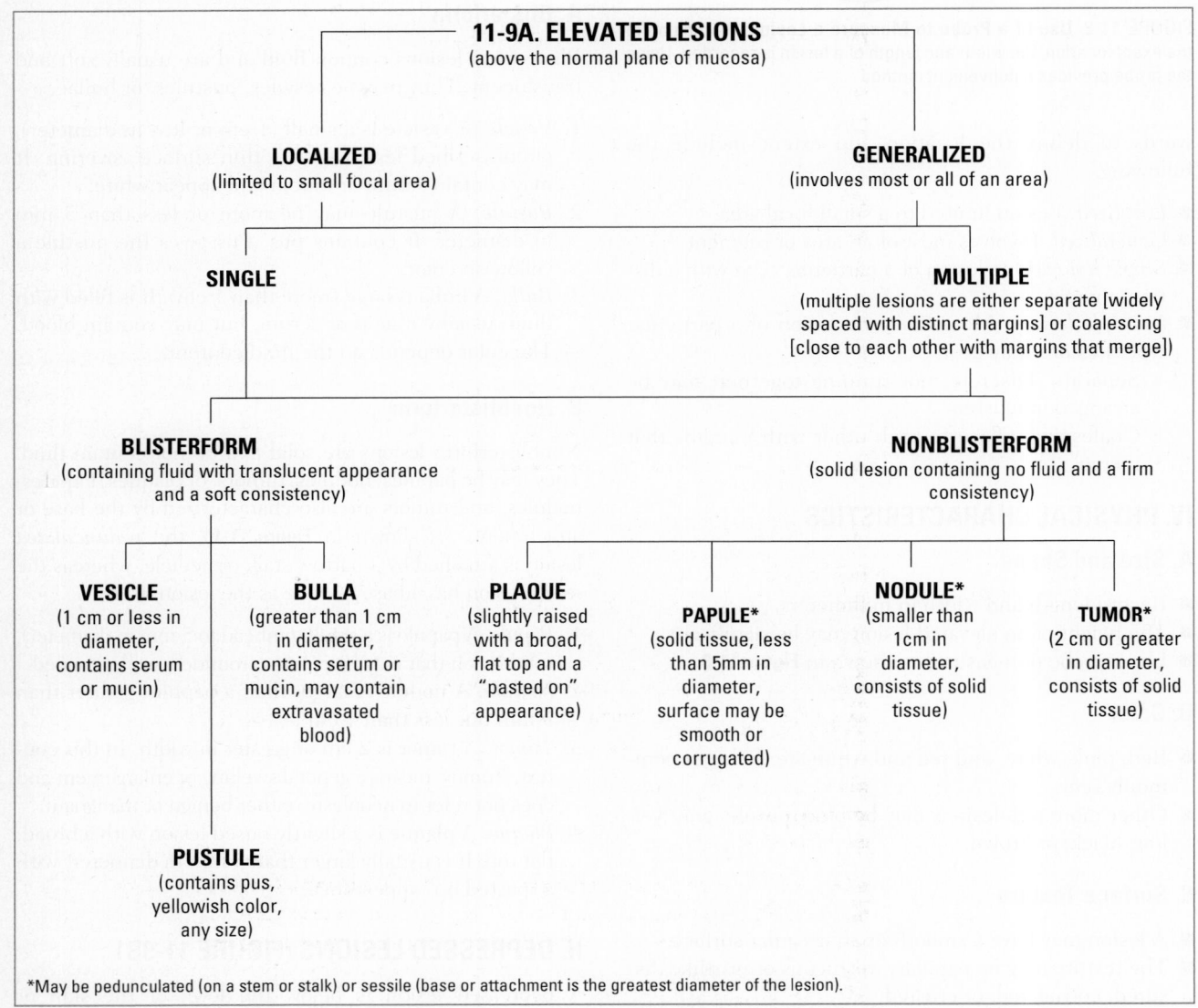

FIGURE 11-9 **A.** Flow Chart: Description of Elevated Soft Tissue Lesions. Elevated lesions are blisterform or nonblisterform. (*continued*)

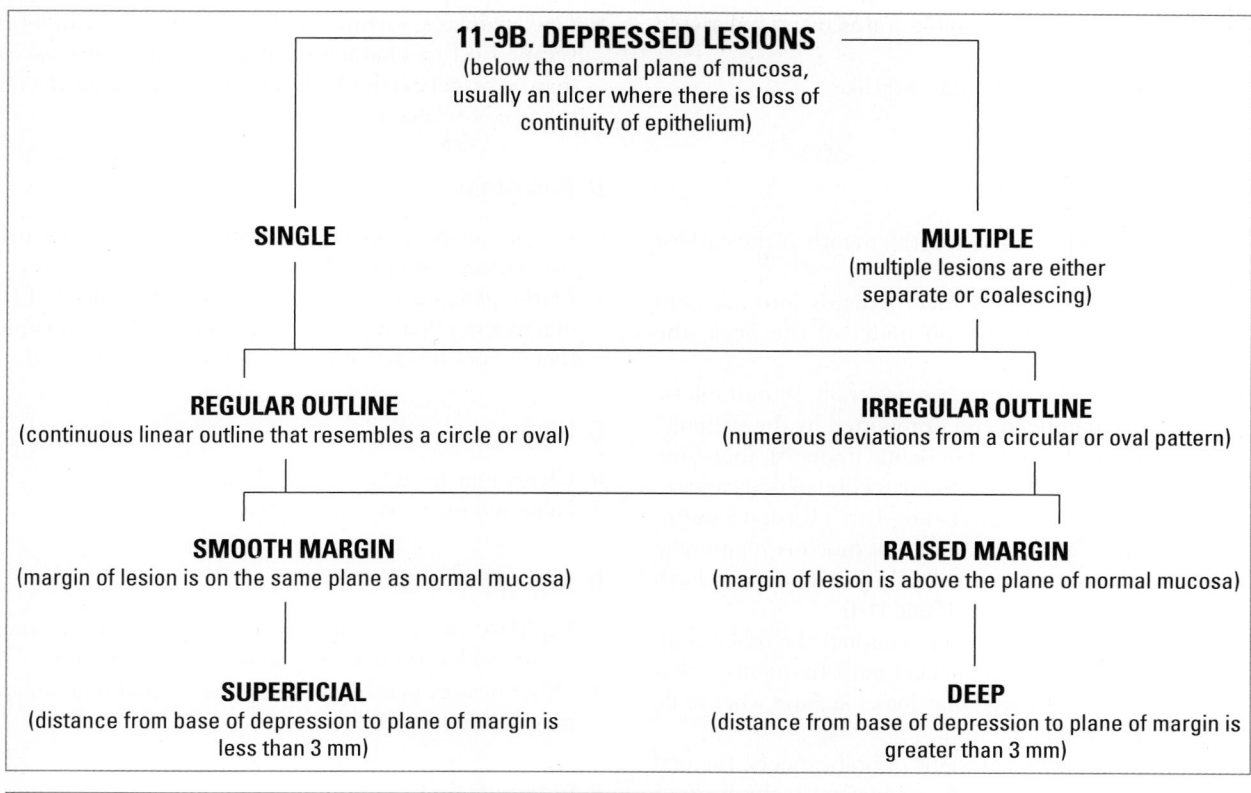

11-9B. DEPRESSED LESIONS
(below the normal plane of mucosa, usually an ulcer where there is loss of continuity of epithelium)

SINGLE

MULTIPLE
(multiple lesions are either separate or coalescing)

REGULAR OUTLINE
(continuous linear outline that resembles a circle or oval)

IRREGULAR OUTLINE
(numerous deviations from a circular or oval pattern)

SMOOTH MARGIN
(margin of lesion is on the same plane as normal mucosa)

RAISED MARGIN
(margin of lesion is above the plane of normal mucosa)

SUPERFICIAL
(distance from base of depression to plane of margin is less than 3 mm)

DEEP
(distance from base of depression to plane of margin is greater than 3 mm)

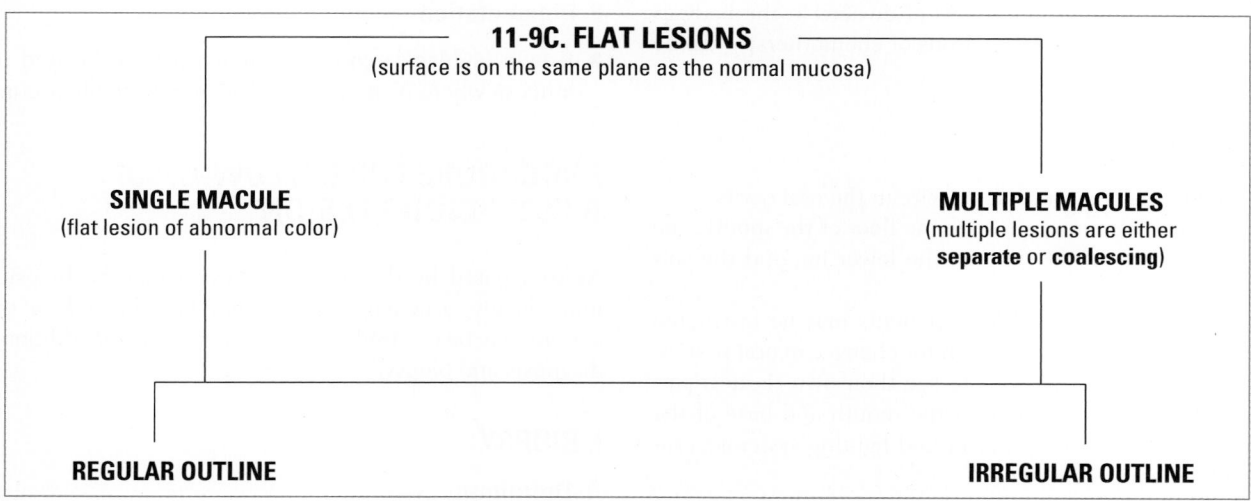

11-9C. FLAT LESIONS
(surface is on the same plane as the normal mucosa)

SINGLE MACULE
(flat lesion of abnormal color)

MULTIPLE MACULES
(multiple lesions are either **separate** or **coalescing**)

REGULAR OUTLINE

IRREGULAR OUTLINE

FIGURE 11-9 (*Continued*) **B.** Flow Chart: Description of Depressed Soft Tissue Lesions. Depressed lesions are below the normal plane of the mucosa, usually an ulcer where there is a loss of continuity of epithelium. **C.** Flow Chart: Description of Flat Soft Tissue Lesions. Flat lesions are on the level normal plane of the mucosa. (A through C reprinted with permission from McCann A. Describing soft tissue lesions of the oral cavity. *Dental Hygienist News.* 1992 Spring;5:9)

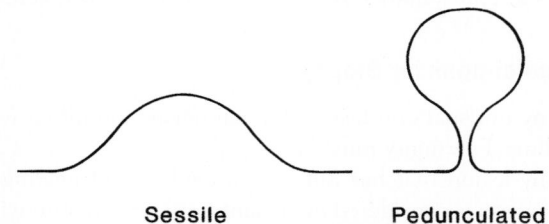

Sessile   Pedunculated

FIGURE 11-10 **Attachment of Nonblisterform Lesions.** The *sessile lesion has a base as wide as the lesion itself; the* pedunculated lesion is attached by a narrow stalk or pedicle.

- *Pseudomembrane.* A loose membranous layer of exudate containing organisms, precipitated fibrin, necrotic cells, and inflammatory cells produced during an inflammatory reaction on the surface of a tissue.
- *Polyp.* Any mass of tissue that projects outward or upward from the normal surface level.
- *Punctate.* Marked with points or dots differentiated from the surrounding surface by color, elevation, or texture.
- *Torus.* Bony elevation or prominence usually found on the midline of the hard palate (torus palatinus) and the

lingual surface of the mandible (torus mandibularis) in the premolar area.

■ *Verrucous* (verrucose). Rough, wartlike.

ORAL CANCER

■ Objective: to detect cancer of the mouth at the earliest possible stage.
■ Discovered later, when cancer extends into adjacent structures and to the lymph nodes of the neck, the prognosis is less favorable.
■ Because the early lesions are generally symptomless, they may go unnoticed and unreported by the patient.
■ Observation by the dentist or dental hygienist, therefore, is the principal method for the detection of oral cancer.
■ The first step in accomplishing this task is to examine the entire face, neck, and oral mucous membrane of each patient at the initial examination and at each maintenance appointment **(Table 11-1)**.
■ It is necessary to know how to conduct the oral examination, where oral cancer occurs most frequently, what an early cancerous lesion may look like, and what to do when such a lesion is found.
■ In addition to the early lesions of oral cancers, the oral manifestations of neoplasms elsewhere in the body as well as the oral manifestations of chemotherapy can be recognized.

I. LOCATION

■ Neoplasms may arise at any site in the oral cavity.
■ The most common sites are the floor of the mouth, the lateral parts of the tongue, the lower lip, and the soft palate complex.
■ Self-examination: although patients may be instructed in self-examination to watch for changes in oral tissues, it is difficult for persons to see their own tissues, particularly the entire floor of the mouth and base of the tongue, by the usual mirror and lighting systems available in a private home.
■ Self-examination needs to be supplemented with professional examination on a scheduled basis.

II. APPEARANCE OF EARLY CANCER

Early oral cancer takes many forms and may resemble a variety of common oral lesions. All types need to be examined with suspicion. Five basic forms are listed here.

A. White Areas

■ White areas vary from a filmy, barely visible change in the mucosa to heavy, thick, heaped-up areas of dry white keratinized tissue.
■ Fissures, ulcers, or areas of induration in a white area are most indicative of malignancy.

■ *Leukoplakia* is a white patch or plaque that cannot be scraped off or characterized as any other disease. It may be associated with physical or chemical agents and the use of tobacco.

B. Red Areas

■ Lesions of red, velvety consistency, sometimes with small ulcers, are identified.
■ *Erythroplakia* is a term used to designate lesions of the oral mucosa that appear as bright red patches or plaques that cannot be characterized as any specific disease.

C. Ulcers

■ Ulcers may have flat or raised margins.
■ Palpation may reveal induration.

D. Masses

■ Papillary masses, sometimes with ulcerated areas, occur as elevations above the surrounding tissues.
■ Other masses may occur below the normal mucosa and may be found only by palpation.

E. Pigmentation

■ Brown or black pigmented areas may be located on mucosa where pigmentation does not normally occur.

PROCEDURE FOR FOLLOW-UP OF A SUSPICIOUS LESION

As designated by the dentist, a lesion may be biopsied immediately, a cytologic smear may be obtained, or the patient may be referred to various specialists for additional diagnosis and biopsy.

I. BIOPSY

A. Definition

Biopsy is the removal and examination, usually by microscope, of a section of tissue or other material from the living body for the purposes of diagnosis. A biopsy is either *excisional*, when the entire lesion is removed, or *incisional*, when a representative section from the lesion is taken.

B. Indications for Biopsy

■ Any unusual oral lesion that cannot be identified with clinical certainty must be biopsied.
■ Any lesion that has not shown evidence of healing in 2 weeks is considered malignant until proven otherwise.
■ A persistent, thick, white, hyperkeratotic lesion and any mass (elevated or not) that does not break through the surface epithelium needs to be biopsied.

■ Any tissue surgically removed is submitted for microscopic examination.

II. CYTOLOGIC SMEAR

A. Definition

The cytologic smear technique is a diagnostic aid in which surface cells of a suspicious lesion are removed for microscopic evaluation.

B. Indications for Smear Technique[5]

■ In general, a lesion for which a biopsy is not planned may be examined by smear. An exception is a keratotic lesion that is not suitable for exfoliative cytology.
■ A lesion that looks like potential cancer is examined by smear if the patient refuses to have a biopsy specimen taken. A positive report from a smear can be used to convince the patient of the need for treatment or biopsy.

C. Applications

■ The smear technique is used for follow-up examination of patients with oral cancer treated by radiation. The treated tissue may heal inadequately and cause persistent ulceration.
■ Cytology is useful for identifying *Candida albicans* organisms in patients with suspected candidiasis (moniliasis).
■ Cytology may be useful in identifying herpesvirus by taking a smear from an intact vesicle.
■ In mass screening programs for cancer detection, smears may be taken. However, all lesions of high suspicion should be referred for biopsy.
■ Research studies to show changes in surface cells, for example, the effects of topical agents, may use a smear technique.

D. Limitations of Smear Technique

■ When a clear-cut lesion, recognized as pathologic, is present, treatment must not be delayed by waiting for cytologic smear analysis.
■ The smear detects only surface lesions.
■ It is difficult or impossible to scrape deep enough to obtain representative cells from a heavily keratinized lesion.
■ Except for candidiasis, treatment cannot be determined by smear technique results only. After a positive smear, a biopsy is needed for definitive diagnosis.
■ Because research has shown that the smear technique is not diagnostically reliable (there can be "false negatives," which turn out to be positive biopsies), a negative report cannot be considered conclusive.

EXFOLIATIVE CYTOLOGY

■ Stratified squamous epithelial cells are constantly growing toward the surface of the mucous membrane where they are exfoliated.

■ Exfoliated cells and the cells beneath them are scraped off, and when these cells are prepared on a slide, changes in the cells can be detected by staining and studying them microscopically.
■ The malignant cells stain differently from normal cells and take on unusual, abnormal forms.

I. PROCEDURE

A. Materials

■ Gauze sponges
■ Glass microscopic slides with frosted end
■ Plain lead pencil
■ Paper clips
■ Blade to scrape lesion (flexible metal spatula)
■ Fixative (70% alcohol)
■ Protective mailing container
■ History form or data sheet

B. Steps

■ *Prepare materials.* Write the patient's name on the frosted ends of two glass slides (two for each lesion) in pencil, and place a paper clip on the end of one slide to prevent contact between the slides when packaged for mailing to the laboratory.
■ *Prepare the lesion.* Irrigate the surface to remove debris. Wipe the surface gently with a wet gauze sponge as needed to remove debris or blood. Do not dry.
■ *Scrape the lesion.* Use a flexible metal spatula. Scrape the entire surface of the lesion firmly several times (all strokes in the same direction) **(Figure 11-11A)**. When a wooden tongue depressor is used, it must be wet before

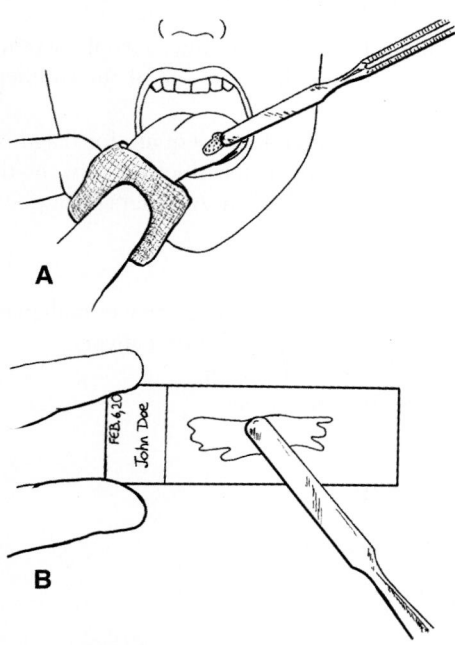

FIGURE 11-11 **Oral Cytology Technique. (A)** Tongue is held out with gauze sponge while a metal spatula is used to scrape a lesion. **(B)** Collected material is spread evenly on a glass slide. See text for details.

taking the sample so the material will not be absorbed into the wood. For intact vesicles, carefully rupture the vesicle so the fluid flows onto the glass slides.

■ *Smear the glass slide.* Spread the collected material on the glass slide. Start at the center of the clear end of the slide and smear evenly across the surface. Cover an area approximately 20 mm wide. Handle all glass slides by their edges to prevent fingerprints or other contamination **(Figure 11-11B)**.

■ *Fix the cells.* Immediately, to prevent drying of the cells, place the slide on a flat surface and flood with generous drops of 70% alcohol or use prepared commercial fixative spray.

■ *Obtain second smear.* Duplicate the previous smear technique. Apply fixing agent immediately.

■ *Complete the fixation.* Leave slides for 30 minutes. After 20 minutes, tip the slide to let remaining alcohol run off. Air-dry where dust or other foreign material cannot contaminate the smear.

■ *Prepare history or data sheet.* Basic information includes the following:
  ■ Dentist. Name and address.
  ■ Patient. Name and address.
  ■ Lesion. Description (size, color, location, shape, consistency, and duration).
  ■ Other. Additional related clinical findings or pertinent history.

■ *Prepare for Mailing.* Wrap slides to prevent breakage. Pack with the history or data sheet. Mailing containers provided by most laboratories list specific instructions.

II. LABORATORY REPORT

The pathologist makes the microscopic examination and classifies the specimen in one of the following categories:

Unsatisfactory: Slide is inadequate for diagnosis. The specimen may have been too thick or thin, or the cells may have dried before fixation. Another smear needs to be made promptly.

■ *Class I:* Normal.
■ *Class II:* Atypical, but not suggestive of malignant cells.
■ *Class III:* Uncertain (possible for cancer).
■ *Class IV:* Probable for cancer.
■ *Class V:* Positive for cancer.

III. FOLLOW-UP

A. Report of Class IV or V

Refer for biopsy.

B. Report of Class III

Reevaluate clinical findings; biopsy usually indicated.

C. Report of Class I or II

■ The patient must not be dismissed until the lesion has healed.
■ When the lesion persists, the dentist either reevaluates the clinical findings and requests a repeat cytologic smear or, preferably, performs a biopsy.

D. Negative Report

■ Either biopsy or smear requires careful follow-up when a negative report is obtained for an oral lesion that appears suspicious by clinical examination.
■ False-negative reports are possible; that is, a malignancy may be present, but the sample examined in the smear or biopsy may not have included cancerous cells.

DOCUMENTATION

Documentation in the permanent record of a patient who needed a biopsy (or smear) because of a questionable cancerous lesion will contain a minimum such as the following:

■ Every detail of the entire oral examination and follow-up procedures with reports from consultants, laboratories, medical follow-up, and outcomes.
■ Recommendations for the frequency of a complete oral examination, at future dental hygiene maintenance appointments.
■ Review of all lifestyle habits that may provide a cause for such an oral lesion to appear in the first place with recommendations for specific preventive methods.
■ A progress note representing the patient's first maintenance appointment following the incident of the biopsy and learning the lesion was not cancerous may be reviewed in **Box 11-2**.

BOX 11-2	Example Progress Note

First-time patient; history and radiographs taken; extra- and intraoral examination revealed a small red area on the side of her tongue about 4 mm wide and 2 mm long. She said that at her last appointment about 3–4 months ago where she used to live, the hygienist mentioned it but didn't make any suggestions except to watch it, and as long as she would be "getting a new dentist where I was moving to, I could find out what was needed." It had not bothered her, but she did come in to start with us so she could find out. She had never seen it, so she couldn't tell whether it changed size. Dr. Joe looked and decided to send her to Dr. Edson (oral surgeon) down the hall for biopsy. We made the appt for her later this pm.

Signed: _____, RDH Date: _____.

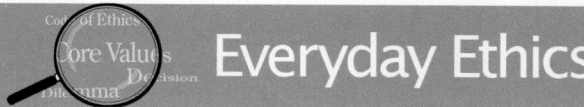

Everyday Ethics

Abby and Sylvia are the two part-time dental hygienists in Dr. Anthony's practice. They practice on different days at the office so rarely see each other except to attend local dental hygiene association meetings. Most patients know both hygienists and may be scheduled with either depending on available time.

Mr. Peters came in for his 3-month maintenance appointment carrying his unlit pipe as usual. This time his appointment was with Abby, and jokes were exchanged about the pipe. During the intraoral examination, Abby found a red lesion on the side of his tongue that was about 4 mm wide. She asked him if he had seen it and his answer was, "Oh yeah, Sylvia mentioned it when I was here last time." Abby glanced at the record and noted that his last date was over 4 months ago. Nothing could be found in the patient's dental record that mentioned any oral lesions.

Questions for Consideration

1. Which of the dental hygiene Code Values (Table II-1, in Section II, Introduction, page 38) are involved here? How?
2. Consider the questions in Table V-1 (in Section V, Introduction, page 362) to help Abby decide which way to go to help Mr. Peters, and improve office policies.
3. Privately, Abby is upset, and she is determined that this needs to be discussed with both Sylvia and Dr. Anthony. Dr. Anthony has never specified a policy for this type of issue. Where and how can she approach them and what recommendations does she need to propose for an office policy?

Factors To Teach The Patient

- Reasons for a careful extraoral and intraoral examination at each maintenance appointment.
- A method for self-examination. Examination includes the face, neck, lips, gingiva, cheeks, tongue, palate, and throat. Any changes are reported to the dentist and the dental hygienist.
- General dietary and nutritional influences on the health of the oral tissues.
- How the oral cavity tends to reflect the general health.
- The Warning Signs of Oral Cancer
  - ☐ A swelling, lump, or growth anywhere, with or without pain.
  - ☐ White scaly patches, or red velvety areas.
  - ☐ Any sore that does not heal promptly (within 2 weeks).
  - ☐ Numbness or tingling.
  - ☐ Excessive dryness or wetness.
  - ☐ Prolonged hoarseness, sore throats, persistent coughing, or the feeling of a "lump in the throat."
  - ☐ Difficulty with swallowing.
  - ☐ Difficulty in opening the mouth.

References

1. National Institute of Dental and Craniofacial Research. *Detecting Oral Cancer: A Guide for Health Care Professionals [Internet]*. Bethesda (MD): National Institutes of Health; [last updated 2010 Jul 2; cited 2011 Mar 15]. [About 9 pages.] Available from: http://www.nidcr.nih.gov/oralhealth/topics/oralcancer/detectingoralcancer.htm
2. Coakley MC. Temporomandibular joint dysfunction (TMJ): the role of the dental hygienist. *J Dent Hyg*. 1988 Nov–Dec;62(10):521–6.
3. McNeill C, Mohl ND, Rugh JD, Tanaka TT. Temporomandibular disorders: diagnosis, management, education, and research. *J Am Dent Assoc*. 1990 Mar;120(3):253, 255, 257.
4. McCann AL, Wesley RK. A method for describing soft tissue lesions of the oral cavity. *Dent Hyg*. 1987 May;61,(5):219–23.
5. Sandler HC, Stahl SS. Exfoliative cytology as a diagnostic aid in the detection of oral neoplasms. *J Oral Surg*. 1958 Sep;16(5):414–18.

Dental Radiographic Imaging

JANET M. GRUBER, RDH, MPA

Chapter Outline

Radiographic images are integral assessment components useful when planning comprehensive care for a patient. They provide the clinician with important diagnostic tools that can be used to detect lesions, diseases, and other conditions of teeth and supporting structures; to localize foreign objects; to assess growth and development; and to document changes in, and progress of, a condition over time.[1]

The dentist is responsible for determining the need for radiographs. Designation of the number and types of dental exposures is made selectively only after a review of the patient's health history and a complete clinical examination.[2] A history of oral and body exposures to radiation is recommended. Excessive dental exposure to low levels of ionizing radiation cannot be justified.[3]

The objective in radiography is to use procedures that expose the patient to the least possible amount of radiation to produce radiographs of the greatest interpretive value. The first consideration is to limit the number of exposures to those that have been deemed necessary.

This chapter provides a summary of terminology and fundamentals of x-ray production. Procedures are included for film exposure and processing, safety factors, analysis of the completed radiographs, and suggestions for patient instruction.

Selected terms used in the study of radiography are listed and defined in **Box 12-1**. **Box 12-2** provides a list of universally used abbreviations.

HOW X-RAYS ARE PRODUCED

X-ray energy is electromagnetic ionizing radiation of very short wavelengths, resulting from the bombardment of a target made of tungsten by highly accelerated electrons in a high vacuum. Electric and magnetic fields positioned at right angles to one another produce the electromagnetic energy.

The various types of energy in the electromagnetic spectrum have similar attributes. The properties of x-rays are listed in **Box 12-3**.

Essential to x-ray production are (1) a source of electrons, (2) a high voltage to accelerate the electrons, and (3) a target to stop the electrons. The parts of the tube and the circuits within the machine are designed to provide these elements.

I. THE X-RAY TUBE (FIGURE 12-1)

A. Protective Tube Housing

Heavy metal enclosure that houses the x-ray tube and reduces the primary radiation to permissible exposure levels.

B. X-Ray Tube

A highly evacuated leaded-glass tube composed of a cathode and anode and surrounded by a specially refined oil with high insulating powers.

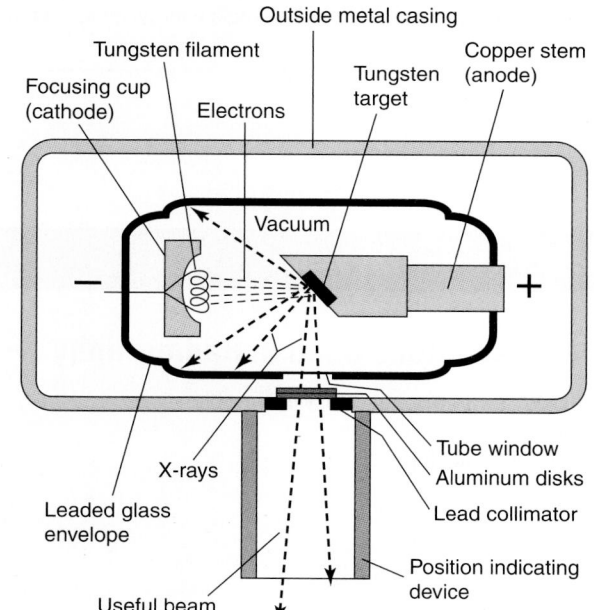

FIGURE 12-1 **X-Ray Tube.** High-speed electrons flowing from cathode to anode hit the tungsten target, create x-ray photons. X-rays exit through the tube window and position-indicating device.

BOX 12-1	Key Words

General Radiography Terms

Ammeter: an instrument for measuring electric current in amperes.

Attenuation: the process by which a beam of radiation is reduced in intensity when passing through some material; the combination of absorption and scattering processes leads to a decrease in flux density of the beam when projected through matter.

Cassette: a light-tight container in which x-ray films are placed for exposure to x-radiation; usually backed with lead to reduce the effect of backscatter radiation; may be made of cardboard, plastic, or of metal with an exposure side of bakelite, aluminum, plastic or magnesium and containing an intensifying screen(s).

Impulse: the burst of radiation generated during a half cycle of alternating current; film exposure time is measured in impulses.

Intensifying screen: a card or plastic sheet coated with fluorescent material positioned singly or in pairs in a cassette. When the cassette is exposed to x-radiation, the visible light from the fluorescent image on the screen adds to the latent image produced directly by x-radiation.

Irradiation: exposure to radiation; one speaks of radiation therapy and of irradiation of a body part.

Latent image: the invisible change produced in an x-ray film emulsion by the action of x-radiation or light from which the visible image is subsequently developed and fixed chemically.

Penumbra: the secondary shadow that surrounds the periphery of the primary shadow; in radiography, it is the blurred margin of an image detail (geometric unsharpness).

Photoelectric effect: the ejection of bound electrons by an incident photon such that the whole energy of the photon is absorbed and transitional or characteristic x-ray emissions are produced.

Photon: a finite bundle of energy of visible light or electromagnetic radiation.

Radiation: the emission and propagation of energy through space or a material medium in the form of waves or particles. Types of radiation are defined in Box 12-4.

Radiograph: a visible image on a radiation-sensitive film emulsion produced by chemical processing after exposure of the film emulsion to ionizing radiation that has passed through an area, region, or substance of interest.

Radiography: the art and science of making radiographs.

Radiologic health: the art and science of protecting human beings from injury by radiation, as well as of promoting better health through beneficial applications of radiation.

Radiology: that branch of science that deals with the use of radiant energy in the diagnosis and treatment of disease.

Radiolucency: the appearance of dark images on a radiograph as a result of the greater amount of radiation that penetrates low-density objects and reaches the film.

Radiopacity: the appearance of light (white) images on a radiograph as a result of the greater amount of radiation that is absorbed by dense objects and does not reach the film.

Rare earth: commonly used to refer to intensifying screens that contain rare earth elements; it may also refer to a screen-film system used for x-ray imaging; the systems are considered "fast" exposure systems.

Rectification: conversion of alternating current (AC) to direct current (DC); a **rectifier** changes AC to DC.

Soma: the entire body with the exclusion of germ cells.

Somatic: adj.

BOX 12-2	Key Words

Abbreviations Used in Radiography

ALARA: as low as reasonably achievable
Gy: gray
HVL: half value layer
kVp: kilovolt peak
mA: milliampere
mAi: milliampere impulse
mAs: milliampere second
mGy: milligray

MPD: maximum permissible dose
mSv: millisievert
PID: position-indicating device
R: roentgen
Rad: radiation absorbed dose
Rem: roentgen equivalent man
Sv: sievert
XCP: extension cone paralleling

BOX 12-3	Properties of X-Rays

Characteristic
- Invisible
- No mass
- No weight

Travel
- In straight line; can be scattered
- At the speed of light

Wavelengths
- Have short wavelengths, high frequency
- Hard x-rays: short wavelengths, high penetration
- Soft x-rays: relatively longer wavelengths; relatively less penetrating; more likely to be absorbed into the tissue

Penetration
- Pass through matter, or
- Absorbed by matter, depending on atomic structure of matter

Causes
- Ionization
- Fluorescence of certain crystals
- Biologic changes in living cells

Produces
- An image on photographic film

C. Cathode (−)

- Tungsten filament, which is a coiled wire heated to generate a cloud of electrons. It is a component of the low-voltage circuit.
- Molybdenum cup around the filament to focus the electrons toward the anode.

D. Anode (+)

A tungsten target embedded in a copper stem, positioned at an angle to the electron beam.

E. Aperture

The window where the useful beam emerges from the tube; covered with a permanent seal of glass.

F. Aluminum Disks

Thin (0.5-mm) sheets of aluminum placed over the aperture to filter out longer-wavelength x-rays.

G. Lead Diaphragm

A lead collimator with a hole to restrict the size of the x-ray beam.

H. Position-Indicating Device (PID)

Open-ended cylinder, or rectangle, that shapes and aims the x-ray beam.

II. CIRCUITS

A circuit is the complete path over which an electrical current may flow. Two circuits are used to produce x-rays. Refer to **Figure 12-2** to examine the electrical circuits in a dental x-ray machine. Two circuits used to produce x-rays are:

- Low-voltage filament circuit
- High-voltage cathode-anode circuit

III. TRANSFORMERS

A transformer increases or decreases the incoming voltage.

A. Autotransformer

A voltage compensator that corrects minor variations in line voltage.

B. Filament Step-Down Transformer

Decreases the line voltage to approximately 3 volts to heat the filament and form the electron cloud.

C. High-Voltage Step-Up Transformer

Increases the current from 110 volts to 60 to 90 kVp (kilovoltage peak) to give electrons the required energy necessary to produce x-ray photons.

IV. MACHINE CONTROL DEVICES

Machines vary, but, in general, when operating an x-ray machine, there are four factors to control: the power switch (to the electrical outlet), the kilovoltage, the milliamperage, and the time.

A. Voltage Control

Voltage is the unit of measurement used to describe the force that pushes an electric current through a circuit.

- *Circuit voltmeter.* Registers line voltage before voltage is stepped up by the transformer (with alternating current, this is 110 volts), or may register the kilovoltage that results after step-up.
- *kVp (selector).* Used to change the line voltage to a selected kilovoltage (60 to 90 kVp).

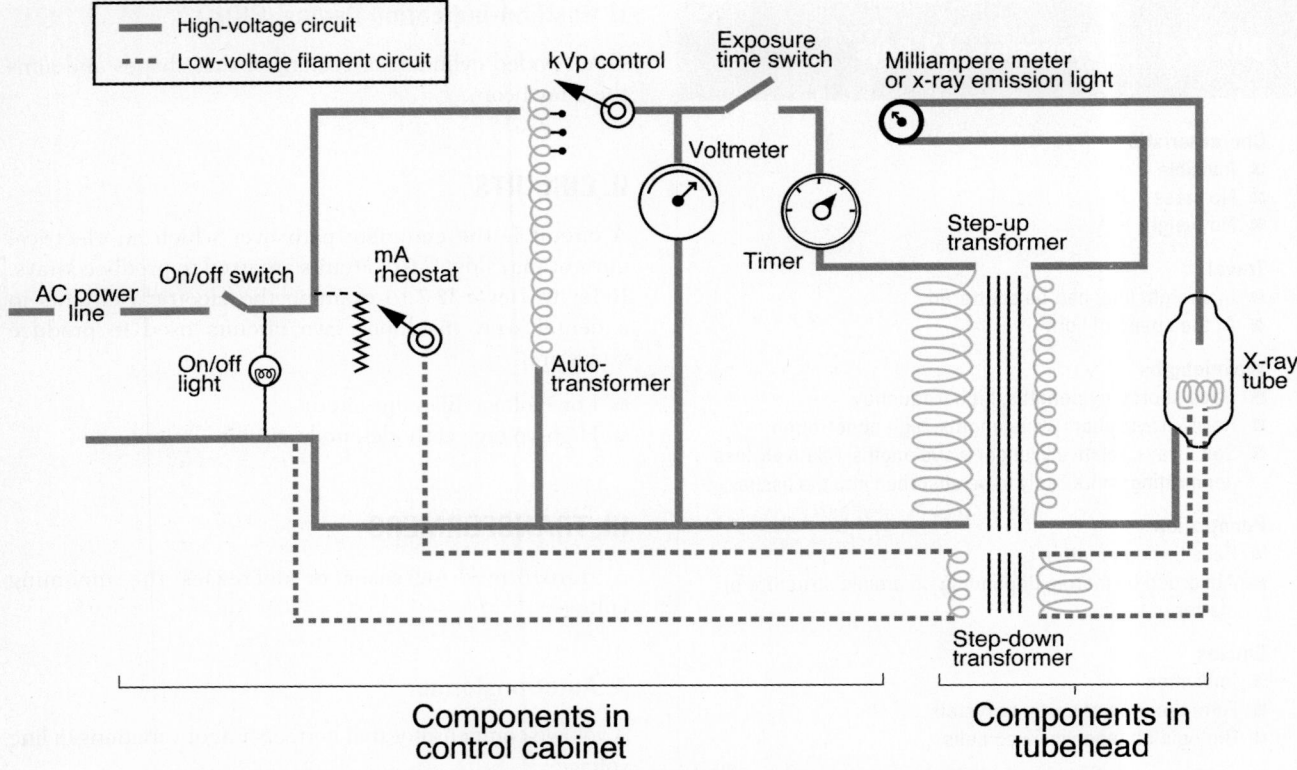

FIGURE 12-2 **Dental X-Ray Machine Circuits.** High- and low-voltage circuits in a dental x-ray machine demonstrating flow of electricity from the on/off switch to the x-ray tube head. (Adapted with permission from Olson SS. Dental radiography laboratory manual. Philadelphia: W.B. Saunders; 1995, 40 p.)

B. Milliamperage Control

■ *Ampere.* The unit of intensity of an electrical current produced by 1 volt acting through a resistance of 1 ohm. A milliampere (mA) is 1/1000 of an ampere.

■ *Milliammeter.* Instrument used to select the actual current through the tube circuit during the time of exposure.

C. Time Control

■ *X-Ray Timer.* A time switch mechanism used to control the length of the exposure time.

■ *Time-Delay Switch.* Mechanism that applies power to the high-voltage circuit once the filament is heated.

■ *Electronic Timer.* Vacuum tube device; resets itself automatically to the last-used exposure time. The timer is calibrated in seconds or in impulses, with 60 *impulses* in each second (in a 60-cycle AC current).

V. STEPS IN THE PRODUCTION OF X-RAYS

X-rays are produced when high-speed electrons are slowed down or stopped suddenly. The many types of radiation produced are defined in **Box 12-4.**

■ Tungsten filament is heated, and a cloud of electrons is produced.

■ Difference in electrical potential is developed between the anode and the cathode.

■ Electrons traveling at a high speed are attracted to the anode from the cathode when the anode is charged positive and the cathode negative. When alternating current is used with a self-rectifying tube, the electrons are attracted back into the tungsten filament.

■ Curvature of the molybdenum cup controls the direction of the electrons and causes them to be projected toward the focal spot.

■ Reaction of the electrons as they strike the tungsten target results in loss of energy.

   A. Approximately 1% of the energy of electrons is converted to x-ray energy (greater percentage at higher kilovoltages).

   B.   Approximately 99% of the energy is converted to heat and is dissipated through the copper anode and oil of the protective tube housing.

■ *General (bremsstrahlung, or braking) radiation* occurs when speeding electrons stop, "brake," or slow down near the tungsten target in the anode. When an electron hits the nucleus of the tungsten atom, all of its kinetic energy is converted into a high-energy x-ray photon. When an electron comes close to but misses the nucleus, an x-ray photon of lower energy is created. General radiation produces x-rays of many different energies.[4]

BOX 12-4	Key Words

Types of Radiation

Bremsstrahlung radiation (white radiation): a distribution of x-rays from very low-energy photons to those produced by the peak kilovoltage applied across an x-ray tube; Bremsstrahlung means "braking radiation" and refers to the sudden deceleration of electrons (cathode rays) as they interact with highly positively charged nuclei, such as tungsten.

Characteristic radiation: the radiation produced by electron transitions from higher energy orbitals to replace ejected electrons of inner electron orbitals; the energy of the electromagnetic radiation emitted is unique or "characteristic" of the emitting atom.

Electromagnetic radiation: forms of energy propagated by wave motion as photons; the radiations differ widely in wavelength, frequency, and photo energy; examples are infrared waves, visible light, ultraviolet radiation, x-rays, gamma rays, and cosmic radiation.

Gamma radiation: short-wavelength electromagnetic radiation of nuclear origin similar to x-rays but usually of higher energy.

Leakage radiation: the radiation that escapes through the protective shielding of the x-ray unit tube head; it may be detected at the sides, top, bottom, or back of the tube head.

Primary radiation: all radiation coming directly from the target of the anode of an x-ray tube.

Scatter radiation: a form of secondary radiation that, during passage through a substance, has been deviated in direction; it may also have been modified by an increase in wavelength.

  Backscatter: radiation deflected by scattering processes at angles greater than 90° to the original direction of the beam of radiation.

  Coherent scattering (Thompson or unmodified): scattering of relatively low-energy x-rays by elastic collisions without loss of photon energy.

  Compton scatter radiation: the incident radiation that has sufficient energy to dislodge a bound electron but attacks a loosely bound electron; the remaining radiation energy proceeds in a different direction as scatter radiation.

Secondary radiation: particles or photons produced by the interaction of primary radiation with matter.

Stray radiation: radiation that serves no useful purpose; it includes leakage, secondary, and scatter radiation.

- *Characteristic radiation* results when a bombarding electron, at 70 kVp or above, displaces an electron from a shell of the target atom, ionizing the atom. Another electron in an outer shell replaces the missing electron, causing a cascading effect. When the displaced electron is replaced, a photon is emitted, resulting in characteristic radiation. Characteristic radiation contributes approximately 10% to the useful beam.
- X-rays leave the tube through the aperture to form the useful beam.
  - A. *Useful beam.* The part of the primary radiation that is permitted to emerge from the tube head aperture and the accessory collimating devices.
  - B. *Central beam* (central ray). The center of the beam of x-rays emitted from the tube.

DIGITAL RADIOGRAPHY

Traditional film-based systems to record radiographic images have been in existence in dentistry since 1895. In the mid to late 1980s, the first direct digital imaging system was introduced and adopted by dental professionals. Digital systems include intraoral, panoramic, and cephalometric imaging. Terminology for digital radiography is listed and defined in **Box 12-5**.

I. DIGITAL IMAGING PRINCIPLES

- Digital radiography requires conventional equipment to generate x-rays.
- The image is captured on sensors or plates of varying sizes, similar to conventional film.
- The information is then recorded as a digital image and displayed as pixels representing some 256 shades of gray.
- The image is subsequently displayed on a computer monitor.
- The image can be enhanced, by changing density and contrast, stored on the hard drive for future reference, and/or electronically sent to other professionals.[5–7]

II. DIGITAL IMAGING AND SENSORS

A. Direct Digital Imaging

- A corded or cordless charge-coupled device (CCD) or complementary-metal-oxide semiconductor (CMOS) sensor in a rigid case is used **(Figure 12-3)**.
- Viewing of the image is possible within seconds of exposure.

B. Indirect or Scanned Digital Imaging

- A cordless photostimuable phosphor plate (PSP plate) is used **(Figure 12-4)**.

BOX 12-5	Key Words

Digital Radiography

Analog: continuous and variable representation of an image as opposed to digital, which is a binary representation (0's and 1's) of an image. An analog image will include all levels of clarity and will not be enhanced as the digital representation.

Charge-coupled device (CCD): a solid-state detector, used in corded intraoral sensors as an image receptor, that converts x-rays to electrons, which are stored in electron wells and then converted to a visible image.

Complementary-metal-oxide semiconductor (CMOS): a corded sensor that has the same characteristics as a CCD, except the individual pixels can be made smaller.

Digital radiography: a filmless imaging system; a method of capturing a radiographic image using a sensor, breaking it into small electronic pieces, and presenting and storing the image using a computer.

Digital subtraction: a method of reversing the gray-scale as an image is viewed; radiolucent (normally black) images appear white and radiopaque (normally white) images appear black.

Digitize: to convert an image into a digital form that can be used by the computer using a grid of pixels.

Direct digital imaging: a filmless method of obtaining a digital image in which an intraoral sensor is directly exposed to x-rays and immediately displays an image, in digital form, on a computer monitor.

Indirect digital imaging: a method of obtaining a digital image in which an existing radiograph is scanned and converted to a digital image or an image is captured intraorally using a photostimulable phosphor plate and then converted from analog to digital by use of a laser scanner. The image is then displayed on a computer monitor.

Photostimuable phosphor plate (PSP): a cordless sensor that converts x-radiation into stored energy. When the PSP is scanned by a laser, the stored energy is released as blue fluorescent light that is converted to digital data and displayed on a computer monitor.

Pixel: The smallest discrete component of an image or picture on a screen that makes up the overall picture; usually dots arranged in rows and columns.

Sensor: a small detector that is placed intraorally to capture a radiographic image.

Storage phosphor imaging: a method of obtaining a digital image in which the image is recorded on phosphor-coated plates and then placed into an electronic processor where a laser scans the plate and produces an image on a computer screen.

- Information on the PSP plate is read by a laser scanner.
- The digital image is displayed on a monitor.
- Traditional films can also be scanned as analog images and converted to digital.

III. STEPS IN THE PRODUCTION OF A DIGITAL RADIOGRAPH

- The sensor, direct or indirect (**Figures 12-3** and **12-4**), is encased in a plastic sleeve (**Figure 12-5**), held in a sensor holder and placed in the patient's mouth.

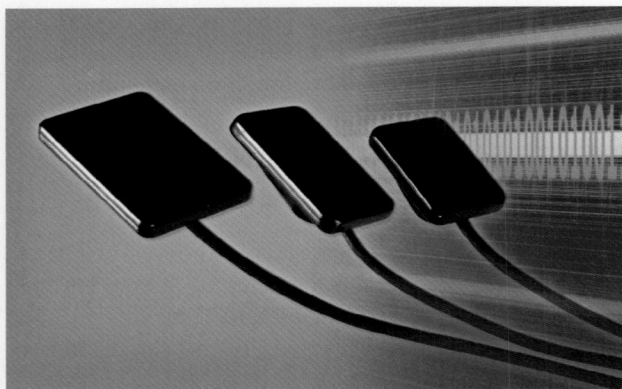

FIGURE 12-3 **Direct Digital Sensors.** Three sensor sizes are shown. CCD or CMOS sensors have integrated circuits made up of a grid of small transistor elements that convert x-rays to electrons in electron wells. Each element represents one pixel in the final image. This information is passed through a cable to the computer for processing.

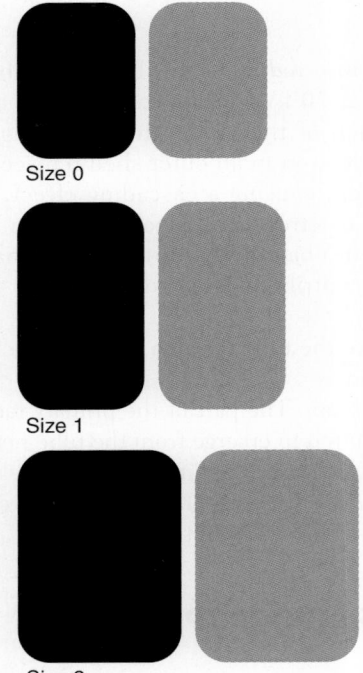

Size 0

Size 1

Size 2

FIGURE 12-4 **Indirect Digital Sensors.** The light blue exposure and black non-exposure sides of three sizes of PSP sensors are shown. PSP sensors are available in intraoral 0–4 sizes, as well as panoramic and cephalometric sizes. The light blue exposure side is covered with phosphor crystals that store x-ray exposure energy. When the sensor is placed in a laser scanner, the energy is released from the phosphor layer and converted to a digital image.

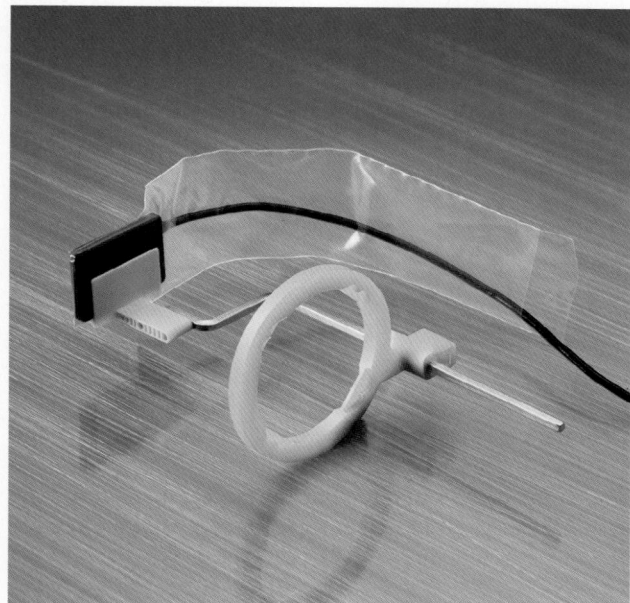

FIGURE 12-5 **Sensor Holder in Plastic Sleeve.** The sensor holder is encased in a plastic sleeve for infection control purposes.

■ When exposed to radiation, an electronic charge is produced on the surface of the sensor.

■ With direct digital imaging, the image is immediately converted from analog form to digital form and displayed on the monitor **(Figure 12-6)**. With indirect digital imaging, the PSP plates store the image until placed in a high-speed laser scanner, by the clinician, that converts the information into a digitized image and displays it on the monitor.

■ The image can then be stored, manipulated, enhanced, retrieved, and transmitted.

■ The CCD or CMOS (direct imaging) sensors can be reused immediately on the same patient, or unwrapped and sanitized, according to the manufacturer's recommendations, for use on another patient. The PSP (indirect imaging) plate is erased by a high-intensity light for approximately 30 seconds.

IV. EVALUATION

A. Advantages of Digital Radiography

■ Reduction of radiation dosage
■ Filmless radiography
■ No darkroom or processing chemistry
■ Immediate feedback for diagnosis
■ Improved diagnostics through software tools
■ Effective patient education tool
■ Ability to send image electronically

B. Disadvantages of Digital Radiography

■ Initial setup costs
■ Direct imaging sensors may be uncomfortable

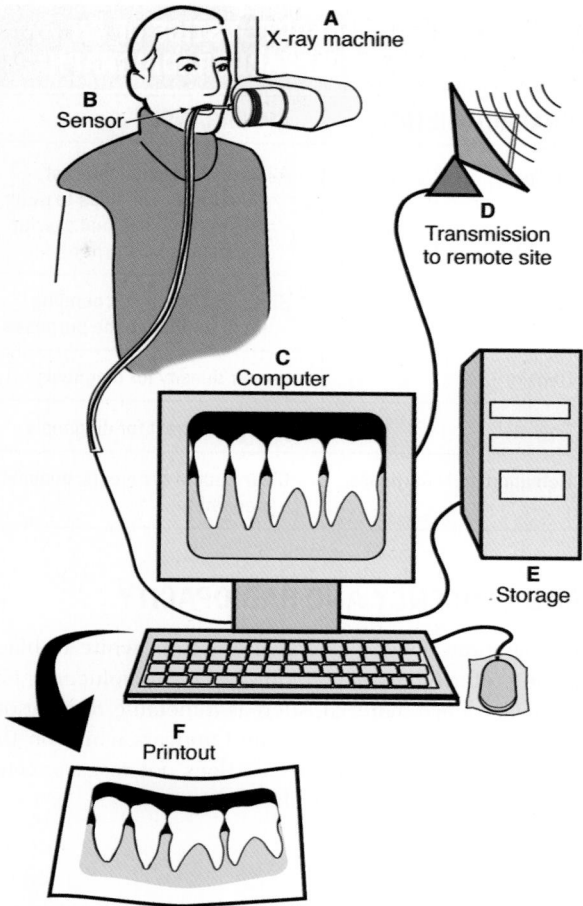

FIGURE 12-6 **Direct Digital Imaging System. (A)** The image is exposed by an x-ray machine, **(B)** captured on a CCD or CMOS sensor in the patient's mouth. **(C)** The signal is transmitted via a cable to the computer, where it is digitized into 256 gray levels. The image is displayed on the computer's monitor, **(D)** transmitted electronically to a remote site, **(E)** stored on a file server, or **(F)** printed on paper.

■ Infection control of sensors: are covered by plastic sleeves as they cannot be heat sterilized

CHARACTERISTICS OF AN ACCEPTABLE RADIOGRAPHIC IMAGE

A *radiographic image* is the visible image on a radiation-sensitive film or a digitized image created by the computer. The image is produced after exposure to ionizing radiation that has passed through an area, or specifically for dentistry, through teeth or a part of the oral cavity. A *radiographic survey* refers to a series of radiographic images.

Before making a radiographic image, it is necessary to know the characteristics that are expected to result in a radiograph of maximum diagnostic value. The basic essentials are the appearance of the image itself, the area covered, and the quality of the processed radiograph. **Table 12-1** provides a list of characteristics of an acceptable radiograph.

TABLE 12-1	CHARACTERISTICS OF AN ACCEPTABLE RADIOGRAPH
CHARACTERISTIC	**APPEARANCE**
Image	All parts of teeth of interest must be shown close to natural size, with minimal overlap and minimal distortion
Area covered	Sufficient tissue surrounding tooth for diagnostic purposes
Density	Proper density for diagnosis
Contrast	Proper contrast for diagnosis
Definition and sharpness	Clear outline of objects; minimal penumbra

I. RADIOLUCENCY AND RADIOPACITY

A radiographic image has gradations from white to black that are referred to as radiopaque or radiolucent. For example, a dense material, such as a metallic restoration, prevents the passage of x-rays and appears white on the processed radiograph. Soft tissue does not resist passage of x-rays and, thus, appears black to gray.

II. RADIOPACITY

The appearance of light (white) images on a radiograph is a result of the lesser amount of radiation that penetrates the structures and reaches the film. A radiopaque structure inhibits the passage of x-rays. Examples include:

- Enamel
- Dentin
- Metallic restorations
- Implants

III. RADIOLUCENCY

The appearance of dark images on a radiograph is a result of the greater amount of radiation that penetrates the structures and reaches the film. A *radiolucent* structure permits the passage of radiation with relatively little attenuation by absorption. Examples include:

- Pulp
- Cysts
- Cavitated dental caries
- Periodontal ligament

FACTORS THAT INFLUENCE THE FINISHED RADIOGRAPH

As the beam leaves the x-ray tube **(Figure 12-1)** it is collimated, filtered, and allowed to travel a designated source–

film (or focal spot–film) distance before reaching the film of a selected speed. The quality or diagnostic usefulness of the finished radiograph, as well as the total exposure of the patient and clinician are influenced by the *kilovoltage, milliampere seconds, time, collimation, filtration, target–film distance, object–film distance,* and *film speed,* as outlined in **Box 12-6.**

Film processing (page 186) also directly influences the quality of the radiograph and indirectly the total exposure. Reexposure would be necessary should the film be rendered inadequate during processing.

I. COLLIMATION

Collimation is the technique for controlling the size and shape of the beam of radiation emitted. A *collimator* is a diaphragm or system of diaphragms made of an absorbing material designed to define the dimensions and direction of a beam of radiation.

A. Purposes

- Eliminate peripheral or more divergent radiation.
- Minimize exposure to patient's face.
- Minimize secondary radiation, which can fog the film and expose the bodies of patient and clinician.

B. Methods

- Lead diaphragm
  A. A diaphragm usually is made of lead with a central aperture of the smallest practical diameter for making radiographic exposure.
  B. It is located between the aluminum filters in the tube head and the position-indicating device (PID).
  C. Recommended thickness of lead: 1/8 inch
  D. Recommended size of aperture: to permit a diameter of the beam of radiation equal to 2.75 inches or 7 cm at the end of the PID next to the patient's face.
- Rectangular collimation
  A. As shown in **Figure 12-7.**
  B. When a rectangular collimator is used, the size of the beam is greatly reduced and patient receives far less unnecessary radiation.
  C. A rectangular beam of radiation's diameter is approximately 11/2 × 2 inches at the skin.
  D. A rectangular collimator is rotated to accommodate films positioned horizontally or vertically.
- Lead-lined cylindrical or rectangular PID
  A. The PID is an open-ended cylinder, or rectangle, to reduce secondary radiation.

C. Relation to Techniques

- Dimensions of the largest periapical film: 11/4 × 15/8 inches.[2]
- Precise angulation techniques are required to eliminate "cone-cut" of film, particularly when rectangular collimation is used.

BOX 12-6	Factors That Influence the Radiographic Image

Kilovoltage Peak
- Affects contrast and density
- Low kVp yields high (short-scale) contrast
- High kVp yields low (long-scale) contrast

Milliamperage
- Affects density
- High mA yields high density
- Low mA yields low density

Time
- Affects density
- Long time yields high density
- Short time yields low density

Collimation
- Shapes the beam
- Not to exceed 2.75 inches or 7 cm at the patient's skin

Lead diaphragm
- PID
- Rectangular
- Cylindrical

Filtration
Types
- Aluminum filters remove low-energy x-rays
- Rare earth filters remove low- and high-energy x-rays

Methods of Filtration
Inherent
- Glass window
- Insulating oil
- Tube head seal

Added
- Aluminum disks
- 1.5 mm for 50 to 69 kVp
- 2.5 for 70 kVp and above

Total filtration
- Combination of inherent and added

Target–film distance
- Longer PID increases resolution of image
- Longer PID decreases scatter of radiation

Object–film distance
- Increased object–film distance achieves parallelism
- Decreased object–film distance decreases penumbra

Film speed
- Faster-speed film decreases definition; image is more grainy

- "Cone-cut" refers to an error of technique that results when the PID is not angled with the central ray centered on the film being exposed.

II. FILTRATION

Filtration is the insertion of absorbers or filters for the preferential attenuation of radiation from a primary beam of x-radiation. Two different types of filters provide filtration in the dental x-ray machine.

A. Types of Filters

- *Aluminum filters* remove low-energy x-ray photons from the x-ray beam.
- *Rare earth filters* selectively remove both low- and high-energy photons from the x-ray beam. Examples of rare earth filters include samarium, erbium, yttrium, niobium, gadolinium, terbium-activated gadolinium oxysulfide, and thulium-activated lanthanum oxybromide.

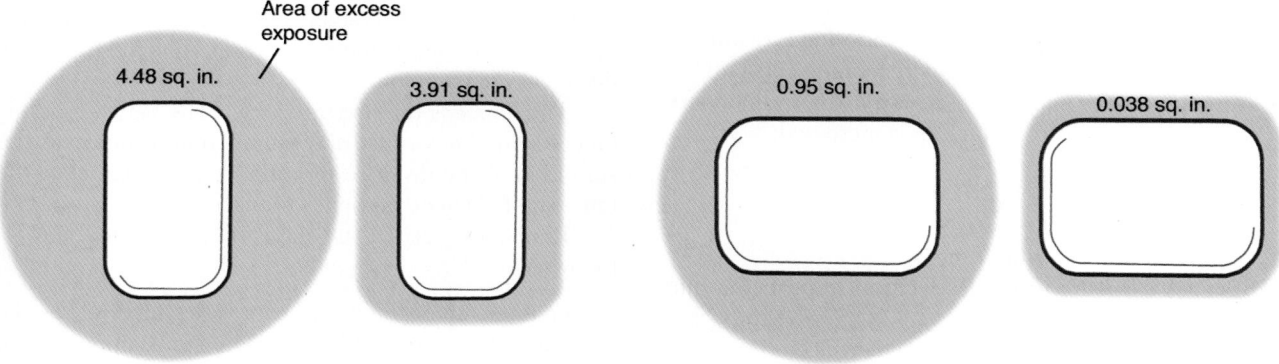

Area of excess exposure

4.48 sq. in.   3.91 sq. in.   0.95 sq. in.   0.038 sq. in.

Size 1 Film   Size 2 Film

FIGURE 12-7 **Cylindrical and Rectangular Position-Indicating Devices.** The useless areas of radiation are greatly lessened when rectangular collimation is used. The patient can be spared exposure to excessive radiation. (Redrawn with permission from Shannon SA. Rectangular versus cylindrical collimation. Dent Hyg. April 1987;61:173. Copyright © 1987 by the American Dental Hygienists' Association.)

B. Purpose

To minimize exposure of the patient's skin to unnecessary radiation.

C. Methods

- *Inherent filtration.* Includes the glass envelope encasing the x-ray tube and the glass window in the tube housing **(Figure 12-1)**.
- *Added filtration.* Thin, pure, aluminum disks inserted between the lead diaphragm and the x-ray tube.
- *Total filtration.* The sum of inherent and added filtration.

The recommended total is the equivalent of 0.5 mm (below 50 kVp), 1.5 mm (50–69 kVp), and 2.5 mm (70 kVp and above) of aluminum.

III. KILOVOLTAGE

Kilovoltage is the potential difference of force that moves electrons between the negative anode and the positive cathode of an x-ray tube. When the kilovoltage is increased, the speed of electrons is increased and the resulting x-rays have a shorter wavelength and more penetrating power. The kVp refers to the crest value (in kilovolts) of the potential difference of a pulsating generator. When only one-half of the wave is used, the value refers to the useful half of the cycle.

A. How kVp Affects the Radiographic Image

- Affects the **contrast**
  - A. Low kilovoltage produces high contrast, with sharp black–white differences in densities between adjacent areas but a small range of distinction between subject thicknesses recorded.
  - B. High kilovoltage produces low contrast, with a wide range of subject thicknesses recorded; greater range of densities from black to white (more gray tones), which provide more interpretive details.
- Affects the **density**: increased kilovoltage results in increased density (other factors remaining constant).
- To maintain the same film **density**: the milliampere seconds is decreased as the kVp is increased.

B. Advantages of High kVp

- Permits shorter exposure time.
- Reduces exposure to tissues lying in front of the film packet.
- Facilitates the detection of bone changes.

C. Disadvantages of High kVp

- Increased radiation to tissues outside the edges of the film.
- More internal scattered radiation at 90 kVp than at 70 kVp.

IV. MILLIAMPERE SECONDS

A. Milliamperage

The measure of the electron current passing through the x-ray tube; it regulates the heat of the filament, which determines the number of electrons available to bombard the target. As the milliamperage is increased, the density of the image is increased.

B. Quantity of Radiation

Quantity of radiation is expressed in milliampere seconds (mAs).

- Definition: mAs is the milliamperes multiplied by the exposure time in seconds; mAi is the milliamperes multiplied by the exposure time in impulses.
- Example: At 10 milliamperes for 1/2 second, the exposure of the film would be 5 mAs. At 10 milliamperes for 15 impulses, the exposure of the film would be 150 mAi.

V. DISTANCE

Several distances are involved in x-ray film exposure. The object–film and the target–film distances are considered for film placement.

A. Object–Film Distance

- Refers to the distance between the object (teeth of interest) and the film.
- With the paralleling technique and the use of a film holder, the object–film distance is greater than it is for the bisecting-angle technique.
- A collimated beam and increased source–film distance compensate to maximize definition and resolution.

B. Target–Film Distance

The PID on the x-ray machine is designed to indicate the direction of the x-ray beam and to serve as a guide in establishing desired target–surface and target–film distances. Techniques using 8-, 12-, and 16-inch target–film distances are common.

The *source* is the *tungsten target*. The target–film distance (sometimes called the source–film distance) is the sum total of the distance from the tungsten target to the film. The PID lightly touches the face.

Principles related to target–film distance are as follows:

- The intensity of the x-ray beam varies inversely as the square of the target–film distance. For example, if two films of the same speed were used, one at a 16-inch target–film distance and one at an 8-inch distance, the film at 16 inches would require four times the exposure (time) to maintain the same density in the finished radiograph.

- The exposure decreases as the distance increases; when the distance is doubled, the radiation exposure to the patient is reduced to one fourth.
- To maintain film density when distance is increased, an increase in mAs, kVp, or time is required.

C. Advantages in the Use of a Long PID

- Increased definition.
- Decreased magnification.
- Decreased skin exposure owing to decreased scatter.

VI. FILMS

With optimum filtration, collimation, and fast film, the skin dose to the face can be reduced significantly. In recent years, the manufacture of very-slow-speed films has been discontinued, the speed of films has been increased, and the use of higher-speed films has gained increased acceptance by the dental profession.

A. Film Composition

A film is a thin, transparent sheet of cellulose acetate coated on both sides with an emulsion of gelatin and silver halide crystals.

- *Film base.* A flexible piece of polyester plastic that is used to provide support for the emulsion.
- *Halide crystals.* Silver bromide and silver iodide crystals are used in dental x-ray film. They are sensitive to radiation and light.
- *Emulsion.* A coating of gelatinous and nongelatinous materials attached to both sides of the film base that keeps the silver halide crystals evenly dispersed in a suspension.
- *Adhesive layer.* A thin layer of adhesive material that covers both sides of the film base and keeps the emulsion on the film base.

B. Film Packet

Sealed paper or plastic envelope that is small, light proof, and moisture resistant, containing an x-ray film (or two), black paper, and a thin sheet of lead foil.

- Two-film packet: useful for processing one film differently from the other to make diagnostic comparisons; for sending to specialist to whom patient may be referred; for legal evidence.
- Purpose of black paper: to protect against light.
- Purposes of lead foil backing: to prevent exposure of the film by scattered radiation that could enter from back of packet and to protect the patient's tissues lying in the path of the x-ray.

C. Film Speed

Film speed or film emulsion speed refers to the sensitivity of the film to radiation exposure. The speed is the amount of exposure required to produce a certain image density. The smaller the grain size, the slower the film speed. The slower the film speed, the less grainy the resulting image.

- *Classification.* Films have been classified by the American National Standards Institute (ANSI) in cooperation with the American Dental Association (ADA). The ANSI/ADA Specification No. 22 designates six groups, A through F. Speed groups A, B, and C, the slowest, are associated with excess radiation exposure and are no longer used.
- *Choice.* F-speed film is recommended for use with rectangular collimation for marked reduction in radiation exposure.

EXPOSURE TO RADIATION

I. IONIZING RADIATION

Ionizing radiation is electromagnetic radiation (e.g., x-rays or gamma rays) or particulate radiation (e.g., electrons, neutrons, or protons) capable of ionizing air directly or indirectly.

The phenomenon of separation of electrons from molecules to change their chemical activity is called ionization. The organic and inorganic compounds that make up the human body may be altered by exposure to ionizing radiation. The biologic effects following irradiation are secondary effects in that they result from physical, chemical, and biologic action set in motion by the absorption of energy from radiation.

Factors that would influence the biologic effects of radiation are outlined in **Box 12-7**. Radiation to *somatic* tissues will affect the irradiated individual only, whereas radiation to *genetic* tissues will affect offspring and possibly future generations.

II. EXPOSURE

A. Types of Exposure

Exposure is a measure of the x-radiation to which a person or object, or a part of either, is exposed at a certain place; this measure is based on its ability to produce ionization.

BOX 12-7	Factors That Influence the Biologic Effects of Radiation

- Quality of the radiation
- Chemical composition of the absorbing medium
- Sensitivity of tissues
- Total dose and dose rate
- Blood supply to the tissues
- Size of the area exposed
- Somatic vs. genetic cells

TABLE 12-2	RADIATION UNITS		
DEFINITION	**TRADITIONAL UNIT**	**S.I. UNIT**[*]	**EQUIVALENT**
Unit of radiation exposure	Roentgen (R)	Coulomb per kilogram (C/kg)	1 R = 2.58 × 10^{-4} C/kg
Unit of absorbed dose	Rad	Gray (Gy)	100 rad = 1 Gy
Unit of dose equivalent	Rem	Sievert (Sv)	100 rem = 1 Sv
Unit of radioactivity	Curie (Ci)	Becquerel (Bq)	1 Ci = 3.7 × 10^{10} Bq

[*]S.I. (System International) is from the French *Système* International d'Unités.

- *Threshold exposure.* The minimum exposure that produces a detectable degree of any given effect.
- *Entrance or surface exposure.* Exposure measured at the surface of an irradiated body, part, or object. It includes primary radiation and backscatter from the irradiated underlying tissue. The term *skin exposure* is used with reference to the exposure measured at the center of an irradiated skin surface area.
- *Erythema exposure.* The radiation necessary to produce a temporary redness of the skin.

B. Exposure Units

The units of absorbed dose are expressed in joules/kilogram (1 rad = 0.01 J/kg). The units shown in **Table 12-2** are the recommendations of the International Commission on Radiation Units and Measurements.[8]

The unit of measurement is the *gray* (Gy). An absorbed dose of 1 Gy is equal to 1 J/kg; therefore, an absorbed dose of 1 Gy is equal to 100 rad.

The unit of biologic equivalence is the *sievert* (Sv). 1 Sv = 100 rem.

C. Dose

The radiation dose is the amount of energy absorbed per unit mass of tissue at a site of interest. The kinds of doses are defined in **Box 12-8**.

D. Permissible Dose

The amount of radiation that may be received by an individual within a specified period without expectation of any significantly harmful result is called the *permissible dose*.

Assumptions on which permissible doses are calculated include the following:

- No irradiation is beneficial.
- There is a dose below which no somatic cellular changes can be produced.

BOX 12-8	Key Words and Abbreviations

Types of Radiation Doses

Absorbed dose: the amount of energy imparted by ionizing radiation to a unit mass of irradiated material at a specific exposure point; the unit of absorbed dose is the gray (Gy).

Cumulative dose: the total dose resulting from repeated exposures to radiation of the same region or of the whole body.

Dose: the amount of energy absorbed per unit mass of tissue at a site of interest.

Dose equivalent: the product of absorbed dose and modifying factors, such as the quality factor, distribution factor, and any other necessary factors; different types of radiation cause differing biologic effects; the unit of dose equivalence is the sievert (Sv).

Dose rate: rate of exposure.

Erythema dose: the minimum quantity of x or gamma radiation that produces the appearance of redness (erythema).

Exit dose: the absorbed dose delivered by a beam of radiation to the surface through which the beam emerges from an object.

Lethal dose: the amount of radiation that is, or could be, sufficient to cause the death of an organism.

LD 50–30: the dose of radiation that is lethal for 50% of a large population in a specified period of time, usually 30 days.

Maximum permissible dose: the maximum dose equivalent that a person (or specified parts of that person) is allowed to receive in a stated period of time; the dose of radiation that would not be expected to produce any significant radiation effects in a lifetime.

Skin dose (surface absorbed dose): the absorbed dose delivered by a radiation beam and backscatter at the point where the central ray passes through the superficial layer of the object.

Threshold dose: the minimum dose that produces a detectable degree of any effect.

TABLE 12-3	MAXIMUM PERMISSIBLE DOSE EQUIVALENT VALUES (MPD)* TO WHOLE BODY, GONADS, BLOOD-FORMING ORGANS, LENS OF EYE		
AVERAGE WEEKLY EXPOSURE†	**MAXIMUM 13-WK EXPOSURE**	**MAXIMUM YEARLY EXPOSURE**	**MAXIMUM ACCUMULATED EXPOSURE‡**
0.1 R	3 R	5 R	5(N–18) R§
0.001 Sv	0.03 Sv	0.05 Sv	0.05(N–18) Sv

*Exposure of persons for dental or medical purposes is not counted against their maximum permissible exposure limits.
†Used only for the purpose of designating radiation barriers.
‡When the previous occupational history of an individual is not definitely known, it shall be assumed that the full dose permitted by the formula 5(N–18) has already been received.
§N = Age in years and is greater than 18. The unit for exposure is the roentgen (R) or sievert (Sv).

- Children are more susceptible than are older people.
- There is a dose below which, even though it is delivered before the end of the reproductive period, the probability of genetic effects is slight.

E. Radiation Hazard

A condition under which persons might receive radiation in excess of the maximum permissible dose. Exposure would be a risk in an area where x-ray equipment is being used or where radioactive materials are stored.

F. National Council on Radiation Protection and Measurements

- *Limits for dentists and dental personnel.* See **Table 12-3**.
- *Limits for patients.* Exposure to radiation shall be kept to the minimum level consistent with clinical requirements for accurate diagnosis based on patient need.[9]

BOX 12-9	Radiation Sensitivity of Tissues and Organs

High
- Bone marrow
- Reproductive cells
- Intestines
- Lymphoid tissue

Moderately High
- Oral mucosa
- Skin

Moderate
- Growing bone
- Growing cartilage
- Small vasculature
- Connective tissue

Moderately Low
- Salivary glands
- Mature bone
- Mature cartilage
- Thyroid gland tissue

Low
- Liver
- Optic lens
- Kidneys
- Muscle
- Nerve

- *ALARA concept.* Radiation exposures are kept As Low As Reasonably Achievable. This concept is accepted and enforced by all regulatory agencies.

III. SENSITIVITY OF CELLS

A. Factors Affecting Cell Sensitivity to Radiation

- *Cell differentiation.* Immature cells are most sensitive. Highly specialized cells are radioresistant.
- *Mitotic activity.* Rapidly reproducing cells are more sensitive; most sensitive when undergoing mitosis.
- *Cell metabolism.* Cells are more sensitive in periods of increased metabolism.

B. Radiosensitive and Radioresistant Tissues

- Radiosensitive: a cell that is sensitive to radiation.
- Radioresistant: a cell that is resistant to radiation.
- Radiation sensitivity of tissues and organs: the relative sensitivities are shown in **Box 12-9**.

C. Tissue Reaction

- *Latent period.* Lapse between the time of exposure and the time when effects are observed. (May be as long as 25 years or relatively shorter, as in the case of the production of a skin erythema.)
- *Cumulative effect*
  A. Amount of reaction depends on dose; the reaction to radiation received in fractional doses is less than the reaction to one large dose.
  B. Partial or total repair occurs as long as destruction is not complete.
  C. Some irreparable damage may be cumulative as, little by little, more radiation is added (e.g., hair loss, skin lesions, falling blood cell count).

RISK OF INJURY FROM RADIATION

The risk of injury from dental diagnostic radiation is extremely low; however, the more radiation received, the higher the chance of cellular injuries. With each exposure to radiation, cellular damage is followed by repair. The effects of radiation exposure are cumulative, and any cellular changes that are not repaired result in damaged tissues. Most of the damage caused by dental diagnostic low-level radiation is repaired within the body cells.

RULES FOR RADIATION PROTECTION

- *Dental x-ray protection,* prepared by the National Council on Radiation Protection and Measurements,[9] provides specific information about radiation barriers, film speed group rating, film badge service sources, x-ray equipment data, and operating procedure regulations.
- To protect the clinician and the patient from excessive radiation, attention is paid to unnecessary radiation that may result from retakes due to inadequate clinical procedures. Perfecting techniques contributes to the accomplishment of minimum exposure for maximum safety.

PROTECTION OF CLINICIAN

I. PROTECTION FROM PRIMARY RADIATION

- Stand behind a protective barrier.
- Avoid the useful beam of radiation.
- Never hand-hold the film during exposure.

II. PROTECTION FROM LEAKAGE RADIATION

- Do not hand-hold the tube housing or the PID of the machine during exposures.
- Test machine for leakage radiation.
- Wear monitoring device for testing exposure.

III. PROTECTION FROM SECONDARY RADIATION

The major sources of secondary radiation are the filter and the irradiated soft tissues of the patient. Other sources may be the leakage from the tube housing or scatter from furniture and walls contacted by the primary beam. Methods of protection are related to these sources.

A. Minimization of Total X-Radiation

- Use high-speed films.
- Have x-ray machines tested frequently for x-ray output and leakage.
- Replace older x-ray machines with modern equipment.

B. Collimation of Useful Beam

Use diaphragms and long PIDs to collimate the useful beam to an area no larger than 2.75 inches or 7 cm in diameter at the patient's skin. Rectangular collimation has

been shown to be more effective than round collimation (**Figure 12-7**).

C. Type of PID

Use a shielded cylinder that is rectangular, long, and open ended, or use some other form of rectangular collimation.

D. Position of Clinician While Making Exposures

The clinician shall stand behind the patient's head behind the major sources of secondary radiation to prevent direct exposure.

- *Exposure of the region of the central incisors.* Stand at a 45° angle to the path of the central ray. This position is approximately behind either the left or the right ear of the patient (**Figure 12-8**).
- *Exposure of other regions.* Stand behind the patient's head and at an angle of 45° to the path of the central ray of the x-ray beam.

E. Distance

- Safety increases with distance.
- The correct position for the clinician is behind an appropriate radiation-resistant barrier wall, preferably with a leaded window to permit a view of the patient during exposures.
- When protective barrier shielding is not available, the clinician shall stand as far as practical from the patient, at least 6 ft (2 m)[10] in the zone between 90° and 135° to the primary central ray, as shown in **Figure 12-8**.

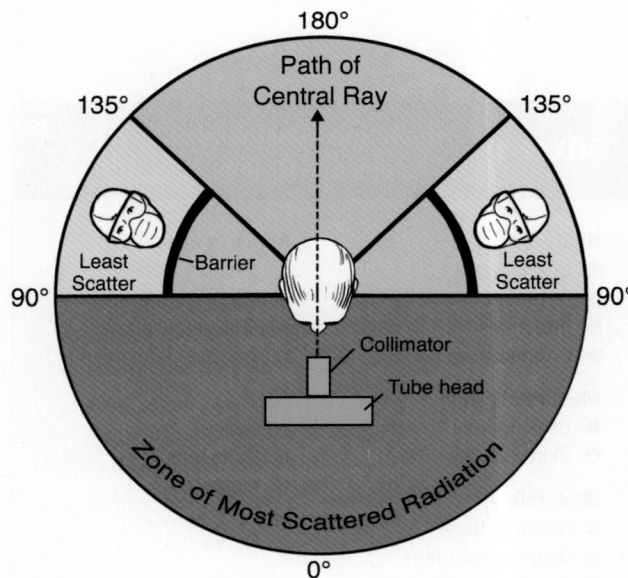

FIGURE 12-8 **Safe Position for Clinician.** While making an exposure, the clinician stands behind the patient's head, between 90° and 135° from the primary beam.

IV. MONITORING

The amount of x-radiation that reaches the dental personnel can be measured economically with a film badge. Badges can be obtained from one of several laboratories. The film badge is:

■ Worn at waist level for 1, 2, or 4 weeks.
■ Returned on a routine basis to the laboratory by mail and processed; its exposure is evaluated.
■ What is used to measure the exposure of the wearer. The wearer is notified by mail of the amount of exposure.
■ Not to be shared with other clinicians.

PROTECTION OF PATIENT

I. FILMS

Use high-speed films. Use the largest intraoral film that can be placed skillfully in the mouth. Maximum coverage is provided in this manner with one exposure, whereas two exposures may be required if smaller films are used to examine the same area of the mouth. This factor is especially important when examining the mouths of children.

II. COLLIMATION

Use diaphragms and an open-ended, shielded (lead lined), rectangular cylinder to collimate the useful beam.

III. FILTRATION

Use filtration of the useful beam to recommended levels (page 167).

IV. PROCESSING

Process films according to the manufacturer's directions. When a choice of two periods of development is offered, the exposure of the patient can be reduced if the longer development time is employed.

V. TOTAL EXPOSURE

Do not expose the patient unnecessarily. Determine a valid reason for each exposure.

VI. PATIENT BODY SHIELDS

The use of leaded or lead-free alloy body shields for each patient is required by law in many states and countries. The purpose of the shield is to absorb scattered rays. An acceptable lead shield contains a minimum of 0.25 mm of lead thickness.

A. Protective Apron
■ *Types*
  ■ General body coverage with extensions over the shoulders and down over the gonadal area.

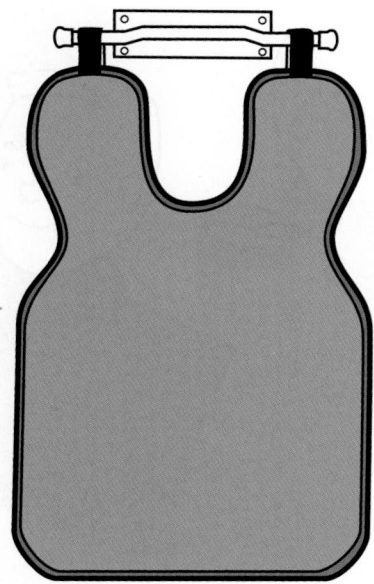

FIGURE 12-9 **Care of Leaded Apron.** The apron can be kept on hooks or a hanging device near the x-ray machine to prevent cracks and prolong the usefulness of the apron.

  ■ Body coverage, with cervical thyroid collar attached.
  ■ Body coverage, with added coverage for the patient's upper back for wear during panoramic radiography.
■ *Care*
  ■ Prevent cracks in leaded shields by hanging **(Figure 12-9)**.
  ■ Disinfect the apron before and after each use.

B. Thyroid Cervical Collar

Thyroid cancer can result from long-term exposure of the gland to x-rays.[11,12] The gland is completely covered during exposure to x-rays. **Figure 12-10** shows the position of a thyroid collar over the neckline of a body apron.

CLINICAL APPLICATIONS

I. ASSESSMENT FOR NEED OF RADIOGRAPHS

■ Review health history.
■ Prepare or review radiation exposure history.
  ■ Medical diagnostic or therapeutic radiation.
  ■ Dates of dental surveys and availability of previous radiographs.
■ Review clinical examination.
■ Obtain dentist's prescription for number and type of radiographs. Refer to the *Guidelines for Prescribing Dental Radiographs* in **Tables 12-4, 12-4A,** and **12-4B.**[2]

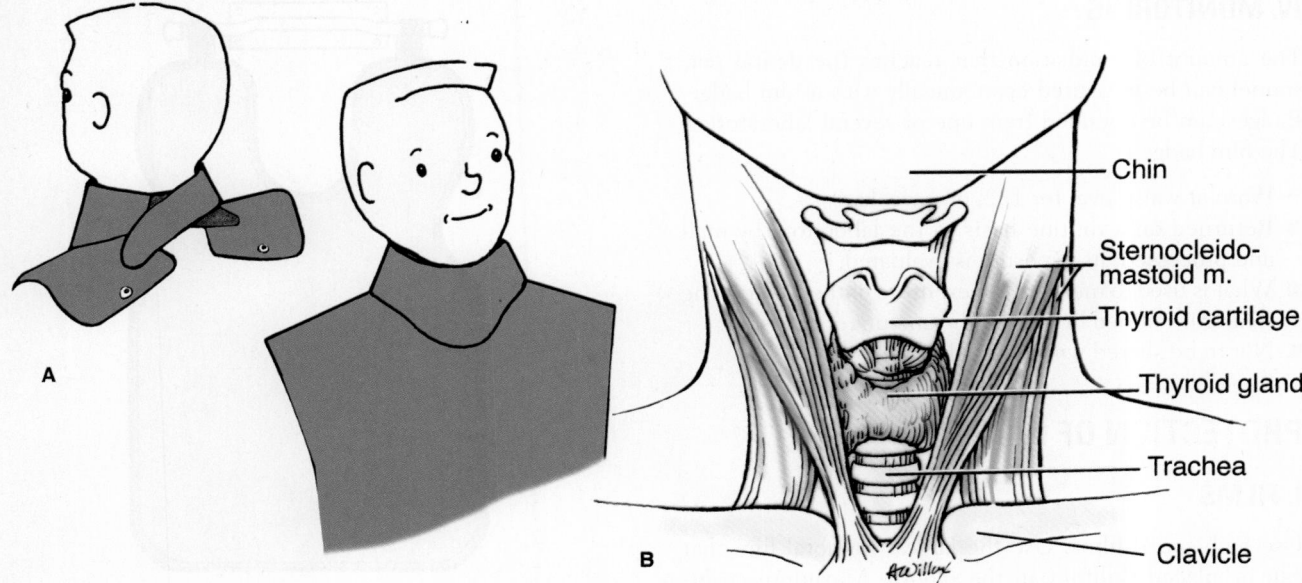

FIGURE 12-10 **Thyroid Cervical Collar. (A)** Thyroid collar in position, covering the neck and overlapping the leaded apron used for general body coverage. Velcro tabs facilitate overlap fastening at back of neck. Collars are available in child and adult sizes. **(B)** The thyroid gland is located over the trachea approximately halfway between the chin and the clavicles. Drawing shows anatomic relationship to the sternocleidomastoid muscle.

II. PREPARATION OF CLINIC FACILITY: INFECTION CONTROL ROUTINE

■ Standard precautions are followed for all radiographic equipment and materials.
■ Use barrier single-use plastic covers for all surfaces to be contacted, including x-ray machine controls.
■ Use disposable materials wherever possible.
■ Wear gloves or overgloves for handling of all radiographic materials.

III. PREPARATION OF CLINICIAN

■ Use full barrier protection that includes a cover-up gown, a mask, protective eyewear, and gloves.
■ Apply standard precautions throughout the radiographic procedure.

IV. PREPARATION OF PATIENT

■ Provide cup for holding removable dental prostheses.
■ For panoramic radiographs, request patient to remove oral and/or facial piercings and all other jewelry worn above the shoulders.
■ Provide antiseptic mouthrinse to lower bacterial contamination of radiographs and aerosols.

V. INTRAORAL EXAMINATION

A. Purpose

To determine necessary adaptations during film placement.

B. Factors of Particular Interest

■ Accessibility, determined by height and shape of palate, flexibility of muscles of orifice, floor of the mouth, possible gag reflex, and size of tongue.
■ Position of teeth and edentulous areas.
■ Apparent size of teeth.
■ Unusual features, such as tori, sensitive areas of the mucous membranes.

VI. PATIENT COOPERATION: PREVENTION OF GAGGING

Gagging may be the result of psychological or physiologic factors. It may present some problem in the placement of all films for molar radiographs and may be initiated in the patient who ordinarily does not gag when techniques are carried out efficiently.

A. Causes of Gagging

■ *Hypersensitive oral tissues.* Particularly common in posterior region of oral cavity.
■ *Anxiety and apprehension*
  A. Fear of unknown, of the film touching a sensitive area.
  B. Previous unpleasant experiences with radiographic techniques.
  C. Failure to comprehend the clinician's instructions.
  D. Lack of confidence in the clinician.
■ *Techniques.* Film moved over the oral tissues or retained in the mouth longer than is necessary.

TABLE 12-4	GUIDELINES FOR PRESCRIBING DENTAL RADIOGRAPHS

The recommendations in this chart are subject to clinical judgment and may not apply to every patient. They are to be used by the dentist only after reviewing the patient's health history and completing a clinical examination. Because every precaution should be taken to minimize radiation exposure, protective thyroid collars and aprons should be used whenever possible. This practice is strongly recommended for children, women of childbearing age and pregnant women.

TYPE OF ENCOUNTER	CHILD WITH PRIMARY DENTITION (before eruption of first permanent tooth)	CHILD WITH TRANSITIONAL DENTITION (after eruption of first permanent tooth)	ADOLESCENT WITH PERMANENT DENTITION (before eruption of third molars)	ADULT, DENTATE OR PARTIALLY EDENTULOUS	ADULT, EDENTULOUS
New Patient (see **Table 12-4A**) being evaluated for dental diseases and dental development	Individualized radiographic exam consisting of selected periapical/occlusal views and/or posterior bitewings if proximal surfaces cannot be visualized or probed. Patients without evidence of disease and with open proximal contacts may not require a radiographic exam at this time	Individualized radiographic exam consisting of posterior bitewings with panoramic exam or posterior bitewings and selected periapical images	Individualized radiographic exam consisting of posterior bitewings with panoramic exam or posterior bitewings and selected periapical images. A full mouth intraoral radiographic exam is preferred when the patient has clinical evidence of generalized dental disease or a history of extensive dental treatment		Individualized radiographic exam, based on clinical signs and symptoms
Recall Patient (see **Table 12-4A**) with clinical caries or at increased risk for caries (see **Table 12-4B**)	Posterior bitewing exam at 6–12 mo intervals if proximal surfaces cannot be examined visually or with a probe			Posterior bitewing exam at 6–18 mo intervals	Not applicable
Recall Patient (see **Table 12-4A**) with no clinical caries and not at increased risk for caries (see **Table 12-4B**)	Posterior bitewing exam at 12–24 mo intervals if proximal surfaces cannot be examined visually or with a probe		Posterior bitewing exam at 18–36 mo intervals	Posterior bitewing exam at 24–36 mo intervals	Not applicable
Recall Patient with periodontal disease (see **Table 12-4A**)	Clinical judgment as to the need for and type of radiographic images for the evaluation of periodontal disease. Imaging may consist of, but is not limited to, selected bitewing and/or periapical images of areas where periodontal disease (other than nonspecific gingivitis) can be identified clinically				Not applicable
Patient for monitoring of growth and development	Clinical judgment as to need for and type of radiographic images for evaluation and/or monitoring of dentofacial growth and development		Clinical judgment as to need for and type of radiographic images for the evaluation an/or monitoring of dentofacial growth and development. Panoramic or periapical exam to assess developing third molars	Usually not indicated	

TABLE 12-4	GUIDELINES FOR PRESCRIBING DENTAL RADIOGRAPHS (*Continued*)				
TYPE OF ENCOUNTER	**CHILD WITH PRIMARY DENTITION** (before eruption of first permanent tooth)	**CHILD WITH TRANSITIONAL DENTITION** (after eruption of first permanent tooth)	**ADOLESCENT WITH PERMANENT DENTITION** (before eruption of third molars)	**ADULT, DENTATE OR PARTIALLY EDENTULOUS**	**ADULT, EDENTULOUS**
Patient with other circumstances including, but not limited to, proposed or existing implants, pathology, restorative/ endodontic needs, treated periodontal disease and caries remineralization	Clinical judgment as to need for and type of radiographic images for evaluation and/or monitoring in these circumstances				

Reprinted from United States Food and Drug Administration, Center for Devices and Radiological Health. The Selection of Patients for Dental Radiographic Examinations [Internet]. Washington, D.C., November, 2004 [updated January 2005, cited November 2005]. Available from http://www.fda.gov/Radiation-EmittingProducts/RadiationEmittingProductsandProcedures/MedicalImaging/MedicalX-Rays/ucm116504.htm

TABLE 12-4A	CLINICAL SITUATIONS FOR WHICH RADIOGRAPHS MAY BE INDICATED FOR NEW AND RECALL PATIENTS

POSITIVE HISTORICAL FINDINGS	POSITIVE CLINICAL SIGNS/SYMPTOMS
1. Previous periodontal or endodontic therapy 2. History of pain or trauma 3. Familial history of dental anomalies 4. Postoperative evaluation of healing 5. Remineralization monitoring 6. Presence of implants or evaluation for implant placement	1. Clinical evidence of periodontal disease 2. Large or deep restorations 3. Deep carious lesions 4. Malposed or clinically impacted teeth 5. Swelling 6. Evidence of dental/facial trauma 7. Mobility of teeth 8. Sinus tract ("fistula") 9. Clinically suspected sinus pathology 10. Growth abnormalities 11. Oral involvement in known or suspected systemic disease 12. Positive neurologic findings in the head and neck 13. Evidence of foreign objects 14. Pain and/or dysfunction of the temporomandibular joint 15. Facial asymmetry 16. Abutment teeth for fixed or removable partial prosthesis 17. Unexplained bleeding 18. Unexplained sensitivity of teeth 19. Unusual eruption, spacing or migration of teeth 20. Unusual tooth morphology, calcification or color 21. Unexplained absence of teeth 22. Clinical erosion

Reprinted from United States Food and Drug Administration, Center for Devices and Radiological Health. The Selection of Patients for Dental Radiographic Examinations [Internet]. Washington, D.C., November, 2004 [updated January 2005, cited November 2005]. Available from http://www.fda.gov/Radiation-EmittingProducts/RadiationEmittingProductsandProcedures/MedicalImaging/MedicalX-Rays/ucm116504.htm

Table 12-4B	HIGH-RISK FACTORS FOR CARIES

1. High level of caries experience or demineralization
2. History of recurrent caries
3. High titers of cariogenic bacteria
4. Existing restoration(s) of poor quality
5. Poor oral hygiene
6. Inadequate fluoride exposure
7. Prolonged nursing (bottle or breast)
8. Frequent high sucrose content in diet
9. Poor family dental health
10. Developmental or acquired enamel defects
11. Developmental or acquired disability
12. Xerostomia
13. Genetic abnormality of teeth
14. Many multisurface restorations
15. Chemo/radiation therapy
16. Eating disorders
17. Drug/alcohol abuse
18. Irregular dental care

Reprinted from United States Food and Drug Administration, Center for Devices and Radiological Health. The Selection of Patients for Dental Radiographic Examinations [Internet]. Washington, D.C., November, 2004 [updated January 2005, cited November 2005]. Available from http://www.fda.gov/Radiation-EmittingProducts/RadiationEmittingProductsandProcedures/MedicalImaging/MedicalX-Rays/ucm116504.htm

B. Preventive Procedures

- Inspire confidence in ability to perform the service.
- Alleviate anxiety; explain procedures carefully. Smile and be cheerful.
- Minimize tissue irritation.
  A. Request patient to swallow before each film placement.
  B. Expose anterior films before posterior as placement is easier to tolerate.
  C. Place film firmly and positively without sliding the film over the tissue, especially the palate.
  D. Rub a finger over the tissues where the film placement is intended to desensitize the tissues.
  E. Instruct patient to breathe through nose with quick breaths; hold the breath during exposure.
  F. Use stick-on film cushions to make film placement more comfortable.
- Use a premedicating agent prescribed by the dentist.
- Use a topical anesthetic (page 573).

PROCEDURES FOR FILM PLACEMENT AND ANGULATION OF RAY

The image projected onto the radiograph is a shadow of the teeth and the surrounding structures. The dental radiographer follows as closely as possible the five principles of shadow casting, listed in **Box 12-10**, when exposing radiographs.

Basic intraoral procedures for periapical, bitewing, and occlusal radiographs are included in this chapter. The principles and uses of panoramic radiographs are also described.

BOX 12-10	Principles of Shadow Casting

1. Place the film as parallel as possible to the object.
2. Use as small an effective focal spot as practical.
3. Use as long a target–object distance as possible.
4. Use as short an object–film distance as possible.
5. Aim the x-ray beam perpendicular to the film.

Two fundamental periapical procedures are used in practice: the *paralleling* or right angle and the *bisecting angle*. The principles for film/sensor placement are shown in **Figure 12-11**.

Clinicians vary in their application of the principles of the two techniques. Basic to both the paralleling technique and the bisecting-angle technique are:

- The primary beam passes through the teeth of interest.
- The film/sensor is placed in relation to the teeth so that all parts of the image are shown as close to their natural size and shape as possible and dimensional distortion is minimized.

The development of a systematic, comfortable, smooth procedure saves time and energy for both patient and clinician. It increases the confidence of the patient, allows for consistency in technique, and leads to the production of good-quality radiographs. A basic objective during radiographic technique is to minimize the length of time the packet or sensor remains in the patient's mouth.

FILM SELECTION FOR INTRAORAL SURVEYS

I. PERIAPICAL SURVEYS

A. Area Covered

To obtain a view of the entire tooth and its periodontal supporting structures.

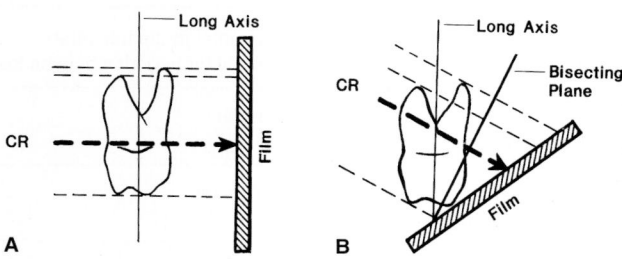

FIGURE 12-11 **Comparison of Paralleling and Bisecting-Angle Techniques. (A)** Paralleling technique. The film is parallel with the long axis of the tooth and the central ray (CR) is directed perpendicularly both to the film and to the long axis of the tooth. **(B)** Bisecting-angle technique. The central ray (CR) is directed perpendicularly to an imaginary line that bisects the angle formed by the film and the long axis of the tooth.

B. Film Sizes

- *Child size.* No. 0 (22 × 35 mm) for primary teeth and small mouths.
- *Anterior.* No. 1 (24 × 40 mm) for anterior regions where width of arch makes positioning of standard film difficult or impossible.
- *Standard.* No. 2 (31 × 41 mm) may be used for all positions.
- *Long bitewing.* No. 3 (27 × 54 mm) infrequently used as periapical film.

C. Sensor Sizes

- No. 0 for primary teeth and small mouths.
- No. 1 for anterior teeth where the width of the arch makes positioning of the size 2 sensor difficult or impossible.
- No. 2 may be used for all positions.
- No. 3 may be used for a long bitewing or periapical.

D. Number of Films or Sensors Used in a Complete Survey

Fourteen to 16 projections plus bitewings depending on the clinician's preferences, the anatomy of the patient's mouth, and the size of the films used.

II. BITEWING (INTERPROXIMAL) SURVEYS

A. Area Covered

1. *Horizontal bitewing radiographic images.* To show:
   - the crowns of the teeth and the alveolar crest in a dentition with normal to slight bone loss
   - proximal surface root caries
   - overhanging restorations

2. *Vertical bitewing radiographic images.* To show:
   - the crowns of the teeth and the alveolar bone level with moderate to severe bone loss
   - proximal surface root caries
   - overhanging restorations

B. Films/Sensors

Refer to **Table 12-5** for film/sensor size and number guidelines.
   The number and size of films/sensors used for bitewing surveys are determined by:

- the size of the dental arch
- the number of teeth present
- patient tolerance

III. OCCLUSAL SURVEYS

A. Purpose

To show large areas of the maxilla, mandible, or floor of the mouth.

B. Film/Sensor

- No. 4 (57 × 76 mm) for use in self-contained packet or in intraoral cassette
- No. 2 (31 × 41 mm) for child or individual areas of adult

DEFINITIONS AND PRINCIPLES

I. PLANES

A. Sagittal or Median

The plane that divides the body in the midline into right and left sides.

TABLE 12-5	BITEWING FILM SURVEYS			
PATIENT	**FILM PLACEMENT**	**FILM SIZE***	**NUMBER OF FILMS**	**REGION**
Adult Posterior survey	Horizontal for dental caries Vertical for periodontal bone loss	2 or 3 2	4	Premolars and molars
Adult Anterior survey	Vertical	1 or 2	3	Centrals, laterals, canines
Child Survey: permanent dentition	Horizontal	2	2	Premolars and molars
Child Survey: mixed dentition	Horizontal	1 or 2	2	Premolars and/or primary molars and permanent molars
Child Survey: all primary teeth	Horizontal	0	2	Primary molars

*Film size is determined by size of dental arch and patient tolerance. Use largest film the patient will tolerate.

B. Occlusal

The mean occlusal plane represents the mean curvature from the incisal edges of the central incisors to the tips of the occluding surfaces of the third molars. The occlusal plane of the premolars and first molar may be considered as the mean occlusal plane.

II. ANGULATION

A. Horizontal

The angle at which the central ray of the useful beam is directed within a horizontal plane. Incorrect horizontal angulation results in *overlapping* or *superimposition* of parts of adjacent teeth in the radiograph and cone-cutting.

B. Vertical

The plane at which the central ray of the useful beam is directed within a vertical plane. Variations:

- Elongation: inadequate vertical angulation
- Foreshortening: excessive vertical angulation

III. LONG AXIS OF A TOOTH

The long axis can be represented by an imaginary line passing longitudinally through the center of the tooth. Because of marked variations in tooth position and root curvature, estimation of the long axis of a tooth is difficult.

PERIAPICAL SURVEY: PARALLELING TECHNIQUE

The paralleling technique is based on the principles that the film/sensor is placed as parallel to the long axis of the tooth as the anatomy of the oral cavity permits, and the central ray is directed at right angles to the film or sensor. In **Figure 12-11A**, the parallel relationship of the film or sensor with the long axis of the tooth and the right-angle direction of the central ray is shown.

- *Maxillary projections.* The film/sensor holder is placed toward the midline of the palate.
- *Mandibular projections.* The film/sensor is placed close to the teeth of interest as long as parallelism is maintained.

I. PATIENT POSITION

As long as the film/sensor is parallel to the long axis of the tooth and the central ray is directed at right angles to the film/sensor, the head may be in any position convenient to the clinician and comfortable for the patient. Slight modification of positioning may be needed for making radiographs in a supine position.

II. FILM/SENSOR PLACEMENT

A. Film/Sensor Position and Angulation of the Central Ray

Instructions for film/sensor placement and angulation are included in this section.

1. *Basic principles.* Principles for film/sensor placement and angulation of the central ray are shown in **Figures 12-12** and **12-13**. The image objective in the completed radiograph is also illustrated.
2. *Horizontal angulation.* The central ray is directed at the center of the film/sensor and through the interproximal area.
3. *Vertical angulation.* The central ray is directed at a right angle to the film/sensor.

B. Film and Sensor-Positioning Holders

The use of a film/sensor holder (film-positioning device) facilitates obtaining the correct angulation of the central ray. Lining up the PID with coordinating parts of the film/sensor holder sets the correct vertical and horizontal angulation so that the central ray is perpendicular to the film/sensor. An example of a disposable film-positioning device is shown in **Figure 12-14**.

- *Purposes.* The use of a beam-guiding, field size-limiting, film/sensor-holding instrument provides:
  A. dose reduction.
  B. improved image quality.
  C. diagnostic radiographs without frequent retakes.
  D. improved infection control.
- *Characteristics.* An effective film/sensor-positioning device has such characteristics as the following:
  A. Simple and adaptable to all positions.
  B. Aids in reducing radiation exposure to patient.
  C. Aids in alignment of x-ray beam.
  D. Comfortable for the patient.
  E. Minimal complexity for learning.
  F. Disposable or conveniently sterilized.
- *Types of film holders* Several types of film holders are listed in **Box 12-11**. Examples of widely used types include the following:
  A. Styrofoam disposable film holder. A disposable bite block used with the paralleling or bisecting-angle techniques **(Figure 12-14)**.
  B. Precision film holder. A stainless steel film holder that offers rectangular collimation for the paralleling technique.
  C. Rinn X-C-P film and sensor holders. A plastic and stainless steel film holder with aiming devices that is used with the paralleling technique.

III. PARALLELING TECHNIQUE: FEATURES

A. Accuracy

The paralleling technique gives a more accurate size and shape of dental structures with less distortion than when the bisecting-angle technique is used.

BOX 12-11	Film-Positioning Devices

Film Holders
Bite blocks, plastic or wooden
Stabe (Styrofoam disposable film holder)
Precision x-ray device
Snap-a-ray
X-C-P (Extension Cone Paralleling)
B-A-I (Bisecting-Angle Instrument)
V.I.P. (versatile intraoral positioner)
Hemostat with rubber bite block

Supplements
Removable denture for stabilization of film holder
Cotton roll to achieve parallelism

■ In **Figures 12-12** and **12-13**, an accurate crown:root ratio is shown with facial and lingual aspects in proper relation to each other.
■ Zygomatic bone can be shown in its normal position above the root apices of the molars and premolars.

B. Horizontal Ray Direction

No rays are directed toward the thyroid, whereas with the bisecting-angle technique, several maxillary radiographs require a relatively steep vertical angulation.

BITEWING SURVEY

I. PREPARATION

A. Patient Position

■ *Traditional.* Sagittal plane perpendicular to the floor and occlusal plane parallel with the floor.
■ *Patient in supine position.* The planes are reversed in their relation to the floor.

B. Vertical Angulation

Set at +8° to +10° for horizontal or vertical bitewings **(Figure 12-15B)**.

C. Patient Instruction

Request patient to practice closing on posterior teeth before positioning film/sensor for posterior bitewing and to practice edge-to-edge closure for anterior bitewing (Figure 18-4 shows edge-to-edge closure in Chapter 18, page 278).

II. FILM/SENSOR PLACEMENT: HORIZONTAL BITEWING SURVEY

Figure 12-15 shows in diagram form the position of the horizontal molar bitewing film/sensor in relation to the teeth, the horizontal and vertical angulation, and the image objective for both the premolar and the molar completed radiographs when standard film/sensor is used.

■ *Molar*
  A. Standard film/sensor in horizontal position.
  B. Center the film/sensor on the second molar to ensure capturing the first and third molars on the radiograph (see **Figure 12-15A**).
■ *Premolar*
  A. Standard film/sensor in horizontal position.
  B. Center the film/sensor over the second premolar.
  C. Place the mesial border of film/sensor at midline of the mandibular canine to include the distal surfaces of maxillary and mandibular canines and a clear view of both the first and second premolars.

III. FILM/SENSOR POSITION: VERTICAL BITEWING SURVEY

■ *Molar*
  A. Standard film/sensor in vertical position.
  B. Center of the film/sensor positioned over the middle of the second molar.
  C. Include at least the distal portion of the first molar and the mesial portion of the third molar.
■ *Premolar*
  A. Standard film/sensor in vertical position.
  B. Position the mesial border of film/sensor at midline of the mandibular canine.
  C. Include the distal portion of maxillary and mandibular canines and a clear view of the first and second premolars. **Figure 12-16** shows in diagram form the image objective for the vertical premolar bitewing, which includes the distal portion of the maxillary and mandibular canines, the first and second maxillary and mandibular premolars, and the mesial portion of the first maxillary and mandibular molars.
■ *Anterior*
  A. Center of film/sensor at proximal space between the lateral and canine for the two canine/lateral bitewings.
  B. Center of film/sensor at midline for central bitewing.

IV. HORIZONTAL ANGULATION (FOR HORIZONTAL AND VERTICAL BITEWINGS)

The horizontal angulation is adjusted to direct the central ray perpendicular to the center of the film/sensor. The central ray passes through the interproximal space or parallel to a line through the interproximal spaces of the teeth of interest.

PERIAPICAL SURVEY: BISECTING-ANGLE TECHNIQUE

The bisecting-angle technique is based on the geometric principle that *the central ray is directed perpendicularly to*

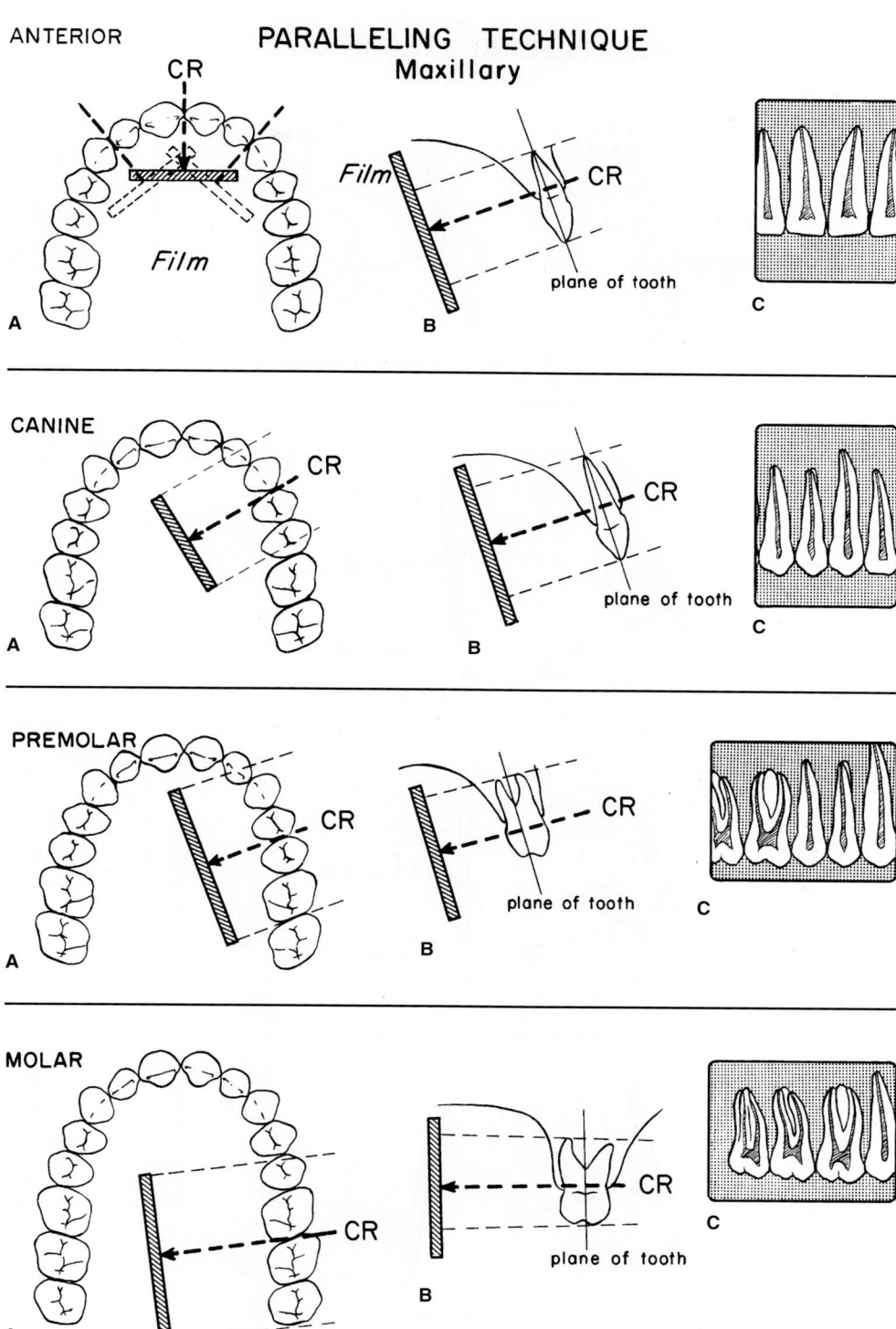

FIGURE 12-12 **Paralleling Technique, Maxillary Arch.** Film positioning for the major maxillary positions. **(A)** Horizontal angulation, with film placed parallel to the long axes of the teeth; central ray (CR) directed parallel with a line through the interproximal space. **(B)** Vertical angulation, with central ray (CR) directed at right angles to the film. **(C)** Image objective for the completed radiograph.

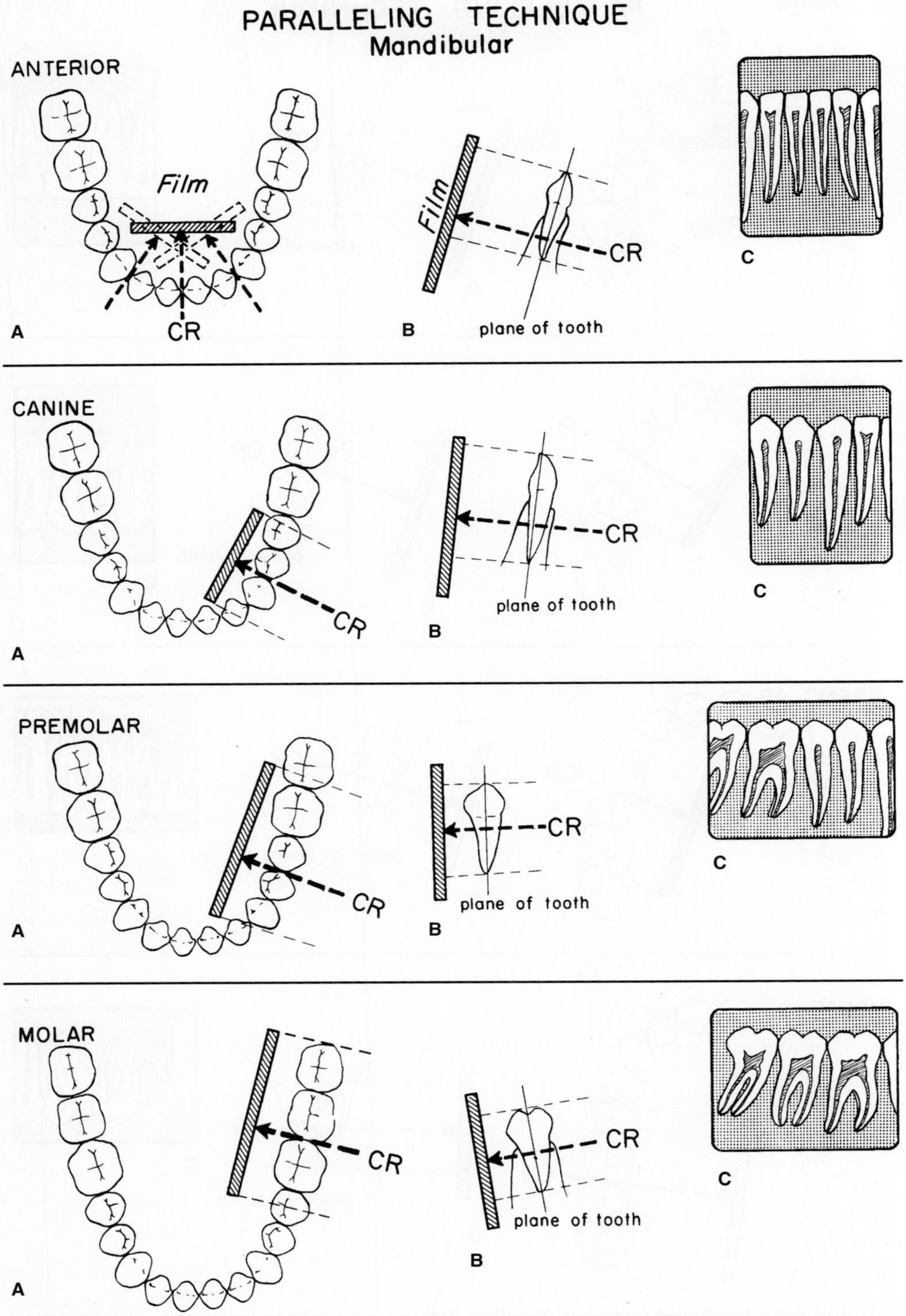

PARALLELING TECHNIQUE
Mandibular

FIGURE 12-13 **Paralleling Technique, Mandibular Arch.** Film positioning for the major mandibular positions. **(A)** Horizontal angulation, with film placed parallel to the long axes of the teeth; central ray (CR) directed through the interproximal space. **(B)** Vertical angulation, with central ray (CR) directed at right angles to the film. **(C)** Image objective for the completed radiograph.

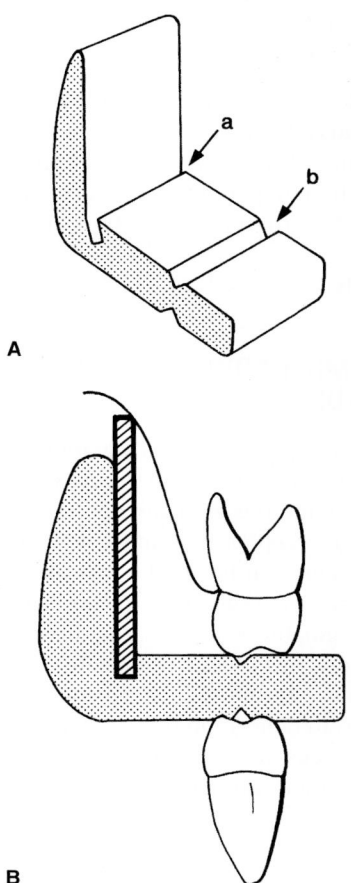

A

B

FIGURE 12-14 **Styrofoam Disposable Film Holder. (A)** Empty holder to show: a, slot for insertion of the film, and b, break-off point to shorten the bite surface for use in the mandibular posterior positions. **(B)** Film placement for maxillary molar radiograph for patient with a high palatal vault.

an imaginary line that is the bisector of the angle formed by the long axis of the tooth and the plane of the film/sensor. **Figure 12-11B** illustrates in diagram form the relationship of the long axis of the tooth, the film/sensor, and the bisector of the angle formed by these two.

Types of film holders:

- *Rinn B-A-I film and sensor holders.* A plastic and stainless steel film/sensor holder with an aiming device that is used with the bisecting-angle technique.
- *Rinn Snap-a-Ray.* A rigid plastic film-holder without a backing plate to prevent film bending, used in both posterior and anterior regions of the mouth. Useful in patients who cannot tolerate the film backing devices of a biteblock.
- *Styrofoam disposable film holder.* A disposable bite block used with the bisecting-angle or paralleling technique.

OCCLUSAL SURVEY

The central midline films for maxillary and mandibular arches are described in this section. A variety of positions for the occlusal films is possible, depending on the area to be examined.

I. USES AND PURPOSES

A. To observe areas not shown on other image projections.
B. To position film when obtaining periapical image projections is impossible.
C. To supplement the angulation provided by other films for such conditions as fractures, impacted teeth, or salivary duct calculi.

II. MAXILLARY MIDLINE TOPOGRAPHIC PROJECTION

A. Position of Patient's Head

The line from the tragus of the ear to the ala of the nose is parallel with the floor.

B. Position of Film

- The stippled side of the film packet is toward the palate.

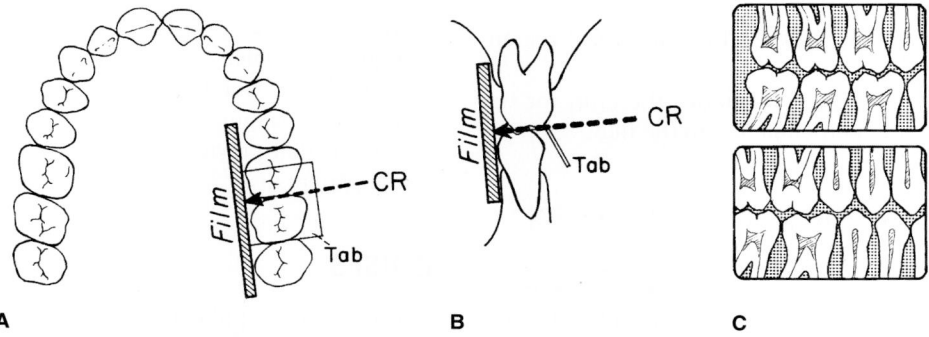

A　　　　　　**B**　　　　　　**C**

FIGURE 12-15 **Horizontal Bitewing Radiograph. (A)** Film/sensor position showing horizontal angulation for molar viewing, with central ray (CR) directed through the interproximal space to the center of the film. Film/sensor is centered over the second molar. **(B)** Vertical angulation set at + 8° to + 10°. **(C)** Image objective for molar (*above*) and premolar (*below*) regions.

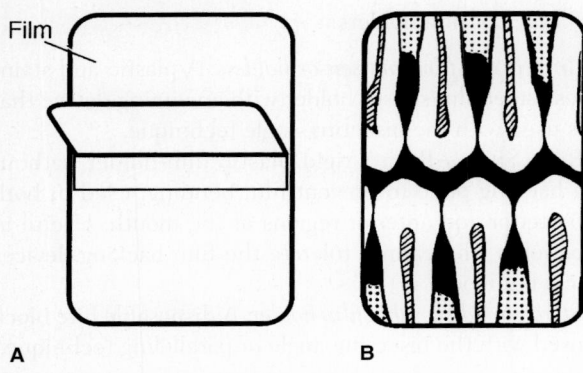

FIGURE 12-16 **Vertical Bitewing Radiograph.** **(A)** Vertical bitewing film with the tab positioned vertically over the center of the film. **(B)** Image objective of maxillary and mandibular premolar regions. Anterior edge of the film is placed behind the midline of the mandibular canine.

■ Posterior border of film is brought back close to the third molar region. Film is held between the teeth with edge-to-edge closure.

C. Angulation

The PID is directed toward the bridge of the nose at a +65° angle.

III. MANDIBULAR TOPOGRAPHIC AND CROSS-SECTIONAL PROJECTION

A. Position of Patient's Head

The head is tilted directly back.

B. Position of Film

The stippled side is toward the floor of the mouth, the posterior border of the film is in contact with the soft tissues of the retromolar area, and the film is held between the teeth in an edge-to-edge bite.

C. Angulation

■ Topographical: Point PID at chin for incisal region: −55° angle.
■ Cross-Sectional: Direct PID under the chin for the floor of the mouth, perpendicular to the film.

PANORAMIC RADIOGRAPHIC IMAGES

Panoramic radiography, or pantomography, refers to methods that produce continuous radiographs showing the maxillary and mandibular arches with adjacent structures on a single radiograph.

The panoramic radiograph is an option to a periapical survey, but it is not a substitute because of the loss of sharpness and detail. The principal advantages of panoramic images are:[13]

■ The broad coverage of facial bones and teeth.
■ Low patient radiation dose.
■ Convenience of the examination for the patient.
■ The short time required to make a panoramic image.
■ Can be used for patients who cannot open their mouths.
■ Visability for patient education.

I. PANORAMIC RADIOGRAPHS AND TECHNIQUE

A panoramic radiograph is a radiographic projection that is positioned outside the mouth during x-ray exposure and is used to examine the maxillary and mandibular jaws in a single image receptor. The movement of the film and tube head produce an image through the process known as tomography. The prefix *tomo* means section; tomography is a radiographic technique that depicts one layer or section of the body in focus while surrounding structures in other planes are blurred. In a panoramic tomograph, the attempt is to radiograph the maxillary and mandibular dentitions in focus in one image receptor. The film/sensor and tube head rotate around the patient's head in opposite directions.

A. Patient Position

Patient positioning depends on the panoramic unit and the patient's height.

■ Seated or standing.
■ The head is stabilized with a chin support or one of several types of head holders characteristic of each machine.
■ Position the patient to ensure that the Frankfort plane (orbitale to tragus of the ear) is parallel to the floor.

B. Cassette

■ Curved or flat.
■ Rigid or flexible.
■ Is marked for the left or right side of the patient.
■ Contains calcium tungstate or rare earth intensifying screens that provide for reduced radiation exposure to the patient.

II. USES

The numerous applications for panoramic radiographic images are outlined in **Box 12-12**. Routine use for patients seeking general oral care cannot be recommended as a substitute for a periapical survey as there is a loss of detail.

BOX 12-12	Uses for Panoramic Images

- Detection and diagnosis of oral pathologic lesions
- Evaluation of impacted teeth
- Examination of the extent of large lesions
- Survey for edentulous patients
- Detection of calcified carotid arteries: potential stroke victims
- Evaluation of growth and development for pedodontic patients
- Evaluation of teeth and jaw position for orthodontic patients
- Detection of fractured jaws and traumatic injuries
- When intraoral films are impossible
  Trismus
  Parkinson's disease
  Cerebral palsy
  Hyperactive gag reflex

III. LIMITATIONS

- There is a loss of definition and detail compared with periapical radiographs.
- Distortion of structures and findings.
- Do not show proximal carious lesions except for large cavities, which can be seen by direct examination.
- Inadequate for examination of periodontal structures.

A. Inferiority of Definition and Detail

Causes of poor definition are:

- Use of intensifying screens.
- Increased object–film/sensor distance.
- Movement of x-ray tube and film/sensor.

B. Distortion

- Magnified images are produced because of increased distance between the film/sensor and object.
- Overlapping. In periapical techniques, each film/sensor is angulated with the central ray so that when a tooth is out of line, adjustment is made to prevent overlapping. With panoramic technique, the head and teeth remain fixed, and the ray and film/sensor are positioned for the average only.

IV. PROCEDURES

Learning to use panoramic equipment is not difficult. Each machine has its own characteristics that can be learned readily from the manufacturer's instructions.

A. Patient Preparation

A thyroid shield cannot be used because of superimposition on the image. A special shield for panoramic radiog-

raphy is available with coverage over the shoulders and partway down the back.

B. Film/Sensor

Film and sensor sizes are usually either 5 × 12 or 6 × 12 inches. Fast-speed film is used to minimize radiation.

C. Processing

Regular processing solutions are used for panoramic film. Special film holders for panoramic films are used during manual processing.

PARACLINICAL PROCEDURES

Supplemental to the chairside clinical procedures are the processing of the films and the mounting of radiographs for diagnostic and clinical use. Standard procedures are outlined in the following sections.

INFECTION CONTROL

I. PRACTICE POLICY

Personnel of each office or clinic can determine a specific protocol appropriate to their facility and the type of processing used. A written policy is necessary for infection control during film exposure, processing, and mounting and during management of the completed radiographs throughout clinical treatment appointments.[14,15]

II. BASIC PROCEDURES

Basic procedures are followed to prevent cross-contamination during transport to the darkroom and during use of the processing equipment.[16,17]

A. Contamination of Films

Films become covered with contaminated saliva and are confined to a disposable cup after exposure.

B. Gloves

Gloved hands fresh from contamination from the patient's mouth do not come into contact with walls, doors, light switches, and other environmental surfaces when transporting a cup of contaminated exposed films to the darkroom.

C. During Processing

- The darkroom work area is prepared by the disinfection of all touch surfaces, and the counter is covered with clean paper.

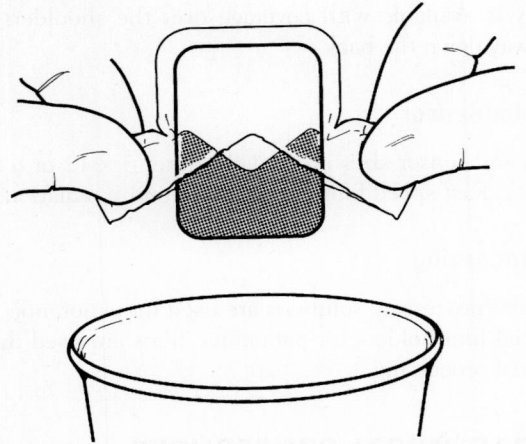

FIGURE 12-17 **Plastic Film Barrier.** Opening plastic film barrier using the no-touch method. Plastic film barriers placed over intraoral film are used to protect film from salivary contamination.

■ Research has shown that bacteria on radiographic film can survive the processing procedures. Processing procedures may reduce the bacterial counts, but the potential for cross-contamination still exists.[17]

D. Waste

Dispose of film wrappers, cups, and contaminated gloves with contaminated waste. Lead foil is disposed of according to environmental waste guidelines.

III. NO-TOUCH METHOD

1. With gloved hands and under appropriate safelight, pull open packets by their tabs or from their barrier envelopes as shown in **Figure 12-17**.
2. Allow films to drop out into a cup or onto the clean barrier-covered surface.
3. Take care not to touch the film. Remove gloves, wash hands, and place films on hangers or into the automatic processor, being careful to touch the films by the edges only.
4. Dispose of waste properly.

Alternative no-touch method.

■ Wear overgloves over powder-free treatment gloves and remove them after dropping film into the cup.
■ Films are then processed while wearing powder-free treatment gloves.

IV. DAYLIGHT LOADER METHOD

Steps for placing films into the daylight loader:

1. With powder-free regloved hands and exposed films in a paper cup, insert films in the daylight compartment.
2. Remove films from packets with the no-touch method, dropping films into a clean cup.

3. Remove gloves. Process films with ungloved hands, being careful to touch film by the edges only.
4. Remove ungloved hands from daylight loader. Don new gloves.
5. Disinfect daylight loader.

FILM PROCESSING

Film processing is the chemical transformation of the latent image, produced in a film emulsion by exposure to radiation, into a stable image visible by transmitted light.

I. STANDARD PROCEDURES

Standardization of processing procedure goes hand-in-hand with standardized exposure techniques if consistently acceptable radiographs are to be prepared. Processing is treated as an exacting chemical procedure in which each step has specific objectives for the finished product.

II. FILM SENSITIVITY

Fast- and extra-fast-speed films are even more sensitive to variations in temperature, light, and processing chemicals than were the medium and slow films formerly in general use.

III. PROCESSING CHEMISTRY

A. Processing Chemicals

In **Table 12-6**, the developer and fixer ingredients are listed with the chemicals involved and their specific reactions.

B. Chemical Reactions

■ Development: selective reduction of affected silver halide salts to metallic silver grains.
■ Fixation: the selective removal of unaffected silver halide crystals.
■ Washing to remove the processing chemicals.

IV. IMAGE PRODUCTION

■ Film emulsion contains crystals of silver halides (bromide and iodide).
■ X-ray exposure changes the silver halides to silver and halide ions.
■ Developer reacts with the halide ions, leaving only the metallic silver in an arrangement corresponding with the radiolucency and radiopacity of the tissue being exposed.
■ Fixer removes only those crystals of silver halide that were not exposed to radiation.
■ End result is a *negative*, showing various degrees of lightness and darkness (microscopic grains of black metallic silver).

TABLE 12-6	PROCESSING CHEMICALS	
DEVELOPER INGREDIENTS	**CHEMICAL**	**ACTIVITY**
Reducing agent	Hydroquinone Elon	Converts exposed silver halide crystals to black metallic silver Generates gray tones in the image
Accelerator	Sodium carbonate	Swells the emulsion and provides an alkaline medium
Restrainers	Potassium bromide	Blocks the action of the reducing agent on the unexposed crystals
Preservative	Sodium sulfite	Slows the oxidation and breakdown of the developer
Solvent	Water	Mixes the chemicals
FIXER INGREDIENTS		
Clearing agents	Ammonium thiosulfate or sodium thiosulfate	Removes all unexposed undeveloped silver halide crystals from emulsion
Acid or activator	Acetic acid Sulfuric acid	Stops development; neutralizes any remaining developer
Hardeners	Potassium alum	Toughens and shrinks the gelatin in the emulsion
Preservative	Sodium sulfite	Slows the oxidation of the fixer
Solvent	Water	Mixes the chemicals

ESSENTIALS OF AN ADEQUATE DARKROOM

The work area is maintained to keep it free from chemicals, water, dust, and other substances that could contaminate the film by either splashing or direct contact should a film touch the bench. The processing room is not used as a storage room or for other dental procedures in which dust or fumes may be produced.

LIGHTING

I. DARKROOM LIGHTING

- Find and eliminate all possible light leaks.
- Conventional safelighting.
  A. 15-watt bulb or less.
  B. Positioned a minimum of 4 feet above the working surface.
  C. Filter is selected according to film type.
  D. GBX2 (red) filters are used for both intraoral and extraoral film.
- LED safelight.
  A. Clusters of 20 red light–emitting diodes.
  B. Twice as much visible light than conventional safelighting.
  C. Lower power consumption than conventional safelight bulb.
  D. LED safelight mounts directly into light socket.

II. SAFELIGHTING TEST

- Unwrap film in the unlit darkroom.
- Place film on work tabletop and place a coin on the film.
- Turn on safelight and leave for 5 minutes.
- Remove coin, process film.
- Observe the radiograph; if any evidence exists of a light circle where the coin was placed, the darkroom safelight is excessive.

AUTOMATED PROCESSING

Automatic film processing refers to the use of equipment designed to transport film mechanically through a series of solutions under controlled conditions. **Figure 12-18** illustrates the film being transported from the entry slot to the developer, the fixer, the water bath, the dryer, and the exit slot.

I. ADVANTAGES OF AUTOMATED PROCESSING

- Consistency of results.
- Conservation of time by dental personnel.
- Finished radiographs in 4–6 minutes.
- Radiographs available for immediate use.

II. PRINCIPLES OF OPERATION

Manufacturer's instructions are followed and routine care and cleaning attended to for maintenance of equipment.

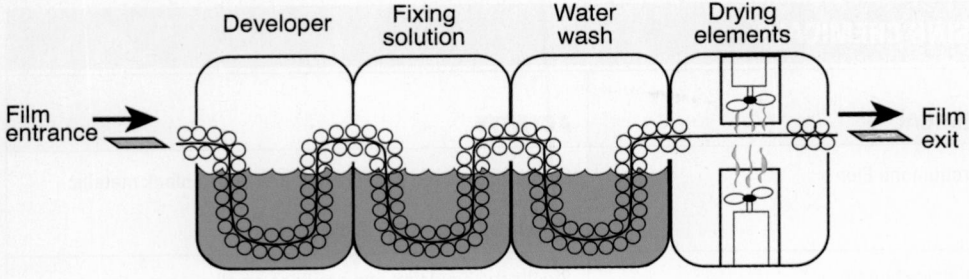

FIGURE 12-18 **Automatic Processor.** Diagram to show an automatic roller transport system that conveys the film over the rollers through the developer, fixer, water bath, and drying elements.

A. Automated Film Transport

Rollers or tracks are used to carry the film through developing, fixing, washing, and drying. Some machines may process only standard intraoral films, whereas others may also accommodate extraoral sizes.

B. High Temperature

Increased temperature decreases processing time.

C. Care of Automatic Processor

The automatic processor requires meticulous routine maintenance. Manufacturer's instructions for each unit are followed routinely.

D. Solution Changes

Large films require more solution and would therefore necessitate more frequent change of the solutions.

MANUAL PROCESSING

The darkroom has three tanks of chemicals and water for processing by hand: the developing tank, fixing tank, and water bath. In most darkrooms, the developer is the left tank, the water bath is in the center tank, and the fixer is in the right tank. The fixer can be identified by a smell similar to vinegar.

I. MANUAL PROCESSING EQUIPMENT

- Developer, water, fixer tanks, and stirring rods
- Accurate, steel-based thermometer; timer
- Safelights and white lights
- Film hangers and drying rod for hangers, or electric dryer
- Processing log

II. PROCESSING TEMPERATURE AND TIMES

The quality of the radiographic image depends greatly on the processing time and temperature, with optimal developing conditions for manual processing being 68°F for 5 minutes.

Higher temperatures would produce films with excessive density; cooler temperatures, too little density. It is necessary to check the developer temperature and recommended time as outlined in **Table 12-7**.

III. STEPS FOR MANUAL PROCESSING

- Check level and temperature of solutions; stir solutions.
- Complete the processing log.
- Turn on safelights and turn off the white lights.
- Load films from the film packet or cassette onto hangers, making sure films are securely fastened.
- Immerse film in the developer; activate timer.
- When timer buzzes, rinse films in circulating water for 30 seconds.
- Immerse the films in the fixer for twice the clearing time.
- Wash the films in circulating water for 10 minutes.
- Dry films until they are no longer tacky.

IV. DISPOSAL OF LIQUID CHEMICALS

Fixer is considered an environmentally hazardous waste material and is disposed of according to governmental regulations.

ANALYSIS OF COMPLETED RADIOGRAPHS

The completed radiographs are mounted and examined at a viewbox with an adequate light source. Interpretation of radiographs is difficult, and the determination of a pathologic condition requires keen evaluation. Attempting to base interpretation on inadequate, insufficient radiographs will result in guesswork rather than in an accurate, timely diagnosis.

I. MOUNTING

- Legibly mark the mount with the name of patient, age, date, name of dentist; printing is preferred.

TABLE 12-7	PROCESSING TEMPERATURES AND TIMES*			
SOLUTION TEMPERATURE	TIME IN DEVELOPER (MINUTES)	RINSE TIME (SECONDS)	TIME IN FIXER (MINUTES)	WASH TIME (MINUTES)
65°F	6			
68°F	5	30 s	2–4 min or twice the clearing time	10 min
70°F	4.5			
72°F	4			
75°F	3			
80°F	2.5			

*These times and temperatures are for D-, E-, or F-speed film and Kodak GBX fixer and developer.

- Handle radiographs only by the edges with clean, dry hands.
- Keep films clean and free from dust, liquids, or other contaminants.
- Arrange radiographs in front of the view box on clean, dry paper.
- The embossed dot near the edge of the negative is the guide to mounting; the raised side of the dot is on the facial side.
- Identify individual negatives by the teeth and other anatomic landmarks.
- Approved mounting system is as follows: Looking at the teeth from outside the mouth, the teeth are viewed and mounted in the same manner as the approved numbering system.

II. ANATOMIC LANDMARKS

A. Definition

An anatomic landmark is an anatomic structure, the image of which may serve as an aid in the localization and identification of the regions portrayed by a radiograph. The teeth are the primary landmarks.

B. Landmarks That May Be Seen in Individual Radiographs

- *Maxillary molar.* Maxillary sinus, zygomatic process, zygomatic (malar) bone, hamular process, coronoid process of the mandible, maxillary tuberosity, lateral pterygoid plate.
- *Maxillary premolar.* Maxillary sinus.
- *Maxillary canine.* Maxillary sinus, junction of the maxillary sinus and nasal fossa (Y-shaped, radiopaque).
- *Maxillary incisors.* Incisive foramen, nasal septum and fossae, anterior nasal spine (V-shaped), median palatine suture, symphysis of the maxillae.

- *Mandibular molar.* Mandibular canal, internal oblique line, external oblique ridge, mylohyoid ridge, submandibular gland fossa.
- *Mandibular premolar.* Mental foramen.
- *Mandibular incisors.* Lingual foramen, mental ridge, genial tubercles, symphysis of the mandible. Nutrient canals are seen most frequently in this radiograph.

III. IDENTIFICATION OF ERRORS IN RADIOGRAPHS

Table 12-8 outlines the more common errors, their causes, and the keys to correction.

A. Causes

Errors may be related to any step in the entire procedure, including film placement, angulation, exposure, processing, and care and handling of the film.

B. Types

Errors appear as problems of improper density or contrast, incomplete or distorted images, fogging, artifacts, or stains.

- *Distortion.* An inaccuracy in the size or shape of an object in the radiograph. Distortion is brought about by misalignment of the PID relative to the object. Vertical distortion produces elongation or foreshortening of the object.
- *Fog.* A darkening of the whole or part of a radiograph by sources other than the radiation of the primary beam to which the film was exposed. Types of fog include chemical, light, and radiation.
- *Artifact.* A blemish or an unintended radiographic image that can result from faulty manufacture, manipulation, exposure, or processing of an x-ray film.

TABLE 12-8	ANALYSIS OF RADIOGRAPHS: CAUSES OF ERRORS	
	ERROR	**CAUSE: FACTORS IN CORRECTION**
Image	Elongation Foreshortening	Insufficient vertical angulation Excessive vertical angulation
	Superimposition (overlapping)	Incorrect horizontal angulation (central ray not directed through interproximal space)
	Partial image	Cone-cut (incorrect direction of central ray or incorrect film placement) Incompletely immersed in processing tank Film touched other film or side of tank during processing
	Blurred or double image	Patient, tube, or packet movement during exposure Film exposed twice
	Stretched appearance of trabeculae or apices	Bent film
	No image	Machine malfunction from time-switch to wall-plug Failure to turn on the machine Film placed in fixer before developer
Density	Too dark	Excessive exposure Excessive developing Developer too warm Unsafe safelight Accidental exposure to white light (may be completely black)
	Too light	Insufficient exposure Insufficient development or excessive fixation Solutions too cool Use of old, contaminated, or poorly mixed solutions Film placement: leaded side toward teeth Film used beyond expiration date
Fog	Chemical fog	Imbalance or deterioration of processing solutions
	Light fog	Unintentional exposure to light to which the emulsion is sensitive, either before or during processing (1) Unsafe safelight (2) Darkroom leak (3) Holding unprocessed films too close to the safelight too long Improper storage of unused film
	Radiation fog	Film exposed before processing
Reticulation	(puckered or pebbly surface)	Sudden temperature changes during processing, particularly from warm solutions to very cold water
Artifacts	Dark lines	Bent or creased film Static electricity (1) Film removed from wrapper with excessive force (2) Wrapper sticking to film when opened with wet fingers, or if there was excessive moisture from patient's mouth Fingernail used to grasp film during placement on hanger
	Herringbone pattern (light film)	Packet placed in mouth backwards with foil next to teeth
Discoloration	Stains and spots	Unclean film hanger Spatterings of developer, fixer, dust Finger marks Insufficient rinsing after developing before fixing Splashing dry negatives with water or solutions Air bubbles adhering to surface during processing (insufficient agitation) Overlap of film on film in tanks or while drying Paper wrapper stuck to film (film not dried when removed from patient's mouth)
	Stains at later date after storage of completed radiographs	Incomplete processing or rinsing Storage in too warm a place Storage near chemicals

IV. INTERPRETATION

Radiographs are used in conjunction with clinical assessment for a complete care program. Periodic radiographs permit continuing evaluation. As part of the permanent record, radiographs help to document the oral condition for comparison as well as for legal and forensic purposes.

The quality of the radiographs determines their usability for diagnostic interpretation. Procedures for the preparation of radiographs are perfected so that the radiographs have maximum interpretability with minimum radiation exposure of the patient.

A. Prerequisites for Interpretation

■ *Mounting.* Mount radiographs in an opaque mount to prevent light between each radiograph from creating glare and producing a blinding effect.
■ *Viewbox.* Use an adequately lighted viewbox. Dimmed room light improves visibility for contrasting radiolucent and radiopaque areas. Holding the radiographs up to view by window, room, or unit light is inadequate, and only gross interpretation can be accomplished. When a viewbox is larger than the mount used, cover the edges to block out peripheral light.
■ *Hand magnifying glass.* Examine radiographs on a viewbox through a magnifying glass. A viewbox is available with a built-on magnifying glass.

B. Systematic Examination

■ Observe one radiographic feature at a time. Examine all of the radiographs in a survey for that feature, rather than taking each radiograph separately to find everything. It is important to note comparisons for each change over the entire survey.
■ When examining a particular tooth, compare the appearance of that tooth in each radiograph in which it appears, including bitewings. At different angulations, different findings may become apparent.

C. Correlation With Clinical Examination

A description of radiographic examination of the teeth may be found on page 267 and of the periodontal tissues on page 240. Correlation of radiographic findings with the clinical examination, using probe and explorer, is basic to an understanding of the true oral condition of the patient.

OWNERSHIP

■ Radiographs belong to the dental practice even though they were paid for by the patient.
■ Patient has a right to a copy of their records and their radiographs.

■ Duplicate originals or use double film packets for exposure.
■ Originals are kept by the dental practice and a duplicate series is to be given to the patient.

DOCUMENTATION

I. RADIATION EXPOSURE HISTORY

■ Inquire whether the patient is receiving or has recently received radiation therapy. It may be necessary to minimize the number of exposures. A consultation with the patient's physician is recommended.
■ Maintain a continuing record for each patient that indicates the date, number of exposures, kVp, mA, time, and area exposed.

II. PATIENT CARE PROGRESS NOTES

Patient care progress notes include the following components:

1. Patient complaint, if applicable, including:
   ■ Location of symptomatic area.
   ■ Duration and severity of symptoms.
2. Clinical findings.
3. Recommended diagnostic procedures.
   ■ Explain to patient necessity of radiographs for accurate diagnosis and treatment.
   ■ Patient has the right to refuse radiographs.
   ■ Obtain the patient's signature to a statement of refusal in the event a legal issue should arise.
4. Type of radiographs (periapical or bitewing), number of exposures and area(s) exposed
5. **Box 12-13** provides an example progress note for the patient who has received dental radiographs.

BOX 12-13	**Example Progress Note When the Patient Has Received Dental Radiographs**

Patient presents with heat sensitivity on tooth #15. Last radiographs were exposed 2 years ago and the patient has several porcelain fused to metal crowns and large amalgam restorations. The patient has recently undergone numerous medical radiographs and requests minimal exposure today. After a complete clinical examination, two premolar and two molar bitewing films along with one periapical film of #15 were exposed.

Signed: _____, RDH Date: _____

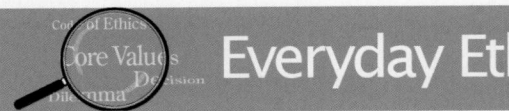

Everyday Ethics

Danielle, a recent dental hygiene graduate, is asked by her employer, Dr. Blum, to limit the number of gloves used to expose and process patients' dental films due to cost constraints. Currently, she uses one pair to expose the patients' radiographs with and removes those gloves to disrobe the patient of the lead shield. She dons a second pair to process the exposed films in an automatic processor and uses a third pair to begin intraoral treatment for her patient. Dr. Blum would like her to wear the same gloves for all the aforementioned procedures. Danielle finds that method unacceptable.

Questions for Consideration

1. List ethical alternatives Danielle has for actions that take both patient safety and employer concerns into consideration. Is there another way to proceed, to limit the number of gloves used per patient?
2. Which Core Values (Table II-1, page 38) are involved as Danielle discussed those alternatives with her employer? Explain why the core values were chosen.
3. What Ethical Theory (Table III-1, page 114) can provide guidance as Danielle tries to resolve this issue? Explain the reason for your choice.

Factors To Teach The Patient

When the Patient Asks About the Safety of Radiation

- Patients ask questions about safety factors, and occasionally a patient may refuse to have any radiographs made. The patient can be reassured with confidence, instructed as to why radiographs are necessary at this time, and informed about how modern equipment and techniques are in accord with radiation standards.
- Adapt the answer to the patient. Certain patients have more fear; others have more knowledge about x-rays. The clinician who expresses confidence aids in allaying fears. Hesitation increases the patient's doubt.
- Radiographs are essential to diagnosis and treatment. Without the information provided, the clinician can only guess at conditions not visible clinically.
- The benefits resulting from the intelligent use of x-rays outweigh any possible negative effects.
- Modern x-ray machines are equipped for safety. Simple details about filtration, collimation, film speed, use of protective shields, and short exposure times can be explained.

Educational Features in Dental Radiographs

- Position of unerupted permanent teeth in relation to primary teeth.
- Detection of early cavitated carious lesions not visible by clinical examination.
- Effects of loss of teeth and the importance of having replacements.
- Periodontal changes and other pathologic conditions appropriate to an individual patient.

References

1. Haring JI, Jansen L. *Dental radiography: principles and techniques.* 2nd ed. Philadelphia: W.B. Saunders; 2000. 4 p.
2. United States Food and Drug Administration; Center for Devices and Radiological Health [Internet]. Washington, D.C.: United States Food and Drug Administration. The selection of patients for dental radiographic examinations; updated 2009 May 6 [cited 2005 Nov]; [about 22 screens]. Available from: http://www.fda.gov/RadiationEmittingProducts/RadiationEmittingProductsandProcedures/MedicalImaging/MedicalX-Rays/ucm116504.htm
3. United States National Research Council, (BEIR-V). *Health effects of exposure to low levels of ionizing radiation.* Washington, D.C.: National Academies Press; 1990.
4. White SC, Pharoah MJ. *Oral Radiology: principles and interpretation.* 5th ed. St. Louis: Mosby; 2004. 11–12 pp.
5. Parks ET, Williamson G. Digital radiography: an overview. *J Contemp Dent Pract.* 2002 Nov15;3(4):23–9.
6. Langland OE, Langlais RP, Preece JW. *Principles of dental imaging.* 2nd ed. Baltimore: Lippincott Williams & Wilkins; 2002. 278–95 pp.
7. Mauriello SM, Platin E. Dental digital radiographic imaging. *J Dent Hyg.* 2001 Fall;75(4):323–31.
8. International Commission on Radiation Units and Measurements (ICRU). *Radiation quantities and units.* ICRU Report No. 33. Washington, D.C.: ICRU; 1980.
9. National Council on Radiation Protection and Measurements. *Radiation protection in dentistry.* NCRP Report No. 145. Washington, D.C.: NCRP; 2003.
10. Haring and Jansen. op. cit., p. 72.
11. White SC. 1992 Assessment of radiation risk from dental radiography. *Dentomaxillofac Radiol.* 1992 Aug;21(3):118–26.
12. Horner K. Review article: radiation protection in dental radiology. *Br J Radiol.* 1994 Nov;67(803):1041–9.
13. White and Pharoah. op.cit., p. 191.
14. American Dental Association, Council on Scientific Affairs. An update on radiographic practices: information and recommendations. *J Am Dental Assoc.* 2001 Feb;132(2):234–238.
15. Haring and Jansen. op. cit., pp. 194–207.
16. Bachman CE, White JM, Goodis HE, Rosenquist, JW. Bacterial adherence and contamination during radiographic processing. *Oral Surg Oral Med Oral Pathol.* 1990 Nov;70(5):669–73.
17. Stanczyk DA, Paunovich ED, Broome JC, Fatone MA. Microbiologic contamination during dental radiographic film processing. *Oral Surg Oral Med Oral Pathol.* 1993 Jul;76(1);112–19.

CHAPTER 13

Study Casts

ESTHER M. WILKINS, BS, RDH, DMD

Chapter Outline

As reproductions of the teeth, gingiva, and adjacent structures, study casts can be useful and frequently indispensable adjuncts in the assessment and care of a patient. Accurate and esthetically acceptable casts have a special use as visual aids for patient instruction.

The study casts, radiographs, and clinical examination with recordings and chartings, together with the medical and dental histories, are utilized in the diagnosis, total care planning, treatment, and subsequent maintenance.

PURPOSES AND USES OF STUDY CASTS

- To serve as a permanent record of the patient's present condition.
- To give sharper delineation to and corroboration of the observations made during the oral examination.
- To observe normal conditions, the variations of and departures from the normal at the outset of treatment and, by comparison with subsequent periodic

casts, to compare and evaluate certain aspects of treatment.

- To be an effective visual aid to use when the oral conditions are explained and the dental and dental hygiene care plans are presented; to enable the patient to visualize and understand the need for the specific care outlined.
- To serve as a guide to clinical treatment procedures.
- To supplement clinical observations when the dental biofilm control program for the patient's daily self-care is explained.
- During charting of the teeth, to note missing teeth; anomalies of size, shape, or number; partial eruption; tooth positions, such as drifting, tilting, rotation, and open or closed contacts.
- During examination of the occlusion, to observe the static relations (Angle's classification, malrelations of groups of teeth, and malpositions of individual teeth) and other features, such as wear patterns and the effects of premature loss of teeth.
- During periodontal charting, to record anatomic features, such as the position, size, and shape of the gingiva and interdental papillae and the position of frena.
- To provide assistance during forensic examination along with radiographs.

STEPS IN THE PREPARATION OF STUDY CASTS

Terms used to describe study casts and their preparation are defined in **Box 13-1**.

Procedures described in this chapter are as follows:

A. Clinical Procedures

1. Assemble materials and equipment.
2. Prepare the patient.
3. Select and prepare the impression trays.
4. Make the interocclusal record for occluding the casts.
5. Make the mandibular impression.
6. Make the maxillary impression.

B. Paraclinical Procedures

1. Assemble materials and equipment.
2. Prepare the impression material for pouring.
3. Pour the casts.
4. Trim and finish the casts.
5. Polish the casts.

CLINICAL PREPARATION

I. ASSEMBLE MATERIALS AND EQUIPMENT

- Coverall (plastic drape), towel, and preprocedural mouthrinse.
- Impression trays.
  - A. Perforated type generally used; small, medium, and large sizes are available.
  - B. Trays for use in the patient's mouth must be disposable or clean, shiny, and sterilized.
- Mixing bowl: clean, dry, flexible rubber or plastic with smooth, unscratched surface. Reserve separate bowls

---

BOX 13-1	Key Words

Study Casts

Alginate: an impression material used for recording minimal detail such as for study casts.

Cast (model): a positive life-size reproduction of the teeth and adjacent tissues usually formed by pouring dental plaster or stone into a matrix or impression.

  Diagnostic or study cast: used in the study of a patient's oral condition in preparation for treatment planning and patient instruction.

  Master cast: used to fabricate a dental restoration or prosthesis.

Centric occlusion or habitual occlusion: the usual maximum intercuspation or contact of the teeth of the opposing arches.

Dental plaster: the beta form of calcium sulfate hemihydrate; a fibrous aggregate of fine crystals with capillary pores that are irregular in shape and porous in character; also referred to as plaster of Paris.

Dental stone: the alpha form of calcium sulfate hemihydrate with physical properties superior to those of the beta form (dental plaster); the alpha form consists of cleavage frag-

ments and crystals in the form of rods and prisms and is therefore more dense than the beta form.

Impression: a negative imprint of an oral structure used to produce a positive replica of the structure; used to make casts for a permanent record or in the production of a dental restoration or prosthesis; usually identified by the type of material used, such as "hydrocolloid impression," "alginate impression," or "rubber base impression."

Interocclusal record: a registration of the positional relationship of the opposing teeth or dental arches made in a plastic material, such as a soft baseplate wax; also called the maxillomandibular relationship record or "wax-bite."

Occlusal plane: the average plane established by the incisal and occlusal surfaces of the teeth; generally not actually a plane, but the planar mean of the curvature of those surfaces.

Polish: to make smooth and glossy usually by friction; the act or process of making a cast smooth and glossy.

Prosthesis: an artificial replacement of an absent part of the human body; a therapeutic device to improve or alter function.

for each dental material: one always for impression material, another kept only for plaster or stone.
- Spatula: clean, dry, stiff, with a smooth, rounded end that reaches every part of the bowl without scraping or cutting its surface.
- Saliva ejector.
- Dental materials.
  A. Soft utility wax for preparation of tray rim (beading).
  B. Alginate: irreversible hydrocolloid with manufacturer's measuring device.
  C. Soft baseplate wax for interocclusal record.
- Water thermometer.

II. CLINICIAN PREPARATION

Standard precautions are observed for all clinic procedures. A mask is always worn when handling powder forms of dental materials to prevent inhalation.

III. PREPARE THE PATIENT
A. History Review

- Review medical and dental histories for possible precautionary needs such as respiratory concerns.
- Plan for impressions when the patient who is at risk for bacteremia has received antibiotic coverage for other procedures and check that the patient has taken the prescription 1 hour before.

B. Explain the Procedure to Be Performed

- The need for, and uses of, study casts are explained as with any procedure not familiar to the patient.
- The reactions of patients who have had an impression made previously may range from indifference to dread, and the conversation and approach can be directed accordingly.

C. Position the Patient

- Position the patient upright for maximum visibility and accessibility and to minimize gagging.
- Stabilize the patient's head on the headrest.

D. Receive Removable Prostheses

- Provide a container with water in which the patient can place removable oral prostheses.

E. Examine the Oral Cavity

- Note facially displaced teeth, height of palate, undercut areas, mandibular tori.
- Note other anatomic features that may influence the size or preparation of the impression tray and the procedures to be carried out during impression making.

F. Free the Mouth of Debris

- When excess, tenacious debris is present, biofilm control instructions are initiated or continued so that debris and biofilm can be removed by the patient with a toothbrush.

G. Provide Preprocedural Mouthrinse

- To aid in the removal of saliva and debris and lessen the numbers of surface microorganisms.
- To lower the surface tension; aids in preventing bubbles in the impression.
- To provide a pleasant taste and feeling for the patient.
- To distract an anxious patient while the trays are being prepared.

H. Dry the Teeth

- Use a cotton roll or compressed air stream to remove saliva from the teeth to prevent irregularities in the surface of the study cast.

I. Prevent Gagging

- General approach
  A. When the radiographic survey has been made for the new patient before the study casts, the clinician will have determined whether precautions to prevent gagging are needed.
  B. With all patients, a calm approach, an exhibition of confidence, a direct and efficient procedure, and a gentle handling of the patient's oral tissues increase rapport and contribute to a satisfactory result.
  C. Other suggestions for prevention of gagging are listed on page 174.
- Technique considerations
  A. Avoid excessive impression material in the tray.
  B. Seat the maxillary tray from posterior to anterior.
  C. Instruct the patient to breathe deeply through the nose before the tray is inserted and to continue after insertion; bring head forward.

THE INTEROCCLUSAL RECORD
I. PURPOSES

- To relate the maxillary and mandibular casts correctly. Many, if not most, maxillary and mandibular casts orient to each other readily in only one position, but when such problems as open bite, crossbite, edentulous areas, or end-to-end or edge-to-edge relations interfere with direct occlusion of the casts, a bite registration is needed.
- To place between the casts during trimming and storage to prevent breakage of the teeth of the cast.

II. PROCEDURE

■ Numerous materials are available to obtain registration, such as wax and quick setting materials. Manufacturer's instructions for use are followed.

■ Request patient to practice opening and closing on the posterior teeth to ensure that the habitual position can be obtained.

■ Warm a shaped piece of soft baseplate wax or mix the bite registration material and place over the occlusal surfaces.

■ Guide patient to close in habitual occlusion.

■ Remove carefully to prevent distortion; chill wax in cold water. Disinfect.

PREPARATION OF IMPRESSION TRAYS

I. SELECTION OF PROPER SIZE AND SHAPE

A. Width

1. Objective: to allow an adequate thickness of impression material on the facial and lingual surfaces of each tooth to provide strength and rigidity to the impression.

2. Tray flanges may be spread to accommodate for extra width in the molar regions, particularly lingual to the mandibular molars in the mylohyoid region.

3. When a tooth is in prominent labioversion, buccoversion, or linguoversion, a minimum thickness of 1/8 to 1/4 inch is suggested, but even then, the fragility of the impression material in that area is increased.

4. Tray: may appear in correct relation to the facial surfaces but may impinge on the lingual or palatal cusps of molars.

B. Length

1. Objectives: To allow coverage of the retromolar area of the mandible and the tuberosity of the maxilla.

2. Anterior: plan for at least 1/4-inch clearance labial to the most protruded incisor without impingement on lingual or palatal gingiva.

II. MAXILLARY TRAY TRY-IN

A. Position of Clinician

At side back of patient.

B. Retraction

1. With index finger of nondominant hand, retract the patient's lip and cheek.

2. At the same time, use the side of the tray to distend the other side of the patient's mouth to gain entry **(Figure 13-1)**.

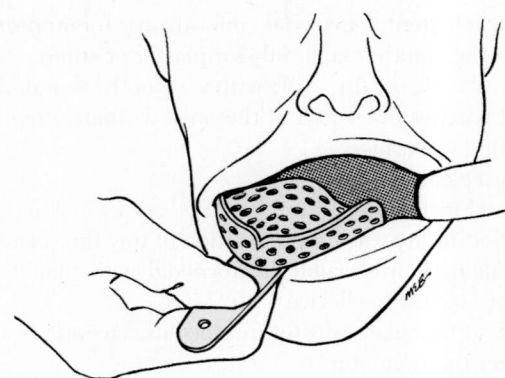

FIGURE 13-1 **Maxillary Tray Insertion.** The patient's lip and cheek are retracted with the fingers of the nondominant hand while the side of the tray is used to distend the other lip and cheek to gain entry. The tray is inserted with a rotary motion. The procedure for the mandibular tray is similar.

C. Insertion

1. With a rotary motion, insert the tray.

2. Orient the tray beneath the arch and center it by using the tray handle and the midline (usually between the central incisors and in line with the middle of the nose) as guides for positioning.

3. Bring the front of the tray to a position 1/4 inch labial to the most labially inclined incisor.

4. Seat the tray by bringing the posterior up before the anterior; retract the lip as the anterior is brought into place.

D. Evaluation of the Tray Size

1. Lower the front of the tray while holding the posterior border in place **(Figure 13-2)**.

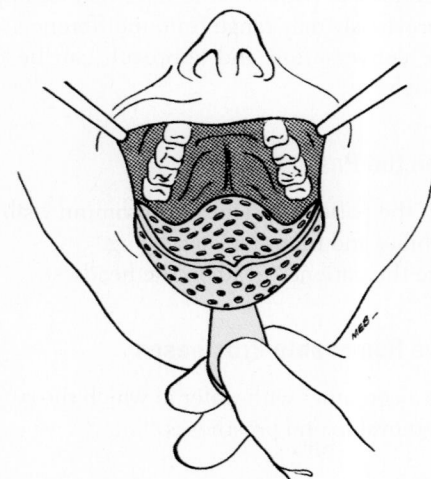

FIGURE 13-2 **Selection of Impression Tray.** Adequate coverage is determined as the posterior border of the tray is held in position while the front of the tray is lowered to observe the relationship of the posterior border to the maxillary tuberosity areas to be covered by the impression. The mandibular tray position is examined by lifting the tray to observe coverage of the retromolar areas.

2. Examine the relationship of the posterior border to the most posterior molars and the tuberosity areas to determine whether the coverage will be ample.
3. Move the tray up and down to observe the relation to the facial surfaces of all teeth, malaligned teeth, protuberances, and other features and thus to assay the space allowed for the impression material.

III. MANDIBULAR TRAY TRY-IN

A. Position of Clinician

At side front of patient.

B. Retraction

1. With index and middle fingers of nondominant hand, retract the patient's lip and cheek.
2. At the same time, use the side of the tray to distend the side of the mouth to gain entry, similar to the procedure illustrated in **Figure 13-1** for the maxillary tray.

C. Insertion

1. With a rotary motion, insert the tray.
2. Orient the tray over the dental arch and center it by using the tray handle and the midline (usually between the central incisors and in line with the center of the chin) as guides for positioning.
3. Bring the tray rim to about 1/4 inch anterior to the most labially positioned incisor; instruct the patient to raise the tongue to permit the lingual flange of the tray to pass by the lateral borders of the tongue without interference.
4. As the tray is lowered, retract the cheeks in the posterior regions to make certain the buccal mucosa is not caught beneath the edge of the tray; hold the lip out to ascertain that there is clearance to the base of the vestibule.

D. Evaluation of Tray Size

1. Lift the tray handle while keeping the posterior border of the tray in position, similar to the procedure illustrated in **Figure 13-2** for the maxilla, to determine whether the coverage will be ample posteriorly to include the retromolar areas and laterally to allow for 1/4-inch thickness of impression material on the facial and lingual aspects of the teeth.
2. Reselect larger or smaller trays as indicated and repeat try-in. When in doubt, use the larger rather than the smaller tray.
3. Note tray sizes used in patient's permanent record for future reference.

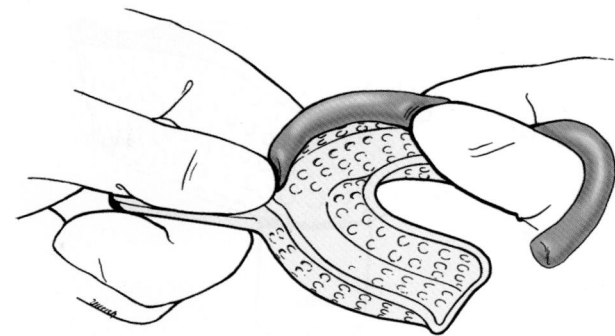

FIGURE 13-3 **Beading the Tray.** A strip of soft utility wax is applied around the periphery of each tray.

IV. APPLICATION OF WAX RIM AROUND BORDERS OF TRAYS (BEADING)

A. Purposes

1. To prevent the metal tray rims from causing discomfort to the soft tissues.
2. To seat the vestibular periphery firmly into position with reduced pressure on the displaced tissues.
3. To prevent penetration of the incisal or occlusal surfaces through the impression material and thus to prevent a defective cast.
4. To provide a slight undercut at the rim as an aid in the retention of the alginate in the tray during placement and removal.
5. To create a posterior palatal seal to aid in preventing excess material from passing into the throat.

B. Procedure

■ Application of wax. Attach a strip of soft utility wax firmly around the entire periphery of each tray **(Figure 13-3)**.
■ Mandibular tray. Add extra layers from cuspid to cuspid labially, and notch the wax to fit about the labial frenum.
■ Maxillary tray
  A. Add extra layers as needed to extend the tray into the vestibule above the anterior teeth, and notch the wax to fit about the labial frenum **(Figure 13-4A)**.
  B. Apply extra thickness across the posterior palatal seal area.
  C. When a patient has a high palatal vault, apply extra wax to support the impression material in that area.
■ Try-in. Try the rimmed trays in the mouth **(Figure 13-4B)**; examine by retraction of the lips and cheeks and by use of a mouth mirror for lingual areas, hold the tray in position.
■ Characteristics of the completed molding. When the tray is held firmly, all borders of the wax will contact the mucous membrane and displace the soft tissue outward and upward. The teeth do not touch the tray.

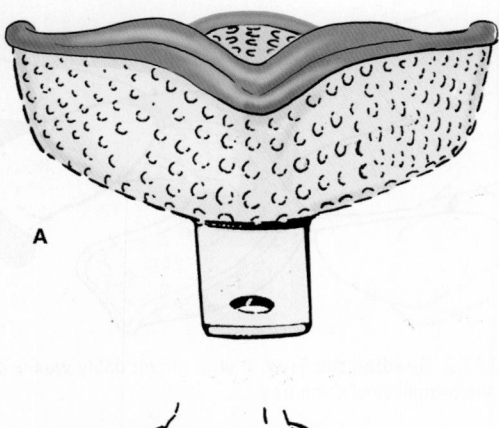

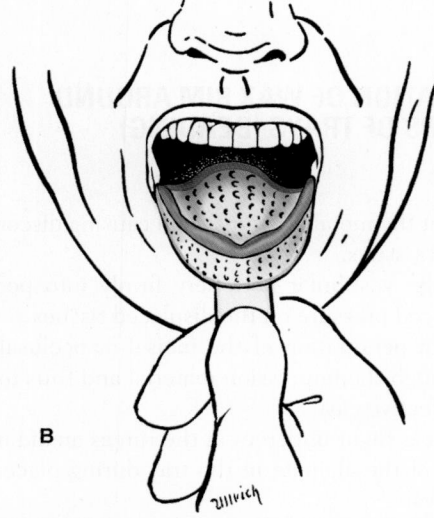

FIGURE 13-4 **Check the Beading Wax. (A)** Tray with double layer of beading wax about the labial frenum. The extra wax extends the tray, protects the soft tissue from the metal rim, and provides a more complete impression of the area. **(B)** Try-in after beading. The wax contacts all borders of the mucous membrane, displaces the soft tissue outward, and prevents the teeth from contacting the tray.

THE IMPRESSION MATERIAL

I. FACTORS RELATED TO THE IMPRESSION MATERIAL THAT CONTRIBUTE TO A SATISFACTORY IMPRESSION

Texts on dental materials can be reviewed for complete information about the irreversible hydrocolloids.[1,2] Properties related to the clinical procedures essential to making an accurate impression are listed here. The manufacturer's directions are followed.

A. Powder

The alginate material deteriorates on standing, particularly at higher temperatures and humidity.

- Keep container tightly closed; store in a cool place.
- Use individually sealed packages to eliminate the problems of heat and moisture.

- Individual package may be refrigerated in hot weather, provided the powder is used immediately on opening. If left exposed, water condenses on the cold powder. The bulk container cannot be refrigerated for that reason.
- Do not agitate powders unnecessarily during mixing. Inhaled dust particles can cause serious irritation to the respiratory system.

B. Water

Temperature controls gelation time.

- At room temperature, 20°–21°C (68°–70°F), an ideal gelation time between 3 and 4 minutes provides adequate working time.
- Temperature of the water is measured with a thermometer at the time of mixing.
- For control in hot, humid weather, use cooler water and refrigerate the bowl and spatula.

C. Strength and Quality

The strength and quality of the finished impression depend on the following factors:

- Powder: water ratio accurately weighed and measured.
- Spatulation (1 minute) to homogenize, to remove bubbles, and to allow chemical reactions to proceed uniformly.
- Holding the impression material in position for an optimum period in accord with manufacturer's specifications. The elasticity of most alginates improves with time; therefore, a superior reproduction can be obtained by waiting. Distortion can result when the impression is left in the mouth too long.

D. Surface Accuracy

The cast must be poured promptly to prevent loss of water from the impression. Permanent distortion can result.

II. MIXING THE IMPRESSION MATERIAL

Follow manufacturer's specifications precisely; total time lapse for mixing and insertion is approximately 2 minutes.

- Place measured water 20°–21°C (68°–70°F, measured with a thermometer) in a clean, dry mixing bowl.
- Sprinkle measured powder (from individually sealed package or premeasured from large container) into the water.
- Quickly incorporate the powder and water using a clean, dry, stiff spatula.
- Mix for 1 minute (clocked) vigorously, incorporating powder into the water, until a smooth, creamy mix is obtained.

III. TRAY PREPARATION

The mandibular impression is made first to introduce the patient to the procedure in an area where discomfort or gagging may be the least likely.

A. Working Time

The working time is 30 seconds.

B. Filling the Tray

- Fill the tray from the posterior, being careful not to trap air bubbles.
- Adapt the material to the tray thoroughly; press slightly through the perforations in the tray.
- Do not overload; fill to a level just below the edge of the wax rim.
- Wet index finger with cold water and pass lightly over the surface of the impression material; smooth the surface and make a slight indent where the teeth will insert.

C. Excess Material

- Quickly gather the excess material from the bowl and bring the material on the spatula near to patient to use for precoating.

THE MANDIBULAR IMPRESSION

I. PRECOAT POTENTIAL AREAS OF AIR ENTRAPMENT

The precoat prevents air bubbles in the finished impression.

- Take a small amount of impression material from the spatula onto the index finger.
- Apply quickly with a positive pressure to:
  A. Undercut areas, such as distal surfaces of teeth adjacent to edentulous areas; cervical areas of erosion or abrasion; and gingival surfaces of fixed partial dentures.
  B. Vestibular areas, particularly anterior areas about the frena.
  C. Occlusal surfaces.

II. STEPS FOR INSERTION OF TRAY

- Follow mandibular tray try-in. In summary, the procedure is as follows:
  A. From 8 o'clock position (4 o'clock for left-handed), retract lip and cheek with fingers of nondominant hand.
  B. Use side of tray to distend the other lip and cheek.
  C. Rotate the tray into position, center it over the teeth, and introduce the tray 1/4-inch anterior to the facial surface of the most anterior incisor.
  D. Instruct patient to raise the tongue while tray is lowered; retract cheeks and lip to clear the way for impression material to reach the base of the vestibule.
- Seat the tray directly downward with a slight vibratory motion to aid in filling all crevices between the teeth.
- Instruct the patient to extrude the tongue briefly to mold the lingual borders of the impression.

- Apply equal bilateral pressure firmly, holding the middle fingers over the premolar regions and using the thumbs to support the mandible; or, if equal pressure can be maintained with one hand, place an index finger over the patient's premolar area on one side and the middle finger over the opposite side, with the thumb under the edge of the mandible for stabilization. Mold cheeks around the tray.
- When the impression tray is held with one hand or when assistance is available, slip the saliva ejector in over the tray and then remove it before the tray is removed.
- When the leftover material on the spatula has lost its surface stickiness (tackiness), hold the impression in position for 2 more clocked minutes.

III. THE COMPLETED IMPRESSION

A. Removal of Impression

1. Hold tray handle with thumb and fingers.
2. Retract cheek and lip with fingers and release the edge of the impression by depressing the buccal mucosa.
3. Do not rock the impression back and forth to release it because these movements may cause permanent distortion of the final impression.
4. Remove the impression with a gentle jerk or snap.

B. Rinse the Impression

Rinse under cool running water to remove saliva, blood, and bacteria. Rinse carefully to prevent splashing contaminated saliva or blood over surroundings.

C. Examine and Evaluate the Impression

Observe surface detail, proper extension over retromolar area, and peripheral roll (rounded border of the impression) generally.

D. Repeat Procedure When Necessary

Correct mistakes rather than be satisfied with a substandard impression.

E. Storage

Disinfect then wrap mandibular impression in a wet towel while making the maxillary impression.

THE MAXILLARY IMPRESSION

I. PREPARATION

A. Request Patient to Rinse

To clear particles left from the mandibular impression and to relax the oral muscles.

B. Examine the Maxillary Teeth

Examine for particles of mandibular impression material and remove. Request patient to use mouth rinse for 2 to 3 minutes.

C. Prepare the Alginate

Fill the tray as described previously for the mandibular impression.

D. Precoat Undercut Areas

Precoat undercut areas, vestibular areas, and occlusal surfaces (see procedure for mandibular impression).

II. STEPS FOR INSERTION OF TRAY

- Follow maxillary tray try-in. In summary, the procedure is as follows:
  A. From 11 o'clock position (1 o'clock if left-handed), retract lip with fingers of nondominant hand.
  B. Use side of tray to distend the lip and cheek.
  C. Insert the tray with a rotary motion; center it over the teeth by using the small gap in the red wax border to relate to the labial frenum.
  D. Introduce the material to the teeth so the wax rim is 1/4 inch facial to the most anterior incisor.
- Seat the tray from posterior to anterior to direct the impression material forward and thus prevent irritation to the soft palate area.
- Retract the lip and bring the tray to place with a slight vibratory motion to allow the material to flow into crevices and proximal areas.
- The middle finger of each hand is placed over the premolar region to support and guide the tray; the index fingers and thumbs hold the lip out.
- Request the patient to form a tight "O" with the lips to mold the impression material.
- Maintain equal pressure on each side of the tray throughout the setting of the alginate. When assistance is available or if the pressure to hold the tray can be maintained with one hand, a saliva ejector can be inserted.
- When the leftover material on the spatula has lost its surface stickiness, hold the impression in place for 2 more clocked minutes.

III. THE COMPLETED IMPRESSION

A. Remove Impression

Hold the tray handle with the thumb and fingers of the dominant hand, and retract the opposite lip and cheek with the fingers of the other hand. Elevate the cheek over the edge of the impression to break the seal, and remove the impression with a sudden jerk.

B. Rinse

Rinse under cool running water to remove saliva, blood, and bacteria. Rinse carefully to prevent dissemination of contaminated saliva and blood.

C. Examine

Examine surface detail and proper extension to include tuberosity areas and a complete reproduction of the height of the vestibule.

D. Repeat Procedure When Necessary

Repeat procedure rather than be satisfied with a substandard impression.

E. Disinfection

Proceed with disinfection for maxillary and mandibular casts.

DISINFECTION OF IMPRESSIONS

To prevent cross-contamination during laboratory procedures, impressions are disinfected in an approved disinfectant after rinsing. When impressions are to be sent to a laboratory, they are isolated in a package. A sealable plastic bag can be used.

- Apply standard precautions; wear protective gloves, eyewear, and mask to handle contaminated impressions.
- Immerse to ensure maximum contact of the agent with all undercut areas. Impression then can be placed in the solution in a sealable plastic bag for 10 to 15 minutes.
- Discard disinfectant solution and rinse the impression under running water.

PARACLINICAL PROCEDURES

Supplemental to the chairside clinical procedures is the laboratory work involved in the production of the study casts from the impressions. These duties may be the responsibility of the dental laboratory technician or other dental team member.

- *The most frequent error in the use of the alginates for impressions is delay in pouring the cast.*
- Undue dehydration or water loss from the alginate causes permanent distortion, an uneven surface, and hence an inaccurate cast.
- Regard for the sensitive properties of the dental materials, precision and practice in laboratory procedures, and pride in the production of neat, smooth,

well-proportioned study casts determine the finished product's appearance, usefulness, and accuracy.

I. EQUIPMENT AND MATERIALS

- Mixing bowl: clean, dry, flexible rubber or plastic, with smooth, unscratched surface. Separate bowls are reserved for each dental material.
- Spatula: clean, dry, stiff, metal with a smooth, rounded end that can reach every part of the bowl without scraping or cutting its surface.
- Plaster knife: sharp.
- Vibrator with protective covering.
- Mechanical mixer.
- Model-base formers, glass or ceramic slab, waxed paper, or other nonabsorbent material.
- Dental materials
  A. Baseplate wax (and wax spatula).
  B. White dental stone.
- Water at room temperature, with measuring container.
- Model trimmer.
- Compass or dividers.
- Plastic ruler.
- Waterproof sandpaper.
- Soap solution.

II. PREPARATION OF THE IMPRESSIONS

- Rinse impressions under cool running water to remove residual disinfectant that may affect the plaster or stone surface after pouring; shake out excess water gently and apply gentle blast of compressed air.
- Create an artificial floor of the mouth in the mandibular impression to facilitate pouring and trimming of the cast.
  A. Trim the lingual impression material all around so that the height is consistent from the occlusal and incisal surfaces to the base of the impression.
  B. Using alginate:
    1. Mix a small portion of alginate.
    2. Hold the mandibular impression upright in the nondominant hand, with the middle and ring fingers extended from under the tray into the tongue area.
    3. Apply alginate over the fingers to form a flat bridge slightly above the lingual flanges of the impression.
    4. Smooth the surface with a finger moistened with cool water; hold until the alginate sets.
    5. When assisted at the chair, the floor of the mandibular impression can be made while the maxillary impression is being held for setting. There is usually sufficient alginate mixed with that for the maxillary impression to use for this purpose.
  C. Using baseplate wax:
    1. Cut a piece of baseplate wax to the shape of the lingual periphery of the impression.

2. Seal into place with a warm spatula, taking care that no heat is applied to the anatomic portions of the impression.
3. Cool under running water.

MIXING THE STONE

I. FACTORS RELATED TO DENTAL STONE THAT CONTRIBUTE TO THE SUCCESSFUL CAST

Texts on dental materials can be reviewed for complete information about gypsum products.[3,4] Some pertinent properties are listed here as reference points.

A. Dental Stone

- Sensitive to changes in the relative humidity of the atmosphere.
- Store in airtight container; close soon after use; do not let water enter the container.
- Keep the spoon or scoop (used to remove the powder) clean and dry.

B. Water

- Controls the strength, rigidity, and hardness of the cast.
- *Temperature.* Generally, cooler water decreases the setting time and warmer water increases it.
- *Quantity.* Follow manufacturer's proportions exactly. Increasing the water over the specifications prolongs the setting time and reduces the strength.

C. Spatulation

Prolonged or very rapid mixing can hasten the chemical reaction and shorten the setting time.

II. THE MIX

- Measure the water and powder by the manufacturer's specifications.
  A. White stone is generally preferred for study casts. Plaster produces a cast more susceptible to breakage.
  B. Ratio of 30–40 ml water to 100 g stone.
- Place measured water (room temperature) in a clean, dry mixing bowl.
- Sift in the powder gradually to prevent air trapping and to allow each particle to become wet.
- Wait briefly until all powder is wet, then vibrate to release large bubbles.
- Use vacuum mixer (follow manufacturer's directions).
- The result is a smooth, homogeneous, creamy mix.

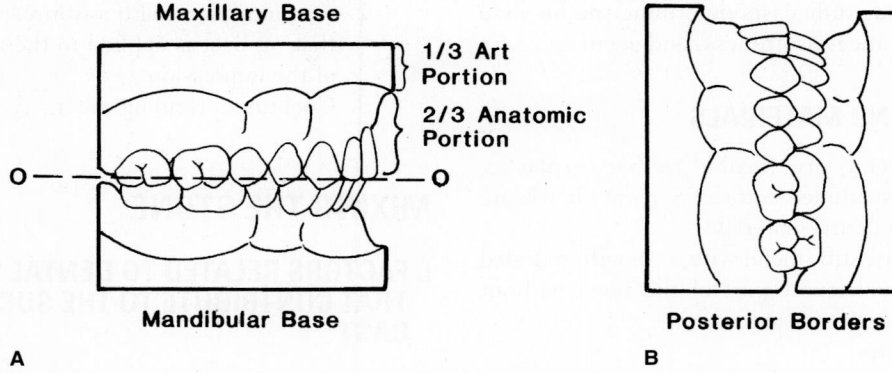

FIGURE 13-5 Finished Study Casts. (A) Proportions and planes. The art portion is one-third and the anatomic portion two-thirds of the total height of the cast. Note parallelism of the maxillary and mandibular bases with the mean occlusal plane (0–0). **(B)** Posterior borders are at right angles to the bases. When the maxillary and mandibular casts are placed on their posterior borders, the teeth intercuspate exactly.

POURING THE CAST

The finished cast has two connected parts, the anatomic portion and the base or art portion **(Figure 13-5)**.

I. POURING THE ANATOMIC PORTION

- Shake water out of the impression.
- Hold the impression tray by the handle and press handle against the vibrator.
- With a small amount of stone mix on the end of the spatula, start at one posterior corner and allow the mix to flow through the impression. Use small amounts and vibrate continually.
  - A. Tip the impression so the material passes into the tooth indentations and flows slowly down the side, across the occlusal surface or the incisal edge, and up the other side of the impression of each tooth.
  - B. Air can be trapped when the process is hurried or when too large a quantity of mix is poured in at one time without attentive control of the flow.
- When all tooth indentations are covered, add larger amounts of mix to fill the impression slightly over the periphery. Vibrate.

II. ONE-STEP METHOD FOR FORMING THE BASE OF THE CAST

- Fill rubber model-base former with the remainder of the mix, or form a mass of stone on a glass or ceramic slab or other nonabsorbent surface (waxed paper on a smooth surface). Add excess stone at the heel areas.
- Invert the poured impression onto the base.
  - A. Use a slight back-and-forth motion to secure the two parts together.
  - B. Avoid the common error of inverting the impression before the stone is firm. The mix can flow out of the impression.

- Adjust tray to proper position.
  - A. Occlusal plane (at premolars) should be parallel with the base of the model-base former or tabletop.
  - B. Midline (anterior as judged by handle of impression tray) centered at the midline of the model-base former.
  - C. Accommodate position so that a tooth in labioversion or buccoversion does not protrude over the trimming line of the art portion **(Figure 13-5)**.
- Add stone on peripheral and heel areas to provide a smooth surface; remove excess so that wax periphery of the tray is visible. When excess stone above the edge of the tray rim is permitted to set, the tray is difficult to separate, and the use of a knife to carve the excess from the tray may damage the cast.
- Final set occurs within 1 hour. Separate 1 hour after pouring to preserve the accuracy and prevent damage to the surface of the cast.

III. OTHER METHODS FOR FORMING THE BASE OF THE CAST

A. Two-Step or Double-Pour Method

- Both maxillary and mandibular impressions are poured and left upright (see "Pouring the Anatomic Portion.")
- Stone is then prepared separately for the bases, and the model-base formers are filled or the mass is placed on the smooth nonabsorbent surface.
- The impression is inverted and held on the surface of the new stone while the sides and periphery are shaped and smoothed.
- An advantage to this method is that there is no danger of inverting the poured impression too soon.
- If the cast is turned before it starts to set, the unset stone can fall away from the occlusal and incisal portions and leave bubbles in strategic places.

B. Boxing Technique

- Objective: to form a wall around the impression before pouring to provide a shape for the base as well as to prevent the need for inverting the poured impression.
- A strip of utility (beading) wax is attached slightly below the periphery of the impression and completely around the impression.
- Boxing wax or baseplate is applied around the strip of utility wax and attached to it by means of a warm spatula at a height that allows for proper thickness of the final cast, about 1/2 inch.
- Care must be taken not to displace the impression dimensionally or to touch the anatomic portions with the warm spatula.
- Pouring is carried out as described previously.
- Work-model formers with side walls to provide the boxing effect are available. Such a mold has a slot through the rubber where the handle of the impression tray can be inserted.

IV. SEPARATION OF THE IMPRESSION AND THE CAST

A. Objective: to remove tray and impression material without breaking the teeth.

B. When model-based former is used, remove it first.

C. Cut away stone from the periphery to free the margin of the tray.

D. Remove the tray by itself.

E. Cut the impression material along the line of the occlusal surfaces and peel off the impression material (with care not to scratch the stone cast during cutting).

F. Direct removal is possible when the teeth are in reasonably normal alignment; remove the tray and the impression material with a straight pull after first releasing the anterior portion by a slight downward and forward movement. When this method is used, do not apply lateral pressures or rock the tray back and forth, because the teeth are broken easily by such forces.

G. Trimming is started promptly, or if delayed, the cast must be thoroughly soaked in water before trimming.

TRIMMING THE CASTS

The exact proportions of the study casts and the steps required to accomplish the trimming and finishing depend on several factors, including the measurements of the patient's dental arches, the positions of the teeth, and the preferences of the dentist. Development of a routine, systematic procedure for trimming can lead to the production of consistent, attractive, and useful diagnostic casts.

I. USE OF MODEL TRIMMER

- Precision-type model trimmer.

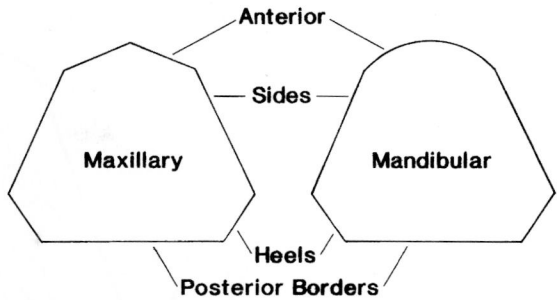

FIGURE 13-6 **Base Shapes for Finished Study Casts.** Maxillary and mandibular casts are trimmed at the labeled areas. See text for procedures.

- Angulators that are available to fit on the table of the model trimmer to give average set angles for trimming the margins of the casts; when these are available, usually directions are supplied by the manufacturer.
- Use protective eyewear and mask while using a model trimmer. Goggles are indicated for laboratory procedures.

II. CHARACTERISTICS OF THE FINISHED CASTS

Before the step-by-step description of the trimming procedures, observe **Figure 13-5** for the overall proportions and planes of ideally finished study casts. **Figure 13-6** outlines the base shapes and **Figure 13-7** shows the occlusal views of the maxillary and mandibular casts.

III. PRELIMINARY STEPS TO TRIMMING THE CAST

A. Casts must be wet; soak at least 5 minutes.

B. Remove bubbles of stone on or about the teeth with a small sharp instrument; use care not to scar the cast.

C. Level down excess stone that is distal to the retromolar area and tuberosity so casts may be occluded. Do not shorten the cast anteriorly to posteriorly at this time.

D. Trim casts conservatively on the sides to make a smooth surface for marking.

IV. TRIMMING THE BASES

A. Objectives

1. To make bases parallel with the mean occlusal plane and to each other.

2. To make correct proportions for the height of the casts; art portion one-third and anatomic portion two-thirds (Figure 13-5A).

B. Mandibular Cast Is Trimmed First

1. Measure the greatest height of the anatomic portion (usually this is from the tip of the canine to the depth of the vestibule) with a plastic ruler (Figure 13-8).

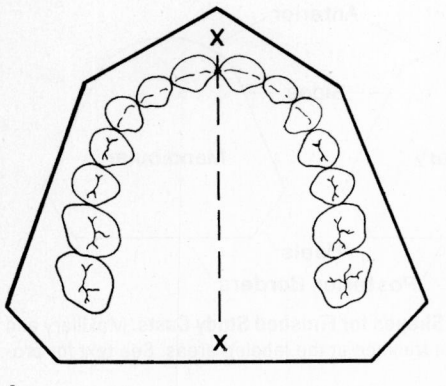
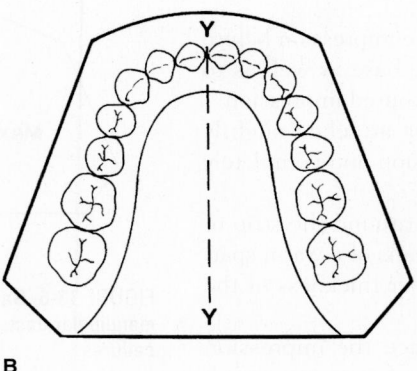

FIGURE 13-7 **Occlusal Views of Finished Casts. (A)** Maxillary. **(B)** Mandibular. The posterior border is perpendicular to the median line from the incisors through the palate (X–X) and the middle of the tongue (Y–Y). The tuberosity of the maxilla and the retromolar areas of the mandible are preserved.

2. Divide by two to obtain the height of the art portion.
3. Add the measured height of the anatomic portion to the height of the art portion for the total height of the cast. Set compass or dividers at this measurement.
4. Place the cast teeth down on a flat surface and mark a line around the art portion at the height calculated in step 3. This line should be parallel with the occlusal plane (line O––O in **Figure 13-8**). Trim the cast at the line.

C. Maxillary Cast Base

1. Measure the greatest depth of the anatomic portion (usually at the canine) and divide by two to obtain the height of the art portion.
2. Relate the two casts (use the wax bite if necessary) and place the mandibular base on the flat surface.
3. Measure from the base of the mandibular cast to the highest point of the maxillary anatomic portion (usually in the vestibule over the canine), and add this figure to the height of the maxillary art portion calculated in the aforementioned step 1.
4. Set the compass at this measurement, and mark a line around the maxillary cast at the total height. The line is parallel with the base of the mandibular cast and with the occlusal plane. Trim.

V. POSTERIOR BORDERS

A. *Select the longest cast to trim first* by measuring from the incisors to points distal to the retromolar and tuberosity areas.

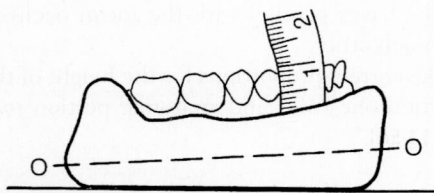

FIGURE 13-8 **Trimming the Base.** Measure the anatomic portion at its greatest height, which is usually from the tip of the canine to the depth of the vestibule. Note ruler in position. One half of the measurement is the height of the art portion. The trimming line (O–O) is parallel with the mean occlusal plane. See text for details.

B. On the longest cast, place the tip of the compass at the gingival border behind the midline anteriorly (usually this is between the central incisors) and mark an arc 1/4-inch distal to the tuberosity (if the maxillary cast) or retromolar area (if the mandibular cast) on each side.
C. Intersect the arc with a line through the central grooves of the molars **(Figure 13-9A)**.
D. Connect the two points across the back of the cast (O––O in **Figure 13-9A**). Check that this line is perpendicular to the median line from the incisors through the palate or the tongue (X–Y in **Figure 13-9B**).
E. With the base of the cast flat on the model trimmer table, trim on the line marked for the posterior border.
F. For the shorter cast, relate the two casts with the wax bite and place flat on the base of the first trimmed cast. Bring them carefully to the cutting surface of the model trimmer, and trim until the two posterior borders are even and parallel.
G. Check by placing the casts on their posterior borders and bringing them together. They relate in their natural intercuspation **(Figure 13-5B)**.

VI. SIDES AND HEELS

■ *Select the widest cast to trim first*; casts are usually widest at the molar region.
■ Mark with a ruler two symmetrical lines 1/4-inch buccal from the buccal bony prominence at the premolar regions and parallel with lines through the central grooves of the premolars **(Figure 13-10A)**.
  A. Check that the lines form equal angles with the posterior border.
  B. Before trimming, make certain that the lines when cut would not remove any vestibular anatomy.
  C. Trim the sides with the base flat on the model trimmer table.
■ Mark trimming lines for the heels; cuts are 1/4-inch wide and parallel with a line through the mesiodistal plane of the opposite canine **(Figure 13-10B)**. Trim with base flat on the model trimmer table.
■ Relate the opposite cast with the wax bite, and trim the sides and heels to match the previously trimmed cast.

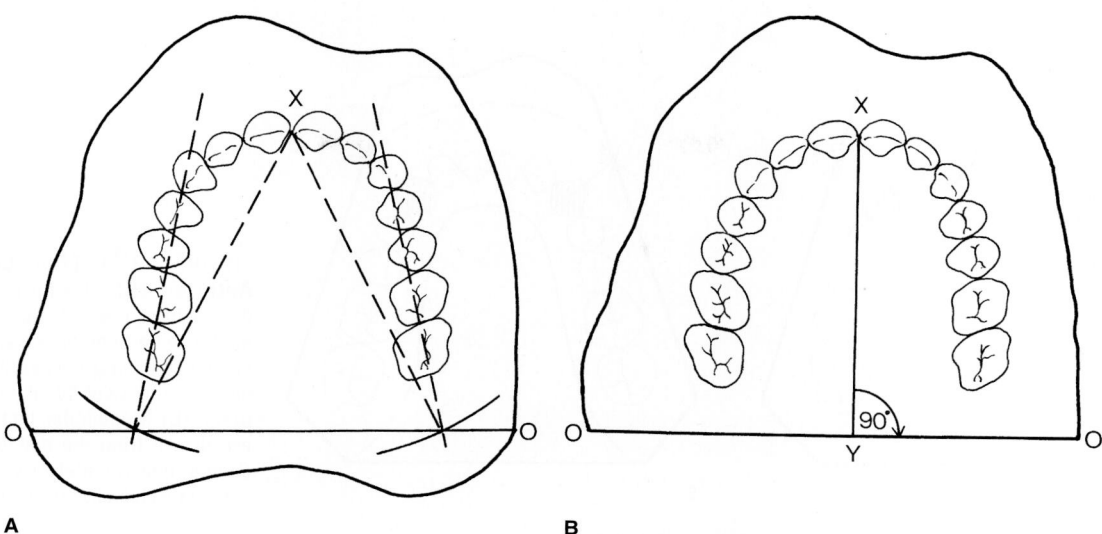

FIGURE 13-9 **Trim Line for Posterior Borders. (A)** On the longest cast, use a compass to draw arcs from the anterior midline point (X) to 1/4-inch distal to the tuberosity (maxilla) or retromolar area (mandible). Intersect the arc with a line through the central grooves of the molars and connect the two points across the cast (O–O).

VII. ANTERIOR

The maxillary cast is trimmed to a point, and the mandibular cast is rounded **(Figure 13-6)**.

A. Maxillary

■ A ruler can be used to draw guidelines for trimming on each side of the midline to the cuspid areas. Note the broken lines in **Figure 13-11A**. The lines need to be 1/4-inch labial to the depth of the mucobuccal fold (vestibule) or to the most labially inclined tooth.

■ Before trimming, check that both sides of the cast are the same length from the intersection of the front cut to the heels.

B. Mandibular

1. Sketch the shape of an arc from canine to canine to conform generally with the curvature of the anterior teeth and approximately 1/4-inch labial to the depth of the mucobuccal fold or the most labially inclined or positioned tooth **(Figure 13-11B)**.

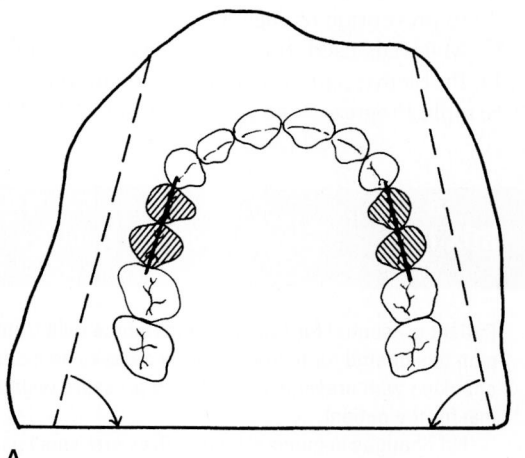
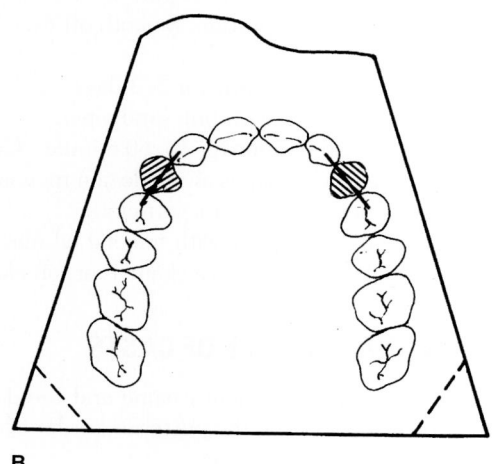

FIGURE 13-10 **Trim Lines for Sides and Heels. (A)** On the widest cast, trim lines for the sides are drawn parallel with lines through the central grooves of the premolars. The two symmetrical lines form equal angles with the posterior border of the cast. **(B)** Mark trim lines for heels 1/4-inch wide and parallel with lines through the mesiodistal plane of the opposite canine. The lines are symmetrical with each other and form equal angles with the posterior border.

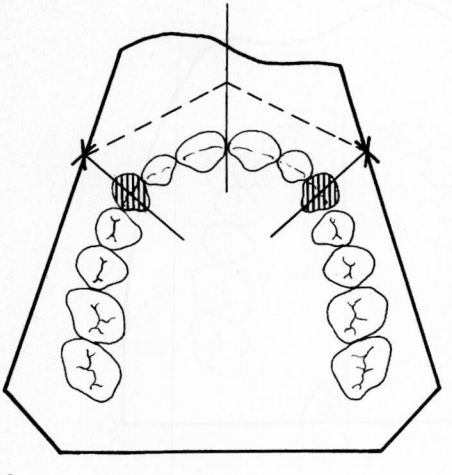

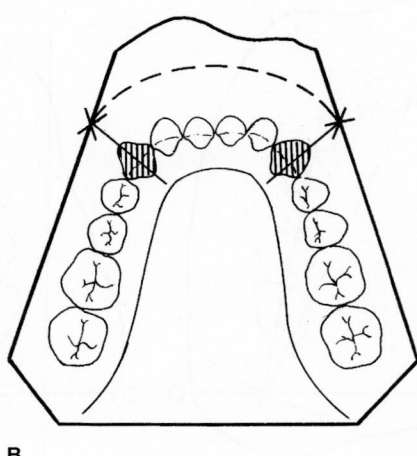

FIGURE 13-11 **Trim Lines for Anterior. (A)** Maxillary lines are drawn from opposite the middle of each canine to meet in a point at the midline and approximately 1/4-inch labial to the most labially positioned tooth. **(B)** Mandibular line forms an arc drawn from the middle of each canine approximately 1/4-inch labial to the most labially positioned tooth.

A

B

2. Before trimming, check that both sides of the cast are the same length from the intersection of the front cut to the heels.

VIII. FINISHING AND POLISHING

■ Trim rough edges and margins of both casts and the lingual portion of the mandibular cast to even off irregularities and make the depth of the vestibule visible. Remaining bubbles are removed.

■ Use waterproof sandpaper and a plaster smoothing stone to remove marks left by the model trimmer on the art portion. Sandpaper is not used on the anatomic portion.

■ Fill any holes in the wet casts with stone applied with a spatula to the flat surfaces of the art portion or a camel's hair brush to the anatomic portion. Smooth off excess.

■ Finish and polish
  A. Allow casts to dry thoroughly for 2–3 days.
  B. Smooth the art portion with fine sandpaper.
  C. Soak in heated soap solution for 30–60 minutes. Concentrated model gloss soap is available commercially.
  D. Rub with chamois, cotton, or a soft cloth.
  E. Talc or baby talcum powder with mineral oil may be used, followed by rubbing with a chamois or soft cloth.

IX. RECORDS AND STORAGE OF CASTS

■ Label each cast with the patient's name and the date. These may be inscribed into the posterior border of the cast before soaping and polishing.

■ Boxes of an appropriate size are available commercially for storage of one or more pairs of casts.

■ Record in the patient's permanent record the size of impression tray used. When casts are made periodically for follow-up, time is saved both in the sterilization of

all sizes for try-in and in the preparation of the wax rim in advance of the patient's appointment.

■ Make a duplicate cast for the permanent record when the dentist uses the original for the design of a prosthesis. The duplicate cast is made by making an impression of the original and pouring it in the same manner as the original.

DOCUMENTATION

■ For the preparation of impressions for study casts a suggested documentation includes:
  A. Date; impressions taken (maxillary, mandibular., or partial); previous experience of patient.
  B. Patient positioning and special advice (e.g., relative to prevention of gagging)
  C. Materials used; trays: size, plastic or metal.
  D. Problems; patient comments; recommendations.

■ Sample Progress Note may be found in **Box 13-2**.

BOX 13-2	Sample Progress Note

Patient presented for routine maintenance with treatment plan designated for follow-up study casts to be made for checking with previous casts. Blood pressure within normal for the patient.

No changes in medical history. Tray size small used as specified. Patient fussed about the discomfort. Next 3-months' appt planned.

Signed: _____, RDH Date: _____

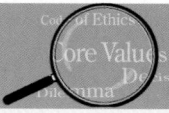

Everyday Ethics

Everyone was rushing around the office trying to finish in time for lunch. Elena was asked to take the impressions for whitening trays for Mrs. Lynch. As Elena places the maxillary tray, the patient begins to gag severely. Mrs. Lynch pushes Elena's arm out of the way and attempts to pull the tray out of her mouth. Elena calls for assistance while forcefully restraining Mrs. Lynch to keep the tray in until the impression material is set.

Questions for Consideration
1. Describe the ethical principle(s) that best describe(s) the actions of Elena.
2. By restraining the patient, were the patient's rights violated? Why or why not? Explain the rationale.
3. Professionally, what choices could Elena have exercised with Mrs. Lynch to improve the outcome?

Factors To Teach The Patient

- Importance and purposes of study casts. Reasons for comparative casts following treatment at a later date.
- Use the unidentified casts of other patients to show effects of treatment or what can happen if the prescribed treatment is not carried out.
- Areas that present difficulty in the dental biofilm control program:
- Show anatomy of gingiva and teeth and demonstrate use of biofilm removal devices on the patient's own study casts.

References

1. Gladwin M, Bagby M. *Clinical aspects of dental materials*. 3rd ed. Philadelphia: Wolters Kluwer/Lippincott Williams & Wilkins; 2009. 111–13, 308–14 pp.
2. Ferracane JL. *Materials in dentistry*. 2nd ed. Philadelphia: Lippincott Williams & Wilkins; 2001. 179, 184–8 pp.
3. Gladwin and Bagby. op.cit., 122–8, 316–28 pp.
4. Ferracane. op.cit., 203–220 pp.

The Periodontium

ESTHER M. WILKINS, BS, RDH, DMD

Chapter Outline

The true test of successful treatment, the real evaluation of the effects of preventive care with patient instruction and nonsurgical instrumentation, is the health of the teeth, the periodontium, the implants, and the periimplant tissues. *The goal of all treatment is to bring the diseased periodontal and periimplant tissues to a state of health that can be maintained by the patient.*

To accomplish this goal, the first steps include learning:

■ To recognize normal, healthy tissue by clinical observation and testing with a periodontal probe,
■ To teach and supervise the patient's necessary daily self-care that must accompany professional care, and

■ To apply the knowledge to the treatment and supervision of the patient until health is attained.

An outline of the clinical features of the periodontal tissues in health and disease is included in this chapter. Information on the clinical features and care of the periimplant tissues is located in Chapter 32, page 469. Key words are defined in **Box 14-1**.

OBJECTIVES FOR ASSESSMENT

The ultimate objective of treatment is to apply knowledge and skill in examination and assessment of the periodontal tissues to patient care so that each patient attains and maintains

| BOX 14-1 | Key Words |

Gingiva and Periodontium

Attachment apparatus: the cementum, periodontal ligament, and the alveolar bone.

Clinical attachment level: the probing depth measured from a fixed point, such as the cementoenamel junction.

Desmosome: cell junction; consists of a dense plate near the cell surface that relates to a similar structure on an adjacent cell, between which are thin layers of extracellular material.

Diastema: a space between two natural adjacent teeth. Plural, diastemata. See also Primate space, in Chapter 18, page 278.

Epithelium: specialized single layer (simple) or multiple (stratified) layers of cells that form on the surface of skin, mucosa, or serous membranes.

    Oral: the tissue serving as a liner for the intraoral mucosal surfaces.

    Squamous: composed of a layer of flat, scalelike cells; or may be stratified.

Fibroblast: fiber-producing cell of the connective tissue; a flattened, irregularly branched cell with a large oval nucleus that is responsible in part for the production and remodeling of the extracellular matrix.

Fibrosis: a fibrous change of the mucous membrane, especially the gingiva, because of chronic inflammation; fibrotic gingiva may appear outwardly healthy, thus masking underlying disease.

Hemidesmosome: half of a desmosome that forms a site of attachment between junctional epithelial cells and the tooth surface.

Hyperkeratosis: abnormal thickening of the keratin layer (stratum corneum) of the epithelium.

Hyperplasia: abnormal increase in volume of a tissue or organ caused by formation and growth of new normal cells.

Hypertrophy: increase in size of tissue or organ caused by an increase in size of its constituent cells.

Keratinization: development of a horny layer of flattened epithelial cells containing keratin.

Marker: identifier; symptoms or signs by which a particular condition can be recognized; for example, clinical and microbiologic markers are used to identify gingival and periodontal infections.

Mastication: act of chewing.

Nonkeratinized mucosa: lining mucosa in which the stratified squamous epithelial cells retain their nuclei and cytoplasm.

Periodontium: tissues surrounding and supporting the teeth; in two sections are the gingival unit, composed of the free and attached gingiva and the alveolar mucosa, and the attachment apparatus, which includes the cementum, periodontal ligament, and alveolar process.

Probing depth: the distance from the gingival margin to the location of the periodontal probe tip inserted for gentle probing at the attachment.

Pus: a fluid product of inflammation that contains leukocytes, degenerated tissue elements, tissue fluids, and microorganisms.

Sharpey's fibers: penetrating connective tissue fibers by which the tooth is attached to the adjacent alveolar bone; the fiber bundles penetrate cementum on one side and alveolar bone on the other.

Stippling: the pitted, orange-peel appearance frequently seen on the surface of the attached gingiva.

Suppuration: formation of pus.

Taste bud: receptor of taste on tongue and oropharynx; goblet-shaped cells oriented at right angles to the surface of the epithelium.

---

optimum oral health. The dental hygienist needs to know when the treatment provided by dental hygiene services is definitive in restoring health and when additional treatment is needed. The patient can be properly informed so that complete treatment by the dentist or periodontist can be provided.

Specific objectives are to be able to:

- Recognize normal periodontal tissues.
- Know the clinical features of the periodontal tissues that are examined for a complete assessment.
- Recognize the markers that are the basic signs of periodontal infections and identify them by degree of severity.
- Identify the dental hygiene treatment and instruction needed.
- Outline the patient's preventive program.

THE TREATMENT AREA

The treatment procedures are applied directly to the teeth, the gingiva, and the gingival sulcus. Detailed knowledge

and understanding of the anatomy and normal clinical appearance of the hard and soft oral tissues are prerequisite to meaningful examination and treatment.

I. THE TEETH

A. Clinical Crown

The part of the tooth above the attached periodontal tissues. It can be considered the part of the tooth where clinical treatment procedures are applied (**Figure 14-1**).

B. Clinical Root

The part of the tooth below the base of the gingival sulcus or periodontal pocket. It is the part of the root to which periodontal fibers are attached.

C. Anatomic Crown

The part of the tooth covered by enamel.

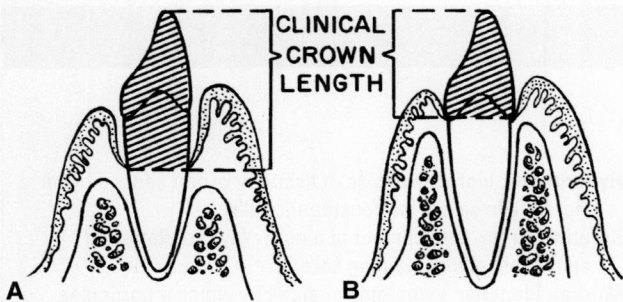

FIGURE 14-1 **Clinical Crown.** The part of the tooth that is above the attached periodontal tissue. **(A)** When the periodontal pocket depth is increased, the clinical crown extends to a position at which the clinical crown length is greater than the clinical root length. The clinical root is that part of the tooth with attached periodontal tissues. **(B)** When the clinical attachment level is at the cementoenamel junction, the clinical crown and the anatomic crown are the same.

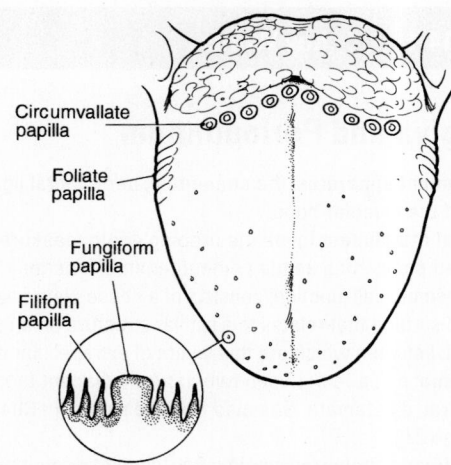

FIGURE 14-2 **Papillae of the Tongue.** Dorsal surface of a human tongue shows the four types of papillae. Inset enlargement shows the shape of filiform and fungiform papillae.

D. Anatomic Root

The part of the tooth covered by cementum.

II. ORAL MUCOSA

The lining of the oral cavity, the oral mucosa, is a mucous membrane composed of connective tissue covered with stratified squamous epithelium. There are three divisions or categories of oral mucosa.

A. Masticatory Mucosa

1. Covers the *gingiva* and the *hard palate,* the areas most used during the mastication of food.
2. Except for the free margin of the gingiva, the masticatory mucosa is firmly attached to underlying tissues.
3. The epithelial covering is generally keratinized.

B. Lining Mucosa

1. Covers the inner surfaces of the lips and cheeks, the floor of the mouth, the underside of the tongue, the soft palate, and the alveolar mucosa.
2. These tissues are not firmly attached to underlying tissue.
3. The epithelial covering is not generally keratinized.

C. Specialized Mucosa

1. Covers the dorsum (upper surface) of the tongue. It is composed of many papillae; some contain taste buds.
2. The distribution of the four types of papillae is shown in **Figure 14-2**.
   - *Filiform:* threadlike keratinized elevations that cover the dorsal surface of the tongue; they are the most numerous of the papillae.

- *Fungiform:* mushroom-shaped papillae interspersed among the filiform papillae on the tip and sides of the tongue. On clinical examination, they appear redder than the filiform papillae and contain variable numbers of taste buds. The inset enlargement in **Figure 14-2** shows the comparative shape and size of the filiform and fungiform papillae.
- *Circumvallate (vallate):* the 10 to 14 large round papillae arranged in a "V" between the body of the tongue and the base. Taste buds line the walls.
- *Foliate:* vertical grooves on the lateral posterior sides of the tongue; also contain taste buds.

III. THE PERIODONTIUM

The periodontium is the functional unit of tissues that surrounds and supports the tooth. The parts are the *periodontal ligament, cementum,* and *bone;* they make up the attachment apparatus.

A. Periodontal Ligament

1. The periodontal ligament is the fibrous connective tissue that surrounds and attaches the roots of teeth to the alveolar bone.
2. The ligament is located in the periodontal space between the cementum and the alveolar bone.
3. It is composed of connective tissue cells and intracellular substance.
4. The fibers that are inserted into the cementum on one side and the alveolar bone on the other are called *Sharpey's fibers.*
5. The two general groups of fibers are the *gingival groups* (around the cervical area within the gingival tissues) and the *principal fiber groups* (surrounding the root).[1]

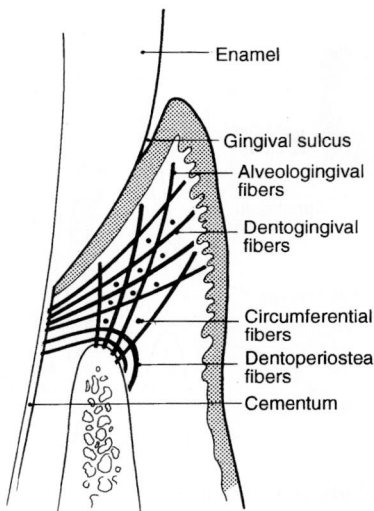

FIGURE 14-3 **Gingival Fiber Groups.** Cross section of the gingiva shows the relation of the gingival fiber groups to the gingival sulcus, the free gingiva, the cementum, and the alveolar bone.

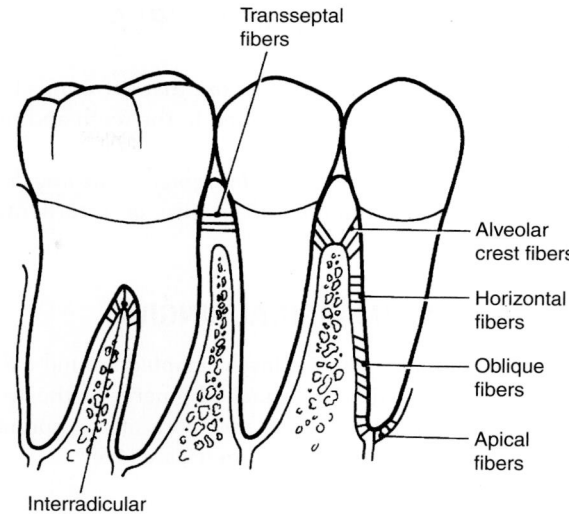
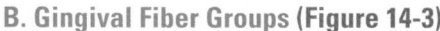

FIGURE 14-4 **Principal Fiber Groups of the Periodontium.** The five principal groups (apical, oblique, horizontal, alveolar crest, and interradicular) are shown. The transseptal fibers of the gingival fiber groups are also shown as they span across from the cervical area of one tooth to the neighboring tooth.

B. Gingival Fiber Groups (Figure 14-3)

1. Dentogingival fibers (free gingiva): from the cementum in the cervical region into the free gingiva to give support to the gingival.
2. Alveologingival fibers (attached gingiva): from the alveolar crest into the free and attached gingiva to provide support.
3. Circumferential fibers (circular): continuous around the neck of the tooth to help to maintain the tooth in position.
4. Dentoperiosteal fibers (alveolar crest): from the cervical cementum over the alveolar crest to blend with fibers of the periosteum of the bone.
5. Transseptal fibers: from the cervical area of one tooth across to an adjacent tooth (on the mesial or distal only) to provide resistance to separation of teeth (**Figure 14-4**).

C. Principal Fiber Groups (Figure 14-4)

The five principal groups of collagen fibers are named for their location on the root and for their direction. They are also called the dentoalveolar fiber groups.
1. Apical fibers: from the root apex to adjacent surrounding bone to resist vertical forces.
2. Oblique fibers: from the root above the apical fibers obliquely toward the occlusal to resist vertical and unexpected strong forces.
3. Horizontal fibers: from the cementum in the middle of each root to adjacent alveolar bone to resist tipping of the tooth.
4. Alveolar crest fibers: from the alveolar crest to the cementum just below the cementoenamel junction to resist intrusive forces.

5. Interradicular fibers: from cementum between the roots of multirooted teeth to the adjacent bone to resist vertical and lateral forces.

D. Cementum

The cementum is a thin layer of calcified connective tissue that covers the tooth from the cementoenamel junction to, and around, the apical foramen.

1. *Functions*
   - To seal the tubules of the root dentin.
   - To provide attachment for the periodontal fiber groups.
2. *Characteristics*
   - Thickness is 50 to 200 μm about the apex; 30 to 60 μm about the cervical area.
   - Vascular and nerve connections are missing; therefore, cementum is insensitive.
   - Relationship of enamel and cementum at the cervical area is shown in Figure 16-2 (page 250).
   - In 10% of the instances, they do not meet and there can be a small area of exposed dentin; in 30%, they meet edge to edge; and in 60%, the cementum overlaps the enamel.

E. Alveolar Bone

1. The alveolar bone consists of the lamina dura, which surrounds the tooth socket, and the supporting bone.
2. When teeth are lost, the alveolar bone is resorbed.
3. The bone functions to support the teeth and provide attachment for the periodontal ligament fibers.

THE PERIODONTAL STRUCTURES

■ The part of the masticatory mucosa that surrounds the necks of the teeth and is attached to the teeth and the alveolar bone.

■ The gingiva is made up of the *free gingiva*, the *attached gingiva,* and the *interdental gingiva* or interdental papilla.

I. FREE GINGIVA (MARGINAL GINGIVA)

In health, the free gingiva is closely adapted around each tooth. It connects with the attached gingiva at the free gingival groove and attaches to the tooth at the coronal portion of the junctional epithelium **(Figure 14-5)**.

A. Free Gingival Groove

1. The free gingival groove is a shallow linear groove that demarcates the free from the attached gingiva. Generally, about one-third of the teeth may show a visible gingival groove when the gingiva is healthy.[2]
2. In the absence of inflammation and pocket formation, the gingival groove runs somewhat parallel with and about 0.5 to 1.5 mm from the gingival margin,[3] and it is approximately at the level of the bottom of the gingival sulcus.

B. Oral Epithelium (Outer Gingival Epithelium, Figure 14-6)

1. Covers the free gingiva from the gingival groove over the gingival margin.
2. Is composed of keratinized stratified squamous epithelium.

C. Gingival Margin (Gingival Crest, Margin of the Gingiva, or Free Margin, Figure 14-5)

1. This is the edge of the gingiva nearest the incisal or occlusal surface.
2. Marks the opening of the gingival sulcus.

II. GINGIVAL SULCUS (CREVICE)

A. Location

The crevice or groove between the free gingiva and the tooth.

B. Boundaries (Figure 14-6)

1. *Inner*: tooth surface. May be the enamel, cementum, or part of each, depending on the position of the junctional epithelium.
2. *Outer*: Sulcular epithelium.
3. *Base*: coronal margin of the attached tissues. The base of the sulcus or pocket is also called the "probing depth," the "depth of the sulcus," or the "bottom of the pocket."

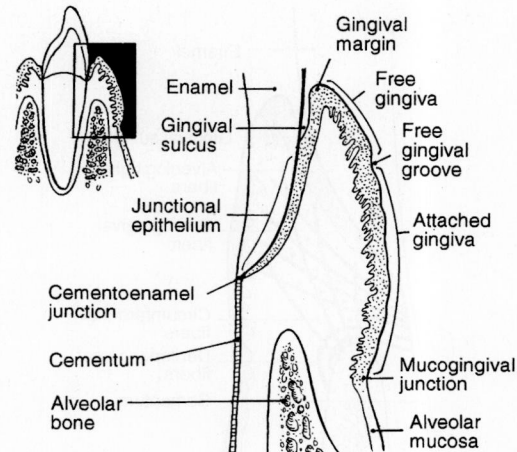

FIGURE 14-5 **Parts of the Gingiva.** Cross-sectional diagram shows the parts of the gingiva and adjacent tissues of a partially erupted tooth. Note that the junctional epithelium is on the enamel.

C. Sulcular Epithelium

The continuation of the oral epithelium covering the free gingiva. Sulcular epithelium is not keratinized.

D. Depth of Sulcus

1. Healthy sulci are shallow and may be only 0.5 mm.
2. The average depth of the healthy sulcus is about 1.8 mm.[4]

E. Gingival Sulcus Fluid (Sulcular Fluid, Crevicular Fluid)

1. A serum-like fluid that seeps from the connective tissue through the epithelial lining of the sulcus or pocket.

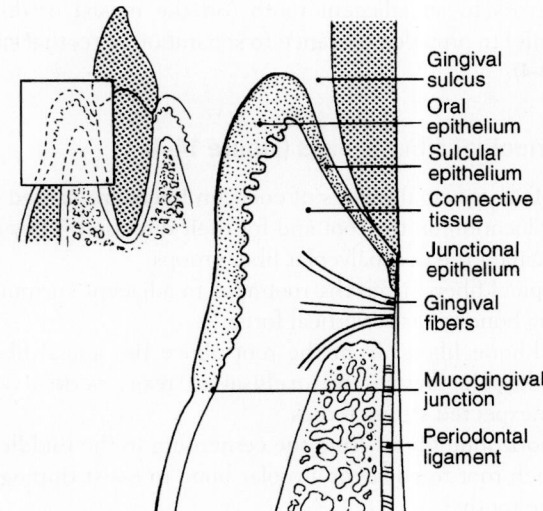

FIGURE 14-6 **The Gingival Tissues.** Cross-sectional diagram shows the histologic relationships of the oral, sulcular, and junctional epithelia and the connective tissue.

2. Occurrence is slight to none in a normal sulcus; increases with inflammation.
3. It is part of the local defense mechanism and is able to transport many substances, including endotoxins, enzymes, antibodies, and certain systemically administered drugs.

III. JUNCTIONAL EPITHELIUM (ATTACHMENT EPITHELIUM)

A. Description

1. The junctional epithelium is a cufflike band of stratified squamous epithelium that is continuous with the sulcular epithelium and completely encircles the tooth.
2. It is triangular in cross section, is widest at the junction with the sulcular epithelium, and narrows down to the width of a few cells at the apical end.
3. The junctional epithelium is not keratinized. It has two basement membranes: one adjacent to the connective tissue and one adjacent to the tooth surface.

B. Size

1. The junctional epithelium may be up to 15 or 20 cells in thickness where it joins the sulcular epithelium and tapers down to 1 or 2 cells in thickness at the apical end.
2. The length ranges from 0.25 to 1.35 mm.

C. Position

■ As the tooth erupts, the attachment is on the enamel; during eruption, the epithelium migrates toward the cementoenamel junction **(Figure 14-7)**.
■ At full eruption, the attachment is usually on the cementum, where it becomes firmly attached **(Figure 14-7D)**.
■ With wear of the tooth on the incisal or occlusal surface and with periodontal infections, the attachment migrates along the root surface **(Figure 14-7E)**.

D. Relation of Crest of Alveolar Bone to the Attached Gingival Tissue

1. The distance between the base of the attachment and the crest of the alveolar bone is approximately 1.0 to 1.5 mm.
2. This distance is maintained in disease when the epithelium moves along the root surface and bone loss occurs.

E. Attachment of the Epithelium to the Tooth Surface

1. The junctional epithelium or attachment epithelium provides a seal at the base of the sulcus.
2. The attachment, or connecting interface between the tooth and the tissue, is accomplished by hemidesmosomes and the basal lamina of the junctional epithelium.

IV. INTERDENTAL GINGIVA (INTERDENTAL PAPILLA)

A. Location

1. In health, the interdental gingiva occupies the interproximal area between two adjacent teeth that are in contact.
2. The tip and lateral borders are continuous with the free gingiva, whereas other parts are attached gingiva.
3. An interproximal area is also called an *embrasure*.
   ■ In Type 1 embrasure, the gingival tissue fills the area.
   ■ In Type 2 embrasure, there is slight to moderate recession of the interdental gingiva.
   ■ In Type 3 embrasure, there is extensive recession or complete loss of the papilla as shown in Figure 28-1 (page 409).

B. Shape

1. *Varies with spacing or overlapping of the teeth:* The interdental gingiva may be flat or saddle-shaped when wide spaces are between the teeth, or it may be tapered and narrow when the teeth are crowded or overlapped.

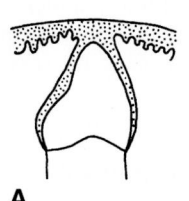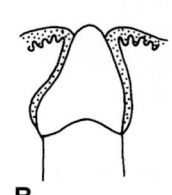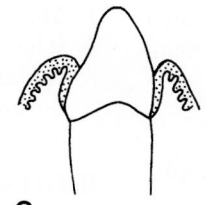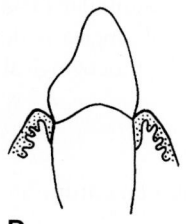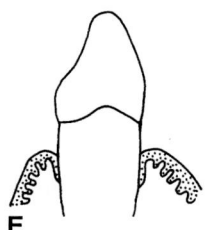

A   **B**   **C**   **D**   **E**

FIGURE 14-7 **Tooth Eruption and the Gingiva. (A)** Before eruption, the oral epithelium covers the tooth. **(B)** As the tooth emerges, the reduced epithelium joins the oral epithelium as the gingival sulcus is formed. **(C)** Partial eruption with the junctional epithelium along the enamel. **(D)** Eruption complete, with junctional epithelium at the cementoenamel junction. **(E)** From disease or other cause, the attachment migrates along the root surface, exposing the cementum.

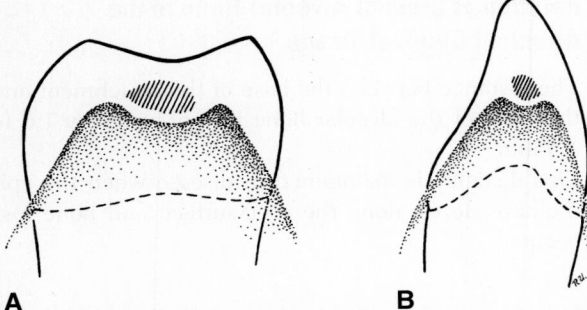

FIGURE 14-8 Col. A col is the depression between the lingual or palatal and the facial papillae under the contact area. The contact area is represented by the striped lines. **(A)** Mesial of mandibular molar to show wide col area. **(B)** Mesial of mandibular incisor to show a narrow col. The col deepens when gingival enlargement occurs.

2. *Between anterior teeth:* pointed, pyramidal.
3. *Between posterior teeth*
   ■ Flatter than anterior papillae because of wider teeth, wider contact areas, and flattened interdental bone.
   ■ Two papillae, one facial and one lingual, connected by a col, are found when teeth are in contact.

C. Col

1. A col is the depression under a contact area between a lingual or palatal and facial papilla that conforms to the proximal contact area as shown in **Figure 14-8**.
2. The center of the col area is not usually keratinized and thus is more susceptible to infection. Most periodontal infection begins in the col area.

V. ATTACHED GINGIVA

A. Extent

1. The attached gingiva is continuous with the oral epithelium of the free gingiva and is covered with keratinized stratified squamous epithelium.
2. Maxillary palatal gingiva is continuous with the palatal mucosa.
3. The attached gingiva of the mandibular facial and lingual gingiva and maxillary facial gingiva is demarcated from the alveolar mucosa by the mucogingival junction.

B. Attachment

Firmly bound to the underlying cementum and alveolar bone.

C. Shape

Follows the depressions between the eminences of the roots of the teeth.

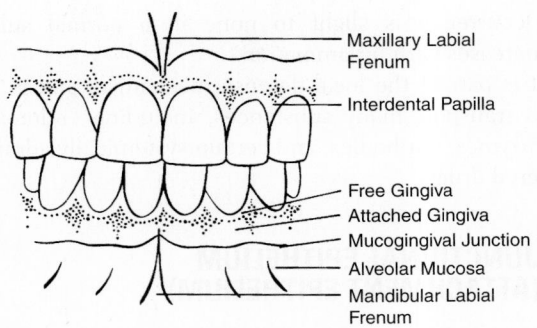

FIGURE 14-9 Parts of the Gingiva. The mucogingival junction for each arch is shown in relation to the attached gingiva, alveolar mucosa, and labial anterior frena.

VI. MUCOGINGIVAL JUNCTION

A. Appearance

1. The mucogingival junction appears as a line that marks the connection between the attached gingiva and the alveolar mucosa.
2. The anterior line is scalloped, but it is fairly straight posterior to the premolars.
3. A contrast can be seen between the pink of the keratinized, stippled, attached gingiva and the darker alveolar mucosa.

B. Location

1. A mucogingival line is found on the facial surface of all quadrants and on the lingual surface of the mandibular arch.
2. There is no alveolar mucosa on the palate. The palatal tissue is firmly attached to the bone of the roof of the mouth.
3. The three mucogingival lines are facial mandibular, lingual mandibular, and facial maxillary.
4. In **Figure 14-9**, the facial maxillary and mandibular mucogingival junctions are shown in relation to the attached gingiva and the alveolar mucosa.

VII. ALVEOLAR MUCOSA

A. Description

1. Movable tissue loosely attached to the underlying bone.
2. It has a smooth, shiny surface with nonkeratinized, thin epithelium. Underlying vessels may be seen through the epithelium.

B. Frena (Singular: Frenum or Frenulum)

1. *Description:* A frenum is a narrow fold of mucous membrane that passes from a more fixed to a movable part, for example, from the attached gingiva at the mucogingival junction to the lip, cheek, or undersurface of the tongue. A frenum serves to check undue movement.

2. *Locations*
   - Maxillary and mandibular anterior frena. At midlines between central incisors. **Figure 14-9** shows diagrammatically the location of the anterior frena.
   - Lingual frenum. From undersurface of the tongue.
   - Buccal frena. In the canine–premolar areas, both maxillary and mandibular.
3. *Attachment of frena in relation to the attached gingiva*
   - Closely associated with the mucogingival junction.
   - When the attached gingiva is narrow or missing, the frena may pull on the free gingiva and displace it laterally. A "tension test" is used to locate frenal attachments and check the adequacy of the attached gingiva (page 233).

THE RECOGNITION OF GINGIVAL AND PERIODONTAL INFECTIONS

I. THE CLINICAL EXAMINATION

The recognition of normal gingiva, gingival infections, and deeper periodontal involvement depends on a disciplined, step-by-step examination.

It is necessary to know the *extent* of the disease:

- *Gingival infections* are confined to the gingiva.
- *Periodontal infections* include all parts of the periodontium, namely, the gingiva, periodontal ligament, bone, and cementum.

A basic examination performed to recognize the signs and effects of inflammation includes information about at least the following markers:

- Gingival tissue changes (color, size, shape, surface texture, position)
- Mucogingival involvement (adequate width of attached gingiva)
- Probing depths; pocket formation (attachment levels)
- Bleeding and exudates
- Furcation involvement
- Dental biofilm (and calculus) present
- Mobility of teeth
- Radiographic evidence

II. SIGNS AND SYMPTOMS

- Patients may or may not have specific symptoms to report because periodontal infections are insidious in development.
- Symptoms the patient notices or feels may include bleeding gingiva, sometimes only while brushing, sometimes with drooling at night, or sometimes spontaneously.
- Other possible symptoms the patient may notice are sensitivity to hot and cold, tenderness or discomfort while eating or pain after eating, food retained between the teeth, unpleasant mouth odors, chronic bad taste, or a feeling that the teeth are loose. Most of these are symptoms of advanced disease.

III. CLINICALLY NORMAL

The terms "clinically normal" or "clinically healthy" may be used to designate gingival tissue that is characterized by the following:

- A shade of pale or coral pink varied by complexion and pigmentation.
- A knife-edged gingival margin that adapts closely around the tooth.
- Stippling, firmness, and minimal sulcus depth with no bleeding when probed.

Although "normal" varies with anatomic, physiologic, and other factors, general characteristics form a baseline for a contrast in the recognition of inflammation.

IV. CAUSES OF TISSUE CHANGES

- Disease changes produce alterations in color, size, position, shape, consistency, surface texture, bleeding readiness, and exudate production.
- To understand the changes that take place in the gingival tissues during the transition from health to disease, first understand inflammation and then what dental biofilm is, the role of biofilm microorganisms in the development of disease, and the inflammatory response by the body.
- When the products of the biofilm microorganisms cause breakdown of the intercellular substances of the sulcular epithelium, injurious agents can pass into the connective tissue, where an inflammatory response is initiated.
- An inflammatory response means that there is increased blood flow, increased permeability of capillaries, and increased collection of defense cells and tissue fluid.
- The changes produce the tissue alterations, such as in color, size, shape, and consistency, that are described in the next section.

V. DESCRIPTIVE TERMINOLOGY

The degree of severity and distribution of a change can be noted when examining the gingiva. When a deviation from normal affects a single area, it can be designated by the number of the adjacent tooth and the surface of the tissue involved, namely, facial, lingual, mesial, or distal.

A. Severity

Severity is expressed as slight, moderate, or severe.

B. Distribution

Terms used for describing distribution are as follows:

1. *Localized:* The gingiva is involved about a single tooth or a specific group of teeth.

2. *Generalized:* The gingiva is involved about all or nearly all of the teeth throughout the mouth. A condition may also be generalized throughout a single arch, the maxillary or mandibular.
3. *Marginal:* A change that is confined to the free or marginal gingiva. This is specified as either localized or generalized.
4. *Papillary:* A change that involves a papilla but not the rest of the free gingiva around a tooth. A papillary change may be localized or generalized.
5. *Diffuse:* Spread out, dispersed; affects gingival margin, attached gingiva, and interdental papillae; may extend into alveolar mucosa. A diffuse condition is more frequently localized, rarely generalized.

VI. EARLY RECOGNITION OF TISSUE CHANGES

1. Marked changes, such as moderate to severe generalized redness, enlargement, sponginess, deep pockets, and definite mobility, are relatively easy to detect even with limited experience, provided there is good light and accessibility for vision.
2. In contrast, when changes are subtle, localized about one or a few teeth, and of a lesser degree of severity, more skillful application of knowledge is needed.
3. *Early recognition and treatment* of gingival and periodontal infections prevents:
   ■ Neglect of conditions that can develop into severe disease.
   ■ Treatment can be less complicated.
   ■ The success of treatment and recovery to healthy tissue is predictable when early recognition makes early treatment possible.

THE GINGIVAL DESCRIPTION

The examination of the gingiva includes evaluation of color, size, shape, consistency, surface texture, position, mucogingival junctions, bleeding, and exudate. These are summarized in **Table 14-1**, which is a clinical reference chart.

I. COLOR

A. Signs of Health

■ *Pale pink.* Darker in people with darker complexions.
■ *Factors influencing color*
  ■ Vascular supply.
  ■ Thickness of epithelium.
  ■ Degree of keratinization.
  ■ Physiologic pigmentation: melanin pigmentation occurs frequently in African Americans, Asians, Indians, and Caucasians of Mediterranean countries.

B. Changes in Disease

1. *In chronic inflammation:* dark red, bluish red, magenta, or deep blue.

2. *In acute inflammation:* bright red.
3. *Extent:* deep involvement can be expected when diffuse color changes extend into the attached gingiva, or from the marginal gingiva to the mucogingival junction, or through into alveolar mucosa.

II. SIZE

A. Signs of Health

1. *Free gingiva:* flat, not enlarged; fits snugly around the tooth.
2. *Attached gingiva*
   ■ Width of attached gingiva varies among patients and among teeth for an individual, from 1 to 9 mm.[5]
   ■ Wider in maxilla than mandible; broadest zone related to incisors, narrowest at the canine and premolar regions.

B. Changes in Disease

1. *Free gingiva and papillae:*
   ■ Become enlarged.
   ■ May be localized or limited to specific areas or generalized throughout the gingiva.
   ■ The col deepens as the papillae increase in size.
2. *Attached gingiva:* decreases in amount as the pocket deepens.

C. Enlargement From Drug Therapy

1. Certain drugs used for specific systemic therapy cause gingival enlargement as a side effect.
2. Examples of such drugs are phenytoin, cyclosporine, and nifedipine.

III. SHAPE (FORM OR CONTOUR)

A. Signs of Health

1. *Free gingiva*
   ■ Follows a curved line around each tooth; may be straighter along wide molar surfaces.
   ■ The margin is knife-edged or slightly rounded on facial and lingual gingiva; closely adapted to the tooth surface.
2. *Papillae*
   ■ Teeth with contact area. Facial and lingual gingiva are pointed or slightly rounded papillae with a col area under the contact (**Figure 14-8**).
   ■ Spaced teeth (with diastemata). Interdental gingiva is flat or saddle shaped.

B. Changes in Disease

1. *Free gingiva:* rounded or rolled.
2. *Papillae:* blunted, flattened, bulbous, cratered (**Figure 14-10**).

	TABLE 14-1	**EXAMINATION OF THE GINGIVAL CLINICAL MARKERS**	

	APPEARANCE IN HEALTH	CHANGES IN DISEASE CLINICAL APPEARANCE	CAUSES FOR CHANGES
Color	Uniformly pale pink or coral pink Variations in pigmentation related to complexion, race	Acute: bright red Chronic: bluish pink, bluish red Attached gingiva: color change may extend to the mucogingival line	Inflammation Capillary dilation Increased blood flow Vessels engorged Blood flow sluggish Venous return impaired Anoxemia Increased fibrosis Deepening of pocket, mucogingival involvement
Size	Not enlarged Fits snugly around the tooth	Enlarged	Edematous: inflammatory fluid, cellular exudate, vascular engorgement, hemorrhage Fibrotic: new collagen fibers
Shape (contour)	Marginal gingiva: knife-edged, flat, follows a curved line about the tooth Papillae: (1) normal contact: papilla is pointed and pyramidal; fills the interproximal area (2) space (diastema) between teeth; gingiva is flat or saddle shaped	Marginal gingiva: rounded rolled Papillae: bulbous flattened blunted cratered	Inflammatory changes: edematous or fibrous Bulbous with gingival enlargement (see edematous and fibrotic, above) Cratered in necrotizing ulcerative gingivitis
Consistency	Firm Attached gingiva firmly bound down	Soft, spongy: dents readily when pressed with probe Associated with red color, smooth shiny surface, loss of stippling, bleeding on probing Firm, hard: resists probe pressure Associated with pink color, stippling, bleeding only in depth of pocket	Edematous: fluid between cells in connective tissue Fibrotic: collagen fibers
Surface Texture	Free gingiva: smooth Attached gingiva: stippled	Acute condition: smooth, shiny gingiva Chronic: hard, firm, with stippling, sometimes heavier than normal	Inflammatory changes in the connective tissue; edema, cellular infiltration Fibrosis
Position of Gingival Margin	Fully erupted tooth: margin is 1–2 mm above cementoenamel junction, at or slightly below the enamel contour	Enlarged gingiva: margin is higher on the tooth, above normal, pocket deepened Recession: margin is more apical; root surface is exposed	Edematous or fibrotic Junctional epithelium has migrated along the root; gingival margin follows
Position of Junctional Epithelium	During eruption along the enamel surface **(Figure 14-7)** Fully erupted tooth: the junctional epithelium is at the cementoenamel junction	Position determined by use of probe, is on the root surface	Apical migration of the epithelium along the root

(*continued*)

TABLE 14-1	EXAMINATION OF THE GINGIVAL CLINICAL MARKERS (*Continued*)		
	APPEARANCE IN HEALTH	**CHANGES IN DISEASE CLINICAL APPEARANCE**	**CAUSES FOR CHANGES**
Mucogingival Junctions	Make clear demarcation between the pink, stippled, attached gingiva and the darker alveolar mucosa with smooth shiny surface	No attached gingiva: (1) Color changes may extend full height of the gingiva; mucogingival line obliterated (2) Probing reveals that the bottom of the pocket extends into the alveolar mucosa (3) Frenal pull may displace the gingival margin from the tooth	Apical migration of the junctional epithelium Attached gingiva decreases with pocket deepening Inflammation extends into alveolar mucosa
Bleeding	No spontaneous bleeding or upon probing	Spontaneous bleeding Bleeding on probing: bleeding near margin in acute condition; bleeding deep in pocket in chronic condition	Degeneration of the sulcular epithelium with the formation of pocket epithelium Blood vessels engorged Tissue edematous
Exudate	No exudate expressed on pressure	White fluid, pus, visible on digital pressure Amount not related to pocket depth	Inflammation in the connective tissue Excessive accumulation of white blood cells with serum and tissue makes up the exudate (pus)

3. *Festoon* ("*McCall's festoon*"): an enlargement of the marginal gingiva with the formation of a lifesaver-like gingival prominence. Frequently, the total gingiva is very narrow, with associated apparent recession, as shown in **Figure 14-10D**.
4. *Clefts*
   - "Stillman's cleft" **(Figure 14-11)**: A localized recession may be V-shaped, apostrophe-shaped, or form a slitlike indentation. It may extend several millimeters toward the mucogingival junction or even to or through the junction.
   - Floss cleft: A cleft created by incorrect floss positioning appears as a vertical linear or V-shaped fissure in the marginal gingiva.[6]
   - Usually occurs at one side of an interdental papilla.
   - The injury can develop when dental floss is curved repeatedly in an incomplete "C" around the line angle so the floss is pressed across the gingiva.

IV. CONSISTENCY

A. Signs of Health

1. Firm when palpated with the side of a blunt instrument (probe).
2. Attached gingiva is bound down firmly to the underlying bone.

B. Changes in Disease

1. *To determine consistency:* Gently press side of probe on free gingiva. Soft, spongy gingiva dents readily; firm, hard tissue resists.
2. *Soft, spongy gingiva:* Related to acute stages of inflammation with increased infiltration of fluid and inflammatory elements.
   - The tissue appears red, may be smooth and shiny with loss of stippling.
   - Has marginal enlargement, and bleeds readily on probing.
3. *Firm, hard gingiva:* Related to chronic inflammation with increased fibrosis.
   - The tissue may appear pink and well stippled.
   - Bleeding, when probed, usually occurs only in the deeper part of a pocket, not near the margin.
4. *Retraction of the margin away from the tooth:* Normally, the free gingiva fits snugly about the tooth.
   - When the margin tends to hang slightly away or is readily displaced with a light air blast.
   - The gingival fibers that support the margin have been destroyed **(Figure 14-3)**.

V. SURFACE TEXTURE

A. Signs of Health

1. *Free gingiva:* smooth

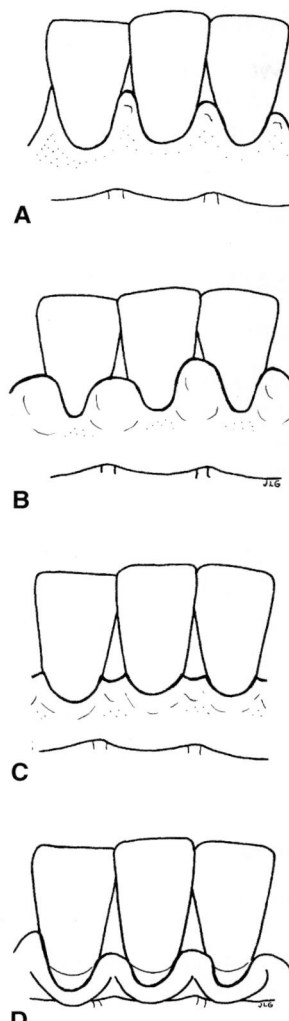

FIGURE 14-10 Gingival Shape or Contour. (A) Blunted papillae. **(B)** Bulbous papillae. **(C)** Cratered papillae. **(D)** Rolled, lifesaver-shaped "McCall's festoons."

2. *Attached gingiva:* stippled (minutely "pebbled" or "orange peel" surface).
3. *Interdental gingiva:* The free gingiva is smooth; the center portion of each papilla is stippled.

B. Changes in Disease

1. *Inflammatory changes:* may be loss of stippling, with smooth, shiny surface.
2. *Hyperkeratosis:* may result in a leathery, hard, or nodular surface.
3. *Chronic disease:* tissue may be hard and fibrotic, with a normal pink color and normal or deep stippling.

VI. POSITION

1. The *actual* position of the gingiva is the level of the attached periodontal tissue. It is not directly visible but can be determined by probing.

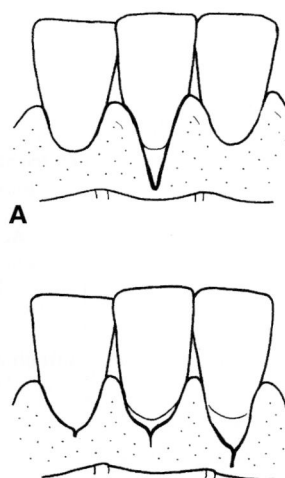

FIGURE 14-11 Gingival Clefts. (A) V-shaped Stillman's cleft. **(B)** Slitlike Stillman's clefts of varying degrees of severity in relation to the mucogingival junction.

2. The *apparent* position of the gingiva is the level of the gingival margin or crest of the free gingiva that is seen by direct observation.

A. Signs of Health

For the fully erupted tooth in an adult, the apparent position of the gingival margin is normally at the level of, or slightly below, the enamel contour or prominence of the cervical third of a tooth.

B. Changes in Disease

1. *Effect of gingival enlargement:* When the gingiva enlarges, the gingival margin may be high on the enamel, partly or nearly covering the anatomic crown.
2. *Effect of gingival recession*
   - Definition: Recession is the exposure of root surface that results from the apical migration of the junctional epithelium **(Figure 14-12)**.
   - Actual recession: The actual recession is shown by the position of the attachment level. The "receded area" is from the cementoenamel junction to the attachment.
   - Visible recession: The visible recession is the exposed root surface that is visible on clinical examination. It is seen from the gingival margin to the cementoenamel junction.
   - Localized recession **(Figure 14-13)**: A localized recession may be narrow or wide, deep or shallow. The root surface is denuded, and the visible recession may extend to or through the mucogingival junction.
   - Measurement: Both actual and visible recession can be measured with a probe from the cementoenamel junction. Total recession is the actual and visible positions added together.

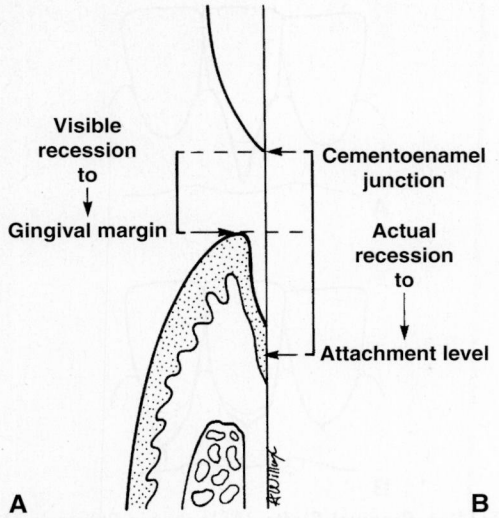

FIGURE 14-12 **Gingival Recession.** (**A**) Clinically visible recession of the gingival margin with root surface apparent to the eye. (**B**) The actual recession exposes the root surface as the periodontal attachment migrates along the root surface.

VII. BLEEDING

A. Signs of Health

1. No bleeding spontaneously or on probing.
2. Healthy tissue does not bleed.

B. Changes in Disease

1. Bleeding occurs spontaneously or when probed.
2. Sulcular epithelium becomes diseased *pocket epithelium.* The ulcerated pocket wall bleeds readily on gentle probing.

VIII. EXUDATE

A. Signs of Health

There is no exudate except slight gingival sulcus fluid. Gingival sulcus fluid cannot be seen by direct observation.

B. Changes in Disease

1. Increased gingival sulcus fluid.
2. Amount of exudate is not an indicator of the extent of disease or the depth of the periodontal pockets.

THE GINGIVA OF YOUNG CHILDREN[7,8]

I. SIGNS OF HEALTH

A. Primary Dentition

1. *Color:* pink or slightly red
2. *Shape:* thick, rounded, or rolled
3. *Consistency:* less fibrous than adult gingiva; not tightly adapted to the teeth; may be easily displaced with a light air jet
4. *Surface texture:* may or may not have stippling; high percentage of patients has shiny gingiva
5. *Attached gingiva:* width of attached gingiva in children aged 3 to 5 years: between 1 and 6 mm.[5]
6. *Interdental gingiva*
   - Anterior: diastemata are frequently present and the papillae are flat or saddle shaped
   - Posterior: col between facial and lingual papillae when teeth are in contact (**Figure 14-8**)

B. Mixed Dentition

1. Constant state of change related to exfoliation and eruption.
2. Free gingiva may appear rolled or rounded, slightly reddened, shiny, and with a lack of firmness.
3. The gingiva covers a varying portion of the anatomic crown, depending on the stage of eruption (**Figure 14-7**).

II. CHANGES IN DISEASE

A. Examination of the periodontal tissues of a child is not different from that of an adult. A complete examination is necessary, including probing around each tooth.

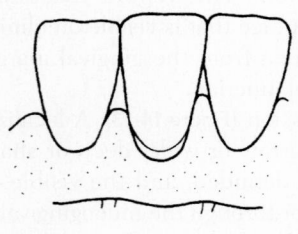
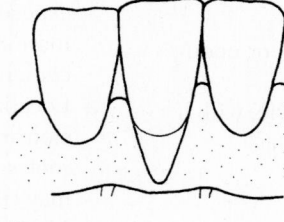
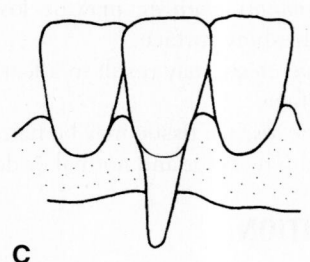

FIGURE 14-13 **Localized Recession.** A single tooth may show narrow or wide, deep or shallow recession. (**A**) Wide, shallow. (**B**) Wide, deep, with narrow attached gingiva. (**C**) Narrow, deep, with missing attached gingiva.

B. Gingivitis occurs frequently in children but is usually reversible without leaving permanent damage.

C. Although relatively rare, periodontitis can occur in primary dentition.

D. Mucogingival problems occur in children.[9,10] The recognition of deficiencies of attached gingiva has particular significance for the child who will need orthodontic treatment.

THE GINGIVA AFTER PERIODONTAL SURGERY

- The characteristics of "normal healthy gingiva" take on different dimensions for the patient who has completed treatment for pockets, bone loss, and other signs of a periodontal infection.
- The junctional epithelium may be apical to the cementoenamel junction.
- After healing, the sulcus depths may be within normal range and no bleeding occurs when probed.
- Depending on the exact treatment performed, examination shows changes from the initial evaluation. For example, where the initial examination showed a deficiency of attached gingiva with frenal pull, mucogingival surgery may have been designed and treatment satisfactorily completed to create new attached gingiva.
- With each maintenance appointment, a thorough, careful examination is necessary to control factors that may permit recurrence of disease.

DOCUMENTATION

The permanent records of a patient who had treatment for a gingival or periodontal condition would have a minimum of the following:

BOX 14-2	Example Progress Note

Patient returned for second quadrant of Scal/Planing. Biofilm poorly removed; said she did get her new electric toothbrush but hadn't had time to open it but would definitely do that this week. I asked her to bring it next appointment so we could go over it together. Said she doubted if she would ever find time to use floss because it took so long. Dr. Roe came and gave anesthesia; scaled maxillary right quad. I believe we can win her over.

Signed: _____, RDH Date: _____.

- Health history with routine follow-up recorded for each visitation.
- Initial charting and descriptive material to show disease symptoms with information to show need for and actual treatment carried out by a series of progress notes defining each appointment with changes identified resulting from specific treatment.
- Individual instruction with biofilm scores from disclosing agent applications. Any personal care products recommended, their demonstration and report of use by the patient. Record of improvements in gingival health noted over the series of appointments.
- Patient's own comments of health change, habits changed, dietary changes, all successes, along with an agreement to a recommended plan for a maintenance program.
- A progress note of an individual patient appointment may be read in **Box 14-2**.

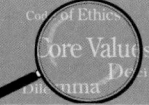

Everyday Ethics

Britain and Nicholas were first-year dental hygiene students just beginning to practice on each other as student partners in the preclinic program. Today their clinical practice was to provide the description of the gingiva; the next session would be learning to use the probe for the pocket/sulcus examination. Nicholas told her his "gums bled when he brushed." As she began, the gingiva seemed soft and loose, but Britain was not sure she understood what is "normal" when she remembered that her instructor had referred to a "range" of normal.

Britain decided to focus on and document the areas that looked pink, and pointed in the interproximal areas. She carefully recorded this information with great detail and then signaled for her instructor to verify the findings. When the instructor reviewed the examination she was pleased with Britain's thoroughness. The instructor provided positive feedback and quickly moved on to the next pair of students. Britain

began to feel uneasy that she hadn't pointed out the gingival tissues that she thought were possibly inflamed.

Questions for Consideration

1. Which of the core values (Table II-1, page 38) have application in this scenario? How and why?

2. Indicate how Nicholas is the center of this dilemma from both the perspective of Britain, a student, and the clinical instructor who finds out from another faculty member who had worked with Britain and Nicholas at an earlier clinical practice session for study cast impressions, that she thinks Nicholas has definite signs of periodontal disease and could use advise about the care he needs.

3. Ethically, what alternatives or actions can Britain take at this time to address the "uneasy" feeling she has about Nicholas' gingival status?

Factors To Teach The Patient

- Characteristics of normal healthy gingiva.
- The significance of bleeding; healthy tissue does not bleed.
- Relationship of findings during a gingival examination to the personal daily care procedures for infection control.
- The special attention needed for an area of gingival recession to prevent abrasion, inflammation, and further involvement.
- How the method of brushing, stiffness of toothbrush filaments, abrasiveness of a dentifrice, and pressure applied during brushing can be factors in gingival recession.

References

1. Avery JK, Steele PF. *Essentials of oral histology and embryology: a clinical approach.* St. Louis: Mosby; 1992. Chapter 9, Dental pulp; pp. 131–4.
2. Ainamo J, Löe H. Anatomical characteristics of gingiva: a clinical and microscopic study of the free and attached gingiva. *J Periodontol.* 1966 Jan–Feb;37(1):5–13.
3. Orban B. Clinical and histologic study of the surface characteristics of the gingiva. *Oral Surg Oral Med Oral Pathol.* 1948 Sep;1(9):827–41.
4. Bhaskar SN, editor. Orban's oral histology and embryology. 11th ed. St. Louis: Mosby; 1991. pp. 323–5.
5. Bowers GM. A study of the width of attached gingiva. *J Periodontol.* 1963 May;34:201–9.
6. Hallman WW, Waldrop TC, Houston GD, Hawkins BF. Flossing clefts: clinical and histologic observations. *J Periodontol.* 1986 Aug;57(8):501–4.
7. Duperon D, Takei HH. Gingival diseases in childhood. In: Newman MG, Takei HH, Klokkevold PR, Carranza FA. *Carranza's clinical periodontics.* 10th ed. St Louis: Saunders; 2006. pp. 404–10.
8. Pinkham JR, editor. Pediatric dentistry: infancy through adolescence. 2nd ed. Philadelphia: Saunders; 1994. Casamassimo PS. Periodontal conditions. pp. 353–7, 607–15.
9. Maynard JG Jr, Ochsenbein C. Mucogingival problems, prevalence and therapy in children. *J Periodontol.* 1975 Sep;46(9):543–52.
10. Andlin-Sobocki A, Marcusson A, Persson M. 3-year observations on gingival recession in mandibular incisors in children. *J Clin Periodontol.* 1991 Mar;18(3):155–9.

CHAPTER 15

Periodontal Examination

ESTHER M. WILKINS, BS, RDH, DMD

Chapter Outline

BOX 15-1	Key Words

Instruments of Examination

Calibration: determination of the accuracy of an instrument by measurement of its variation from a standard (calibration between examiners).

Clinical attachment level: probing depth as measured from the cementoenamel junction (or other fixed point) to the location of the probe tip at the coronal level of attached periodontal tissues.

Explorer: a slender stainless steel instrument with a fine flexible, sharp point used for examination of the surfaces of the teeth to detect irregularities.

Fremitus: a vibration perceptible by palpation.

Periodontometer: instrument used to measure mobility.

Probe: smooth, slender instrument usually round in diameter with a rounded tip designed for examination of the teeth and soft tissues; except for a few probes made only for blunt examination, probes are calibrated in millimeter increments to facilitate recordings for comparison with periodic assessments.

Probing depth: the distance from the gingival margin to the location of the periodontal probe tip at the coronal border of attached periodontal tissues.

Tactile: pertaining to the touch.

Tactile discrimination: the ability to distinguish relative degrees of roughness and smoothness, for example, on a tooth surface, using an explorer or a periodontal probe; also called tactile sensitivity.

Tension test: application of tension at the mucogingival junction by retracting cheek, lip, and tongue to tighten the alveolar mucosa and test for the presence of attached gingiva; area of missing attached gingiva is revealed when the alveolar mucosa and frena are connected directly to the free gingiva.

Parts of the gingival and dental clinical examinations are made by direct visual observation, whereas other parts require *tactile* examination using a probe and/or an explorer. These two types of instruments, assisted by a mouth mirror, are key instruments in patient examination and assessment. Considerable skill is required for accurate and efficient probing and exploring.

General principles of instrumentation are described on pages 594 to 596. **Box 15-1** contains definitions for key words associated with this chapter.

I. PRECAUTION

- A probe or an explorer is not applied to the teeth and gingiva until an initial review of information from the patient history has been made.
- Of particular significance is knowledge of a patient's susceptibility to the effects of bacteremia.
- Patients at risk must receive prophylactic antibiotic premedication before instrumentation.

II. BASIC SETUP

Tray arrangements for all patients with permanent teeth need a basic setup composed of at least a mouth mirror, probes to include a furcation probe, and explorers to include a subgingival explorer.

THE MOUTH MIRROR

I. DESCRIPTION

A. Parts

The mirror has three parts: the handle, shank, and working end, which is the mounted mirror or mirror head.

B. Types of Mirror Surfaces

- *Plane (flat):* may produce a double image.
- *Concave:* magnifying.
- *Front surface:* The reflecting surface is on the front of the lens rather than on the back as with plane or magnifying mirrors. The front surface eliminates "ghost" images.

C. Diameters

- Mirror diameters vary from 5/8 to 1 1/4 inches. In addition, special examination mirrors are available in 1½- to 2-inch diameters.

D. Attachments

- Mirrors may be threaded plain stem or cone socket to be joined to a handle.
- Because mirrors tend to become scratched, replacement of the working end is possible without purchasing new handles.

E. Handles

- Thicker handles contribute to a more ergonomically comfortable grasp and greater control.
- Light weight provides decreased fatigue.

F. Disposable Mirrors

- Plastic mirrors can be useful for screening or other short examination procedures.
- Take-home mirrors for patient instruction. Patient may observe lingual and posterior aspects where biofilm may be difficult to remove.

II. PURPOSES AND USES

A mouth mirror is used to provide indirect vision, indirect illumination, transillumination, and retraction.

A. Indirect Vision

- Needed for all surfaces where direct vision is not possible.
- Examples are the distal surfaces of posterior teeth and lingual surfaces of anterior teeth.

B. Indirect Illumination

- Reflection of light from the dental overhead light or headlight worn by the clinician to any area of the oral cavity can be accomplished by adapting the mirror.

C. Transillumination

- Transillumination refers to reflection of light through the teeth.
- Mirror is held to reflect light from the lingual aspect while the teeth are examined from the facial.
- Mirror is held for indirect vision on the lingual while light from the overhead dental light passes through the teeth. Translucency of enamel can be seen clearly, whereas dental caries or calculus deposits appear opaque.

D. Retraction

The mirror is used to protect or prevent interference by the cheeks, tongue, or lips.

III. PROCEDURE FOR USE

A. Grasp and Rest

Use modified pen grasp with finger rest on a tooth surface wherever possible:

- To provide stability and control.
- To assist in retraction of lips and cheek.
- Exercises for gaining skill in control of instruments are described on page 625.

B. Retraction

- Use a water-based lubricant on dry or cracked lips and corners of mouth.
- Adjust the mirror position so that the angles of the mouth are protected from undue pressure of the shank of the mirror.
- Insert and remove mirror carefully to avoid hitting the teeth because this can be very disturbing to the patient.

C. Maintain Clear Vision

- Warm mirror with water; rub along buccal mucosa to coat mirror with thin transparent film of saliva, and request patient to breathe through the nose to prevent condensation of moisture on the mirror. Use a detergent or other means for keeping a clear surface.
- Discard scratched mirrors.

IV. CARE OF MIRRORS

- Dismantle mirror and handle for sterilization.
- Examine carefully after ultrasonic cleaning before sterilization to ensure removal of debris around back, shank, and rim of reflecting surface.
- Handle carefully during sterilization procedures to prevent other instruments from scratching the reflecting surface.
- Consult manufacturer's specifications for sterilizing or disinfecting procedures that may cloud the mirror, particularly the front surface type.

APPLICATION OF AIR

I. PURPOSES AND USES

With appropriate, timely application of air to clear saliva and debris and/or dry the tooth surfaces, the following can be accomplished:

A. Improve and Facilitate Examination Procedures

- Make a thorough, more accurate examination.
- Dry supragingival calculus to facilitate exploring and scaling. Small deposits may be light in color and not visible until they are dried. Dried calculus appears chalky and presents a contrast to tooth color.
- Deflect the free gingival margin for observation into the subgingival area. Subgingival calculus usually appears darker than supragingival.
- Make identification of areas of demineralization and carious lesions easier.
- Recognize location and condition of restorations, particularly tooth-color restorations.

B. Improve Visibility of the Treatment Area During Instrumentation

- Dry area for finger rest to provide stability during instrumentation.
- Facilitate positive scaling techniques.
- Minimize appointment time.
- Evaluate complete removal of supragingival calculus after instrumentation.

C. Prepare Teeth and/or Gingiva for Certain Procedures

Examples are to dry surfaces for:
- Application of caries-preventive agents when indicated.
- Make impression for study cast.
- Apply topical anesthetic.

II. COMPRESSED AIR SYRINGE

A. Description

1. *Air Source.* Air compressor with tubing attachment to syringe.
2. *Air Tip.* Has angled working end that can be turned for maxillary or mandibular application. Tip may be disposable or removable for sterilization.

B. Procedure for Use

1. Use palm grasp about the handle of the syringe; place thumb on release lever or on button on handle.
2. Test the air flow so that the strength of flow can be controlled.
3. Make controlled, relatively short, gentle applications of air.
4. Supplement air drying with use of saliva ejector and folded gauze sponge placed in vestibule.

C. Precautions

- Avoid sharp blasts of air on sensitive cervical areas of teeth or open carious lesions. Such areas may be dried by blotting with a gauze sponge or cotton roll to avoid patient discomfort.
- Avoid applying air directly into a pocket. Subgingival biofilm may be forced into the tissues and may create a bacteremia.
- Avoid forceful application of air, which can direct saliva and debris out of the oral cavity, contaminate the working area and clinician, and create aerosols. Air directed toward the posterior region of the patient's mouth may cause coughing.
- Avoid startling the patient; forewarn when air is to be applied.

PROBE

- Early in the patient examination, the patient's periodontal disease status is determined. The probe determinations provide major information for determining disease status of the periodontal tissues.
- Treatment planning varies depending on whether the condition is gingivitis, which may be reversible, or periodontitis with periodontal pockets, bone loss, and root surface involvement, which require more extensive therapy.

I. TYPES OF PROBES

- Two general types of probes available are the traditional or standard manual probes and the controlled force or automated probes.

- Automated probes were developed and researched in an attempt to overcome the problems in obtaining consistent readings with traditional probes.

II. PURPOSES AND USES

A probe is used for the following purposes:

A. Assess the Periodontal Status for Preparation of a Treatment Plan

- Classify the disease as gingivitis or periodontitis by determining whether bone loss has occurred and whether the pockets are gingival or periodontal. A systematic screening method can be used (PSR, in Chapter 22, page 321).
- Determine the extent of inflammation in conjunction with the overall gingival examination. Bleeding on probing is an early sign of inflammation in the gingiva.

B. Make a Sulcus and Pocket Survey

- Examine the shape, topography, and dimensions of sulci and pockets.
- Measure and record probing depths.
- Evaluate tooth-surface pocket wall.
- Chart calculus location and severity.
- Record other root surface irregularities discerned by the probe.

C. Determine Clinical Attachment Level (Clinical attachment level is described on page 231 and illustrated in Figure 15-8.)

D. Make a Mucogingival Examination

- Determine relationship of gingival margin, attachment level, mucogingival junction, and frena.
- Measure the width of the attached gingiva (**Figure 15-11**).

E. Make Other Gingival Determinations

- Evaluate gingival bleeding on probing and prepare a gingival bleeding index.
- Measure the extent of visible gingival recession.
- Determine the consistency of the gingival tissue.

F. Guide Treatment

- Summarize gingival characteristics, including probing depth, bleeding, and consistency (all determined using a probe), to provide a basis for patient instruction as part of the total treatment.
- Define probing depth of sulcus or pocket for application of instruments for scaling, root planing and maintenance debridement, and define depth for use of an explorer for evaluation of these procedures.
- Detect anatomic configuration of roots, subgingival deposits, and root irregularities that complicate instrumentation. For this, the probe is used in conjunction with the explorer.

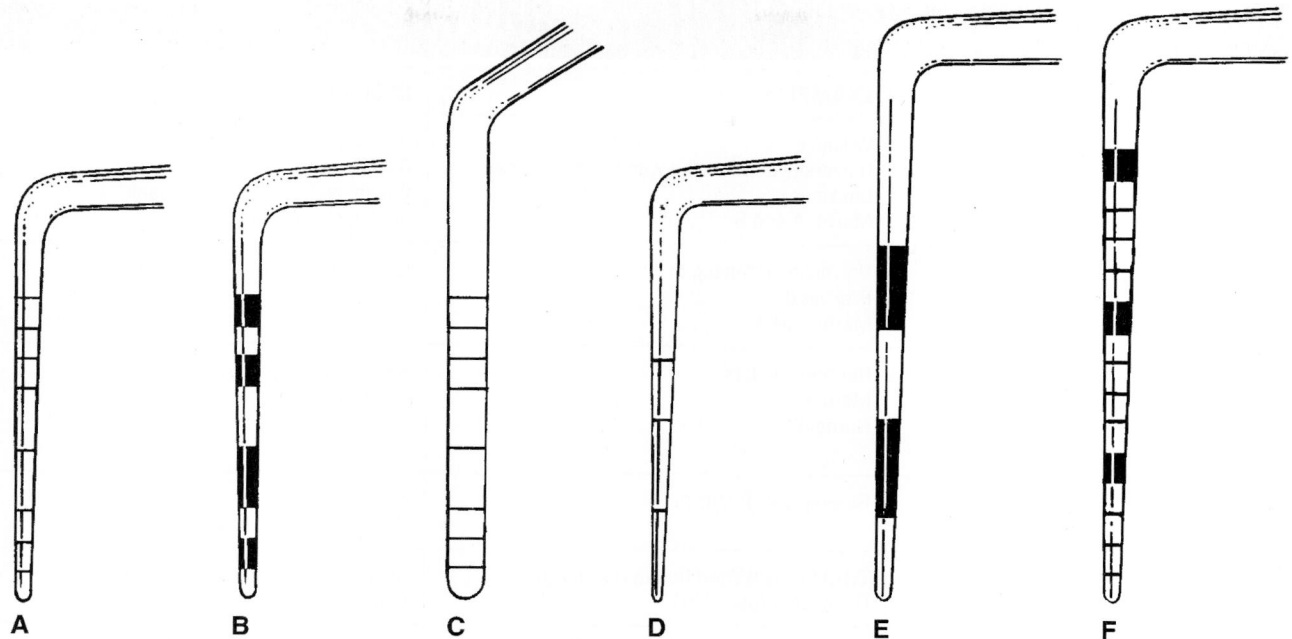

FIGURE 15-1 **Examples of Probes.** Names and calibrated markings shown are (**A**) Williams (1-1-1-2-2-1-1-1), (**B**) Williams, color-coded, (**C**) Goldman-Fox (1-1-1-2-2-1-1-1), (**D**) Michigan O (3-3-2), (**E**) Hu-Friedy or Marquis Color-coded (3-3-3-3 or 3-3-2-3), and (**F**) Hu-Friedy PCPUNC 15 (each millimeter to 15), color coded at 5-10-15. See Table 15-1 for additional data on probes.

G. Evaluate Success and Completeness of Treatment

- Evaluate posttreatment tissue response to professional treatment on an immediate, short-term basis, as well as at periodic maintenance examinations.
- Evaluate patient's self-treatment through therapeutic disease control procedures.
- Identify signs of continued health revealed by the probing effects of the following:
  - No bleeding; healthy tissue does not bleed.
  - Reduced probing depth; comparison of pretreatment and posttreatment probing depth.
  - Tissue is firm, as shown by application of the probe to the surface of the free gingiva.

H. Evaluation at Maintenance Appointments

- At each maintenance appointment, a reevaluation with complete probing is needed
- To ensure continued self-care by the patient.
- To identify early disease changes that require additional professional treatment.

III. DESCRIPTION OF MANUAL PROBES

- A probe is a slender instrument with a smooth, rounded tip designed for examination of the depth and topography of a gingival sulcus or periodontal pocket.
- A probe has three parts: the handle, the angled shank, and the working end, which is the probe itself.

A. Materials

- Stainless steel.
- Plastic: for screenings and titanium implant probing.

B. Characteristics

- *Straight working end*
  - Tapered, round, flat, or rectangular in cross section with a smooth rounded end.
  - Calibrated in millimeters at intervals specific for each kind of probe; some have color coding. **Figure 15-1** shows a comparison of a few typical markings; **Table 15-1** lists probe markings with examples.
- *Curved working end:* Paired furcation probes have a smooth, rounded end for investigation of the topography and anatomy around roots in a furca. Examples are the Nabers 1N and 2N probes **(Figure 15-9B)**.

C. Selection

- The probe chosen for use by a clinician is frequently the instrument first used when a particular technique was learned, or one that provides comfort and ease of manipulation.
- Regular use of the same type of probe results in greater consistency of readings.
- Analysis of a probe and comparison with other probes are recommended. Important features to be considered in probe selection are:

TABLE 15-1	TYPES OF PROBES	
PROBE MARKINGS (mm)	**EXAMPLES**	**DESCRIPTION**
Marks at 1-2-3-5-7-8-9-10	Williams University of Michigan with Williams marks Glickman Merritt A and B	Round, tapered (available with color-code) Round, narrow diameter, fine Round, with longer lower shank Round, single bend to shank
Marks at 3-3-2	University of Michigan 0 Premier 0 Marquis M-1	Round, fine, tapered, narrow diameter

Marks at
   3-6-9-12
   3-6-8-11
   (and other variations)
	Hu-Friedy QULIX
	Marquis
	Nordent
		Round, tapered, fine
		Color-coded

Marks at each mm to 15	Hu-Friedy PCPUNC 15	Round Color-coded at 5-10-15
Marks at 3.5-5.5-8.5-11.5	WHO Probe (World Health Organization) Figure 22-7 (page 321)	Round, tapered, fine, with ball end Color-coded
No marks	Gilmore Nabers 1N, 2N	Tapered, sharper than other probes Curved, with curved shank for furcation examination

- *Adaptability.* The probe needs to be adaptable around the complete circumference of each tooth, both posterior and anterior, so that no millimeter of probing depth can be neglected. Flat probes require more attention to adaptation and are useful primarily on facial and lingual surfaces.
- *Markings.* Markings need to be easy to read so that probing depth can be readily identified and measured, and no disease area is overlooked. Color coding contributes to readability.

- The level of attached tissue assumes a varying position around the tooth.
- The gingival margin varies in its position on the tooth.
- Proximal surfaces are approached by entering from both the facial and lingual aspects of a tooth.
  - Gingival and periodontal infections begin in the col area more frequently than in other areas (col area, Figure 14-8, page 214).

GUIDE TO PROBING

A pocket is a diseased gingival sulcus. The use of a probe is the only accurate, dependable method to locate, assess, and measure sulci and pockets.

I. POCKET CHARACTERISTICS

- A pocket is measured from the base of the pocket (top of attached periodontal tissue) to the gingival margin. **Figure 15-2** shows two probing depths beneath gingival margins that are at the same level.
- The pocket (or sulcus) is continuous around the entire tooth, and the entire pocket or sulcus needs to be measured. "Spot" probing is inadequate for a thorough evaluation for diagnosis for treatment planning.
- The depth varies around an individual tooth; probing depth rarely measures the same all around a tooth or even around one side of a tooth.

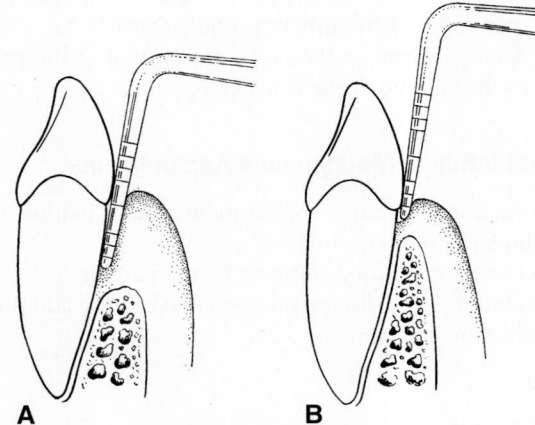

FIGURE 15-2 **Probing Depth.** A pocket is measured from the gingival margin to the attached periodontal tissue. Shown is the contrast of probe measurements with gingival margins at the same level. (**A**) Deep periodontal pocket (7 mm) with apical migration of attachment. (**B**) Shallow pocket (2 mm) with the attachment near the cementoenamel junction.

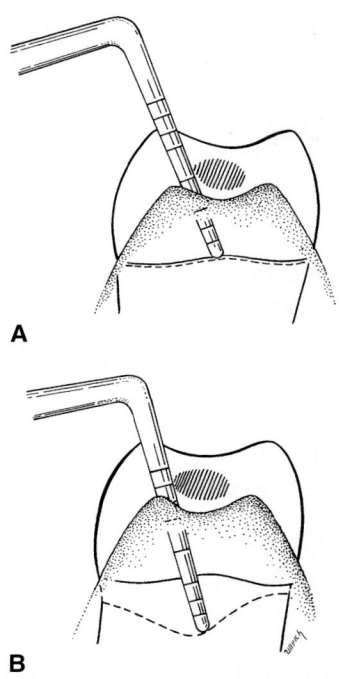

A

B

FIGURE 15-3 **Proximal Surface Probing. (A)** Probe must be applied more than half way across from facial to overlap with probing from the lingual. **(B)** Probe in area of crater formation. Probing is usually deeper on the proximal surface under the contact area than on the facial or lingual surfaces.

- ▨ Probing depth may be deepest directly under the contact area because of crater formation in the alveolar bone **(Figure 15-3)**.
- ■ Anatomic features of the tooth surface wall of the pocket influence the direction of probing. Examples are concave surfaces, anomalies, shape of cervical third, and position of furcations.

II. EVALUATION OF TOOTH SURFACE

- ■ During the movement of the probe, calculus and tooth surface irregularities can be felt and evaluated.
- ■ The information obtained is used to plan the scaling and root planing appointments.

III. FACTORS THAT AFFECT PROBE DETERMINATIONS

- ■ The general objectives of probing are accuracy and consistency so that recordings are dependable for comparison with future probings as well as with colleagues in practice together.
- ■ At the same time, patient discomfort and trauma to the tissues must be minimal.
- ■ Probing is influenced by many factors, such as those described in the following topics.

A. Severity and Extent of Periodontal Disease

- ■ With application of light pressure and a secure finger or hand rest, the probe is inserted under the gingival

margin, held against the tooth as it is passed along the tooth surface to the attached tissue level.
- ■ Diseased tissue offers less resistance, so that with increased severity of inflammation, the probe inserts to a deeper level.[1]
- ■ Average levels show that the probe is stopped as follows:
  - ▨ *Normal healthy tissue:* The probe is at the base of the sulcus or crevice, at the coronal end of the junctional epithelium.
  - ▨ *Gingivitis and early periodontitis:* The probe tip is within the junctional epithelium.
  - ▨ *Advanced periodontitis:* The probe tip passes through the junctional epithelium to reach attached connective tissue fibers.

B. The Probe Itself

- ■ *Calibration:* Must be accurately marked, otherwise readings cannot be accurate.
- ■ *Thickness:* A thinner probe slips through a narrow pocket more readily.
- ■ *Readability:* Aided by the markings and color-coding.

C. Technique Applied

- ■ *Grasp:* Appropriate for maximum tactile sensitivity.
- ■ *Finger rest:* Placed on nonmobile tooth with uniformity.
- ■ *Pressure applied:* Only enough pressure to maintain the probe against the tooth surface wall of the pocket is required. Tactile sensitivity to the texture, deposits, elevations (calculus) or depressions on the tooth surface is needed.

D. Placement Problems

- ■ *Anatomic variations:* tooth contours, furcations, contact areas, anomalies.
- ■ *Interferences:* calculus, irregular margins of restorations, fixed dental prostheses.
- ■ *Accessibility, visibility:* obstructed by tissue bleeding, limited opening by patient, macroglossia.

PROBING PROCEDURES

I. PROBE INSERTION

- ■ Grasp probe with modified pen grasp.
- ■ Establish finger rest on a neighboring tooth, preferably in the same dental arch.
- ■ Hold side of instrument tip flat against the tooth near the gingival margin. The cervical third of a primary tooth is more convex **(Figure 15-4)**.
- ■ Gently slide the tip under the gingival margin.
  - ▨ *Healthy or firm fibrotic tissue:* Insertion is more difficult because of the close adaptation of the tissue to the tooth surface; underlying gingival fibers are strong and tight.

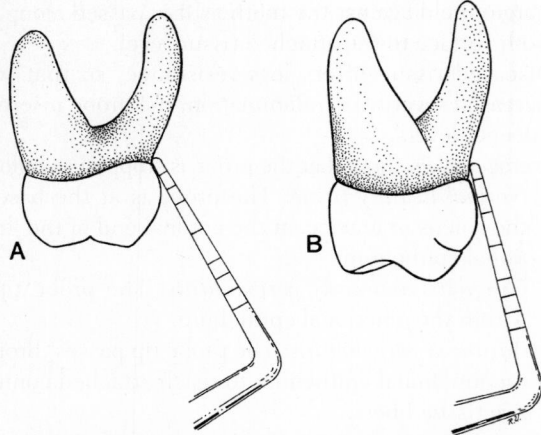

FIGURE 15-4 **Primary and Permanent Maxillary Molars. (A)** Accentuated convexity of the cervical third and widespread roots of the primary molar complicate probe placement. Probe may encounter the root. **(B)** Permanent tooth with less convexity of the cervical third and roots that are less widely spread.

- *Spongy, soft tissue:* Gingival margin is loose and flabby because of the destruction of underlying gingival fibers. Probe inserts readily, and bleeding can be expected on gentle probing.

II. ADVANCE PROBE TO BASE OF POCKET

- Hold side of probe tip flat against the tooth surface; probe is parallel with long axis of the tooth for vertical insertion. Widespread roots of primary molars may make this probe position difficult unless the tissue is unduly distended by the probe **(Figure 15-4)**.
- Slide the probe along the tooth surface vertically down to the base of the sulcus or pocket.
  - Maintain contact of the side of the tip of the probe with the tooth.
  - Gingival pocket: Side of probe is on enamel.
  - Periodontal pocket: Side of probe is on the cemental or dentinal surface when inserted to a level below the cementoenamel junction.

- As the probe is passed down the side of the tooth, roughness may be felt (calculus?). Evaluation of the topography and nature of the tooth surface is essential to instrumentation.
- When obstruction by a hard bulky calculus deposit is encountered, lift the probe away from the tooth and follow over the edge of the calculus until the probe can move vertically into the pocket again.
- The base of the sulcus or pocket feels soft and elastic (compared with the hard tooth surface and calculus deposits), and with slight pressure, the tension of the attached periodontal tissue at the base of the pocket can be felt.
- Use only the pressure needed to detect by tactile means the level of the attached tissue, whether junctional epithelium or deep connective tissue fibers. A light pressure of 10 g, or of no more than 20 g, is ample.
- Position the probe for reading.
  - Bring the probe to position as nearly parallel with the long axis of the tooth as possible for reading the depth.
  - Interference of the contact area does not permit placing the probe parallel for the measurement directly beneath the contact area. Hold the side of the shank of the probe against the contact to minimize the angle **(Figure 15-3)**.

III. READ THE PROBE

- Measurement for a probing depth is made from the gingival margin to the attached periodontal tissue.
- Count the millimeters that show on the probe above the gingival margin and subtract the number from the total number of millimeters marked on the particular probe being used. A comparison of pocket measurement using probes with different calibrations is shown in **Figure 15-5**.
- When the gingival margin appears at a level between probe marks, use the higher mark for the final reading.
- Dry the area being probed to improve visibility for specific reading.

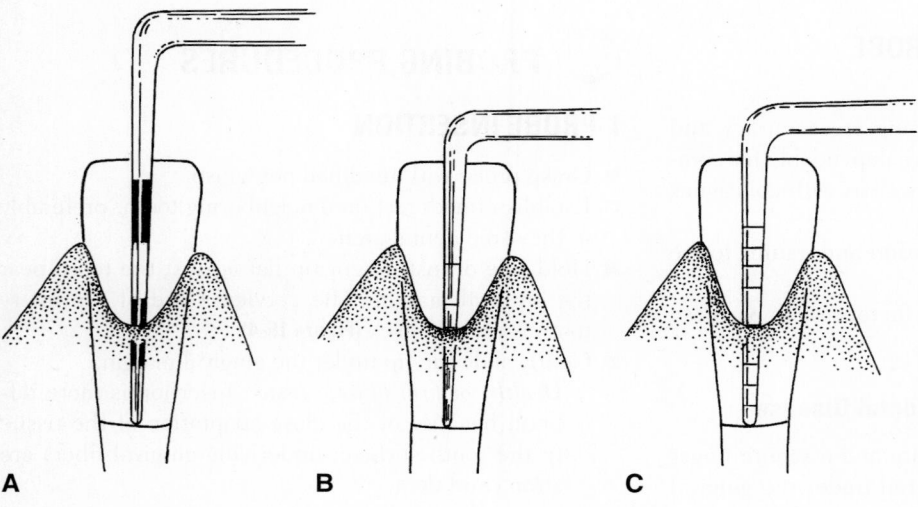

A   B   C

FIGURE 15-5 **Comparison of Probe Readings.** Measurement of same 5-mm pocket with three different probes. **(A)** Color-coded, **(B)** Michigan O, **(C)** Williams.

IV. CIRCUMFERENTIAL PROBING

A. Probe Stroke

Maintain the probe in the sulcus or pocket of each tooth as the probe is moved in a walking stroke **(Figure 15-6)**.

- It is not necessary to remove the probe and reinsert it to make individual readings. Use a continuous probing to avoid missing a deep pocket area.
- Repeated withdrawal and reinsertion cause unnecessary trauma to the gingival margin and hence increase posttreatment discomfort.

B. Walking Stroke

- Hold the side of the tip against the tooth at the base of the pocket.
- Slide the probe up (coronally) about 1 to 2 mm and back to the attachment in a "touch . . . touch . . . touch . . ." rhythm **(Figure 15-6)**.
- Observe probe measurement at the gingival margin at each touch.
- Advance millimeter by millimeter along the facial and lingual surfaces into the proximal areas.

V. ADAPTATION OF PROBE FOR INDIVIDUAL TEETH

A. Molars and Premolars

- Orient the probe at the distal line angle for both facial and lingual application.
- Insert the probe at the distal line angle and probe in a distal direction; adapt the probe around the line angle; probe across the distal surface until the side of the probe contacts the contact area, then slant the probe to continue under the contact area **(Figure 15-3)**.

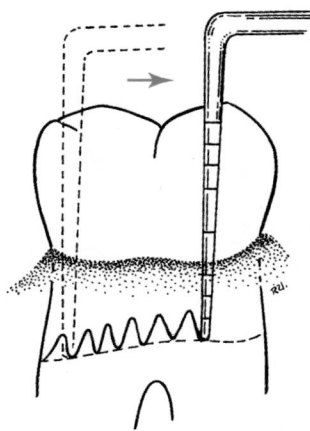

FIGURE 15-6 **Probe Walking Stroke.** The side of the tip of the probe is held in contact with the tooth. From the base of the pocket, the probe is moved up and down in 1- to 2-mm strokes as it is advanced in 1-mm steps. The attached periodontal tissue at the base of the pocket is contacted on each down stroke to identify probing depth in each area.

- Note the probing depth and slide the probe back to the distal line angle. Proceed in the mesial direction around the mesial line angle and across the mesial surface.
- *When the side of the probe touches the contact area, the probe is slanted to continue measurements over half way across the mesial surface.*

B. Anterior Teeth

- Initial insertion may be at the distal line angle or from the midline of the facial or lingual surfaces.
- Proceed around the distal line angle and across the distal surface; reinsert and probe the other half of the tooth.

C. Proximal Surfaces

- Continue the walking stroke around each line angle and onto the proximal surface.
- Roll the instrument handle between the fingers to keep the side of the probe tip adapted to the tooth surface at line angles and as the tooth contour varies.
- Continue the strokes under the contact area. Overlap strokes from facial surface with strokes from lingual surface to ensure full coverage **(Figure 15-3)**. **Make sure that the col area under each contact has been thoroughly examined.**

VI. RECORD OF PROBING MEASUREMENTS

- Six measurements are recorded for each tooth, 3 from the facial, and 3 from the lingual or palatal as shown in **Figure 15-7**.
- For each of the six areas, the deepest probing measurement is recorded.
- Two recordings each are made for proximal areas: Numbers 3 and 6 for the mesial, and 1 and 4 for the distal in **Figure 15-7**. Frequently the deepest probing will be in the col, directly under the contact area.
- Additional recordings may be needed for furcations, mucogingival involvements, or other special areas.
- Recordings of probing depths are part of the total periodontal charting.

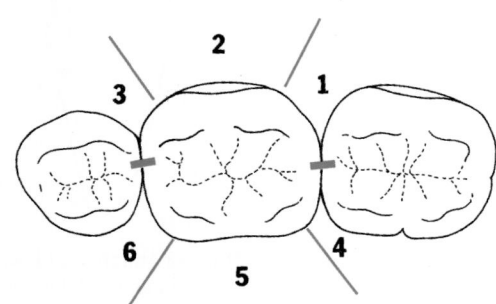

FIGURE 15-7 **Charting Probing Depths.** The pocket/sulcus is measured completely around each tooth. Record the deepest measurement for each of the six areas around the tooth. Areas 1, 3, 4, and 6 extend from the line angle to under the contact area.

■ Figure 8-4 (page 106) illustrates a typical chart form in which boxes are provided for recording probing depth, clinical attachment level, and mobility for each tooth.

CLINICAL ATTACHMENT LEVEL

■ Attachment level refers to the position of the periodontal attached tissues at the base of a sulcus or pocket.
■ It is measured from a fixed point to the attachment, whereas the probing depth is measured from a changeable point (the crest of the free gingiva) to the attachment **(Figure 15-8A)**.

I. RATIONALE

■ A loss of attachment occurs in disease as the junctional epithelium migrates toward the apex.
■ Stability of attachment is characteristic in health, and treatment procedures may be aimed to obtain a gain of attachment.
■ Evaluation can be made of the outcome of periodontal treatment and the stability of the attachment during maintenance examinations.
■ When periodontal disease is active, pocket formation and migration of the attachment along the cemental surface continue.

II. PROCEDURE

A. Selecting a Fixed Point

■ Cementoenamel junction usually is used.
■ Margin of a permanent restoration.
■ For animal research, a notch may be made in the tooth; in human research studies, a template or splint may be made for each patient.

B. Measuring in the Presence of Visible Recession

■ Cementoenamel junction is visible directly.
■ Measure from the cementoenamel junction to the attachment **(Figure 15-8B)**.
■ The clinical attachment level is greater than the probing depth when there is visible recession.

C. Measuring When the Cementoenamel Junction Is Covered by Gingiva

■ Slide the probe along the tooth surface, into the pocket, until the cementoenamel junction is felt **(Figure 15-8C)**.
■ Remove the calculus when it covers the cementoenamel junction.
■ Measure from the gingival crest to the cementoenamel junction.
■ Subtract the millimeters from cementoenamel junction to gingival crest from the total probing depth to the attachment.
■ Probing depth is greater than the clinical attachment level when the cementoenamel junction is covered by the free gingiva.

D. Measuring When the Free Gingival Margin Is Level With the Cementoenamel Junction

■ Apply the probe to measure the probing depth.
■ With the gingival margin at the cementoenamel junction, that measurement is the same as the probing depth
■ The probing depth equals the clinical attachment level when the free gingival margin is level with the cementoenamel junction **(Figure 15-8D)**.

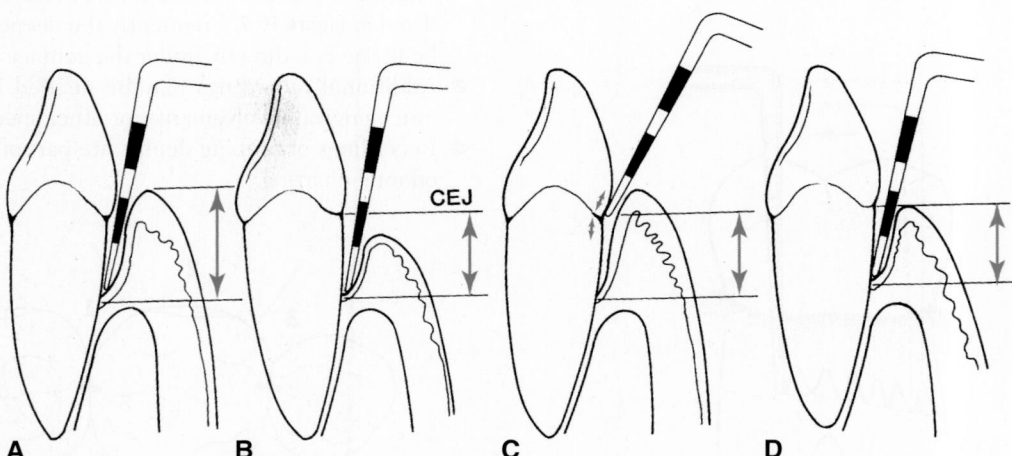

FIGURE 15-8 **Clinical Attachment Level. (A)** Probing depth: the pocket is measured from the gingival margin to the attached periodontal tissue. **(B)** Clinical attachment level in the presence of gingival recession is measured directly from the cementoenamel junction (CEJ) to the attached tissue. **(C)** Clinical attachment level when the gingival margin covers the cementoenamel junction: first the cementoenamel junction is located as shown, and then the distance to the cementoenamel junction is measured and subtracted from the probing depth. **(D)** The clinical attachment level is equal to the probing depth when the gingival margin is at the level of the cementoenamel junction.

FURCATION EXAMINATION

When a pocket extends into a furcation area, special adaptation of the probe must be made to determine the extent and topography of the furcation involvement.

I. ANATOMIC FEATURES

A. Bifurcation (Teeth With Two Roots)

1. *Mandibular molars:* The furcation area is accessible for probing from the facial and lingual surfaces **(Figure 15-9)**.
2. *Maxillary first premolars:* The furcation area is accessible from the mesial and distal aspects, under the contact area.
3. *Primary mandibular molar.* Widespread roots.

B. Trifurcation (Teeth With Three Roots)

1. *Maxillary molars:* A palatal root and two buccal roots, the mesiobuccal and the distobuccal roots. Access for probing is from the mesial, buccal, and distal surfaces.
2. *Maxillary primary molars:* Widespread roots **(Figure 15-4)**.

II. EXAMINATION METHODS

A. Early Furcation

1. Measure probing depth.
2. Examine the area by adapting the probe closely to the tooth surface and moving the end of the probe over the anatomic curvatures of the roots.
3. Check radiograph for signs of furcation involvement **(Figure 15-17)**.

B. Points of Access

1. Measure probing depths at points of access for each bifurcation or trifurcation area.

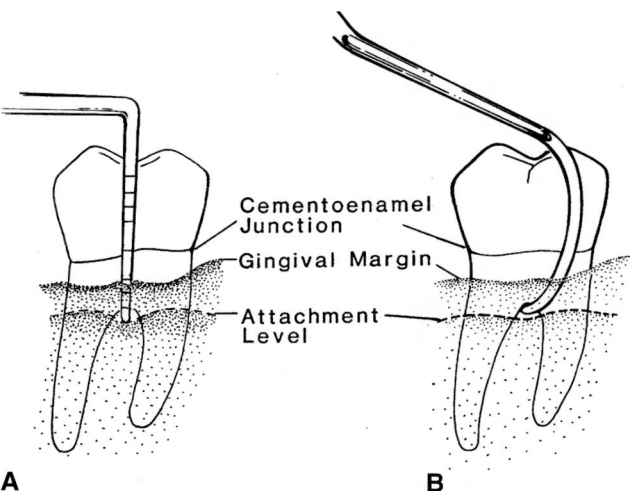

A   **B**

FIGURE 15-9 **Furcation Examination. (A)** Limited access of a straight probe to examine a furcation. Williams probe inserted into bifurcation in area of gingival recession shows probing depth of 3 mm. **(B)** Nabers furcation probe used to examine the topography of the furcation area.

2. Position of gingival margin will vary. **Figure 15-9A** shows apparent recession and 3-mm pocket at the level of the bifurcation.

C. Probe Adaptation

Use probe in diagonal or horizontal position to examine between roots when there is gingival recession or a flexible, short, soft pocket wall that permits access.

D. Use of Furcation Probe

Use a furcation probe, such as a Nabers 1N or 2N, to examine advanced furcation **(Figure 15-9B)**.

E. Complications

Anatomic variations that complicate furcation examination are fused roots; anomalies, such as extra roots; or low or high furcations.

MUCOGINGIVAL EXAMINATION

I. TENSION TEST[2]

A. Purposes

- To detect adequacy of the width of the attached gingiva.
- To locate frenal attachments and their proximity to the free gingiva.
- To identify promptly the mucogingival junction.

B. Procedures

- *Facial*
  1. Retract cheeks and lips laterally by grasping the lips with the thumbs and index fingers. Watch at the mucogingival junction.
  2. Move the lips and cheeks up and down and across, creating tension at the mucogingival junction.
  3. Follow around from the molar areas on the right to molar areas on the left, both maxillary and mandibular. Observe frenal attachments.
- *Lingual (mandible)*
  1. Hold a mouth mirror to tense the mucosa of the floor of the mouth, gently retracting the side of the tongue, so that the mucogingival junction is clearly visible.
  2. Request patient to move the tongue to the left, to the right, and up to touch the palate.

C. Observations

- Blanching at the mucogingival junction.
- Frenal attachments.
- Area(s) of apparent recession where there is very little keratinized gingiva and the base of the sulcus or pocket is near the mucogingival junction.

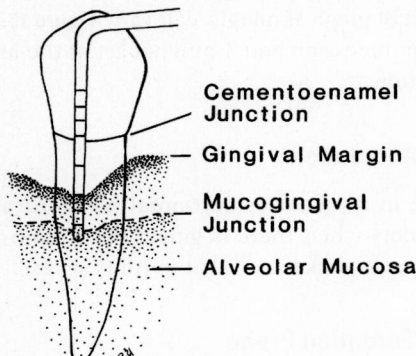

FIGURE 15-10 **Mucogingival Examination.** Probe in position for measuring probing depth where attached gingiva is missing. Absence of attached gingiva permits the probe to pass through the mucogingival junction into the alveolar mucosa.

■ Area where color, size, loss of stippling, smooth shininess, or other characteristic indicates the need for careful probing to determine the amount of attached gingiva.
■ Area where tension pulls the free gingiva away from the tooth, thereby indicating no attached gingiva.

II. GINGIVAL TISSUE EXAMINATION

■ When inflammation is present and a pocket extends to or through the mucogingival junction, a streak of color (red, bluish-red) that shows the inflammatory changes from the gingival margin to the mucogingival junction may be apparent.
■ When such an area does not pull away during a tension test or does not permit passage of a probe through to the alveolar mucosa, the area is noted in the record for examination after elimination of inflammation.

III. PROBING

■ When a pocket extends to or beyond the mucogingival junction, the probe may pass through the pocket directly into the alveolar mucosa (**Figure 15-10**).
■ The absence of attached gingiva indicates that mucogingival involvement is present.

IV. MEASURE THE AMOUNT OF ATTACHED GINGIVA

■ Place the probe (no pressure) on the external surface of the gingiva and measure from the mucogingival junction to the gingival margin to determine the width of the total gingiva (**Figure 15-11A**).
■ Insert the probe and measure probing depth (**Figure 15-11B**).
■ Subtract the probing depth from the total gingival measurement to get the width of the attached gingiva.
■ Record findings.

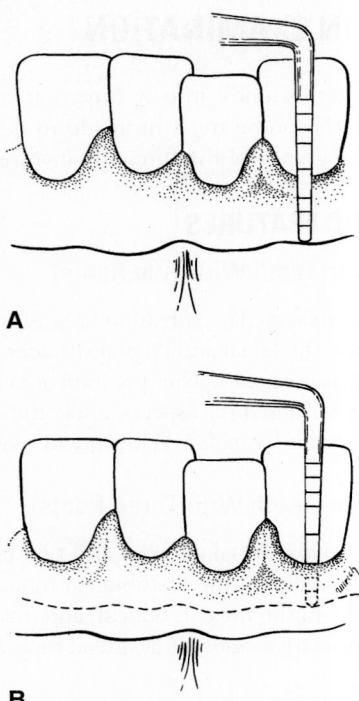

FIGURE 15-11 **Measuring Attached Gingiva. (A)** Measure the total gingiva by laying the probe over the surface of the gingiva and measuring from the free margin to the mucogingival junction. **(B)** Measure the probing depth. Dotted line represents the base of the pocket. Subtract the probing depth **(B)** from the total gingiva **(A)** to obtain the width of attached gingiva. The area illustrated shows 2 mm of attached gingiva.

EXPLORERS

I. GENERAL PURPOSES AND USES

An explorer is used for the following:

A. Detect, by Tactile Sense, the Texture and Character of the Tooth Surfaces

■ For calculus defects or irregularities in the surfaces and margins of restorations, and other irregularities that are not apparent to direct observation.
■ An explorer is used to confirm direct observation. Do not use an explorer on remineralizing potentially dental carious lesions.

B. Define the Extent of Instrumentation Needed and Guide Techniques

■ For scaling and root planing.
■ Removing an overhanging filling.

C. Evaluate the Completeness of Treatment

■ For periodontal nonsurgical treatment as shown by the smooth tooth surface.
■ For removal of an overhanging filling by the smooth margins of the restoration.

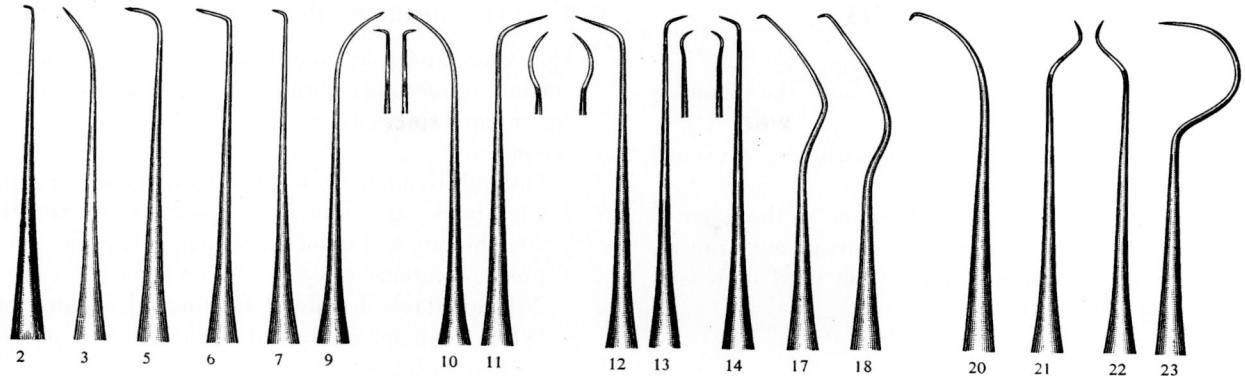

FIGURE 15-12 **Explorers.** This series from Nos. 2 through 23 shows standard shapes of explorer tips. Nos. 2 through 7, 17, 18, 20, and 23 are single instruments. Nos. 9 and 10, 11 and 12, 13 and 14, and 21 and 22 are paired instruments. (Courtesy of the S.S. White Company, Philadelphia, PA.)

II. DESCRIPTION

A. Working End

- Slender, wirelike, metal *tip* that is circular in cross section and tapers to a fine sharp *point*.
- Design
  1. Single: A single instrument may be universal and adaptable to any tooth surface, or it may be designed for specific groups of surfaces. In **Figure 15-12**, Nos. 2 through 7, 17, 18, 20, and 23 are single instruments.
  2. Paired: Paired instruments are mirror images of each other, curved to provide access to contralateral tooth surfaces. In **Figure 15-12**, Nos. 9 and 10, 11 and 12, 13 and 14, and 21 and 22 are paired.
  3. Design of a balanced instrument: Middle of the working end is centered over the long axis of the handle (**Figure 15-13**).

B. Shank

1. *Straight, curved, or angulated:* Whether a shank is straight, curved, or angulated depends on the use and adaptation for which the explorer was designed. In **Figure 15-12**, compare the straight shanks of Nos. 2, 5, 6, 7, 13, and 14 with the others in the series, which are not straight. A curved shank may facilitate application of the instrument to proximal surfaces, particularly of posterior teeth.
2. *Flexibility:* The slender, wirelike explorers have a degree of flexibility that contributes to increased tactile sensitivity for the clinician.

C. Handle

1. *Weight:* For increased tactile sensitivity, a lightweight handle is more effective.
2. *Diameter:* A wider diameter with serrations for friction while grasping can prevent finger cramping from too tight a grasp. With a lighter grasp, tactile sensitivity can be increased.

D. Construction

1. *Single-ended:* A single-ended instrument has one working end on a separate handle.
2. *Double-ended:* A double-ended instrument has two working ends, one on each end of a common handle. Most paired instruments are available double-ended. Other double-ended instruments combine two single instruments, for example, two unpaired explorers or an explorer with a probe.

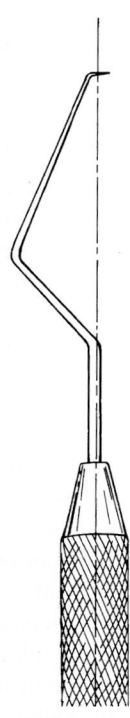

FIGURE 15-13 **Balanced Explorer Design.** With the middle of the tip centered over the long axis of the handle (shown by broken line from tip), the explorer can be positioned in a sulcus or pocket with ease and does not cause trauma to the gingival tissue. Shown is the balanced TU-17 explorer.

III. PREPARATION OF EXPLORERS

- Sharpen and retaper a dull explorer tip.
- With the explorer tip sharp and tapered, the following can be expected:
  - Increased tactile sensitivity with less pressure required.
  - Prevention of unnecessary trauma to the gingival tissue, because less pressure allows greater control.
  - Decreased instrumentation time with increased patient comfort.

IV. SPECIFIC EXPLORERS AND THEIR USES

- A variety of explorers is available, as shown by the examples in **Figure 15-12**.
- The function of each type is related to its adaptability to specific surfaces of teeth at particular angulations.
- Certain explorers can be used effectively for detection of dental caries in pits and fissures, and others are designed to be adapted to examine proximal surfaces for calculus or dental caries.
- Certain ones are designed for use subgingivally, whereas others cannot be adapted subgingivally without inflicting damage to the sulcular epithelium. Therefore, such explorers are limited to supragingival adaptation only.

A. Explorers for Deep Pockets and Inside Furcations

- Several explorers designed for very deep pockets and inside furcation areas are in current use.
- Examples: Orban 20; TU-17; Number 3A (shown in **Figure 15-12**); OD 11/12 designed like Gracey 11/12 curet.

B. Subgingival Explorer: The Pocket Explorer

- *Shape:* The pocket explorer has an angulated shank with a short tip **(Figure 15-13)**. The tip can be measured to ensure that it is less than 2 mm. A longer tip cannot be adapted to the line angles of narrow roots.
- *Features for subgingival root examination*
  1. Back of tip can be applied directly to the attached periodontal tissue at the base of the pocket without lacerating, as shown in **Figure 15-14**. When a straight or sickle explorer is directed toward the base of the pocket, the sharp tip can pass into the epithelium without resistance.
  2. The short tip can be adapted to rounded tooth surfaces and line angles. Long tips of other explorers have a tangential relationship with the tooth and cause distention and trauma to sulcular or pocket epithelium.
  3. Narrow short tip can be adapted at the base where the pocket narrows without undue displacement of the pocket soft tissue wall.
- *Supragingival use of No. TU-17:* It may be adapted to all surfaces and is especially useful for proximal surface examination. It is not adaptable to pits and fissures.

C. Sickle or Shepherd's Hook (No. 23 in **Figure 15-12**)

1. *Use:* examining pits and fissures and supragingival smooth surfaces; examining surfaces and margins of restorations and sealants.
2. *Adaptability*
   - Difficult to apply to proximal surfaces because the wide hook can contact an adjacent tooth and the straight long section of the tip can pass over a small proximal carious lesion.
   - Not adaptable for deep subgingival exploration. When the point is directed to the base of a pocket, trauma to the attachment area can result. In the attempt to prevent such damage, the clinician may not explore to the base of the pocket, thus providing incomplete service.

D. Pigtail or Cowhorn (Nos. 21 and 22 in **Figure 15-12**)

1. *Use:* proximal surfaces for calculus, dental caries, or margins of restorations
2. *Adaptability:* as paired, curved tips, they are applied to opposite tooth surfaces

BASIC PROCEDURES FOR USE OF EXPLORERS

- Development of ability to use an explorer and a probe is achieved first by learning the anatomic features of each tooth surface and the types of irregularities that may be encountered on the surfaces.
- The second step is repeated practice of careful and deliberate techniques for application of the instruments.
- The objective is to adapt the instruments in a routine manner that relays consistent comparative information about the nature of the tooth surface.
- Concentration, patience, attention to detail, and alertness to each irregularity, however small it may seem, are necessary.

I. USE OF SENSORY STIMULI

- Both explorers and probes can transmit tactile stimuli from tooth surfaces to the fingers.
- A fine explorer usually gives a more acute sense of tactile discrimination to small irregularities than does a thicker explorer.
- Probes vary in diameter; the narrow types may provide greater sensitivity.

II. TOOTH SURFACE IRREGULARITIES

- Three basic tactile sensations can be distinguished when probing or exploring.

■ These may be grouped as normal tooth surface, irregularities created by excess or elevations in the surface, and irregularities caused by depressions in the tooth surface. Examples of these are listed here.

A. Normal

1. *Tooth structure:* the smooth surface of enamel and root surface that has been planed; anatomic configurations, such as cingula, furcations
2. *Restored surfaces:* smooth surfaces of metal (gold, amalgam) and the softer feeling of plastic; smooth margin of a restoration

B. Irregularities: Increases or Elevations in Tooth Surface

1. *Deposits:* calculus
2. *Anomalies:* enamel pearl
3. *Restorations:* overcontoured, irregular margins (overhangs)

C. Irregularities: Depressions, Grooves

1. *Tooth surface:* demineralized or carious lesion, abrasion, erosion, pits such as those caused by enamel hypoplasia, areas of cemental resorption on the root surface.
2. *Restorations:* deficient margin, rough surface.

III. TYPES OF STIMULI

During exploring and probing, distinction of irregularities can be made through auditory and tactile means.

A. Tactile

■ Tactile sensations pass through the instrument to the fingers and hand and to the brain for registration and action.
■ Tactile sensations, for example, may be the result of catching on an overcontoured restoration, dropping into a carious lesion, hooking the edge of a restoration or lesion, encountering an elevated deposit, or simply passing over a rough surface.

B. Auditory

■ As an explorer or probe moves over the surface of enamel, cementum, a metallic restoration, a plastic restoration, or any irregularity of tooth structure or restoration, a particular surface texture is apparent. With each contact, sound may be created.
■ The clean smooth enamel is quiet; the rough cementum or calculus is scratchy or noisy. Sometimes a metallic restoration may "squeak" or have a metallic "ring." With experience, differentiations can be made.

EXPLORERS: SUPRAGINGIVAL PROCEDURES

I. USE OF VISION

■ Supragingival exploration for defects of the tooth surface differs from subgingival in that when a surface is dried, much of the actual exploration is performed to confirm visual observation.
■ The exceptions are the proximal areas near and around contact areas that cannot be directly observed.
■ Unnecessary exploration can be avoided. With adequate light and a source of air, proper retraction, and use of a mouth mirror, dried supragingival calculus can generally be seen as either chalky white or brownish-yellow in contrast to tooth color. A minimum of exploration can confirm the finding.

II. FACIAL AND LINGUAL SURFACES

■ Adapt the tip so that the side of the point is always on the tooth surface.
■ Move the instrument in short walking strokes over the surface being examined, or direct the side of the tip gently over a suspected carious lesion.
■ An intact surface where remineralization can be going on must not be vigorously explored. Careful noninvasive examination can be made using the side of the tip of a probe gently to test whether the demineralized area has slight roughness. As described in Chapter 26, on page 378, picking or scratching the surface can prevent further remineralization.

III. PROXIMAL SURFACES

■ Lead with the tip onto a proximal surface, rolling the handle between the fingers to ensure adaptation around the line angle. Keep the side of the point of the explorer in contact with the tooth surface at all times.
■ Explore under the proximal contact area when there is recession of the papilla and the area is exposed. Overlap strokes from facial and lingual surfaces to ensure full coverage.

EXPLORERS: SUBGINGIVAL PROCEDURES

I. ESSENTIALS FOR DETECTION OF TOOTH SURFACE IRREGULARITIES

1. Definite but light grasp.
2. Consistent finger rest with light pressure.
3. Definite contact of the side of the sharp tip with the tooth.
4. Light touch as the instrument is moved over the tooth surface.

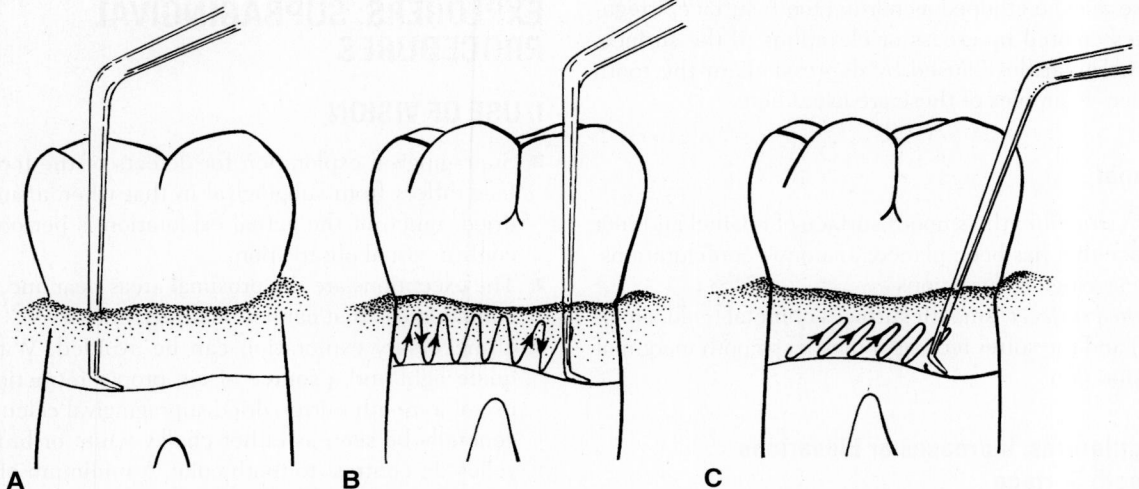

FIGURE 15-14 Use of Subgingival Explorer. (A) The lower shank (next to tip) is held parallel with the long axis of the tooth. The explorer is passed into the pocket and lowered until the back of the working tip meets resistance from the attached periodontal tissue at the base of the pocket. **(B)** Vertical walking stroke. With the side of the tip in contact with the tooth surface at all times, the explorer is moved over the surface. **(C)** Diagonal walking stroke. Complete exploration of the surface is needed; therefore, groups of strokes are overlapped.

II. STEPS FOR USE OF THE SUBGINGIVAL EXPLORER (FIGURE 15-14)

1. With the tip in contact with the tooth supragingivally, hold the lower shank (the part of the shank that is next to the tip) parallel with the long axis of the tooth.
2. Gently slide the tip under the gingival margin into the sulcus or pocket.
3. Keep the point in contact with the tooth at all times to prevent unnecessary trauma to the pocket or sulcular epithelium. Adapt the tip closely to the tooth surface by applying the side of the point.
4. Slide the explorer tip over the tooth surface to the base of the pocket until, with the back of the tip, the resistance of the soft tissue of the attached periodontal tissue is felt **(Figure 15-14A)**.
5. Calculus deposits may obstruct direct passage of the instrument to the base of the pocket. Lift the tip slightly away from the tooth surface and follow over the deposit to proceed to the base of the pocket.
6. Use a "walking" stroke **(Figure 15-14B)**.
7. Lead with the tip. Move it ahead as the instrument progresses.
8. Length of stroke depends on the depth of a pocket.
   - Shallow sulcus: The stroke may extend the entire depth.
   - Deep pocket: Controlled strokes 2- to 3-mm long can allow improved adaptation of the instrument.
   - Explore a deep pocket in sections. First explore the apical area next to the base of the pocket, then move up to a higher section.
9. Do not remove the explorer from the pocket for each stroke on a particular surface because
   - Trauma to the gingival margin caused by repeated withdrawal and reinsertion can cause the patient posttreatment discomfort.

- Concentration on the texture of the tooth surface is interrupted.
10. Proximal surface.
    - Lead with tip of instrument; do not "back into" an area.
11. Continue the strokes around the line angle. Roll the instrument handle between the fingers to keep the tip closely adapted as the tooth contour changes.
12. Continue strokes under the contact area. Overlap strokes from facial and lingual aspects for full coverage.

RECORD FINDINGS

I. SUPRAGINGIVAL CALCULUS

A. Distribution

- Supragingival calculus is generally localized.
- It is most commonly confined to the lingual surfaces of the mandibular anterior teeth and the facial surfaces of the maxillary first and second molars, opposite the openings to the salivary ducts.

B. Amount

Indicate a subjective measurement of slight, moderate, heavy.

II. SUBGINGIVAL CALCULUS

A. Distribution

Subgingival calculus can be either localized or generalized. Record in relation to pocket probing depth on a chart or form to show exact locations.

B. Amount

Indicate a subjective measurement of slight, moderate, heavy.

III. OTHER IRREGULARITIES OF TOOTH SURFACE

Note on the chart or in the record any other deviation from normal detected.

MOBILITY EXAMINATION

- Because of the nature and function of the periodontal ligament, teeth have a slight normal mobility.
- Mobility can be considered abnormal or pathologic when it exceeds normal.
- Increased mobility can be a clinical sign of periodontal trauma from occlusion as described in Chapter 18 (page 279).

I. PROCEDURE FOR DETERMINATION OF MOBILITY

1. Position the patient for clear visibility with maximum light and ready accessibility through convenient retraction.
2. Stabilize the head: Request the patient to press the head against the headrest. Motion of the head, lips, or cheek can interfere with a true evaluation of tooth movement.
3. Use two single-ended metal instruments with wide blunt ends, held with a modified pen grasp. Use of wooden tongue depressors or plastic mirror handles is not recommended because of their flexibility. Testing with the fingers without the metal instruments can be misleading because the soft tissue of the fingertips can move and give an illusion of tooth movement.
4. Apply specific, firm finger rests (fulcrums): A standardized finger rest pressure contributes increased consistency to the determinations. The teeth may be dried with air or sponge to prevent slipping of the instruments or the finger on the finger rest.
5. Apply the blunt ends of the instruments to opposite sides of a tooth, and rock the tooth to test horizontal mobility. Keep both instrument ends on the tooth as pressure is applied first from one side and then the other.
6. Test vertical mobility (depression of the tooth into its socket) by applying, on the occlusal or incisal surface, pressure with one of the mirror handles.
7. Test each primary abutment tooth of a fixed partial denture.
8. Move from tooth to tooth in a systematic order.

II. RECORD DEGREE OF MOVEMENT

A. Scale

N, 1, 2, 3 or I, II, III are frequently used, sometimes with a plus sign (+) to indicate mobility between numbers.

B. Recording

Although subjective, interpretation may be considered as follows.[3]

N = normal, physiologic
1 = slight mobility, greater than normal
2 = moderate mobility, greater than 1 mm displacement
3 = severe mobility, may move in all directions, vertical as well as horizontal.

C. The Letter N Means *Normal Mobility*

All teeth that have a periodontal ligament have normal mobility. No tooth has zero mobility except in a condition, such as ankylosis, in which there is no periodontal ligament.

D. Chart Form

A chart form such as Figure 8-4 (page 106) can provide for a place to record mobility. Preferably more than one space can be reserved so that comparative readings may be recorded at successive maintenance appointments.

FREMITUS

I. DEFINITION

- Fremitus means palpable vibration or movement.
- In dentistry, fremitus refers to the vibratory patterns of the teeth. A tooth with fremitus has excess contact, possibly related to a premature contact. Usually, the tooth also demonstrates some degree of mobility because the excess contact forces the tooth to move.
- The test is used in conjunction with occlusal analysis and adjustment.
- Because fremitus depends on tooth contact, determination is made only on the maxillary teeth.

II. PROCEDURE FOR DETERMINATION OF FREMITUS

1. Seat the patient upright with the head stabilized against the headrest; the occlusal biting plane is parallel with the floor.
2. Press an index finger on each maxillary tooth at about the cervical third **(Figure 15-15)**.
3. Request the patient to "click the back teeth" repeatedly but gently.
4. Start with the most posterior maxillary tooth on one side, and move the index finger tooth by tooth around the arch.
5. Record by tooth number the teeth where vibration is felt and the teeth where actual movement is noted.

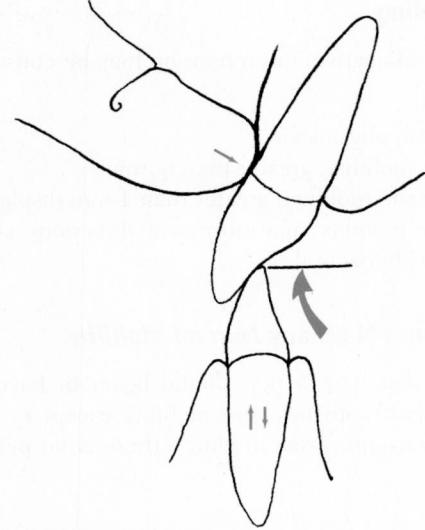

FIGURE 15-15 **Fremitus.** With the patient seated upright and the head stabilized against the headrest, an index finger is placed firmly over the cervical third of each maxillary tooth in succession starting with the most posterior tooth on one side and moving around the arch. The patient is requested to click the posterior teeth.

The degree recorded may be subjective, but the following range has been suggested.

  N = normal (without vibration or movement).
  + = One-degree fremitus; only slight vibration can be felt.
  ++ = Two-degree fremitus; the tooth is clearly palpable but movement is barely visible.
  +++ = Three-degree fremitus; movement is clearly observed visually.

RADIOGRAPHIC EXAMINATION

■ Radiographs provide essential information to aid and supplement clinical findings.
■ During the examination, and especially during probing, the radiographs are placed available for viewing in conjunction with examination.
■ When the radiographs have not been prepared (or processed) at the time of initial probing, areas needing special confirmation can be marked on the record for review at the next appointment.
■ Selection of radiographs: For observing evidence of periodontal involvement, *periapical* radiographs are needed.
■ *Horizontal bitewing* radiographs do not show the complete periodontal tissues that extend around the roots. When bone loss is moderate to severe, the crest of the bone may be seen in a *vertical bitewing* survey, which is useful in checking during the maintenance phase.
■ Viewing the radiographs: The need for radiographs free from errors of technique and viewed with magnification on an adequately lighted viewbox or on the computer cannot be overemphasized.

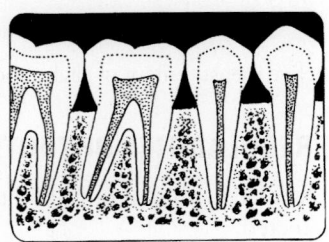

FIGURE 15-16 **Normal Bone Level.** Drawing of a radiograph to show normal bone level, 1 to 1.5 mm from the cementoenamel junction.

RADIOGRAPHIC CHANGES IN PERIODONTAL INFECTIONS

I. BONE LEVEL

A. Normal Bone Level

The crest of the interdental bone appears from 1.0 to 1.5 mm from the cementoenamel junction (**Figure 15-16**).

B. Bone Level in Periodontal Disease

The height of the bone is lowered progressively as the inflammation is extended and bone is destroyed.

II. SHAPE OF REMAINING BONE

A. Horizontal Bone Loss

■ When the crest of the bone is parallel with a line between the cementoenamel junctions of two adjacent teeth, the term *"horizontal bone loss"* is used (**Figures 15-17 and 15-18**).
■ When inflammation is the sole destructive factor, the bone loss usually appears horizontal.
■ When the amount of remaining bone is fairly evenly distributed throughout the dentition, the condition may be described as *generalized horizontal bone loss.* It may be designated either by millimeters from the position of the normal bone level or by percentage. When making estimates, referral to the table of average root lengths can be helpful (Appendix V, page 116).

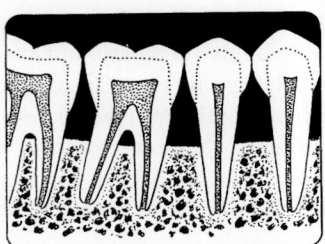

FIGURE 15-17 **Horizontal Bone Loss (1).** Bone level in periodontal disease is more than 1 to 1.5 mm from the cementoenamel junction. When bone loss is horizontal, the crest of the alveolar bone is parallel with a line between the cementoenamel junctions of adjacent teeth. Note early furcation involvement in the second molar and moderate furcation involvement in the first molar.

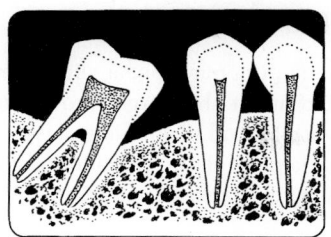

FIGURE 15-18 **Horizontal Bone Loss (2).** Second molar has drifted mesially into the space created when the first molar was removed. Note that the level of the crestal bone is parallel with a line between the cementoenamel junctions of the second premolar and the tipped second molar.

- When bone loss is confined to specific areas, the condition is described as *localized* horizontal bone loss.

B. Angular or Vertical Bone Loss

- Reduction in height of crestal bone that is irregular; the bone level is not parallel with a line joining the adjacent cementoenamel junctions. Note in **Figure 15-19** that the V-shaped mesial bone loss on the mesial of the first molar has lost its white lining of lamina dura. It is a true "vertical" or "angular" bone loss possibly related to trauma from occlusion. Contrast this area with the molar in **Figure 15-18** where the lamina dura is an intact clear white line. The V-shaped area in this radiograph shows a tipped tooth due to extraction of the adjacent supporting tooth. No trauma or disease was involved.
- Angular bone loss is more commonly *localized*; rarely generalized.
- When inflammation and trauma from occlusion are combined in causing the destruction and irregular shape of the bone, the bone may appear with "*angular defects*" or with "*vertical bone loss.*"

III. CRESTAL LAMINA DURA

A. Normal

White, radiopaque; continuous with and connects the lamina dura about the roots of two adjacent teeth;

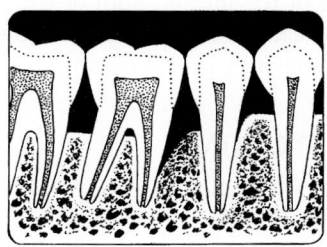

FIGURE 15-19 **Angular or Vertical Bone Loss; Mesial of the First Molar.** The level of the crestal bone between the second premolar and the first molar is not parallel with a line between the cementoenamel junctions of the same teeth.

covers the interdental bone of the two premolars in **Figure 15-16**.

B. Evidence of Disease

The crestal lamina dura is indistinct, irregular, radiolucent, fuzzy (**Figure 15-19**, mesial of first molar).

IV. FURCATION INVOLVEMENT

A. Normal

Bone fills the area between the roots (**Figure 15-16**).

B. Evidence of Disease

- Radiolucent area in the furcation.
- Early furcation involvement may appear as a small radiolucent black area or as a slight thickening of the periodontal ligament space. It can be confirmed by probing. Early furcation involvement is shown in the second molar in **Figure 15-17**.
- Furcation involvement of maxillary molars may become more advanced before radiographic evidence can be seen. Superimposition of the palatal root may mask a small area of involvement. When the proximal bone level in the radiograph appears at the level where the furcation is normally located, furcation involvement should be suspected and probed for confirmation.
- Maxillary first premolar furcation involvement cannot be seen in a radiograph except at an unusual angulation or unusual position of the tooth. With correct vertical and horizontal angulation, the roots are superimposed.
- Early furcations may show at one angulation but not at another; variations in technique can obscure a furcation involvement. All furcations must be carefully probed.

V. PERIODONTAL LIGAMENT SPACE

A. Normal

- The periodontal ligament is connective tissue and, hence, appears radiolucent in a radiograph. It appears as a fine black radiolucent line next to the root surface. On its outer side is the lamina dura, the bone that lines the tooth socket and appears radiopaque. A normal ligament shows clearly around the molar roots in **Figure 15-20**, whereas a widened black ligament space is evident in the premolars of the same radiograph.

B. Evidence of Disease

Widening or thickening.

- *Angular thickening or triangulation:* The space is widened only near the coronal third, near the crest of the interdental bone.

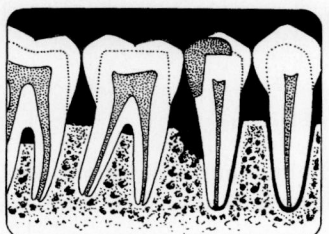

FIGURE 15-20 **Periodontal Ligament Space.** First and second molars have a normal periodontal ligament space, which appears as a fine black line about the roots. The first premolar shows thickening of the ligament space about the entire root, and the second premolar has thickening only about the mesial surface of the root.

■ *Complete periodontal ligament thickened along an entire side of a root to the apex, or around the root* (Figure 15-20): When viewed at different angulations (in the various radiographs of a complete survey), the ligament space may reveal varying thicknesses, thus showing that the disease involvement is not consistent around the entire root or that other structures are superimposed.

EARLY PERIODONTAL DISEASE

■ The real preventive service is to recognize *early signs* of periodontal involvement so that treatment can be initiated to arrest the disease and prevent more severe involvement, which could lead to tooth loss.
■ The recognition of severe bone loss, advanced furcation involvement, and marked thickening of the periodontal ligament space is not difficult after a basic understanding has been gained.
■ The difficult part is to watch carefully for incipient, often isolated indications of early periodontal disease. These changes can be seen in all age groups, from young children to elderly patients.

I. EARLIEST SIGNS

■ The earliest signs of periodontal involvement are not evident in a radiograph.
■ Only after the inflammation has extended from the soft tissue (gingivitis) to the supporting periodontal tissues and bone resorption has become sufficient does radiographic evidence appear.

II. INITIAL BONE DESTRUCTION

■ The usual interproximal pathway of inflammation from gingivitis to periodontitis is directly from the inflamed gingival connective tissue into the crest of the interdental bone.
■ Initial bone destruction most frequently can be observed in a radiograph at the crest of the interdental bone in the crestal lamina dura.

III. RADIOGRAPHIC EVIDENCE

■ Crestal lamina dura may appear slightly irregular, fuzzy, and radiolucent. At this stage, the radiograph is best examined with a hand magnifying glass.
■ Angular thickening of the periodontal ligament space (triangulation) may also be apparent.

OTHER RADIOGRAPHIC FINDINGS

■ Any other radiographic findings that may be related directly or indirectly to periodontal involvement and its contributing factors are noted in the record.
■ Certain findings have a direct relation to dental hygiene care and instruction, particularly local factors that contribute to food impaction or biofilm retention.

I. CALCULUS

■ Gross deposits, primarily those on proximal surfaces, may be seen in radiographs.
■ Observing these may be helpful, but the probe and explorer are needed to define the exact location and extent.
■ The density and contrast of the radiograph influence whether calculus is seen. Because all deposits are not visible, the use of radiographs has very limited value for specific calculus detection.

II. OVERHANGING RESTORATIONS

■ Some proximal overhanging margins may be seen on radiographs.
■ The use of an explorer is necessary to detect irregular margins and to examine all proximal margins that do not reveal irregularities in the radiographs.
■ Superimposition can mask an overhanging margin in a radiograph.

III. RELATIONSHIP TO POCKETS

■ Radiographs do not show pockets; soft tissue does not show in a radiograph.
■ Because a pocket is measured from the gingival margin to the base of the pocket, both of which are soft tissue, pockets cannot be seen on a radiograph. Probing is necessary to identify pocket depth.

DOCUMENTATION

Documentation in the permanent record for a patient with a gingival or periodontal condition needs to include a minimum of the following:

■ Findings by clinical observation and the use of a periodontal probe: sulcus and probing depths,

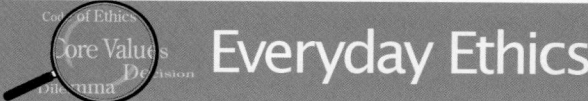

Everyday Ethics

Mrs. Claren, a neat-appearing lady in her 50s, was new to the practice. After a careful history recording, Doris, the dental hygienist, started the gingival examination and continued into the routine probing. Many of the probing depths were 3 and 4 mm, and some even 5 mm. Doris could feel subgingival calculus as she probed, and there was bleeding from her gentle probing.

Doris was nearly finished and was recording findings when the patient raised her head and said, "You aren't cleaning my teeth. What is it you are doing?" Suddenly Doris realized that this lady may never have had a complete periodontal examination and was unaware of her moderate to severe chronic periodontitis with generalized subgingival calculus.

Questions for Consideration

1. Which of the dental hygiene core values in Section II, Introduction (Table II-1, page 38) come into play in this scenario with Doris and Mrs. Claren? Think of each of the core values in relation to a first-time patient compared with a long-time patient.

2. Review the Legal and Ethical concepts described in Section IV, Introduction Table IV-1 (page 339) with thoughts of how they may be of help to Doris as she thinks over how to answer Mrs. Claren. Make a list of choices on the explanations Doris will decide as most pertinent.

3. How is this a simple need to explain office policy to a new patient or is informed consent the priority here?

attachment levels, status of furcations, leading to the dental hygiene diagnosis.

- Mobility, fremitus, occlusal problems, and other findings that will tie the complete oral plan for dental hygiene care into the overall major treatment plan for dental care by a dentist.
- A sample progress note for a dental hygiene appointment is found in **Box 15-2.**

BOX 15-2	Example Progress Note

Patient starting 5th year; our routine 5-year complete history and examination with "like new" records; patient was prepared with a book to read. Mable (dental assistant) made the complete radiographic survey.

Intra–extra oral no unusual tissue changes; gingiva good color; probing showed a few over 3 mm but in general with no bleeding on probing; mobility, fremitus, ok; plaque score nearly perfect; some calculus mand anteriors to remove as with a usual maintenance. Our efforts with Cambra have paid off, no evidence new demineralization: patient has not needed a restoration in 2 years, Still talking about whitening, especially # 9 and said she might even do an implant there this year (believe she will do whitening; believes it too much to take out a perfectly good tooth).

Appointment for regular 3 months maintenance when Dr. R will review the 5-year exam with the radiographs.

Signed: _____, RDH Date: _____.

Factors To Teach The Patient

- The need for a careful, thorough examination if treatment is to be complete and effective.
- Information about the instruments and how their use makes the examination complete. Examples are the complete radiographic survey, probing 360° around each tooth, and exploring each subgingival tooth surface.
- Why bleeding can occur when probing. Healthy tissue does not bleed.
- Relation of probing depth measurements to normal sulci.
- Significance of mobility.

References

1. Listgarten MA. Periodontal probing: what does it mean? *J Clin Periodontol.* 1980 Jun;7(3):165–76.
2. Kopczyk RA, Saxe SR. Clinical signs of gingival inadequacy: the tension test. *ASDC J Dent Child.* 1974 Sep–Oct;41(5):352–5.
3. Miller SC. *Textbook of periodontia.* 3rd ed. Philadelphia: Blakiston Co; 1950. p. 125.

Periodontal Disease Development

ESTHER M. WILKINS, BS, RDH, DMD

Chapter Outline

Early in the process of case assessment in preparation for care planning, the presence and severity of periodontal infection is determined. Is the patient's disease limited to the gingival tissue without loss of periodontal attachment? Does the patient have bone loss, pocket formation, or other signs of periodontitis?

■ When the disease is limited to the gingiva, the possibility of reversal of the infection is considered first in the care planning objectives.
■ Can the patient be guided to learn new habits of self-treatment through daily infection control supple-

mented by periodic professional scaling and other dental hygiene care?
■ When there is apical positioning of the periodontal attachment with alveolar bone loss and other indications of periodontitis, can conservative procedures of *nonsurgical periodontal therapy* provide sufficient professional treatment? Is more complex periodontal therapy required?
■ Individual differences and the particular clinical features of each patient are identified. The oral tissues need treatment to bring them to a state of maximum health that can be maintained by the patient.

DETERMINATION OF CASE DIAGNOSIS

■ The patient history, clinical examination, radiographs, and other data from the assessment are put together to determine the initial diagnosis which may range from early gingivitis to advanced periodontal involvement.

■ Except in cases of advanced periodontitis, the need for additional treatment after initial nonsurgical periodontal therapy is rarely possible to predict. Reassessment of the treated tissues is built into the care plan. At the outset, the patient is given a clear understanding of the purpose of such a reevaluation.

■ In this chapter the classification of gingival and periodontal diseases is included **(Tables 16-1** and **16-2)**. Local and systemic contributing and risk factors that affect the development of the gingival and periodontal infections are identified. Key words are defined in **Box 16-1**.

DEVELOPMENT OF GINGIVAL AND PERIODONTAL INFECTIONS

The stages of development of gingivitis and periodontitis are divided into the *initial lesion,* the *early lesion, the established lesion,* and the *advanced lesion.*[1] With an accumulation of dental biofilm on the cervical tooth surface adjacent to the gingival margin, an inflammatory reaction is set up, and the natural defense mechanisms respond.

I. THE INITIAL LESION

A. Inflammatory Response to Dental Biofilm

1. Occurs within 2 to 4 days of irritation from bacterial accumulation.
2. Migration and infiltration of white blood cells into the junctional epithelium and gingival sulcus result from the natural body response to infectious agents.

TABLE 16-1	CLASSIFICATION OF GINGIVAL AND PERIODONTAL DISEASES AND CONDITIONS: GINGIVAL DISEASES

I. GINGIVAL DISEASES
  A. **Dental Plaque-Induced Gingival Diseases***
    1. Gingivitis associated with dental plaque only
      a. Without other local contributing factors
      b. With local contributing factors
    2. Gingival diseases modified by systemic factors
      a. Associated with the endocrine system
        1. Puberty-associated gingivitis
        2. Menstrual cycle-associated gingivitis
        3. Pregnancy associated
          a. Gingivitis
          b. Pyogenic granuloma
        4. Diabetes mellitus-associated gingivitis
      b. Associated with blood dyscrasias
        1. Leukemia-associated gingivitis
        2. Other
    3. Gingival diseases modified by medications
      a. Drug-influenced gingival diseases
        1. Drug-influenced gingival enlargements
        2. Drug-influenced gingivitis
          a. Oral contraceptive-associated gingivitis
          b. Other
    4. Gingival diseases modified by malnutrition
      a. Ascorbic acid-deficiency gingivitis
      b. Other
  B. **Non-Plaque-Induced Gingival Lesions**
    1. Gingival diseases of specific bacterial origin
      a. *Neisseria gonorrhea*–associated lesions
      b. *Treponema pallidum*–associated lesions
      c. Streptococcal species-associated lesions
      d. Other
    2. Gingival diseases of viral origin
      a. Herpesvirus infections
        1. Primary herpetic gingivostomatitis
        2. Recurrent oral herpes
        3. Varicella zoster infections
      b. Other

    3. Gingival diseases of fungal origin
      a. *Candida*-species infections
        1. Generalized gingival candidosis
      b. Linear gingival erythema
      c. Histoplasmosis
      d. Other
    4. Gingival lesions of genetic origin
      a. Hereditary gingival fibromatosis
      b. Other
    5. Gingival manifestations of systemic conditions
      a. Mucocutaneous disorders
        1. Lichen planus
        2. Pemphigoid
        3. Pemphigus vulgaris
        4. Erythema multiforme
        5. Lupus erythematosus
        6. Drug-induced
        7. Other
      b. Allergic reactions
        1. Dental restorative materials
          a. Mercury
          b. Nickel
          c. Acrylic
          d. Other
        2. Reactions attributable to
          a. Toothpastes/dentifrices
          b. Mouthrinses/mouthwashes
          c. Chewing gum additives
          d. Foods and additives
        3. Other
    6. Traumatic lesions (factitious, iatrogenic, accidental)
      a. Chemical injury
      b. Physical injury
      c. Thermal injury
    7. Foreign body reactions
    8. Not otherwise specified (NOS)

*Can occur on a periodontium with no attachment loss or on a periodontium with attachment loss that is not progressing.
Source: Reprinted with permission from 1999 International Workshop for a Classification of Periodontal Diseases and Conditions. Papers. Oak Brook, Illinois, October 30–November 2, 1999. *Ann Periodontol.* 1999 Dec;4(1):2,3.

TABLE 16-2	CLASSIFICATION OF GINGIVAL AND PERIODONTAL DISEASES AND CONDITIONS: PERIODONTAL DISEASES

II. CHRONIC PERIODONTITIS†
- A. Localized
- B. Generalized

III. AGGRESSIVE PERIODONTITIS
- A. Localized
- B. eneralized

IV. PERIODONTITIS AS A MANIFESTATION OF SYSTEMIC DISEASES
- A. Associated with hematological disorders
  1. Acquired neutropenia
  2. Leukemias
  3. Other
- B. Associated with genetic disorders
  1. Familial and cyclic neutropenia
  2. Down's syndrome
  3. Leukocyte adhesion deficiency syndromes
  4. Papillon–Lefévre syndrome
  5. Chediak–Higashi syndrome
  6. Histiocytosis syndromes
  7. Glycogen storage disease
  8. Infantile genetic agranulocytosis
  9. Cohen's syndrome
  10. Ehlers–Danlos syndrome (Types IV and VIII)
  11. Hypophosphatasia
  12. Other
- C. Not otherwise specified (NOS)

V. NECROTIZING PERIODONTAL DISEASES
- A. Necrotizing ulcerative gingivitis (NUG)
- B. Necrotizing ulcerative periodontitis (NUP)

VI. ABSCESSES OF THE PERIODONTIUM
- A. Gingival abscess
- B. Periodontal abscess
- C. Pericoronal abscess

VII. PERIODONTITIS ASSOCIATED WITH ENDODONTIC LESIONS
- A. Combined periodontic-endodontic lesions

VIII. DEVELOPMENTAL OR ACQUIRED DEFORMITIES AND CONDITIONS
- A. Localized tooth-related factors that modify or predispose to plaque-induced gingival diseases or periodontitis
  1. Tooth anatomic factors
  2. Dental restorations/appliances
  3. Root fractures
  4. Cervical root resorption and cemental tears
- B. Mucogingival deformities and conditions around teeth
  1. Gingival/soft tissue recession
     a. Facial or lingual surfaces
     b. Interproximal (papillary)
  2. Lack of keratinized gingiva
  3. Decreased vestibular depth
  4. Aberrant frenum/muscle position
  5. Gingival excess
     a. Pseudopocket
     b. Inconsistent gingival margin
     c. Excessive gingival display
     d. Gingival enlargement
  6. Abnormal color
- C. Mucogingival deformities and conditions on edentulous ridges
  1. Vertical and/or horizontal ridge deficiency
  2. Lack of gingiva/keratinized tissue
  3. Gingival/soft tissue enlargement
  4. Aberrant frenum/muscle position
  5. Decreased vestibular depth
  6. Abnormal color
- D. Occlusal trauma
  1. Primary occlusal trauma
  2. Secondary occlusal trauma

*Can be further classified on the basis of extent and severity.
Source: Reprinted with permission from 1999 International Workshop for a Classification of Periodontal Diseases and Conditions. Papers. Oak Brook, Illinois, October 30–November 2, 1999. *Ann Periodontol.* 1999 Dec;4(1):2,3.

3. Increased flow of gingival sulcus fluid.
4. Early breakdown of collagen of the supporting gingival fiber groups (Figure 14-3, page 211).
5. Fluid fills the spaces in the connective tissue.

B. Clinical Appearance

- No clinical evidence of change may appear in the earliest phases.
- Slight marginal redness with enlargement due to the fluid collection follows as the infection develops.

II. THE EARLY LESION

A. Increased Inflammatory Response

- Dental biofilm becomes older and thicker (7 to 14 days; time reflects individual differences).

- Infiltration of fluid, lymphocytes, and neutrophils with a few plasma cells into the connective tissue.
- Breakdown of collagen fiber support to the gingival margin.
- *Epithelium proliferates:* Epithelial extensions and rete ridges are formed.

B. Clinical Appearance

- Early signs of gingivitis become apparent with slight gingival enlargement; will become an established lesion if undisturbed.
- Early gingivitis is reversible when biofilm is controlled and inflammation is reduced. Healthy tissue may be restored.
- Susceptibility of individuals varies; time before lesion becomes established varies.

BOX 16-1	Key Words

Disease Development

Cicatrix: the fibrous tissue left after the healing of a wound; cicatricial: adj.

Collagen: white fibers of the connective tissue.

Collagenase: enzyme that catalyzes the degradation (hydrolysis) of collagen.

Desquamation: shedding of the outer epithelial layer of the stratified squamous epithelium of skin or mucosa.

Diastema: a space or abnormal opening; as a dental term, it is a space between two adjacent teeth in the same dental arch.

Edema: an accumulation of excessive fluid in cells, tissues, or a serous cavity.

Enzyme: a protein secreted by body cells that acts as a catalyst to induce chemical changes in other substances but remains unchanged itself.

Food impaction: forceful wedging of food into the periodontium by occlusal forces.

Gingivitis: inflammation of the gingival tissues.

Iatrogenic: resulting from treatment by a professional person.

Infiltration: the diffusion or accumulation in a tissue or cells of substances not normal to it or in amounts in excess of normal.

Lesion: any pathologic or traumatic discontinuity of tissue or loss of function of a part; broad term including wounds, sores, ulcers, tumors, and any other tissue damage.

Nonsurgical periodontal therapy: includes dental biofilm removal and biofilm control (by patient); supragingival and subgingival scaling; root planing; and the adjunctive use of chemotherapeutic agents for control of bacterial infection, desensitizing hypersensitive exposed root surfaces, and dental caries prevention as related to the health of the periodontium.

Periodontitis: inflammation in the periodontium affecting gingival tissues, periodontal ligament, cementum, and supporting bone.

Permeable: permitting passage of a fluid.

Refractory: not readily responsive to treatment.

Toxin: a poison; protein produced by certain animals, higher plants, and pathogenic bacteria.

> **Bacterial toxin:** poison produced by bacteria; includes exotoxins, endotoxins, and toxic enzymes.

Xerostomia: dryness of the mouth from a lack of normal secretions.

III. THE ESTABLISHED LESION

A. Progression From the Early Lesion

1. Fluid and leukocyte migration into tissues and sulcus increase; plasma cells are related to areas of chronic inflammation.
2. Formation of *pocket epithelium.*
   - Proliferation of the junctional and sulcular epithelium continues in an attempt to wall out the inflammation.
   - Pocket epithelium is more permeable; areas of ulceration of the lining epithelium develop.
   - Early pocket formation with bleeding on probing.
3. Collagen destruction continues; connective tissue fiber support lost.
4. Progression to early periodontal lesion may occur, or some established lesions may remain stable for extended periods of time.

B. Clinical Appearance

Clear evidence of inflammation is present with marginal redness, bleeding on probing, and spongy marginal gingiva. Later, chronic fibrosis develops.

IV. THE ADVANCED LESION

A. Extension of Inflammation

1. Bacteria from supragingival biofilm enter the sulcus and provide the source for subgingival biofilm.

2. Biofilm microorganisms produce irritants.
3. *Alveolar bone destruction*
   - Inflammation spreads through the loose connective tissue along (beside) the blood vessels to the alveolar bone.[2]
   - Most commonly, the inflammation enters the bone through small vessel channels in the alveolar crest.
   - Inflammation spreads through the bone marrow and out into the periodontal ligament.

B. Progressive Destruction of Connective Tissue

1. Connective tissue fibers below the junctional epithelium are destroyed; the epithelium migrates along the root surface.
2. Coronal portion of junctional epithelium becomes detached.
3. Exposed cementum where Sharpey's fibers were attached becomes altered by inflammatory products of bacteria and the sulcus fluid.
4. Diseased cementum contains a thin superficial layer of endotoxins from the bacterial breakdown.
5. Without treatment, the pocket becomes progressively deepened.

C. Characteristics of the Advanced Lesion

1. Pocket formation, mobility, bone loss; all signs of periodontitis.

2. Persistence of the chronic inflammatory process; plasma cells predominate.
3. Junctional epithelium continues to migrate; lesion extends through connective tissue.
4. Periods of inactivity alternating with periods of activity can be expected.

V. CLASSIFICATION

- *Periodontal disease* is not a single pathologic entity.
- It is a term used to describe a variety of inflammatory and degenerative diseases that affect the supporting structures of the teeth.
- A widely used system for classifying the types and severity of periodontal disease is shown in **Tables 16-1** and **16-2**.

GINGIVAL AND PERIODONTAL POCKETS

- A pocket is a diseased sulcus.
- The area of the sulcus and the pocket is the treatment area where calculus collects and instrumentation for nonsurgical periodontal therapy is applied.
- It is the presence or absence of infection that distinguishes a pocket from a sulcus and the level of attachment on the tooth that distinguishes a gingival pocket from a periodontal pocket.
- A pocket has an *inner wall (the tooth surface),* and an *outer wall (the sulcular epithelium or pocket epithelium)* of the free gingiva. The two walls meet at the base of the pocket.
- The base of the pocket is the coronal margin of the attached periodontal tissues. Histologically, the base of a healthy sulcus is the coronal border of the junctional epithelium, whereas the base of a pocket (diseased sulcus) may be at the coronal border of the connective tissue attachment.

- Pockets are divided into *gingival* and *periodontal* types to clarify the degree of anatomic involvement. Periodontal pockets are then further categorized by their position in relation to the alveolar bone, that is, whether their pocket base is suprabony or intrabony **(Figure 16-1)**.

I. GINGIVAL POCKET

- *Definition*: A pocket formed by gingival enlargement without apical migration of the junctional epithelium **(Figure 16-1B)**.
- The margin of the gingiva has moved toward the incisal or occlusal without the deeper periodontal structures becoming involved.
- The tooth wall is enamel.
- During eruption, the base of the sulcus is at various levels along the enamel. The base of the sulcus of a fully erupted tooth is near the cementoenamel junction.
- All gingival pockets are suprabony, that is, the base of the pocket is coronal to the crest of the alveolar bone.

II. PERIODONTAL POCKET

- *Definition*: A pocket formed as a result of disease or degeneration that caused the junctional epithelium to migrate apically along the cementum.
- The periodontal deeper structures (attachment apparatus) are involved, that is, the cementum, periodontal ligament, and bone.
- The tooth wall is cementum or partly cementum and partly enamel.
- The base of the pocket is on cementum at the level of attached periodontal tissue.
- Periodontal pockets may be suprabony or intrabony.
  A. *Suprabony:* Pocket in which the base of the pocket is coronal to the crest of the alveolar bone **(Figure 16-1C)**.

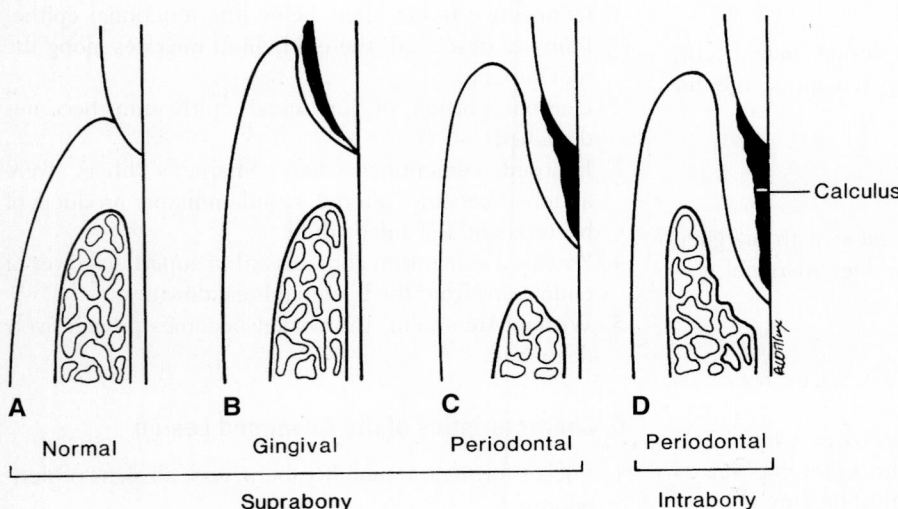

A — Normal
B — Gingival
C — Periodontal
Suprabony
D — Periodontal
Intrabony

Calculus

FIGURE 16-1 Types of Pockets. (A) Normal relationship of the gingival tissue and the cementoenamel junction in a fully erupted tooth. **(B)** Gingival pocket showing attachment at the cementoenamel junction and the pocket formed by enlarged gingival tissue. There is no bone loss. **(C)** Periodontal pocket showing attachment on cementum with root surface exposed. Gingival tissue has enlarged. **(D)** Periodontal intrabony pocket with the bottom of the pocket within the bone. See the text for further description of each type of pocket.

B. *Intrabony*: Pocket in which the base of the pocket is below or apical to the crest of the alveolar bone **(Figure 16-1D)**. "Intra" means located within the bone. The term "infrabony" is used in some texts. "Infra" means under or beneath.

TOOTH SURFACE POCKET WALL

I. TOOTH STRUCTURE INVOLVED

- A sulcus or a pocket has a gingival side, which is the sulcular epithelium, and a tooth side.
- In gingival pockets, the tooth surface wall is enamel, whereas in periodontal pockets, the tooth surface wall is either cementum or a combination of cementum and enamel.
- The positions of the periodontal attachment and the gingival margin determine whether the tooth surface wall is cementum or enamel. Pockets may be the same depth when measured with a probe, but because of the location of the attachment on the tooth surface, the tooth surface pocket wall varies.

II. CONTENTS OF A POCKET

A. Pocket Size

- A pocket is narrow, and the pocket epithelial lining is adjacent to and follows the contour of the tooth.
- When calculus deposits are present, the pocket wall follows the contour of the calculus. The firmness of the free gingiva is influential in confining and shaping the subgingival calculus deposit.
- Access of the opening of the pocket to the oral cavity provides an opportunity for dental biofilm to collect. The deeper the pocket, the less it can be cleaned by toothbrushing or other biofilm control devices.

B. Substances Found in a Pocket

Subgingival biofilm is described in Chapter 19 on page 289. The following may be inside a pocket in contact with the tooth surface on one side and with the surface of the pocket epithelium on the other side:

- *Microorganisms and their products*: enzymes, endotoxins, and other metabolic products.
- Gingival sulcus fluid.
- Desquamated epithelial cells.
- Leukocytes, the numbers of which increase with increased inflammation in the tissues.
- Purulent exudate made up of living and broken down leukocytes, living and dead microorganisms, and serum.

III. NATURE OF THE TOOTH SURFACE

Knowledge of the characteristics and quality of the tooth surface pocket wall is of prime importance in instrumentation. During the examination of the tooth surface with probe and explorer, the various irregularities are differentiated. The manner in which the irregularities came into existence is important for interpretation and understanding.

A. Pocket Development Factors

- The pocket deepens as a result of continuing action of the irritants and destructive agents from dental biofilm.
- The periodontal ligament fibers become detached, and the junctional epithelium migrates apically.
- The cementum becomes exposed to the open pocket and the oral fluids.
- Physical, structural, and chemical changes alter the cementum.
- Surface changes occur as a result of the exchange of minerals with oral fluids and exposure to biofilm bacteria and their products. On different surfaces of the same teeth or different teeth in the same mouth, any of the following can occur[3]:
  - Hypermineralization of the surface cementum
  - Demineralization
  - Calculus formation
  - Dental biofilm and debris collection

B. Tooth Surface Irregularities

- Surface irregularities are detected supragingivally by drying the surface and observing under adequate direct or indirect light; an explorer is used as needed.
- Subgingivally, examination is dependent, for the most part, on tactile and auditory sensitivity transmitted by a probe and an explorer.
- Causes of surface roughness include the following on the enamel surface
  1. Structural defects: cracks and grooves.
  2. Demineralization; cavitated dental caries.
  3. Calculus deposits and heavy stain deposits.
  4. Erosion, abrasion.
  5. Pits and irregularities from hypoplasia.
- Irregularities at the *cementoenamel junction*
  1. Cementum overlaps enamel in 60% to 65% of teeth.
  2. Cementum and enamel meet directly in 30%.
  3. A small zone of dentin may be between the cementum and enamel in 5% to 10%.[4]
  4. The relationships of enamel and cementum at the cementoenamel junction are shown in **Figure 16-2**.

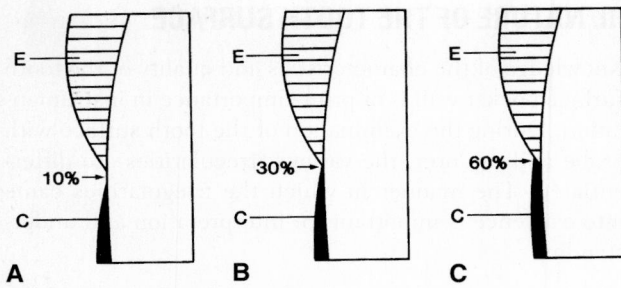

FIGURE 16-2 **Cementoenamel Junction.** The possible relationships of the enamel and the cementum of the cementoenamel junction. **(A)** The cementum and the enamel do not meet and there is a small zone of dentin exposed in 10% of teeth. **(B)** The cementum meets the enamel in approximately 30% of teeth. **(C)** The cementum overlaps the enamel in about 60% of teeth.

- *Root surface* irregularities
    1. Diseased altered cementum
    2. Cemental resorption
    3. Root caries
    4. Abrasion
    5. Calculus
    6. Deficient or overhanging filling
    7. Grooves from previous incomplete instrumentation

COMPLICATIONS OF POCKET FORMATION

I. FURCATION INVOLVEMENT

Furcation involvement means that the clinical attachment level and bone loss have extended into the furcation area, or furca, the area between the roots of a multirooted tooth.

A. Types of Furcations

Furcation involvement is usually classified by the amount of a furcation that has been exposed by periodontal bone destruction.

The four general classes, as shown in **Figure 16-3**, are as follows:

- *Class I*: early, beginning involvement. A probe can enter the furcation area, and the anatomy of the roots on either side can be felt by moving the probe from side to side.
- *Class II*: moderate involvement. Bone has been destroyed to an extent that permits a probe to enter the furcation area but not to pass through between the roots.
- *Class III*: severe involvement. A probe can be passed between the roots through the entire furcation.
- *Class IV*: Same as Class III, with exposure resulting from gingival recession, especially after periodontal therapy.

B. Clinical Observations

1. When the gingiva over the furcation has not receded, the following may be seen:
    - The furcation is covered by the gingival tissue pocket wall.
    - No differences in color, size, or other tissue changes may exist to differentiate the area from adjacent gingiva, but when color changes do exist, they provide clues to supplement probe examination.
2. When the gingiva over a molar buccal furcation is receded, the root division may be seen directly (**Figure 16-3**, Class IV).

C. Detection

A suggested procedure for probing furcations is described on page 232.

II. MUCOGINGIVAL INVOLVEMENT

A pocket that extends to or beyond the mucogingival junction and into the alveolar mucosa is described as *mucogingival involvement*. There is no attached gingiva in the area, and a probe can be passed through the pocket and beyond the mucogingival junction into the alveolar mucosa.

A. Significance of Attached Gingiva

1. *Functions of attached gingiva*
    - Give support to the marginal gingiva.
    - Withstand the frictional stresses of mastication and toothbrushing.

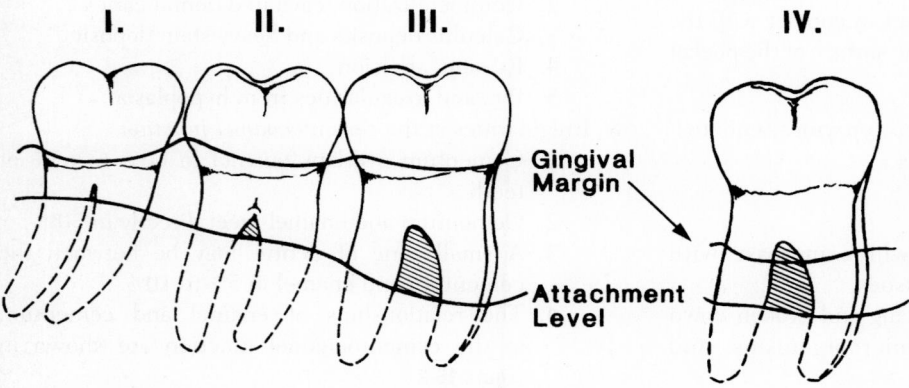

FIGURE 16-3 **Classification of Furcations. (I)** Early, beginning involvement. **(II)** Moderate involvement, in which the furcation can be probed but not through and through. **(III)** Severe involvement, when the bone between the roots is destroyed and a probe can be passed through. **(IV)** Same as III, with clinical exposure resulting from gingival recession.

■ Provide attachment or a solid base for the movable alveolar mucosa for the action of the cheeks, lips, and tongue.

2. *Barrier to passage of inflammation*
   ■ Without attachment, inflammation from a pocket area can extend to the alveolar mucosa.
   ■ The junctional epithelium (epithelial attachment) acts as a barrier to keep infection outside the body.
   ■ With destruction of the connective tissue and periodontal ligament fibers under the junctional epithelium, the epithelium migrates along the root. A pocket is created.
   ■ In mucogingival involvement, the bottom of the pocket extends into the alveolar mucosa. There, the unconfined inflammation can spread more rapidly in the loose connective tissue.

B. Clinical Observations

1. Color changes, tension test, and probe measurements are used during assessment of the mucogingival areas.
2. *Width of attached gingiva:* A narrow zone of gingiva from gingival margin to mucogingival junction, caused by recession or occurring naturally without recession, is more susceptible to developing mucogingival involvement because there is less attached gingiva at the start.
3. *Base of pocket at mucogingival junction:*
   ■ When the probe measures only 1 to 2 mm and there is no bleeding on probing, but the tip of the probe is at the mucogingival junction, the area is recorded and reevaluated at each successive maintenance review.
   ■ A patient with such an area needs specific instruction in biofilm control procedures for preventive maintenance.
4. When an area of minimal attached gingiva (1 to 2 mm) is placed under stress by restorative, prosthetic, or orthodontic treatment procedures, an assessment is made of the need for periodontal treatment to increase the zone of attached gingiva.

LOCAL CONTRIBUTING FACTORS IN DISEASE DEVELOPMENT

■ Dental biofilm is the primary etiologic factor in the development of gingival and periodontal diseases. A variety of other factors predispose some patients to the retention of bacterial deposits and hence to the development of disease in the soft tissues.
■ Factors described in this section relate to dental biofilm retention. Although loose debris can be cleared away by self-cleansing, dental biofilm adheres firmly to the tooth surface and cannot be removed completely by self-cleansing.
■ Retentive areas relate to rough surfaces of teeth and restorations, tooth contour and position, and gingival size, shape, and position.

■ Iatrogenic causes, that is, factors created by professionals during patient treatment or neglect of treatment, are significant.
■ Factors, such as mastication, saliva, the tongue, cheeks, lips, oral habits, and personal biofilm control procedures, contribute.
■ The patient's study casts can be especially useful for observing the physical factors. Irregularities, contour, position, malocclusion, and contact areas of the teeth, as well as features of the gingiva, may be partially or wholly noted. Problem areas can be explained to the patient by demonstration on the study casts. Changes in the patient's habits and daily personal care routine can be encouraged.

I. FACTORS INVOLVED

Complicating and risk factors for disease development may be etiologic, predisposing, or contributing. They are delineated as follows:

■ *Etiologic factor:* a factor that is the actual cause of a disease or condition.
■ *Predisposing factor:* a factor that renders a person susceptible to a disease or condition.
■ *Contributing factor:* a factor that lends assistance to, supplements, or adds to a condition or disease.
■ *Risk factor:* an exposure that increases the probability that disease will occur.

Etiologic, predisposing, and contributing factors may be local or systemic, defined as follows:

■ *Local factor:* a factor in the immediate environment of the oral cavity or specifically in the environment of the teeth or periodontium.
■ *Systemic factor:* a factor that results from or is influenced by a general physical or mental disease or condition.

II. DENTAL FACTORS

A. Tooth Surface Irregularities

Pellicle and biofilm microorganisms attach to defective or rough surfaces, including the following:

■ Pits, grooves, cracks
■ Calculus
■ Exposed altered cementum with irregularities
■ Demineralization and cavitated dental caries
■ Iatrogenic
   ■ Rough or grooved surfaces left after scaling
   ■ Inadequately contoured and polished dental restorations **(Figure 16-4B)**

B. Tooth Contour

Altered shape may interfere with self-cleansing mechanisms and make personal care procedures difficult.

- *Congenital abnormalities*
  A. Extra or missing cusps
  B. Bell-shaped crown with prominent facial and lingual contours tends to provide deeper retentive area in cervical third.
- Teeth with flattened proximal surfaces have faulty contact with adjacent teeth, thus permitting debris to wedge between.
- Occlusal and incisal surfaces altered by attrition interrupt normal excursion of food during chewing. Marginal ridges have worn down.
- Areas of erosion and abrasion
- Carious lesions
- Heavy calculus deposits; biofilm retained on rough surface.
- Overcontoured and undercontoured restorations

C. Tooth Position

- *Malocclusion:* Irregular alignment of a single tooth or groups of teeth leaves areas conducive to collection of microorganisms for biofilm formation.
  - Crowded or overlapped
  - Rotated
  - Deep anterior overbite (Figure 18-10, page 275).
    - Mandibular teeth force food particles against maxillary lingual surface.
    - Lingual inclination of mandibular teeth allows maxillary teeth to force food particles against mandibular facial gingiva.
- Tooth adjacent to edentulous area may be inclined or migrated; contact missing.
- Opposing tooth missing; tooth may extrude beyond the line of occlusion.
- *Related to eruption*
  - Incomplete eruption: below line of occlusion
  - Partially erupted impacted third molar
- Lack of function or use of teeth eliminates or decreases effectiveness of natural cleansing.
  - Lack of opposing teeth
  - Open bite
  - Marked maxillary anterior protrusion

- Crossbite with limited lateral excursion
- Unilateral chewing
- *Food impaction*
  - Created by the combined effect of tooth contour, missing proximal contact, proximal carious lesions, irregular marginal ridge relationship.
  - Inclination related to loss of adjacent tooth, and a plunger cusp from the opposite arch **(Figure 16-4A)**
- *Defective contact area*
  - Restoration margin is faulty, and the contact area is missing, improperly located, or unnaturally wide **(Figure 16-4B)**.
  - Inclined tooth with irregular marginal ridge relation **(Figure 16-4C)**.

D. Dental Prostheses

- Orthodontic appliances provide retentive areas.
- Fixed partial denture with deficient margin of an abutment tooth or an unusually shaped pontic.
- Removable partial denture with inadequately adapted clasps.

III. GINGIVA

A. Position

Deviations from normal provide retentive areas for biofilm.

- *Receded:* depressed area is left at cementoenamel junction.
- *Enlarged:* extended to or over the height of contour.
- Reduced height of interdental papilla leaves open interdental area.
- Tissue flap over occlusal surface of erupting tooth.
- Periodontal pocket
  - Free gingiva cannot adhere to tooth.
  - Shape of pocket conducive to dental biofilm collection.
  - Depth of pocket not available to toothbrush and cleaning aids.
  - Calculus provides rough retentive surface.

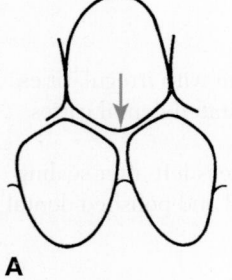 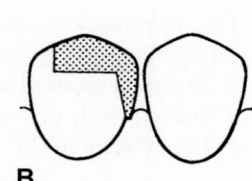 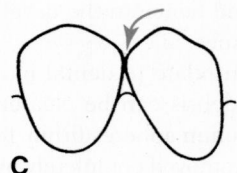 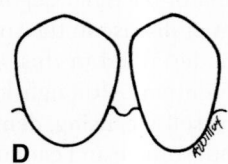

FIGURE 16-4 Effect of Tooth Position. (A) Food impaction area, shown by plunger cusp (*with arrow*) directing pressure between lower teeth with open contact area. **(B)** Inadequate restoration without proximal contact and with overhang. **(C)** Tipped tooth leaving irregular marginal ridge relation. **(D)** Natural open contact (diastema) with saddle-shaped gingival margin.

B. Size and Contour

- Deviation of shape of enlarged gingiva: rolled, bulbous, cratered.
- Combination with presence of irregular restorations or dental prosthesis can result in marked biofilm retention.

C. Effect of Mouth Breathing

Dehydration of oral tissues in anterior region leads to changes in size, shape, surface texture, and consistency.

IV. OTHER FACTORS

A variety of factors may predispose or contribute to the progression of periodontal infections. Some of the items listed here may have an indirect effect, whereas others have a direct effect on the oral tissues.

A. Personal Oral Care

- *Neglect:* Neglect can lead to generalized dental biofilm accumulation and disease promotion.
- *Faulty biofilm control techniques:* Incorrect use of brush, abrasive dentifrice, and the effects of other harmful, detrimental procedures are described in Chapter 27 on page 457.
- *Awareness of oral cleanliness:* Cleansing habits, including both self-cleansing mechanisms and mechanical biofilm removal, depend in part on an individual's perception and feeling of debris through taste and tongue activity.

B. Diet and Eating Habits

- Soft foods tend to adhere more than fibrous, firm foods.
- Cariogenic food selection.
- Masticatory deficiencies limit diet selection. Missing teeth, ill-fitting partial dentures, and various occlusal deficiencies alter diet selection and eating habits.

SELF-CLEANSING MECHANISMS

The teeth, by their anatomy, alignment, and occlusion, function with the gingiva, tongue, cheeks, and saliva in a relationship called the self-cleansing mechanism of the oral cavity. A summary of the natural self-cleansing mechanisms during and following mastication is included here.

The following steps are described for food particles, but the same processes apply to any substances that enter the mouth and influence oral cleanliness and the formation of deposits on the teeth.

I. FOOD ENTERS THE MOUTH

Food is carried by the tongue, assisted by the lips and cheeks, to the occlusal surfaces for grinding.

- Salivary flow increases as a result of sensory reflex stimulation.
- Saliva begins lubrication of food and oral tissues.

II. THE TEETH ARE BROUGHT TOGETHER FOR CHEWING

The food moves over the occlusal surfaces.

- Marginal ridges tend to force particles toward occlusal surfaces, away from the proximal region.
- Contact areas prevent interdental entrance.

III. FOOD IS FORCED OUT BY PRESSURE OF BITE

Food passes over the smooth facial and lingual surfaces.

- Embrasures provide spillways for the escape of particles.
- Cervical enamel ridges deflect particles away from the free gingiva onto the attached gingiva.
- Gingival crest prevents retention of particles by its position at a point below the height of contour of the cervical enamel ridge, by its knife-edge shape, and by its close adherence to the tooth surface.
- Interdental papilla fills the interproximal area and prevents particles from entering.

IV. FOOD PARTICLES ARE BROUGHT BACK BY THE TONGUE TO THE OCCLUSAL SURFACES FOR ADDITIONAL CHEWING

The process is repeated until the food is ready for swallowing.

- Salivary flow continues to be stimulated by repeated masticatory movements.
- Saliva moistens food and oral mucosa and thus reduces the adhering capacity of the food.

V. FOOD PARTICLES REMAINING ON THE TEETH ARE REMOVED

- Tip of tongue explores and attempts to dislodge remaining particles.
- Lips and cheeks in conjunction with tongue aid in natural rinsing process by forcing saliva over and between the teeth.
- Saliva continues to flow in increased amounts during rinsing and swallowing of particles, then gradually returns to its normal flow.

RISK FACTORS FOR PERIODONTAL DISEASES

- Identification of risk factors for periodontal diseases can provide significant insight for the assessment and care planning for an individual patient.

- The various periodontal pathogenic microorganisms do not affect all people with the same degree of severity. It is clear that host factors play a significant role.
- Certain risk factors are related to lifestyle, habits, treatable systemic diseases, and other controllable factors.
- Factors derived from genetic predisposition, congenital immunodeficiencies, or other systemic conditions require a greater effort for the control of periodontal problems.

I. EFFECT OF CERTAIN DRUGS

Medications for specific systemic conditions can lead to gingival enlargement.[5,6] The enlarged tissue encourages dental biofilm retention, thus increasing the potential for periodontal infections.

- *Phenytoin-induced gingival enlargement:* Phenytoin is a drug used to control seizures.
- *Cyclosporine-induced gingival enlargement:* Cyclosporine is an immunosuppressant drug used for patients with organ transplants to prevent rejection.
- *Nifedipine-induced gingival enlargement:* Nifedipine is used in the treatment of angina and ventricular arrhythmias.

II. TOBACCO

- Use of tobacco, any form, is a major risk factor for periodontal involvement.

- Smokers, especially cigarette users, have increased bone loss. An association between periodontal disease and all forms of tobacco use has been shown.[7,8]
- Users of smokeless tobacco products experience oral effects, including predisposition to oral cancer. Periodontal lesions with severe recession and root exposure occur where the quid is held.[9]

III. DIABETES[10]

- Increased susceptibility to periodontal infections.
- Periodontal treatment improves the metabolic control of diabetes, as described in Chapter 68 (page 1029).
- Patient with well-controlled diabetes and healthy periodontal tissues is not at greater risk for susceptibility to infections, including periodontal.

IV. OTHER SYSTEMIC CONDITIONS

A. Osteoporosis[11]

Many risk factors for osteoporosis are also risk factors for periodontitis, including cigarette smoking, nutritional deficiencies, corticosteroid use, and immune dysfunction.

- Greater periodontal attachment loss in patients with osteoporosis.
- Loss of alveolar bone results from osteopenia.

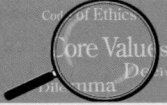 # Everyday Ethics

Basic records for Gloria, who was new to the office, were completed at a previous appointment. On her medical history form, Gloria had written "early diabetes" but did not supply the name and phone number of her current physician and said that she would bring it the next time. There were no radiographs taken at the initial appointment because Gloria said she had full x-rays taken less than a year ago and she would request them from her previous dentist. As she rushed out of office, Gloria made her dental hygiene appointment for one week later during her lunch hour from work.

Gloria arrived late for her scheduled appointment and said she had to be back at work in less than 1 hour. Tina, the dental hygienist, asked if she had eaten and she hadn't; Tina hesitated knowing that a basic rule about patients with diabetes is to make sure that they have eaten prior to the dental appointment. The care plan that had been developed for Gloria included 4 quadrants of scaling and root planing with anesthesia because of the significant amount of calculus and the fact that some periodontal pockets were deep enough to bleed and be sensitive; but Gloria refused the anesthesia. She also stated that her dental hygiene maintenance appointment should only take one hour for whole mouth as it had with the dental hygienist at her previous dental office.

Tina felt that there were so many wrong things about the whole situation: the radiographs had not yet arrived from the other dentist; Dr. Nedham had not been in the office that week and had not yet approved the complete treatment plan; and the short time the patient was allowing for Tina to complete a moderately heavy scaling without anesthesia was questionable. Tina told Gloria that the appointment should be rescheduled for another day, but Gloria insisted that her dental hygiene maintenance care be completed at this appointment. Tina was barely able to remove all of the calculus completely as possible from one quadrant, without providing any personal care instruction, before Gloria got out of the chair and rushed off.

Questions for Consideration

1. Which of the dental hygiene core values have application in this scenario? Explain how each of the ones selected apply.
2. Is this situation either an ethical issue or a dilemma for Tina? Explain your answer.
3. Use the questions in Table V-1 (Section V Introduction, page 362) to determine what different actions Tina could have taken at this appointment and to plan what she can do next regarding future planning for Gloria's dental hygiene care.

B. Psychosocial Factors

■ Higher levels of social strain are found in patients with periodontal infections.[12]

■ Stress is considered a factor in the etiology of necrotizing ulcerative gingivitis.

DOCUMENTATION

Documentation for a patient with need for periodontal therapy includes at least the following in the patient's permanent record along with radiographs, physician's approvals for therapy, and other correspondence of record.

■ Initially a complete history : medical, dental, former periodontal therapy, current symptoms and current complaint or problem, and clinical examination with charting of periodontal findings, and of the teeth; summary of prognosis and diagnosis.

■ At each appointment a complete record of treatment accomplished, and patient instruction, oral findings and changes on the way to health.

■ A sample progress note may be reviewed in **Box 16-2**.

BOX 16-2	Example Progress Note

New patient (Ms. Box) arrived late for first quadrant scaling/root planing with anesthesia. Refused anesthesia. Started brief instruction in recommended personal daily care but patient said she "knew all that." It was apparent that Ms. Box had not had this type of treatment; calculus was very hard and difficult to remove. Explained to her that next appointment I would recheck this area and advised very thorough brushing and flossing at least twice but better also at noon or chew xylitol gum after lunch. She wanted a name for a good mouthrinse, and I advised plain fluoridated water for now until we see the response when we finish the other quadrants.

Signed: _____, RDH Date: _____

Factors To Teach The Patient

■ What a pocket is and how it forms.
■ How a pocket is measured with a probe and that, until the sulci and pockets are probed, it is not possible to tell whether disease is present and how far it has progressed. Probing depth must be checked regularly all around every tooth to be sure nothing is developing insidiously.
■ Factors that contribute to disease development and progression.
■ What a risk factor is and the importance of planning personal and professional care to include risk factor problems.

References

1. Newman MG, Takei HH, Klokkevold PR, Carranza FA. *Clinical periodontology.* 10th ed. St. Louis: Saunders; 2006. Chapter 21, Gingival inflammation; p. 355–61.
2. Weinmann JP. Progress of gingival inflammation into the supporting structures of the teeth. *J Periodontol.* 1941 Jul;12:71.
3. Selvig KA. Biological changes at the tooth-saliva interface in periodontal disease. *J Dent Res.* 1969 Sep–Oct;48(5):846–55.
4. Bhaskar SN, editor. *Orban's oral histology and embryology.* 11th ed. St. Louis: Mosby; 1991. p. 192.
5. Fattore L, Stablein M, Bredfeldt G, Semla T, Moran M, Doherty-Greenberg JM. Gingival hyperplasia: a side effect of nifedipine and diltiazem. *Spec Care Dentist.* 1991 May–Jun;11(3):107–09.
6. Payne JB. The facts about gingival hyperplasia. *Dent Teamwork.* 1992 Sep–Oct;5(5):22–4.
7. Akef J, Weine FS, Weissman DP. The role of smoking in the progression of periodontal disease: a literature review. *Compendium.* 1992 Jun;13(6):526, 528–31.
8. Haber J, Wattles J, Crowley M, Mandell R, Joshipura K, Kent RL. Evidence for cigarette smoking as a major risk factor for periodontitis. *J Periodontol.* 1993 Jan;64(1):16–23.
9. Johnson R, Herzog A. Oral effects of smokeless tobacco use. *Dent Hyg.* 1987 Aug;61(8):354–59.
10. American Academy of Periodontology, Committee on Research, Science and Therapy. Position paper: diabetes and periodontal diseases. *J Periodontol.* 1999 Aug;70(8):935–49.
11. Wactawski-Wende J, Grossi SG, Trevisan M, Genco RJ, Tezal M, Dunford RG, Ho AW, Hausman E, Hreshchyshyn MM. The role of osteopenia in oral bone loss and periodontal disease. *J Periodontol.* 1996 Oct;67(10 Suppl):1076–84.
12. Moss ME, Beck JD, Kaplan BH, Offenbacher S, Weintraub JA, Koch GG, Genco RJ, Machtei EE, Tedesco LA. Exploratory case-control analysis of psychosocial factors and adult periodontitis. *J Periodontol.* 1996 Oct;67(10 Suppl):1060–69.

The Teeth

ESTHER M. WILKINS, BS, RDH, DMD

Chapter Outline

Clinical examination and assessment of the teeth is essential before treatment to provide guidelines for treatment planning, instrumentation, instruction, and follow-up evaluation.

■ In general, patients may tend to be more concerned about their teeth than about the periodontium, the supporting structures that maintain the teeth in their positions.

■ The reasons may be related to personal appearance; level of knowledge, which may be greater about teeth than about gingiva; and sensitivity and pain associated with ailments of the teeth they may have experienced.

BOX 17-1	Key Words

Teeth

Accessory root canal: a secondary canal extending from the pulp to the surface of the root; frequently found near the apex of a root but may occur higher and provide a connection to a periodontal pocket.

Amelogenesis: production and development of enamel.

Avulsion: the tearing away or forcible separation of a structure or part. Tooth avulsion is the traumatic separation of a tooth from the alveolus.

Bruxism: an oral habit of grinding, clenching, or clamping the teeth; involuntary, rhythmic, or spasmodic movements outside the chewing range; may damage teeth and attachment apparatus.

Cariogenic: adj. conducive to dental caries.

Carious: adj. used to define a carious lesion.

Cementicle: a calcified spherical body, composed of cementum, lying free within the periodontal ligament, attached to the cementum or imbedded within the cementum.

Dental caries: disease of the mineralized structures of the teeth characterized by demineralization of the hard components and dissolution of the organic matrix.

> **Arrested caries:** carious lesion that has become stationary and does not show a tendency to progress further; frequently has a hard surface and takes on a dark brown or reddish-brown color.
>
> **Primary caries:** occurs on a surface not previously affected; also called initial caries; early lesion may be referred to as incipient caries.
>
> **Rampant caries:** widespread formation of chalky white areas and incipient lesions that may increase in size over a comparatively short time.
>
> **Recurrent caries:** occurs on a surface adjacent to a restoration; may be a continuation of the original lesion; also called secondary caries.

Dentition: the natural teeth in the dental arch.

> **Primary (deciduous) dentition:** the first teeth; normally will be shed and replaced by permanent teeth.

Permanent dentition: the natural 32 teeth that serve throughout life.

Mixed dentition: combination of primary and permanent teeth between ages 6 and 12 when primary teeth are being replaced; starts with the eruption of the first permanent tooth.

Succedaneous: the permanent teeth that erupt into the positions of exfoliated primary teeth.

Edentulous: without teeth; referred to as partially edentulous when some, but not all, teeth are missing.

Electrolyte: a conductor; a substance that, in solution, dissociates into electrically charged particles (ions) and thus is capable of conducting an electric current.

Etiology: the science or study of the cause of a disease or disorder.

Exfoliation: loss of primary teeth following physiologic resorption of root structure.

Facet: a small flattened surface on a hard body, such as a tooth; a wear facet can result from attrition or repeated parafunctional contact.

Hypoplasia: incomplete development or underdevelopment of a tissue or organ.

> **Enamel hypoplasia:** incomplete or defective formation of the enamel of either primary or permanent teeth. The result may be an irregularity of tooth form, color, or surface.

Idiopathic: denoting a condition of unknown cause.

Incipient: beginning; coming into existence.

pH: the symbol of hydrogen ion concentration expressed in numbers corresponding to the acidity or alkalinity of an aqueous solution; the range is from 14 (pure base) to 0 (pure acid); neutral is at 7.0.

> **Critical pH:** the pH at which demineralization occurs; for enamel, pH 4.5 to 5.5; for cementum, pH 6.0 to 6.7.

Resorption: removal of bone or tooth structure; gradual dissolution of the mineralized tissue; may be internal or external; occurs during exfoliation of a primary tooth and from the pressure of orthodontic treatment.

- Background study of dental anatomy, oral histology, and oral pathology is essential to this phase of clinical practice.
- Key words are defined in **Box 17-1**.

THE DENTITIONS

The three divisions are the primary dentition, the mixed dentition, and the permanent dentition.

I. Primary Dentition
   A. Formation of the primary teeth begins *in utero.*
   B. Table 49-6 (page 761) shows the weeks *in utero* when each primary tooth begins to mineralize and the average months after birth when the enamel is completely formed before the date of eruption.

II. Mixed Dentition
   A. The mixed dentition, when primary teeth are being exfoliated and permanent teeth move in to take their places, occurs between the ages of 6 and 12 years.
   B. **Figure 17-1** illustrates the mixed dentition of a child approximately 6 years of age just before the permanent teeth start to erupt.

III. Permanent Dentition
   A. Mineralization of the permanent teeth starts at birth and continues into adolescence. The chronology of development and eruption of the permanent teeth appears in **Table 17-1**.
   B. Roots normally are completed by 3 years after eruption.

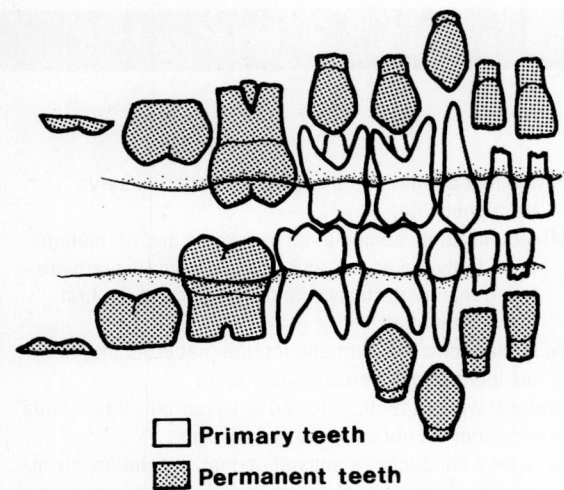

☐ Primary teeth
▦ Permanent teeth

FIGURE 17-1 **Mixed Dentition at Approximately Age 6 Years.** The average child has 20 primary teeth in place, and root resorption of the incisors has started as the developing permanent incisors move into position. The first permanent molars are partially erupted.

DEVELOPMENTAL AND NONCARIOUS DENTAL LESIONS

ENAMEL HYPOPLASIA

Enamel hypoplasia is a defect that occurs as a result of a disturbance in the formation of the organic enamel matrix.

I. TYPES AND ETIOLOGY

A. Hereditary

Enamel is partly or wholly missing. An example is amelogenesis imperfecta, described in Chapter 21 on page 310.

B. Systemic (Environmental)

Factors that may contribute to enamel hypoplasia during tooth development include severe nutritional deficiency, particularly rickets; fever-producing diseases, such as measles, chickenpox, and scarlet fever; congenital syphilis; hypoparathyroidism; birth injury; prematurity; Rh hemolytic disease; fluorosis.

C. Local

A single tooth can be affected; trauma or periapical inflammation about a primary tooth can injure the adjacent developing permanent tooth.

II. APPEARANCE

A. Hereditary

The teeth may appear brown.

B. Systemic

Also called "chronologic hypoplasia" because the lesions are found in areas of those teeth where the enamel was forming during the systemic disturbance.

TABLE 17-1	TOOTH DEVELOPMENT AND ERUPTION: PERMANENT TEETH				
		HARD TISSUE FORMATION BEGINS	**ENAMEL COMPLETED (YEARS)**	**ERUPTION (YEARS)**	**ROOT COMPLETED (YEARS)**
Maxillary	Central incisor	3–4 mo	4–5	7–8	10
	Lateral incisor	10 mo	4–5	8–9	11
	Canine	4–5 mo	6–7	11–12	13–15
	First premolar	1 1/2–1 3/4 y	5–6	10–11	12–13
	Second premolar	2–2 1/4 y	6–7	10–12	12–14
	First molar	at birth	2 1/2–3	6–7	9–10
	Second molar	2 1/2–3 y	7–8	12–13	14–16
	Third molar	7–9 y	12–16	17–21	18–25
Mandibular	Central incisor	3–4 mo	4–5	6–7	9
	Lateral incisor	3–4 mo	4–5	7–8	10
	Canine	4–5 mo	6–7	9–10	12–14
	First premolar	1 3/4–2 yr	5–6	10–12	12–13
	Second premolar	2 1/4–2 1/2 yr	6–7	11–12	13–14
	First molar	at birth	2 1/2–3	6–7	9–10
	Second molar	2 1/2–3 yr	7–8	11–13	14–15
	Third molar	8–10 yr	12–16	17–21	18–25

Source: Logan WH, Kronfield R. Development of the human jaws and surrounding structures from birth to age fifteen. *JADA.* 1933 or 35;20:379–424; Orban B. Oral histology and embryology. St. Louis: Mosby; 1944. Schour I, McCall JO. Chronology of the human dentition. p. 240.

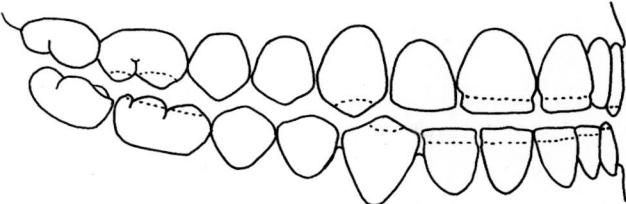

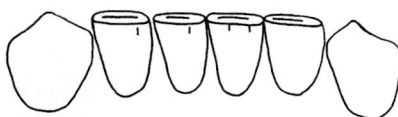

FIGURE 17-4 Attrition. Attrition of the incisal surfaces of mandibular anterior teeth has extended to expose the dentin. Dentin usually appears as a brown line or ring.

FIGURE 17-2 Enamel Hypoplasia. Chronologic hypoplasia, usually in the form of grooves or pits, appears in the enamel at a level corresponding with the stage of development of the teeth. For this patient, the disturbance in enamel development occurred at approximately 10 months of age.

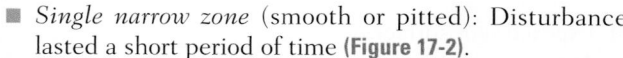

B. Age Factor

Increases with age (but not because of age) as bruxism continues over time. More attrition is seen in men than in women of comparable age.

II. ETIOLOGY

A. Bruxism

Predisposing factors may be psychological, tension, or occlusal interferences.

B. Usage

Wear of surfaces on each other. Predisposing factors may be coarse foods, chewing tobacco, culturally related chewing habits, or abrasive dusts associated with certain occupations.

III. APPEARANCE

A. Initial Lesion

Small polished facet on a cusp tip or ridge, or slight flattening of an incisal edge.

B. Advanced

Gradual reduction in cusp height; flattening of incisal or occlusal plane **(Figure 17-4)**.

C. Staining of Exposed Dentin

Discoloration may occur; stain usually is brown.

D. Radiographic

The pulp chamber and canals may be narrowed and sometimes obliterated as the result of formation of secondary dentin.

- *Single narrow zone* (smooth or pitted): Disturbance lasted a short period of time **(Figure 17-2)**.
- *Multiple:* Disturbance to the ameloblast occurred over a period of time, or several times.
- *Teeth most frequently affected:* First molars, incisors, canines, because the disturbances generally occur during the first year when those teeth are mineralizing.

C. Hypoplasia of Congenital Syphilis

- Transmission of syphilis from mother to fetus after the 16th week of pregnancy may alter the development of the tooth germs.
- **Figure 17-3** illustrates tooth forms that may result. The mesiodistal width may be reduced, and incisors are frequently narrowed at the incisal third.

D. Local Enamel Hypoplasia

A single tooth with a yellow or brown intrinsic stain.

ATTRITION

Attrition is the wearing away of a tooth as a result of tooth-to-tooth contact **(Figure 17-4)**.

I. OCCURRENCE

A. Location

May be found on occlusal, incisal, and proximal surfaces.

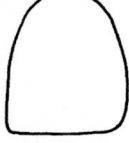
Normal

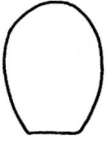
Screwdriver Notched
Hutchinson's incisors

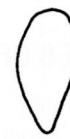
Peg
lateral

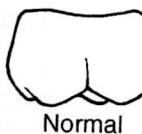
Normal

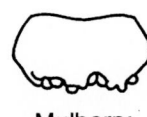
Mulberry
molar

FIGURE 17-3 Crown Forms of Enamel Hypoplasia. Hutchinson's incisors and mulberry molars are typical crown forms that result from congenital syphilis. The central incisors are narrowed at the incisal third, and the lateral incisors may be conical or peg-shaped.

EROSION

Erosion is the loss of tooth substance by a chemical process that does not involve known bacterial action.

I. OCCURRENCE

A. Location

Facial or lingual surfaces, depending on cause.

B. Usually Involves Several Teeth

II. ETIOLOGY

The lesions are caused by some form of chemical dissolution.

A. Chronic Vomiting

Acid of chronic vomiting affects lingual surfaces, particularly anterior teeth.

- Pregnancy.
- Eating disorder, such as bulimia as described in Chapter 63 (page 962).

B. Extrinsic

- *Industrial:* Workers' teeth can be exposed to atmospheric acids.
- *Dietary:* Facial surfaces are more frequently affected.
- Carbonated beverages.
- Lemons or other citrus fruit sucked frequently.

C. May Be Idiopathic (Unknown)

III. APPEARANCE

- Smooth, shallow, hard, shiny (in contrast to dental caries, in which appearance is soft and discolored).
- Shape varies from shallow saucerlike depressions to deep wedge-shaped grooves; margins are not sharply demarcated.
- May progress to involve the dentin and stimulate secondary dentin.
- May occur in combination with dental caries, calculus, or dental restorations.[1]

ABRASION

Abrasion is the mechanical wearing away of tooth substance by forces other than mastication.

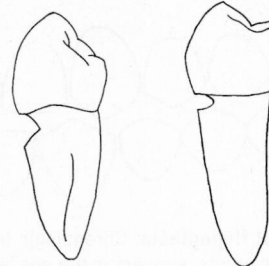

FIGURE 17-5 Abrasion. Profile view of the facial surface of mandibular premolars shows shape of abrasion on the root. Note that the area of abrasion undermines the enamel.

I. OCCURRENCE

- Exposed root surfaces.
- At incisal edge or on occlusal surface.

II. ETIOLOGY

- The lesion originates from a mechanical abrasive activity.
- The action of microorganisms is not essential for the development of abrasion. Dental caries may occur in the abraded area as a secondary lesion.
- *Abrasive agent:* A common cause is an abrasive dentifrice applied with vigorous horizontal toothbrushing. **Figure 17-5** shows the effect on the root surface.
- *Occupational causes:* These include, for example, tacks held by carpenters, pins by dressmakers.
- Pipe held between teeth; may be held in the same place over many years.

III. APPEARANCE

- V- or wedge-shaped with hard, smooth, shiny surface and clearly defined margins.
- Except for incisal biting habits, the lesions occur initially on exposed cementum, then extend into the dentin.

FRACTURES OF THE TEETH

- Trauma to the face may involve fractured bones and teeth in addition to soft tissue injuries. Fractured jaw and methods of treatment are described in Chapter 69 on page 1081.
- Emergency care for a forcibly displaced tooth is found in Table 69-5 on page 1081.

I. CAUSES OF TOOTH FRACTURES

- Automobile, bicycle, and diving accidents
- Contact sports when mouth protectors are not worn
- Blows incurred while fighting
- Falls

II. DESCRIPTION

A. Line of Fracture

■ May be horizontal, diagonal, or vertical
■ **Figure 17-6** illustrates fractures of a central incisor

B. Radiographic Signs of Recent Trauma

■ Widened periodontal ligament space
■ Radiolucent fracture line
■ Radiopaque areas where fracture segments overlap
■ Tooth displacement

III. CLASSIFICATION: WORLD HEALTH ORGANIZATION[12]

Classification provided by the World Health Organization is numbered as a special section of the *International Classification of Diseases*. Both primary and permanent dentitions are included. **Figure 17-6** illustrates fractures of a central incisor.

873.60 Fracture of enamel of tooth only. Includes chipping and incomplete fractures (cracks).

873.61 Fracture of crown of tooth without pulpal involvement.

873.62 Fracture of crown with pulpal involvement.

873.63 Fracture of root of tooth.

873.64 Fracture of crown and root of tooth with or without pulpal involvement.

873.65 Fracture of tooth, unspecified.

873.66 Luxation (dislocation) of tooth. This category may involve concussion, subluxation, and luxation. A tooth with concussion is sensitive to percussion but is not loosened or displaced. Loosening without displacement is subluxation, and loosening with displacement is luxation.

873.67 Intrusion or extrusion of tooth. Intrusion into the alveolar bone is usually accompanied by fracture of the alveolar socket. Extrusion from the socket is a partial displacement.

873.68 Avulsion of tooth. Avulsion is the complete displacement of the tooth out of its socket.

Emergency care for a tooth forcibly displaced is found in Table 69-5, page 1081.

DENTAL CARIES

The World Health Organization has defined dental caries as a "localized, posteruptive, pathologic process of external origin involving softening of the hard tooth tissue and proceeding to the formation of a cavity."[2] Dental caries is a preventable disease.

I. DEVELOPMENT OF DENTAL CARIES

Requirements for the development of a carious lesion are microorganisms, carbohydrate, and a susceptible tooth surface. Figure 34-4 (page 506) is a diagram that shows four overlapping circles to illustrate the essential factors in dental caries initiation.

■ Dental biofilm may contain numerous types of acid-forming bacteria. Mutans steptococcus in the initiation and lactobacillus in the progression of the lesion have been specifically implicated.
■ The role of dental biofilm and the many factors involved are described on page 291.

II. CLASSIFICATION

A. G.V. Black's Classification[4]

■ The standard method for classifying dental caries was developed by Dr. G.V. Black, a noted dental educator who divided the categories into classes according to surfaces of the teeth; each class is represented by a Roman numeral.
■ The categories customarily are used for carious lesions, cavity preparations, and finished restorations. **Figure 17-7** defines and illustrates the classifications.

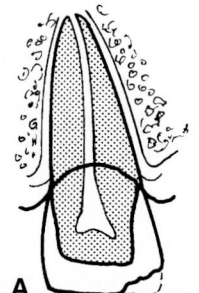 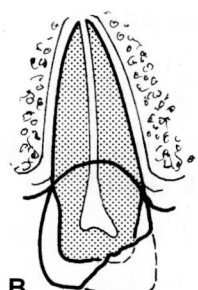 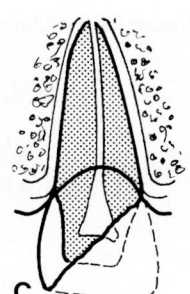 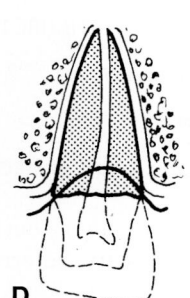 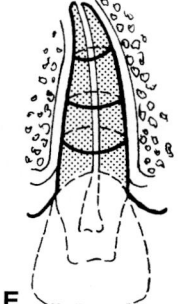

FIGURE 17-6 **Fractures of Teeth. (A)** Enamel fracture. **(B)** Crown fracture without pulpal involvement. **(C)** Crown fracture with pulpal involvement. **(D)** Fracture of crown and root near neck of tooth. **(E)** Root fractures involving cementum, dentin, and the pulp may occur in the apical, middle, or coronal third of the root.

CLASSIFICATION: LOCATION	APPEARANCE	METHOD OF EXAMINATION
Class I. Cavities in pits or fissures a. Occlusal surfaces of premolars and molars b. Facial and lingual surfaces of molars c. Lingual surfaces of maxillary incisors	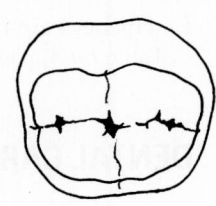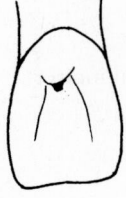	Direct or indirect visual Radiographs not useful
Class II. Cavities in proximal surfaces of premolars and molars	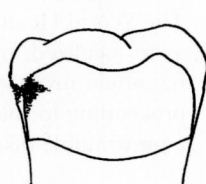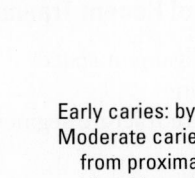	Early caries: by radiographs only Moderate caries not broken through from proximal to occlusal: Visual by color changes in tooth and loss of translucency Extensive caries involving occlusal: direct visual

Class III.
Cavities in proximal surfaces of incisors and canines that do not involve the incisal angle
	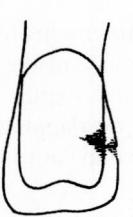	Early caries: by radiographs or transillumination
		Moderate caries not broken through to lingual or facial:
		  1. Visual by tooth color change
		  2. Radiograph
		Extensive caries; direct visual

Class IV. Cavities in proximal surfaces of incisors or canines that involve the incisal angle	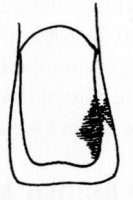	Visual Transillumination
Class V. Cavities in the cervical 1/3 of facial or lingual surfaces (not pit or fissure)	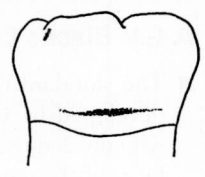	Direct visual: dry surface for vision Dull probe to distinguish demineralization: whether rough or hard and unbroken Areas may be sensitive to touch
Class VI. Cavities on incisal edges of anterior teeth and cusp tips of posterior teeth	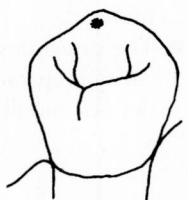	Direct visual May be discolored

FIGURE 17-7 Dental Caries: Classification of Cavities.

B. Nomenclature by Surfaces

- *Simple cavity:* involves one tooth surface. Example: occlusal cavity.
- *Compound cavity:* involves two tooth surfaces. Example: mesio-occlusal cavity, referred to as an "M-O" cavity.
- *Complex cavity:* involves more than two tooth surfaces. Example: mesio-occlusal-distal, referred to as an "M-O-D" cavity.

ENAMEL CARIES

I. STEPS IN THE FORMATION OF A CARIOUS LESION

A. Phase I: Incipient Lesion

- *Subsurface demineralization:* Acid products from cariogenic dental biofilm pass through microchannels (pores) from the surface of the enamel to the subsurface area in the dentin.

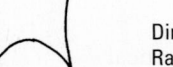

■ *Visualization:* The area of demineralization is not visible by clinical observation during initial changes; a thin layer of enamel remains over the surface.

■ *First clinical evidence:* White area appears with no breakthrough to enamel surface; with time, area may turn brown from food, beverages, or tobacco use.

■ *Remineralization:* Low concentrations of fluoride applied frequently during the early phase can provide sources for uptake by the demineralized zone. The porous demineralized area readily takes up fluoride from dentifrice, mouthrinse, fluoridated drinking water, and all possible sources.

■ Figure 35-3 (page 521) shows examples of levels of concentration of fluoride in surface enamel and in a white demineralized area.

B. Phase II: Untreated Incipient Lesion

■ *Breakdown of enamel over the demineralized area:* Visible to observation and irregular to the gentle application of the side of an explorer tip or blunt probe.

■ *Progression of carious lesion:* Follows general direction of enamel rods.

■ *Spread of carious lesion:* Spreads at dentinoenamel junction; continues along the dentinal tubules (Figure 17-8).

II. TYPES OF DENTAL CARIES (DESCRIBED BY LOCATION)

A. Pit and Fissure

■ Caries begins in a minute fault in the enamel.

■ Pit or fissure irregularity occurs where three or more lobes of the developing tooth join; closure of the enamel plates is imperfect. Examples: occlusal pits of molars and premolars.

■ Occurs at the endings of grooves of the teeth. Example: the buccal groove of a mandibular molar.

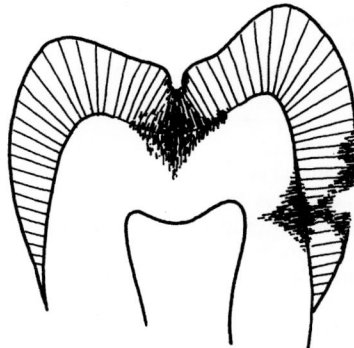

FIGURE 17-8 **Dental Caries.** Cones of dental caries in a pit and fissure and on a smooth tooth surface. Dental caries follows the general direction of the enamel rods, spreads at the dentinoenamel junction, and then continues along the dentinal tubules.

B. Smooth Surface

■ Caries begins in smooth surfaces where there is no pit, groove, or other fault.

■ It occurs in areas where dental biofilm is protected from removal, such as proximal tooth surfaces, protected near a contact area, cervical thirds of teeth, and other difficult-to-clean areas.

EARLY CHILDHOOD CARIES[5,6]

■ Early childhood caries (ECC) is a form of caries found in very young children. Common causes are the routine use of a nursing bottle (with milk or sweetened beverage) when going to sleep or prolonged at-will breast-feeding. More information about ECC is located in Chapter 49 (page 768).

■ Other names for the same condition are nursing bottle mouth, baby bottle syndrome, baby bottle caries, and prolonged nursing habit.

I. ETIOLOGY

A. Microbiology

■ High levels of *Mutans streptococci* have been cultured from the saliva and dental biofilm from the teeth of children with early childhood caries.[7,8]

■ *Lactobacilli* also are found in large numbers in the biofilm.

B. Risk Factors

■ Teaching the parents about the cause and effects of early childhood caries is a significant part of anticipatory guidance, as shown in Tables 49-1 and 49-2 (pages 756–757).

■ Significant risk factors include the nursing bottle that contains sweetened milk or other fluid sweetened with sucrose; the pacifier dipped or filled with a sweet agent, such as honey; and prolonged at-will breast-feeding. Early childhood caries risk factors are listed in Table 49-9 on page 764.

II. EFFECTS

■ Maxillary anterior teeth and primary molars are the first to be affected (Figure 49-6, page 768).

■ As the baby falls asleep, pools of sweet liquid can collect about the teeth. While the sucking is active, the liquid passes beyond the teeth.

■ The nipple covers the mandibular anterior teeth; hence, they are rarely affected.

III. RECOGNITION

■ Children need to be seen for an examination no later than 6 months after eruption of the first tooth.[9]

TABLE 17-2	EXAMINATION OF THE TEETH

FEATURE	TO OBSERVE	DENTAL HYGIENE IMPLICATION
Morphology	Number of teeth (missing teeth verified by radiographic examination) Size, shape Arch form Position of individual teeth Injuries: fractures of the crown (root fractures observed in radiographs)	Selection and adaptation of instruments Areas prone to dental caries initiation, particularly the difficult-to-reach areas during biofilm control Pulp test for vitality may be indicated
Development	Anomalies and developmental defects Pits and white spots	Distinguish hypoplasia and dental fluorosis from demineralization Identify pits for sealants
Eruption (Table 17-1)	Sequence of eruption: normal, irregular Unerupted teeth observed in radiographs	Care in using floss in the col area where the epithelium is usually less mature in young children Orthodontic needs Procedures for preservation of primary teeth
Deposits (Table 17-1) **Food debris** **Biofilm** **Calculus** **Supragingival** **Subgingival**	Overall evaluation of self-care and biofilm-control measures Relation of appearance of teeth to gingival health Extent and location of biofilm, debris, and calculus Calculus and the tooth surface pocket wall	Need for instruction and guidance Frequency of follow-up and maintenance appointments
Stains **(pages 306 to 310)** **Extrinsic** **Intrinsic**	Extrinsic: colors relate to causes Intrinsic: dark, grayish Tobacco stain	Need for test for pulp vitality Stain removal procedures; selection of polishing agent Dentifrice recommendation Biofilm-control emphasis for biofilm-related stains Provide information concerning the oral effects of tobacco use Tobacco cessation program (page 489)
Regressive Changes	Attrition: primary and permanent Abrasion: physical agents that may be a cause Erosion	Evaluate causes and treat or counsel for prevention Dietary analysis: for finding foods that may be related Selection of nonabrasive dentifrice Habit evaluation
Exposed Cementum	Relation to gingival recession, pocket formation Areas of narrow attached gingiva Hypersensitivity	Special care areas where only slight attached gingiva remains Nonabrasive dentifrice advised Measures to prevent root-surface caries Care during instrumentation Indication for application of desensitizing agent
Dental Caries	Areas of demineralization Stages of carious lesions Proximal lesions observed in radiographs Arrested caries Root caries	Charting Treatment plan Cavitated vs. Noncavitated Preventive program for caries control, fluoride, dietary factors Follow-up and frequency of maintenance
Restorations	Contour of restorations, overhangs Proximal contact (see separate heading later in this table) Surface smoothness Staining	Chart and correct inadequate margins Selection of instruments and polishing agents Dentifrice selection to prevent discoloration

(continued)

TABLE 17-2	EXAMINATION OF THE TEETH (Continued)	
FEATURE	**TO OBSERVE**	**DENTAL HYGIENE IMPLICATION**
Factors Related to Occlusion	Health of supporting structures; observation of radiographs for signs of trauma from occlusion	Need for study of bruxism and other parafunctional habits
Tooth Wear	Facets; worn-down cusp tips	Chart inadequate contacts for corrective measures
Proximal Contacts	Use of floss to find open contact areas Areas of food retention	Use of floss by patient
Mobility	Degree; comparison of chartings Possible causes	Need for reduction of inflammatory factors that may be related Dentist will identify and treat factors related to trauma from occlusion
Classification	Position of teeth Angle's classification	Relationship to orthodontic treatment needs
Habits	Nail or object biting; lip or cheek biting Observe effects on lip, cheek, teeth Tongue thrust; reverse swallow	Guidance for habit correction when indicated
Edentulous Areas	Radiographic evaluation for impacted, unerupted teeth, retained root tips, other deviations from normal	Supplemental fulcrum selection during instrumentation Applied biofilm-control procedures for abutment teeth

Replacement for Missing Teeth
    Dentures
    Partial dentures
    Implants
	Teeth and tissue that support a prosthesis
	Cleanliness of a prosthesis
	Factors that contribute to food and debris retention
		Preventive measures for harm to supporting teeth and soft tissues
		Instruction in personal care of fixed and removable dentures; use of floss under fixed partial denture; other appropriate care

Saliva	Amount and consistency Dryness of mouth	Relation to instruction for prevention of dental caries: more caries can be expected in a dry mouth Use of saliva substitute; fluoride

- Demineralization may be noted along the cervical third of the maxillary anterior teeth. The source of the problem may be detected and preventive procedures initiated through parental counseling.
- At a later stage the lesions appear dark brown. Eventually, the crowns may be destroyed to the gingival margin, abscesses may develop, and the child may suffer severe pain and discomfort (Figure 49-3, page 761).

ROOT CARIES

- Root caries is a soft, progressive lesion of cementum and dentin that involves bacterial infection and invasion. It is also called cemental caries, cervical caries, or radicular caries.
- The incidence of root caries increases with age, but not because of age. Gingival recession is necessary for root

caries, and gingival recession is related to periodontal infections that lead to recession.

I. STEPS IN THE FORMATION OF A ROOT SURFACE LESION

- Gingival recession exposes the cemental surface. Caries does not form in the root surface while periodontal fibers are still attached.
- Dental caries starts near the cementoenamel junction. Cementum is thin and is soon destroyed; dentin is invaded.
- Enamel is not involved except by extension or when it is undermined. Root caries occurs in a mildly acidic environment. If the pH were lower, enamel would become carious.
- The critical pH for enamel is 4.5 to 5.0; for cementum, 6.0 to 6.7.[10]

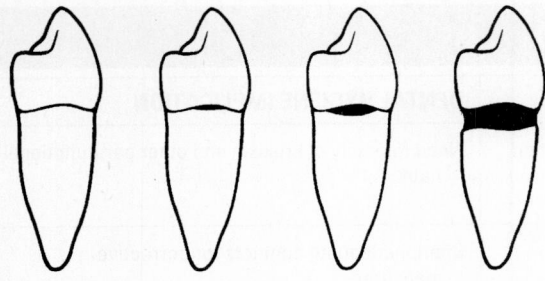

FIGURE 17-9 Root Caries. A root surface lesion starts near the cementoenamel junction after gingival recession has exposed the root surface. The lesion is progressive, undermines the enamel, and may eventually surround the cervical third of the cementum. (*Source:* Banting DW, Courtright PN. Distribution and natural history of carious lesions on the roots of the teeth. *Dent J.* 1975 Jan;41(1):45–9.)

- *M. streptococci* and *lactobacilli* are primary organisms associated with root caries. Antibody levels to *Streptococcus mutans* are elevated.[11,12]

II. EFFECTS

- Low levels of root caries incidence has been shown to be directly related to the fluoride concentration in the drinking water.[13]
- Lifelong residence in a community with near-optimum levels of fluoride in the water was shown to be associated with at least an average 30% decrease in the incidence of root caries compared with that associated with lifelong residence in a nonfluoridated community.[14]

III. CLINICAL RECOGNITION

Root caries cavitated lesions are described as soft, leathery, or hard. Active lesions are soft or leathery, whereas inactive or arrested lesions are hard.

- Soft, shallow, ill-defined lesion.
- Increases laterally to coalesce with other small lesions and eventually may extend completely around the tooth with undermining of the enamel **(Figure 17-9)**.
- Yellowish, light brown, dark brown to black.
- Leathery in texture when explored (active lesion). Do not pick with a sharp explorer when remineralization is taking place; remineralization process can be arrested.
- Arrested root caries displays cavitation and discoloration.

IV. RISK FACTORS FOR ROOT CARIES

Risk factors are shown in **Box 17-2**. Prevention and control of root caries depend on control of risk factors.

| BOX 17-2 | Risk Factors: Root Caries |

- Periodontal infection: Root surfaces exposed
  All factors that contribute to bone loss and attachment loss.
- Microorganisms: Caries-producing; potential transmission
- Local/behavioral
  Inadequate personal hygiene
  Dental biofilm accumulations
  Poor compliance
- Diet: Frequent use of cariogenic foods
- Low fluoride exposure
  Outside fluoridated community water supply
    Insufficient daily self-application (dentifrice, mouthrinse, frequency)
- Xerostomia
  Medications with side effects
  Radiation to head/neck
  Salivary gland dysfunction
- History of dental caries
  Many restorations: coronal and root
  Overhanging margins, open contact areas, and other biofilm traps
  Poor compliance for dental care
- Prosthetic devices
  Inadequate biofilm removal daily
  Overdentures, clasps, provide biofilm-retentive areas
- Tobacco use: sugar content of smokeless tobacco

CLINICAL EXAMINATION OF THE TEETH

I. FACTORS TO OBSERVE

- **Table 17-4** lists factors to observe during the examination of the teeth and suggests relationships to appointment procedures.
- Attention to examination for the stages of dental caries is described on page 379. Careful identification of cavitated versus noncavitated lesions is essential to avoid exploring a remineralizing area.
- Information about hypoplasia, attrition, erosion, abrasion, and other tooth irregularities are recorded for the total patient history.

II. RECOGNITION OF CARIOUS LESIONS

Both visual and exploratory examination with dull probe only are used to identify cavitated and noncavitated lesions.

A. Preparation

- Dry each tooth or group of teeth with compressed; adjust mouth mirror for indirect light and vision.
- Carefully inspect each surface, first visually and then, only when necessary, gently with a blunt explorer as necessary to confirm visual findings (page 379).

■ Avoid using a sharp pointed explorer in a potentially remineralizing area. Review Chapter 26 pages 377 to 385 for complete description.

B. Visual Examination

■ Characteristic changes in the color and translucency of tooth structure may be observed.

■ Changes either are definite signs of dental caries progress or may lead to a suspicion of dental caries, which can then be studied in the radiograph or recorded for future review.

■ Variations in color and translucency include the following:
  ▪ Chalky white areas of demineralization.
  ▪ Grayish-white discoloration of marginal ridges caused by dental caries of the proximal surface underneath.
  ▪ Grayish-white color spreading from margins of restorations.
  ▪ In relation to an amalgam restoration, dental caries may appear translucent in outer portions and white and opaque adjacent to the amalgam.
  ▪ Open carious lesions may vary in color from yellowish brown to dark brown.
  ▪ Discoloration is generally less severe when dental caries progresses rapidly than when it progresses slowly.
  ▪ Dull, flat white, opaque areas under direct light show loss of translucency, particularly of the enamel.
  ▪ Dark shadow on a proximal surface may be shown by transillumination.
  ▪ Transillumination is especially useful for anterior teeth and unrestored posterior teeth.

C. Exploratory Examination

A. Smooth Surface Caries

■ *Technique:* Adapt the side of the tip of the probe or blunt explorer closely to the tooth surface, as described on page 379. Examine for roughness versus smoothness and continuity of tooth surface versus breaks in continuity. *Do not use pressure or break the surface when checking an area that may be remineralizing.*

■ *Restorations:* Follow the margins of all restorations around with an explorer. Overhanging margins may or may not appear in the radiographs, depending on superimposition. Chart all irregularities of existing restorations.

B. Pit and Fissure Caries

■ When a pit or fissure is discolored, one may not determine visually whether dental caries is present.

When the objective is to distinguish the pit for a sealant and the decision is made to place a sealant, the explorer can then be used to clean out the pit of debris in preparation for sealant placement.

■ An obvious cavity does not need to be explored.

III. RADIOGRAPHIC EXAMINATION

■ During the clinical examination, information revealed by radiographs is utilized for supplementation and confirmation.

■ Neither clinical nor radiographic examination is complete without the other. A few principal items to be seen in a radiographic examination of the teeth include: anomalies, impactions, fractures, internal and root resorption, and periapical radiolucencies.

■ *Dental caries:* For coronal caries use a horizontal bitewing survey; for root caries use a vertical bitewing survey.

■ Periodontal radiographic findings are described in Chapter 15 starting on page 240. Vertical bitewing radiographs are needed for evaluation of periodontal bone levels.

■ Panoramic, extraoral, or occlusal radiographs are needed for detecting or defining anomalies and pathologic lesions outside the scope of periapical radiographs.

TESTING FOR PULPAL VITALITY

■ Any tooth suspected of being nonvital needs to be tested for pulpal vitality or degree of vitality.

■ The two basic types of pulp testing are thermal and electric.

■ Diagnosis of vitality is made not only on the basis of a pulp test but also on consideration of all data from the patient history and clinical and radiographic examinations.

I. CAUSES OF LOSS OF VITALITY

■ A tooth may become nonvital from bacterial causes, particularly invasion of the pulp from dental caries or periodontal diseases.

■ Physical causes may be mechanical or thermal injuries. Examples of mechanical injuries are trauma, such as a blow, or iatrogenic dental procedures, such as cavity preparation or too-rapid orthodontic movement.

II. OBSERVATIONS THAT SUGGEST LOSS OF VITALITY

A. Clinical

■ Intrinsic discoloration of a tooth crown (intrinsic stains, page 309).

- Fracture (part of the crown may be missing, **Figure 17-6**).
- Large carious lesion or large restoration.
- Fistula with opening into the oral cavity over the apical region of a tooth.

B. Radiographic

- Apical radiolucency, which may indicate a granuloma, cyst, or abscess.
- Bone loss with a widened periodontal ligament space extending to the apex.
- Fractured root.
- Large carious lesion or restoration that appears closely related to the pulp chamber.

III. RESPONSE TO PULP TESTING

A. Rationale

- Pulp testing is based on the knowledge that a stimulus can create pain to which a patient can react. The pulp tester, therefore, determines the conduction of stimuli to the sensory receptors.
- The vitality of the pulp depends on its blood supply and not on its nerve supply. For that reason, a positive or negative pulp test may not always show the true condition of the pulp.

B. Factors That Influence a Patient's Response to a Pulp Test

- *Degree of pulpal degeneration or inflammation:* A necrotic pulp gives no response at all, whereas an acutely or chronically inflamed pulp responds at varying degrees between no response and full normal response.
- *Pain threshold:* The pain threshold is the lowest intensity of pain caused by a threshold stimulus. A threshold stimulus is the minimum stimulus necessary to induce patient response.
- *Reaction to pain:* May vary with a patient's attitude, age, sex, emotional security, fatigue, drugs used, as well as the size of the pulp and thickness of the dentin, particularly the amount of secondary dentin.
- *Nerve transmission blocks:* injuries or lesions of nerves, and anesthetics.
- *Adjacent metal:* restorations or continuous bridgework.

C. Responses

An electric tester reveals only whether a pulp is vital or nonvital. Using thermal testing may show the following:

- No response: necrotic pulp.

- Lingering pain after removal of stimulus: irreversible pulpitis.
- Pain subsides promptly: reversible pulpitis.

IV. THERMAL PULP TESTING

Cold or hot stimuli may be used. For all methods, a control test is performed on a healthy tooth on the opposite side of the arch. Inform the patient in advance about the procedure and what to expect.

A. Cold Test

- *Materials:* Cold testing may be accomplished with an air blast, cold drink, ice stick, ethyl chloride in a spray or on a cotton swab, or a carbon dioxide dry-ice stick. Isolate the test teeth and dry with a gauze sponge.
- *Preparation of ice stick:* Small icicles may be prepared by freezing water in anesthetic needle covers.
- *Dry-ice stick:* Made from carbon dioxide and delivered using a special holder with a plunger.

B. Heat Test

- *Temporary stopping:* Warm temporary stopping (gutta-percha). Apply to a tooth dried with cotton sponge.
- *Water:* Warm to hot water. Isolate tooth and bathe in very warm water.

V. ELECTRICAL PULP TESTER

A. Types

- *Battery-operated*
  A. Advantages: Hand held so a clinician can work alone; portable.
  B. Disadvantage: Battery can run down. Some types have a light to indicate current in circuit.
- *Plug-in*
  A. Advantage: Is more dependable than battery-operated.
  B. Disadvantage: Is not self-contained; requires house-current plug.
  C. Newer models have grounding connection for patient to hold.

B. Precaution

- The application of an electrical current to a patient with a cardiac pacemaker or any electronic life-support device by the use of a pulp tester, ultrasonic scaler, desensitizing equipment, or electrosurgical instrument may interfere with the function of the life-support device and may constitute a serious health hazard.[15]

- A review of the patient history and consultation with the patient's cardiologist are necessary before application of a pulp tester.

C. Preparation and Use of Equipment

- Manufacturer's instructions are provided for each pulp tester and are followed carefully. When the tester rheostat is separate from the applicator tip, an assistant is needed.
- Consistency of procedures is essential to obtain consistent readings. The same pulp tester is used for a particular patient at continuing comparative tests. Notes in a patient's record can indicate specific directions for that patient.

D. General Procedures

- Assemble equipment.
- Explain briefly to the patient what is to be done, but avoid detailed description, which could create anxiety or apprehension.
- Dry the teeth to be tested to prevent the current from passing to the gingiva; isolate with cotton rolls and insert a saliva ejector, or use a rubber dam.
- Moisten the end of the tip of the tester with a small amount of toothpaste. Another electrolyte (conductor) may be used if its consistency allows it to remain where placed and prevents it from flowing over the tooth surface.
- Instruct the patient to signal when a sensation is felt; suggest raising a hand or making a sound.
- Apply tester tip. The patient lightly holds the handle to complete the circuit.
- Apply first to at least one tooth other than the one in question, preferably an adjacent tooth and the same tooth on the contralateral side. Such a procedure determines a normal response for the patient.
- Place *without pressure* but with definite contact on sound tooth structure in a consistent location on the middle or gingival third. The middle third of the crown of a single-rooted tooth and the middle third of each cusp of a multirooted tooth are frequently used **(Figure 17-10)**.

E. Readings

- Avoid contact with gingival or other soft tissues. A low-resistance circuit can be formed, thus allowing the circuit to by-pass the tooth.
- Avoid contact with metallic restorations. The metal forms a more rapid conductor than does tooth structure. When approximal restorations are in contact, the circuit can be transmitted across to the adjacent tooth. The reading obtained would not pertain to the tooth in question

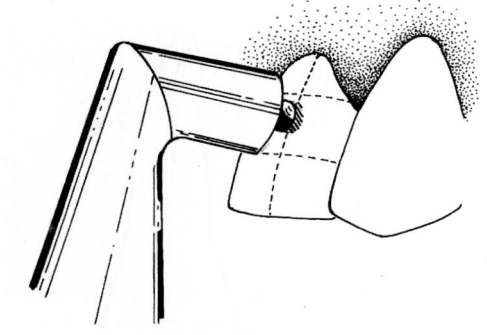

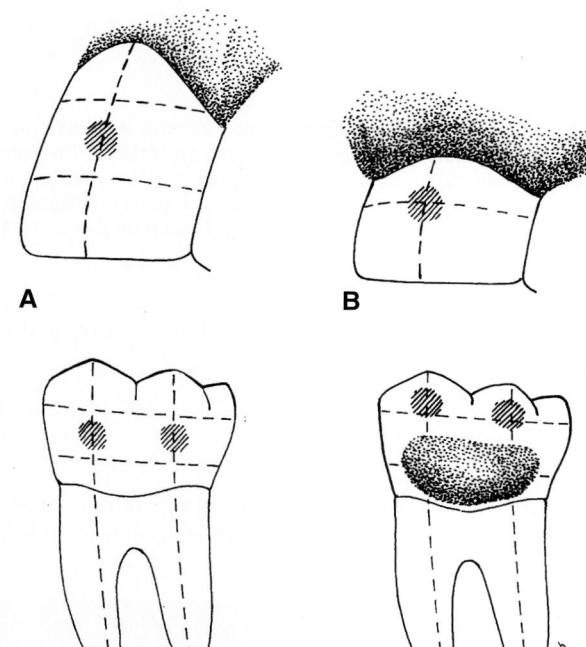

FIGURE 17-10 Pulp Tester in Position. (A) Correct contact point for tip of pulp tester is within the middle third of the crown. Avoid contact with gingiva or restorations. **(B)** Adjustment of position of contact point because of gingival enlargement. **(C)** Contact points on multirooted tooth. Place tip of pulp tester in the middle third over each root. **(D)** Adjustment of position of contact points because of large Class V restoration.

(Figure 17-11). A nonconductive clear plastic matrix strip may be inserted to separate the two metallic restorations.
- Test each tooth at least twice. Average the readings.
- Record on patient's record the average number at which a minimal stimulus induced a response. Record for all teeth tested, not only the tooth in question.

F. Reasons for False-Negative Responses[15]

- Patient premedicated with analgesics, tranquilizers, narcotics, or alcohol.
- Recently traumatized tooth.
- Pulp canal narrow and calcified.

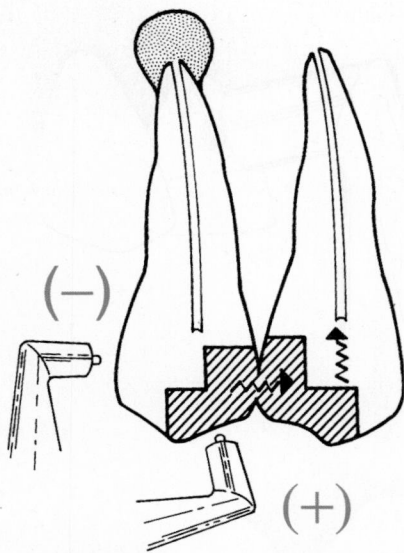

FIGURE 17-11 **Use of Pulp Tester.** False-positive response can result when the tester is placed on a metallic restoration. The current can be transmitted across a contact area to give a reading for the adjacent tooth rather than for the tooth in question. (*Source:* Antel J, Christie WJ. Electrical pulp testing. *J Can Dent Assoc.* 1979 Nov;45(11):597–600.)

- Newly erupted tooth with incomplete closure at the apex; immature tooth.

DOCUMENTATION

The official permanent records of a patient who requires treatment of individual teeth needs at least the following included:

- Patient histories reviewed in total at least every year, but questioned at each maintenance appointment; complete oral radiographic survey with the initial examination and repeated at intervals in keeping with treatment planning.
- Emphasis in each entry of the patient's efforts in biofilm control and diet to lessen the potential for new dental caries activity.
- A sample progress note is included in **Box 17-3**.

BOX 17-3	**Sample Progress Note**

Patient maintenance appt rather routine. Vitals no changes; intra-extraoral exam tissue clear except for cheekbite left side near molars; dental exam found 3 new small carious lesions. Introduced a Cambra-like plan with emphasis only on the snacks and especially pop drinks which Joyce said she did use a lot of; brief review of sugary rinses too often, (could she use a glass of nice fluoridated water, etc; tried to be careful that I didn't sound critical, or dump too much on at one time) Asked if she would fill out a questionnaire for me (the risk factor questionnaire) saying I really would like to help prevent so many new cavities. She ended up with "I thought everyone has cavities every time they go to the dentist." But she seemed sincerely interested.

Signed:_____, RDH Date:_____.

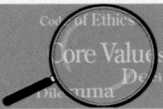 **Everyday Ethics**

Barbara, the dental hygienist, has just finished a thorough review of oral hygiene instruction with Mrs. Canavan when she is called out of the treatment room. In today's examination, Barbara had charted two possible carious lesions that will need to be restored. Barbara wanted Mrs. Canavan to realize all the things she could do to prevent dental caries. Her 9-year-old daughter, Millie, had several restorations today at her appointment with the dentist in another treatment room, had finished first, and was waiting for her mom.

When Barbara returned she could overhear Mrs. Canavan talking with her daughter and explaining how she got all the cavities. She described biofilm as painful and how "that's what happens when you eat a lot of candy and drink a lot of soft drinks instead of milk." Barbara stopped to watch quietly. Apparently Millie seemed to understand that it is the biofilm that causes all her cavities, but she was not getting accurate information on the mechanism of action. Mrs. Canavan seemed to be threatening her daughter.

Questions for Consideration

1. Which of the core values (Table II-1, in Section II Introduction, page 38) of dental hygiene are in effect in this situation? Would it be ethical for Barbara to join the conversation and attempt to clarify for both of them? How could she help them both understand the real prevention plan?
2. Describe the positive and negative effects that may occur if Barbara corrects the mother in front of the daughter, or instead, if she asks the daughter to go back to the reception room, and then tries to discuss daily biofilm removal and food selection again with Mrs. Canavan.
3. Using the questions of Table V-1 in Section V (page 362) what alternative approaches will Barbara be able to use to help Mrs. Canavan understand the daily personal needs for prevention of carious lesions?

Factors To Teach The Patient

- The cause and process of enamel or root caries formation and development for the patient at risk.
- A description of the hardness of the enamel and of why a cavity in a tooth crown is sometimes larger in the dentin before there is evidence from the external surface.
- Why radiographs are needed to detect proximal incipient caries.
- Reasons for preservation of primary teeth.
- Frequency of complete oral examination in relation to a continuing preventive program.
- Preventive measures for control and prevention of tooth abrasion, such as dentifrice selection and correction of brush selection and use.
- Dietary factors related to erosion.
- Methods for prevention of dental caries, such as fluorides, biofilm prevention and control, and control of cariogenic foods in the diet.
- Methods for prevention of early childhood caries. Nothing but plain water is used in bedtime or naptime nursing bottles. Avoid the use of a sweetener on a pacifier.
- Medicines or vitamin preparations made with heavy syrup (sucrose) have been shown to cause dental caries. Parents must learn to clean (rinse, not brush) children's teeth after sugar exposures.[16]
- Discuss accident prevention procedures, such as always wearing a mouthguard for contact sports and wearing seat belts.

References

1. Sognnaes RF, Wolcott RB, Xhonga FA. Dental erosion. 1. Erosion-like patterns occurring in association with other dental conditions. *J Am Dent Assoc.* 1972 Mar;84(3):571–576.

2. World Health Organization. Application of the International Classification of Diseases to dentistry and stomatology. 2nd ed. ICD-DA. 1978:88–89.

3. World Health Organization. The etiology and prevention of dental caries. *World Health Organ Tech Rep Ser.* 1972;494:1–19.

4. Blackwell RE. *G.V. Black's operative dentistry.* Volume 2. 9th ed. Milwaukee: Medico-Dental Publishing Co.; 1955. pp. 1–4.

5. Ripa LW. Nursing caries: a comprehensive review. *Pediatr Dent.* 1988;10(4):268–82.

6. Brice DM, Blum JR, Steinberg BJ. The etiology, treatment, and prevention of nursing caries. *Compend Cont Educ Dent.* 1996 Jan;17(1):92, 94:96–8.

7. Van Houte J, Gibbs G, Butera C. Oral flora of children with "nursing bottle caries." *J Dent Res.* 1982 Feb;61(2):382–5.

8. Berkowitz RJ, Turner J, Hughes C. Microbial characteristics of the human dental caries associated with prolonged bottle-feeding. *Arch Oral Biol.* 1984;29(11):949–51.

9. American Academy of Pediatric Dentistry. Oral health policies. *Pediatr Dent.* 1998 Nov;20(6):22–5.

10. Hoppenbrouwers PM, Driessens FC, Borggreven JM. The mineral solubility of human tooth roots. *Arch Oral Biol.* 1987;32(5):319–22.

11. van Houte J, Lopman J, Kent R. The predominant cultivable flora of sound and carious human root surfaces. *J Dent Res.* 1994 Nov;73(11):1727–34.

12. Zambon JJ, Kasprzak SA. The microbiology and histopathology of human root caries. *Am J Dent.* 1995 Dec;8(6):323–8.

13. Burt BA, Ismail AI, Eklund SA. Root caries in an optimally fluoridated and a high-fluoride community. *J Dent Res.* 1986 Sep;65(9):1154–8.

14. Stamm JW, Banting DW, Imrey PB. Adult root caries survey of two similar communities with contrasting natural water fluoride levels. *J Am Dent Assoc.* 1990 Feb;120(2):143–9.

15. Sognnaes RF, Wolcott RB, Xhonga FA. Dental erosion. 1. Erosion-like patterns occurring in association with other dental conditions. *J Am Dent Assoc.* 1972 Mar;84(3):571–6.

16. World Health Organization. Application of the International Classification of Diseases to dentistry and stomatology. 2nd ed. ICD-DA. 1978:88–9.

17. Cohen S, Burns RC, editors. *Pathways of the pulp.* 7th ed. St. Louis: Mosby; 1998. Chapter 1, Diagnostic procedures; pp. 13–4.

18. Rekola M. In vivo acid production from medicines in syrup form. *Caries Res.* 1989 Nov–Dec;23(6):412–16.

The Occlusion

ESTHER M. WILKINS, BS, RDH, DMD

Chapter Outline

Occlusion is the relationship of the teeth in the mandibular arch to those in the maxillary arch as they are brought together. The occlusion is examined and recorded as part of the oral examination. Knowledge of the occlusion of each patient can contribute significantly to complete care and instruction. Recognition of malocclusion assists in the referral of patients to the orthodontist, gives many valuable points of reference for patient instruction, and determines necessary adaptations in techniques. **Box 18-1** defines key words relating to occlusion and occlusal factors.

Recognizing a patient's occlusion and understanding the oral health problems of malocclusion can aid in accomplishing the following:

■ Providing information for the comprehensive assessment and planning dental hygiene care.
■ Planning personalized instruction in relation to such factors as oral habits, masticatory efficiency, personal oral care procedures, and predisposing factors to dental and periodontal infections.
■ Adapting techniques of instrumentation to malpositioned teeth or groups of teeth.
■ Planning the frequency of maintenance appointments for professional care on the basis of deposit retention areas, particularly those that are difficult to reach in routine personal care.
■ Providing the general features of malocclusion to consider when orthodontic referral is discussed with the patient.

BOX 18-1	**Key Words**

Occlusion

Ankylosis: union or consolidation of two similar or dissimilar hard tissues previously adjacent but not attached.

Dental ankylosis: rigid fixation of a tooth to the surrounding alveolus as a result of ossification of the periodontal ligament; prevents eruption and orthodontic movement.

Centric occlusion: the maximum intercuspation or contact of the teeth of the opposing arches; also called habitual occlusion.

Centric relation: the most unstrained, retruded physiologic relation of the mandible to the maxilla from which lateral movements can be made.

Cephalometer: an orienting device for positioning the head for radiographic examination and measurement.

Cephalometric analysis: the process of evaluating dental and skeletal relationships by way of measurements obtained directly from the head or from cephalometric radiographs and tracings made from the radiographs.

Cephalostat: a head-holding instrument used to obtain cephalometric radiographs; head is held in a precisely defined position relative to the film and to the central ray of the x-ray source.

Diastema: a space between two adjacent teeth in the same arch.

Facet: A facet is a shiny, flat, worn spot on the surface of a tooth, frequently on the side of a cusp.

Occlusal guard: a removable dental appliance usually made of plastic that covers a dental arch and is designed to minimize the damaging effects of bruxism and other oral habits; also called bite guard, mouth guard, or night guard.

Occlusal prematurity: any contact of opposing teeth that occurs before the desirable intercuspation.

Orthodontic and dentofacial orthopedics: the specialty area of dentistry concerned with the diagnosis, supervision, guidance, and treatment of the growing and mature dentofacial structures; includes conditions that require movement of teeth and the treatment of malrelationships and malformations of the craniofacial complex.

Orthopedics: correction of abnormal form or relationship of bone structures; may be accomplished surgically (orthopedic surgery) or by the application of appliances to stimulate changes in the bone structure through natural physiologic response (orthopedic therapy); orthodontic therapy is orthopedic therapy.

Parafunctional: abnormal or deviated function, as in bruxism.

Pathologic migration: the movement of a tooth out of its natural position as a result of periodontal infection; contrasts with mesial migration, which is the physiologic process maintained by tooth proximal contacts in the normal dental arches.

Tongue thrust: the infantile pattern of suckle-swallow movement in which the tongue is placed between the incisor teeth or alveolar ridges; may result in an anterior open bite, deformation of the jaws, and abnormal function.

Trauma from occlusion: injury to the periodontium that results from occlusal forces in excess of the reparative capacity of the attachment apparatus; also called occlusal traumatism.

STATIC OCCLUSION

Static occlusal relationships are seen when the jaws are closed in centric occlusion. The static occlusion can be efficiently observed in occluded study casts and seen directly in the oral cavity when the lips and cheeks are retracted. Classification of malocclusion and the variations that occur with each category are described here.

I. NORMAL (IDEAL) OCCLUSION

The ideal mechanical relationship between the teeth of the maxillary arch and the teeth of the mandibular arch is as follows:

A. All teeth in the maxillary arch are in maximum contact with all teeth in the mandibular arch in a definite pattern.

B. Maxillary teeth slightly overlap mandibular teeth on the facial surfaces.

II. MALOCCLUSION

Any deviation from the physiologically acceptable relationship of the maxillary arch and/or teeth to the mandibular arch and/or teeth.

III. TYPES OF FACIAL PROFILES (FIGURE 18-1)

A. Mesognathic

Having slightly protruded jaws, which give the facial outline a relatively flat appearance (straight profile).

B. Retrognathic

Having a prominent maxilla and a mandible posterior to its normal relationship (convex profile).

C. Prognathic

Having a prominent, protruded mandible and normal (usually) maxilla (concave profile).

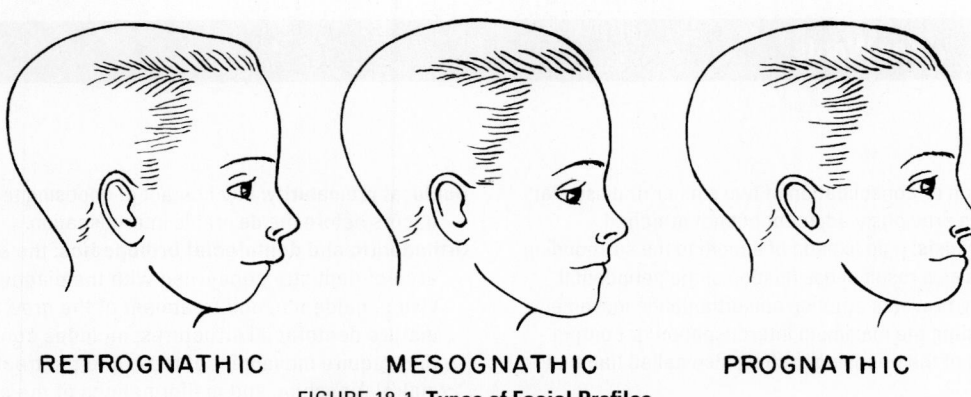

RETROGNATHIC   MESOGNATHIC   PROGNATHIC

FIGURE 18-1 **Types of Facial Profiles.**

IV. MALRELATIONS OF GROUPS OF TEETH

A. Crossbites

■ *Posterior.* Maxillary or mandibular posterior teeth are either facial or lingual to their normal position. This condition may occur bilaterally or unilaterally (**Figure 18-2**).
■ *Anterior.* Maxillary incisors are lingual to the mandibular incisors (**Figure 18-3**).

B. Edge-to-Edge Bite

Incisal surfaces of maxillary teeth occlude with incisal surfaces of mandibular teeth instead of overlapping as in normal occlusion (**Figure 18-4**).

C. End-to-End Bite

Molars and premolars occlude cusp-to-cusp as viewed mesiodistally (**Figure 18-5**).

D. Open Bite

Lack of occlusal or incisal contact between certain maxillary and mandibular teeth because either or both have failed to reach the line of occlusion. The teeth cannot be brought together, and a space remains as a result of the arching of the line of occlusion (**Figure 18-6**).

E. Overjet

The horizontal distance between the labioincisal surfaces of the mandibular incisors and the linguoincisal surfaces

of the maxillary incisors (**Figure 18-7**). One way to measure the amount of overjet is to place the tip of a probe on the labial surface of the mandibular incisor and, holding it horizontally against the incisal edge of the maxillary tooth, read the distance in millimeters.

F. Underjet

Maxillary teeth are lingual to mandibular teeth. Measurable horizontal distance between the labioincisal surfaces of the maxillary incisors and the linguoincisal surfaces of the mandibular incisors (**Figure 18-8**).

G. Overbite

Overbite, or vertical overlap, is the vertical distance by which the maxillary incisors overlap the mandibular incisors.

■ *Normal overbite:* An overbite is considered normal when the incisal edges of the maxillary teeth are within the incisal third of the mandibular teeth, as shown in **Figure 18-9** in side view and in **Figure 18-11A** in anterior view.
■ *Moderate overbite:* An overbite is considered moderate when the incisal edges of the maxillary teeth appear within the middle third of the mandibular teeth (**Figure 18-11B**).
■ *Deep (severe) overbite*
   A. Deep (severe): When the incisal edges of the maxillary teeth are within the cervical third of the mandibular teeth (**Figure 18-11C**).
   B. Very deep: When in addition the incisal edges of the mandibular teeth are in contact with the maxillary

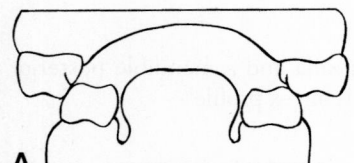 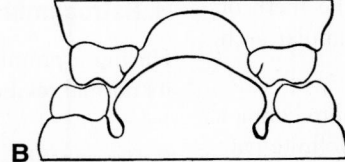 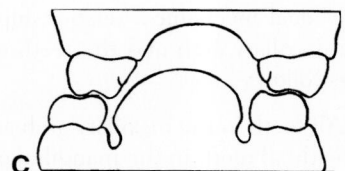

A   B   C

FIGURE 18-2 **Posterior Crossbite. (A)** Mandibular teeth lingual to normal position. **(B)** Mandibular teeth facial to normal position. **(C)** Unilateral crossbite: right side, normal; left side, mandibular teeth facial to normal position.

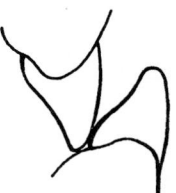

FIGURE 18-3 **Anterior Crossbite.** Maxillary anterior teeth are lingual to mandibular anterior teeth. Anterior crossbite occurs in Angle's Class III malocclusion.

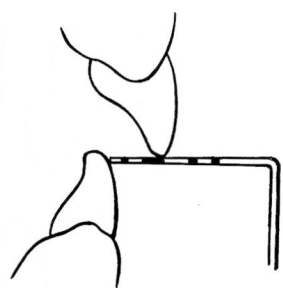

FIGURE 18-7 **Overjet.** Maxillary incisors are labial to the mandibular incisors. Measurable horizontal distance is evident between the incisal edge of the maxillary incisors and the incisal edge of the mandibular incisors. A periodontal probe can be used to measure for recording the distance.

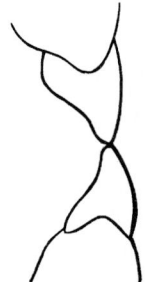

FIGURE 18-4 **Edge-to-Edge Bite.** Incisal surfaces occlude.

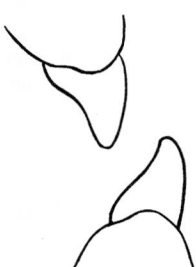

FIGURE 18-8 **Underjet.** Maxillary incisors are lingual to the mandibular incisors. Measurable horizontal distance is evident between the incisal edges of the maxillary incisors and the incisal edges of the mandibular incisors.

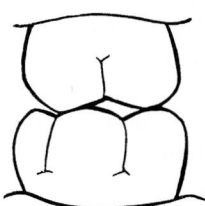

FIGURE 18-5 **End-to-End Bite.** Molars in cusp-to-cusp occlusion as viewed from the facial.

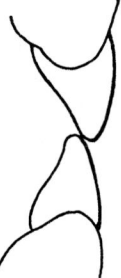

FIGURE 18-9 **Normal Overbite.** Profile view to show the position of the incisal edge of the maxillary tooth within the incisal third of the facial surface of the mandibular incisor.

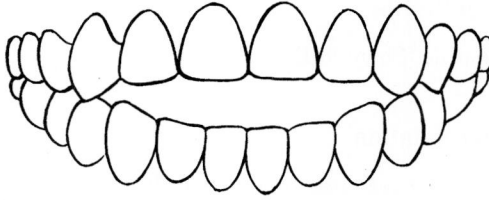

FIGURE 18-6 **Open Bite.** Lack of incisal contact. Posterior teeth in normal occlusion.

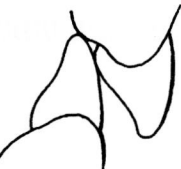

FIGURE 18-10 **Deep (Severe) Anterior Overbite.** Incisal edge of the maxillary tooth is at the level of the cervical third of the facial surface of the mandibular anterior tooth. See the facial view in Figure 18-11C.

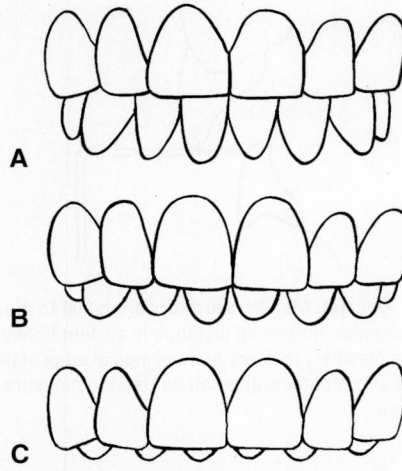

FIGURE 18-11 Overbite, Anterior View. (A) Normal overbite: incisal edges of the maxillary teeth are within the incisal third of the facial surfaces of the mandibular teeth. **(B)** Moderate overbite: incisal edges of maxillary teeth are within the middle third of the facial surfaces of the mandibular teeth. **(C)** Severe overbite: the incisal edges of the maxillary teeth are within the cervical third of the facial of the mandibular teeth. When the incisal edges of the mandibular teeth are in contact with the maxillary lingual gingival tissue, the overbite is considered very severe. See the profile view in Figure 18-10.

lingual gingival tissue. A side view of very deep over-bite is shown in **Figure 18-10**.

■ *Clinical examination of overbite*
1. Direct observation: With the posterior teeth closed together, the lips can be retracted and the teeth observed, as in **Figure 18-11**. The degree of anterior overbite is judged by the position of the incisal edge of the maxillary teeth:
   A. Normal (slight), within the incisal third of the mandibular incisors **(Figure 18-11A)**.
   B. Moderate overbite, within the middle third **(Figure 18-11B)**.
   C. Severe overbite, within the cervical third **(Figure 18-11C)**.
2. Mirror view: By placing a mouth mirror under the incisal edge of the maxillary teeth, one can sometimes see the mandibular teeth in contact with the maxillary palatal gingiva. When contact is not visible, an examination of the lingual gingiva may reveal teeth prints or at least enlargement and redness from the contact.

V. MALPOSITIONS OF INDIVIDUAL TEETH

A. Labioversion

A tooth that has assumed a position labial to normal.

B. Linguoversion

Position lingual to normal.

C. Buccoversion

Position buccal to normal.

D. Supraversion

Elongated above the line of occlusion.

E. Torsiversion

Turned or rotated.

F. Infraversion

Depressed below the line of occlusion, for example, primary tooth that is submerged or ankylosed.

DETERMINATION OF THE CLASSIFICATION OF MALOCCLUSION

The determination of the classification of occlusion is based on the principles of Edward H. Angle, presented in the early 1900s. He defined normal occlusion as "the normal relations of the occlusal inclined planes of the teeth when the jaws are closed"[1] and based his system of classification on the relationship of the first permanent molars.

■ Although authorities have since agreed that the maxillary first permanent molars do not occupy a fixed position in the dental arch, Angle's system serves to provide an acceptable basis for a useful classification.
■ A more comprehensive picture of malocclusion is made by the orthodontist, who studies the relationships of the position of the teeth to the jaws, the face, and the skull.
■ Three general classes of malocclusion are described in the following sections. These classes are designated by Roman numerals.
■ Because the mandible is movable and the maxilla is stationary, the classes describe the relationship of the mandible to the maxilla. For example, in distoclusion (Class II) the mandible is distal, whereas in mesioclusion (Class III) the mandible is mesial to the maxilla, as compared to the normal position.

I. NORMAL (IDEAL) OCCLUSION (FIGURE 18-12)

A. Facial Profile

Mesognathic **(Figure 18-1)**.

B. Molar Relation

The mesiobuccal cusp of the maxillary first permanent molar occludes with the buccal groove of the mandibular first permanent molar.

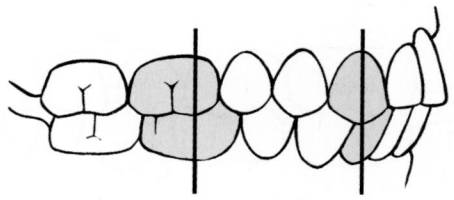

Normal (Ideal) Occlusion
Molar relationship: mesiobuccal cusp of maxillary first permanent molar occludes with the buccal groove of the mandibular first permanent molar.

Malocclusion
Class I: Neutroclusion.
Molar relationship: same as Normal, with malposition of individual teeth or groups of teeth.

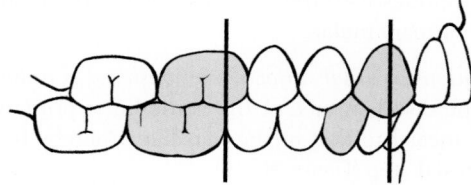

Class II: Distoclusion.
Molar relationship: buccal groove of the mandibular first permanent molar is distal to the mesiobuccal cusp of the maxillary first permanent molar by at least the width of a premolar.
Division 1: mandible is retruded and all maxillary incisors are protruded.

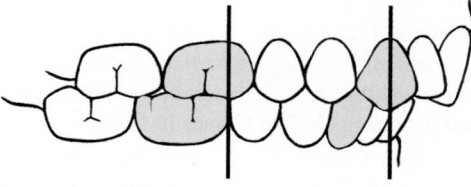

Class II: Distoclusion.
Division 2: mandible is retruded and one or more maxillary incisors are retruded.

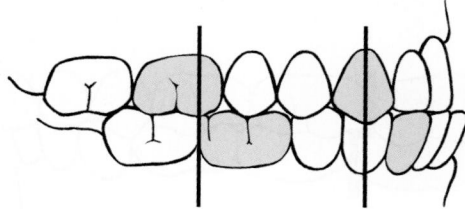

Class III: Mesioclusion.
Molar relationship: buccal groove of the mandibular first permanent molar is mesial to the mesiobuccal cusp of the maxillary first permanent molar by at least the width of a premolar.

FIGURE 18-12 **Normal Occlusion and Classification of Malocclusion.**

C. Canine Relation

The maxillary permanent canine occludes with the distal half of the mandibular canine and the mesial half of the mandibular first premolar.

II. MALOCCLUSION

A. Class I or Neutroclusion (Figure 18-12)

- *Facial profile:* Same as normal occlusion.
- *Molar relation:* Same as normal occlusion.
- *Canine relation:* Same as normal occlusion.
- *Malposition of individual teeth or groups of teeth.*
- *General types of conditions that frequently occur in Class I*
  - Crowded maxillary or mandibular anterior teeth
  - Protruded or retruded maxillary incisors
  - Anterior crossbite
  - Posterior crossbite
  - Mesial drift of molars resulting from premature loss of teeth

B. Class II or Distoclusion (Figure 18-12)

- *Description:* mandibular teeth posterior to normal position in their relation to the maxillary teeth.
- *Facial profile:* retrognathic; maxilla protrudes; lower lip is full and often rests between the maxillary and mandibular incisors; the mandible appears retruded or weak (**Figure 18-1**, retrognathic).
- *Molar relation*
  - The buccal groove of the mandibular first permanent molar is distal to the mesiobuccal cusp of the maxillary first permanent molar by at least the width of a premolar.
  - When the distance is less than the width of a premolar, the relation can be classified as "tendency toward Class II."
- *Canine relation*
  - The distal surface of the mandibular canine is distal to the mesial surface of the maxillary canine by at least the width of a premolar.
  - When the distance is less than the width of a premolar, the relation can be classified as "tendency toward Class II."
- *Class II, Division 1*
  - Description: The mandible is retruded and all maxillary incisors are protruded.
  - General types of conditions that frequently occur in Class II, Division 1 malocclusion: deep overbite, excessive overjet, abnormal muscle function (lips), short mandible, or short upper lip.
- *Class II, Division 2*
  - Description: The mandible is retruded, and one or more maxillary incisors are retruded.
  - General types of conditions that frequently occur in Class II, Division 2 malocclusion: Maxillary lateral

incisors protrude while both central incisors retrude, crowded maxillary anterior teeth, or deep overbite.
■ *Subdivision:* One side is Class I, the other side is Class II (may be Division 1 or 2).

C. Class III or Mesiocclusion (Figure 18-12)

■ *Description:* Mandibular teeth are anterior to normal position in relation to maxillary teeth.
■ *Facial profile:* prognathic; lower lip and mandible are prominent **(Figure 18-1).**
■ *Molar relation*
  ■ The buccal groove of the mandibular first permanent molar is mesial to the mesiobuccal cusp of the maxillary first permanent molar by at least the width of a premolar.
  ■ When the distance is less than the width of a premolar, the relation can be classified as "tendency toward Class III."
■ *Canine relation*
  ■ The distal surface of the mandibular canine is mesial to the mesial surface of the maxillary canine by at least the width of a premolar.
  ■ When the distance is less than the width of a premolar, the relation can be classified as "tendency toward Class III."
■ *General types of Conditions that frequently occur in Class III malocclusion*
  ■ True Class III: Maxillary incisors are lingual to mandibular incisors in an anterior crossbite **(Figure 18-3).**
  ■ Maxillary and mandibular incisors are in edge-to-edge occlusion.
  ■ Mandibular incisors are very crowded but lingual to maxillary incisors.

OCCLUSION OF THE PRIMARY TEETH[2]

I. NORMAL (IDEAL) OCCLUSION

A. Primary Canine Relation

Same as permanent dentition.

■ *With primate spaces*[*]
  ■ Mandibular: between mandibular canine and first molar **(Figure 18-13A).**
  ■ Maxillary: between maxillary lateral incisor and canine **(Figure 18-13B).**
■ *Without primate spaces:* Closed arches.

---

[*]*Primate space:* a diastema or gap in the tooth row occasionally observed in the human primary dentition. It is characteristic of nearly all species of primates except man. The maxillary primate spaces accommodate the mandibular canines, and the mandibular primate spaces accommodate the maxillary canines when the teeth are in occlusion. As a reduction in the length of canines accompanied man's evolution, the canines no longer protruded beyond the occlusal level. The diastema (primate space) was no longer functional.

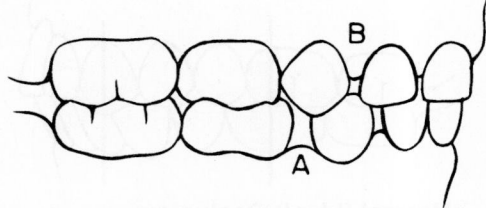

FIGURE 18-13 **Primary Teeth With Primate Spaces. (A)** Mandibular primate space between the canine and the first molar. **(B)** Maxillary primate space between the lateral incisor and the canine.

B. Second Primary Molar Relation

The mesiobuccal cusp of the maxillary second primary molar occludes with the buccal groove of the mandibular second primary molar.

■ *Variations in distal surfaces relationships:* Terminal step.
  ■ The distal surface of the mandibular primary molar is mesial to that of the maxillary, thereby forming a mesial step **(Figure 18-14A).**
  ■ Morphologic variation in molar size; maxillary and mandibular primary molars have approximately the same mesiodistal width.
■ *Variation:* Terminal plane.
  ■ The distal surfaces of the maxillary and mandibular primary molars are on the same vertical plane **(Figure 18-14B).**
  ■ The maxillary molar is narrower mesiodistally than the mandibular molar (occurs in many patients).
■ *Effects on occlusion of first permanent molars*
  ■ Terminal step: First permanent molar erupts directly into proper occlusion **(Figure 18-14A).**
  ■ Terminal plane: First permanent molars erupt end to end. With mandibular primate space, early mesial shift of primary molars into the primate

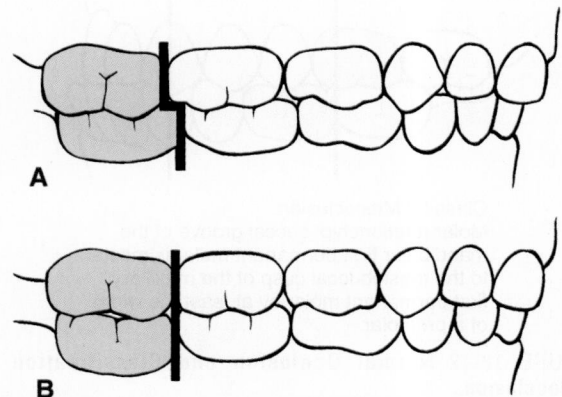

FIGURE 18-14 **Eruption Patterns of the First Permanent Molars. (A)** Terminal step. The distal surface of the mandibular second primary molar is mesial to the distal surface of the maxillary primary molar. **(B)** Terminal plane. The distal surfaces of the mandibular and maxillary second primary molars are on the same vertical plane; permanent molars erupt in end-to-end occlusion.

space occurs, and the permanent mandibular molar shifts into proper occlusion. Without primate spaces, late mesial shift of permanent mandibular molar into proper occlusion occurs, following exfoliation of second primary molar **(Figure 18-14B)**.

II. MALOCCLUSION OF THE PRIMARY TEETH

Same as permanent dentition.

FUNCTIONAL OCCLUSION

In contrast to static occlusion, which pertains to the relationship of the teeth when the jaws are closed, functional occlusion consists of all contacts during chewing, swallowing, or other normal action. Functional occlusion is associated with performance:

- Pressures or forces created by the muscles of mastication are transmitted from the teeth, after contact, to the periodontium.
- Such forces are necessary to maintain the occlusal relationship of the teeth and guide the teeth during eruption.
- The forces are also necessary to provide functional stimulation for the preservation of the health of the attachment apparatus, namely, the periodontal ligament, the cementum, and the alveolar bone.

I. TYPES OF OCCLUSAL CONTACTS

A. Functional Contacts

Functional contacts are the normal contacts that are made between the maxillary teeth and the mandibular teeth during chewing and swallowing. Each contact is momentary, so the total contact time is only a few minutes each day.

B. Parafunctional Contacts

Parafunctional contacts are those made outside the normal range of function.

- They result from occlusal habits and neuroses.
- They are potentially injurious to the periodontal supporting structures, but only in the presence of dental biofilm and inflammatory factors.
- They create wear facets and attrition on the teeth.
- They can be divided into the following:
  - Tooth-to-tooth contacts: Bruxism, clenching, tapping.
  - Tooth-to-hard-object contacts: Nail biting; occupational use of such objects as tacks or pins; use of smoking equipment, such as a pipe stem or hard cigarette holder.
  - Tooth-to-oral-tissues contacts: Lip or cheek biting.

II. PROXIMAL CONTACTS

Proximal contacts serve to stabilize the position of teeth in the dental arches and to prevent food impaction between the teeth. Attrition or wear of the teeth occurs at the proximal contacts.

A. Drifting

- When proximal contact is lost, teeth can drift into spaces created by unreplaced missing teeth.
- There is a natural tendency for mesial migration of teeth toward the midline.
- In the absence of disease, the surrounding periodontal tissues adapt to repositioned teeth.

B. Pathologic Migration

- With destruction of the supporting structures of a tooth as a result of periodontal infection, and with a force to move a tooth weakened by disease and bone loss, migration of the tooth can result.
- Pathologic migration occurs when disease is present; in contrast, drifting is migration with a healthy periodontium.

TRAUMA FROM OCCLUSION

Periodontal tissue injury caused by repeated occlusal forces that exceed the physiologic limits of tissue tolerance is called *trauma from occlusion*. Other names are periodontal traumatism, occlusal traumatism, and periodontal trauma.

I. TYPES OF TRAUMA FROM OCCLUSION

- Primary trauma from occlusion results when the following happens:
  - Excessive occlusal force is exerted on a tooth with normal bone support.
  - Example: the effect of a new restoration placed above the line of occlusion.
- Secondary trauma from occlusion occurs when the following happens:
  - Excessive occlusal force is exerted on a tooth with bone loss and inadequate alveolar bone support.
  - The ability of the tooth to withstand occlusal forces is impaired.
  - A tooth has lost the support of the surrounding bone; even the pressures of what are usually considered normal occlusal forces may create lesions of trauma from occlusion.

II. EFFECTS OF TRAUMA FROM OCCLUSION

The attachment apparatus (periodontal ligament, cementum, and alveolar bone) has as its main purpose the maintenance of the tooth in the socket in a functional state. In a healthy situation, occlusal pressures and forces during chewing and swallowing are readily dispersed or absorbed and no unusual effects are produced.

A. Excess Forces

■ When the forces of occlusion are greater than can be taken care of by the attachment apparatus, damage can result.

■ Circulatory disturbances, tissue destruction from crushing under pressure, bone resorption, and other pathologic processes are initiated.

B. Relation to Inflammatory Factors

■ *Trauma from occlusion does not cause gingivitis, periodontitis, or pocket formation.* The steps in the development of inflammatory disease and pockets are outlined in Chapter 16 on page 248.

■ In the presence of inflammatory disease, the existing periodontal destruction may be aggravated or promoted by trauma from occlusion.

III. METHODS OF APPLICATION OF EXCESS PRESSURE

To understand the nature of the occlusal forces that can cause periodontal trauma from occlusion, it is helpful to recognize types of tooth contacts that can overburden a tooth or a group of teeth.[3]

A. Individual Teeth That Touch Before Full Closure

The contact is premature and may put excessive force on an individual tooth.

B. Two or Only a Few Teeth in Contact During Movement of the Jaw

The teeth involved receive a disproportionate amount of force.

C. Initial Contacts on Inclined Planes of Cusps

Following the initial contact, when the teeth are brought together in a closed position, there may be excess pressure on the teeth where initial contact was made.

D. Heavy Forces Not in a Vertical or Axial Direction

■ Normal occlusal relationships imply a direct cusp-to-fossa position during closure, with the force of

occlusion in a vertical direction toward the tooth apex and parallel with the long axis.

■ When pressures are exerted laterally or horizontally, excess force is placed on the periodontal attachment apparatus.

E. Increased Frequency, Intensity, and Duration of Contacts

In the presence of parafunctional habits, such as bruxism, clenching, tapping, or biting objects, many more than the usual number of tooth contacts are made each day, and the intensity and duration are altered.

IV. RECOGNITION OF SIGNS OF TRAUMA FROM OCCLUSION

No one clinical or radiographic finding clearly defines the presence of trauma from occlusion. Diagnosis of the condition is complex. The possible observations listed as follows are looked for specifically and recorded for evaluation and correlation with the patient history and all other clinical determinations.

A. Clinical Findings That May Occur in Trauma From Occlusion

■ Tooth mobility
■ Fremitus
■ Sensitivity of teeth to pressure and/or percussion
■ Pathologic migration
■ Wear facets or atypical incisal or occlusal wear
■ Open contacts related to food impaction
■ Neuromuscular disturbances in the muscles of mastication (In severe cases, muscle spasm can occur.)
■ Temporomandibular joint symptoms

B. Radiographic Findings

Characteristics that may occur in trauma from occlusion include:

■ Widened periodontal ligament spaces, particularly angular thickening (triangulation). This finding frequently occurs in conjunction with tooth mobility.
■ Angular (vertical) bone loss in localized areas (see Figure 15-19, page 241).
■ Root resorption.
■ Furcation involvement.
■ Thickened lamina dura. Although related to occlusal forces, thickened lamina dura cannot be considered a detrimental or destructive effect of trauma from occlusion. It may be a defense reaction to strengthen tooth

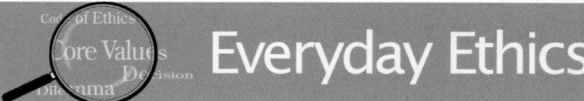

Everyday Ethics

Many of the first-year dental hygiene students struggled to learn the specific classifications of malocclusion and how to recognize them in their patients. The problem was often a locker room discussion item, and it was agreed that they noticed that the instructors didn't always look for the details of a patient's occlusion when the record was checked.

One clinic day Roxanne was confused, and she decided to write just anything down on the patient's chart. When the instructor came to check the oral examination, she questioned why Roxanne had the classification of the occlusion documented as a Class II Distoocclusion. Roxanne just shrugged her shoulders and said, "I don't know."

Questions for Consideration

1. Summarize the ethical concerns related to Roxanne's deciding to "just write down anything" rather than look up the information she needs to provide an accurate assessment of the patient's condition.
2. What legal issues might be connected with inaccurate documentation of information in the patient's permanent record? For an example, use a forensic examination team seeking help from a dental office record.
3. Discuss why this situation can be regarded as both an ethical issue and an ethical dilemma.
   Refer to Section V Introduction, Table V-1 (page 362) for assistance.

---

support against occlusal forces. Thickened lamina dura is frequently associated with teeth that have undergone orthodontic treatment.

RECOMMENDATIONS FOR THE PATIENT WITH ORTHODONTIC NEEDS

- Observe the facial profile as the patient enters and is seated in the dental chair to estimate the classification of occlusion before examination of the teeth.

BOX 18-2	Example Progress Note

11-yr-old Ellen came for routine maintenance and examination. She always tried to hide her smile (rotated lateral and crowded mand anteriors); this time she was full of questions about having ortho because several of her friends were wearing appliances, and her mother said she could ask me and Dr. Spry about who to go to for hers. When Dr. Spry came in to check her he told her what a good idea it was and gave her the card of an orthodontist of his choice for her. I explained how we would be seeing her on a regular basis, and that I would help her learn how to care for her mouth with the appliances on.

Signed: _____, RDH Date: _____.

- Avoid mention of a dentofacial deformity that would make the patient feel self-conscious.
- Avoid suggesting to the patient or a parent the possible procedures the orthodontist may use in treatment because complications become known only after the complete diagnosis.
- Closing to centric relation can be performed most effectively by instructing the patient to curl the tongue and to try to hold the tip of the tongue as far back as possible while closing.
- When a small child has difficulty in occluding, the clinician may firmly but gently press the cushions of the thumbs on the mucous membrane over the pterygomandibular raphe, holding the thumbs between the cheek and buccal surfaces of the teeth as the patient is requested to close.
- Prepare mouth guards for patients in contact sports.
- Study the occlusion of the patient with removable dentures with the dentures in and out of the mouth.

DOCUMENTATION

Documentation for the occlusion of every patient needs to include a minimum of the following:

- Basic classification of the occlusion with variations noted.
- Record occlusal habits including bruxism, clenching, or other parafunctional habits.
- Previous orthodontic treatment; dates, patient report of satisfaction.
- A progress note of a patient's appointment when seeking information about the need for orthodontic treatment may be read in **Box 18-2**.

Factors To Teach The Patient

- Interpretation of the *general* purposes of orthodontic care (function and esthetics) to patients referred by the dentist to an orthodontist.
- Dependence of masticatory efficiency on the occlusion of the teeth.
- Influence of masticatory efficiency on food selection in the diet.
- Influence of masticatory efficiency and diet on the nutritional status of the body and oral health.
- Interpretation of the dentist's suggestions for the correction of oral habits.
- The space-maintaining function of the primary teeth in prevention of malocclusion of permanent teeth.
- The role of malocclusion as a predisposing factor for dental biofilm retention in the formation of dental caries and periodontal infections.
- Dental biofilm removal methods for reducing dental calculus and soft deposit retention in areas where teeth are crowded, displaced, or otherwise not in normal occlusion.
- The relation of the occlusion and the position of the teeth to the patient's personal oral care procedures.
  - Selection of the proper type of toothbrush.
  - Application of thorough toothbrushing method or methods.
  - Use of dental floss.
- Specific reasons for frequency of maintenance examinations when related to malocclusion and while in the process of having orthodontic therapy.

References

1. Angle EH. *Malocclusion of the teeth.* 7th ed. Philadelphia: S.S. White Manufacturing; 1907. pp. 50–7.
2. Baume LJ. Physiological tooth migration and its significance for the development of the occlusion. I. The biogenetic course of the deciduous dentition. *J Dent Res.* 1950 Apr;29(2):123–32; II. The biogenesis of the accessional dentition. *J Dent Res.* 1950 Jun;29(3):331–7; III. The biogenesis of the successional dentition. *J Dent Res.* 1950 Jun;29(3):338–48; IV. The biogenesis of overbite. *J Dent Res.* 1950 Aug;29(4):440–7.
3. Allen DL, McFall WT, Jenzano JW. *Periodontics for the dental hygienist.* 4th ed. Philadelphia: Lea & Febiger; 1987. pp. 85–6.

CHAPTER 19

Dental Biofilm and Other Soft Deposits

ESTHER M. WILKINS, BS, RDH, DMD

During the clinical examination of the teeth and surrounding soft tissues, the soft and hard deposits that accumulate on the teeth and within the sulci or pockets are recognized and assessed. From the findings, an initial preventive care plan can be formulated on the basis of the individual needs of the patient. Key words are defined in Box 19-1.

■ The soft deposits are acquired pellicle or cuticle, dental biofilm, materia alba, and food debris, each of which is an entity.

■ The hard, calcified deposit on teeth is dental calculus, which is described in Chapter 20.

■ A classification with definitions of the dental deposits is presented in **Table 19-1**.[1]

ACQUIRED PELLICLE

■ The acquired pellicle is a tenacious membranous layer that is amorphous, acellular, and organic.

■ It forms over exposed tooth surfaces, as well as over restorations and dental calculus.

■ Its thickness, which varies from 0.1 to 0.8 μm, usually is greatest near the gingival margin.

I. FORMATION

■ Within minutes after all external material has been removed from the tooth surfaces, the acquired pellicle begins to form.

BOX 19-1	Key Words

Dental Biofilm

Acellular: not made up of or containing cells.

Adsorption: attachment of one substance to the surface of another; the action of a substance in attracting and holding other materials or particles on its surface.

Aerobe: heterotrophic microorganism that can live and grow in the presence of free oxygen; some are obligate, others facultative; *adj.* aerobic.

Anaerobe: heterotrophic microorganism that lives and grows in complete (or almost complete) absence of oxygen; some are obligate, others facultative; *adj.* anaerobic.

Biofilm: matrix-enclosed bacterial populations adherent to each other and/or to surfaces or interfaces.

Calculogenesis: formation of calculus.

   Calculogenic: adjective applied to dental biofilm that is conducive to the formation of calculus.

Cariogenesis: development of dental caries.

   Cariogenic: adjective to indicate a conduciveness to the initiation of dental caries, such as a cariogenic biofilm or a cariogenic food.

Facultative: able to live under more than one specific set of environmental conditions; contrast with obligate.

Flora: the collective organisms of a given locale.

   Oral flora: the various bacteria and other microscopic organisms that inhabit the oral cavity. The mouth has an indigenous flora, meaning those organisms that are native to that area of the body. Certain organisms specifically reside in certain parts, for example, on the tongue, on the mucosa, or in the gingival sulcus.

Food impaction: the forceful wedging of food into the periodontium by occlusal forces.

Heterotrophic: not self-sustaining; feeding on others.

Intermicrobial matrix: material present between bacteria in dental biofilm; derived from saliva, gingival exudate, and microorganisms.

Infection: invasion and multiplication of a microorganism in body tissues.

Leukocyte: white blood corpuscle capable of amoeboid movement; functions to protect the body against infection and disease. (For a description of the various white blood cells, see page 1027 and Figure 67-1.)

Materia alba: white or cream-colored cheesy mass that can collect over dental biofilm on unclean, neglected teeth; it is composed of food debris, mucin, and bacteria.

Maturation: stage or process of attaining maximal development; become mature.

Microbiota: the microscopic living organisms of a region.

Microorganism: minute living organisms, usually microscopic; includes bacteria, rickettsiae, viruses, fungi, and protozoa.

Mycoplasma: pleomorphic, gram-negative bacteria that lack cell walls; many are regular oral cavity residents; some are pathogenic.

Obligate: ability to survive only in a particular environment; opposite of facultative.

Parasite: plant or animal that lives upon or within another living organism and draws its nourishment therefrom; may be obligate or facultative; *adj.* parasitic.

Pathogen: disease-producing agent or microorganism; *adj.* pathogenic.

Planktonic: free floating bacteria such as in saliva or sulcular (crevicular) fluid.

Pleomorphism: assumption of various distinct forms by a single organism or within a species; *adj.* pleomorphic.

Saprophyte: any organism, such as bacteria, that lives upon dead or decaying organic matter.

■ It is composed primarily of glycoproteins from the saliva that are selectively adsorbed by the hydroxyapatite of the tooth surface.

■ The adsorbed material becomes a highly insoluble coating over the teeth, calculus deposits, restorations, and complete and partial dentures.

II. TYPES OF PELLICLES[2]

A. Surface Pellicle, Unstained

■ The unstained pellicle is clear, translucent, insoluble, and not readily visible until a disclosing agent has been applied.

■ When stained with a disclosing agent, it appears thin, with a pale staining that contrasts with the thicker, darker staining of dental biofilm.

B. Surface Pellicle, Stained

■ Unstained pellicle can take on extrinsic stain and become brown, grayish, or other colors, as described in Chapter 21 on page 309 with other stains.

C. Subsurface Pellicle

■ Surface pellicle is continuous with subsurface pellicle that is embedded in tooth structure, particularly where the tooth surface is partially demineralized.[3]

III. SIGNIFICANCE OF PELLICLE

A. Protective

Pellicle appears to provide a barrier against acids; thus, it may aid in reducing a dental caries attack.[3]

TABLE 19-1	TOOTH DEPOSITS		
CATEGORY	**TOOTH DEPOSIT**	**DESCRIPTION**	**DERIVATION**
Nonmineralized	Acquired pellicle	Translucent, homogeneous, thin, unstructured film covering and adherent to the surfaces of the teeth, restorations, calculus, and other surfaces in the oral cavity	Supragingival: saliva Subgingival: gingival sulcus fluid
	Microbial (bacterial) biofilm	Dense, organized bacterial systems embedded in an intermicrobial matrix that adhere closely to the teeth, calculus, and other surfaces in the oral cavity Water irrigation removes only the outer layer of loose organisms	Colonization of oral microorganisms
	Materia alba	Loosely adherent, unstructured, white or grayish-white mass of oral debris and bacteria that lies over dental biofilm Vigorous rinsing and water irrigation can remove materia alba	Incidental accumulation
	Food debris	Unstructured, loosely attached particulate matter Self-cleansing activity of tongue and saliva and rinsing vigorously remove debris	Food retention following eating
Mineralized	Calculus	Calcified dental biofilm; hard, tenacious mass that forms on the clinical crowns of the natural teeth and on dentures and other appliances	Biofilm mineralization
	a. Supragingival	Occurs coronal to the margin of the gingiva; is covered with dental biofilm	Source of minerals is saliva
	b. Subgingival	Occurs apical to the margin of the gingiva; is covered with dental biofilm	Source of minerals is gingival sulcus fluid

Source: From Schroeder HE. *Formation and inhibition of dental calculus.* Vienna: Hans Huber; 1969. p. 14–5.

B. Lubrication

Pellicle keeps surfaces moist; prevents drying.

C. Nidus for Bacteria

Pellicle participates in biofilm formation by aiding the adherence of microorganisms.

D. Attachment of Calculus

One mode of calculus attachment is by the acquired pellicle (in Chapter 20, page 299).

DENTAL BIOFILM

- Dental biofilm is a dense, nonmineralized, complex mass of colonies in a gel-like intermicrobial matrix.
- It adheres firmly to the acquired pellicle and hence to the teeth, calculus, and fixed and removable restorations.
- Dental biofilm contains many types of microorganisms, primarily bacteria. More than 600 distinct microbial species are found in dental biofilm. Morphologic forms of bacteria are shown in **Figure 19-1**.

- Other organisms included may be yeasts, protozoa, and viruses. Characteristics of supragingival and subgingival biofilms are shown in **Table 19-2**.

I. STAGES IN THE FORMATION OF BIOFILM

Biofilm is formed in three basic steps, namely, pellicle formation, bacterial colonization, and biofilm maturation **(Figure 19-2)**. Biofilm formation does not occur randomly but involves a series of complex interactions.

A. Formation of a Pellicle

- The pellicle forms on the tooth surface by selective adsorption of protein components from the saliva.
- Initial attachment of bacteria to the pellicle is by selective adherence of specific bacteria from the oral environment.
- Innate characteristics of the bacteria and the pellicle determine the adhesive interactions that cause a particular organism to adhere to a particular pellicle.

B. Bacterial Multiplication and Colonization

- Microcolonies form in layers as the bacterial colonies multiply.

TABLE 19-2	CHARACTERISTICS OF SUPRAGINGIVAL AND SUBGINGIVAL BIOFILM	
CHARACTERISTIC	**SUPRAGINGIVAL BIOFILM**	**SUBGINGIVAL BIOFILM**
Location	Coronal to the margin of the free gingiva	Apical to the margin of the free gingiva
Origin	Salivary glycoprotein forms pellicle Microorganisms from saliva are selectively attracted to pellicle	Downgrowth of bacteria from supragingival biofilm

Distribution	Starts on proximal surfaces and other protected areas
	Heaviest collection on
	    Areas not cleaned daily by patient
	    Cervical third, especially facial
	    Lingual mandibular molars
	    Proximal surfaces
	Pit and fissure biofilm
		Shallow pocket: similar to supragingival biofilm
		Undisturbed; held by pocket wall
		Attached biofilm covers calculus
		Unattached biofilm extends to the periodontal attachment

Adhesion	Firmly attached to acquired pellicle, other bacteria, and tooth surfaces Surface bacteria (unattached): loose; washed away by saliva or swallowed	Adheres to tooth surface, subgingival pellicle, and calculus Subgingival flora: loose, floating, motile organisms in deep pocket do not adhere; they are between adherent biofilm on tooth and the pocket epithelium
Retention	Rough surfaces of teeth or restorations Malpositioned teeth Carious lesions	Pocket holds biofilm against tooth Overhanging margins of fillings that extend into pockets hold biofilm
Shape and Size	Friction of tongue, cheeks, lips, limits shape and size Thickness: thicker at the cervical third and on proximal surfaces Healthy gingiva: thin biofilm, 15–20 cells thick Chronic gingivitis: thick biofilm, 100–300 cells thick	Molded by pocket wall to shape of the tooth surface Follows form created by subgingival calculus May become thicker as the diseased pocket wall becomes less tight
Structure	Adherent, densely packed microbial layer over pellicle on tooth surface Intermicrobial matrix Onset: small isolated colonies 2–5 d; colonies merge to form a covering of biofilm	Three layers (Figure 19-4) 1. Tooth-surface-attached biofilm: many gram-positive rods and cocci 2. Unattached biofilm in middle: many gram-negative, motile forms; spirochetes; leukocytes 3. Epithelium-attached biofilm: gram-negative, motile forms predominate; many leukocytes migrate through epithelium
Microorganisms	Early biofilm: primarily gram-positive cocci Older biofilm (3–4 d): increased numbers of filaments and fusiforms 4–9 d undisturbed: more complex flora with rods, filamentous forms 7–14 d: vibrios, spirochetes, more gram-negative organisms	Environment conducive to growth of anaerobic population Diseased pocket: primarily gram-negative, motile, spirochetes, rods
Sources of Nutrients for Bacterial Proliferation	Saliva Ingested food	Tissue fluid (gingival sulcus fluid) Exudate Leukocytes

Significance	Etiology of
	    Gingivitis
	    Supragingival calculus
	    Dental caries (Figure 19-6)
		Etiology of
		    Gingivitis
		    Periodontal infections
		    Subgingival calculus

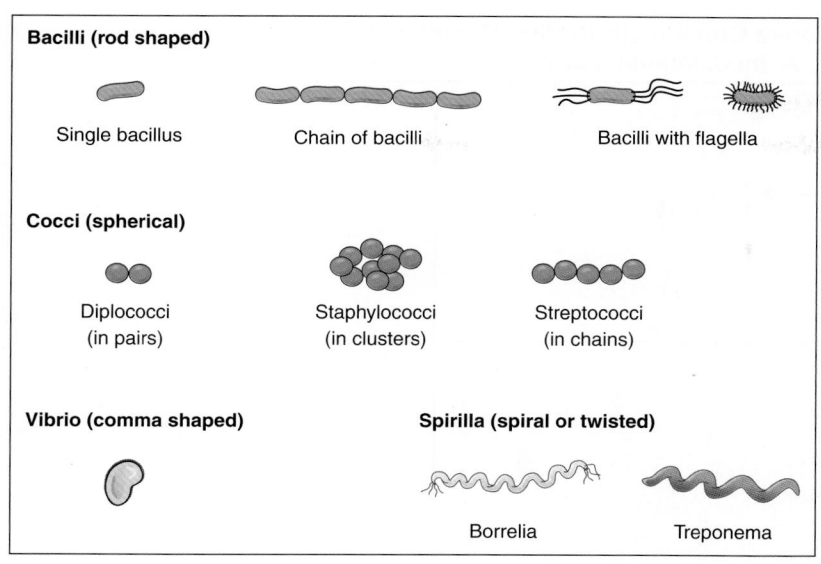

FIGURE 19-1 **Bacteria shapes: cocci, bacilli, spiral.** (Reprinted with permission from Sakai J. *Practical Pharmacology for the Pharmacy Technician*. Baltimore, MD: Lippincott Williams & Wilkins; 2008.)

- With increased size, colonies meet and coalesce to form a continuous bacterial mass.
- Organisms of the first few hours are primarily gram-positive cocci and rods.

C. Biofilm Growth and Maturation

- The increase in the mass and thickness of biofilm results from bacterial multiplication.

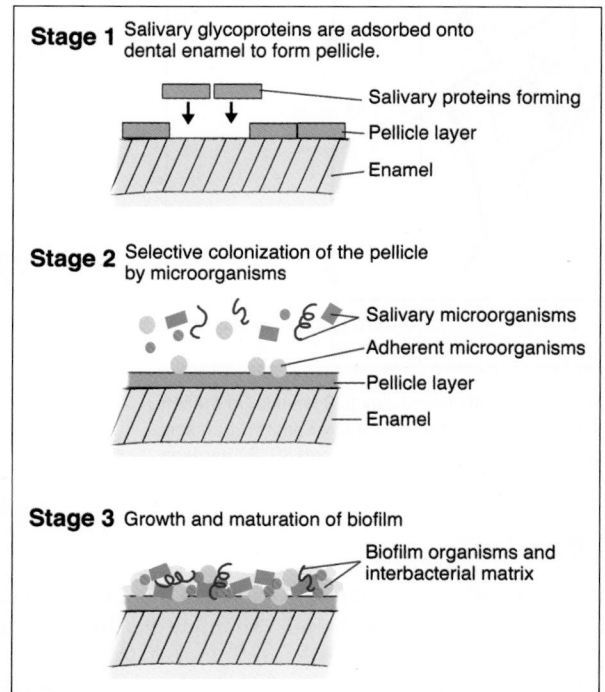

FIGURE 19-2 **Stages of Biofilm Formation.** Diagrammatic representation of the three stages of dental biofilm formation. (Adapted with permission from Katz S, McDonald JL, Stookey GK. Preventive dentistry. Upper Montclair, NJ: DCP Publishing; 1977.)

- Left undisturbed, there is continuous adherence of bacteria to the biofilm surface.

D. Matrix Formation

- The intermicrobial substance is derived mainly from saliva for supragingival biofilm and from gingival sulcus fluid and exudate for subgingival biofilm.
- Other components of the intermicrobial substance are the polysaccharides, glucans, and fructans or levans produced by certain bacteria from dietary sucrose. The polysaccharides are sticky and contribute to the adhesion of the biofilm to the teeth.

II. CHANGES IN BIOFILM MICROORGANISMS

- Dental biofilm consists of a complex mixture of microorganisms that occur primarily as microcolonies. The population density is very high and it increases as biofilm ages.
- The probability of the development of dental caries and/or gingivitis increases as the number of microorganisms increases.
- Changes in the types of organisms occur within biofilm as the biofilm matures.
- When personal oral hygiene practices are discontinued, the numbers of bacteria increase rapidly.
- The changes in oral flora follow a pattern such as that shown in **Figure 19-3**. The changes can be described as follows[4]:

A. Days 1 to 2

- Early biofilm consists primarily of gram-positive cocci.
- Streptococci, which dominate the bacterial population, include *Streptococcus mutans* and *Streptococcus sanguis*.

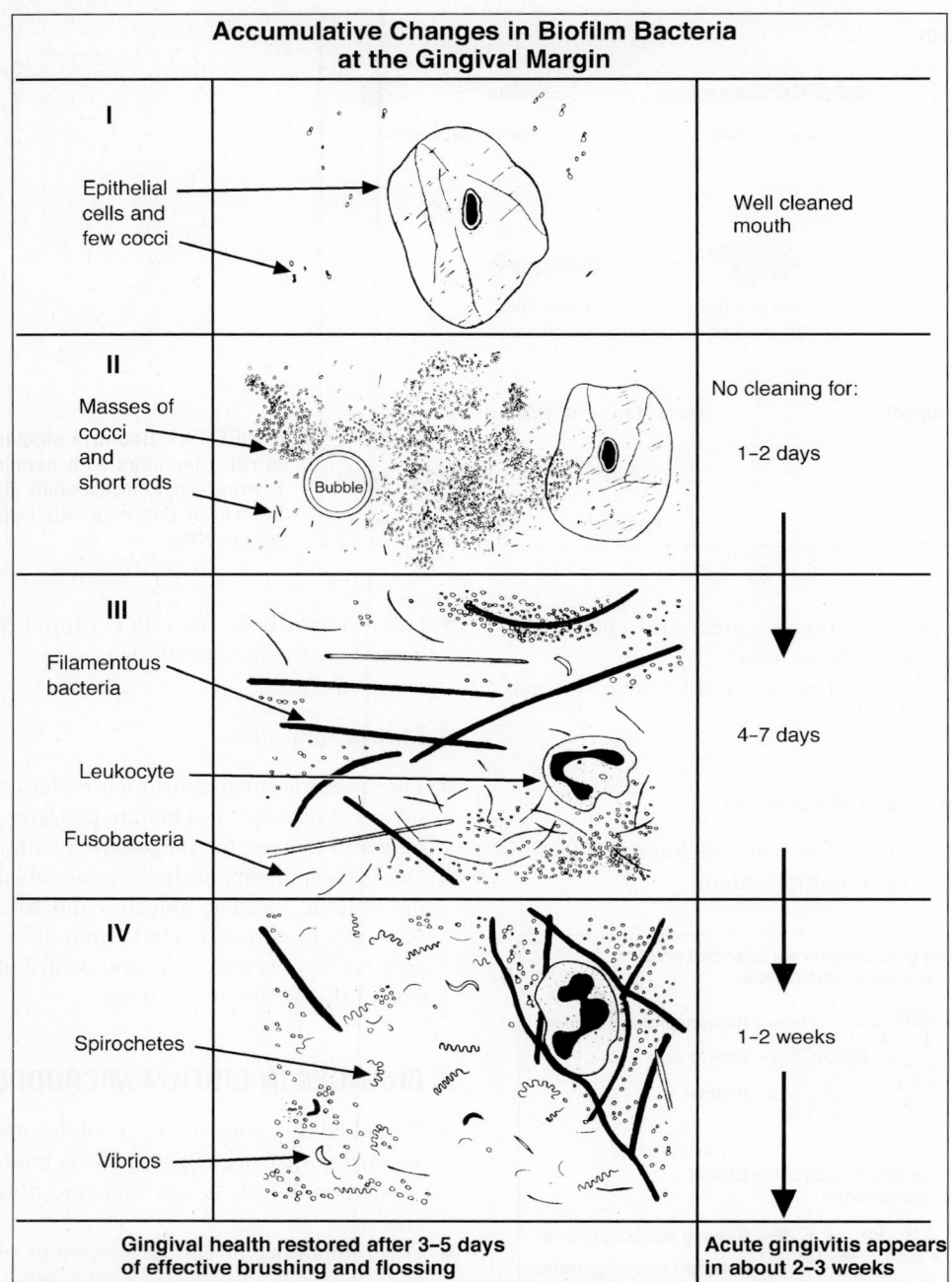

Accumulative Changes in Biofilm Bacteria at the Gingival Margin

I — Epithelial cells and few cocci — Well cleaned mouth

II — Masses of cocci and short rods / Bubble — No cleaning for: 1–2 days

III — Filamentous bacteria / Leukocyte / Fusobacteria — 4–7 days

IV — Spirochetes / Vibrios — 1–2 weeks

Gingival health restored after 3–5 days of effective brushing and flossing

Acute gingivitis appears in about 2–3 weeks

FIGURE 19-3 **Biofilm Microorganisms.** On the right are the time intervals from 1 day to 3 weeks. On the left are the changes in the biofilm content that take place as biofilm ages. As the numbers of microorganisms increase, the numbers of defense cells (leukocytes) also increase. (From Barton RE, Matteson SR, Richardson RE (eds.). *The dental assistant.* 6th ed. Philadelphia: Lea & Febiger; 1988. Crawford JJ. Microbiology.)

B. Days 2 to 4

- The cocci still dominate, and increasing numbers of gram-positive filamentous forms and slender rods may be seen on the surface of the cocci colonies.
- Gradually, the filamentous forms grow into the cocci layer and replace many of the cocci.
- Slow biofilm formers continue to form biofilm comprised primarily of cocci for a longer time than do fast biofilm formers.

C. Days 4 to 7

- Filaments increase in numbers, and a more mixed flora begins to appear with rods, filamentous forms, and fusobacteria.
- Biofilm near the gingival margin thickens and develops a more mature flora, with gram-negative spirochetes and vibrios.
- As biofilm spreads coronally, the new biofilm has the characteristic coccal forms.

D. Days 7 to 14

- Vibrios and spirochetes appear, and the number of white blood cells increases.
- As biofilm matures and thickens, more gram-negative and anaerobic organisms appear.
- During this period, signs of inflammation are beginning to be observed in the gingiva.

E. Days 14 to 21

- Vibrios and spirochetes are prevalent in older biofilm, along with cocci and filamentous forms.
- The densely packed filamentous microorganisms arrange themselves perpendicular to the tooth surface in a palisade.
- Gingivitis is evident clinically.

III. EXPERIMENTAL GINGIVITIS[4]

- Gingivitis develops in 2 to 3 weeks when biofilm is left undisturbed on the tooth surfaces.
- Most gingivitis is reversible, and when the gingiva is treated by biofilm removal procedures, the gingiva can return to health within a few days.
- An experimental gingivitis program to demonstrate the effect of biofilm can be conducted as follows:
  - Observe and record characteristics of the healthy gingiva at the outset. Record a gingival index (page 326), a biofilm index (pages 315 to 321), and a bleeding index (pages 325 to 327).
  - Withhold all biofilm control procedures for a period of 3 weeks.
  - Repeat clinical observations of tissues and record indices at least weekly during the test period. Note initial evidence of gingivitis.
  - Reinstate biofilm removal measures after final recordings at 3 weeks. Make daily observations relative to gingival bleeding and indications that healing is taking place. In 1 week, repeat gingival and biofilm indices.

SUBGINGIVAL DENTAL BIOFILM

I. SOURCE

- Subgingival biofilm results from the apical proliferation of microorganisms from supragingival biofilm.
- In the early stages of gingivitis and periodontitis, the supragingival biofilm is a strong influence on the accumulation and pathogenic features of the subgingival biofilm.

II. MICROORGANISMS

- The flora of the subgingival biofilm differs from that of the supragingival biofilm.

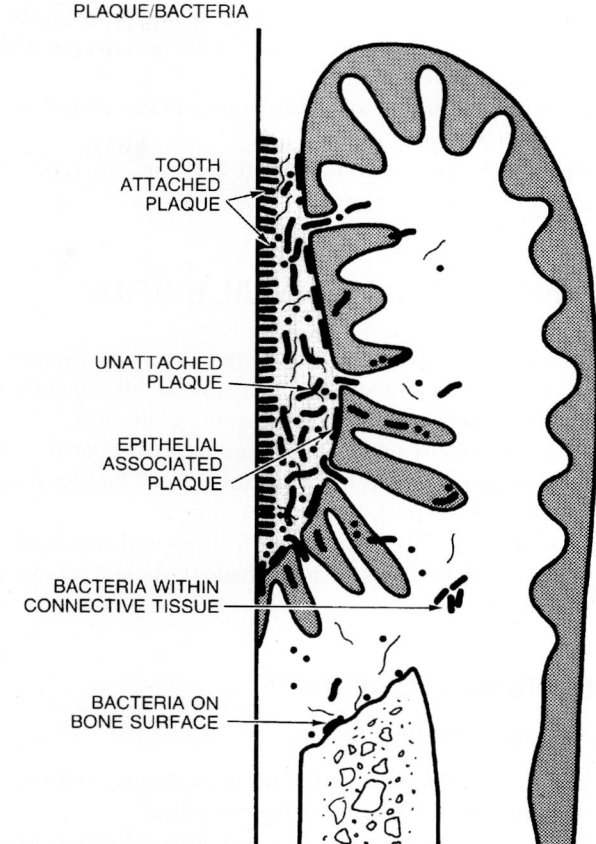

PLAQUE/BACTERIA

TOOTH ATTACHED PLAQUE

UNATTACHED PLAQUE

EPITHELIAL ASSOCIATED PLAQUE

BACTERIA WITHIN CONNECTIVE TISSUE

BACTERIA ON BONE SURFACE

FIGURE 19-4 Bacterial Invasion. Diagram of a periodontal pocket shows bacteria of attached and unattached biofilm bacteria within the pocket epithelium, in the connective tissue, and on the surface of the bone. (Adapted with permission from Carranza FA. *Clinical periodontology.* 8th ed. Philadelphia: Saunders; 1996. 89 p.)

- The subgingival biofilm includes more anaerobic and motile organisms, and they are predominantly gram-negative.

III. ORGANIZATION OF SUBGINGIVAL BIOFILM (FIGURE 19-4)

A. Tooth-Surface-Attached Biofilm

- Over the pellicle, which covers the tooth surface, is a layer of densely packed microorganisms.
- The biofilm of this area is associated with calculus formation, root caries, and root resorption.

B. Unattached Biofilm

- Between the two layers of attached biofilm are many planktonic, motile, gram-negative organisms. The planktonic "free-floating" biofilm contains many white blood cells.

C. Epithelium-Associated Biofilm

- Loosely attached to the pocket epithelium are many gram-negative microorganisms and numerous white

blood cells. Many virulent pathogenic organisms in this layer may be considered a focus for the advancement of periodontal infection.
- From this layer, microorganisms invade the underlying connective tissue.
- **Figure 19-4** shows bacteria within the connective tissue and on the bone surface.[5]

COMPOSITION OF DENTAL BIOFILM

- Biofilm is composed of microorganisms and intermicrobial matrix. Organic and inorganic solids constitute approximately 20%, and water accounts for 80%.
- Microorganisms make up at least 70% to 80% of the solid matter, which is higher in subgingival biofilm than in the supragingival.
- Composition differs among individuals and among different tooth surfaces of an individual. As biofilm ages, it changes.

I. INORGANIC ELEMENTS[6,7]

A. Calcium and Phosphorus

- The concentration of calcium, phosphorus, and magnesium is higher in biofilm than in saliva.
- During the mineralization and demineralization processes, saliva transports the minerals.

B. Fluoride

- The concentration of fluoride in biofilm is higher when fluoridated water is used, and it increases following professional topical applications of fluoride and the use of fluoride-containing dentifrices and mouth rinses.

II. ORGANIC COMPONENTS

The organic intermicrobial substance surrounds the microorganisms of biofilm and contains primarily carbohydrates and proteins, with small amounts of lipids.

A. Carbohydrates

- Carbohydrates include glucans and fructans or levans made from dietary sucrose. Dextran is a type of glucan.
- Carbohydrates contribute to the adherence of microorganisms to each other and to the tooth.

B. Proteins

- Supragingival biofilm contains proteins derived from saliva.
- Subgingival biofilm contains proteins from gingival sulcus fluid.

CLINICAL ASPECTS

I. DISTRIBUTION OF BIOFILM

A. Location

1. *Supragingival Biofilm:* Biofilm is coronal to the gingival margin.
2. *Gingival Biofilm:* Biofilm forms on the external surfaces of the oral epithelium and attached gingiva.
3. *Subgingival Biofilm:* Biofilm is located between the periodontal attachment and the gingival margin, within the sulcus or pocket.
4. *Fissure Biofilm:* Biofilm that also develops in pits and fissures.

B. By Surfaces

- *During Formation*
  - Supragingival biofilm formation begins at the gingival margin, particularly on proximal surfaces, and increases rapidly when left undisturbed.
  - It spreads over the gingival third and on toward the middle third of the crown.
- *Tooth Surfaces Involved*
  - Biofilm occurs most frequently on proximal surfaces and around the gingival third, associated with protected areas **(Figure 19-5)**.
  - The least amounts occur where self-cleansing activities are in effect as described in Chapter 16, page 253.

Palatal surfaces of maxillary teeth may have the least biofilm because of the activity of the tongue.

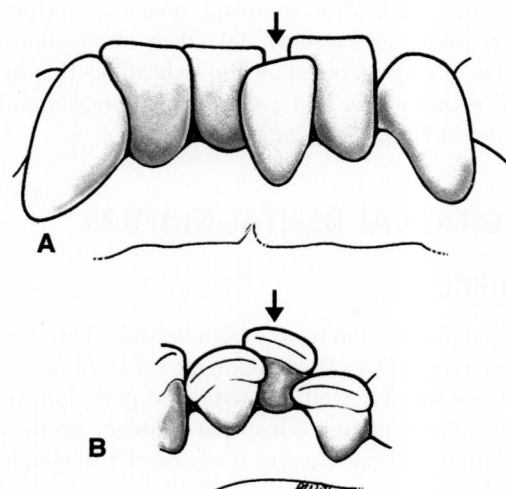

FIGURE 19-5 **Biofilm Accumulation in Protected Areas.** Crowded mandibular anterior teeth demonstrate dental biofilm after use of a disclosing agent. The thickest biofilm is on the proximal surfaces and at the cervical thirds of the teeth. Note the central incisors in facial view **(A)** and lingual view **(B)**, with thick extensive biofilm on the less accessible protected surfaces.

C. Factors Influencing Biofilm Accumulation

1. *Crowded Teeth:* **Figure 19-5** illustrates the accumulation of dental biofilm around crowded mandibular anterior teeth. Research has shown that when personal biofilm removal efforts are made conscientiously, biofilm accumulation around crowded teeth is not greater than that around teeth in good alignment.[8] In **Figure 19-5**, for example, the thick biofilm shown on the lingual of the crowded mandibular left central incisor, could be removed using a toothbrush in a vertical position (Figure 27-12, page 401).
2. *Rough Surfaces:* More rapid collection occurs on rough surfaces of teeth, restorations, and calculus.
3. *Difficult to Clean:* Thick, dense deposits usually collect in difficult-to-clean areas, such as under overhanging margins of crowns or fillings, under ledges of calculus, and in areas associated with carious lesions.
4. *Out of Occlusion:* Deposits may extend over an entire crown of a tooth that is unopposed, out of occlusion, or not used during mastication.
5. *Bacterial Multiplication:* The thickness of biofilm results from constant cell division of the bacteria within the biofilm.

II. DETECTION OF BIOFILM

A. Direct Vision

1. *Thin Biofilm:* May be translucent and therefore not visible until disclosed.
2. *Stained Biofilm:* May acquire extrinsic stains that make it visible, for example, yellow, green, tobacco, as described in Chapter 21 on pages 306 to 309.
3. *Thick Biofilm:* The tooth may appear dull, dingy, with a matted fur-like surface. Materia alba or food debris may collect over the biofilm.

B. Use of Explorer or Probe

1. *Tactile Examination:* When calcification has started, biofilm may feel slightly rough; otherwise, the surface may feel only somewhat slippery because of the coating of soft, slimy biofilm.
2. *Removal of Biofilm:* When no biofilm is visible, it may be detected by passing the side of the tip of a probe over the suspected tooth surface. When present, biofilm adheres to the probe tip.

C. Use of Disclosing Agent

- When a disclosing agent is applied, biofilm takes on the color and becomes readily visible **(Figure 19-5)**.
- Disclosing agent is not to be applied until the evaluation of the oral mucosa and gingival color has been recorded.

D. Clinical Record

1. Record biofilm by location and extent (slight, moderate, or heavy). An index or biofilm score is recommended in Chapter 22, pages 315 to 321.
2. Biofilm recordings and indices are kept for comparison in conjunction with the instructional plan for biofilm control by the patient, for both current and maintenance appointments.
3. Biofilm evaluation records are included with permanent records of the complete charting and oral examination.

SIGNIFICANCE OF DENTAL BIOFILM

- Microbial biofilm plays a major role in the initiation and progression of both dental caries and periodontal infections.
- Periodontal diseases and dental caries are infectious, transmissible diseases caused by pathogenic microorganisms found in microbial biofilms.
- Biofilm is significant in the formation of dental calculus. Calculus is essentially mineralized dental biofilm.
- General oral cleanliness depends on the daily removal of dental biofilm deposits. The accumulation of dental biofilm on the teeth and tongue contributes to an unpleasant personal esthetic appearance as well as to halitosis.

DENTAL CARIES

- Dental caries is a disease of the dental calcified structures (enamel, dentin, and cementum) that is characterized by demineralization of the mineral components and dissolution of the organic matrix.
- Clinical characteristics and types of cavitated dental caries are described in Chapter 17 on pages 261 to 266.
- The process of dental caries from the initial noncavitated demineralized area to the cavitated carious lesion is described in Chapter 26 on page 378.
- The sequence of events leading to demineralization and dental caries is shown in **Figure 19-6**.

I. MICROORGANISMS IN BIOFILM[9]

- Mutans streptococci (*S. mutans* and *Streptococcus sobrinus,* predominantly) and other acid-forming bacteria are initially the etiologic agents.
- Lactobacilli have a significant role in the progression of a carious lesion and mutans streptococci are prominent in the initiation of the carious process.
- Decreased salivary flow (xerostomia) and increased frequency of dietary carbohydrate promote the growth of mutans streptococci and lactobacilli in dental biofilm.

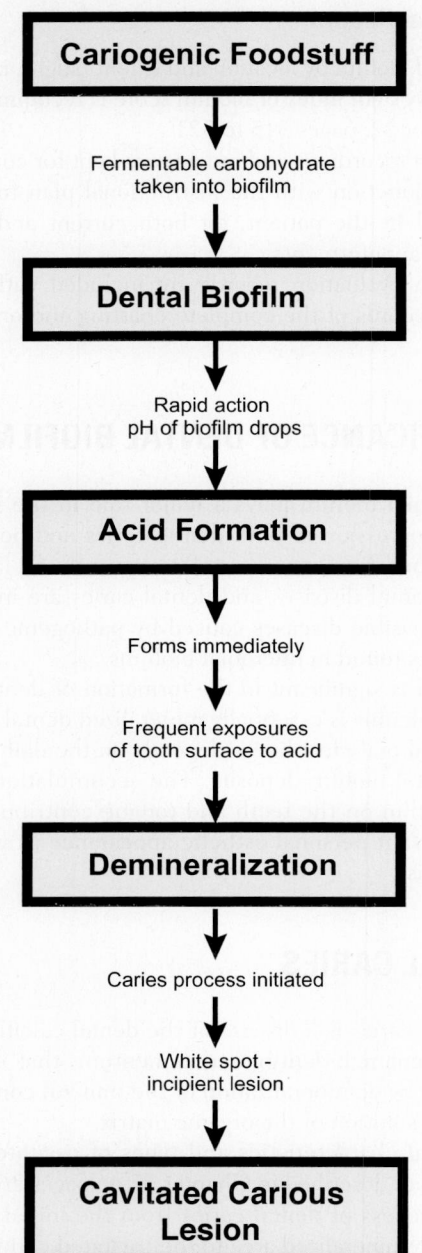

FIGURE 19-6 **Development of Dental Caries.** Flowchart shows the step-by-step action within the microbial biofilm on the tooth surface.

II. THE pH OF BIOFILM

- Acid formation begins *immediately* when the cariogenic substance is taken into the biofilm.
- The pH of the biofilm is lowered promptly, and 1 to 2 hours are required for the pH to return to a normal level, assuming the biofilm is left undisturbed.
- Biofilm pH before eating ranges from 6.2 to 7.0; it is lower in the caries-susceptible person and higher in the caries-resistant person.
- Immediately following sucrose intake into biofilm, a rapid drop in the pH of the biofilm occurs.[10,11]

- Critical pH for enamel demineralization averages 4.5 to 5.5, below which the enamel demineralizes. The critical pH for root surface demineralization is approximately 6.0 to 6.7.[12]
- The amount of demineralization depends on the length of time and the frequency with which the acid with a pH below the critical pH is in contact with the tooth surface.
- With each meal or snack that contains sucrose, the pH of the biofilm is lowered (Figure 34-8, page 513).
- Large amounts of sucrose eaten at mealtimes can be expected to be less cariogenic than small amounts eaten at frequent intervals during the day.[13]
- These and other related facts could be presented to the patient when the diet is discussed as part of a total dental caries control program with dietary assessment.

III. THE CARIOUS LESION

- The incipient carious lesion begins as subsurface demineralization. Acid from bacterial action on the tooth surface passes through microchannels in the enamel, demineralization occurs, and eventually a white spot can be seen clinically.
- Early and continuous use of fluoride for remineralization is necessary. Dental caries formation is described in Chapter 26 on page 378 and the use of fluoride in remineralization is included on page 383 in Chapter 26.

EFFECT OF DIET ON BIOFILM

I. CARIOGENIC FOODS

A. Dental Caries

- The relationship of the cariogenic food content of the diet and its frequency of use to the development of dental caries is well defined in research and clinical application. Dental caries initiation is outlined in **Figure 19-6**.

B. Effect of Sucrose on Amount and pH of Biofilm

- When a cariogenic diet is used, biofilm forms and grows more profusely.[14]
- Patients who were fed sucrose by stomach tube had a less acidogenic biofilm than the patients who were fed sucrose by mouth.[15]

II. FOOD INTAKE

- Food particles are not needed in the mouth for biofilm to form.
- In one study, neither varying the number of meals nor feeding by stomach tube affected the development of biofilm.[16]
- In another study, less biofilm developed in a group of stomach-fed patients compared with those fed by mouth.[15]

III. TEXTURE OF DIET

- The friction of mastication has been shown to affect only the occlusal and incisal thirds of the crowns of teeth.
- Biofilm on the gingival third collected in spite of a normal diet that included coarse bread and fresh fruit[4] or chewing raw carrots three times daily as the only methods for personal care.[17]
- Chewing apples did not affect moderate amounts of biofilm, but it did tend to remove food debris in a group of 12-year-olds.[18]

PERIODONTAL INFECTIONS

- Certain microorganisms of dental biofilm and their toxic products are responsible for periodontal infectious diseases.
- The pathogens exist in biofilms. Biofilms provide protection and give the organisms increased resistance to antibiotics. The biofilm plays an important role in periodontal therapy.

I. BACTERIA OF HEALTHY VERSUS DISEASED PERIODONTAL TISSUES

- The microbiota of the healthy gingival sulcus differs from the bacteria of the diseased pocket. Table 39-1 (page 611) lists the characteristics of the diseased periodontal pocket in comparison with the healthy and the treated pocket.
- In health, there is a majority of aerobic, gram-positive organisms. The total number of organisms and white blood cells is low compared with a diseased pocket.

II. THE DISEASE PROCESS

- The biofilm of each of the various periodontal diseases (chronic, aggressive, and the others defined in Table 16-2, page 246) has its own microbial complex of subgingival pathogenic microorganisms.[19,20]
- Major microorganisms implicated in destructive periodontal infections are shown in **Box 19-2**.

III. PERIODONTAL INFECTION AND TOTAL BODY HEALTH

- Subgingival invasive pathogens initiate periodontal infections that lead to destruction of the periodontal supporting tissues including the periodontal ligament, the cementum, and alveolar bone.
- Through the diseased periodontal pockets that develop, bacteria and the toxic products they produce have access to the circulation of the human body, and carry the diseased materials to major systems throughout the body.
- The link of inflammatory factors from periodontal infection has been connected with systemic diseases and conditions. There are risk factors in common.

| **BOX 19-2** | **Pathogens in Destructive Periodontal Diseases** |

Strong evidence for etiology
- *Aggregatibacter actinomycetemcomitans*
- *Porphyromonas gingivalis*
- *Tannerella forsythensis*

Moderate evidence for etiology
- *Campylobacter rectus*
- *Eubacterium nodatum*
- *Fusobacterium nucleatum*
- *Prevotella intermedia*
- *Parvimonas micra*
- *Treponema denticole*

Source: [No authors listed] Consensus report. Periodontal diseases: pathogenesis and microbial factors. *Ann Periodontol.* 1996 Nov; 1:928.

Interactions have been identified between a wide variety of systemic diseases and conditions, including atherosclerotic disease, adverse pregnancy outcomes, diabetes and complications of diabetes, pulmonary diseases, and stroke.[21]

MATERIA ALBA

- Materia alba is a loosely adherent mass of bacteria and cellular debris that frequently occurs on top of dental biofilm where biofilm removal is neglected.

I. CLINICAL APPEARANCE AND CONTENT

- Materia alba ("white material") distinguishes itself clinically as a bulky, soft deposit that is clearly visible without application of a disclosing agent. It is white, or grayish white, and characteristically may resemble cottage cheese.
- Materia alba is a product of informal accumulation of living and dead bacteria, desquamated epithelial cells, disintegrating leukocytes, salivary proteins, and possibly a few particles of food debris.

II. EFFECTS

- Surface bacteria in contact with the gingiva contribute to gingival inflammation.
- Tooth surface demineralization and early noncavitated lesions are seen frequently under materia alba.

III. PREVENTION

- Materia alba can be removed with a water spray or oral irrigator, whereas dental biofilm cannot.

■ Clinical distinction of materia alba, food debris, and dental biofilm is necessary, but patient instruction for the removal of all three involves the same basic biofilm control procedures.

FOOD DEBRIS

■ Loose food particles collect about the cervical third and proximal embrasures of the teeth.
■ Cariogenic foods contribute to dental caries because liquefied carbohydrate diffuses rapidly into the biofilm and hence to the acid-forming bacteria.
■ *Food impaction:* When there are open contact areas, mobility of teeth, or irregularities of occlusion such as plunger cusps, food may be forced between the teeth during mastication. This could result in vertical food impaction.
■ Horizontal or lateral food impaction occurs in facial and lingual embrasures, particularly when the interdental papillae are reduced or missing.
■ Food debris adds to a general unsanitary condition of the mouth. Some self-cleansing through the action of the tongue, lips, saliva, and related factors may take place.
■ Debris removal by toothbrushing, flossing, and other aids constitutes a total biofilm control program. Cleansing of food debris from about fixed prostheses and orthodontic appliances is necessary in the plan for oral sanitation.

DOCUMENTATION

The permanent records for each patient will include information about the soft deposits on the teeth with a suggested minimum of the following:

BOX 19-3   Example Progress Note

Appt for third quadrant scaling with anesthesia. Patient still not doing adequate biofilm removal and other hygiene procedures; discussed and showed her disclosed dentition where most proximal surfaces showed red and bled with probing. Demonstrated how to work the power toothbrush in between; she said she doesn't use her power brush much. When asked why, she shrugged and said it was a nuisance to care for it; tried to make some suggestions, with emphasis that it would help her gingiva get healthy sooner; I asked if this week she would use it and include all four quadrants, especially the next one we will do next (max. left) so we can see the difference from my scaling. She said she would try.

Signed: _____, RDH Date: _____

■ Clinical description of appearance of the teeth relative to the biofilm, materia alba, or food debris as indications of the personal oral care on a daily basis.
■ Patient's understanding of biofilm and the significance of various deposits.
■ Patient's description of the methods used daily: brush teeth, tongue, floss, rinse, and exactly what products are used at each mouthcare episode (specified for the scheduled times, that is, morning after breakfast, chew xylitol gum after lunch, etc.).

A sample progress note for a patient's appointment may be reviewed in **Box 19-3**.

Everyday Ethics

Daria was particularly excited to begin her patient schedule today because a student from the local community college was coming to observe her. Daria had graduated from the same dental hygiene program 4 years earlier and had volunteered to participate in the program for students to observe practitioners.

Roland, a second-year student, presented promptly at the receptionist's window 15 minutes prior to the first patient. Daria was already busily preparing her treatment room, and she quickly introduced herself to the student. She invited Roland to ask her any questions but not in front of a patient. She said she would introduce him to the patient at the beginning of each appointment, and would request verbal approval from the patient for his presence; he would scrub up and assist. Roland was impressed with Daria's professionalism.

After the first appointment was completed, Roland asked Daria why she was still using the term "plaque" during patient

instruction instead of "biofilm" and why she didn't disclose the teeth before the selective polishing procedures. "Oh," Daria replied, "Is this something new you learned in school? I've only been to one continuing education course since I left school but I didn't hear anything about—what is it? Biofilm?"

Questions for Consideration
1. Role-play the dialogue that might take place regarding use of the term "plaque" versus "biofilm," which was a new concept for Daria.
2. Ethically, how is Daria violating/not violating any ethical principles relative to total patient care by not using disclosing agent to identify the biofilm? In what ways may terminology be important in practice?
3. Which of the dental hygiene core values (Table II-1, in Section II, Introduction, page 38) are in action in this scenario? Describe how each one selected was in action.

Factors To Teach The Patient

■ Location, composition, and properties of dental biofilm, with emphasis on its role in dental caries and periodontal infections.

■ The cause and prevention of dental caries.

■ Effects of personal oral care procedures in the prevention of dental biofilm.

■ Biofilm control procedures with special adaptations for individual needs.

■ Sources of cariogenic foodstuff in the diet, with suggestions for control.

■ Relationship of frequency of eating cariogenic foods to dental caries.

References

1. Schroeder HE. *Formation and inhibition of dental calculus.* Vienna: Hans Huber Publishers; 1969. p. 14–5.

2. Meckel AH. Formation and properties of organic films on teeth. *Arch Oral Biol.* 1965 Jul–Aug;10(4):585–98.

3. Meckel AH. The nature and importance of organic deposits on dental enamel. *Caries Res.* 1968;2(2):104–14.

4. Löe H, Theilade E, Jensen SB. Experimental gingivitis in man. *J Periodontol.* 1965 May–Jun;36:177–87.

5. Saglie R, Newman MG, Carranza FA, Pattison GL. Bacterial invasion of gingiva in advanced periodontitis in humans. *J Periodontol.* 1982 Apr;53(4):217–22.

6. Mandel ID. Relation of saliva and plaque to caries. *J Dent Res.* 1974 Mar–Apr;53(2):246–66.

7. Grøn P, Yao K, Spinelli M. A study of inorganic constituents in dental plaque. *J Dent Res.* 1969 Sep–Oct;48(5):799–805.

8. Årtun J, Osterberg SK. Periodontal status of secondary crowded mandibular incisors: long-term results after orthodontic treatment. *J Clin Periodontol.* 1987 May;14(5):261–6.

9. Van Houte J, Sansone C, Joshipura K, Kent R. Mutans streptococci and non-mutans streptococci acidogenic at low pH, and in vitro acidogenic potential of dental plaque in two different areas of the human dentition. *J Dent Res.* 1991 Dec;70(12):1503–7.

10. Stephan RM. Intra-oral hydrogen-ion concentrations associated with dental caries activity. *J Dent Res.* 1944 Aug;23:257.

11. Rosen S, Weisenstein PR. The effect of sugar solutions on pH of dental plaques from caries-susceptible and caries-free individuals. *J Dent Res.* 1965 Sep–Oct;44(5):845–9.

12. Hoppenbrouwers PM, Driessens FC, Borggreven JM. The mineral solubility of human tooth roots. *Arch Oral Biol.* 1987;32(5):319–22.

13. Gustafsson BE, Quensel CE, Lanke LS, Lundquist C, Grahnèn H, Bonow BE, Krasse B. The vipeholm dental caries study: the effect of different levels of carbohydrate intake on caries activity in 436 individuals observed for five years. *Acta Odontol Scand.* 1954 Sep;11(3–4):232–64.

14. Carlsson J, Egelberg J. Effect of diet on early plaque formation in man. *Odontol Revy.* 1965;16(1):112–25.

15. Littleton NW, Carter CH, Kelley RT. Studies of oral health in persons nourished by stomach tube. I. Changes in the pH of plaque material after the addition of sucrose. *J Am Dent Assoc.* 1967 Jan;74(1):119–23.

16. Egelberg J. Local effect of diet on plaque formation and development of gingivitis in dogs. III. Effect of frequency of meals and tube feeding. *Odontol Revy.* 1965;16(1):50–60.

17. Lindhe J, Wicén PO. The effects on the gingivae of chewing fibrous foods. *J Periodont Res.* 1969;4(3):193–200.

18. Birkeland JM, Jorkjend L. The effect of chewing apples on dental plaque and food debris. *Community Dent Oral Epidemiol.* 1974;2(4):161–2.

19. Socransky SS, Haffajee AD, Cugini MA, Smith C, Kent RL Jr. Microbial complexes in subgingival plaque. *J Clin Periodontol.* 1998 Feb;25(2):134–44.

20. Haffajee AD, Socransky SS. Microbial etiological agents of destructive periodontal diseases. *Periodontol 2000.* 1994 Jun;5:78–111.

21. Garcia RI, Henshaw MM, Krall EA. Relationship between periodontal disease and systemic health. *Periodontology 2000.* 2001;25:21–36.

Calculus

ESTHER M. WILKINS, BS, RDH, DMD

Chapter Outline

Dental calculus is mineralized dental biofilm that is filled with crystals of various calcium phosphates. It is covered with a layer of nonmineralized dental biofilm containing viable, active bacteria. The hard, tenacious mass forms on the clinical crowns of the natural teeth and dental implants, dentures, and other dental prostheses. Terms and key words associated with calculus are defined in **Box 20-1**.

OBJECTIVES FOR DENTAL HYGIENE PRACTICE

■ A major objective in nonsurgical periodontal therapy is to prepare the teeth, through complete calculus removal, to have biologically acceptable smooth surfaces.

■ *Clinical Care:* Comprehensive understanding of the characteristics, origin, development, and methods of prevention of calculus is essential to patient examination, assessment, treatment, and instruction.

■ *Patient Learning:* For successful treatment and prevention, the patient needs to know the interrelationship between biofilm, calculus, and oral health; the need for complete removal of calculus; and the reasons for the painstaking manner in which scaling procedures must be carried out.

CLASSIFICATION AND DISTRIBUTION OF CALCULUS

Dental calculus is classified by its location on a tooth surface as related to the adjacent free gingival margin, that is, supragingival and subgingival (**Figure 20-1**).

BOX 20-1	**Key Words**

Calculus

Amorphous: without definite shape or visible differentiation in structure.

Apatite: crystalline mineral component of bones and teeth that contains calcium and phosphate.

Calculus: abnormal concretion composed of mineral salts, usually occurring within the hollow organs or their passages; also called stones, such as gallstones or kidney stones.

Denture calculus: mineralized dental biofilm that occurs on a dental prosthesis.

Ectopic: out of place; arising or produced at an abnormal site or in a tissue where it is not normally found.

Ectopic oral calcification: examples are pulp stones, denticles, and salivary calculi.

Germfree: free of microorganisms; a germfree animal in research is reared under completely sterile conditions.

Matrix: intercellular or intermicrobial substance of a tissue, or the tissue from which a structure develops, gains support, and is held together.

Mineralization: addition of mineral elements, such as calcium and phosphorus, to the body or a part thereof with resulting hardening of the tissue.

Nidus: nucleus, focus, point of origin.

Pyrophosphate: inhibitor of calcification that occurs in parotid saliva of humans in variable amounts; anticalculus component of "tarter-control" dentifrices.

Saturated: holding all of a substance (solute) that can be dissolved in the solution.

Supersaturated: a solution containing more of an ingredient than can be held in solution permanently.

I. SUPRAGINGIVAL CALCULUS

A. Location

- On the clinical crown coronal to the margin of the gingiva.
- On implants, complete and partial dentures.

B. Distribution: Most Frequent Sites

- On the lingual surfaces of mandibular anterior teeth and the facial surfaces of maxillary first and second molars, opposite the openings of the ducts of the salivary glands.
- On the crowns of teeth out of occlusion; nonfunctioning teeth; or teeth that are neglected during daily biofilm removal (toothbrushing, flossing, or other personal care).

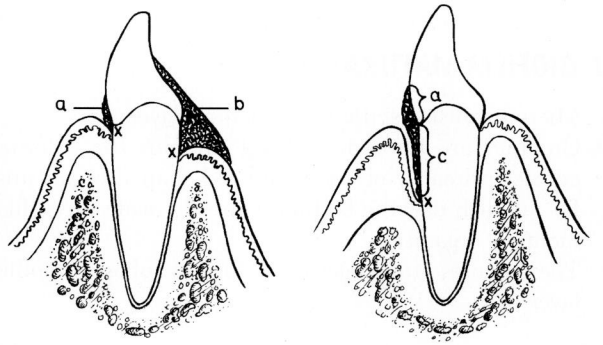

FIGURE 20-1 **Dental Calculus.** (a) Supragingival calculus on cervical third of a mandibular anterior tooth extends slightly subgingivally. (b) Supragingival calculus over crown, exposed root surface, and the margin of the gingiva. (c) Subgingival calculus along root to the bottom of a periodontal pocket. (x) Bottom of pocket.

- On surfaces of dentures, dental prostheses, and tongue piercings' barbells.

C. Other Names for Supragingival Calculus

- Supramarginal.*
- Extragingival.
- Coronal, indicating that the calculus is on the anatomic crown.
- Salivary, a term indicating that the source of the minerals is the saliva.

II. SUBGINGIVAL CALCULUS

A. Location

- On the clinical crown apical to the margin of the gingiva and extending nearly to the clinical attachment on the root surface.
- On dental implants.

B. Distribution

- May be generalized or localized on single teeth or a group of teeth.
- Heaviest deposits are related to areas most difficult for the patient to access during personal oral biofilm removal procedures.

---

*The terms supragingival and subgingival are at present probably the most widely used. Supramarginal and submarginal are more specific in their definition because the margin of the free gingiva is the dividing line between the two categories. The gingiva includes free and attached.

C. Other Names for Subgingival Calculus

- Submarginal.*
- Serumal, a term indicating that the source of the minerals is the blood serum.

COMPOSITION

- Calculus is made up of inorganic and organic components and water.
- The percentages vary depending on the age and hardness of a deposit and the location from which the sample for analysis is taken.
- Mature calculus usually contains inorganic components between 70 and 90%; the rest is organic components and water.
- The chemical content of supragingival and subgingival calculus is similar.[1-3]

I. INORGANIC CONTENT

A. Major Inorganic Components

- The main components are calcium (Ca), phosphorus (P), carbonate (CO_3), sodium (Na), magnesium (Mg), and potassium (K).

B. Trace Elements

- Various trace elements have been identified.
- Trace elements include chlorine (Cl), zinc (Zn), strontium (Sr), bromine (Br), copper (Cu), manganese (Mn), tungsten (W), gold (Au), aluminum (Al), silicon (Si), iron (Fe), and fluorine (F).

C. Fluoride in Calculus

- The concentration of fluoride in calculus varies and is influenced by the amount of fluoride received from fluoride in the drinking water, topical applications,[4] dentifrices,[5,6] or any form that is received by contact with the external surface of the calculus.

D. Crystals

- At least two-thirds of the inorganic matter of calculus is crystalline, principally apatite.
- Predominating is hydroxyapatite, which is the same crystal present in enamel, dentin, cementum, and bone.
- Calculus also contains varying amounts of brushite, whitlockite, and octacalcium phosphate.[7]

E. Calculus Compared With Teeth and Bone

- Dental enamel is the most highly mineralized tissue in the body and contains 96% inorganic salts; dentin contains 65% and cementum and bone contain 45 to 50%.[8]
- Mature calculus has approximately 70 to 90% inorganic content.
- A comparison of calculus with the tooth parts provides insight into the effects of instrumentation, the difficulty of distinguishing calculus from cementum or dentin when scaling subgingivally, and the modes of attachment of calculus to the tooth surface.

II. ORGANIC CONTENT

- The organic proportion of calculus consists of various types of microorganisms, desquamated epithelial cells, leukocytes, and mucin from the saliva.
- Substances identified in the organic matrix include cholesterol, cholesterol esters, phospholipids, and fatty acids in the lipid fraction; reducing sugars and carbohydrate–protein complexes in the carbohydrate fraction; and keratins, nucleoproteins, and amino acids in the protein portion.[9,10]

CALCULUS FORMATION[11]

Calculus results from the deposition of minerals into a biofilm organic matrix. Calculus formation occurs in three basic steps: *pellicle formation, biofilm formation,* and *mineralization.* Mineralization of supragingival and subgingival calculus is essentially the same, although the source of the elements for mineralization is not the same.

I. PELLICLE FORMATION

- The pellicle, or cuticle, is composed of mucoproteins from the saliva and is an acellular material.
- The pellicle begins to form within minutes after all deposits have been removed from the tooth surface.

II. BIOFILM MATURATION

- Microorganisms settle in the pellicle layer.
- Colonies are formed. In early calculus the colonies consist primarily of cocci and rod-shaped organisms. By the fifth day, the biofilm is mostly made up of filamentous organisms.
- The colonies grow together to form a cohesive biofilm layer.

III. MINERALIZATION

A. Early Calculus Formation

- Mineralization foci (centers) form.

---

*The terms supragingival and subgingival are at present probably the most widely used. Supramarginal and submarginal are more specific in their definition because the margin of the free gingiva is the dividing line between the two categories. The gingiva includes free and attached.

- Undisturbed, within 24 to 72 hours, more and more mineralization centers develop close to the underlying tooth surface. Eventually, the centers grow large enough to touch and unite.
- Mineralization first occurs within the intermicrobial matrix. The filamentous microorganisms provide the matrix for the deposition of minerals.
- As the deposit ages, mineralization within the bodies of the bacteria occurs.

B. Germfree Animal Studies

- A calculus-like deposit has been observed on the teeth of germfree animals that have no biofilm.[12–14]
- It may indicate that other organic substances, such as the pellicle, may mineralize.
- The pellicle is between the dental biofilm and the tooth surface. Since the attachment of calculus is very strong, it is expected that the pellicle must mineralize to create such a firm bond.

C. Sources of Minerals

- *Supragingival Calculus.* The source of elements for supragingival calculus is the saliva.
- *Subgingival Calculus.* The gingival sulcus fluid and the inflammatory exudate supply the minerals for the subgingival deposits. Because the amount of sulcus fluid and exudate increases with increases in inflammation, more minerals are available for mineralization of subgingival biofilm.

D. Crystal Formation

- Mineralization consists of crystal formation, namely, hydroxyapatite, octacalcium phosphate, whitlockite, and brushite, each with a characteristic developmental pattern.
- The crystals form in the intercellular matrix and on the surface of bacteria and finally within the bacteria.[15,16]

E. Mechanism of Mineralization[17]

- The mineralization process is considered the same for both supragingival and subgingival calculus.
- Heavy calculus formers have higher salivary levels of calcium and phosphorus than do light calculus formers.[18]
- Light calculus formers have higher levels of parotid pyrophosphate.[19]
- Pyrophosphate is an inhibitor of calcification and is used in anticalculus dentifrices.
- The process by which minerals, mainly calcium and phosphate, become incorporated from the saliva or gingival sulcus fluid into the biofilm matrix is still not completely understood.
- Research studies point to the probability that calcification of calculus may involve the same phenomena as those of other ectopic calcifications (such as urinary or renal calculi) and may be similar to normal calcification of bone, cartilage, enamel, or dentin.

IV. STRUCTURE OF CALCULUS

A. Layers

- Calculus forms in layers that are more or less parallel with the tooth surface.
- The layers are separated by lines that appear to be pellicle that was deposited over the previously formed calculus, and as mineralization progressed, the pellicle became imbedded.
- The lines between the layers of calculus can be called "incremental lines." They form around the tooth in supragingival calculus, but they form irregularly from crown to apex on the root surface in subgingival calculus. The lines are evidence that calculus grows or increases by apposition of new layers.

B. Surface

- The surface of a calculus mass is rough and can be detected by use of an explorer or probe.

C. Outer Layer

- The outer layer of subgingival calculus is partly calcified.
- On the surface is a thick, matlike, soft layer of dental biofilm. The outer surface of the biofilm on the subgingival calculus is in contact with the diseased pocket epithelial lining.

V. FORMATION TIME

- Formation time means the average number of days required for the primary soft deposit to change to the mature mineralized stage.
- The average time is about 12 days, within a range from 10 days for rapid calculus formers to 20 days for slow calculus formers.[18] Mineralization can begin as early as 24 to 48 hours when a patient's personal daily oral hygiene is neglected.
- Formation time depends on individual tendency, but it is strongly influenced by the roughness of the tooth surface and the care and character of personal biofilm control measures.
- Estimation of the approximate formation time for an individual can be helpful when planning instruction and counseling as well as treatment planning for professional care and frequency of maintenance appointments.

ATTACHMENT OF CALCULUS

- Calculus is more readily removed from some tooth surfaces than from others.

- The ease or difficulty of removal can be related to the manner of attachment of the calculus to the tooth surface.
- Several modes of attachment have been observed by conventional histologic techniques and electron microscopy. On any one tooth and in any one area, more than one mode of attachment may be found.
- When studying the attachment types, the character of the hard, smooth enamel surface and that of the rough, porous, cemental surface can be compared.
- Three general modes of attachment can be identified.[20]

I. ATTACHMENT BY MEANS OF AN ACQUIRED PELLICLE

- The pellicle is a thin, acellular, homogeneous layer positioned between the calculus and the tooth surface.
- Calculus attachment is superficial because no interlocking or penetration occurs.
- Pellicle attachment occurs most frequently on enamel and newly scaled and planed root surfaces.
- Calculus may be removed readily because of the smooth attachment.

II. ATTACHMENT TO MINUTE IRREGULARITIES IN THE TOOTH SURFACE BY MECHANICAL LOCKING INTO UNDERCUTS

- Enamel irregularities include cracks, lamellae, and carious defects.
- Cemental irregularities include tiny spaces left at previous locations of Sharpey's fibers, resorption lacunae, scaling grooves, and cemental tears.
- Difficult to be certain all calculus is removed when it is attached by this method because calculus becomes locked into the irregularities.

III. ATTACHMENT BY DIRECT CONTACT BETWEEN CALCIFIED INTERCELLULAR MATRIX AND THE TOOTH SURFACE

- Interlocking of inorganic crystals of the tooth with the mineralizing dental biofilm.
- Distinction between calculus and cementum is difficult during root debridement.

SIGNIFICANCE OF DENTAL CALCULUS

Calculus has long been considered to have an important role in the development, promotion, and recurrence of gingival and periodontal infections.

- Calculus is significant in the progression of inflammatory periodontal diseases.
- The disease-producing bacteria held in the rough surface of the calculus perpetuate the inflamed state supragingivally for gingivitis and subgingivally close to the pocket lining epithelium to promote periodontitis.

- The control of biofilm deposits by the patient on a daily basis, supplemented by complete professional calculus removal, can reduce or eliminate gingival inflammation.

I. RELATION TO DENTAL BIOFILM

- Subgingival biofilm develops as a result of downgrowth of supragingival biofilm bacteria.
- Subgingival biofilm contains pathogenic bacteria that cause inflammation and destruction in the soft tissue and lead to loss of attachment to the tooth surface and development and deepening of the pocket.

II. RELATION TO ATTACHMENT LOSS AND POCKET FORMATION

- With increased pocket depth, greater amounts of biofilm can accumulate with increased numbers of pathogenic organisms. Irritation to the pocket lining stimulates greater flow of gingival sulcus fluid, which contains minerals for subgingival calculus formation.
- Calculus is mineralized biofilm. The biofilm bacteria next to the tooth surface are mineralized first.
- Subgingival calculus is always covered by masses of active biofilm bacteria. The bacterial mass is in contact with the diseased pocket epithelium and promotes gingivitis and periodontitis.
- With its rough surface, permeable structure, and porosity, calculus can act as a reservoir for endotoxins and tissue breakdown products.
- Calculus is a predisposing factor in pocket development in that it provides a haven for the collection of bacterial masses on the rough surface of the calculus deposit.

CLINICAL CHARACTERISTICS

Identification of calculus prior to removal depends on knowledge of its appearance, consistency, and distribution. Appointment planning, selection of instruments, and techniques depend on understanding the texture, morphology, and mode of attachment of calculus. **Table 20-1** provides a summary of clinical characteristics.

I. SUPRAGINGIVAL EXAMINATION

A. Direct Examination

Supragingival deposits may be seen directly or indirectly, using a mouth mirror.

B. Use of Compressed Air

- Small amounts of calculus may be invisible when they are wet with saliva.
- With light and drying with air, small deposits usually can be seen.

TABLE 20-1	CLINICAL CHARACTERISTICS OF DENTAL CALCULUS	
CHARACTERISTIC	**SUPRAGINGIVAL CALCULUS**	**SUBGINGIVAL CALCULUS**
Color	White, creamy yellow, or gray May be stained by tobacco, food, or other pigments Slight deposits may be invisible until dried with compressed air	Light to dark brown, dark green, or black Stains derived from blood pigments from diseased pocket
Shape	Amorphous, bulky Gross deposits may (1) Form interproximal bridge between adjacent teeth (Figure 20-1B) (2) Extend over the margin of the gingiva Shape of calculus mass is determined by the anatomy of the teeth, contour of gingival margin, and pressure of the tongue, lips, cheeks	Flattened to conform with pressure from the pocket wall Combination of the following calculus formations occur* (1) Crusty, spiny, or nodular (2) Ledge or ringlike (3) Thin, smooth veneers (4) Finger- and fernlike (5) Individual calculus islands
Consistency and Texture	Moderately hard Newer deposits less dense and hard Porous surface covered with nonmineralized biofilm	Brittle, flintlike Harder and more dense than supragingival calculus Newest deposits near bottom of pocket are less dense and hard Surface covered with dental biofilm
Size and Quantity	Quantity has direct relationship to (1) Personal oral care procedures and biofilm control measures (2) Physical character of diet (3) Individual tendencies (4) Function and use Increased amount in tobacco smokers	Related to pocket depth Increased amount with age because of accumulation Quantity is related to personal care, diet, and individual tendency as it is with supragingival Subgingival is primarily related to the development and progression of periodontal infection
Distribution on Individual Tooth	Coronal to margin of gingiva May cover a large portion of the visible clinical crown, or may form fine thin line near gingival margin	Apical to margin of gingiva Extends to bottom of the pocket and follows contour of soft tissue attachment With gingival recession, subgingival calculus may become supragingival and become covered with typical supragingival calculus
Distribution on Teeth	Symmetrical arrangement on teeth except when influenced by (1) Malpositioned teeth (2) Unilateral hypofunction (3) Inconsistent personal care (4) Abrasion from food Occurs with or without associated subgingival deposits Location related to openings of the salivary gland ducts: (1) Facial surface of maxillary molars (2) Lingual surface of mandibular anterior teeth	Heaviest on proximal surfaces, lightest on facial surfaces Occurs with or without associated supragingival deposits

*Everett FG, Potter GR. Morphology of submarginal calculus. *J Periodontol.* 1959 Jan;30(1):27–31.

II. SUBGINGIVAL EXAMINATION

A. Visual Examination

- Dark edge of calculus may be seen at or just beneath the gingival margin.
- Gentle air blast can deflect the margin from the tooth for observation into the pocket.
- Using transillumination, a dark, opaque, shadowlike area seen on a proximal tooth surface may be subgingival calculus. Without calculus, stain, or thick soft deposit, the enamel is translucent.

B. Gingival Tissue Color Change

- Dark calculus may reflect through a thin margin and suggest the presence of subgingival calculus.

C. Tactile Examination

- *Probe.* While probing for sulcus/pocket characteristics, a rough subgingival tooth surface can be felt when calculus is present.
- *Explorer.* A fine subgingival explorer is needed that can be adapted close to the root surface all the way to the bottom of a pocket. Figure 15-14 (page 238) illustrates the use of the subgingival explorer.
- Each subgingival area needs to be examined carefully to the bottom of the pocket, completely around each tooth.

D. Radiographic Examination

- Radiographic examination is not useful for calculus detection because of highly mineralized tooth structure superimposed over calculus deposits.
- Thick, highly mineralized calculus may be detected on proximal tooth surfaces except when there is overlapping.

E. Perioscopy

- The use of dental endoscopy in deep pockets and furcations can show otherwise undetectable calculus, especially burnished calculus.[21]

PREVENTION OF CALCULUS

- Dental calculus can be a serious periodontal health problem.
- Patients at risk for calculus formation need personalized counseling.
- Risk factors related to calculus formation are similar to those for dental biofilm formation and relate to biofilm removal during the patient's personal daily oral care.

- There are several methods for coping with the problem of calculus including patient instruction and daily care and professional clinical nonsurgical periodontal therapy.

I. PERSONAL DENTAL BIOFILM CONTROL

A. Objective

- Removal of dental biofilm by appropriately selected brushing, flossing, and supplementary methods is a major factor in the control of dental calculus reformation.

B. Instruction

- The patient needs to understand the necessity for individual daily biofilm removal and be motivated to spend time each day.
- The dental hygienist first needs to teach and demonstrate the best choices of equipment and the correct procedures for the individual mouth; then second, patiently follow up over continuing appointments to commend the patient's successes and reteach as necessary.

C. Regular Professional Supervision

- Professional maintenance appointments on a regular basis can supplement the personal care.

II. PROFESSIONAL REMOVAL OF CALCULUS

- Thorough removal of calculus provides a smooth tooth surface in an environment conducive to gingival healing.
- The smooth surfaces can be easier for the patient to maintain.
- With emphasis on good oral hygiene and routine professional removal, low levels of supragingival and subgingival calculus have been demonstrated on a long-term basis.[22]

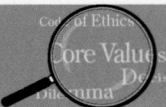

Everyday Ethics

Coronal polishing legislation had just been passed at the state level. Certified dental assistants (CDA) were now eligible to take a short course and then begin polishing procedures on a patient after the dentist or the dental hygienist removes all calculus deposits. Mindy, the CDA in the office, completed the course and was ready to polish. As the hygienist in the office, Hilary was basically unaffected by the change in the dental practice act and continued to treat her patients in all aspects of the preventive protocol.

However, Dr. Bell found that additional services could be offered to his patients at the time of their restorative appointment by removing the calculus and then having Mindy finish with the polish. One day, as Hilary was on her way to find Dr. Bell to check her patient, she saw Mindy using

a curet to remove what she stated as "slight subgingival deposits that didn't come off with the polishing cup."

Questions for Consideration

1. Which of the dental hygiene core values (Table II-1 in Section II, Introduction, page 38) enter into the actions of this scenario? Explain the relationship of each of the selected ones.
2. Would you consider what the hygienist observed the dental assistant doing as an ethical issue or dilemma? Explain your answer.
3. If Dr. Bell dismisses the fact that Mindy was using instruments to remove calculus, what choices of action could Hilary pursue?

III. ANTICALCULUS DENTIFRICE AND MOUTHRINSE

A. Objective

- Calculus-control dentifrices currently available aim to inhibit calculus crystal growth, which in turn should lessen the amount of calculus deposited on the teeth.
- The dentifrices do not have an effect on existing calculus deposits and are offered as a preventive measure against the formation of new supragingival calculus.
- For a patient who cannot control supragingival calculus, and hence cannot achieve optimum gingival tissue health, an anticalculus dentifrice may provide motivation, as well as a supplement to mechanical biofilm removal efforts.[23]

B. Chemotherapeutic Anticalculus Agents

- Agents used in "tartar-control" mouth rinses or dentifrices include pyrophosphates, zinc citrate or zinc chloride, and triclosan.[24]
- Soft tissue irritation or dentinal hypersensitivity has contraindicated their use by selected patients.

DOCUMENTATION

The permanent record of the patient subject to formation of calculus needs to include a minimum of the following:

- Calculus deposits are described in the initial examination record: charted to show location for reference during the clinical removal and during teaching personal care for prevention.
- The extent of supragingival and subgingival deposits (slight, moderate, or heavy) is designated for diagnosis, treatment planning, and for reference during instrumentation.

BOX 20-2	Example Progress Note

Patient for routine maintenance. No changes in health history; blood pressure 128/80; extraoral/intraoral nothing remarkable; probing: no bleeding on probing except distal #17 with probing depth at 4 mm with rough surface (calculus removed); demonstrated flossing and angle for toothbrush to get way back there. She blamed it on being left-handed and difficulty to turn brush. (She reminded me that it has been nearly 4 y since she first came. She believes we saved her teeth and thanked us all.)

Signed: _____, RDH Date: _____

- Personal patient care procedures demonstrated; preventive measures discussed; and frequency of continuing care appointments recommended.
- A sample patient progress note may be reviewed in **Box 20-2.**

Factors To Teach The Patient

- Good oral hygiene and frequent professional care for complete scaling are consistent with low levels of supragingival and subgingival calculus.
- What calculus is and how it forms from dental biofilm.
- The effect of calculus on the health of the periodontal tissues and, therefore, on the general health of the oral cavity.
- Properties of calculus that explain the need for detailed, meticulous scaling procedures.
- Reasons for producing a calculus-free smooth tooth surface during scaling.
- Biofilm control measures that the patient may carry out to minimize calculus deposits.
- What to expect from use of an anticalculus dentifrice.
- Only selecting products with an ADA Seal of Acceptance.

References

1. Mandel ID. Biochemical aspects of calculus formation. *J Periodont Res.* 1974;9(1):10–7.
2. Glock GE, Murray MM. Chemical investigation of salivary calculus. *J Dent Res.* 1938 Aug;17:257.
3. Mandel ID, Levy BM. Studies on salivary calculus. I. Histochemical and chemical investigations of supra- and subgingival calculus. *Oral Surg Oral Med Oral Pathol.* 1957 Aug;10(8):874–84.
4. Schait A, Mühlemann HR. Fluoride uptake by calculus following topical application of fluorides. *Helv Odont Acta.* 1971 Oct;15(2):132–3.
5. Kinoshita S, Schait A, Schroeder HE, Mühlemann HR. Origin of fluoride in early dental calculus. *Helv Odont Acta.* 1965 Oct;9(2):141–7.
6. Mühlemann HR, Schait A, Schroeder HE. Salivary origin of fluorine in calcified dental plaques. *Helv Odont Acta.* 1964 Oct;8:128.
7. Grøn P, van Campen GJ, Lindstrom I. Human dental calculus. Inorganic chemical and crystallographic composition. *Arch Oral Biol.* 1967 Jul;12(7):829–37.
8. Melfi RC. *Permar's oral embryology and microscopic anatomy.* 9th ed. Philadelphia: Lea & Febiger; 1994. 85 p.
9. Mandel ID, Levy BM, Wasserman BH. Histochemistry of calculus formation. *J Periodontol.* 1957 Apr;28:132.
10. Mandel ID. Histochemical and biochemical aspects of calculus formation. *Periodontics.* 1963 Mar–Apr;1:43.
11. Mandel ID. Calculus update: prevalence, pathogenicity and prevention. *J Am Dent Assoc.* 1995 May;126(5):573–80.
12. Fitzgerald RJ, McDaniel EG. Dental calculus in the germ-free rat. *Arch Oral Biol.* 1960 Aug;2:239–40.
13. Gustafsson BE, Krasse B. Dental calculus in germfree rats. *Acta Odontol Scand.* 1962;20(2):135–42.
14. Theilade J, Fitzgerald RJ, Scott DB, Nylen MU. Electron microscopic observations of dental calculus in germfree and conventional rats. *Arch Oral Biol.* 1964 Jan–Feb;9:97–100.
15. Gonzales F, Sognnaes RF. Electron microscopy of dental calculus. *Science.* 1960 Jan;131:156–8.

16. Zander HA, Hazen SP, Scott DB. Mineralization of dental calculus. *Proc Soc Exp Biol Med.* 1960 Feb;103:257–60.

17. Ingram GS, Edgar WM. Calcium salt precipitation and mechanisms of inhibition under oral conditions. *Adv Dent Res.* 1995 Dec;9:427.

18. Schroeder HE. *Formation and inhibition of dental calculus.* Vienna: Hans Huber Publishers; 1969. pp. 73–4.

19. Vogel JJ, Amdur BH. Inorganic pyrophosphate in parotid saliva and its relation to calculus formation. *Arch Oral Biol.* 1967 Jan;12(1):159–63.

20. Canis MF, Kramer GM, Pameijer CM. Calculus attachment. Review of the literature and new findings. *J Periodontol.* 1979 Aug;50(8):406–15.

21. Geisinger ML, Mealey BL, Schoolfield J, Mellomig JT. The effectiveness of subgingival scaling and root planing: An evaluation of therapy with and without the use of the periodontal endoscope. *J Periodontol.* 2007 Jan;78(1):22–8.

22. Anerud A, Löe H, Boysen H. The natural history and clinical course of calculus formation in man. *J Clin Periodontol.* 1991 Mar;18(3):160–70.

23. Tilliss TS. A closer look at tartar control dentifrices. *J Dent Hyg.* 1989 Oct;63(8):364–6, 368.

24. Mariotti AJ, Burrell KH. Mouthrinses and dentifrices. In: *ADA/PDR guide to dental therapeutics.* 4th ed. Chicago: ADA and Thomson; 2006. pp. 264–5, 267–9, 273–4.

CHAPTER 21

Dental Stains and Discolorations

ESTHER M. WILKINS, BS, RDH, DMD

Chapter Outline

Discolorations of the teeth and restorations occur in three general ways: (1) stain adheres directly to the surfaces, (2) stain contained within calculus and soft deposits, and (3) stain incorporated within the tooth structure or the restorative material. Instructional and clinical procedures apply to all three. The first two types may be removed by scaling or polishing. Certain stains may be prevented by the patient's routine personal care.

SIGNIFICANCE

- The significance of stains is primarily the appearance or cosmetic effect.
- In general, any detrimental effect on the teeth or gingival tissues is related to the dental biofilm or calculus in which the stain occurs.
- Thick deposits of stain conceivably can provide a rough surface on which dental biofilm can collect and irritate the adjacent gingiva.

- Certain stains provide a means of evaluating oral cleanliness and the patient's habits of personal care.
- Key words that relate to dental stains and discolorations are defined in **Box 21-1**.

I. CLASSIFICATION OF STAINS

A. Classified by Location

- *Extrinsic:* Extrinsic stains occur on the external surface of the tooth and may be removed by procedures of toothbrushing, scaling, and/or polishing.
- *Intrinsic:* Intrinsic stains occur within the tooth substance and cannot be removed by techniques of scaling or polishing.

B. Classified by Source

- *Exogenous.* Exogenous stains develop or originate from sources outside the tooth. Exogenous stains may be

Dental Stains and Discolorations

Amelogenesis imperfecta: imperfect formation of enamel; hereditary condition in which the ameloblasts fail to lay down the enamel matrix properly or at all.

Chlorophyll: green plant pigment essential to photosynthesis.

Chromogenic: producing color or pigment.

Chronologic: arranged in order of time.

Dentinogenesis imperfecta: hereditary disorder of dentin formation in which the odontoblasts lay down an abnormal matrix; can occur in both primary and permanent dentitions.

Endogenous: produced within or caused by factors within.

Exogenous: originating outside or caused by factors outside.

Extrinsic: derived from or situated on the outside; external.

Hypoplasia: incomplete development or underdevelopment of an organ or a tissue.

Intrinsic: situated entirely within.

extrinsic and stay on the outer surface of the tooth or intrinsic and become incorporated within the tooth structure.

■ *Endogenous.* Endogenous stains develop or originate from within the tooth. Endogenous stains are always intrinsic and usually are discolorations of the dentin reflected through the enamel.

II. RECOGNITION AND IDENTIFICATION

More than one type of stain may occur and more than one etiologic factor may cause the stains of an individual's dentition. A differential diagnosis may be needed.

A. Medical and Dental History

■ Developmental complications, medications, use of tobacco, and fluoride histories all contribute necessary information.

■ Accurately prepared medical and dental histories can provide information to supplement clinical observations.

B. Food Diary

■ Assessment of a patient's food diary may aid in identifying certain contributing factors.

C. Oral Hygiene Habits

■ The history of personal biofilm removal with the type and frequency of use of toothbrush, floss, and other supplemental materials and devices may help explain the presence of certain stains.

■ The state of oral hygiene and oral cleanliness is significant to the occurrence of dental stains.

III. APPLICATION OF PROCEDURES FOR STAIN REMOVAL

A. Stains Occurring Directly on the Tooth Surface

■ Stains that are directly associated with the biofilm or pellicle on the surface of the enamel or exposed cementum are removed as much as possible during toothbrushing by the patient.

■ Certain stains can be removed by scaling, whereas others require polishing.

■ When stains are tenacious, excessive polishing is avoided. As mild an abrasive agent as possible is used. Precautions are taken to prevent the following:

　■ Abrasion of the tooth surface or gingival margin

　■ Removal of a layer of fluoride-rich tooth surface

　■ Overheating with a power-driven polisher

B. Stains Incorporated Within Tooth Deposits

■ When stain is included within the substance of a soft deposit or calculus, it is removed with the deposit.

EXTRINSIC STAINS

The most frequently observed stains, yellow, green, black line, and tobacco, are described first; descriptions of the less common orange, red, and metallic stains follow.

I. YELLOW STAIN

A. Clinical Appearance

■ Dull, yellowish discoloration of dental biofilm.

B. Distribution on Tooth Surfaces

■ Yellow stain is associated with the presence of dental biofilm.

C. Occurrence

■ Common to all ages.

■ More evident when personal oral care procedures are neglected.

D. Etiology

■ Usually food pigments.

II. GREEN STAIN

A. Clinical Appearance

■ Light or yellowish green to very dark green.

- Embedded in dental biofilm.
- Occurs in three general forms:
  - Small curved line following contour of facial gingival crest.
  - Smeared irregularly, may even cover entire facial surface.
  - Streaked, following grooves or lines in enamel.
- The stain is frequently superimposed by soft yellow or gray debris (materia alba and food debris).
- Dark green may become embedded in surface enamel and be observed as an exogenous intrinsic stain when superficial layers of deposit are removed.
- Enamel under stain is sometimes demineralized as a result of cariogenic biofilm. The rough demineralized surface encourages biofilm retention, demineralization, and recurrence of green stain.

B. Distribution on Tooth Surfaces

- Primarily facial; may extend to proximal.
- Most frequently facial cervical third of maxillary anterior teeth.

C. Composition

- Chromogenic bacteria and fungi.
- Decomposed hemoglobin.
- Inorganic elements include calcium, potassium, sodium, silicon, magnesium, phosphorus, and other elements in small amounts.[1]

D. Occurrence

- May occur at any age; primarily found in childhood.
- Collects on both permanent and primary teeth.

E. Recurrence

- Recurrence depends on fastidiousness of personal care procedures.

F. Etiology

- Green stain results from oral uncleanliness, chromogenic bacteria, and gingival hemorrhage.
- Chromogenic bacteria or fungi are retained and nourished in dental biofilm where the green stain is produced.
- Blood pigments from hemoglobin are decomposed by bacteria.
- Predisposing factors are related to the lack of personal oral care, the presence of means for retention of dental biofilm and retained food debris.

G. Clinical Approach

- Do not scale the area. Often, an area of demineralized tooth structure underlies the stain and soft deposits.

- Ask the patient to remove the soft deposits during a dental biofilm control lesson. Initiate a daily fluoride remineralization program.

H. Other Green Stains

- In addition to the clinical entity known as "green stain" that was just described, dental biofilm and acquired pellicle may become stained a green color by a variety of substances.
- Differential distinction may be determined by questioning the patient or from items in the medical or dental histories. Green discoloration may result from the following:
  - Chlorophyll preparations
  - Metallic dusts of industry
  - Certain drugs. The stain from smoking marijuana may appear grayish-green.

III. BLACK-LINE STAIN

Black-line stain is a highly retentive black or dark brown calculus-like stain that forms along the gingival third near the gingival margin. It may occur on primary or permanent teeth.

A. Other Names

- Pigmented dental biofilm, brown stain, black stain.

B. Clinical Features

- Continuous or interrupted fine line, 1 mm wide (average), no appreciable thickness.
- May be a wider band or even occupy entire gingival third in severe cases (rare).
- Follows contour of gingival crest about 1 mm above crest.
- Usually demarcated from gingival crest by clear white line of unstained enamel.
- Appears black at bases of pits and fissures.
- Heavy deposits slightly elevated from the tooth surface may be detected by the gentle application of an explorer. Black-line stain has been compared to a calculus deposit.
- Gingiva is firm, with little or no tendency to bleed.
- Teeth are frequently clean and shiny, with a tendency to lower incidence of dental caries.

C. Distribution on Tooth Surfaces

- Facial and lingual surfaces; follows contour of gingival crest onto proximal surfaces.
- Rarely on facial surface of maxillary anterior teeth.
- Most frequently: lingual and proximal surfaces of maxillary posterior teeth.

D. Composition and Formation[2,3]

- Black-line stain, like calculus, is composed of microorganisms embedded in an intermicrobial substance.
- The microorganisms are primarily gram-positive rods, with other bacteria, including cocci, in smaller percentages.
- The composition of black-line stain is different from the composition of supragingival calculus, in which cocci predominate.
- Attachment to the tooth of black-line stain is by a pellicle-like structure.[4]
- Mineralization in black-line stain is similar to the formation of calculus.

E. Occurrence

- All ages; more common in childhood.
- More common in female patients.
- Frequently found in clean mouths.

F. Recurrence

- Black-line stain tends to form again despite regular personal care.
- Quantity may be less when biofilm control procedures are meticulous.

G. Predisposing Factors

- None apparent, except a natural tendency.

IV. TOBACCO STAIN

A. Clinical Appearance

- Light brown to dark leathery brown or black.
- Shape
  - Diffuse staining of dental biofilm.
  - Narrow band that follows contour of gingival crest, slightly above the crest.
  - Wide, firm, tarlike band may cover cervical third and extend to central third of crown.
- Incorporated in calculus deposit.
- Heavy deposits (particularly from smokeless tobacco) may penetrate the enamel and become exogenous intrinsic.

B. Distribution on Tooth Surface

- Cervical third, primarily.
- Any surface, as well as pits and fissures.
- Most frequently on lingual surfaces.

C. Composition

- Tar and products of combustion.
- Brown pigment from smokeless tobacco.

D. Predisposing Factors

- Natural tendencies. The quantity of stain is not necessarily proportional to the amount of tobacco used.
- Personal oral care procedures: increased deposits occur with neglect.
- Extent of dental biofilm and calculus available for adherence.

V. OTHER BROWN STAINS

A. Brown Pellicle

- The acquired pellicle is smooth and structureless and recurs readily after removal.[5]
- The pellicle can take on stains of various colors that result from chemical alteration of the pellicle.[6]

B. Stannous Fluoride[7–9]

- Light brown, sometimes yellowish, stain forms on the teeth in the pellicle after repeated use of a stannous fluoride gel or other product.
- The brown stain results from the formation of stannous sulfide or brown tin oxide from the reaction of the tin ion in the fluoride compound.

C. Foodstuffs

- Tea, coffee, and soy sauce are often implicated in the formation of a brownish-stained pellicle.
- As with other brown pellicle stains, less stain occurs when the personal oral hygiene and biofilm control are excellent.

D. Anti-Biofilm Agents[10,11]

- Chlorhexidine and alexidine are used in mouthrinses and are effective against biofilm formation.
- A brownish stain on the tooth surfaces may result, usually more pronounced on proximal and other surfaces less accessible to routine biofilm control procedures.
- The stain also tends to form more rapidly on exposed roots than on enamel. Tooth staining has been considered a significant side effect.

E. Betel Leaf[12]

- Betel leaf chewing is common among people of all ages in eastern countries. Betel has a caries-inhibiting effect.
- The discoloration imparted to the teeth is a dark mahogany brown, sometimes almost black. It may become thick and hard, with partly smooth and partly rough surfaces.
- Microscopically, the black deposit consists of microorganisms and mineralized material with a laminated

pattern characteristic of subgingival calculus. It can be removed by gentle scaling.

VI. ORANGE AND RED STAINS

A. Clinical Appearance

■ Orange or red stains appear at the cervical third.

B. Distribution on Tooth Surfaces

■ More frequently on anterior than on posterior teeth.

C. Occurrence

■ Rare (red more rare than orange).

D. Etiology

■ Chromogenic bacteria.

VII. METALLIC STAINS

A. Metals or Metallic Salts From Metal-Containing Dust of Industry

1. *Clinical appearance.* Examples of colors on teeth:
   ▨ Copper or brass: green or bluish-green.
   ▨ Iron: brown to greenish-brown.
   ▨ Nickel: green.
   ▨ Cadmium: yellow or golden brown.
2. *Distribution on tooth surfaces*
   ▨ Primarily anterior; may occur on any teeth.
   ▨ Cervical third more commonly affected.
3. *Manner of formation*
   ▨ Industrial worker inhales dust through mouth, bringing metallic substance in contact with teeth.
   ▨ Metal imparts color to biofilm.
   ▨ Occasionally, stain may penetrate tooth substance and become exogenous intrinsic stain.

B. Metallic Substances Contained in Drugs

1. *Clinical appearance.* Examples of colors on teeth:
   ▨ Iron: black (iron sulfide) or brown.
   ▨ Manganese (from potassium permanganate): black.
2. *Distribution on tooth surfaces*
   ▨ Generalized, may occur on all.
3. *Manner of formation*
   ▨ Drug enters biofilm substance, imparts color to biofilm and calculus.
   ▨ Pigment from drug may attach directly to tooth substance.
4. *Prevention*
   ▨ Use a medication through a straw or in tablet or capsule form to prevent direct contact with the teeth.

ENDOGENOUS INTRINSIC STAINS

Stains incorporated within the tooth structure may be related to the period of tooth development.

I. PULPLESS TEETH

Not all pulpless teeth discolor. Improved endodontic procedures have contributed to the prevention of many discolorations formerly associated with that cause.

A. Clinical Appearance

■ A wide range of colors exists; stains may be light yellow-brown, slate gray, reddish-brown, dark brown, bluish-black, or black. Others have an orange or greenish tinge.

B. Manner of Formation

■ Blood and other pulp tissue elements may be made available for breakdown as a result of hemorrhages in the pulp chamber, root canal treatment, or necrosis and decomposition of the pulp tissue.
■ Pigments from the decomposed hemoglobin and pulp tissue penetrate the dentinal tubules.

II. TETRACYCLINES

■ Tetracycline antibiotics, used widely for combating many types of infections, have an affinity for mineralized tissues and are absorbed by the bones and teeth. They can be transferred through the placenta and enter fetal circulation.
■ Discoloration of the teeth of a child can result when the drug is administered to the mother during the third trimester of pregnancy or to the child in infancy and early childhood.
■ Color of teeth may be light green to dark yellow, or a gray-brown. The discoloration depends on the dosage, the length of time the drug was used, and the type of tetracycline. After eruption, the teeth may fluoresce under ultraviolet light, but that property is lost with age and exposure.[13,14]
■ Discoloration may be generalized or limited to specific parts of individual teeth that were developing at the time of administration of the antibiotic. Reference to the Table of Tooth Development, Table 17-1, Permanent teeth (page 258); Table 49-8, Primary teeth (page 762) can assist in determining the patient's age at the time the drug was administered, and the patient's medical history at that age may reveal the illness for which the antibiotic was prescribed.

III. IMPERFECT TOOTH DEVELOPMENT

Defective tooth development may result from factors of genetic abnormality or environmental influences during tooth development.

A. Hereditary: Genetic[15]

- *Amelogenesis imperfecta:* The enamel is partially or completely missing because of a generalized disturbance of the ameloblasts. Teeth are yellowish-brown or gray-brown.
- *Dentinogenesis imperfecta ("Opalescent dentin"):* The dentin is abnormal as a result of disturbances in the odontoblastic layer during development. The teeth appear translucent or opalescent and vary in color from gray to bluish-brown.

B. Enamel Hypoplasia

- *Systemic hypoplasia* (chronologic hypoplasia resulting from ameloblastic disturbance of short duration): Teeth erupt with white spots or with pits. Over a long period, the white spots may become discolored from food pigments or other substances taken into the mouth.
- *Local hypoplasia* (affects single tooth): White spots may become stained as in systemic hypoplasia.

C. Dental Fluorosis

- Dental fluorosis was originally called "brown stain." Later, Dr. Frederick S. McKay, who studied the condition and described it in the dental literature, named it "mottled enamel."

    A. *Manner of formation*
- Enamel hypomineralization results from ingestion of excessive fluoride ion in drinking water (more than 2 parts per million) during the period of mineralization. The enamel alterations are a result of toxic damage to the ameloblasts.
- When the teeth erupt, they have white spots or areas that later become discolored from oral pigments and appear light or dark brown.

- Severe effects of excess fluoride during development may produce cracks or pitting; the discoloration concentrates in these. This condition and appearance led to the name mottled enamel.

    B. *Classification*
- Dean provided the original definitions for five grades of fluorosis (in Chapter 22, page 331). They ranged from "questionable" (a few white flecks or spots) to "severe" (marked brown staining and pitting of the enamel surfaces).[16]
- More specific classifications have been developed for clinical and research purposes,[17,18] such as the Tooth Surface Index of Fluorosis (TSIF; in Chapter 22, page 332).

IV. OTHER SYSTEMIC CAUSES

- Several types of tooth discolorations may result from blood-borne pigments.
- Pigments circulating in the blood are transmitted to the dentin from the capillaries of the pulp. For example, prolonged jaundice early in life can impart a yellow or greenish discoloration to the teeth.
- Erythroblastosis fetalis (Rh incompatibility) may leave a green, brown, or blue hue to the teeth.

EXOGENOUS INTRINSIC STAINS

- When intrinsic stains come from an outside source, not from within the tooth, the stain is called exogenous intrinsic.
- Extrinsic stains, such as tobacco and green stains, can provide stain that becomes intrinsic.
- Restorative materials cause staining of teeth, as described in the section that follows.
- Tooth-color restorations may become stained from the various extrinsic staining substances.

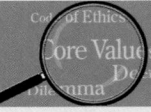

Everyday Ethics

Everyday EthicsDaniel returned to the dental office of Dr. Windum after 3 years of working on the East Coast. At the age of 32, Daniel was exhibiting signs of early periodontitis with gingival inflammation and increased subgingival calculus. Ruthie, the dental hygienist, immediately began talking to Daniel about biofilm and suggesting improvements for his personal daily brushing and flossing to change his personal care of his gingival tissues. After she completed a quadrant of scaling with local anesthesia, she suggested that rinsing with chlorhexidine after brushing before going to bed would help the healing.

Dr. Windum confirmed Ruthie's recommendation and wrote the prescription. Daniel left the office only to call a few days later to complain about the "awful brown stain on his teeth and horrible taste of the mouthrinse." He further indicated that he had stopped using the product and wanted to come in and have the stain removed immediately.

Questions for Consideration

1. Which of the dental hygiene core values (in Section II, Introduction, Table II-1, page 38) have application in this scenario? How does each core value selected enter the picture?
2. Daniel seems more concerned about the tooth staining and flavor of the chlorhexidine rinse than about the health of his gingival tissues while Ruthie's concerns are for improving his gingival health. What ethical principles may be in effect here?
3. Using the questions in Table V-1 (in Section V, Introduction, (page 362) help Ruthie work out a more favorable response to her choice of therapy for her patient's poor gingival health.

Patient in for second quadrant scaling/planning with anesthesia.

Personal care was poor; time was spent reviewing the methods the patient was using to keep the staining down from her tobacco habit. She claimed only to smoke one-half pack per day but the staining seemed greater than that. I suggested using a whitening dentifrice after lunch in addition to her usual morning and bedtime. She didn't act interested. Explained that her gingiva needed the third brushing even if she didn't mind the staining.

Signed: _____, RDH Date: _____

Factors To Teach The Patient

■ Predisposing factors that contribute to stain accumulation.
■ Personal care procedures that can aid in the prevention or reduction of stains.
■ Advantages of starting a smoking cessation program.
■ Reasons for not using an abrasive dentifrice with vigorous brushing strokes to lessen or remove stain accumulation.
■ The need to avoid tobacco, coffee, tea, and other beverages or foodstuffs that can stain, to prevent discoloration of new restorations.
■ Reasons for the difficulty of removing certain extrinsic stains during scaling and polishing.
■ Effect of tetracyclines on developing teeth. Need to avoid use during pregnancy and by children to age 12.

I. RESTORATIVE MATERIALS

A. Silver Amalgam

■ Silver amalgam can impart a gray to black discoloration to the tooth structure around a restoration.
■ Metallic ions migrate from the amalgam restoration into the enamel and dentin.
■ Silver, tin, and mercury ions eventually contact debris at the junction of the tooth and the restoration and form sulfides, which are products of corrosion.

B. Copper Amalgam

■ Copper amalgam used for filling primary teeth may impart a bluish-green color.

II. ENDODONTIC THERAPY

■ Silver nitrate: bluish-black.
■ Volatile oils: yellowish-brown.
■ Strong iodine: brown.
■ Aureomycin: yellow.
■ Silver-containing root canal sealer: black.

III. STAIN IN DENTIN

Discoloration resulting from a carious lesion is an example.

DOCUMENTATION

The permanent record of a patient with staining on the teeth needs explanations in the record of which stains, their location and other information of a descriptive nature.

■ Record color, type, extent, and location of stains with the patient's examination and assessment.
■ Make additions to the dental history as information is gained concerning the origin of stains such as those related to tooth development, systemic disease, occupations, or medications.
■ A sample progress note may be found in **Box 21-2**.

References

1. Shay DE, Haddox JH, Richmond JL. An inorganic qualitative and quantitative analysis of green stain. *J Am Dent Assoc.* 1955 Feb;50(2):156–60.
2. Theilade J, Slots J, Fejerskov O. The ultrastructure of black stain on human primary teeth. *Scand J Dent Res.* 1973;81(7):528–32.
3. Slots J. The microflora of black stain on human primary teeth. *Scand J Dent Res.* 1974;82(7):484–90.
4. Theilade J. Development of bacterial plaque in the oral cavity. *J Clin Periodontol.* 1977 Dec;4(5):1–12.
5. Meckel AH. The formation and properties of organic films on teeth. *Arch Oral Biol.* 1965 Jul–Aug;10(4):585–98.
6. Eriksen HM, Nordbø H. Extrinsic discoloration of teeth. *J Clin Periodontol.* 1978 Nov;5(4):229–36.
7. Horowitz HS, Chamberlin SR. Pigmentation of teeth following topical applications of stannous fluoride in a nonfluoridated area. *J Public Health Dent.* 1971 Winter;31(1):32–7.
8. Shannon IL. Stannous fluoride: does it stain teeth? How does it react with tooth surfaces? A review. *Gen Dent.* 1978 Sep–Oct; 26(5):64–71.
9. Leverett DH, McHugh WD, Jensen ØE. Dental caries and staining after twenty-eight months of rinsing with stannous fluoride or sodium fluoride. *J Dent Res.* 1986 Mar;65(3):424–7.
10. Flötra L, Gjermo P, Rölla G, Waerhaug J. Side effects of chlorhexidine mouth washes. *Scand J Dent Res.* 1971 Apr;79(2):119–25.
11. Formicola AJ, Deasy MJ, Johnson DH, Howe EE. Tooth staining effects of an alexidine mouthwash. *J Periodontol.* 1979 Apr;50(4):207–11.
12. Reichart PA, Lenz H, König H, Becker J, Mohr U. The black layer on the teeth of betel chewers: a light microscopic, microradiographic, and electronmicroscopic study. *J Oral Pathol.* 1985 Jul;14(6): 466–75.
13. Ehrlich A, Torres HO. *Essentials of dental assisting.* Philadelphia: Saunders; 1992. Chapter 20, Restorative dentistry; p. 389–93.
14. Robinson HB, Miller AS. *Color atlas of oral pathology.* 5th ed. Philadelphia: Lippincott; 1990. p. 55.
15. Robinson op.cit., p. 41.
16. Moulton FR, editor. *Fluorine and dental health.* Washington: American Association for the Advancement of Science; c1942. Dean HT. Investigation of physiological effects by epidemiological method.
17. Thylstrup A, Fejerskov O. Clinical appearance of dental fluorosis in permanent teeth in relation to histologic changes. *Community Dent Oral Epidemiol.* 1978 Nov;6(6):315–28.
18. Horowitz HS, Driscoll WS, Meyers RJ, Heifetz SB, Kingman A. A new method for assessing the prevalence of dental fluorosis—the Tooth Surface Index of Fluorosis. *J Am Dent Assoc.* 1984 Jul;109(1):37–41.

CHAPTER

Indices and Scoring Methods

CHARLOTTE J. WYCHE, RDH, MS

Chapter Outline

Chapter 22 provides an introduction to scoring methods used by clinicians, researchers, and community practitioners to evaluate indicators of oral health status. It is not possible to explain all of the many dental indices that have been used in a variety of settings, but several well-known and widely used indices and scoring methods are described in this chapter. **Box 22-1** defines related terminology.

TYPES OF SCORING METHODS

Indices and scoring methods are used in clinical practice and by community programs to determine and record the oral health status of individuals and groups. Familiarity with the various types of indices is useful to distinguish between different evaluation criteria needed for an individual oral health assessment and a group oral health survey.

BOX 22-1	Key Words

Indices and Scoring Methods

Calibration: agreement with a set standard of performance; determination of accuracy and consistency between examiners to standardize procedures and gain reliability of recorded findings. Examiners who collect dental index data for epidemiological research or community health assessment are trained to measure the index in exactly the same way each time.

Community oral health assessment: a multifaceted process of identifying factors that affect the oral health status of a selected population.

Data: pieces of information collected using measurements and/or counts.

Data collection: the process of gathering information (through the use of tools such as dental indices).

Epidemiology: the study of the relationships of various factors that determine the frequency and distribution of diseases in the human community; study of health and disease in populations.

Incidence: the rate at which a certain event occurs, as the number of new cases of a specific disease occurring during a certain period of time.

Index: a graduated, numeric scale with upper and lower limits; scores on the scale correspond to a specific criterion for individuals or populations; *pl.* indices or indexes.

Dental index: describes oral status by expressing clinical observations as numeric values.

Indicator: a factor that typically characterizes a disease or health condition; a factor measured and analyzed to describe health status. Dental indices described in this chapter measure oral health indicators.

Pilot study: a trial run of a planned study using a small sample to pretest an instrument, survey, or questionnaire.

Placebo: an inactive substance or preparation with no intrinsic therapeutic value given to satisfy a patient's symbolic need for drug therapy; used in controlled research studies in a form identical in appearance to the material being tested.

Prevalence: the total number of cases of a specific disease or condition in existence in a given population at a certain time.

Ramfjord Index Teeth: teeth used for epidemiologic studies of periodontal diseases: the maxillary right and mandibular left first molars, maxillary left and mandibular right first premolars, and maxillary left and mandibular right central incisors.

Reliability: ability of an index or test procedure to measure consistently at different times and under a variety of conditions; reproducibility; consistency.

Sample: a portion or subset of an entire population.

Screening: assessment of many individuals to disclose certain characteristics or diseases in a population.

Individual screening: brief assessment for initial evaluation and classification of need for additional examination and treatment planning.

Status: refers to the state or condition of an individual or population.

Surveillance: the ongoing systematic collection, analysis, and interpretation of outcome-specific data for use in planning, implementing, and evaluating the effect of public health programs and practices.

Validity: ability of an index or test procedure to measure what it is intended to measure.

I. INDIVIDUAL ASSESSMENT SCORE

A. Purpose

In clinical practice, an index, biofilm record, or scoring system for an individual patient can be used for education, motivation, and evaluation.

■ The effects of personal disease control efforts, the progress of healing between professional treatments, and the maintenance of health over time can be monitored.

■ An example is the "Plaque-Free Score," in which a patient is able to measure the effects of personal daily care efforts by the changes in the scores.

B. Uses

■ To provide individual assessment to help a patient recognize an oral problem.

■ To reveal the degree of effectiveness of present oral hygiene practices.

■ To motivate the patient during preventive and professional care for the elimination and control of oral disease.

■ To evaluate the success of individual and professional treatment over a period of time by comparing index scores.

II. CLINICAL TRIAL

A. Purpose

A clinical trial is planned to determine the effect of an agent or procedure on the prevention, progression, or control of a disease.

■ The trial is conducted by comparing an experimental group with a control group that is similar to the experimental group in every way except for the variable being studied.

■ Examples of indices used for clinical trials are the Plaque Index (PL I)[1] and the Patient Hygiene Performance (PHP).[2]

B. Uses

■ To determine baseline data before experimental factors are introduced.
■ To measure the effectiveness of specific agents for the prevention, control, or treatment of oral conditions.
■ To measure the effectiveness of mechanical devices for personal care, such as toothbrushes, interdental cleaning devices, or irrigators.

III. EPIDEMIOLOGIC SURVEY

A. Purpose

The word *epidemiology* denotes the study of disease characteristics of populations. Epidemiologic surveys provide information on the trends and patterns of oral health and disease in populations.

■ An example is the DMFT (decayed, missing, and filled teeth) Index[3] that has been used with populations around the world to determine the extent of dental caries.
■ Such a survey was designed for evaluation of groups of people rather than an individual patient.

B. Uses

■ To determine the prevalence and incidence of a particular condition occurring within a given population.
■ To provide baseline data on indicators that show existing dental health status in populations. The Surgeon General's Report on *Oral Health in America*[4] uses epidemiologic data to identify oral health disparities in certain populations.
■ To provide data to support recommendations for public health interventions to improve the health status of populations, such as those provided in the United States *Healthy People 2020* document.[5]

IV. COMMUNITY SURVEILLANCE

A. Purpose

Community surveillance of oral health indicators and determinants can be accomplished at many levels.

■ Government agencies, local community-based service-providing agencies, and professional associations are examples of groups that collect data to determine oral health status by conducting oral health screenings.
■ The techniques for conducting community-based oral screenings are similar to those used when conducting epidemiologic surveys, but there is usually a practical application in mind of planning for local community-based oral health services or education.

■ An example of a system designed to be used by a community-based group is the Association of State and Territorial Dental Directors' (ASTDD) Basic Screening Survey.[6]

B. Uses

■ To assess the needs of a community.
■ To provide information to help plan community-based health promotion/disease prevention programs.
■ To compare the effects or evaluate the results of community-based programs.

INDICES

An index is an expression of clinical observations in numeric values. It is used to describe the status of the individual or group with respect to a condition being measured. The use of a numeric scale and a standardized method for interpreting observations of a condition results in an index score that is more consistent and less subjective than a word description of that condition.

I. DESCRIPTIVE CATEGORIES OF INDICES

A. General Categories

■ *Simple Index:* measures the presence or absence of a condition. An example is an index that measures the presence of dental biofilm without evaluating its effect on the gingiva.
■ *Cumulative Index:* measures all the evidence of a condition, past and present. An example is the DMFT Index for dental caries (page 327).

B. Types of Simple and Cumulative Indices

■ *Irreversible:* measures conditions that will not change. An example is an index that measures dental caries.
■ *Reversible:* measures conditions that can be changed. Examples are indices that measure dental biofilm.

II. SELECTION CRITERIA

A useful and effective index:

■ is simple to use and calculate.
■ requires minimal equipment and expense.
■ uses a minimal amount of time to complete.
■ does not cause patient discomfort nor is otherwise unacceptable to a patient.
■ has clear-cut criteria that are readily understandable.
■ is as free as possible from subjective interpretation.

- is reproducible by the same examiner or different examiners.
- is amenable to statistical analysis; has validity and reliability.

INDICES THAT MEASURE ORAL HYGIENE STATUS (BIOFILM, DEBRIS, CALCULUS)

Indices that measure oral hygiene status can be used in a clinical setting to educate and motivate an individual patient. When data is collected in a community setting, such as a nursing home, the findings can help determine how daily oral care is being provided and monitor the results of oral hygiene education programs.

I. "PLAQUE INDEX" (PL I)[1,7]

A. Purpose

To assess the thickness of biofilm at the gingival area.

B. Selection of Teeth

The entire dentition or selected teeth can be evaluated.

- *Areas Examined:* Examine four gingival areas (distal, facial, mesial, lingual) systematically for each tooth.
- *Modified Procedures:* Examine only the facial, mesial, and lingual areas. Assign double score to the mesial reading, and divide the total by 4.

C. Procedure

- Dry the teeth and examine visually using adequate light, mouth mirror, and probe or explorer.
- Evaluate dental biofilm on the cervical third; pay no attention to biofilm that has extended to the middle or incisal thirds.
- Use probe to test the surface when no biofilm is visible. Pass the probe or explorer across the tooth surface in the cervical third and near the entrance to the sulcus. When no biofilm adheres to the probe tip, the area is scored 0. When biofilm adheres, a score of 1 is assigned.
- Use a disclosing agent, if necessary, to assist evaluation for the 0 to 1 scores. When the Pl I is used in conjunction with the Gingival Index (GI), the GI must be completed first because the disclosing agent masks the gingival characteristics.
- Include biofilm on the surface of calculus and on dental restorations in the cervical third in the evaluation.

- Criteria.

"PLAQUE INDEX" (PL I)	
SCORE	**CRITERIA**
0	No biofilm.
1	A film of biofilm adhering to the free gingival margin and adjacent area of the tooth. The biofilm may be recognized only after application of disclosing agent or by running the explorer across the tooth surface.
2	Moderate accumulation of soft deposits within the gingival pocket that can be seen with the naked eye or on the tooth and gingival margin.
3	Abundance of soft matter within the gingival pocket and/or on the tooth and gingival margin.

D. Scoring

- *Pl I for Area*
  Each area of a tooth (distal, facial, mesial, lingual, or palatal) is assigned a score from 0 to 3.
- *Pl I for a Tooth*
  Scores for each area are totaled and divided by 4.
- *Pl I for Groups of Teeth*
  Scores for individual teeth may be grouped and totaled and divided by the number of teeth. For instance, a Pl I may be determined for specific teeth or groups of teeth. The right side of the dentition may be compared with the left.
- *Pl I for the Individual*
  Add the scores for each tooth and divide by the number of teeth examined. The Pl I ranges from 0 to 3.
- *Suggested Range of Scores for Patient Reference*

RATING	**SCORES**
Excellent	0
Good	0.1–0.9
Fair	1.0–1.9
Poor	2.0–3.0

- *Pl I for a group*
  Add the scores for each member of a group and divide by the number of individuals.

II. "PLAQUE CONTROL RECORD"[8]

A. Purpose

To record the presence of dental biofilm on individual tooth surfaces to permit the patient to visualize progress while learning biofilm control.

B. Selection of Teeth and Surfaces

- All teeth are included. Missing teeth are identified on the record form by a single thick horizontal line.

- Four surfaces are recorded: facial, lingual, mesial, and distal.
- Six areas may be recorded. The mesial and distal segments of the diagram may be divided to provide space to record proximal surfaces from the facial separately from the lingual or palatal surfaces **(Figure 22-1)**.[9]

C. Procedure

- Apply disclosing agent or give a chewable tablet. Instruct patient to swish and rub the solution over the tooth surfaces with the tongue before rinsing.
- Examine each tooth surface for dental biofilm at the gingival margin. No attempt is made to differentiate quantity of biofilm.
- Record by making a dash or coloring in the appropriate spaces on the diagram **(Figure 22-1)** to indicate biofilm on facial, lingual, palatal, mesial, and/or distal surfaces.

D. Scoring

- Total the number of teeth present; multiply by 4 (or 6 if modification is used) to obtain the number of available surfaces. Count the number of surfaces with biofilm.
- Multiply the number of biofilm-stained surfaces by 100 and divide by the total number of available surfaces to derive the percentage of surfaces with biofilm.
- Compare scores over subsequent appointments as the patient learns and practices biofilm control. Ten percent or less biofilm-stained surfaces can be considered a good goal, but if the biofilm is regularly left in the same areas, special instruction is indicated.

Calculation: **Example for "Plaque Control Record"**
Individual findings: 26 teeth scored; 8 surfaces with biofilm

- Multiply the number of teeth by 4: $26 \times 4 = 104$ surfaces
- Percent with biofilm =

$$\frac{\text{Number of surfaces with biofilm} \times 100}{\text{Number of available tooth surfaces}} = \frac{8 \times 100}{104}$$

$$= \frac{800}{104}$$

$$= 7.6\%$$

Interpretation
Although 0% is ideal, less than 10% biofilm-stained surfaces has been suggested as a guideline in periodontal therapy. After initial therapy and when the patient has reached a 10% level of biofilm control or better, necessary additional periodontal and restorative procedures may be initiated.[8] In comparison, a similar evaluation using a biofilm-free score would mean that a goal of 90% or better biofilm-free surfaces would have to be reached before the surgical phase of treatment could be undertaken.

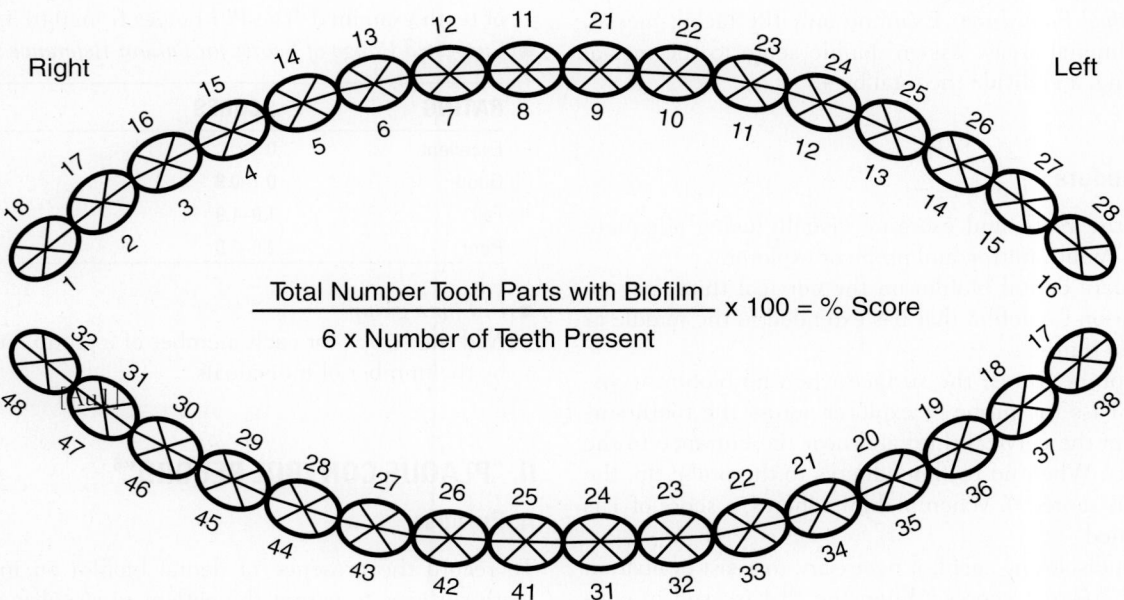

Total Number Tooth Parts with Biofilm / 6 x Number of Teeth Present x 100 = % Score

FIGURE 22-1 "Plaque Control Record." Diagrammatic representation of the teeth includes spaces to record biofilm on six areas of each tooth. The facial surfaces are on the outer portion and the lingual and palatal surfaces are on the inner portion of the arches. Teeth are numbered by the ADA System on the inside and by the FDI System on the outside. (*Source:* Adapted with permission from Ramfjord SP, Ash MM. *Periodontology and periodontics.* Philadelphia: WB Saunders Co.; 1979. 273 p. and from O'Leary TJ, Drake RB, Naylor JE. *J. Periodontol.* 1972;43:38.)

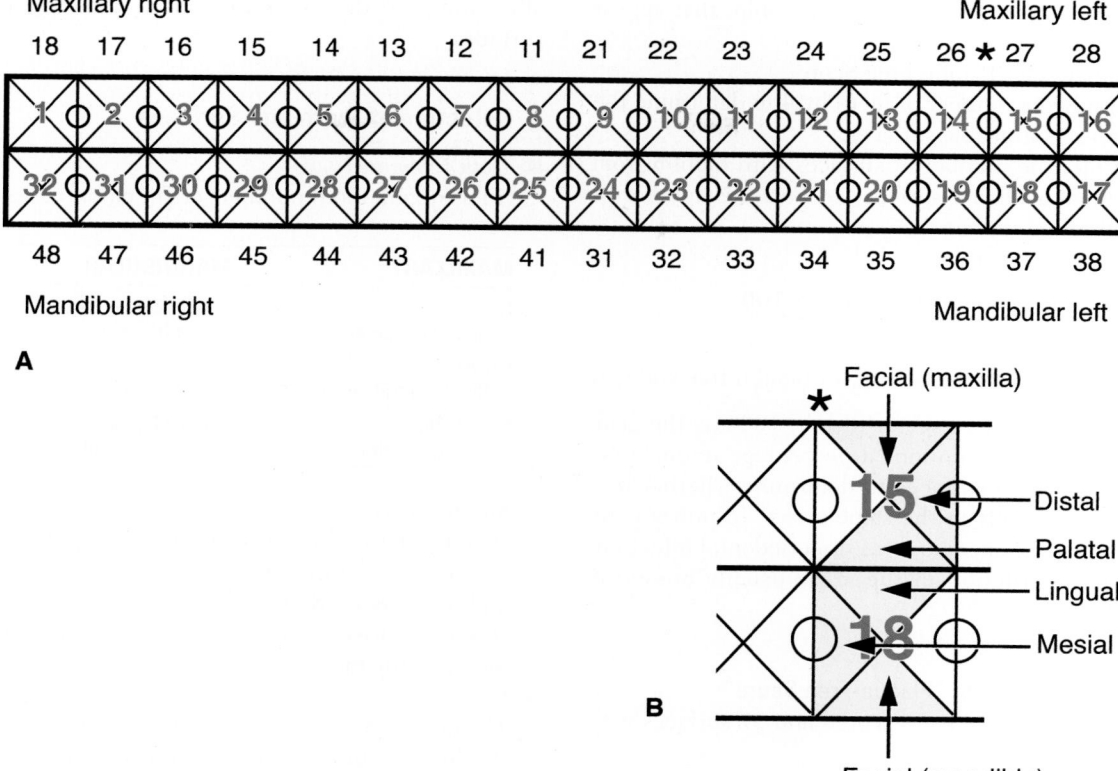

FIGURE 22-2 **"Plaque-Free Score."** **(A)** Diagrammatic representation of the teeth used to record biofilm and papillary bleeding. **(B)** Enlargement of one section of the diagram shows tooth surfaces. Teeth are numbered by the ADA System inside each block and by the FDI System outside each block. (*Source:* Adapted with permission from Grant DA, Stern IB, Listgarten MA. *Periodontics*. 6th ed. St. Louis: Mosby; 1988. 613 p.)

III. "PLAQUE-FREE SCORE"[10]

A. Purpose

To determine the location, number, and percentage of biofilm-free surfaces for individual motivation and instruction. Interdental bleeding can also be documented.

B. Selection of Teeth and Surfaces

- All erupted teeth are included. Missing teeth are identified on the record form by a single thick horizontal line through the box in the chart form.
- Four surfaces are recorded for each tooth: facial, lingual or palatal, mesial, and distal.

C. Procedure

- *"Plaque-Free Score"*
  A. Apply disclosing agent or give chewable tablet. Instruct patient to swish and rub the solution over the tooth surfaces with the tongue before rinsing.

  B. Examine each tooth surface for evidence of biofilm. Use adequate light and a mouth mirror for visualizing all surfaces. The patient needs a hand mirror to see the location of the biofilm that has been missed during personal hygiene procedures.
  C. Record in red the surfaces showing biofilm. Use an appropriate tooth chart form or a diagrammatic form, such as that shown in **Figure 22-2**. Red ink for recording the biofilm is suggested when a red disclosing agent is used to help the patient associate the location of the biofilm in the mouth with the recording.
- *Papillary Bleeding on Probing*
  A. The small circles between the diagrammatic tooth blocks in **Figure 22-2** are used to record proximal bleeding on probing.
  B. Improvement in the gingival tissue health will be demonstrated over a period of time as fewer bleeding areas are noted.

D. Scoring: "Plaque-Free Score"

- Total the number of teeth present

- Total the number of surfaces with biofilm that appear in red on the tooth diagram
- To calculate the "Plaque-Free Score"
  - Multiply the number of teeth by 4 to determine the number of available surfaces.
  - Subtract the number of surfaces with biofilm from the total available surfaces to find the number of biofilm-free surfaces.
  - Biofilm-free score =

$$\frac{\text{Number of biofilm-free surfaces} \times 100}{\text{Number of available surfaces}}$$

$$= \text{Percentage of biofilm-free surfaces}$$

- Evaluate biofilm-free score: Ideally, 100% is the goal. When a patient maintains a percentage under 85%, check individual surfaces to determine whether biofilm is usually left in the same areas. To prevent the development of specific areas of periodontal infection, remedial instruction in the areas usually missed is indicated.

Calculation: Example for "Plaque-Free Score"

Individual findings: 24 teeth scored and 37 surfaces with biofilm

- Multiply the number of teeth by 4: 24 × 4 = 96 available surfaces.
- Subtract the number of surfaces with biofilm from total available surfaces: 96 − 37 = 59 biofilm-free surfaces.
- Percentage of biofilm-free surfaces =

$$\frac{59 \times 100}{96} = 61.5\%$$

Interpretation

On the basis of the ideal 100%, 61.5% is poor. More personal daily oral care instruction is indicated.

E. Scoring: Papillary Bleeding on Probing

- Total the number of small circles marked for bleeding. A patient with 32 teeth has 30 interdental areas. The mesial or distal surface of a tooth adjacent to an edentulous area is probed and counted.
- Evaluate total interdental bleeding. In health, bleeding on probing does not occur.

IV. PATIENT HYGIENE PERFORMANCE[2]

A. Purpose

To assess the extent of biofilm and debris over a tooth surface. Debris is defined for the PHP as the soft foreign material consisting of dental biofilm, materia alba, and food debris that is loosely attached to tooth surfaces.

B. Selection of Teeth and Surfaces

- *Teeth Examined*
  (FDI System tooth numbers are in parentheses.)

MAXILLARY	MANDIBULAR
No. 3 (16) Right first molar	No. 19 (36) Left first molar
No. 8 (11) Right central incisor	No. 24 (31) Left central incisor
No. 14 (26) Left first molar	No. 30 (46) Right first molar

- *Substitutions*
  When a first molar is missing, is less than three-fourths erupted, has a full crown, or is broken down, the second molar is used. The third molar is used when the second is missing. The adjacent central incisor is used for a missing incisor.
- *Surfaces*
  The facial surfaces of incisors and maxillary molars and the lingual surfaces of mandibular molars are examined. These surfaces are the same as those used for the Simplified Oral Hygiene Index (see **Figure 22-4**).

C. Procedure

Apply disclosing agent. Instruct the patient to swish for 30 seconds and expectorate, but not rinse.

- Examination is made using a mouth mirror.
- Each tooth surface to be evaluated is subdivided (mentally) into five sections **(Figure 22-3A)** as follows:
  A. Vertically. Three divisions-mesial, middle, and distal.
  B. Horizontally. The middle third is subdivided into gingival, middle, and occlusal or incisal thirds.

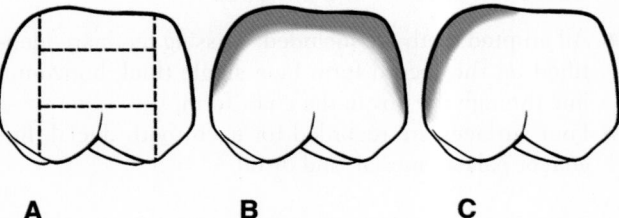

A　　　　**B**　　　　**C**

FIGURE 22-3 **Patient Hygiene Performance (PHP). (A)** Oral debris is assessed by dividing a tooth into 5 subdivisions, each of which is scored 1 when debris is shown to be present after use of a disclosing agent. **(B)** Example of debris score of 3. Shaded portion represents debris stained by disclosing agent. **(C)** Example of debris score of 1. (*Source:* Podshadley AG, Haley JV. A method for evaluating oral hygiene performance. *Public Health Rep* 1968 Mar;83(3):259–64.)

■ Each of the five subdivisions is scored for the presence of stained debris as follows:

PHP	
SCORE	**CRITERIA**
0	No debris (or questionable).
1	Debris definitely present.
M	When all three molars or both incisors are missing.
S	When a substitute tooth is used.

D. Scoring

■ *Debris Score for Individual Tooth*
   Add the scores for each of the five subdivisions. The scores range from 0 to 5. Examples are shown in **Figure 22-3B** and **C**.

■ *PHP for the Individual*
   Total the scores for the individual teeth and divide by the number of teeth examined. The PHP ranges from 0 to 5.

■ *Suggested Range of Scores for Evaluation*

RATING	**SCORES**
Excellent	0 (no debris)
Good	0.1–1.7
Fair	1.8–3.4
Poor	3.5–5.0

Calculation: Example for an Individual

TOOTH	**DEBRIS SCORE**
No. 3 (16)	5
No. 8 (11)	3
No. 14 (26)	4
No. 19 (36)	5
No. 24 (31)	2
No. 30 (46)	3
Total	22

$$\frac{\text{Total debris score}}{\text{Number of teeth scored}} = \frac{22}{6} = 3.66$$

Interpretation
According to the suggested range of scores, this patient with a PHP of 3.66 would be classified as exhibiting poor hygiene performance.

■ *PHP for a Group*
   To obtain the average PHP score for a group or population, total the individual scores and divide by the number of people examined.

V. SIMPLIFIED ORAL HYGIENE INDEX (OHI-S)[11,12]

A. Purpose

To assess oral cleanliness by estimating the tooth surfaces covered with debris and/or calculus.

B. Components

The OHI-S has two components, the Simplified Debris Index (DI-S) and the Simplified Calculus Index (CI-S). The two scores may be used separately or may be combined for the OHI-S.

C. Selection of Teeth and Surfaces

■ *Identify the Six Specific Teeth* (**Figure 22-4**)
   ■ *Posterior:* The facial surfaces of the maxillary molars and the lingual surfaces of the mandibular molars are scored. Although usually the first molars are examined, the first fully erupted molar distal to each second premolar is used if the first molar is missing.

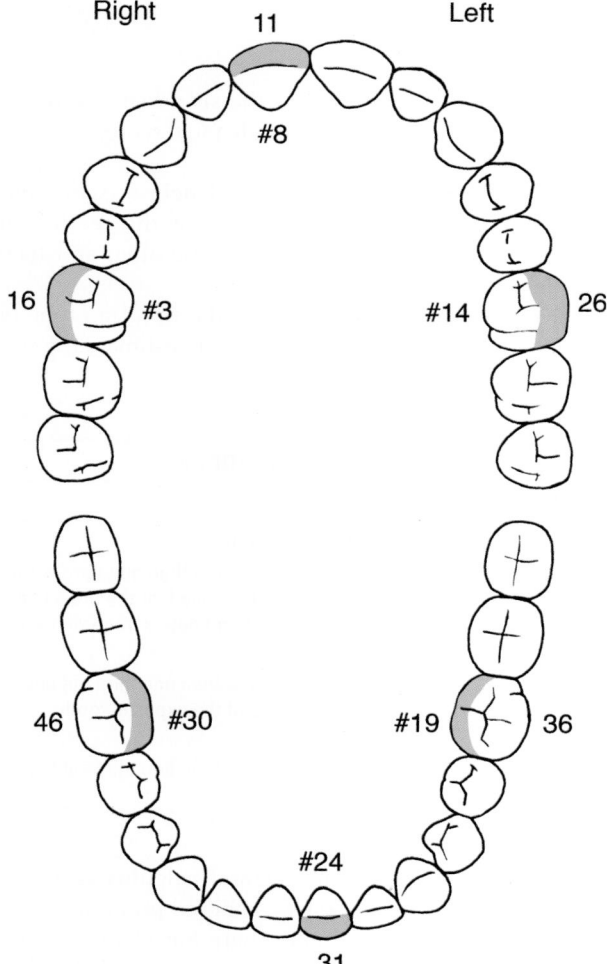

FIGURE 22-4 **Simplified Oral Hygiene Index (OHI-S).** Six tooth surfaces are scored as follows: facial surfaces of maxillary molars and of the maxillary right and mandibular left central incisors, and the lingual surfaces of mandibular molars. Teeth are numbered by the ADA System on the lingual surface and by the FDI System on the facial surface.

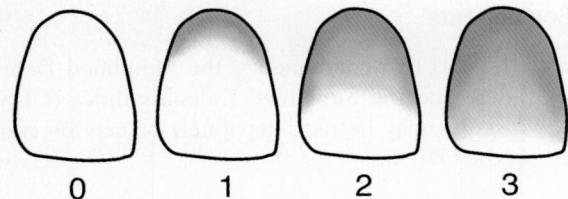

FIGURE 22-5 Simplified Oral Hygiene Index. For the Debris Index, 6 teeth (Figure 22-4) are scored. Scoring of 0 to 3 is based on tooth surfaces covered by debris as shown.

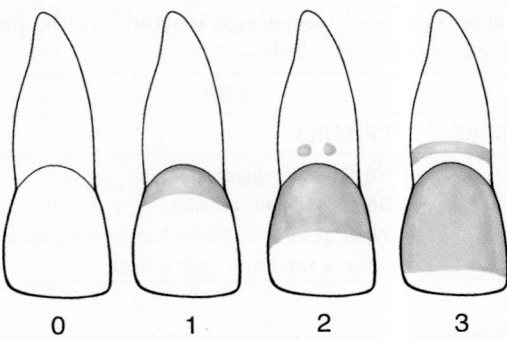

FIGURE 22-6 Simplified Oral Hygiene Index. For the Calculus Index, 6 teeth (Figure 22-4) are scored. Scoring of 0 to 3 is based on location and tooth surface area with calculus as shown. Note slight subgingival calculus recorded as 2 and more extensive subgingival calculus as 3.

- *Anterior:* The facial surfaces of the maxillary right and the mandibular left central incisors are scored. When either is missing, the adjacent central incisor is scored.
- *Extent*
    - Either the facial or lingual surfaces of the selected teeth are scored, including the proximal surfaces to the contact areas.

D. Procedure

- *Qualification:* At least two of the six possible surfaces are examined to calculate an individual score.
- *Record Six Debris Scores*
    - Definition of oral debris: Oral debris is the soft foreign matter on the surfaces of the teeth that consists of dental biofilm, materia alba, and food debris.
    - Examination: Run the side of the tip of a probe or explorer across the tooth surface to estimate the surface area covered by debris.
    - Criteria (**Figure 22-5**)

DEBRIS INDEX (DI-S)	
SCORE	**CRITERIA**
0	No debris or stain present.
1	Soft debris covering not more than one third of the tooth surface being examined, or the presence of extrinsic stains without debris, regardless of surface area covered.
2	Soft debris covering more than one third but not more than two thirds of the exposed tooth surface.
3	Soft debris covering more than two thirds of the exposed tooth surface.

- *Record Six Calculus Scores*
    - Definition of calculus: Dental calculus is a hard deposit of inorganic salts composed primarily of calcium carbonate and phosphate mixed with debris, microorganisms, and desquamated epithelial cells.
    - Examination: Use an explorer to estimate surface area covered by supragingival calculus deposits. Identify subgingival deposits by exploring and/or probing. Record only definite deposits of hard calculus.

- Criteria: Location and tooth surface areas scored are illustrated in **Figure 22-6**.

CALCULUS INDEX (CI-S)	
SCORE	**CRITERIA**
0	No calculus present.
1	Supragingival calculus covering not more than one third of the exposed tooth surface being examined.
2	Supragingival calculus covering more than one third but not more than two thirds of the exposed tooth surface, or the presence of individual flecks of subgingival calculus around the cervical portion of the tooth.
3	Supragingival calculus covering more than two thirds of the exposed tooth surface or a continuous heavy band of subgingival calculus around the cervical portion of the tooth.

E. Scoring

- *OHI-S Individual Score*
    - Determine separate Simplified Debris Index (DI-S) and Simplified Calculus Index (CI-S).
        1. Divide each total score by the number of sextants.
        2. DI-S and CI-S values range from 0 to 3.
    - Calculate the Simplified Oral Hygiene Index (OHI-S).
        1. Combine the DI-S and CI-S.
        2. OHI-S value ranges from 0 to 6.
- *Suggested Range of Scores for Evaluation*[12]

INDIVIDUAL DI-S AND CI-S	
RATING	**SCORES**
Excellent	0
Good	0.1–0.6
Fair	0.7–1.8
Poor	1.9–3.0

OHI-S (COMBINED DI-S AND CI-S)	
RATING	**SCORES**
Excellent	0
Good	0.1–1.2
Fair	1.3–3.0
Poor	3.1–6.0

Calculation: Example for an Individual

TOOTH	DI-S	CI-S SCORE
No. 3 (16)	2	2
No. 8 (11)	1	0
No. 14 (26)	3	2
No. 19 (36)	3	2
No. 24 (31)	2	1
No. 30 (46)	2	2
Total	**13**	**9**

$$\text{DI-S} = \frac{\text{Total debris score}}{\text{Number of teeth scored}} = \frac{13}{6} = 2.17$$

$$\text{CI-S} = \frac{\text{Total calculus scores}}{\text{Number of teeth scored}} = \frac{9}{6} = 1.50$$

$$\text{OHI-S} = \text{DI-S} + \text{CI-S} = 2.17 + 1.50 = 3.67$$

Interpretation
According to the suggested range of scores, the score for this individual (3.67) indicates a poor oral hygiene status.

- *OHI-S Group Score*
  Compute the average of the individual scores by totaling the scores and dividing by the number of individuals.

INDICES THAT MEASURE GINGIVAL AND PERIODONTAL HEALTH

Measurements for gingival and periodontal indices have varied over the years. Two indices, not completely described here, are of historic interest.

- The P-M-A (Papillary-Marginal-Attached) Index, attributed to Schour and Massler[13] and later revised by Massler,[14] was used to assess the extent of gingival changes in large groups for epidemiologic studies.
- The Periodontal Index (PI) of Russell,[15] another acclaimed contribution to the study of disease incidence, was a complex index that accounts for both gingival and periodontal changes. Its aim was to survey large populations.
- For patient instruction and motivation, several bleeding indices and scoring methods have been developed.
- Bleeding on gentle probing or flossing is an early sign of gingival inflammation and precedes color changes and enlargement of the gingival tissues.[16,17]
- On the basis of the principle that healthy tissue does not bleed, testing for bleeding has become a significant procedure for evaluation prior to treatment planning, after therapy to show the effects of treatment, and at

maintenance appointments to determine continued control of gingival inflammation.

I. PERIODONTAL SCREENING AND RECORDING (PSR)[18,19]

A. Purpose

To assess the state of periodontal health of an individual patient.

- A modified form of the original CPITN index.[20]
- Designed to indicate periodontal status in a rapid and effective manner and to motivate the patient to seek necessary complete periodontal assessment and treatment.
- Used as a screening procedure to determine the need for comprehensive periodontal evaluation.

B. Selection of Teeth

The dentition is divided into sextants. Each tooth is examined. Posterior sextants begin distal to the canines.

C. Procedure

- *Instrument:* Probe originally designed for World Health Organization surveys **(Figure 22-7)**.

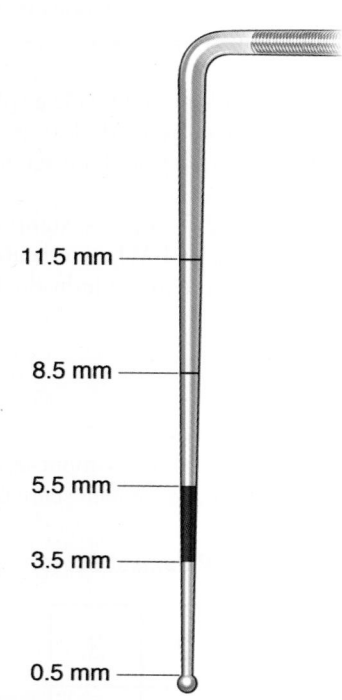

11.5 mm

8.5 mm

5.5 mm

3.5 mm

0.5 mm

FIGURE 22-7 **WHO Periodontal Probe.** The specially designed WHO probe measures 3.5-, 5.5-, 8.5-, and 11.5-mm intervals. This probe is used to make determinations for the Periodontal Screening and Recording (PSR) and the Community Periodontal Index (CPI). (*Source:* Fédération Dentaire Internationale. A simplified periodontal examination for dental practices. Based on the Community Periodontal Index of Treatment Needs—CPITN. *Aus. Dent* J. 1985 Oct;30(5):368-70.)

- Markings: At intervals from tip: 3.5, 2.0, 3.0, and 3.0 mm (total 11.5 mm).
  - Working tip: A ball 0.5 mm in diameter. The functions of the ball are to aid in the detection of calculus, rough overhanging margins of restorations, and other tooth surface irregularities and to facilitate assessment at the probing depth and reduce risk of over-measurement.
  - Color-coded between 3.5 and 5.5 mm.
- *Probe Application*
  - Insert probe gently into a sulcus until resistance is felt.
  - Apply a circumferential walking step to probe systematically about each tooth through each sextant.
  - Observe color-coded area of the probe for prompt identification of probing depths.
  - Each sextant receives one code number corresponding to the deepest position of the color-coded portion of the probe.
- *Criteria*
  - Five codes and an asterisk are used. **Figure 22-8** shows the clinical findings, code significance, and patient management guidelines.
  - Each code may include conditions identified with the preceding codes; for example, Code 3 with probing depth from 3.5 to 5.5 mm also may include calculus, an overhanging restoration, and bleeding on probing.
  - One need not probe the remaining teeth in a sextant when a Code 4 is found. For Codes 0, 1, 2, and 3, the sextant is completely probed.
- *Recording*
  - Use a simple six-box form to provide a space for each sextant. The form can be made into peel-off stickers or a rubber stamp to facilitate recording in the patient's permanent record.
  - One score is marked for each sextant; the highest code observed is recorded. When indicated, an asterisk is added to the score in the individual space with the sextant code number.

D. Scoring

- *Follow-up Patient Management*
  Patients are classified into assessment and treatment planning needs by the highest coded score of their PSR.

Calculation: Example 1 PSR Sextant Score

4_*	2	3
3	2_*	4_*

Interpretation
With Codes 3 and 4, a comprehensive periodontal examination is indicated. Asterisks in this example

indicate furcation involvement in two sextants, and a possible mucogingival involvement in the mandibular anterior sextant. When the patient has not been aware of the presence of periodontal involvement, counseling is important if cooperation and compliance are to be obtained.

Calculation: Example 2 PSR Sextant Score

2	1	2
2	1_*	2_*

Interpretation
An overall Code 2 can indicate calculus and overhanging restorations that must be removed. All restorations must be checked for recurrent dental caries. Appointments for instruction in dental biofilm control are of primary concern. In this example, the asterisks in two sextants indicate a notable clinical feature such as minimal attached gingiva.

II. COMMUNITY PERIODONTAL INDEX (CPI)[21]

A. Purpose

To screen and monitor the periodontal status of populations.

- Originally developed as the CPITN index that included a code to indicate an individual and group-summary recording of treatment needs. However, because of changes in the management of periodontal disease, the treatment needs portion of the index has been eliminated.
- One component of a complete oral health survey[21] designed by the World Health Organization that includes the assessment of many oral health indicators including mucosal lesions, dental caries, fluorosis, prosthetic status, and dentofacial anomalies.
- Later modified to form the PSR index for scoring individual patients.

B. Selection of Teeth

- The dentition is divided into sextants for recording on the assessment form.
- Posterior sextants begin distal to canines.

Adults (20 years and older)

- A sextant is examined only if there are two or more teeth present that are not indicated for extraction.
- Ten index teeth are examined.

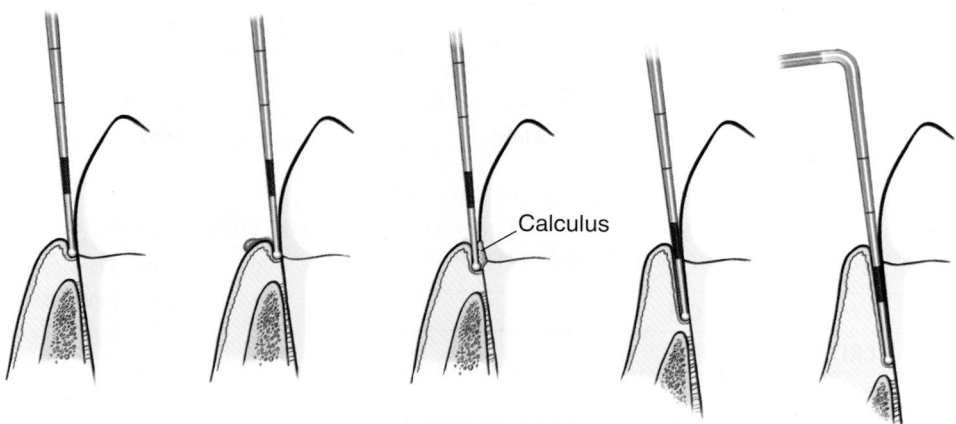

PSR and CPI sextant scores	Code 0	Code 1	Code 2	Code 3	Code 4
CPI description	• Entire black band of the probe is visible	• Entire black band of the probe is visible, but bleeding is present after gentle probin	• Entire black band is visible, but calculus is present • Bleeding may or may not be present.	• 4 to 5 mm pocket depth • Black band on probe partially hidden by gingival margin	• 6 mm or greater pocket depth • Black band of probe completely hidden by gingival margin
PSR sextant code description	• Colored area of probe completely visible • No calculus, defective restoration margins or bleeding	• Colored area of probe completely visible • No calculus or defective restoration margins • Bleeding after gentle probing	• Colored area of probe completely visible • Supra or subgingival rough surface or calculus • Defective restoration margins	• Colored area of probe only partially visible • Calculus, defective restorations, and bleeding may or may not be present	• Colored area of probe completely disappears (probing depth of 5.5 mm or greater)
PSR management guidelines	• Biofilm control instruction • Preventive care	• Biofilm control instruction • Preventive care	• Biofilm control instruction • Complete preventive care • Calculus removal • Correction of defective restoration margins	• Comprehensive periodontal assessment and treatment plan is indicated	• Comprehensive periodontal assessment and treatment plan is indicated

FIGURE 22-8 **Community Periodontal Index CPI) and Periodontal Screening and Recording (PSR) Codes.** (*Sources:* World Health Organization. *Oral health surveys: basic methods.* 4th ed. Geneva: WHO; 1997. 27, 38 pp. and American Dental Association[19] and American Academy of Periodontology.[18])

- The first and second molars in each posterior sextant. If one is missing, no replacement is selected and the score for the remaining molar is recorded.
- The maxillary right central incisor and mandibular left central incisor.
- If no index teeth or tooth is present in the sextant, then all remaining teeth in the sextant are examined and the highest score is recorded.

Children and Adolescents (7 to 19 years of age)

- Six index teeth are examined; the first molar in each posterior quadrant and the maxillary right and the mandibular left incisors.
- For children under the age of 15, pocket depth is not recorded to avoid the deepened sulci associated with erupting teeth. Only bleeding and calculus are considered.

C. Procedure

- *Instrument:* A specially designed probe **(Figure 22-7)** is used to record both the CPI and PSR. The probe is described in **Figure 22-7**.
- *Criteria:* CPI score
  A. Five codes are used to record bleeding, calculus, and pocket depth. The criteria for the codes are similar to the criteria for the PSR, as illustrated in **Figure 22-8**.

CPI

CODE	CRITERIA
0	Healthy periodontal tissues.
1	Bleeding after gentle probing; entire colored band of probe is visible.
2	Supragingival or subgingival calculus present; entire colored band of probe is visible.
3	4- to 5-mm pocket; colored band of probe is partially obscured.
4	6-mm or deeper; colored band on the probe is not visible.

- *Criteria:* Loss of attachment code
  In conjunction with the CPI, the WHO probe is also used to record loss of attachment (LOA). The five LOA codes used are illustrated in **Figure 22-9**. Loss of attachment is not recorded for individuals less than 15 years of age.

LOA CODE	CRITERIA
0	0 to 3 mm loss of attachment
1	4 to 5 mm loss of attachment
2	6 to 8 mm loss of attachment
3	9 to 11 mm loss of attachment
4	12 mm or greater loss of attachment

III. SULCUS BLEEDING INDEX (SBI)[16]

A. Purpose

To locate areas of gingival sulcus bleeding and color changes in order to recognize and record the presence of early (initial) inflammatory gingival disease.

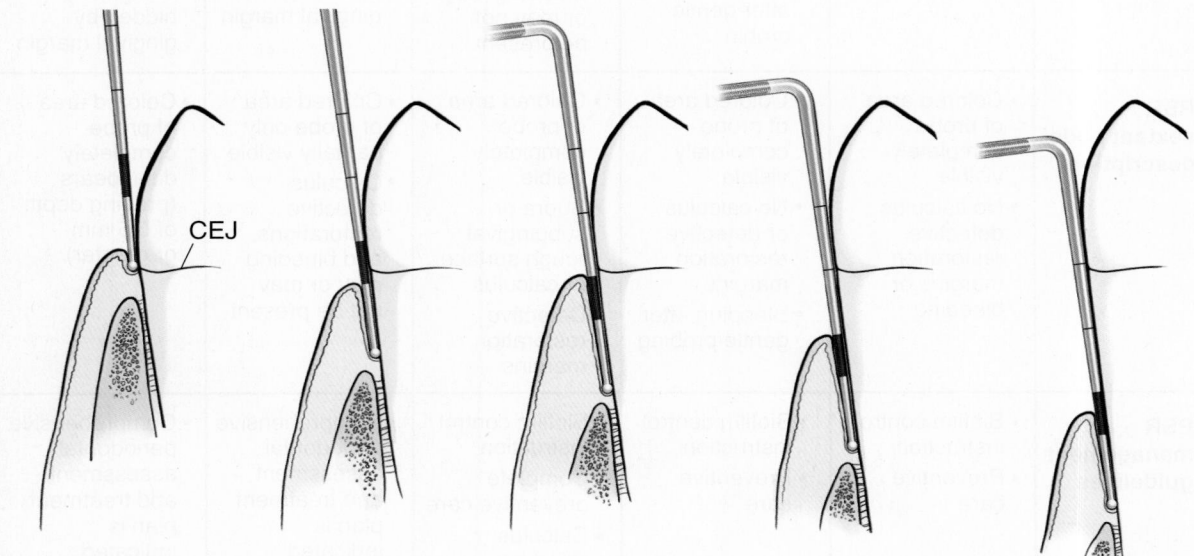

Code 0	Code 1	Code 2	Code 3	Code 4
• 0 to 3 mm loss of attachment • Cementoenamel junction (CEJ) is covered by gingival margin and CPI score is 0 to 3. If CEJ is visible, or if CPI score is 4, LOA codes 1 to 4 are used.	• 3.5 to 5.5 mm loss of attachment • CEJ is within the black band on the probe	• 6 to 8 mm loss of attachment CEJ is between the top of the black band and the 8.5 mm mark on the probe	• 9 to 11 mm loss of attachment • CEJ is between the 8.5 mm and 11.5 mm marks on the probe	• 12 mm or greater loss of attachment • CEJ is beyond the highest (11.5 mm) marks on the probe

FIGURE 22-9 **Loss of Attachment Codes.** (*Source:* World Health Organization. *Oral health surveys: basic methods.* 4th ed. Geneva: WHO; 1997. 27, 39 pp.)

B. Areas Examined

Four gingival units are scored systematically for each tooth: the labial and lingual marginal gingiva (M units), and the mesial and distal papillary gingiva (P units).

C. Procedure

- Use standardized lighting while probing each of the four areas.
- Walk the probe to the base of the sulcus, holding it parallel with the long axis of the tooth for M units, and directed toward the col area for P units.
- Wait 30 seconds after probing before scoring apparently healthy gingival units.
- Dry the gingiva gently if necessary to observe color changes clearly.
- Criteria

SBI	
CODE	**CRITERIA**
0	Healthy appearance of P and M, no bleeding on sulcus probing.
1	Apparently healthy P and M showing no change in color and no swelling, but bleeding from sulcus on probing.
2	Bleeding on probing and change of color caused by inflammation. No swelling or macroscopic edema.
3	Bleeding on probing and change in color and slight edematous swelling.
4	(1) Bleeding on probing and change in color and obvious swelling or (2) Bleeding on probing and obvious swelling.
5	Bleeding on probing and spontaneous bleeding and change in color, marked swelling with or without ulceration.

D. Scoring

- *SBI for Area*
  Score each of the four gingival units (M and P) from 0 to 5.
- *SBI for Tooth*
  Total scores for the 4 units and divide by 4.
- *SBI for Individual*
  Total the scores for individual teeth and divide by the number of teeth. SBI scores range from 0 to 5.

IV. GINGIVAL BLEEDING INDEX (GBI)[22]

A. Purpose

To record the presence or absence of gingival inflammation as determined by bleeding from interproximal gingival sulci.

B. Areas Examined

Each interproximal area has two sulci, which are scored as one interdental unit or individually.

- Certain areas may be excluded from scoring because of accessibility, tooth position, diastemata, or other factors, and if exclusions are made, a consistent procedure should be followed for an individual and for a group if a study is to be made.
- A full complement of teeth has 30 proximal areas. In the original studies, third molars were excluded, and 26 interdental units were recorded.[23]

C. Procedure

- *Instrument*
  Unwaxed dental floss is used. Floss has the advantages of being readily available, disposable, and usable by the instructed patient.
- *Steps*
  1. Pass the floss interproximally first on one side of the papilla and then on the other.
  2. Curve the floss around the adjacent tooth, and bring the floss below the gingival margin.
  3. Move the floss up and down for one stroke, with care not to lacerate the gingiva. Adapt finger rests to provide controlled, consistent pressure.
  4. Use a new length of clean floss for each area.
  5. Retract for visibility of bleeding from both facial and lingual aspects.
  6. Allow 30 seconds for reinspection of an area that does not show blood immediately either in the area or on the floss.
- *Criteria*
  Bleeding indicates the presence of disease. No attempt is made to quantify the severity of bleeding because no bleeding represents health.

D. Scoring

The numbers of bleeding areas and scorable units are recorded. Patient participation in observing and recording over a series of appointments can increase motivation.

V. EASTMAN INTERDENTAL BLEEDING INDEX (EIBI)[23,24]

A. Purpose

To assess the presence of inflammation in the interdental area as indicated by the presence or absence of bleeding.

B. Areas Examined

Each interdental area around the entire dentition.

C. Procedure

- *Instrument*
  Triangular wooden interdental cleaner.

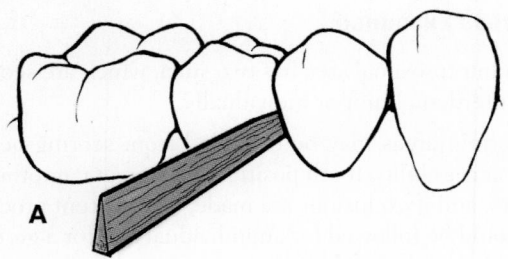

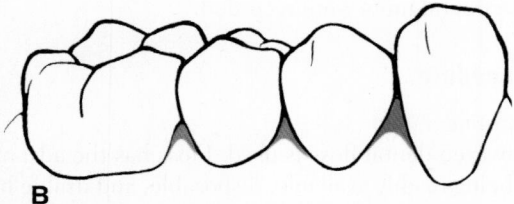

FIGURE 22-10 **Eastman Interdental Bleeding Index.** The test for interdental bleeding is made by inserting a wooden interdental cleaner into each interdental space. **(A)** Wooden interdental cleaner inserted in a horizontal path, parallel with the occlusal surfaces. **(B)** The presence or absence of bleeding is noted within a quadrant 15 seconds after final insertion. Bleeding indicates the presence of inflammation.

- *Steps*
  1. Insert gently, then immediately remove, a wooden cleaner into each interdental area in such a way as to depress the papilla 1 to 2 mm **(Figure 22-10)**.
  2. Make the path of insertion horizontal (parallel to the occlusal surface), taking care not to angle the point in an apical direction.
  3. Insert and remove four times; move to next interproximal area.
  4. Record the presence or absence of bleeding within 15 seconds for each area.

D. Scoring

- *Number of Bleeding Sites*
  The number may be totaled for an individual score for comparison with scores over a series of appointments.
- *Percentage Scores*
  Index is expressed as a percentage of the total number of sites evaluated. Calculations can be made for total mouth, quadrants, or maxillary versus mandibular.
- *Calculation Example*
  An adult with a complete dentition has 15 maxillary and 15 mandibular interproximal areas. The EIBI revealed 13 areas of bleeding. To calculate percentage:

$$\frac{\text{Number of bleeding areas}}{\text{Total number of areas}} \times 100 = \text{Percent bleeding area}$$

$$\frac{13}{30} \times 100 = 43\%$$

VI. GINGIVAL INDEX (GI)[7]

A. Purpose

To assess the severity of gingivitis based on color, consistency, and bleeding on probing.

B. Selection of Teeth and Gingival Areas

A gingival index may be determined for selected teeth or for the entire dentition.

- *Areas Examined*
  Four gingival areas (distal, facial, mesial, lingual) are examined systematically for each tooth.
- *Modified Procedure*
  The distal examination for each tooth can be omitted. The score for the mesial area is doubled, and the total score for each tooth is divided by four.

C. Procedure

- Dry the teeth and gingiva; under adequate light, use a mouth mirror and probe.
- Use the probe to press on the gingiva to determine the degree of firmness.
- Slide the probe along the soft tissue wall near the entrance to the gingival sulcus to evaluate bleeding **(Figure 22-11)**.

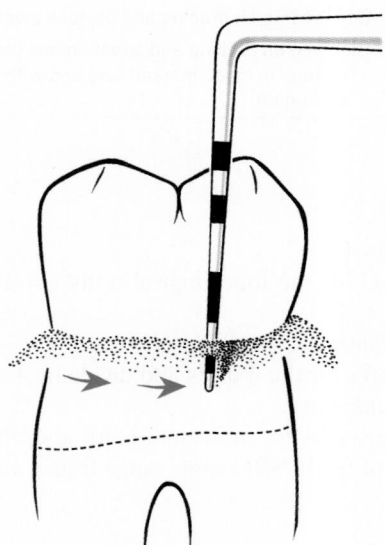

FIGURE 22-11 **Gingival Index (GI).** Probe stroke for bleeding evaluation. The broken line represents the level of attachment of the periodontal tissues. The probe is inserted a few millimeters and moved along the soft tissue pocket wall with light pressure in a circumferential direction. The stroke shown here is in contrast with the walking stroke used for probing depth evaluation and measurement.

■ Criteria

GI CODE	CRITERIA
0	Normal gingiva.
1	Mild inflammation-slight change in color, slight edema. *No bleeding* on probing.
2	Moderate inflammation-redness, edema, and glazing. *Bleeding* on probing.
3	Severe inflammation-marked redness and edema. Ulceration. Tendency to *spontaneous bleeding.*

D. Scoring

■ *GI for Area*
Each of the four gingival surfaces (distal, facial, mesial, lingual) is given a score of 0 to 3.

■ *GI for a Tooth*
Scores for each area are totaled and divided by four.

■ *GI for Groups of Teeth*
Scores for individual teeth may be grouped and totaled, and divided by the number of teeth. A GI may be determined for specific teeth, group of teeth, quadrant, or side of mouth.

■ *GI for the Individual*
Scores for each tooth are added up and divided by the number of teeth examined. Scores range from 0 to 3.

■ *Suggested Range of Scores for Patient Reference*

RATING	SCORES
Excellent (healthy tissue)	0
Good	0.1–1.0
Fair	1.1–2.0
Poor	2.1–3.0

Calculation: Example for an Individual

Using six teeth for an example of screening; teeth selected are known as the Ramfjord Index Teeth.[25]

TOOTH NO.	M	F	D	L	
3 (16)	3	1	3	1	
9 (21)	1	0	1	1	
12 (24)	2	1	2	0	
19 (36)	3	1	3	3	
25 (41)	1	1	1	1	
28 (44)	2	1	2	0	
Total	12	5	12	6	= 35

$$\text{Gingival index} = \frac{\text{Total score}}{\text{Number of surfaces}} = \frac{35}{24} = 1.45$$

Interpretation
According to the suggested range of scores, the score for this individual (1.45) indicates only fair gingival health (moderate inflammation). The ratings for each gingival area or surface can be used to help the patient compare gingival changes and improve oral hygiene procedures.

■ *GI for a Group*
Add the individual GI scores and divide by the number of individuals examined.

INDICES THAT MEASURE DENTAL CARIES EXPERIENCE

Dental caries experience data are most useful when measuring the prevalence of dental disease in groups rather than individuals. The population scores can document such information as the number of persons in any age group who are affected by dental caries, the number of teeth that need treatment, or the proportion of teeth that have been treated.

I. PERMANENT DENTITION: DECAYED, MISSING, AND FILLED TEETH (DMFT) OR SURFACES (DMFS)[3,26]

A. Purpose

To determine total dental caries experience, past and present, by recording either the number of affected teeth or tooth surfaces.

B. Selection of Teeth and Surfaces

■ The DMFT is based on 28 teeth.
■ The DMFS is based on surfaces of 28 teeth; 128 surfaces.
  ■ 16 posterior teeth × 5 surfaces (facial, lingual, mesial, distal, and occlusal) = 80 surfaces.
  ■ 12 anterior teeth × 4 surfaces (facial, lingual, mesial, and distal) = 48 surfaces.
  ■ Teeth that are missing due to dental caries are recorded using 5 surfaces for posterior and 4 surfaces for anterior teeth.
■ Teeth not counted
  ■ Third molars.
  ■ Unerupted teeth. A tooth is considered erupted when any part projects through the gingiva. Certain types of research may require differentiation between clinical emergence, partial eruption, and full eruption.
  ■ Congenitally missing and supernumerary teeth.
  ■ Teeth removed for reasons other than dental caries, such as an impaction or during orthodontic treatment.
  ■ Teeth restored for reasons other than dental caries, such as trauma (fracture), cosmetic purposes, or use as a bridge abutment.

■ Primary tooth retained with the permanent successor erupted. The permanent tooth is evaluated because a primary tooth is never included in this index.

C. Procedures

■ *Examination*
  ■ Examine each tooth in a systematic sequence.
  ■ Observe teeth by visual means as much as possible.
  ■ Use adequate light.
  ■ Review the stages of dental caries on page 379.
■ *Criteria for Recording*[26]
  ■ Each tooth is recorded once when using the DMFT index.
  ■ 5 surfaces for posterior teeth and 4 surfaces for anterior teeth are recorded when using the DMFS index.
  ■ DMF indices use a dichotomous scale (present or absent) to record decay.

DMF RATING	CRITERIA
Decayed (D)	Visible dental caries is present or both dental caries and a restoration are present.
Missing (M)	A tooth has been extracted because of dental caries or when it is carious, nonrestorable, and indicated for extraction.
Filled (F)	Any permanent or temporary restoration is present or a defective restoration without evidence of dental caries is present.

D. Scoring

■ *Individual DMF*
  ■ Total each component separately.
  ■ Total D + M + F = DMF
  Example: An individual presents with dental caries on the mesial and occlusal surfaces of a posterior tooth, caries on the mesial surface of an anterior tooth, a molar tooth and an anterior tooth are missing because of dental caries, and there is an amalgam restoration on the mesial-distal-occlusal surfaces of a posterior tooth.
  DMFT = 2 + 2 + 1 = 5
  DMFS = 3 + 9 + 3 = 15
■ A DMF score may have different derivations. For example, an individual with a DMF score of 15 who had regular dental care may have a distribution such as D = 0, M = 0, F = 15.
■ *Group DMF*
  ■ Total the DMFs for each individual examined.
  ■ Divide the total DMFs by the number of individuals in the group.

Calculation: **Example**
A population of 20 individuals with individual DMF scores of 0,0,0,0,2,2,3,3,3,4,9,9,9,10,10,10,11,11,12, and 16 equals a group total DMF of 124.

$$\frac{124}{20} = 6.2 = \text{the average DMF for the group}$$

This DMF average represents accumulated dental caries experience for the group.

■ The differences in caries experience between two groups of individuals within this population are notable and influence interpretation of the results. For the first 10 individuals, the group average is $\frac{17}{10} = 1.7$ and for the second 10 individuals the average DMF is $\frac{107}{10} = 10.7$. Scores for these two groups can be presented separately because of the wide difference.
■ Average DMF scores can also be presented by age group.
■ *Specific Treatment Needs of a Group*
  ■ To calculate the percentage of DMF teeth that need to be restored, divide the total D component by the total DMF.

Calculation: **Example 1**
To calculate the *percent of DMF teeth* that need to be restored, divide the total D component by the total number of DMF teeth.

D = 175, M = 55, F = 18
Total DMFT = 248

$$\frac{D}{DMF} = \frac{175}{248} = 0.70 \text{ or } 70\% \text{ of the teeth need restorations}$$

Calculation: **Example 2**
The same type of calculations can be used to determine the *percent of all teeth* in a group of individuals that are missing.

20 individuals have 28 × 20 = 560 permanent teeth.

$$D = 175, M = 55, F = 18$$

$$\frac{M}{\text{Total \# of teeth}} = \frac{55}{560} = 0.098 \text{ or nearly } 10\% \text{ of all their}$$

teeth lost because of dental caries.

II. PRIMARY DENTITION: DECAYED, INDICATED FOR EXTRACTION, AND FILLED (df AND def) [27]

A. Purpose

To determine the dental caries experience for the primary teeth present in the oral cavity by evaluating teeth or surfaces.

B. Selection of Teeth or Surfaces

- deft or dft: 20 teeth evaluated.
- defs or dfs: 88 surfaces evaluated.
  - *Posterior teeth:* Each has five surfaces: facial, lingual or palatal, mesial, distal, and occlusal. (8 teeth × 5 surfaces = 40 surfaces.)
  - *Anterior teeth:* Each has four surfaces: facial, lingual or palatal, mesial, and distal. (12 teeth × 4 surfaces = 48 surfaces.)
- Teeth not counted
  - Missing teeth, including unerupted and congenitally missing.
  - Supernumerary teeth.
  - Teeth restored for reasons other than dental caries are not counted as f.

C. Procedure

- *Instruments and Examination*
  Same as for DMF.
- *Criteria*

df OR def

RATING	CRITERIA
d	Primary teeth (or surfaces) with dental caries but not restored.
e	Primary teeth (or number of surfaces) that are ***indicated for extraction*** because of dental caries.
f	Primary teeth (or surfaces) that do not have dental caries. Each tooth (or surface) is scored once only, recurrent caries around a restoration receive a "d" score.

- *Difference between deft/defs and dft/dfs*
  In the deft and defs, both "d" and "e" are used to describe teeth with dental caries. Thus, d and e are sometimes combined, and the index becomes the dft or dfs.

D. Scoring

Calculation: Example 1 Individual dft
A 2½-year-old child has 18 teeth. Teeth A (55) and J (65) are unerupted. There is no sign of dental caries in teeth M (73), N (72), O (71), P (81), Q (82), and R (83). All other teeth have two carious surfaces each, except tooth B (54), which is broken down to the gum line.

Summary:

Total number of teeth = 18
Number of "d" teeth = 12
Number of "f" teeth = 0
dft = d + f = 12 + 0 = 12

Interpretation
Twelve of 18 teeth (67%) with carious lesions indicates a serious need for dental treatment and a caries management program for the child.

Calculation: Example 2 Individual dfs
Using the same 2½-year-old child to calculate dfs:

Eleven teeth each have two carious surfaces: 11 × 2 = 22 carious surfaces

Tooth B has 1 × 5 = 5 carious surfaces
Total dfs: d + f = 27 + 0 = 27

Interpretation
The child has 48 total anterior surfaces (12 teeth × 4 surfaces) and 30 total posterior surfaces (6 teeth × 5 surfaces) to total 78 surfaces.

$$\frac{\text{dfs}}{\text{Number of surfaces}} = \frac{27}{78}$$

= 0.34 or 34% of the surfaces in need of dental treatment

E. Mixed Dentition

A DMFT or DMFS and a deft or defs are never added together.

III. PRIMARY DENTITION: DECAYED, MISSING, AND FILLED (dmft AND dmfs)[27]

A. Purpose

To determine dental caries experience for children. Only primary teeth are evaluated.

B. Selection of Teeth or Surfaces

- dmft: 12 teeth evaluated (8 primary molars; 4 primary canines).
- dmfs: 56 surfaces evaluated.
  A. *Primary molars:* 8 × 5 surfaces each = 40
  B. *Primary canines:* 4 × 4 surfaces each = 16
- Each tooth is counted only once. When both dental caries and a restoration are present, the tooth or surface is scored as "d."

C. Procedure

- Instruments and examination are the same as for DMF or df.
- Criteria for dmft or dmfs

dmf RATING	CRITERIA
d	Primary molars and canines (or surfaces) that are carious.
m	Primary molars and canines (or surfaces) that are missing. A primary molar or canine is presumed missing because of dental caries when it has been lost before normal exfoliation.
f	Primary molars and canines (or surfaces) that have a restoration but are without caries.

D. Scoring

Calculation: Example 1 Individual dmf

A 7-year-old boy has all primary molars and canines present. Examination reveals two carious surfaces on one molar tooth, one missing canine tooth, and one two-surface amalgam filling on a molar tooth.

dmft = 1 + 1 + 1 = 3
dmfs = 2 + 4 + 2 = 8

E. Mixed Dentition

Permanent and primary teeth are evaluated separately. A DMFT or DMFS and a dmft or dmfs are never added together.

IV. EARLY CHILDHOOD CARIES (ECC AND S-ECC) [28]

A. Purpose

To provide case definitions that determine caries status of children 5 years of age or younger.

B. Selection of Teeth or Surfaces

Each surface (mesial, distal, facial, lingual, occlusal) of each tooth visible in the child's mouth is evaluated. Only primary teeth are scored.

C. Procedure

■ Visual examination of all surfaces of each erupted tooth.
■ Criteria for case definition are included in **Table 22-1**.

D. Scoring

■ A designation of ECC or S-ECC for a particular individual relates the age of the child with the status of decayed, missing, and filled tooth surfaces observed.
■ Community-based surveys identify the percentage of a population with ECC and/or S-ECC.

V. ROOT CARIES INDEX (RCI) [29]

A. Purpose

To determine total root caries experience for individuals and groups and provide a direct, simple method for recording and making comparisons.

B. Selection of Teeth

■ Up to four surfaces (mesial, distal, facial, lingual/palatal) are counted for each tooth.
■ Only surfaces with visible gingival recession are counted.
■ Teeth with multiple roots with extreme recession, though rare, could present with two or three lesions on the same surface. In this case, the most severe lesion is selected for recording and each surface is counted only once.

C. Procedure

■ *Examination*
   A. Use adequate retraction and light to examine each tooth to determine where gingival recession has occurred and root surfaces are directly visible. Visible recession is shown in Figure 14-12 on page 220.
   B. Apply current knowledge of the stages of dental caries to prevent damage to remineralizing areas during examination. Only cavitated lesions are recorded.

TABLE 22-1	EARLY CHILDHOOD CARIES CASE DEFINITION			
AGE	**BIRTH TO 3 YEARS (0–35 MONTHS)**	**3–4 YEARS (36–47 MONTHS)**	**4–5 YEARS (48–59 MONTHS)**	**5–6 YEARS (60–71 MONTHS)**
Early Childhood Caries (ECC)	1 or more teeth with decayed (either cavitated or non-cavitated), missing, or filled surfaces			
Severe Early Childhood Caries (S-ECC)	■ 1 or more teeth with decay (either cavitated or non-cavitated) or fillings present on SMOOTH surface enamel OR ■ 1 or more teeth missing due to caries.	■ 1 or more cavitated or filled smooth surfaces in primary maxillary anterior teeth ■ 1 or more missing teeth due to caries OR ■ dmfs* score ≥4	■ 1 or more cavitated or filled smooth surfaces in primary maxillary anterior teeth ■ 1 or more missing teeth due to caries OR ■ dmfs* score ≥5	■ 1 or more cavitated or filled smooth surfaces in primary maxillary anterior teeth ■ 1 or more missing teeth due to caries OR ■ dmfs* score ≥6

*dmfs = total number of decayed missing and filled surfaces.
Source: Drury TF, Horowitz AM, Ismail AI, Maertens MP, Rizier RG, Selwitz RH. Diagnosing and reporting early childhood caries for research purposes. *J Public Health Dent.* 1999 Summer; 59(3):192–7.

■ *Record a Rating for Each Root Surface.*

RCI RATING	CRITERIA
No R	Root surface with a covered cementoenamel junction and no visible recession (R = recession).
R-D	Root surface with recession present and root caries present (D = decay).
R-F	Root surface with recession present and the surface is restored (F = filled).
R-N	Root surface with recession, but no caries or restoration is present.
M	The tooth is missing.

D. Scoring

Calculation: Formula

$$\frac{R\text{-}D + R\text{-}F}{R\text{-}D + R\text{-}F + R\text{-}N} \times 100 = RCI$$

Calculation: Example Individual RCI
A man, aged 70, presents with 23 natural teeth (23 × 4 = 92 surfaces). Clinical examination reveals:

$$R\text{-}D = 26$$
$$R\text{-}F = 8$$
$$R\text{-}N = 58$$

$$RCI = \frac{26 + 8}{26 + 8 + 58} = \frac{37}{92} \times 100 = 36.9\%$$

Interpretation
A score of 36.9% for the individual means that of all tooth surfaces with visible gingival recession, 36.9% have cavitated carious lesions or have been previously restored.

■ *Group or Community RCI*
The R-D, R-F, and R-N scores for all individuals in the group are added together and the RCI formula is calculated using the total scores.

INDICES THAT MEASURE DENTAL FLUOROSIS

Dental indices such as the Thylstrup–Fejerskov Index,[30] the Fluorosis Risk Index,[31] and the Developmental Defects of Dental Enamel Index[32,33] have been used to investigate the effects of fluoride concentration on dental enamel. The two indices described here are the most commonly used for community-based assessment.

I. DEAN'S FLUOROSIS INDEX[34]

A. Purpose

To measure the prevalence and severity of dental fluorosis.

■ Originally developed in the 1930s and refined in 1942 to relate the severity of hypomineralization of dental enamel to concentration of fluoride in the water supply.
■ Considered less sensitive than some other measures of fluorosis, but still recommended for use in community studies.

B. Selection of Teeth

The smooth surface enamel of all teeth is examined.

C. Procedure

Each tooth is visually examined for signs of fluorosis and assigned a numerical score using the descriptive categories shown in **Table 22-2**.

D. Scoring

■ An individual fluorosis score is assigned using the highest numerical score recorded for two or more teeth.
■ Community levels of fluorosis are indicated by the percentage of individuals in the sample or population that receive scores in each category.

TABLE 22-2	SCORING SYSTEM FOR DEAN'S FLUOROSIS INDEX	
CATEGORY	**DESCRIPTION**	**NUMERICAL SCORE**
Normal	Smooth, creamy white tooth surface	0
Questionable	Slight changes from normal transparency	1
Very Mild	Small, scattered opaque areas; less than 25% of tooth surface	2
Mild	Opaque areas; less than 50% of tooth surface	3
Moderate	Significant opaque and/or worn areas; may have brown stains	4
Severe	Widespread, significant hypoplasia, pitting, brown staining, worn areas, and/or a corroded appearance	5

Source: Moulton FR (ed). Fluorine and dental health. Washington DC: American Association for the Advancement of Science; 1942. Dean HT. The investigation of physiological effect by the epidemiological method. p. 23–71.

TABLE 22-3	SCORING SYSTEM FOR TOOTH SURFACE INDEX OF FLUOROSIS (TSIF)

DESCRIPTION	NUMERICAL SCORE
No evidence of fluorosis	0
Areas with parchment-white color; less than 1/3 of visible tooth surface; includes fluorosis confined to anterior incisal edges and posterior cusp tips.	1
Parchment-white color on at least 1/3 but less than 2/3 of visible tooth surface.	2
Parchment-white color on at least 2/3 of visible tooth surface.	3
Staining (from light to very dark brown) in conjunction with parchment white areas as described above in levels 1, 2, or 3.	4
Discrete stained and rough pitted areas; but no staining on intact enamel surfaces.	5
Discrete pitting plus staining of intact enamel surfaces.	6
Confluent pitting over large areas of tooth surface; anatomy of tooth may be altered; dark-brown stain usually present.	7

Source: Horowitz HS. Driscoll WS, Meyers RJ, Heifetz SB, Kingman AK. A new method for assessing the prevalence of dental fluorosis—The tooth surface Index of fluorosis. *J Am Dent Assoc.* 1984 Jul;109(1):37–41.

II. TOOTH SURFACE INDEX OF FLUOROSIS (TSIF)[35]

A. Purpose

- To measure the prevalence and severity of dental fluorosis.
- More sensitive than Dean's Index in identifying the mildest signs of fluorosis.

B. Selection of Teeth

The smooth surface enamel, cusp tips, and incisal edges of all teeth are examined.

C. Procedure

Each tooth is examined visually and assigned a numerical score using the criteria in **Table 22-3**.

D. Scoring

TSIF data are presented as a distribution citing the percent of the population with each numerical score, rather than as mean scores for the entire group.

INDICES FOR COMMUNITY-BASED ORAL HEALTH SURVEILLANCE

Community oral health screenings can be performed at every level; local, national, and worldwide. Data collected by such screenings are useful for monitoring health status and determining population access to or need for oral health services.

I. WORLD HEALTH ORGANIZATION BASIC SCREENING SURVEY[21]

A. Purpose

To collect comprehensive data on oral health status and dental treatment needs of a population. This system is suitable for surveying both adults and children.

B. Tissues/Areas Examined

Survey categories include the following:

- Orofacial (intraoral and extraoral) lesions and anomalies
- Temporomandibular joint status
- Periodontal status
- Dentition status and treatment need
- Prosthetic status and need
- Need for immediate care/referral

C. Procedures

- Standardized assessment form with boxes for data entry identifies the codes and descriptive criteria for each data collection category.
- Standardized codes facilitate computerized data entry and analysis.
- Photographs in the training manual provide examples of criteria for each code.

| TABLE 22-4 | ASSOCIATION OF STATE AND TERRITORIAL DENTAL DIRECTORS BASIC SCREENING SURVEY (BSS) SCORING CRITERIA |

	SCORE	PRESCHOOLERS	SCHOOLCHILDREN	ADULTS
Untreated Caries (≥ ½ mm discontinuity in tooth surface)	0 = no untreated caries 1 = untreated caries	✓	✓	✓
Caries Experience (ever had a cavity)	0 = no caries experience 1 = caries experience	✓	✓	
Early Childhood Caries (ECC) (3 years old with one or more upper front teeth that were ever decayed, filled, or missing due to caries)	0 = no ECC 1 = ECC	✓		
Treatment Urgency	0 = no obvious problem (routine dental care indicated) 1 = early dental care (within two weeks) 2 = urgent care (as soon as possible—presents with pain, swelling, etc.)	✓	✓	✓
Sealants on Permanent Molars	0 = no sealants 1 = sealants		✓	
Natural Teeth	0 = no natural teeth 1 = at least one natural tooth			✓

A ✓ mark indicates that the oral condition category is scored in that particular age group. Some categories (i.e., sealants) are not scored in all age groups.
Source: Association of State and Territorial Dental Directors. *Basic screening surveys: An approach to monotoring community oral health.* Columbus: ASTDD; 2003. pp. 33–42.

D. Scoring

- Data can be analyzed by survey team or arrangements can be made for data entry forms to be analyzed by the World Health Organization.

II. ASSOCIATION OF STATE AND TERRITORIAL DENTAL DIRECTORS BASIC SCREENING SURVEY (BSS)[6]

A. Purpose

- *To provide oral screening for adult, school age, and/or preschool populations.*
  - Data levels are consistent with monitoring the United States Public Health Service national health objectives.
  - Data collected can easily be compared with data collected by other communities and states using the data collection techniques.
- *The system was designed to be used by screeners with or without dental background because:*
  - Sometimes nondental personnel have better access to some population groups.

- Some communities have little access to dental public health professionals.

B. Selection of Teeth

All teeth are examined, but each individual patient receives one score for each category **(Table 22-4)**.

C. Procedure

- Oral screening can be combined with an optional questionnaire that collects additional data on demographics and access to dental care.
- Screeners are trained and calibrated. They record oral findings using photographs and detailed descriptions of associated criteria.

D. Scoring

- **Table 22-4** outlines the scoring criteria and categories recorded for each age group.
- Data from each indicator can be compiled and expressed in frequency graphs or tables as a percentage of the population that exhibits a specific category trait.

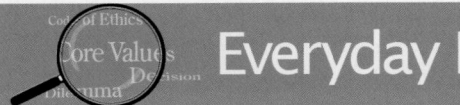

Everyday Ethics

Susanna began practicing in the team clinic at the dental school and found the work to be very challenging. As a hygienist, she was not only performing preventive treatment for maintenance patients but was also responsible for data collection for several research projects. Suddenly, the importance of understanding and calculating the various indices became critical. In particular, Susanna found herself reviewing the procedures for the OHI-S, bleeding indices, and the DMFT.

Susanna had always enjoyed her clinical interactions with patients, but now scoring and recording information on each and every tooth was beginning to cause her some stress. Generally Susanna practiced without an assistant and found it difficult to do both examining and recording. Near the end of one day when she was organizing the day's work for

Dr. Lowe's caries study, she discovered that she had omitted several surfaces in one quadrant. This was the patient's final visit to the dental school. Susanna contemplated what to do when she realized the data was missing.

Questions for Consideration

1. Discuss how ADHA's roles for dental hygienists (page 10) apply to Suzanna's daily duties.
2. Can Susanna "defend" her actions to Dr. Lowe by submitting the data she does have on the patient? Explain your rationale.
3. Which of the core values (page 10) or principles of ethical behavior come into play in collecting research data such as described in this scenario?

DOCUMENTATION

Factors related to dental indices to document in the patient records include:

- Name of the index or indices used
- Score calculated for the index
- Objective statement that provides an interpretation of the index score
- Follow-up instructions provided to the patient
- An example progress note appears in **Box 22-2**.

Factors To Teach Patient or Members of The Community

- How an index is used and calculated, and what the scores mean.
- Purpose for the selection of the particular index being used.
- Correlation of index scores with current oral health practices and procedures.
- Procedures to follow to improve index scores and bring the oral tissues to health.

BOX 22-2	**Examples of Components in a Progress Note: When a Dental Index Has Been Used During Patient Assessment**

Month, Day, Year
Patient presents for reassessment of biofilm and bleeding levels 14 days following oral hygiene instructions that were provided during dental hygiene maintenance visit. "Plaque-Free Score" = 89%; SBI score = 2. "Plaque-Free Score" compared to previous score of 22%; SBI score compared to previous score of 5. Significant improvement noted in scores except on maxillary facial surfaces. Patient congratulated on areas of success. Additional instruction provided specifically related to biofilm removal on posterior facial and proximal tooth surfaces. Patient observed while brushing and flossing maxillary molar areas using a mirror. Next visit: 3 months reevaluation.

Signed: _____, RDH Date: _____

References

1. Silness J, Löe H. Periodontal disease in pregnancy. II. Correlation between oral hygiene and periodontal condition. *Acta Odontol Scand*. 1964 Feb;22:121–35.
2. Podshadley AG, Haley JV. A method for evaluating oral hygiene performance. *Public Health Rep*. 1968 Mar;83(3):259–64.
3. Klein H. Palmer CE, Knutson JW. Studies on dental caries. I. Dental status and dental needs of elementary school children. *Public Health Rep*. 1938 May 13;53(19):751–65.
4. United States Department of Health and Human Services. Oral health in America: a report of the surgeon general. Rockville. US Department of Health and Human Services, National Institute of Dental and Craniofacial Research, National Institutes of Health. 2000 May. p. 63–89.
5. United States Department of Health and Human Services. Healthy people 2020: Topics and objectives: oral health [Internet]. Washington, DC, U.S. Department of Health and Human Services; launched 2010 Dec 2 [cited 2011 Feb 8]; [1 screen]. Available from: http://www.healthypeople.gov/2020/topicsobjectives2020/objectiveslist.aspx?topicid = 32
6. Association of State and Territorial Dental Directors. Basic screening surveys: an approach to monitoring community oral health. Columbus, OH. ASTDD. 2003. [cited 2005, June 20]. pp. 33-42. Available from: http://www.astdd.org
7. Löe H. The gingival index, the plaque index and the retention index systems. J Periodontol. 1967 Nov-Dec;38(6):Suppl:610–6.
8. O'Leary TJ, Drake RB, Naylor JE. The plaque control record. *J Periodontol*. 1972 Jan;43(1):38.

9. Ramfjord SP, Ash MM. Periodontology and periodontics. Philadelphia: WB Saunders Co; 1979. 273 p.

10. Grant DA, Stern IB, Everett FG. Periodontics. 5th ed. St. Louis: Mosby; 1979. pp. 529–31.

11. Greene JC, Vermillion JR. The simplified oral hygiene index. *J Am Dent Assoc.* 1964 Jan;68:7–13.

12. Greene JC. The oral hygiene index-development and uses. *J Periodontol.* 1967 Nov–Dec;38(6):Suppl:625–37.

13. Schour I, Massler M. Prevalence of gingivitis in young adults (abstract #33 in: IADR: scientific proceedings). *J Dent Res.* 1948 Dec;27(6):733.

14. Massler M. The P-M-A index for the assessment of gingivitis. *J Periodontol.* 1967 Nov–Dec;38(6):Suppl:592–601.

15. Russell AL. A system of classification and scoring for prevalence surveys of periodontal disease. *J Dent Res.* 1956 Jun;35(3):350–9.

16. Mühlemann HR, Son, S. Gingival sulcus bleeding-a leading symptom in initial gingivitis. *Helv Odontol Acta.* 1971 Oct;15(2):107–13.

17. Meitner SW, Zander HA, Iker HP, Polson AM. Identification of inflamed gingival surfaces. *J Clin Periodontol.* 1979 Apr;6(2):93–7.

18. American Academy of Periodontology. Parameter on comprehensive periodontal examination. *J Periodontol.* 2000 May;71(5 Suppl):847–8.

19. Khocht A, Zohn H, Deasy M, Chang KM. Assessment of periodontal status with PSR and traditional clinical periodontal examination. *J Am Dent Assoc.* 1995 Dec;126(12):1658–65.

20. Ainamo J, Barmes D, Beagrie G, Cutress T, Martin J, Sardo-Infirri J. Development of the World Health Organization (WHO) community periodontal index of treatment needs (CPITN). *Int Dent J.* 1982 Sep;32(3):281–91.

21. World Health Organization. Oral health surveys: basic methods. Geneva: World Health Organization; 1997. pp. 26–39.

22. Carter HG, Barnes GP. The gingival bleeding index. *J Periodontol.* 1974 Nov;45(11):801–5.

23. Abrams K, Caton J, Polson A. Histologic comparisons of interproximal gingival tissues related to the presence or absence of bleeding. *J Periodontol.* 1984 Nov;55(11):629–32.

24. Caton JG, Polson, AM. The interdental bleeding index: a simplified procedure for monitoring gingival health. *Compend Contin Educ Dent.* 1985;6(2):88, 90–92.

25. Ramfjord SP. Indices for prevalence and incidence of periodontal disease. *J Periodontol.* 1959 Jan;30:51.

26. United States Department of Health and Human Services, Public Health Service, National Institutes of Health. Oral health surveys of the National Institute of Dental Research, diagnostic criteria and procedures, NIH Publication No. 91-2870. Bethesda, MD: National Institute of Dental Research; 1991.

27. Gruebbel AO. A measurement of dental caries prevalence and treatment service for deciduous teeth. *J Dent Res.* 1944 Jun;23:163.

28. Drury TF, Horowitz AM, Ismail AI, Maertens MP, Rizier RG, Selwitz RH. Diagnosing and reporting early childhood caries for research purposes. *J Public Health Dent.* 1999 Summer;59(3):192–7.

29. Katz RV. Assessing root caries in populations: the evolution of the root caries index. *J Public Health Dent.* 1980 Winter;40(1):7–16.

30. Thylstrup A, Fejerskov O. Clinical appearance of sental fluorosis in permanent teeth in relation to histologic changes. *Community Dent Oral Epidemiol.* 1978 Nov;6(6):315–28.

31. Pendrys DG. The fluorosis risk index: a method for investigating risk factors. *J Public Health Dent.* 1990 Fall;50(5):291–8.

32. Fédération Dentaire Internationale, Commission on Oral Health, Research and Epidemiology. An epidemiological index of developmental defects of dental enamel (DDE Index). *Int Dent J.* 1982 Jun;32(2):159–67.

33. Clarkson J, O'Mullane, D. A modified DDE Index for use in epidemiological studies of enamel defects. *J Dent Res.* 1989 March;68(3):445–50.

34. Moulton FR (ed). Fluorine and dental health. Washington, DC: American Association for the Advancement of Science; 1942. Dean HT. The investigation of physiological effect by the epidemiological method. pp. 23–71.

35. Horowitz HS, Driscoll WS, Meyers RJ, Heifetz SB, Kingman AK. A new method for assessing the prevalence of dental fluorosis-the tooth surface index of fluorosis. *J Am Den.* 1984 Jul;109(1):37–41.

Dental Hygiene Diagnosis and Care Planning

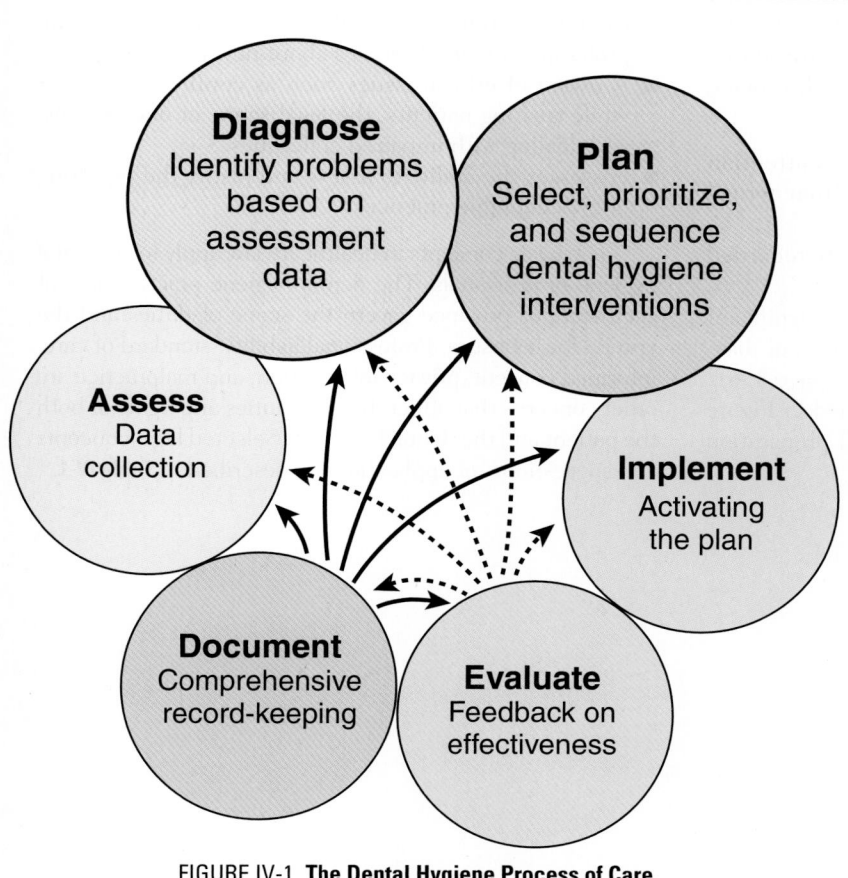

FIGURE IV-1 **The Dental Hygiene Process of Care.**

INTRODUCTION

After the initial assessment is completed as described in Section III, the data are assembled, sequenced, and analyzed in preparation for planning dental hygiene treatment and education interventions that help the patient acquire and maintain optimum oral health. A formal written care plan is used to educate the patient, secure informed consent for treatment, and communicate planned dental hygiene interventions with other oral care team members.

THE DENTAL HYGIENE PROCESS OF CARE

Figure IV-1 on the previous page shows the position of diagnosis and care planning in the total Dental Hygiene Process of Care.

I. DIAGNOSE

The diagnosis segment of the Dental Hygiene Process of Care is related to analyzing the assessment data that has been collected. Dental hygiene diagnosis statements identify patient needs that can be met by implementing treatment and education interventions that are within the scope of dental hygiene practice. Dental diagnoses, on the other hand, are directed at those diseases and conditions for which the dentist will provide treatment.

■ Dental hygiene diagnosis statements focus attention on behavioral aspects as well as deviations from normal oral health.
■ Chartings, radiographs, histories, and all recorded patient data are analyzed together.
■ Each diagnostic statement identifies with a significant oral hygiene problem of the patient. Examples of diagnostic statements are shown in Table 24-2 (page 356).
■ A blueprint care plan, such as that designed in Figure 24-1 (page 354), clarifies thinking toward preparation of diagnostic statements.

II. PLAN

After analyzing the assessment data, the next step in the Dental Hygiene Process of Care is to develop a plan for patient care.

■ The dental hygiene care plan selects interventions that are based on analysis of assessment data that has been consolidated into diagnostic statements that define patient needs.
■ The care plan is developed to conform to and be integrated with the total treatment plan of the patient.
■ The overall objectives of the dental health care team focus on the oral health of the patient. The ultimate goal will be the control of oral diseases.

ETHICAL APPLICATIONS

The potential for an ethical situation arises anytime a dental hygienist interacts with a patient, with members of the dental team, or with individuals involved in the special needs of the patient, such as family, caregivers, or members of specialty practices. A dental hygienist who provides ethical patient care:

■ Is cognizant of the respect each patient deserves.
■ Maintains communication among all parties responsible for dental and dental hygiene treatment.
■ Attains a knowledge of current standards of care through continuing education coursework and reading professional journal articles about new research.
■ Is aware of ethical issues such as conflict of interest while treating patients, the legal scope of one's duties, and dealing with impaired colleagues.
■ Possesses the ability to assess and justify the reporting of unacceptable practices.

The basic concepts in healthcare law apply to all dental hygiene professionals. The dental hygiene practice acts of each state or province govern the scope of duties and the criteria for licensure. Professional liability, standard of care, informed consent, privacy information, and malpractice are other concerns that affect the daily duties and rights of both the patient and the dental hygienist. Selected legal concepts and suggestions for application are described in **Table IV-1**.

TABLE IV-1	LEGAL AND ETHICAL CONCEPTS	
LEGAL CONCEPT	**EXPLANATION**	**APPLICATION EXAMPLES**
Professional Liability	A licensed professional is legally accountable for all actions; bound by the law.	Scope and duties of the dental hygienist are defined in each state's Dental Hygiene Practice Act.
Scope of Practice	A dental hygienist is legally bound to provide care within the dental hygiene scope of practice.	Adherence to dental hygiene licensure requirements and performance of functions defined as legal within in each state's Dental Hygiene Practice Act.
Standard of Care	A professional uses the ordinary and reasonable skill that is commonly used by other reputable dental hygienists when caring for patients; involves prudent judgment and use of all available resources.	Evaluating the patient's charting and examination data before determining which radiographs are needed according to individualized maintenance intervals.
Informed Consent	Voluntary affirmation by a patient to allow examination or treatment by authorized dental hygienist or other member of the dental team.	Involves the ongoing process of communicating and educating a patient about oral health treatment options, not only a printed form to sign.
Negligence/Malpractice	Failure to perform professional duties according to the accepted standard of care. Patient who has a complaint must show that the dental hygienist has a "duty" to the patient, was "derelict" and breached that duty, and provide evidence of "direct cause," and that "damages" resulted.	Not performing circumferential probing and informing/referring a patient when periodontal concerns exist can be considered negligence.

Planning for Dental Hygiene Care

CHARLOTTE J. WYCHE, RDH, MS

Chapter Outline

In the dental hygiene process of care described in Chapter 1 and illustrated in **Figure IV-1**, assessment data are used to formulate the dental hygiene diagnosis. Then, using an evidence-based approach, a dental hygiene care plan and appointment sequence can be formalized. Terms and key words used in conjunction with these steps are defined in **Box 23-1**.

ASSESSMENT FINDINGS

Assessment includes the gathering of details regarding the health status of the patient, followed by analysis and synthesis of the data. The application of clinical judgment and critical thinking skills is necessary to arrive at a dental hygiene diagnosis. Assessment procedures are described in detail in Chapters 9 through 22.

I. THE CHIEF COMPLAINT

The patient's statement regarding the reason for seeking dental and dental hygiene care is considered when planning. If a patient has a significant concern, such as pain, this need is addressed before initiating dental hygiene treatment.

II. RISK FACTORS

Whether or not the patient presents for dental hygiene care with current oral disease, several risk factors can be noted that increase the patient's potential for diminished oral health status. When a patient presents for dental hygiene care exhibiting one or more risk factors, it is essential to develop a care plan that provides anticipatory guidance through preventive education and counseling.

Planning for Dental Hygiene Care

ADLs (Activities of Daily Living): a measure of the ability to carry out the basic tasks needed for self-care.

IADLs (Instrumental Activities of Daily Living): a measure of the ability to perform more of the complex tasks necessary to function in our society; tasks that require a combination of physical and cognitive ability.

Anticipatory guidance: patient education and oral hygiene instructions that anticipate potential oral and systemic health problems associated with risk factors identified during patient assessment.

ASA: American Society of Anesthesiologists; originally developed the ASA Classifications to determine modifications necessary to provide general anesthetic to patients during surgical procedures.

Assessment: the critical analysis and evaluation or judgment of a particular condition, situation, or other subject of appraisal.

Chief complaint: the patient's concern as stated during the initial health history preparation; may be the reason for seeking professional care; a complaint such as pain or discomfort may require emergency dental diagnosis.

Compromised therapy: initial therapy and continued periodontal maintenance provided as the therapeutic end point in cases where the severity and extent of the disease or the age and health of the patient preclude optimal results of periodontal therapy.

Definitive care: complete care; end point at which all treatment required at the time has been completed.

Diagnose: to identify or recognize a disease or problem.

Diagnosis: a statement of the problem; a concise technical description of the cause, nature, or manifestations of a condition, situation, or problem; identification of a disease or deviation from normal condition by recognition of characteristic signs and symptoms.

Dental hygiene diagnosis: identification of an existing or potential oral health problem that a dental hygienist is qualified and licensed to treat.

Differential diagnosis: identification of which one of several diseases or conditions may be producing the symptoms.

Evidence-based care: providing oral care based on relevant, scientifically sound research.

OSCAR: a mnemonic that stands for **O**ral, **S**ystemic, **C**apability, **A**utonomy, and **R**eality. Developed by the American Academy of Oral Medicine to provide a convenient, systematic approach to identifying dental, medical/pharmacologic, functional, ethical, and fiscal factors that need to be evaluated and weighed when planning treatment for geriatric individuals or those with disabilities.

Prognosis: prediction of outcome; a forecast of the probable course and outcome of a disease and the prospects of recovery as expected by the nature of the specific condition and the symptoms of the case.

Dental hygiene prognosis: a judgment regarding the results (outcomes) expected to be achieved from oral treatment provided by a dental hygienist.

Risk factor: an attribute or exposure that increases the probability of disease, such as an aspect of personal behavior, environmental exposure, or an inherited characteristic associated with health-related conditions.

Modifiable risk factor: a determinant that can be modified by intervention, thereby reducing the probability of disease.

A. Risk Factors for Periodontal Infections or Poor Response to Periodontal Therapy[1–8]

- Behavioral factors (inadequate biofilm removal, diet, noncompliance with dental hygiene recommendations)
- Tobacco use
- Systemic conditions (diabetes, decreased immune factors, osteoporosis, osteopenia)
- Hormonal considerations (pregnancy, menopause)
- Nutritional status
- Iatrogenic factors (overhangs, open contacts, residual calculus)
- Genetic factors

B. Periodontal Disease As a Risk Factor for Systemic Conditions[9–14]

Current research suggests that the presence of periodontal infection is a contributing factor to a variety of systemic conditions.

- Infective endocarditis
- Cardiovascular disease (CVD) and atherosclerosis
- Diabetes mellitus
- Respiratory disease
- Adverse pregnancy outcomes

C. Risk Factors for Dental Caries[15]

- Behavioral factors (inadequate biofilm removal)
- Dietary factors (frequent use of cariogenic foods/beverages)
- Low fluoride
- Tooth morphology and position (deep occlusal pits and fissures, exposed root surfaces, rotated positioning)
- Xerostomia
- Personal and family history of dental caries/restorative dentistry
- Developmental factors (modifications of dental enamel)
- Genetic factors (immune response)

C. Risk Factors for Oral Cancer[16,17]

- Tobacco use
- Alcohol use
- Sun exposure (lips and face)

III. PATIENT'S OVERALL HEALTH STATUS

A. Physical Status

The extent of the patient's medical, physical, and psychological risk determines modifications necessary during treatment. Patient positioning, sequence and timing of treatments, and prevention of medical complications need consideration.

The American Society of Anesthesiologists' (ASA) Classification System[18] **(Table 23-1)** and the OSCAR Planning Guide[19] **(Table 23-2)** are two examples of systematic approaches used to help determine modifications necessary when providing patient care.

B. Tobacco Use

The patient's use of tobacco will affect oral status and dental hygiene treatment outcomes. Information on planning dental hygiene interventions for the patient who uses tobacco is found in Chapter 33 on pages 487 to 489.

IV. ORAL HEALTHCARE KNOWLEDGE LEVEL OF THE PATIENT

Before planning individualized patient care, an attempt is made to assess the patient's oral health knowledge level. From that baseline, planned educational interventions can build on current knowledge rather than provide information too far above or below the patient's current understanding.

V. THE PATIENT'S SELF-CARE ABILITY

The patient's ability to manipulate a toothbrush and floss and to comply with suggested oral care regimens

TABLE 23-1	ASA* PHYSICAL STATUS CLASSIFICATION SYSTEM		
ASA CLASSIFICATION		**EXAMPLES OF PHYSICAL OR PSYCHOSOCIAL MANIFESTATIONS**	**DENTAL HYGIENE TREATMENT CONSIDERATIONS**
ASA I	Without systemic disease; a normal, healthy patient with little or no dental anxiety	Able to walk one flight of stairs with no distress ADL/IADL level = 0	No modifications necessary
ASA II	Mild systemic disease or extreme dental anxiety	Must stop after walking one flight of stairs because of distress Well-controlled chronic conditions Upper respiratory infections Healthy pregnant woman Allergies ADL/IADL level = 1	Minimal risk; minor modifications to treatment and/or patient education may be necessary
ASA III	Systemic disease that limits activity but is not incapacitating	Must stop en route walking one flight of stairs Chronic cardiovascular conditions Controlled insulin-dependent diabetes Chronic pulmonary diseases Elevated blood pressure ADL/IADL level = 2 or 3	Elective treatment is not contraindicated, but serious consideration of treatment and/or patient/caregiver education modifications may be necessary
ASA IV	Incapacitating disease that is a constant threat to life	Unable to walk up one flight of stairs Unstable cardiovascular conditions Extremely elevated blood pressure Uncontrolled epilepsy Uncontrolled insulin-dependent diabetes	Conservative, noninvasive management of emergency dental conditions; more complex dental intervention may require hospitalization during treatment; caregiver training for daily oral care may be necessary
ASA V	Patient is moribund and not expected to survive	End-stage renal, hepatic, infectious disease, or terminal cancer	Only palliative treatment is delivered; caregiver training for daily oral care may be necessary.

*American Society of Anesthesiologists.
Source: ASA Physical Status Classification System [Internet]. Park Ridge, IL:American Society of Anesthesiologists; updated 2008 [cited 2010 Mar 4];[1 screen]. Available from: http://www.asahq.org/clinical/physicalstatus.htm and Malamed SF. Medical emergencies in the dental office, 5th ed. St. Louis:Mosby;2000. pp. 41–4.

TABLE 23-2	TREATMENT PLANNING WITH OSCAR

A systematic approach to identifying factors to evaluate when planning dental hygiene care.

ISSUE	FACTORS OF CONCERN
Oral	Teeth, restorations, prostheses, periodontium, pulpal status, oral mucosa, occlusion, saliva, tongue, alveolar bone
Systemic	Normative age changes, medical diagnoses, pharmacologic agents, interdisciplinary communication
Capability	Functional ability, self-care, caregivers, oral hygiene, transportation to appointments, mobility within the dental office
Autonomy	Decision-making ability, dependence on alternative or supplemental decision makers
Reality	Prioritization of oral health, financial ability or limitations, significance of anticipated life span

Reprinted with permission from Ship JA, Mohammad AR (eds). The clinician's guide to oral health in gereatric patients. Baltimore: American Academy of Oral Medicine; 1999. p. 21.

will determine the success of planned interventions. Patients with disabilities or physical limitations will require modification to ensure adequate daily dental biofilm removal.

An Activities of Daily Living (ADL)[20] classification level, described in **Table 23-3**, can provide a guide to determine whether adaptive aids or caregiver training for personal oral care procedures is necessary.

VI. DOCUMENTATION OF ASSESSMENT DATA

Complete and accurate records are essential. When data entry is not computerized, all entries are recorded in the patient record in ink. Standardized abbreviations are used to document all findings. Misunderstandings can lead to legal involvement.

THE PERIODONTAL DIAGNOSIS

Planning for the number and length of appointments in a treatment sequence will be determined by both the dental and dental hygiene periodontal diagnosis.

I. CURRENT PERIODONTAL STATUS

A description of past and current periodontal conditions, as well as risk factors that affect the progress of disease, determine a patient's current periodontal status.

II. CASE TYPE

For purpose of determining the sequences and number of appointments required for initial nonsurgical

TABLE 23-3	MEASURES OF PATIENT FUNCTIONING*	

EXAMPLES OF ACTIVITIES OF DAILY LIVING (ADLs)	EXAMPLES OF INSTRUMENTAL ACTIVITIES OF DAILY LIVING (IADLs)	LEVELS
Brushing *Flossing* *Applying interdental aids* Feeding Ambulation (Walking) Bathing Continence Communication Dressing Toileting Transfer (from bed to toilet) Grooming	*Maintaining self-care regimens* *Ability to make and keep dental appointments* Writing Cooking Shopping Climbing stairs Managing medication Reading Cleaning Using telephone	*Level 0* Ability to perform the task without assistance *Level 1* Ability to perform the task with some human assistance; may need a device or mechanical aid but or still independent *Level 2* Ability to perform the task with partial assistance *Level 3* Requires full assistance to perform the task; totally dependent

*This scale provides a simple means of summarizing a person's ability to carry out the basic tasks needed for self-care.
Source: Resnic B. Care of the older patient. In: Nettina SM (ed). The Lippincott manual of nursing practice. 7th ed. Phidelphia: Lippincott Williams & Wilkins; 2001. pp. 167–8.

periodontal therapy, it is useful to divide the periodontal diagnosis into case types as the following:

Type 1: Gingival Disease

Inflammation of the gingiva characterized by changes in color, form, size, position of margin, with bleeding on probing.

Type 2: Early Periodontitis

Progression of inflammation into the deeper periodontal structures with slight bone loss and connective tissue attachment; subgingival calculus and measurable pocket depth with bleeding on probing.

Type 3: Moderate Periodontitis

A more advanced state of the preceding type, with increased destruction of the periodontal structures, increased probing depths with bleeding, noticeable loss of bony support with early to moderate furcation invasions; mobility and fremitus.

Type 4: Advanced Periodontitis

Further progression of periodontal inflammation with increased probing depths with bleeding, major loss of bony support, furcation invasions, and possible evidence of trauma from occlusion with increased tooth mobility and fremitus, and other signs and symptoms, as described in Chapter 18, page 272.

III. CLASSIFICATION OF PERIODONTAL DISEASE

The extent, severity, and chronic or aggressive nature of the patient's periodontal disease can be characterized as listed in Table 23-4.

IV. PARAMETERS OF CARE

Clinical diagnosis, therapeutic goals, treatment considerations, and outcomes assessment for periodontal disease are outlined in the periodontal Parameters of Care.[21] Planning considerations are graded by the severity of infection. Examples are listed in **Table 23-4**.

DENTAL CARIES RISK LEVEL

Treatment for dental caries is provided by the dentist; however, the plan for dental hygiene care includes interventions aimed at managing risk factors for dental caries. A Caries Management by Risk Assessment (CAMBRA) protocol, which helps to determine an adult patient's caries risk level and suggests possible interventions to address risk factors is found in Table 26-1 on page 381. A

CAMBRA assessment tool (Table 49-9) and a treatment guidelines protocol (Table 49-10) for children 0–5 years old are found on pages 764 and 766.

THE DENTAL HYGIENE DIAGNOSIS

I. BASIS FOR DIAGNOSIS

- Patient interview data (chief complaint, identification of oral problems, and comprehensive personal/social, medical, and dental health histories)
- Physical assessment data (vital signs, extraoral and intraoral tissue examination, and dental and periodontal chartings)
- Treatment or education needs that may be addressed by providing oral care services within the dental hygienist's legal scope of practice
- Treatment needs that may be addressed by consultation with another licensed healthcare professional

II. DIAGNOSTIC STATEMENTS

- Provide the basis for planning interventions that are within the scope of dental hygiene practice.
- Reflect expected outcomes of dental hygiene interventions.
- Identify patient responses that are changeable by dental hygiene interventions.
- Exclude diagnoses that require treatments legally defined as dental practice.
- For examples of dental hygiene diagnostic statements, see Table 24-2, page 356.

III. DIAGNOSTIC MODELS[22–26]

Medical and dental models of diagnosis classify diagnostic statements according to disease processes. In contrast, dental hygiene models have been developed more like nursing models that encompass a broader focus. These models:

- Address health functioning and behaviors.
- Describe actual or potential health problems that dental hygienists are educated and licensed to treat.
- The dental hygiene diagnosis models, described in **Table 23-5**, give direction and a scientific basis from which to determine dental hygiene interventions and formulate patient care plans.

THE DENTAL HYGIENE PROGNOSIS

Prognosis means a look ahead to an anticipated outcome or end point. The dental hygiene prognosis is a statement of the possible outcomes that can be expected from the dental hygiene intervention selected for an individual patient.

(continued on page 347)

TABLE 23-4	PARAMETERS OF CARE		

CLINICAL DIAGNOSIS	THERAPEUTIC GOALS	TREATMENT CONSIDERATIONS	
Biofilm-Induced Gingivitis	■ To establish gingival health through elimination of etiologic factors	*Dental Treatment Plan* ■ The dental treatment plan may indicate surgical correction of gingival deformities.	*Dental Hygiene Care Plan* ■ Customized patient education ■ Supra- and subgingival debridement ■ Antimicrobial agents, and correction of biofilm-retentive factors
Chronic Periodontitis ■ With slight to moderate loss of periodontal support.	■ To arrest progression of disease and prevent recurrence ■ To preserve health, comfort, and function.	*Dental Treatment Plan* ■ If resolution of the condition does not occur, consider periodontal surgery.	*Dental Hygiene Care Plan* ■ Elimination and control of systemic risk factors ■ Biofilm control ■ Supra- and subgingival scaling and root planing ■ Adjunctive antimicrobial agents ■ Elimination of contributing local factors
Chronic Periodontitis ■ With advanced loss of periodontal support.	■ To alter or eliminate microbial etiology and contributing risk factors ■ To arrest the progression of disease	*Dental Treatment Plan* ■ May include regeneration of periodontal attachment following the completion and evaluation of initial therapy	*Dental Hygiene Care Plan* ■ Initial therapy as described above *Compromised Therapy* ■ Severity/extent of disease, or the age/health of the patient preclude optimal results ■ Initial therapy and continued periodontal maintenance become the endpoint
Periodontal Maintenance	■ To minimize the recurrence and progression of the disease ■ To reduce the incidence of tooth loss		*Dental Hygiene Care Plan* ■ Comparison of clinical data to previous baseline measurements ■ Assessment of personal oral hygiene status and compliance with maintenance intervals ■ Oral hygiene reinstruction or modification ■ Counseling on control of risk factors
Acute Periodontal Diseases Includes ■ Gingival abscess ■ Periodontal abscess ■ Necrotizing diseases ■ Herpetic gingivostomatitis ■ Pericoronitis ■ Periodontal-endodontic lesions	■ To eliminate acute signs and symptoms of the condition as soon as possible	*Dental Treatment Plan* ■ Treatment considerations depend on the presenting condition	*Dental Hygiene Care Plan* ■ Collaborate with the attending dentist to prioritize treatment for the immediate need

(continued)

TABLE 23-4	PARAMETERS OF CARE (*Continued*)		
CLINICAL DIAGNOSIS	**THERAPEUTIC GOALS**	**TREATMENT CONSIDERATIONS**	
Aggressive Periodontitis	■ To alter or eliminate microbial etiology and contributing risk factors ■ To arrest or slow the progression of the disease	***Dental Treatment Plan may include*** ■ General medical evaluation and consultation ■ Microbial identification ■ Antibiotic sensitivity testing ■ Alternative antimicrobial agents or delivery systems ■ Evaluation/counseling of family members	***Dental Hygiene Care Plan*** ■ Care parameters planned for chronic periodontitis
Mucogingival Conditions ■ Deviations from normal anatomic relationship between gingival margin and mucogingival junction	■ To maintain and restore function and esthetics	***Dental Treatment Plan*** ■ May include surgical treatment	***The Dental Hygiene Care Plan*** ■ Careful comparison of baseline and follow-up findings, control of inflammation through biofilm control, scaling and root planing, and/or antimicrobial agents

Source: American Academy of Periodontology. Parameters of Care. *J Periodontol.* 2000 May;71(5 Suppl):i–ii, 847–83.

TABLE 23-5	DIAGNOSTIC MODELS USED IN PLANNING DENTAL HYGIENE CARE
MODEL NAME	**DIAGNOSTIC STATEMENTS**
Dental Hygiene Diagnostic Model[22,23]	Developed by following six steps that form the process of diagnostic decision making: (1) Initial review (2) Hypothesis formation (3) Inquiry strategy (4) Problem synthesis (5) Diagnostic decision making (6) Learning from the process Recorded in patient treatment records using the notation "DHDX" and accompanied by a treatment plan or treatment goal statement
The Human Needs Model[24]	Based on whether specific criteria defining eight human needs are met or unmet by the patient's current oral health status Written by outlining goals to be obtained for resolving each observed deficit
The Dental Hygiene Process Model[25]	Identify patient's problem in terms of response rather than need and state the possible etiology Classified into several categories, which include general systemic, soft tissue, periodontal, oral hygiene, and dental categories Written by stating the problem and the etiologic factor joined by the phrase "related to"
The Oral Health-Related Quality of Life (OHRQL) Model[26]	Diagnostic statements for individuals/populations are based on the assessment of domains related to health/preclinical disease; biological/physiological dis-ease; and the broad-based sequelae to disease, such as symptom status, function status, health perceptions, and overall quality of life Dental hygiene actions are formulated for each domain, incorporating a multidisciplinary approach to care

I. CRITERIA FOR VARIOUS PROGNOSES

Prognosis is expressed in general terms for either an individual tooth or the overall prognosis for the patient's teeth. The criteria for various prognoses are listed in **Box 23-2**.

II. FACTORS THAT DETERMINE PROGNOSIS

■ Assessment data regarding current disease status
■ The patient's risk factors
■ The patient's commitment to personal care and preventive regimens
■ Interventions with the potential to reverse a patient's oral problem
■ Treatment alternatives selected
■ Evidence from the scientific literature

III. EXPECTED OUTCOMES

The identification of results expected following dental hygiene interventions is based on treatment and self-care behavior goals set by the clinician with the patient during the planning phase of care. Examples of potential outcomes from dental hygiene interventions in a three-part care plan are listed in Chapter 24 on page 356.

CONSIDERATIONS FOR PROVIDING CARE

I. ROLE OF THE PATIENT

A. Purpose

The willingness and/or ability of the patient to participate in reducing risk factors and changing oral health behaviors will be the key to reaching goals set during planning.

B. Procedure

■ Determine the patient's level of understanding of dental diseases, risk factors, and oral health behaviors.
■ Determine the patient's physical ability to manipulate recommended oral care aids.
■ Determine lifestyle factors that impact the patient's ability to comply with oral health recommendations.
■ Educate patients regarding the importance of their role in eliminating modifiable risk factors, setting oral health goals and complying with recommendations.

II. TISSUE CONDITIONING

Preparation or conditioning of the gingival tissue for scaling can be of particular significance when there is spongy, soft tissue that bleeds on slight provocation, and when the area is generally septic from dental biofilm and debris accumulation.

A. Purpose

Anticipated outcomes of a tissue-conditioning program include:

■ Gingival healing
  A. Tissues become less edematous.
  B. Bleeding is minimized.
  C. Scaling procedures are facilitated.
■ Reduced bacterial accumulation
  A. Less likelihood that bacteremias will be produced during scaling.

BOX 23-2	Criteria for Various Prognoses	
Prognosis is assigned by the presence of one or more of the following factors.		
Good	■ Adequate control of etiologic factors ■ Adequate patient self-care ability ■ Adequate periodontal support	
Fair	■ Adequate control of etiologic factors ■ Adequate patient self-care ability ■ Less than 25% attachment loss ■ Class I or less furcation involvement	
Poor	■ Greater than 50% attachment loss with Class II furcation ■ Patient self-care difficult due to location and depth of furcation	
Questionable	■ Greater than 50% attachment loss with poor crown-to-root ratio ■ Poor root form: Instrumentation access ■ Inaccessible Class II furcation or Class III furcation ■ Greater than 2+ mobility ■ Significant root proximity	
Hopeless	■ Inadequate attachment to maintain the tooth	

Modified with permission from: McGuire, M.K.: Prognosis vs Outcome: Predicting Tooth Survival, *Compend. Contin. Educ. Dent., 21,217,* March, 2000.

B. Contamination is reduced in the aerosols produced.

■ Learning by the patient

While conditioning the tissue for scaling, the patient can do the following:

■ Practice oral health behaviors
■ Experience the benefits of a clean mouth
■ From lifetime habits for continued maintenance

B. Procedure

■ Initiate a pretreatment program of daily biofilm removal.
■ Recommend daily use of an antibacterial rinse after thorough brushing and flossing before going to bed.
■ Select affected quadrants for scaling only after patient cooperation has been demonstrated.

III. PREPROCEDURAL ANTIMICROBIAL RINSING

A. Purpose

Preprocedural removal of dental biofilm will lower the bacterial count in aerosols and decrease the potential for bacteremia.

B. Procedure

■ The first choice is patient brushing and flossing.
■ Vigorous rinsing with an antibacterial mouthwash is beneficial.[27]
■ Forcing the fluid between the teeth for 1–2 minutes can remove loose debris and surface bacteria approximately 1 mm below the gingival margin.[28]
■ Even rinsing with water will have some effect on bacteria; however, chlorhexidine rinses have the most substantivity.[29]

IV. PAIN AND ANXIETY CONTROL

A. Purpose

■ Control of discomfort during treatment procedure.
■ More consistent patient compliance with recommended interventions and need to return for additional scheduled appointments.

B. Procedures

1. When there is a patient complaint of pain or discomfort, treat those areas first unless tissue conditioning is required.

2. Treat either the quadrant with the fewest teeth or the least severe periodontal infection first to ensure the following:
   ■ Make the first scaling less complicated.
   ■ Help orient an anxious patient to clinical procedures.
3. Patient posttreatment discomfort is minimized to select a maxillary and mandibular quadrant on the same side when two quadrants are to be treated at the same appointment.
4. The need for anesthesia is determined by:
   ■ the patient's previous pain control experiences
   ■ severity of the periodontal infection
   ■ depth of pockets
   ■ consistency and distribution of calculus
   ■ potential patient discomfort during scaling
   ■ sensitivity of the patient's tissues

V. MAINTENANCE DURING DENTAL THERAPY

A. Purpose

When restorative, prosthetic, or orthodontic, treatment extends over a long period of time, periodic appointments with the dental hygienist are needed for monitoring the continued success of the patient's self-care.

B. Procedure

Dental hygiene care provided during extended dental therapy follows the dental hygiene process of care and includes:

■ gingival tissue assessment
■ probing to determine bleeding
■ biofilm check with disclosing agent
■ reinforcement of daily oral care measures
■ scaling and root planing to remove calculus
■ additional instruction for care of new prostheses
■ motivational encouragement

VI. FOUR-HANDED DENTAL HYGIENE

A. Purpose

Planning patient care while practicing with a dental assistant increases the dental hygienist's efficiency through the use of:

■ flexible scheduling.[30]
■ two treatment chairs in an overlapping time frame.
■ assistance with patient management.

B. Procedure

A well-trained dental hygiene assistant can be delegated such duties as:

■ patient reception and seating
■ medical history update before confirmation by the dental hygienist

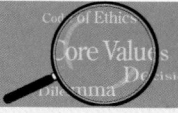

Everyday Ethics

Victoria, the dental hygienist, is discussing the assessment findings for her patient, Mr. Rush, with the rest of the dental team. Mr. Rush has stated that he has already been told at his general dental practice that he has extensive active periodontal disease. He was referred to this practice because he wants all of the most compromised teeth extracted and dental implants placed.

Mr. Rush has a number of risk factors, such as poorly controlled diabetes and smoking. Because his dental insurance is running out in 3 months, everyone is in a rush to get the treatment started, and the potential for a poor prognosis has not been discussed. In fact, Victoria's concerns about the patient's risk factors are being pushed aside.

Question for Consideration

1. Is this an ethical issue or an ethical dilemma?
2. What is Victoria's obligation (duty) to make sure that Mr. Rush understands how his risk factors compromise the prognosis of his treatment plan? What action can Victoria take if her concerns continue to be ignored and treatment progresses without interventions that address the risk factors involved in Mr. Rush's case?
3. How can Victoria proceed to obtain informed consent from Mr. Rush and ensure that his rights to optimal care are maintained?

- radiographs (following individual state certification guidelines)
- reinforcement of oral hygiene instruction
- chairside assistance during sealant placement and ultrasonic scaling
- cleanup/disinfection of the treatment room in preparation for the next patient

EVIDENCE-BASED SELECTION OF DENTAL HYGIENE PROTOCOLS

Dental hygiene interventions are planned using scientific evidence of efficacy and efficiency. Scientific evidence from dental and medical literature can improve opportunities for achieving successful outcomes from dental hygiene treatment. The patient can benefit if the dental hygienist has developed skills in accessing and evaluating the scientific literature.

THE WRITTEN DENTAL HYGIENE CARE PLAN

Chapter 24 outlines specific procedures for preparation and documentation of a formal written dental hygiene care plan.

DOCUMENTATION

- All assessment findings are documented before developing a formal written, care plan.
- A suggested format for documenting a formal, written dental hygiene care plan is found in Chapter 24 on page 354.
- An example progress note for an assessment appointment before developing a dental hygiene care plan, is found in **Box 23-3**.

BOX 23-3	**Example Progress Note Related to Assessment Before Developing a Dental Hygiene Care Plan**

Patient presents for initial patient visit. Completed assessment data collected and documented, including vital signs, medical, social and dental histories, intraoral and extraoral examination findings, and dental radiographs, in preparation for developing a formal written dental hygiene care plan. Complete plan for both dental and dental hygiene treatment will be presented to patient at next appointment, scheduled in 2 weeks.

Signed: _____, RDH Date: _____.

 **Factors To Teach The Patient**

- A clear explanation of how assessment data are used in planning dental hygiene care.
- The importance of using scientific evidence of success in the selection of patient-specific therapeutic and preventive interventions.
- Why disease control measures are learned before and in conjunction with scaling.
- Facts of oral disease prevention and oral health promotion relevant to the patient's current level of healthcare knowledge and individual risk factors.
- The long-term positive effects of comprehensive continuing care.

References

1. Molloy J, Wolff LF, Lopez-Guzman A, Hodges JS. The association of periodontal disease parameters with systemic medical conditions and tobacco use. *J Clin Periodontol.* 2004 Aug;31(8):625–32.

2. Fisher MA, Taylor GW, Tilashalski KR. Smokeless tobacco and severe active periodontal disease, NHANES III. *J Dent Res.* 2005 Aug;84(8):705–10.

3. Takayanagi H. Inflammatory bone destruction and osteoimmunology. *J Periodont Res.* 2005 Aug; 40(4):287–93.

4. Mulligan R, Sobel S. Osteoporosis: diagnostic testing, interpretation, and correlations with oral health-implications for dentistry. *Dent Clin North Am.* 2005 Apr;49(2):463–84.

5. Mascarenhas P, Gapski R, Al-Shammari K, Wang HL. Influence of sex hormones on the periodontium. *J Clin Periodontol.* 2005 Aug; 30(8):671–81.

6. Schifferle RE. Nutrition and periodontal disease. *Dent Clin North Am.* 2005 Jul;49(3):595–610.

7. Matthews DC, Tabesh M. Detection of localized tooth-related factors that predispose to periodontal infections. *Periodontol 2000.* 2004;34:136–50.

8. Tatakis DN, Kumar PS. Etiology and pathogenesis of periodontal diseases. *Dent Clin North Am.* 2005 Jul;49(3):491–516.

9. Daly CG, Mitchell DH, Highfield JE, Grossberg DE, Stewart, D. Bacteremia due to periodontal probing: a clinical and microbial investigation. *J Periodontol.* 2001 Feb;72(2):210–14.

10. Okuda K, Kato T, Ishihara K. Involvement of periodontopathic biofilm in vascular diseases. *Oral Dis.* 2004 Jan;10(1):5–12.

11. Iacopino IM. Periodontitis and diabetes interrelationships: role of inflammation. *Ann Periodontol.* 2001 Dec;6(1):125–37.

12. Holmstrup P, Poulsen AH, Andersen L, Skuldbol T, Fiehn NE. Oral infections and systemic diseases. *Dent Clin North Am.* 2003 Jul; 47(3):575–98.

13. Offenbacher S, Lieff S, Boggess KA, Murtha AP, Madianos PN, Champagne CM, McKaig RG, Jared HL, Mauriello SM, Auten RL Jr, Herbert WN, Beck JD. Maternal periodontitis and prematurity. Part I: obstetric outcome of prematurity and growth restriction. *Ann Periodontol.* 2001 Dec;6(1):164–74.

14. Moore S, Ide M, Coward PY, Randhawa M, Borkowska E, Baylis R, Wilson RF. A prospective study to investigate the relationship between periodontal disease and adverse pregnancy outcomes. *Br Dent J.* 2004 Sep 1;197(5):251–8.

15. Rethman J. Trends in preventive care: caries risk assessment and indications for dental sealants. *J Am Dent Assoc.* 2000 Jun; 131 Suppl:8S–12S.

16. Scully C, Newman L, Bagan JV. The role of the dental team in preventing and diagnosing cancer: 2. Oral cancer risk factors. *Dent Update.* 2005 Jun;32(5), 261–2, 264–6, 269–70.

17. Perea-Milla Lopez E, Minarro-Del Moral RM, Martinez-Garcia C, Zanetti R, Rosso S, Serrano S, Aneiros JF, Jimenez-Puente A, Redondo M. Lifestyles, environmental and phenotypical factors associated with lip cancer: a case-control study in southern spain. *Br J Cancer.* 2003 Jun 2;88(11):1702–7.

18. ASA Physical Status Classification System [Internet]. Park Ridge, IL:American Society of Anesthesiologists; updated 2008 [cited 2010 Mar 4];[1 screen]. Available from: http://www.asahq.org/clinical/physicalstatus.htm

19. Ship JA, Mohammed A.R, editors. *The clinician's guide to oral health in geriatric patients.* Baltimore: American Academy of Oral Medicine; 1999. 21 p.

20. Resnick B. Care of the Older Patient. In: Nettina SM, editor. *The Lippincott manual of nursing practice.* 7th ed. Philadelphia:Lippincott Williams & Wilkins;2001. 167–168 pp.

21. American Academy of Periodontology. Parameters of care. *J Periodontol.* 2000 May;71(5 Suppl):i–ii, 847–83.

22. Gurenlian JR. Diagnostic decision making. In: Woodall IR editor. *Comprehensive dental hygiene care.* 4th ed. St. Louis:Mosby;1993. 361–70 pp.

23. Gurenlian JR. Recording the dental hygiene diagnosis. *Access.* 1994 Nov;8:15.

24. Darby ML, Walsh MM. Application of the human needs conceptual model to dental hygiene practice. *J Dent Hyg.* 2000 Summer;74(3):230–7.

25. Mueller-Joseph L, Petersen M. *Dental hygiene process: diagnosis and care planning.* Albany:Delmar;1995. 46–63 pp.

26. Williams KB, Gadbury-Amyot CC, Bray KK, Manne D, Collins P. Oral health-related quality of life: a model for dental hygiene. *J Dent Hyg.* 1998 Spring;72,(2):19–26.

27. Fine DH, Korik I, Furgang D, Myers R, Olshan A, Barnett ML, Vincent, J. Assessing pre-procedural subgingival irrigation and rinsing with an antiseptic mouthrinse to reduce bacteremia. *J Am Dent Assoc.* 1996 May;127(5):641–2, 645–6.

28. Veksler AE, Kayrouz GA, Newman MG. Reduction of salivary bacteria by pre-procedural rinses with chlorhexidine 0.12%. *J Periodontol.* 1991 Nov;62(11):649–51.

29. Wunderlich RC, Singleton M, O'Brien WJ, Caffesse RG. Subgingival penetration of an applied solution. *Int J Periodontics Restorative Dent.* 1984;4(5):64–71.

30. Blitz P, Wright V. It takes two. *RDH,* 1994 Sep;14(9):18, 21, 23, 25.

The Dental Hygiene Care Plan

CHARLOTTE J. WYCHE, RDH, MS

Chapter Outline

A written dental hygiene care plan is an essential part of the integrated components of the dental hygiene process of care illustrated in Figure IV-1 (page 339). Terms and key words for this chapter are defined in **Box 24-1**.

PREPARATION OF A DENTAL HYGIENE CARE PLAN

Dental hygiene care is planned to address the needs of the entire oral cavity. The care plan is based on assessment of the oral mucosa, teeth, periodontal supporting structures, and health factors that influence the oral environment. A care plan that integrates a basic three-part plan to care for all of the patient's dental hygiene needs has a major influence on the future oral health of the patient.

I. PARTS OF A CARE PLAN

A. Periodontal/Gingival Health

■ The primary objective of the dental hygiene plan for periodontal therapy is to restore and maintain health of the periodontal tissues.
■ Additional attention is paid to interventions that can reduce individualized risk factors for developing periodontal disease or for complications related to the associations between systemic disease and periodontal disease.

B. Dental Caries Control

■ The plan for caries control includes a remineralization program, fluorides, dental sealants, and dietary control of fermentable carbohydrates based on an individualized assessment of caries risk.

BOX 24-1	Key Words

Planning Dental Hygiene Care

Consent: voluntary agreement to an action proposed by another.

Informed consent: a patient's voluntary agreement to a treatment plan after details of the proposed treatment have been presented and comprehended by the patient.

Informed refusal: a patient's decision to refuse recommended treatment after all options, potential risks, and potential benefits have been thoroughly explained.

Intervention: to happen or take place between other events; to intervene, as with a specific treatment.

Prioritize: to arrange in order of importance.

Sequence: a continuous or related series of things (such as dental hygiene interventions) following in a certain order or succession.

Total treatment plan: sequential outline of the essential services and procedures that must be carried out by the dentist, the dental hygienist, and the patient to eliminate disease and restore the oral cavity to health and normal function.

Dental hygiene care plan: the services within the framework of the total treatment plan to be carried out by the dental hygienist.

■ Even when the patient's caries risk level is low, the plan includes a minimum frequency of recall examination to monitor risk factors and preventive recommendations such as daily use of fluoride toothpaste.

C. Other

A plan for preventive care starts with the patient's personal daily bacterial control and includes interventions that eliminate modifiable risk factors for oral disease such as tobacco cessation counseling, desensitizing exposed dentin, resolving halitosis, and much, much more.

II. DESCRIPTION

The written care plan is a prioritized sequence of evidence-based dental hygiene interventions that are:

■ Predicated on the dental hygiene diagnosis.
■ Composed of integrated plans for the care and control of periodontal disease, dental caries control, management of risk factors, and other preventive interventions.
■ Integrated into a total treatment plan that encompasses the patient's restorative and surgical needs, as shown in **Table 24-1**.
■ Contained within the scope of dental hygiene practice as defined by each practice act.

III. RATIONALE

A written dental hygiene care plan will help to:

■ Focus on individualized patient needs and risk factors when selecting dental hygiene interventions.
■ Prioritize the sequence of planned treatment and education.
■ Provide a checklist to ensure that all planned interventions are accomplished.

IV. OBJECTIVES

A well-prepared dental hygiene care plan includes the following:

■ Plans care for patient needs based on assessment data collected.
■ Is flexible and realistic.
■ Contains treatment and education goals that address problems and risk factors identified during the assessment phase.
■ Provides interventions and recommendations based on current scientific evidence.

COMPONENTS OF A WRITTEN CARE PLAN

A dental hygiene care plan may be written using a variety of formats. Components of a well-written care plan are described in this section. **Figure 24-1** is a suggested template for a patient-specific care plan that follows the dental hygiene process of care. The recommended components of a written care plan are described in this section.

I. DEMOGRAPHIC DATA

■ Patient name, date of birth (age), and gender.
■ A designation of initial or maintenance therapy.
■ The name of the student or clinician who prepared the written plan.
■ The date that the written plan was prepared.
■ Notation of the patient's chief complaint or statement indicating the patient's reason for presenting for treatment.

II. ASSESSMENT FINDINGS AND RISK FACTORS

This section of the plan contains a thorough, summarized description of significant findings.

TABLE 24-1	COMPONENTS OF A MASTER TREATMENT PLAN	
PHASE	**PROCEDURES**	**INCLUDED IN THE DENTAL HYGIENE CARE PLAN**
Preliminary phase	■ Assessment data collection ■ Emergency care (pain, biopsy)	✔
Phase I therapy	■ Dental biofilm control ■ Introduction of additional preventive measures (diet changes, fluorides, mouthguard) ■ Calculus removal ■ Correction of restorative and prosthetic irritants (biofilm traps, overhangs) ■ Restorative carles control	✔ ✔ ✔
Outcomes evaluation of phase I	■ Probing depths ■ Clinical signs of inflammation ■ Dental biofilm control ■ Patient's participation	✔ ✔ ✔ ✔
Phase II surgical	■ Periodontal ■ Endodontic ■ Implant placement	
Phase III restorative	■ Final restorations ■ Fixed/removable prostheses	
Evaluation of overall outcomes	■ Periodontal response to restorations/implants ■ Other response to restorations	✔
Phase IV maintenance	■ Appointments for continuing care and supervision ■ Refining biofilm control techniques	✔ ✔

A. Medical History

■ Systemic diseases and conditions: current and past
■ Medications
■ Overall health status
■ Functional assessment

B. Social and Dental History

■ Treatment history
■ Oral health knowledge and behaviors
■ Cultural factors

C. Clinical Examination

■ Extraoral and intraoral
■ Soft and hard tissue

D. Link to Risk Factors

■ Risk for increased oral disease
■ Increased risk of systemic disease due to oral infection
■ Potential for compromised treatment outcomes

III. PERIODONTAL DIAGNOSIS AND STATUS

■ The periodontal diagnosis formulated by the dentist is included in the dental hygiene care plan.
■ Guidelines for noting the periodontal diagnosis/case type and Parameters of Care, useful for planning dental hygiene treatment interventions, are listed in Table 23-4 on page 345.

IV. CARIES RISK STATUS

■ CAMBRA, a caries risk assessment tool that provides guidelines for identifying caries risk status and selecting dental hygiene interventions based on risk factor assessment is detailed in Table 26-1 (page 381) for adult patients for children 0–5 years old in Table 49-9 (page 764).
■ Understanding of a patient's individualized risks for dental caries can guide the plan for oral health education and counseling as well as treatment interventions, such as dental sealants or fluoride recommendations to enhance remineralization.

(continued on page 356)

Patient Specific Dental Hygiene Care Plan

Patient name _____ Age _____ Gender: M ☐ F ☐   Initial therapy ☐

Provider name _____ Date _____   Maintenance ☐

Chief complaint: Re-evaluation ☐

Assessment Findings

Medical history	At Risk For
Systemic disease	
Other conditions	
Medications	
ASA classification	
ADL/IADL level	
Social and dental history	
Treatment history	
Dental knowledge	
Health behaviors	
Cultural factors	
Dental examination	
Extraoral examination	
Intraoral examination	
Teeth/restorations	
Periodontal examination	

Periodontal Diagnosis/Case Type and Status:	Caries Management Risk Assessment (CAMBRA) level: Low ☐ Moderate ☐ High ☐ Extreme ☐

Dental Hygiene Diagnosis

Problem	Related to (Risk Factors and Etiology)
Extraoral	
Intraoral	
Restorative/caries risk	
Periodontal status or risk	
Systemic health	
Self-care ability	

FIGURE 24-1 **Patient-Specific Dental Hygiene Care Plan.** The written care plan includes a summary of assessment findings, the dental hygiene diagnosis, planned dental hygiene interventions, expected outcomes, and an appointment plan that sequences treatment procedures and education interventions for each appointment. (Modified with permission from a care plan model, based on the *Dental Hygiene Process of Care,* that was originally provided by Dr. Laura Mueller-Joseph.) (*continued*)

Planned Interventions
(to arrest or control disease and regenerate, restore or maintain health)

Clinical	Education/Counseling	Oral Hygiene Instruction/Home Care

Expected Outcomes

Goals	Evaluation Methods	Time Frame
1		
2		
3		
4		

Appointment Plan
(sequence of planned intrventions)

Appt #	Plan for Treatment and Services	Plan for Education, Counseling and Oral Hygiene Instruction
1	Quadrant	
2		
3		
4		

Re-evaluation Findings

Re-treat ☐   Refer ☐   Continuing care interval _____

Description of post-treatment outcomes:

FIGURE 24-1 (*Continued*)

TABLE 24-2	EXAMPLES OF DENTAL HYGIENE DIAGNOSTIC STATEMENTS
PROBLEM	**RISK FACTORS AND ETIOLOGY**
Hypersensitivity	*Related to:* Exposed cementum/gingival recession
Gingival bleeding	*Related to:* Biofilm accumulation causing inflammation
Increased caries risk (CAMBRA level = EXTREME)	*Related to:* Previous history of dental caries and consumption of sugar-sweetened soft drinks frequently throughout each day
Biofilm Control Record score = fair to poor score	*Related to:* Limited ability to perform oral self care tasks (ADL level 3)

V. DIAGNOSTIC STATEMENTS

Table 24-2 contains examples of dental hygiene diagnostic statements that:

- link observed or potential oral health problems identified during the patient assessment to probable etiology or risk factors.
- relate to problems and solutions that can be addressed within the dental hygiene scope of practice.

VI. PLANNED INTERVENTIONS

Dental hygiene interventions are measures applied to regenerate, restore, or maintain oral health. Selected interventions are specific to the individual patient's assessment findings and include the following:

- Clinical treatments, such as scaling, root planing, and debridement, selected for the purpose of arresting or controlling existing disease.
- Preventive measures, such as dental sealants, that maintain tooth integrity.
- Education and counseling in such topics as etiology and progression of oral disease and elimination of risk factors.
- Individualized oral hygiene instructions and personal daily oral care regimens based on patient needs and abilities.

VII. EXPECTED OUTCOMES

A plan for treatment or personal oral care outcomes, created in consultation with the patient, contains:

- At least one goal for each oral health problem identified in the dental hygiene diagnosis.
- A realistic time frame for measuring success.

VIII. EVALUATION METHODS

Evaluation of clinical outcomes is discussed more completely on pages 727. Evaluation methods identified in the dental hygiene care plan:

- Include assessment data collection and comparison with initial assessment findings.
- Clearly identify how progress toward each goal will be measured.

An example of an evaluation method that could be identified in the written care plan is the use of periodontal probing to determine reduction in pocket depths.

IX. THE APPOINTMENT PLAN

An appointment plan for multiple appointments:

- Outlines interventions sequenced in order of clinical performance.
- Can be adapted at each appointment to respond to new information or immediate patient need.
- Properly prioritized and sequenced treatment and education interventions will be:
  - More comfortable for the patient.
  - More effective in reaching planned oral health goals.

X. REEVALUATION

At the reevaluation appointment:

- New assessment data are collected and analyzed.
- A determination is made regarding whether expected outcomes of the care plan have been met.
- Maintenance appointment interval is determined.

SEQUENCING AND PRIORITIZING PATIENT CARE

I. OBJECTIVES

Reasons for preparing a well-sequenced dental hygiene care plan are:

A. To Provide Evidence-Based, Individualized Patient Care

- Determined by analysis of assessment data.
- Based on documented evidence of success.

- Enhanced by the clinician's ability to assess the value of information available in the scientific literature.

B. To Eliminate or Control Etiologic and Predisposing Disease Factors

- The principal etiologic agents in both dental caries and periodontal and gingival diseases are the microorganisms of dental biofilm.
- Dental hygiene interventions can modify a variety of risk factors that predispose the patient to oral disease.

C. To Eliminate the Signs and Symptoms of Disease

Measures to eliminate signs of infection such as gingival bleeding and probing depths are included in the care plan.

D. To Promote Oral Health and Prevent Recurrence of Disease

Methods used to achieve optimum oral health are as follows:

- Education on the etiology of oral disease.
- Counseling on prevention measures and elimination of risk factors.
- Instruction and supervision in daily self-care techniques.
- Encouragement of regularly scheduled maintenance follow-up for dental hygiene care.

II. FACTORS AFFECTING SEQUENCE OF CARE

Treatment sequence defines the order in which the parts of an individual appointment are to be carried out. Sequence planning involves:

- identification of overall treatment and education patterns appropriate for an individual patient's needs.
- outline of a series of appointments, with specific services, treatment procedures, and educational interventions included.

The sequence of care for an individual patient is determined by numerous factors.

A. Urgency

Discomfort or pain that requires first attention could apply to:

- an area of the gingiva that is particularly difficult to clean because of inaccessibility.
- an area with a periodontal abscess or with necrotizing ulcerative gingivitis (NUG).

B. Existing Etiologic Factors

In patients with gingival or periodontal infection or risk for dental caries, success of the treatment depends on thorough, daily biofilm removal. Biofilm control measures are introduced and success is evaluated before additional dental hygiene interventions will be effective.

C. Severity and Extent of the Condition

The number and length of appointments and the sequencing of procedures planned are affected by the severity of the condition. Findings that indicate the severity of gingival or periodontal infection include:

- changes in color, size, shape, or consistency of the gingiva.
- probing depths.
- bleeding on probing.
- mobility of the teeth.
- clinical and radiographic signs of attachment or bone loss.

D. Individual Patient Requirements

When writing the actual plan, each patient is considered individually. Items from the patient history that may require adaptation in appointment length, spacing, or sequencing when planning dental hygiene care include the following:

1. Antibiotic premeditation
   - Current recommended standard prophylactic regimens and a list of conditions that require antibiotic premedication appear on page 131.
   - All instrumentation, including probing and exploring, as well as mobility determination, is accomplished under antibiotic coverage.
   - Because bacteremias can occur, initial instruction and practice of biofilm-removing procedures are carried out while the patient is premedicated. Early introduction of biofilm control measures in the care plan is imperative.
   - Efficient use of appointment time and/or spacing of appointment dates will avoid unnecessary extra antibiotic coverage.
2. Systemic diseases.
   - Chronic disease will influence the content and length of appointments.
3. Physical disability.
   - Physical limitations, such as those described in Chapter 58 starting on page 885, will require adaptation of the appointment plan.
4. Other considerations.
   - An outline for maintenance appointments can be found in Chapter 47 on page 735.
   - A treatment sequence for a patient with necrotizing ulcerative gingivitis is found in Chapter 41 on page 654.

■ A suggested outline for conducting a biofilm control program using a series of lessons is found in Chapter 25 on page 367.

PRESENTING THE DENTAL HYGIENE CARE PLAN

Before treatment is begun, the care plan is discussed with the dentist and explained to the patient.

I. PRESENTING THE PLAN TO THE DENTIST

A. Purpose

■ To integrate the dental hygiene care plan into the patient's total treatment plan.
■ To provide a coordinated dental and dental hygiene statement to the patient regarding oral health needs.

B. Procedure

■ Follow sequence on the patient's written care plan.
■ Summarize demographic data.
■ Summarize major systemic and dental health assessment findings.
■ Summarize risk factors.
■ Indicate planned intervention strategies, goals, and expected outcomes.
■ Outline planned appointment sequence and services to be provided.
■ Be prepared to give detail and answer questions.

II. EXPLAINING THE PLAN TO THE PATIENT

■ A clinician with good verbal communication skills and the ability to build a trusting relationship can influence patient acceptance of treatment needs and compliance with recommendations.[1]
■ Use of an intraoral camera during presentation of the plan for care provides visual documentation of need for oral health interventions.
■ Motivational interviewing techniques, outlined in Chapter 3 on page 29, will help the dental hygienist to determine and respond to the patient's readiness to change health behaviors that increase risk for oral disease.

A. Purpose

■ To provide the patient with information needed to give informed consent for treatment.
■ To reinforce the patient's role in setting and reaching oral health goals outlined in the plan.

B. Procedure

■ Position the patient in an upright position, face to face with clinician.

■ Use terminology that is appropriate to the patient's level of understanding.
■ Educate the patient regarding systemic and dental health assessment findings and their link to oral disease.
■ Educate the patient regarding planned interventions, appointment sequence, dental hygiene services, and expected outcomes.
■ Present information using visual aids such as the patient's own radiographs, dental models, drawings or pictures, videotapes, brochures, or an intraoral camera.
■ Engage the patient in planning and setting goals.
■ Be prepared to give detail and answer questions.
■ Obtained signed informed consent.

INFORMED CONSENT

It is every patient's right to possess knowledge that will allow shared decision making with the oral care provider while treatment is being planned.

■ Informed consent is a legal concept that can exist even without a written document.
■ Informed consent can be lacking even when a document has been signed if the patient has not had the opportunity to comprehend and evaluate the risks and benefits of the suggested treatment.
■ "Expressed consent" is given either orally or in writing.
■ "Implied consent," granted by the patient's presence in the dental chair, only applies to data collection procedures, data analysis, and treatment planning.[2]

I. INFORMED CONSENT PROCEDURES

Box 24-2 provides information for obtaining informed consent.

■ The patient is informed of all treatment options available and consents to follow the recommendations in the agreed-upon care plan.
■ When potential risks, complications, or failure are associated with therapy, consent is obtained in writing prior to beginning treatment.[3]
■ Informed consent includes recommendations for referral to other healthcare providers as necessary.[3]
■ If necessary, use forms written in simpler terms, larger print, or the patient's primary language.[4]
■ Create a duplicate copy for the patient to take home.[4]

II. INFORMED REFUSAL

The patient's right to autonomy in making decisions regarding oral treatment requires that practitioners respect a patient's decision to refuse treatment.[5] Refusal of care as well as any recommended treatment options are documented in the patient's permanent record.

BOX 24-2	Informed Consent

Information to Disclose

- *Diagnosis:* description of patient's problem(s)
- *Treatment:* nature and rationale for the proposed treatment(s)
- *Alternatives:* viable alternatives to the proposed treatment(s)
- *Consequences:* risks and benefits of all proposed treatment alternatives, including physical and psychological effects, costs, and potential resulting problems
- *Prognosis:* expected outcome with treatment(s), with alternative treatment(s), and without treatment

Principles of Informing

- Assess the patient's ability to give informed consent.
- Simplify the terminology so that the patient can understand.
- Encourage the patient and family to ask questions.
- Continue to assess the patient's understanding and reeducate as often as necessary.
- Document all relevant factors and include the signed form in patient record.

BOX 24-3	Example Progress Note: Present Care Plan and Obtain Informed Consent for Dental Hygiene Care

Patient presents for discussion of formal dental hygiene care plan related to periodontal therapy and quadrant scaling and root planing. Explained all assessment findings and risk factors, discussed dental hygiene diagnosis statement, planned interventions and expected outcomes of treatment. Responded to numerous questions related to the rationale for scheduling multiple treatment appointments. Patient stated that all questions had been answered, then signed/dated the informed consent form. Next visit: begin treatment as described for appointment #1 on the care plan form.

Signed: _____, RDH Date: _____.

- Age or disability-related cognitive impairment may require consultation with a caregiver or legal guardian as well as the patient.[8]

III. ADDITIONAL CONSIDERATIONS

- Cultural differences of individual patients require special effort to obtain informed consent. Careful exploration of language skills, and potentially conflicting health beliefs and values can enhance communication.[6,7]

DOCUMENTATION

- A written dental hygiene care plan documents all information related to each component of the formal plan as described in this chapter and illustrated in **Figure 24-1**.
- An example progress note for a patient appointment to explain the dental hygiene care plan and obtain informed consent is found in **Box 24-3**.

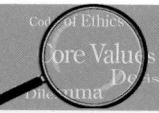 Everyday Ethics

Ellen is responsible for explaining two alternative treatment plans to Mrs. Kwan, who is new to the practice. Mrs. Kwan must decide between several extractions, which would require crown and bridge or implant replacement, and treatment of periodontally involved teeth with poor prognosis. The decision must be made today if she is to begin treatment early next week, when there are several open appointments available.

English is not Mrs. Kwan's first language, and no one in the practice speaks her language. Ellen has explained the information carefully, using pictures and patient-appropriate words, and she has gone over both treatment alternatives several times. When Ellen asks Mrs. Kwan to summarize her understanding of the care plan she just nods her head, smiles, and says, "I'll sign whatever you say."

Questions for Consideration

1. Does it appear that Mrs. Kwan understands her treatment alternatives and is informed sufficiently to give consent? What alternatives can Ellen consider so that informed consent is ensured?

2. Does Ellen have an ethical responsibility, as the knowledgeable professional, to select the choice of treatments as Mrs. Kwan requests? Why or why not?

3. In what ways does the pressure of making a timely decision reflect paternalistic treatment of Mrs. Kwan?

Factors To Teach The Patient

- Why a dental hygiene care plan is made.
- Why patient input into the final care plan is important.
- Which parts of the plan are to be carried out by the patient.
- How the roles of patient and members of the dental team are interrelated in eliminating the patient's oral problems.
- The patient's rights and responsibilities regarding informed consent.

References

1. Goldie G. Enhance verbal skills to get patients to accept what they need. *Contemp Oral Hyg* 2002 May–Jun;2:14.
2. Schoen DH, Dean M-C. *Contemporary periodontal instrumentation*. Philadelphia:WB Saunders;1996. p. 208.
3. Greenwell H. Committee on Research, Science, and Therapy. The American Academy of Periodontology. Position paper: Guidelines for periodontal therapy. *J Periodontal*. 2001 Nov;72(11):1624–8.
4. Pape T. Legal and ethical considerations of informed consent. *AORN J*. 1997 Jun;65(6):1122–7.
5. Odom JG, Bowers DF. Informed consent and refusal. In: Weinstein BD. *Dental ethics*. Philadelphia: Lea & Febiger; 1993. 65–80 pp.
6. Sprague PS, Winslow GR. Cultural expectations and dental care. *Gen Dent*. 2001 Jan;50(1)26–8.
7. Fitch P. Cultural competence and dental hygiene care delivery: integrating cultural care into the dental hygiene process of care. *J Dent Hyg*. 2004 Winter;78(1)11–21.
8. Yellowitz JA. Cognitive function, aging, and ethical decisions: recognizing change. *Dent Clin North Am*. 2005 Apr;49(2):389–410.

Implementation: Prevention

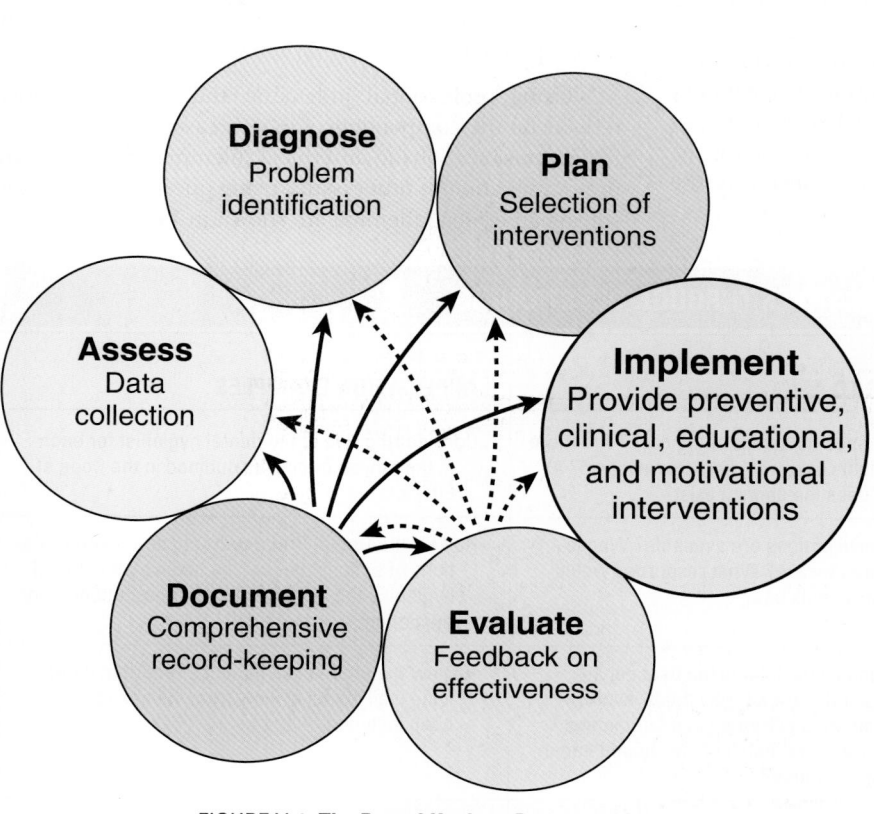

FIGURE V-1 **The Dental Hygiene Process of Care**

INTRODUCTION

Implementation of the prevention care plan is a significant component of both the dental hygiene care plan and the total treatment plan. The aim of health promotion and disease prevention is to help each patient learn to accept the responsibility for health practices and daily oral self-care regimens that prevent oral disease on a lifelong basis. The influence of oral health on total body health may be a new concept for many patients.

The focus of chapters in Section V is prevention. In the sequence of patient treatment, introduction to preventive measures occurs first, before treatment interventions are implemented.

THE DENTAL HYGIENE PROCESS OF CARE

The implementation phase of the Dental Hygiene Process of Care, illustrated in **Figure V-1**, is about providing the dental hygiene interventions identified in a patient's dental hygiene care plan. Dental hygiene interventions, selected using individualized patient assessment data, are designed to meet oral health goals that have been developed in concert with the patient. Interventions implemented by the dental hygienist are typically either educational or clinical in nature.

Patient education and counseling provide the basis for health promotion and disease prevention. The patient's commitment to self care on a daily basis before and after treatment is essential to keep the teeth and gingival tissues free from new or recurrent disease caused by the microorganisms of dental biofilm.

The dental hygienist has the responsibility to:

- Consider each patient's current oral health practices, cultural factors, physical abilities, and life circumstances when implementing the preventive care plan.
- Implement dental hygiene interventions for each patient that attain and maintain oral health and contribute to systemic health.
- Educate about oral disease and prevention modalities based on individualized patient needs.
- Identify an approach that will motivate each patient to accept and adhere to recommended preventive procedures and self-care protocols.

ETHICAL APPLICATIONS

As ethical issues and dilemmas in the dental setting become more complex, other approaches to ethical decision making can be utilized. While a situation involving patient treatment may appear to be routine in nature, the ethically competent dental hygienist can:

- Understand how the patient feels.
- View a concern from various perspectives.
- Determine who is responsible.
- Document and share clear, concise, and objective evidence.
- Communicate clearly with all parties involved in the situation.
- Act within acceptable moral standards to determine an acceptable decision.

Using professional judgment, the dental hygienist reflects on the components of moral reasoning when making a decision. Solving an ethical dilemma often leads to the examination of other issues using questions. Steps for solving an ethical dilemma are shown in **Table V-1**.

TABLE V-1	DECISION ALTERNATIVES THROUGH QUESTIONING	
ETHICAL DECISION CONCEPT	**QUESTIONS TO ASK**	**APPLICATION EXAMPLES**
Recognize Conflict	What are the specific details of the case? Are there issues of rights or moral character involved? At what level does the conflict exist?	Consider the role of the dental hygienist for each of the ethical principles outlined in the Code of Ethics.
Accumulate Possible Options	What alternative actions are available? Whose interests are at stake? What resources would other professionals use?	Review the Dental Practice Act to determine limitations of actions that can be taken by the dental hygienist, the dentist, and other practitioners for the patient.
Evaluate the Alternatives	Which decision would lead to the best consequences overall? Are all individuals involved being respected and treated in a fair manner? Which alternative(s) could be developed into a general rule to follow?	Review the entries in a patient's record to determine if all points of view from the case have been included.
Reflect on the Decision	Can the action taken be justified as the best choice? What alternative actions could be selected?	Discuss a similar situation at the next office/ staff meeting to enhance responsiveness in ethical protocols to evaluate the course of action.

CHAPTER 25

Patient Learning for Health Behavioral Change

ESTHER M. WILKINS, BS, RDH, DMD

The dental hygienist is a primary care provider of preventive services. As a specialist in oral health care, the dental hygienist is involved at all levels of prevention: primary, secondary, and tertiary.

■ Within the process of dental hygiene care, the needs of a patient are assessed from the histories and clinical findings, a dental hygiene diagnosis is made, and the care plan is outlined.

■ When planning the sequence of treatment for the patient, initiation of preventive measures precedes clinical services except in an emergency.

■ One important reason is that the patient must learn and practice procedures of daily self-care if oral health is to be attained and maintained.

■ Box 25-1 defines key terms related to health promotion and disease prevention for the individual patient.

STEPS IN A PREVENTIVE PROGRAM

Each patient needs a preventive care plan. To plan and carry out a preventive program takes a cooperative effort by the patient and members of the dental team.

| BOX 25-1 | Key Words |

Health Promotion and Disease Prevention

Behavior: manner in which an individual acts or performs.

Behavior modification: approach to correct undesirable behavior through systematic manipulation of environmental and behavioral variables; treatment procedure for certain mental and physical disorders.

Communication: verbal or nonverbal interaction or interchange; nonverbal, without spoken words, may be accomplished through pictures, gestures, facial expressions, or posture.

Compliance: extent to which a person's health behaviors coincide with dental/medical health advice; also called **adherence.**

Dental health education: the provision of oral health information to people in such a way that they can apply it in everyday living.

Dysphagia: difficulty in swallowing.

Evaluation: appraisal of changes in a patient's behavior or oral health status that have resulted from interventions by the professional healthcare personnel.

Halitophobia: imaginary halitosis; constant fear of having bad breath; sometimes related to an underlying psychiatric condition.

Health education: combination of learning opportunities planned to facilitate and reinforce voluntary behavior conducive to the health of the individual or group.

Health promotion: planned combination of educational, economic, organizational, or environmental support for actions conducive to health of individuals or groups.

Learning: acquiring knowledge or skills through study, instruction, or experience; true learning means that knowledge acquired is applied in everyday living.

  Affective domain: the domain of learning concerned with attitudes, interests, and appreciations.

  Cognitive domain: the domain of learning concerned with knowledge outcomes and intellectual abilities.

  Psychomotor domain: the domain of learning concerned with levels of motor skills.

Marketing: the task of establishing, maintaining, and enhancing patient relationships so that the goals of the patient, the group, or the community can be achieved.

Motivation: inner driving force that prompts an individual to act to satisfy a need or desire or to accomplish a particular goal.

Noncompliance: failure to carry out a prescribed healthcare plan, for example, failure to take medications as prescribed.

Organoleptic: stimulating any of the organs of sensation; susceptible to a sensory stimulus.

Preventive dental hygiene: sum total of the efforts to promote, restore, and maintain the oral health of the individual.

Putrefaction: enzymatic decomposition, especially of proteins with the production of foul-smelling compounds, such as hydrogen sulfide, ammonia, and mercaptans.

Volatile sulfur compounds (VSCs): hydrogen sulfide; methyl mercaptan; and, to a lesser extent, dimethyl sulfide and dimethyl disulfide produced by microbial metabolism and which create oral malodor.

Xerogenic: producing or causing dry mouth.

I. ASSESS THE PATIENT'S NEEDS

1. Review all information from the histories, radiographic and clinical examinations, and chartings.
2. Identify the presence and severity of infection and the risk factors for oral health.
3. Utilize indices to rate the extent of the needs and provide a baseline for continuing comparisons. For most patients, a dental biofilm score can be helpful for showing the patient the extent of the gingival problem, and a dietary record along with the charting of carious lesions help show the dental problem.
4. Does the patient show willingness and readiness to learn? How may cultural values and beliefs promote or block the patient's response and compliance?

II. PLAN FOR INTERVENTION

1. Apply information about the patient, such as educational level, occupation, socioeconomic background, cultural influences, and attitudes toward oral health and oral care.

2. Determine the current personal oral care procedures carried out by the patient and the frequency.
3. Note factors that may affect the patient's dexterity when using oral cleaning devices, such as an occupation that requires manual or digital skill.
4. Recognize the influence of age and physical and mental disabilities. Will another person (parent or other caregiver) be needed to carry out the necessary procedures?
5. Outline the procedures needed and work out goals with the patient.
6. Explain what can occur if the patient does not follow the care plan.

III. IMPLEMENTATION

1. How can the patient best be helped to be aware of personal oral health problems and to learn and practice more effective health behaviors?
2. Provide motivating demonstration and supervision for daily self-care, dental biofilm removal, self-applied fluoride, and other applicable preventive measures.

3. Introduce tobacco use cessation when indicated.
4. Show methods for self-evaluation.
5. Spread instruction over several appointments while clinical procedures are being completed. Learning takes time and reinforcement.

IV. PERFORM CLINICAL PREVENTIVE SERVICES

1. Scaling for complete calculus removal and biofilm debridement.
2. Apply caries-preventive agents: fluoride, sealants.

V. EVALUATE PROGRESSIVE CHANGES

1. Can the patient demonstrate the procedures for self-care?
2. Do the teeth and gingiva show the benefits of learning?
3. Record a dental biofilm score at each appointment and compare previous recordings with the patient.
4. At appropriate intervals, probe to note improvement in tissue quality, bleeding on probing, and probing depths.
5. Provide preventive counseling for corrective action when goals are not met.

VI. PLAN SHORT- AND LONG-TERM MAINTENANCE

1. Determine appropriate maintenance intervals.
2. Reevaluate to monitor continuance of preventive practices.
3. Provide supplemental care for the patient who does not respond to basic therapy.

PATIENT COUNSELING

- Personalized patient counseling contributes first to the knowledge, attitudes, and practices of the individual and then, through the individual, to the family and the community.
- Periodontal infections and dental caries can be prevented or controlled, and, therefore, teeth can be preserved throughout the lifetime of the individual.
- First attention is given to the intra- and extraoral examination to recognize possible pathologic areas to identify for exfoliative cytology and/or biopsy.
- For most patients, major attention is placed on prevention and control of dental caries and/or periodontal infection, with emphasis on dental biofilm control and tobacco use cessation.
- Attention needs to be paid to prevention of oral accidents such as those related to mouth protectors for contact sports, safety belts for automobiles, and children's accidents that lead to fractured anterior teeth.

- Knowledge of and belief in health facts are not enough. Benefits result only when knowledge is put into action.
- *Learning occurs when an individual changes behavior and when beneficial changes are incorporated into everyday living.*

MOTIVATION

- An individual is motivated to practice behavior that leads to achievement of goals that are valued.
- Instruction can be effective if the patient considers oral health a valuable asset.
- Stimulation of behavior, or motivation, stems from basic physiologic or social needs.
- Peer group approval and the need to conform to group standards, as well as the fear of disapproval or rejection when, for example, appearance of the teeth or odor of the breath is unacceptable, are frequently much stronger motivating factors than is a health reason, such as freedom from infection or the ability to chew food.

THE LEARNING PROCESS

I. PRINCIPLES OF LEARNING

1. Learning is more effective when an individual is physiologically and psychologically ready to learn.
2. Individual differences must be considered if effective learning is to take place.
3. Motivation is essential for learning.
4. What an individual learns in a given situation depends on what is recognized and understood.
5. Transfer of learning is facilitated by recognition of similarities and dissimilarities between past experiences and the present situation.
6. An individual learns what is actually used.
7. Learning takes place more effectively in situations from which the individual derives feelings of satisfaction.
8. Evaluation of the results of instruction is essential to determine whether learning is taking place.

II. THE LEARNING LADDER[1]

- **Figure 25-1** illustrates the six steps from learner unawareness to habit formation.
- When beginning to help a patient learn about oral health and what the individual's needs are, one must determine where the patient stands on the ladder and start from there.

  Briefly, the ladder steps are as follows:

1. Unawareness

Many patients have little concept of the new information about dental and periodontal infections and how they are prevented or controlled.

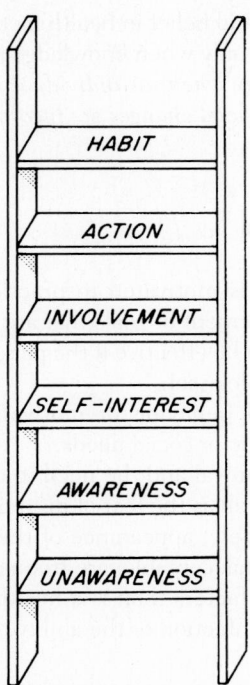

FIGURE 25-1 The Learning Ladder. Learning takes place in a series of steps from unawareness through interest and involvement to habit formation. See the text for the description of each step on the ladder. (Adapted with permission from Harris NO, Christen AG. Primary preventive dentistry. 4th ed. Norwalk (CT): Appleton & Lange; Reprinted by permission of Pearson Education, Inc., Upper Saddle River, NJ.)

2. Awareness

Patients may have a good knowledge of the scientific facts, but they do not apply the facts to personal action.

3. Self-interest

Realization of the application of facts/knowledge to the well-being of the individual is an initial motivation.

4. Involvement

With awareness and application to self, the response to action is forthcoming when attitude is influenced.

5. Action

Testing new knowledge and beginning of change in behavior may lead to an increased awareness that a real health goal is possible to attain.

6. Habit

Self-satisfaction in the comfort and value of sound teeth and healthy periodontal tissues helps to make certain practices become part of a daily routine. Ultimate motivation is finally reached.

INDIVIDUAL PATIENT PLANNING

- Instruction for most new patients will start during the assessment when they first find out there is evidence of periodontal inflammation and dental caries.
- Each patient will have individual requirements.
- Individual instruction for most new patients will start with personal biofilm removal procedures to begin the self-care lifetime program for disease control.
  - The patient is shown the oral condition, changes and benefits that can be expected are explained, and cooperation is solicited.
  - The influence of oral health on systemic general health (and vice versa, the influence of a systemic condition on oral health) is emphasized early, particularly if any of the patient's own systemic conditions are among the known risk factors with oral risk factors.
- With a clear definition of the needs of a patient, a recommended regimen or program can be outlined.
- All of the factors that apply to an individual patient are matched with the available dental biofilm control procedures. These include the selection of a toothbrush, toothbrushing method, interdental care devices and methods, dentifrice, and applied techniques for implants and fixed and removable dental prostheses.
- In this framework, the patient helps to formulate the goals that must be accomplished.

I. WHEN TO TEACH

The initial instruction is best given *first*, before any clinical treatment. Instruction provided before clinical treatment can be more effective because:

- Emphasis is placed on the importance of self-care.
- In any individual appointment, instruction time is not limited by the end of the appointment time.
- The patient's gingiva are not sensitive from instrumentation.
- Healing progresses more favorably if not immediately disturbed by practicing oral hygiene techniques.
- The patient can be more receptive to instruction at the beginning of the appointment because he/she is not tired and anxious to leave.

II. THE SETTING

A. Teaching Facility

- A specific area may be set aside and furnished for biofilm control instruction in a dental office or clinic. Such an area can be planned with mirrors for the patient to use to observe the appearance of the teeth covered with disclosing agent, and be able to see placement of the toothbrush and floss in all areas of the mouth.
- Sitting upright in the dental chair can also be used effectively. Instruments and other dental equipment can be moved away to create an atmosphere conducive to learning.

PRESENTATION, DEMONSTRATION, PRACTICE

- A suggested outline for conducting the dental biofilm control program follows. Various adaptations can be applied to tailor the plan to individual patients.
- Each of the "lessons" described in the following outline is meant to represent the opening few minutes of each appointment before instrumentation for scaling, when a quadrant with anesthesia plan is used for each appointment.
- A biofilm index or score and/or a bleeding index are made at the start. The index or score is understood by the patient, and new and review instructions are provided as indicated.

I. FIRST LESSON

A. Objective

- Orientation to dental biofilm removal.

B. Description

- Describe the formation and composition of dental biofilm, its relationship to oral disease (dental caries and periodontal infection), and specifically the relationship to the patient's present condition.
- Present an overview of the biofilm control program, what it can accomplish, and its purposes in relation to professional treatment.

C. Evaluate With the Patient

- Show the patient using mirror and probe.
- Too long a "lecture" with too many facts and details at one time may mean the patient cannot absorb any of them.
- *Patient with gingivitis:* Show and explain the formation of dental calculus and how periodontal disease can develop if gingivitis is left untreated.
- *Patient with periodontitis:* introduce pocket formation and the reasons for pocket elimination.
- *Patient whose most severe problem is dental caries:* When a food record for assessment is to be prepared, orientation to the preparation of the food diary precludes discussion of biofilm, cariogenic foods, and dental caries until the dietary record is obtained.

D. Demonstration

- While the patient observes in a mirror, a healthy area of gingiva and an inflamed area can be compared.
- Use the probe to show a gingival sulcus and/or increased pocket depth related to periodontal involvement. Bleeding on probing is an important indicator of disease and is recorded.

- Remove a sample of biofilm with a curet to demonstrate the thickness and consistency of biofilm and to use for a phase microscope demonstration when available.

E. Application of a Disclosing Agent

- *Explain its purpose:* Discoloration of biofilm shows where the masses of bacteria accumulate.
- *Examine the teeth with the patient:* Point out the stained biofilm and explain how the bacteria must be removed to control inflammation.
- *Record biofilm score or index* (in Chapter 22, page 315). Explain the score to the patient and save it to compare at future evaluations.

F. Instruction

- *Keep instruction simple:* Select a soft brush and ask the patient to remove the stained biofilm. After brushing, examine the teeth with the patient. The patient will see where accessible biofilm was removed.
- Divide instruction over several appointments.
- The use of a toothbrush is the most effective means of biofilm removal for facial and lingual surfaces. Dental floss and other interdental devices are needed for the proximal tooth surfaces.
- *Additional devices: care of fixed prostheses and implants:* Instruction for care of a new prosthesis is provided at the same appointment as its placement. Follow-up can be necessary to prevent the problem of overloaded lessons impossible for a patient to absorb. Dental implants need special attention in the same manner, with repeats during successive appointments (page 470 in Chapter 32).

G. Summary of Lesson I

- At the first lesson, a specific toothbrushing method is not necessarily presented.
- The exceptions are as follows:
  - The patient who demonstrates an acceptable brushing technique and whose mouth has been kept reasonably clean and shows no signs of detrimental brushing may only need to be shown a few special adaptations for the difficult-to-reach areas or other improvements.
  - The patient who demonstrates a brushing method that is detrimental, such as a vigorous horizontal stroke or a haphazard scrub-brush method, and whose teeth and/or gingiva show the effects of harmful brushing needs an introduction to a less destructive method.

H. Instruction at End of Appointment

- Encourage use of disclosing agent at home; provide patient with tablets or instructions for purchasing. Suggest using a tablet for biweekly biofilm checks.

- Emphasize the need for cleaning regularly for complete daily dental biofilm removal. Discuss carrying a tooth-brush and dental floss for use when not at home.
- Write down the specific name (number) of the brush for the patient to purchase for home use; advise maintaining two brushes, not replaced at the same time so they are not both old at the same time (Chapter 27, page 405).

II. SECOND LESSON

A. Objectives

- To evaluate the patient's success to date and to review and expand the knowledge content of the previous lesson.

B. Evaluation

1. Ask the patient for comments and questions.
2. *Examine the gingival tissue with the patient:* Evaluate and compare with progress notes recorded from previous examination. Changes in color, size, and bleeding on probing are noted and recorded.
3. *Apply the disclosing agent:* Evaluate the biofilm as the patient self-evaluates, using a hand mirror. Chart biofilm index or other record and compare, with the patient, with previous score or index.
4. Review brushing and flossing where disclosing agent revealed missed biofilm.

C. Review and Extension of Knowledge

1. Invite questions from patient concerning biofilm formation and gingival and periodontal infections to determine how clearly information from the previous lesson was understood and retained.
2. Always commend and compliment the patient for successes and improvements, however small.
3. Discuss dentifrice and floss recommendations.
4. Relate self-care biofilm removal to the professional treatment phase of oral care.

III. CONTINUOUS INSTRUCTION

A. Number of Lessons

- It is not possible to predict in advance the number of specific teaching sessions a patient will need to demonstrate mastery of the recommended procedures and to show by the appearance of the teeth and health of the gingiva that the practices have been carried out daily.
- When additional supervision is indicated after professional treatment has been completed, short appointments may be scheduled in conjunction with dental appointments.
- One learning experience is rarely adequate. When a patient has been able to maintain relatively clean teeth and clinically healthy gingiva and can demonstrate an acceptable toothbrushing method, a review of difficult-to-reach areas can be made and reevaluated at a follow-up appointment.

B. Relationship to Gingival Health

- When areas of gingival marginal redness and sponginess persist, tooth surfaces are checked carefully for residual calculus, and scaling and planing are completed as indicated.
- When a patient consistently fails to remove dental biofilm in certain areas, a reevaluation of the program is made. Perhaps the selected procedures are too difficult for the patient to accomplish, or perhaps supplementary measures are needed.

C. Maintenance

- After the initial instruction series, a follow-up is scheduled after a short interval for the first maintenance appointment.
- One must evaluate the patient's ability to continue adequate self-care and determine whether true learning has resulted and new habits have been adopted.
- *Learning means that a change in behavior has occurred.*
- At each maintenance appointment, a biofilm score or index is recorded, and the patient can evaluate the progress made.

IV. INSTRUCTION ADAPTABILITY

- The methods for presentation, demonstration, practice, and evaluation described in the previous pages can be adapted readily to various age levels.
- Awareness of the changing motivation and interests of the young to the elderly, and adaptations of terminology with respect for the patient's level of understanding, ease the transition from patient to patient.
- Others for whom instruction is provided are the caregivers who attend to patients who are unable to care for themselves. In Section VIII, the various chapters that pertain to patients with disabilities include suggestions for patient care.

THE PRESCHOOL CHILD

- The establishment of positive health habits and attitudes in the adult has its beginnings in childhood.
- Even before birth and during the first year after birth, the parent's education for prevention of dental caries and gingival infection begins.
- After birth, regular daily systemic fluoride in the absence of fluoridation, as well as attention to the control of cariogenic foods, can mean a great deal to the future oral health of the child.

- Oral health during the preschool years is considered in detail in Chapter 49.
- Anticipatory Guidance for parents is described in Tables 49-1 and 49-2 on pages 756 and 757.

THE TEACHING SYSTEM

- A simple, direct approach, such as has been described, with specific content and unembellished material focuses the attention of the patient on the central theme: control of oral biofilm.
- The more practical, realistic, and goal centered the components of instruction can be, the more effective the outcomes will be in terms of treatment and prevention of recurrence of infection.

I. REEVALUATION

- A teaching system is reevaluated from time to time, particularly as new research reveals new aspects of prevention and treatment.
- New devices for biofilm removal and gingival care may become available, and these are studied before recommendations to patients can be made.
- The teaching system presented in this chapter has a built-in evaluation of patient learning.
- The outcomes of learning are shown by examination and demonstration: examination for the gingival characteristics consistent with health; demonstration of disclosable biofilm, and demonstration of the patient's ability to use floss and brush for biofilm removal without harm to the oral tissues.
- The patient's own interest, enthusiasm over personal accomplishments, and pleasure over a cleaner, healthier mouth is an evaluation in itself.

II. OUTCOMES

- Because the ultimate objective of biofilm control is to prevent dental caries and periodontal infections, the oral health history of the patient over several years can be used to document a true evaluation.
- The teaching system involves development of the patient's attitudes relative to continuing professional supervision and regular appointments for examination and treatment.
- An *informed,* knowledgeable patient will have reasons for *practicing* appropriate, scientifically based, self-care measures.

EVALUATION OF TEACHING AIDS

I. GENERAL CHARACTERISTICS

Evaluation of teaching aids involves consideration of the following:

A. Simplicity

- Ease of management, readily obtainable, inexpensive or disposable if not cleaned and disinfected.
- Simplify the presentation for understanding by the patient.

B. Content

Practical, evidence-based, meaningful.

C. Cultural and Linguistic Appropriateness

- Accommodation for all patients.
- Printed materials available in various languages.

D. Level of Orientation

Appropriate for the individual patient.

E. Durability

- If reusable, the teaching aids need to maintain their cleanliness and freshness.
- Washable materials can be selected when available.

F. Cost

- Reasonable. Cost relates to their essential value in reaching goals.

G. Objectives

- Objective of a teaching aid must be clear and readily understood by the patient.
- In teaching, activities need to be reality centered, not fantasy centered. A well-intentioned visual aid may provide entertainment rather than education and have no transfer value to the behavioral pattern of the patient, in terms of the actual oral health lesson.

II. READING MATERIAL FOR THE PATIENT

A. Selection

- Effectively presented informational books and leaflets can supplement and reinforce individually presented instruction.
- Selected with a purpose, a booklet or other printed material may be presented to the patient to read while at the appointment, or it may be given for "homework."
  - The booklet's contents are reviewed with the patient; particular sections may be marked to personalize the instruction and encourage reading.
- Select educational materials written in the patient's own language; use "plain language" publications; or provide handouts with explanatory pictures.
- Indiscriminate distribution of printed materials is pointless.

B. The Teacher: The Dental Hygienist

- Obtaining copies of and reviewing newly available materials are essential parts of a dental hygienist's work, even as a teacher reviews new textbooks and materials for possible use in a classroom.
- Instruction sheets and leaflets can be custom-made with the cooperation and recommendations of the dentist. It is especially helpful to have postcare instructions and biofilm control procedures outlined so that the patient can have a reference for home use.
- Materials can be personalized by writing the patient's name on them with special procedures or reminders.

III. USE OF MODELS

A. Patient's Study Cast

- The cast can be useful to explain oral conditions or restorations, such as the need to replace missing teeth.
- With certain patients, aspects of dental biofilm control can be demonstrated, provided the patient is properly oriented to associate the cast with the teeth in the mouth.

B. Commercially Available Models

- Although plastic models (dentoforms) have been used extensively for teaching toothbrushing methods, their meaningfulness to the patient has not been demonstrated.
- When a toothbrush is available for demonstration directly in the mouth and for a patient to use to practice brushing under supervision, the need for taking the time to demonstrate on a model first may be questioned.
- When teaching is by means of the model and brush only, and particularly when the oversized model is used, the patient's learning needs careful evaluation.
- All three of the patient evaluation methods described in this chapter (gingival status after using the recommended care procedures, disclosed biofilm, and ability of patient to demonstrate an appropriate brushing method) can be utilized.
- The model and the large toothbrush do not necessarily represent a problem to the patient, and most patients can imitate the motions of the toothbrush on the model accurately when asked.
- The difficulty comes in transferring the motions to the mouth and relating such motions to the bacterial collections on the teeth. The more complex the technique, the greater the difficulty of transfer.

USE OF DISCLOSING AGENTS

- A disclosing agent is a preparation in liquid, tablet, or lozenge form that contains a dye or other coloring agent.
- In dental hygiene, a disclosing agent is used to identify dental biofilm deposits for instruction, evaluation, and

---

BOX 25-2	Key Words

Disclosing Agents

Diffusion: process of being widely spread.

Diffusibility: refers to the ability of a disclosing agent to spread readily over a tooth surface and flow into the interproximal areas.

Disclosing agent: selective dye in solution, tablet, or lozenge form used to visualize and identify dental biofilm on the surfaces of the teeth.

Eosin: rose-colored dye used for preparing histologic specimens for microscopic study; companion dye with hematoxylin for the well-known "H & E" that stains nuclei blue and the cytoplasm pink.

Erythrosin: red-colored dye used in solution or tablet form for a disclosing agent in the identification of dental biofilm on teeth.

F.D.&C. (Food Drug & Cosmetic): United States Food, Drug, and Cosmetic Act regulates the packaging, labeling, importing, and exporting of such products as disclosing agents.

Fluorescein: bright yellow fluorescing dye effective for disclosing dental biofilm on teeth; used in ophthalmology to reveal corneal lesions of the eye.

---

research. Key words related to disclosing agents are defined in **Box 25-2**.

- Dental biofilm may be nearly colorless unless stained by foods, beverages, or tobacco. After use of a disclosing agent, the soft deposits pick up and hold the color of the agent **(Figure 25-2)**.
- After staining, the deposits that can be seen distinctly provide a valuable visual aid for patient instruction. Such a procedure can demonstrate dramatically to the patient the presence of deposits and the areas that need special attention during personal oral care.

I. PURPOSES

A disclosing agent clearly demarcates soft deposits that might otherwise be invisible and therefore facilitates the following:

- Personalized patient instruction in the location of soft deposits and the techniques for removal.
- Self-assessment by the patient on a daily basis during initial instruction and periodic checks thereafter.
- Continuing evaluation of the effectiveness of the instruction for the patient will provide the following:
  - Evidence of the need for revisions of the biofilm control procedures.
  - Long-term effects over successive maintenance appointments contribute to evidence of periodontal health maintenance.

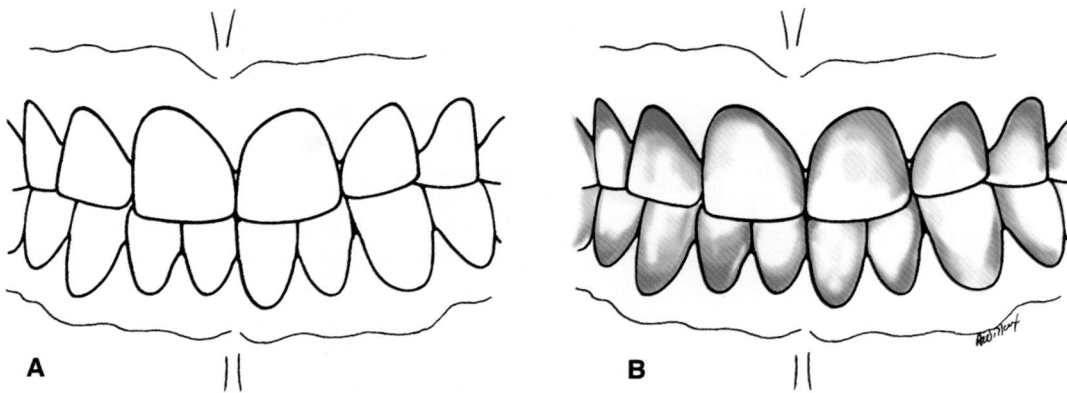

FIGURE 25-2 **Use of Disclosing Agent. (A)** Appearance of the teeth before application of a disclosing agent. Dental biofilm and pellicle are usually invisible. **(B)** After use of a disclosing agent on the same teeth as those shown in A, dental biofilm and pellicle take on the color of the dye used in the disclosing agent. As noted, soft deposits are extensive, and are especially thick on the proximal surfaces.

■ Conducting research studies to gain new information about the incidence and formation of deposits on the teeth, the effectiveness of specific devices for dental biofilm control, and antibiofilm agents and to evaluate clinical and instructional group health programs.

II. PROPERTIES OF AN ACCEPTABLE DISCLOSING AGENT

A. Intensity of Color

A distinct staining of deposits is evident. The color contrasts with normal colors of the oral cavity.

B. Duration of Intensity

The color does not rinse off immediately with ordinary rinsing methods and is not removable by the saliva for the period of time required to complete the instruction or clinical service. The color is removed from the gingival tissue and lips by the completion of the appointment, however, as the patient may have a personal reaction to color retained for a longer period of time.

C. Taste

The patient is not made uncomfortable by an unpleasant or highly flavored substance. The main reason for using the disclosant is to motivate the patient; therefore, the use of the agent needs to be pleasant and encourage cooperation.

D. Irritation to the Mucous Membrane

The patient is questioned concerning the possibility of an idiosyncrasy to an ingredient. When this information is obtained, it is entered on the patient's permanent history record. Because of the possibility of allergy, more than one type of disclosing agent can be available for use.

E. Diffusibility

A solution is thin enough so it can be applied readily to the exposed surfaces of the teeth, yet thick enough to impart an intense color to dental biofilm.

F. Astringent and Antiseptic Properties

The application of an antiseptic before scaling frequently is recommended, and if an antiseptic disclosing agent is used, one solution can serve a dual purpose.

A disclosant may inhibit the growth of microorganisms. In quantitative biofilm research studies, therefore, disclosing agents without antibacterial properties are used.

III. FORMULAE

A variety of disclosing agents has been used. Skinner's iodine solution was formerly the most classic and widely used. In general, iodine solutions are less desirable because of their unpleasant flavor.

Aniline dyes have been shown to have carcinogenic potential. Therefore, the use of basic fuchsin and beta rose (flavored basic fuchsin) has been discouraged.

The formulae of a few disclosing agents are included in this chapter. Other well-known agents are Skinner's, Buckley's, Berwick's, Talbot's iodoglycerol, Easlick's Bismarck Brown, and Metaphen solutions.

A. Mercurochrome Preparations

■ *Mercurochrome solution* (5%)
  ■ Mercurochrome 1.5 g
  ■ Water (distilled) to make 30.0 ml
■ *Flavored mercurochrome disclosing solution*
  ■ Mercurochrome 13.5 g
  ■ Water (distilled) 3.0 l

- Oil of peppermint 3 drops
- Artificial noncariogenic sweetener

B. Erythrosin

- *Concentrate for application by rinsing*
  - F.D.&C. Red No. 3 or No. 28 6.0 g
  - Water (distilled) to make 100.0 ml
- *For direct topical application*
  - Erythrosin 0.8 g
  - Water (distilled) 100.0 ml
  - Alcohol (95%) 10.0 ml
  - Oil of peppermint 2 drops
- *Tablet*[2]
  - F.D.&C. Red No. 3 15.0 mg
  - Sodium chloride 0.747%
  - Sodium sucaryl 0.747%
  - Calcium stearate 0.995%
  - Soluble saccharin 0.186%
  - White oil 0.124%
  - Flavoring 2.239%
  - Sorbitol to make a 7-grain tablet

C. Fast Green

- F.D.&C. Green No. 3.5% or 2.5%

D. Fluorescein[3]

- F.D.&C. Yellow No. 8 (used with a special ultraviolet light source to make the agent visible)

E. Two-Tone[4]

- F.D.&C. Green No. 3
- F.D.&C. Red No. 3
- Thicker (older) biofilm stains blue; thinner (newer) biofilm stains red.

IV. METHODS FOR APPLICATION

Complete the gingival tissue evaluation before application because disclosing agent masks tissue colors.

A. Solution for Direct Application (Painting)

1. Have patient rinse and swish with water to remove food particles and heavy saliva.
2. Apply water-based lubricant generously to prevent staining of the lips.
3. Dry the teeth with compressed air, retracting cheek or tongue.
4. Use swab or small cotton pellet to carry the solution to the teeth.
5. Apply solution generously to the crowns of the teeth only.

6. Direct the patient to spread the agent over all surfaces of the teeth with the tongue.
7. Examine the distribution of agent and request the patient to rinse if indicated.

B. Rinsing

1. A few drops of a concentrated preparation are placed in a paper cup and water is added for the appropriate dilution.
2. Instruct the patient to rinse and swish the solution over all tooth surfaces.

C. Tablet or Wafer

The patient chews the wafer (one half may be sufficient for some patients), swishes it around for 30 to 60 seconds, and rinses.

V. INTERPRETATION OF FINDINGS

- Clean tooth surfaces do not absorb the coloring agent; when pellicle and dental biofilm are present, they absorb the agent and are disclosed **(Figure 25-2)**.
- Pellicle stains as a thin, relatively clear covering, whereas dental biofilm appears darker, thicker, and more opaque.
- *Two-tone*
  - Red biofilm: Newly formed, thin, usually supragingival.
  - Blue biofilm: Thicker, older, more tenacious; usually is seen at and just below gingival margin, especially on proximal surfaces and where brush or floss is not easily applied; may be associated with calculus deposits.

VI. PATIENT INSTRUCTION

Because biofilm and pellicle are frequently invisible to a patient, a disclosing agent can provide a visual method for patient instruction.

A. Explain Dental Biofilm

The patient needs to be informed about the composition and effect of biofilm in the production of gingival and periodontal infections, with particular reference to the individual mouth.

B. Show Location and Distribution of Biofilm

- With a mirror, the patient can observe the teeth before and compare with the disclosed dental biofilm.
- A disposable mouth mirror is needed to show the lingual surfaces and posterior facial areas. Wash the disposable mouth mirror and give to the patient to view the teeth at home.
- Show the special areas of concern. Relate the tinted areas to the health of the gingiva.

C. Demonstrate Methods for Daily Biofilm Removal

A plan for instruction is outlined earlier in this chapter. The techniques for toothbrushing and interdental care are described in Chapters 27 and 28.

TECHNICAL HINTS FOR DISCLOSING AGENTS

1. Avoid using disclosing or antiseptic solutions on teeth that have tooth-color restorations because these materials may become stained by the coloring agents.
2. Do not apply a disclosing agent before a sealant is to be placed.
3. Purchase solutions in small quantities. Do not keep solutions containing alcohol longer than 2 or 3 months because the alcohol will evaporate and render the solution too highly concentrated.
4. Use small bottles with dropper caps for solutions. Transfer solution to a dappen dish for use. Do not contaminate the solution by dipping cotton pliers with pellet directly into the container bottle.
5. Request local druggist to stock disclosing tablets for patients to purchase. Advise patients of the stores where the agents may be purchased.

XEROSTOMIA

Saliva has many functions in the oral cavity relating to the maintenance of health of the teeth and soft tissues.

- Saliva is protective in its functions of lubrication and cleansing.
- It contains immunoglobulins, electrolytes, and other substances that aid in resistance to disease (Box 25-3).

BOX 25-3	Functions of Saliva

Lubrication of membranes, gingiva, teeth
Cleansing in self-cleansing mechanism
Tasting
Digestion: Food breakdown: chewing
           Food bolus formation
           Swallowing
Protection against diseases
   Antibacterial
   Antifungal
   Antiviral
Buffering: pH control
Remineralization
   Protection against demineralization
Speech
Carrier of antibodies, hormones, enzymes
   Provide data for diagnostic testing

- *Xerostomia* means dryness of the mouth. It is caused by absence or diminished quantity of saliva.
- Lack of saliva and the resulting dry mouth are significant contributing factors to oral discomfort and disease, particularly dental caries.
- Xerostomia is a symptom, not a disease entity.

I. CAUSES OF XEROSTOMIA

- *Radiation to head and neck for cancer therapy:* permanent damage to the salivary glands can result.
- *Surgical removal of glands:* The glands may be removed because of neoplasm.
- *Sjögren's syndrome*[5]: The syndrome is an autoimmune disorder of the salivary and lacrimal glands with symptoms of polyarthritis, enlarged parotid glands, marked xerostomia, and dryness of the eyes.
- *Pharmacologically induced xerostomia:* Many drugs that are common prescription items produce dry mouth as a side effect.[6]
- Box 25-4 shows a partial list of the classes of drugs that decrease salivary function.
- Temporary dry mouth occurs in diseases accompanied by high fever with dehydration or fluid loss; with control of certain diseases, such as diabetes or hyperthyroidism, salivary flow returns to normal.

II. EFFECTS OF XEROSTOMIA

During patient examination and history preparation, questions and clinical observations can point to the existence of dry mouth even when a patient does not complain of the symptoms.

A. Clinical Symptoms

1. Feeling of oral dryness; tongue sticks to palate.
2. Difficulty with mastication, swallowing, or speech.
3. Impaired taste.
4. Thirst, with resultant increased use of fluids; licking of lips.
5. Smarting, burning, and soreness of mucosa and tongue.

BOX 25-4	Partial List of Classes of Drugs That Decrease Salivary Function

Anticholinergics
Antihistamines
Antihypertensives
Antianxiety
Anticonvulsants
Diuretics
Narcotics
Antidepressants (tricyclic)

B. Oral Effects

1. Heavy dental biofilm, materia alba, and debris accumulation can lead to increased severity of periodontal infection and demineralization of tooth surface.
2. Predisposition to dental caries, particularly root caries.
3. Problems of denture wearing.
4. Dietary changes because of discomfort during eating; may use large quantities of liquid to soften food for swallowing.

III. MANAGEMENT OF XEROSTOMIA[7,8]

A. Pilocarpine Therapy[8,9]

- Pilocarpine acts to increase salivary output.
- Patients with Sjögren's syndrome or other causes of xerostomia can get relief.

B. Prevention of Dental Caries

- Severe, rampant dental caries related to any cause needs prompt counseling and treatment.
- One example is radiation therapy. Even before the radiation treatments are started, oral hygiene and caries prevention instruction start, and a fluoride program is initiated.

C. Personal Care Program

- Rigorous biofilm control effort by the patient for dental biofilm removal.
- Multiple fluorides may be recommended: use of dentifrice, rinse, and brush-on gel (or tray).
- Advise patient to avoid tobacco and alcohol and to use foods that are noncariogenic.

D. Environmental Factors

- Patient may need to adjust air humidification in living quarters.

E. Use of a Saliva Substitute[9]

- A saliva substitute is a preparation with physical and chemical properties similar to those of real saliva.
- The ideal substitute is able to coat the mucosa and teeth to keep them moist, reduce enamel solubility, and remineralize the surface, as well as to help prevent accumulation of dental biofilm.
- Saliva substitutes contain carboxymethylcellulose (CMC) and the minerals calcium and phosphorous, fluoride, and other ions typical of normal human saliva.
- A small amount is placed into the mouth and distributed over all surfaces with the tongue. Patients can use the preparation at will, as needed for comfort.

F. Early Recognition

- Dental hygienists are often the first to observe dry mouth (during the intraoral examination) and the first to hear the complaints of the patient of the discomforts caused.
- Early diagnosis and early treatment of Sjögren's syndrome or other causes of xerostomia can provide a major contribution to the general and oral health as well as comfort of the patient.

HALITOSIS

Halitosis, an unpleasant odor of exhaled air, is a symptom of importance in the complete consideration of health promotion and disease prevention. The sources or causes may be local or systemic. Bad breath can be a health concern.

- The effects on the individual may be to create a sensitivity leading to a social handicap that can impair general daily living and personal relationships.
- When a patient asks about the breath, the request for help must be taken seriously.
- Halitosis is also known as oral malodor, fetor ex ore, or just bad breath. It is sometimes called by names related to the cause such as "hunger breath," "menstrual breath," "tobacco breath," or "garlic breath."

I. ETIOLOGY

At least 90% of all malodor originates in the oral cavity, whereas the remaining 10% has systemic or nonoral causes.

A. Oral Causes and Contributing Factors

- *Periodontal infections:* odor from subgingival dental biofilm
- Tongue coating harbors microorganisms
- Xerostomia
- Faulty restorations retaining food and bacteria
- Unclean dentures
- Oral pathologic lesions: carcinomas
- Throat infection
- Cleft palate

B. Systemic and Non-Oral Factors[10]

- Renal or hepatic failure
- Carcinomas
- Diabetes
- Upper respiratory; nasal passages
- Cirrhosis of the liver

II. ASSESSMENT

- The normal breath of a healthy person with healthy oral tissues is nonodiferous or mildly sweet smelling. Suggestions for the assessment are included here.
- The list of predisposing and etiologic factors provide a guide to specific areas of concern.

A. Medical, Dental, and Personal History[11]

- Systemic influences: relate to list of causes.
- Medications history: side effects of dry mouth
- Tobacco use
- Diet, eating habits

B. Extraoral Examination

- *Organoleptic.* Smelling of the exhaled air is the simplest and most common method for identification.
- *Detection oral source.* When the odor is detected from the open mouth, but not from the nose when the mouth is closed, it can be assumed that the odor has an oral origin.

C. Intraoral Examination

- Tongue coating
- Evidence of mouth breathing
- Xerostomia: dry mucosa

D. Complete Periodontal Examination

- General personal care: state of oral hygiene
- Probing for attachment levels, probing depths; periodontal status
- Evidence of neglect; history of dental hygiene care

E. Measurement of Oral Malodor[12]

- *Composition*
  - The majority of malodor arises in the mouth from microbial metabolism.

- Volatile sulphur compounds (VSCs) are produced consisting of hydrogen sulfide, methyl mercaptan, and lesser amounts of dimethyl sulfide and dimethyl disulfide.
  - The VSCs are much higher in patients with periodontal diseases.[13]
- *Instrumental examination*
  - A VSC monitor has been developed especially for use in research to test the effects of mouthrinses and other products on oral malodors.
  - A portable sulfide monitor (halimeter) is available for obtaining either or both oral or nasal readings to differentiate the sources of malodor.[14]

III. INTERVENTIONS

A. Dental Hygiene Care Plan

- Objectives are based on achieving optimum gingival and periodontal health.
- Daily dental biofilm control and cleaning of all fixed and removable prostheses and implants are mandatory.
- All potential sources of biofilm retention need to be removed and carious lesions restored.

B. Plan for Instruction

- For patients who want to use a mouthrinse to help produce pleasant oral odors, advise that mouthrinses have only temporary effects on malodor.
- Rinses with alcohol, glycerin, or strong oxidizing agents that can have detrimental effects on the oral tissues when used extensively are avoided.

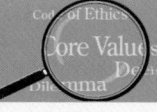 # Everyday Ethics

Jeremy, now 15 years old, has been a patient of Tressa, the dental hygienist, since he was 3 years old. Jeremy had undergone extensive restorative work as a young child because he had collided on a swing set with an older sibling, which resulted in trauma to both maxillary and mandibular incisors and permanent tooth buds. Jeremy had received a "fair plus" on his oral homecare report card at the last few visits. However, this time when Tressa went to greet him in the waiting room, Jeremy's mother asked her to "really get on him" about brushing his teeth every day.

During her oral assessment, Tressa noted extremely heavy biofilm on all teeth, generalized bleeding on probing, staining on the anterior restorations, and a distinctly unpleasant odor. "Jeremy," she lectured, "you must take better care of your teeth! Your breath smells really bad. And you are jeopardizing all of that expensive dental work your parents have paid for." Turning very red, Jeremy pulled his cap over his eyes, crossed his arms, and refused to reply. As she continued to provide patient education, Jeremy was clearly

not paying attention and Tessa became annoyed. She commented that she was going to speak to his mother about his poor attitude.

In a final attempt to turn his attention to prevention, Tressa showed Jeremy intraoral photographs she taken that morning of a patient with extreme periodontal disease. "Is that what you want to look like?" she asked.

Questions for Consideration

1. Describe how Tressa's approach to prevention violates Jeremy's rights, even though he is technically still a child and in spite of his mother's request.
2. Explain why showing Jeremy another patient's intraoral photographs violates ethical standards of dental hygiene practice.
3. What core values and ethical principles can guide Tressa as she reflects on her communication style and develops an alternative approach to prevention that is both ethical and effective?

BOX 25-5	Example Progress Note

JOE came for regular maintenance. He told about going to Dr. Rogers for the halitosis tests we had recommended. (Our office communication with Dr. Rogers is in this permanent record. He had confirmed our diagnosis of periodontal infection causes, and advised that JOE have complete "pocket treatment" with chlorhexidine rinsing.) Oral exam revealed that JOE already is doing his home care better and brushing more. Today: instruction with new brush with tongue cleaner on the back of the handle; followed by mand. right quadrant scale/debride with anesthesia. next quadrant in one week.

Signed: _____, RDH Date: _____.

Factors To Teach The Patient

- The relationship between preventive measures and clinical services.
- Why particular preventive measures were selected for the particular patient.
- Self-assessment and methods for determining health of gingiva; assessment of dental biofilm after use of a disclosing agent.
- Objectives for dental biofilm infection control.
- Treatment measures for xerostomia, such as diet, personal care, and where to obtain and how to use a saliva substitute.
- Purposes for use of disclosing agents; the appearance of stained dental biofilm and the methods of daily care necessary to keep biofilm controlled.
- For the parent, method of application of a disclosing agent to a small child's teeth to evaluate the presence of biofilm.

C. Tongue Cleaning

Brushing and cleaning of the dorsal surface of the tongue is a daily requirement. The tongue is a major source of the organisms producing VSCs.[15]

DOCUMENTATION

Routine documentation for a patient's personal oral care needs to include a minimum of the following

- All patient assessment in preparation for selection of teaching content and methods.
- Methods, procedures, patient progress, and problems are recorded following each appointment.
- Special references to salivary factors, xerostomia, halitosis, include causes and methods of detection, as well as modes of treatment and prevention with patient instruction included.
- The documented record needs review before each appointment as a guide to continuing instruction.
- A sample progress note may be reviewed in **Box 25-5**.

References

1. Christen AG, Katz CA. Understanding human motivation. In: Harris NO Christen AG. *Primary preventive dentistry.* 4th ed. Norwalk (CT): Appleton & Lange; 1995. pp. 393–6.
2. Arnim SS. Use of disclosing agents for measuring tooth cleanliness. *J Periodontol.* 1963 May;34:227.
3. Lang NP, Ostergaard E, Löe H. A fluorescent plaque disclosing agent. *J Periodont Res.* 1972 Nov;7(1):59–67.
4. Block PL, Lobene RR, Derdivanis JP. A two-tone dye test for dental plaque. *J Periodontol.* 1972 July;43(7):423–6.
5. Fox PC, Brennan M, Pillemer S, Radfar L, Yamano S, Baum BJ. Sjögren's syndrome: a model for dental care in the 21st century. *J Am Dent Assoc.* 1998 Jun;129(6):719–28.
6. Felder RS, Millar SB, Henry RH. Oral manifestations of drug therapy. *Spec Care Dent.* 1988 May–Jun;8(3):119–24.
7. Fox PC. Management of dry mouth. *Dent Clin North Am.* 1997 Oct;41(4):863–75.
8. Lockhart PB, Fox PC, Gentry AC, Acharya R, Norton J. Pilot study of controlled-release pilocarpine in normal subjects. *Oral Surg Oral Med Oral Pathol Oral Radiol Endod.* 1996 Nov;82(5):517–24.
9. Yagiela J. Agents affecting salivation. In: American Dental Association, Council on Scientific Affairs. *ADA/PDR guide to dental therapeutic.* 4th ed. Chicago: ADA and Thomson Publishing; 2006. pp. 251–62.
10. Preti G, Clark L, Cowart BJ, Feldman RS, Lowry LD, Weber E, Young IM. Non-oral etiologies of oral malodor and altered chemosensation. *J Periodontol.* 1992 Sep;63(9):790–6.
11. Bosy A. Oral malodor: philosophical and practical aspects. *J Can Dent Assoc.* 1997 Mar;63(3):196–201.
12. Rosenberg M, McCulloch CA. Measurement of oral malodor: current methods and future prospects. *J Periodontol.* 1992 Sep;63(9):776–92.
13. Yaegaki K, Sanada K. Biochemical and clinical factors influencing oral malodor in periodontal patients. *J Periodontol.* 1992 Sep;63(9):783–9.
14. Ratcliff R. Current concepts in the causes and treatment of halitosis. *J Pract Hyg.* 1997 July/Aug;6:47.
15. De Boever EH, Loesche WJ. Assessing the contribution of anaerobic microflora of the tongue to oral malodor. *J Am Dent Assoc.* 1995 Oct;126(10):1384–93.

CHAPTER 26

Protocols for Prevention and Control of Dental Caries

ESTHER M. WILKINS, BS, RDH, DMD

Chapter Outline

THE DENTAL CARIES PROCESS

Dental caries is an infectious, transmissible, communicable disease. As such, it is first, preventable, and when primary prevention has not been effective, the infection is controllable. Most patients have limited knowledge of the complex activity on the surfaces of their teeth that causes the teeth to develop cavities. Many patients take for granted the fact that they have a few cavities every year. Dental hygienists have new information from current research to impart to their patients.

- On the tooth surface, a constant process of demineralization and remineralization is going on.
- All ages are susceptible.
- Each step in the caries process has significance in the protocol for prevention and/or control that is planned with an individual patient.

- The basic caries process starts with certain acidogenic bacteria in dental biofilm acting to metabolize the fermentable carbohydrates ingested by the patient.[1]
- Acids are formed that in turn act to demineralize the enamel, cementum, and/or dentin and lead to cavity formation.
- Figure 34-4 (page 506) shows the interrelation of the caries process.
- Terminology to describe dental caries is defined in Box 26-1.

I. ACIDOGENIC BACTERIA

- Specific bacteria in the biofilm on the tooth surfaces metabolize acid from the fermentable carbohydrates ingested by the individual.
- *Mutans streptococci* are infectious organisms that colonize the teeth and help to form the dental biofilm

BOX 26-1	Key Words

Dental Caries

Acidogenic bacteria: bacteria in dental biofilm capable of metabolizing fermentable carbohydrates into acids.

Buffer: a substance that by its presence in solution is capable of neutralizing alkali or acid.

Caries risk assessment: procedure to predict future dental caries development before the clinical onset of the disease.

Cariology: science and study of dental caries.

Cavitation: process in the formation of cavities; final stage in the caries process.

Cavity: a hole; the final stage of demineralization and breakdown of tooth structure. The classification of cavities by tooth surfaces and anatomic location is defined on page 261.

Demineralization: major stage in the dental caries process in which minerals, primarily calcium and phosphorous, are removed from tooth structure by acids formed by acidogenic bacteria, primarily *Mutans streptococci* and Lactobacilli.

Dental caries: infectious disease of teeth caused by acidogenic bacteria with dissolution of enamel and dentin (coronal caries) and cementum and dentin (root caries).

Arrested caries: after remineralization, the caries process is halted; the area usually becomes discolored with a brownish tinge, darker with age and in a tobacco user.

Cavited carious lesion: advanced lesion with break through the tooth surface; contrast with **noncavitated carious lesion,** when a dull probe passed over a white demineralized area detects no roughness or breakthrough.

Rampant caries: rapidly progressive caries occurring in many teeth simultaneously; also called acute caries in contrast to chronic caries (slow developing).

Secondary caries: carious lesions at the margin of an existing restoration; also called recurrent caries.

Remineralization: healing process in which minerals are redeposited in the demineralized tooth structure; accomplished by the protective factors of the saliva and the action of fluoride to inhibit demineralization and interfere with the enzymatic requirements of bacteria.

through their ability to create a sticky environment for survival and multiplication.

■ Although there are many acid-forming bacteria present, two groups of bacteria predominate in the caries process: the *Mutans streptococci* (including both *Streptococcus mutans* and *Streptococcus sobrinus*) and the *Lactobacillus* species.

■ *Mutans streptococci* are most active during the initial stages of demineralization and cavity formation, whereas the lactobacilli are more active during the progression of the cavity.

■ Permanent colonization of a child's teeth with *Mutans streptococci* can take place soon after tooth eruption. Transmission of the acid-forming organisms is usually from close family members, particularly the mother.[2]

II. FREQUENT FERMENTABLE CARBOHYDRATES

■ Fermentable carbohydrates included are sucrose, glucose, fructose, and cooked starch.

■ Acids produced during the metabolic processes include acetic, lactic, formic, and proprionic.

■ *Frequency* of ingestion of sugary foods by the patient has a strong influence on the amount of acid produced and the extent of tooth destruction.

III. ACID PRODUCTION

■ The acid formed passes rapidly into the tiny diffusion channels between the enamel rods or into the exposed root surfaces.

■ The acid dissolves the calcium and phosphate mineral in the subsurface of the enamel or dentin structure.

■ The subsurface initial carious lesion is formed as shown in Figure 35-3 (page 521). It is observed clinically as a white area.

IV. DEMINERALIZATION

■ Demineralization is the process by which the minerals of the tooth structure are dissolved out by the organic acids produced from the fermentable carbohydrate by the acidogenic bacteria.

■ With repeated bathing of the tooth surface with the acids produced in the course of a day, the tooth demineralization can progress in time to the final stage of dental caries, the dental cavity.

■ Smooth surface caries as well as pits and fissures can result when cariogenic nutrients are available.

V. REMINERALIZATION

Remineralization can take over to halt or arrest the demineralization process. Saliva and fluoride provide protective factors in promoting remineralization. Fluoride therapy is an essential part of the protocol in dental caries control.[3]

A. Saliva

■ Protective factors of the saliva can balance or reverse the destruction of the tooth structure.

■ Saliva has many properties and functions, particularly to buffer the acids and to supply minerals to replace those calcium and phosphate ions dissolved from the tooth during demineralization.

■ Saliva is a continuing source for fluoride transport to the tooth surfaces. Saliva derives fluoride from all of its contacts, including fluoride from fluoridated water, fluoride products used by the patient (dentifrice, mouthrinse) and fluoride products for professional application (varnish, topical fluorides).

B. Fluoride Mechanisms of Action[3]

- *Inhibits demineralization:* When fluoride is present in the fluid of the biofilm around the enamel crystals (or dentin of the root), it will pass through the diffusion channels with the acid and increase the fluoride of the subsurface lesion to prevent the continued dissolution of the minerals.
- *Enhances remineralization:* As the saliva flows over the biofilm, its buffering properties neutralize the acid produced by the bacteria. The pH rises toward neutral and prevents further dissolution of the minerals. Minerals in the saliva can go back into the tooth for remineralization.
- *Inhibits bacteria in the biofilm:* Fluoride can change to HF (hydrogen fluoride) when it is contacted by the acid produced by the bacteria from the carbohydrates in the patient's diet. In the HF form, it can then diffuse over the cell membrane of the acidogenic bacteria. Inside it dissociates again and the fluoride ions interfere with essential enzyme activity within the bacterial cell.

DENTAL CARIES DIAGNOSIS AND DETECTION[4]

- Formerly the term "dental caries" referred only to the destructive lesion of the tooth structure that made a break in the tooth surface and created a cavity.
- Dental caries made its way through enamel and into dentin (coronal caries Figure 17-7, page 262) or through the cementum and into the dentin (root caries).
- Diagnosis meant detection of decay with loss of tooth substance.
- When unrestored, dental caries continued into the pulp, created a toothache, and required a root canal treatment or extraction. Patients went for their dental hygiene "recall" regularly to find out where their new cavities were.
- Now that dental caries is treated as an infection, the *end-stage* of the infection is the hole or cavity that requires therapy for restoration.
- The diagnosis of dental caries as an infection has transformed what formerly was detection of *cavities-to-be-filled* to identification of each stage of the disease.
- The earliest stages of dental caries are usually eligible for remineralization of the natural tooth structure.

I. PREREQUISITES FOR CARIES DETECTION[5]

- Adequate lighting.
- Sharp eyes.

- Blunt probes: no sharp explorers used: Remineralizing surfaces must not be scratched or altered in any way.
- Tri-syringe for viewing teeth wet and dry.
- Reproducible bitewing radiographs for showing coronal caries; *vertical bitewings* for root caries detection.

II. THE STAGES OF DENTAL CARIES

A. Initial Infection: Invisible Lesion

Mutans streptococci and other acid-forming bacteria infect the tooth by the following:

- Clinging to the smooth tooth surface.
- Creating a biofilm.
- Producing acid from available fermentable carbohydrate.
- The acid produced diffuses through the microchannels between the enamel rods, dissolves the tooth minerals, and creates the subsurface lesion (Figure 35-3, page 521).

B. Early Subsurface Infection

- Generally invisible

C. White Area Lesion

- Examination with air under bright light can show the white area of subsurface demineralization.
- Surface smooth, with blunt probe run lightly over the surface.
- Careful examination: Surface must not be broken or scratched.
- Picking or scratching a mineralizing surface can prevent further mineralization.[6,7]
- Remineralization process starts with saliva action and increased fluoride.

D. White Area: Later Stage

- Examination: Run blunt probe gently over the surface with no pressure.
- When there is slight surface roughness, beginning breakdown: Do not scratch the surface.
- Remineralization may still be effective and allowed to continue.

E. Cavitation

- *Visual examination*
  - Observation: open cavity can be observed directly.
  - Open cavity with no intact tooth structure over the surface may be seen without exploration.
  - Gentle air blast may be sufficient to clear loose biofilm and debris for direct vision.
- *Instrumental*
  - Avoid picking or scratching a surface undergoing remineralization.

- Probe or explorer not needed if visual examination of the occlusal, facial, palatal, or lingual identifies a cavity.
- Small proximal caries at the contact area needs radiograph for confirmation of depth.
- *Radiographic examination*
  - Bitewing views: for cavities on proximal surfaces primarily; vertical bitewings for root caries detection.
  - Early caries not extending into dentin: radiograph cannot reveal true depth because of tooth density.
  - Large cavities do not need radiographic examination for detection, only for extension to pulpal involvement.
  - Treatment plan for definite cavitation: appoint with a dentist for restoration.

III. PREVIOUS MANAGEMENT OF DENTAL CARIES

- In the early half of the past century, the history of dental caries management shows many restorations placed, but also many diseased teeth removed and prosthetic replacements provided.
- Reductions in caries of 40 to 60% since 1945 in the United States were observed for those fortunate enough to live in the communities with fluoridation of the water supply.
- Recent history has shown reductions in dental caries prevalence generally related to the widespread home use of fluoride dentifrices and mouthrinses as well as professional topical applications of solutions, gels, and varnishes.
- Although the decline of dental caries in the general population has tapered off in more recent years, dental caries is still a major problem in the health and welfare of adults as well as children.

SELECTIVE CARE PLANNING

- The dental hygienist is challenged to select a management strategy for the individual patient to cover all needs.
- The care plan will need to provide for treatment of existing nonreversible carious lesions but also will open up a changed pattern of personal care previously unrealized by the patient so that new lesions can be prevented.
- A variety of patients present for dental hygiene care. On the one side will be the patient with no current new dental caries, but a few simple questions may reveal that here is a patient with irregular habits of diet and personal oral care that could lead to serious problems later.
- At the opposite extreme is the need for as early recognition as possible of the lesions that have gone out of control and present as definite cavities in need of dental restorative care.

I. OBJECTIVES FOR CARIES MANAGEMENT

A. Determine Restorative Treatment Needs

- Chart existing restorations and sealants.
- Chart cavitated dental carious lesions (final stage of caries process in need of restoration).
- Chart secondary (recurrent) lesions.
- Chart sealants in need of repair.
- Chart demineralized areas for future observation.

B. Determine Areas That Require Remineralization

- Chart white areas and white cervical lines.
- Outline appropriate strategies for the patient.

C. Define Steps for Remineralization Program

- Explain needs and corrective methods for patient understanding.
- Prepare and explain risk assessment for the individual.
- Select and demonstrate procedures that must be followed.
- Plan for evaluation and reevaluation at continuing maintenance appointments.

II. RISK FACTORS

- Risk factors are habits, behaviors, lifestyles, or conditions that, when present, increase the probability of a disease occurring.
- The risk factors in **Table 26-1** apply primarily to adult patients (including teenage). Table 49-1 (page 756) and Table 49-2 (page 757) list risk factors selected especially for the oral health of early childhood.
- Caries management begins with risk factor assessment so that specific needs of the individual patient can be identified.

III. RISK ASSESSMENT

A. Purposes and Uses of Individual Patient Risk Assessment

- The use of a patient's own list of risk factors can be a significant educational experience for the patient.
- Enlighten the patient of the existing individual oral problems.
- Provide factual information about the development and transmissibility of caries.
- Relate the patient's cavitated carious lesions to behavioral and lifestyle habits that will need to change to arrest demineralization and initiate remineralization.
- Encourage the patient to apply caries preventive methods to family and other closely related individuals.
- Be a guide for the management of a caries preventive plan for reversing demineralizing lesions.

TABLE 26-1	CARIES MANAGEMENT BY RISK ASSESSMENT (CAMBRA)

RISK FACTORS AND MANAGEMENT GUIDELINES FOR PATIENTS AGE 6 AND OLDER

	CAMBRA RISK LEVEL			
	LOW RISK	**MODERATE RISK**	**HIGH RISK**[*]	**EXTREME RISK**[†]
Risk Factors	The number and extent or severity of risk factors are taken into consideration to determine an individual caries risk level for each patient.			
Social History	Dentally aware. Regularly scheduled dental visits. Low caries rate in family members.	Low knowledge of dental disease. Irregular or nonexistent dental visits. Family history of caries and generally poor oral health. Personal history of recreational drug use.		
Medical History	No serious medical problems. No or few medications. Normal salivary flow. No physical problems or handicaps.	Medically compromised. Disabled/handicapped. Xerostomia (side effect of medications or systemic disease). Radiation therapy.		
Use of Fluoride	Drinks fluoridated water. Lived in a fluoridated community as a child. Uses fluoride dentifrice and/or fluoride mouthrinse regularly.	Does not drink fluoridated water. Did not live in a fluoridated community as a child. Irregular or nonexistent use of fluoridated dentifrice or fluoride rinses. Irregular personal oral care habits.		
Dietary Habits	Infrequent sugar intake. Rarely snacks between meals. Uses xylitol gum when chews gum.	Frequent sugar intake. Snacks frequently. Not familiar with Food Guide Pyramid. Uses chewing tobacco frequently.		
Clinical/Oral	Regular brushing at least 2 times daily. Daily interdental cleansing. No prostheses, orthodontics, or other special care requirement. Good hand dexterity; no handicap. Low biofilm scores.	History of previous caries experience. Current cavitated lesions. Noncavitated (white) lesions. Multiple restorations. Unsealed deep pits and fissures. Exposed root surfaces; previously restored root surfaces.		
MANAGEMENT GUIDELINES	**LOW RISK**	**MODERATE RISK**	**HIGH RISK**	**EXTREME RISK**
Bitewing Radiographs Vertical Bitewings for Root Caries	Every 24–36 mo	Every 18–4 mo	Every 6–18 mo	Every 6 months until no cavitated lesions are observed.
Frequency of Caries Recall Exam	Every 6 mo	Every 4–6 mo	Every 3–4 mo	Every 3 mo
Chemotherapeutic Management	OTC fluoride dentifrice Optional NaF varnish if root exposure or sensitivity	OTC fluoride toothpaste 0.05% NaF rinse daily Initial 1–2 application of NaF varnish, plus application at 4–6 mo recall Xylitol gum or candy 4× daily Optional: calcium phosphate topical paste if excessive root exposure	Fluoride varnish every 3–4 mo 1.1% NaF toothpaste used 2× daily 0.05% NaF rinse 2× daily Initial 1–3 application of NaF varnish, plus application at 3–4 mo recall Chlorhexidine rinse one minute daily for 1 wk each month Xylitol gum or candy 4× daily Optional: calcium phosphate topical paste	Fluoride varnish every 3 mo 1.1% NaF toothpaste used 2× daily 0.05% NaF rinse 2× daily Initial 1–3 application of NaF varnish, plus application at 3 mo recall Chlorhexidine rinse one minute daily for 1 wk each month Xylitol gum or candy 4× daily Acid-neutralizing rinses as needed if mouth feels dry Required: calcium phosphate topical paste 2× daily
Sealants	Optional	Recommended	Recommended	Recommended

[*]Patients with one or more cavitated lesions are assigned a *high* risk level
[†]When xerostomia, is present in addition to cavitated lesions, the *extreme* risk level is assigned.
Adapted with permission from Jenson L, Budnez AW, Featherstone JD, Ramos-Gomez FJ, Spolsky VW, Young DA. Clinical protocols for caries management by risk assessment. *J Calif Dent Assoc.* 2007 Oct;35(10):714–23.

B. Sources and Selection of Risk Factors

■ *From the patient's medical, dental, and social histories*[8]
1. The regular history form can show answers to questions pertinent to a caries control program.
2. The patient's *perception of needs* is guided by past dental experiences, family, and cultural influences.
3. Immediate considerations of a patient that could show personal *value placed on oral health* often emphasize appearance, cost implications, and personal time involved.
4. *Past dental experience* as shown by primary prevention, including sealants, secondary prevention by restorations, and tertiary prevention by extraction and replacement of teeth.
5. *Fluoride history* showing residences and availability of community water supply fluoridation throughout life and currently. Other exposures to fluoride, including home dentifrice used over the years, and professional applications.

6. *Success in changing habits,* such as the person who was a tobacco user but was able to cease use completely can be very indicative of the patient's ability to turn around caries-producing habits.

■ *Questioning the patient directly*
1. Brief introductory checklist to show current daily care and fluoride.
2. Example: **Box 26-2** may introduce conversation and stimulate interest to encourage the patient to look at current habits as causes of oral problems.

■ *Food diary*
1. For analysis of sugar exposures Figure 34-7 (page 511).
2. Food diary form is described in Chapter 34 on page 508.

IV. APPLICATION

■ The preparation and procedure for introducing a protocol for caries prevention or control with emphasis on

---

BOX 26-2	Patient's Checklist

ORAL HEALTH CHECK SHEET

Name: _____

PLEASE CHECK "YES" OR "NO" OR FILL IN OTHER

	Yes	No	Other (please write)
1. Fluoride in your drinking water as a small child?			
2. Fluoride in your drinking water where you live now?			
3. Use toothpaste with fluoride in it now? Favorite kind? _____			
4. Brush at least twice each day?			
5. Use dental floss every day?			
6. Wear orthodontic appliances?			
7. Use sugar-free chewing gum when you chew gum?			
8. Have dry mouth most of the time?			
9. Sip on beverages other than water throughout the day? Mostly what?_____			
10. Snack frequently? Mostly what?_____			
Date: _____			

- remineralization of early, noncavitated lesions can lay the groundwork for a successful program.
- Most patients will learn very little about the seriousness of their problem if handed a checklist of things to be done every day.
- Participation in the process of selection can inform the patient (and parents) of the needs and ways of coping with change.
- Using the list in **Box 26-2**, help patients check off the topics that apply to their personal lifestyle and oral health habits.
- Beside each risk factor, the patients can identify possible changes to make to prevent future cavities.

V. THE PATIENT WITH NO DENTAL CARIES

- Primary prevention remains a top priority.
- The objective is to provide the patient with positive care and education so that dental health will be maintained indefinitely.
- A review is made with the patient of all the factors that classify the patient as "low risk." Such an understanding by the patient can encourage ideal personal daily biofilm removal.
- Supervision at routine maintenance appointments: necessary to prevent introduction of habit changes that can lead to caries infection.

A PROTOCOL FOR REMINERALIZATION[9,10]

- A first approach to treating dental caries as an infectious disease is to eliminate as many of the causative factors as possible.
- That applies primarily to removal daily of the acid-forming bacteria and the fermentable carbohydrates that allow the harmful bacteria to survive and multiply.
- At the same time that the infectious agents are being reduced in numbers, consideration for the contagious aspect of the microorganisms is needed.
- When possible, close personal contacts with the patient and caregivers can be checked, advised relative to the potential communicability, have their own teeth checked, and cavitated carious lesions restored.

I. REMOVE THE NIDUS OF INFECTION

A. Restoration of All Real Cavities

- Dental carious lesions contain large numbers of acidogenic bacteria, especially *Mutans streptococci* and lactobacilli.
- Well-placed restorations with marginal seal will help lower the bacterial counts in the oral cavity.
- Use of restorative materials containing fluoride is recommended wherever possible.

B. Placement of Sealants

- Closing off the pits and fissures where microorganisms can live, multiply, and contribute to carious lesions.
- Live microorganisms cannot survive when sealed into a pit or fissure.

C. Family Members

- Encourage family members and other close contacts to have necessary restorative dentistry completed and to adopt measures for personal dental care that ensure optimum oral health.

II. SYSTEMIC DISEASE FACTORS

- Identify diseases and medications with a side effect of dry mouth.
- Selected medically or nutritionally compromised patients may be at risk for dental caries and need additional preventive measures to be recommended.

III. INITIATE DAILY PREVENTIVE MEASURES

A. Personal Fluoride Use

- Use fluoridated water; fill personal drinking bottles from faucets giving fluoridated water.
- Fluoride-containing dentifrice 2–3 times per day with brushing at least 3 minutes.
- Non–alcohol-containing fluoride mouthrinse daily; may recommend daily gel tray.
- Fluoride 1.1% dentifrice before bed with no further eating or drinking.

B. Dietary Modifications

- Fermentable carbohydrate exposures eliminated between meals and at the ends of meals.
- Select snacks from noncarbohydrate foods; avoid sweetened beverages.

C. Chew Sugar-Free Gum at Ends of Meals

- Use sugar-free chewing gum, with xylitol.[11]
- Xylitol reduces levels of *Streptococcus mutans* and promotes remineralization.

IV. PROFESSIONAL APPLICATIONS

- After brushing before retiring, use prescription chlorhexidine rinse: one 16-ounce bottle (0.12%); 2 to 3 minute rinse with swish between teeth; no eating after. just before going to bed; concentration remains high all night due to its substantivity.[12]
- Chlorhexidine is highly effective against *Mutans streptococcus* infections.
- Fluoride 1.1% dentifrice brush-on to start when the chlorhexidine short-term rinse is completed in approximately 10 days.

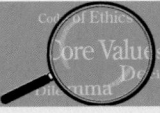

Everyday Ethics

Sophie and Helen were two sisters who had been Dr. Newbury's patients for the past 30 years. Now in their 70s, they were experiencing new concerns with restorations and crowns that showed signs of occlusal wear and recurrent caries. Many margins of amalgam restorations had catches with the explorer upon examination.

Ken, the dental hygienist, continued to stress the importance of more frequent maintenance visits, but Sophie curtly reminded him that she "has been coming to the dentist since before he was born!" Ken suspected they did not want to hear about crowns that should be replaced or make decisions about the restorations that needed replacement.

A progress note in Helen's chart read, "the patient was not open to new homecare education techniques or interested in a proposed treatment plan to replace amalgam restorations in teeth 15, 18, 19, 30, and 31."

Questions for Consideration

1. What ethical principles and dental hygiene Core Values are involved as Ken thinks about how to help these patients understand the need for treatment that they have stated they do not want?
2. Does the entry in the patient's chart provide sufficient information to document informed refusal? Why or why not? Explain your rationale using legal and ethical concepts in Table IV-1 in Section IV Introduction, page 339.
3. Consult the Decision Alternatives Through Questioning steps in Table V-1 in Section V Introduction on page 362 to determine at least two alternative approaches Ken might pursue in order to deliver a professional standard of care for these patients without compromising their rights.

■ Fluoride varnish applications at frequent dental hygiene appointments.[13]

MAINTENANCE CARE PLANNING

Planning for maintenance is to monitor all of the special procedures for dental caries control. Frequent contact with the patient through telephone and e-mail messages during the first month can help to show the concern of the dental hygienist for the patient and the oral health problems.

■ Biofilm control check: Use disclosing agent and record the biofilm score.
■ Clinical detection for demineralization areas, need for sealants, margins of restorations.
■ Radiographs are never routine; only use when specifically indicated by findings.

Patient came for broken restoration in #14 just to see if it would be all right to wait; asked could the dental hygienist smooth the sharp edge. She had been told on telephone that the dentist was not in that day.
On exam, found large part of a distobuccal amalgam restoration cracked off.

Polished off rough margin and patient tried it with her tongue and was pleased. Appointment made for the dentist but will call if an earlier date opens up.

Signed: _____, RDH Date: _____.

■ Discuss details of the continuation of the remineralization program.
■ Patient compliance with fluoride details and all personal oral care.
■ Need for repeat short-term chlorhexidine rinse schedule determined by other positive or negative results of the protocol thus far.
■ Fluoride varnish application repeat.

DOCUMENTATION

Documentation for the patient with a caries risk management program such as the CAMBRA requires detailed records checking the risk factors and all progress being made.

■ Initial planning: Record all instruction and survey report from the analysis of risk factors.
■ Specific oral care and dietary changes recommended and follow-up successes noted.
■ Patient comments on the individual efforts: likes and dislikes; what can continue.
■ Evaluation of teeth and periodontal tissues with probing and visual examinations.
■ A sample progress note may be found in **Box 26-3**.

Factors To Teach The Patient

■ What causes cavities and how they develop.
■ Early dental caries is not a cavity: what demineralization means.
■ How remineralization can be helped by using fluoride toothpaste and drinking fluoridated water daily.
■ Using fluorides is necessary throughout life.

References

1. Featherstone JD. The science and practice of caries prevention. *J Am Dent Assoc.* 2000 Jul;131(7):887–99.
2. Caufield PW, Cutter GR, Dasanayake AP. Initial acquisition of *Mutans streptococci* by infants: evidence for a discrete window of infectivity. *J Dent Res.* 1993 Jan;72(1):37–45.
3. Featherstone JD. Prevention and reversal of dental caries: role of low-level fluoride. *Community Dent Oral Epidemiol.* 1999 Feb; 27(1):31–40.
4. Pitts NB. Clinical diagnosis of dental caries: a European perspective. *J Dent Educ.* 2001 Oct;65(10):972–8.
5. Kidd EA. Caries management. *Dent Clin North Am.* 1999 Oct; 43(4):743–64.
6. Van Dorp CS, Exterkate RA, Cate JM. The effect of dental probing on subsequent enamel demineralization. *ASDC J Dent Child.* 1988 Sep-Oct;55(5):343–7.
7. Warren JJ, Levy SM, Wefel JS. Explorer probing of root caries lesions: an in vitro study. *Spec Care Dentist.* 2003;23(1):18–21.
8. Brown JP. Indicators for caries management from the patient history. *J Dent Educ.* 1997 Nov;61(11):855–60.
9. American Dental Association, Council on Access, Prevention and Interprofessional Relations. Caries diagnosis and risk assessment. *J Am Dent Assoc.* 1995 Jun;126 Suppl:1S–24S.
10. Hildebrandt GH. Caries risk assessment and prevention for adults. *J Dent Educ.* 1995 Oct;59(10):972–9.
11. Hayes C. The effect of non-cariogenic sweeteners on the prevention of dental caries: a review of the evidence. *J Dent Educ.* 2001 Oct;65(10):1106–9.
12. Anderson MH, Bales DJ, Omnell KA. Modern management of dental caries: the cutting edge is not the dental bur. *J Am Dent Assoc.* 1993 Jun;124(6):36–44.
13. Anusavice KJ. Chlorhexidine, fluoride varnish, and xylitol chewing gum: underutilized preventive therapies? *Gen Dent.* 1998 Jan–Feb;46(1):34–8, 40.

Oral Infection Control: Toothbrushes and Toothbrushing

KAREN A. RAPOSA, RDH, MBA

Chapter Outline

The personal oral health care plan for prevention interventions is determined from each patient's oral health needs, dental caries risk factors, periodontal infection risk factors, and the patient's ability to perform self-care procedures. The dental hygienist has a professional ethical obligation to review current research and select appropriate methods and oral care devices that each patient or the responsible parent or caretaker is capable of learning.

An objective for the dental hygienist is to teach and motivate each patient and the responsible caregiver to maintain the oral cavity in a clean healthy state. Personal daily care requires the following sequence of procedures at least two times each day:

- Use dental floss first to remove biofilm from proximal surfaces and debris that may have collected in the interproximal embrasures.
- Flossing before brushing allows access of the proximal tooth surfaces and interdental gingiva to fluoride and other agents in the toothpaste for dental caries prevention and gingival health.
- Toothbrushing follows flossing to remove the adhering biofilm from tooth surfaces and to apply the preventive agents to the gingival tissues and teeth.
- A final step in oral cleanliness and health is to clean the tongue.

The toothbrush is the principal instrument in general use for removal of dental biofilm and is a necessary part of oral disease control. Many different designs of both manual and power toothbrushes and supplementary devices have been manufactured and promoted. Uses of the toothbrush are as follows:

- Biofilm removal
- Application of treatment or preventive agents
- Contribute to halitosis control
- Sanitation of oral cavity

Patients who have not previously received professional advice concerning the best brush for their particular oral conditions probably have used brushes selected on the basis of cost, availability, advertising claims, family tradition, or habit. Because of the variety of brushes currently available, and the constant development of new brushes, dental professionals need to maintain a high level of knowledge on these products to advise patients appropriately.

Key words relating to toothbrushes are listed in **Box 27-1** with their definitions.

DEVELOPMENT OF TOOTHBRUSHES

Crudely contrived toothpicks, presumably used for relief from food impaction, are believed to be the earliest implements devised for the care of the teeth. Excavations in Mesopotamia uncovered elaborate gold toothpicks used by the Sumerians about 3000 B.C.

BOX 27-1	Key Words

Toothbrushes

Abrasion (gingiva): lesion of the gingiva that results from mechanical removal of the surface epithelium.

Abrasion (tooth): loss of tooth structure produced by a mechanical cause (such as a hard-bristled toothbrush used with excessive pressure and an abrasive dentifrice); abrasion contrasts with erosion, which involves a chemical process.

Angled: a nylon filament that is placed in the brush head at an angle.

Bristle: individual short, stiff, natural hair of an animal; historically, toothbrush bristles were taken from a hog or wild boar, but current toothbrush bristles are made of nylon and are called filaments.

End-rounded: characteristic shape of each toothbrush filament; a special manufacturing process removes all sharp edges and provides smooth, rounded ends to prevent injury to gingiva or tooth structure during use.

Filament: individual synthetic fiber; a single element of a tuft fixed into a toothbrush head.

Mechanical biofilm control: oral hygiene methods for removal of dental biofilm from tooth surfaces using a toothbrush and selected devices for interdental cleaning; contrasts with chemotherapeutic biofilm control in which an antimicrobial agent is used.

Power toothbrush: a brush driven by electricity or battery; also called power-assisted, automatic, electric, or mechanical (in contrast with manual).

Sonic: a term used to describe a power toothbrush that operates in the audible range of human hearing.

Stiffness: the reaction force exerted per unit area of the brush during deflection; the term stiffness is used interchangeably with firmness of toothbrush bristles or filaments; the stiffness depends primarily on the length and diameter of the filaments.

Sulcular brushing: a method in which the end-round filament tips are directed into the gingival sulcus at approximately 45° for the purpose of loosening and removing dental biofilm from both the gingival sulcus and the tooth surface just below the gingival margin.

Toothbrush head: the part of the toothbrush composed of the tufts and the stock (extension of the handle where the tufts are attached).

Tuft: a cluster of bristles or filaments secured together in one hole in the head of a toothbrush.

The earliest record of the "chewstick," which has been considered the primitive toothbrush, dates back in the Chinese literature to about 1600 B.C. The care of the mouth was associated with religious training and ritual: the Buddhists had a "toothstick," and the Mohammedans used the "miswak" or "siwak." Chewsticks, made from various types of tasty woods by crushing an end and spreading the fibers in a brushlike manner, are still used in several regions of the world.[1]

The *Ebers Papyrus*, compiled about 1500 B.C. and dating probably to about 4000 B.C., contained reference to conditions similar to periodontal diseases and to preparations used as mouthwashes and dentifrices. The writings of Hippocrates (about 300 B.C.) include descriptions of diseased gums related to calculus and of complex preparations for the treatment of unhealthy mouths.[1-4]

I. EARLY TOOTHBRUSHES

It is believed that the first brush made of hog's bristles was mentioned in the early Chinese literature. Pierre Fauchard in 1728 in *Le Chirurgien Dentiste* described many aspects of oral health. He condemned the toothbrush made of horse's hair because it was rough and destructive to the teeth and advised the use of sponges or herb roots. Fauchard recommended scaling of teeth and developed instruments and splints for loose teeth, as well as dentifrices and mouthwashes.

One of the earlier toothbrushes made in England was produced by William Addis about 1780. By the early 19th century, craftsmen in various European countries constructed handles of gold, ivory, or ebony in which replaceable brush heads could be fitted. The first patent for a toothbrush in the United States was issued to H. N. Wadsworth in the middle of the 19th century.

Many new varieties of toothbrushes were developed around 1900, when celluloid was available for the manufacture of toothbrush handles. In 1919, the American Academy of Periodontology defined specifications for toothbrush design and brushing methods in an attempt to standardize professional recommendations.[5]

Nylon came into use in toothbrush construction in 1938. World War II complications prevented Chinese export of wild boar bristles, and synthetic materials were substituted for natural bristles. Since then, synthetic materials have been improved and manufacturers' specifications standardized. Most toothbrushes are made exclusively of synthetic materials. Power toothbrushes, although developed earlier, were not actively promoted until the 1960s.

II. EARLY BRUSHING METHODS

Historically, the purpose of brushing was to provide *massage* to increase the resistance of the gingival tissue. Massage or friction from a hard-bristled brush was believed to *increase keratinization*, which, in turn, resulted in the resistance to bacterial invasion.[5]

BOX 27-2	Historical Perspective on Proper Toothbrushing Instruction

Koecker, in 1842,[6] wrote that after the dentist has scaled off the tartar, the patient will clean the teeth every morning and after every meal with a hard brush and an astringent powder. For the inner surfaces, he recommended a conical-shaped brush of fine hog's bristles. For the outer surfaces, he believed in an oblong brush made of the "best white horse-hair." He instructed the patient to press hard against the gums so the bristles go between the teeth and "between the edges of the gums and the roots of the teeth. The pressure of the brush is to be applied in the direction from the crowns of the teeth towards the roots, so that the mucus, which adheres to the roots under the edges of the gums, may be completely detached, and after that, removed by the friction in a direction towards the grinding surfaces."

As quoted in **Box 27-2**, Koecker described, in 1842, a "new" method for daily care of teeth.[6] This early work proved to be the forerunner of contemporary oral care.

MANUAL TOOTHBRUSHES

I. CHARACTERISTICS OF AN EFFECTIVE TOOTHBRUSH[7]

A. Conforms to individual patient requirements in size, shape, and texture.

B. Is easily and efficiently manipulated.

C. Is readily cleaned and aerated; impervious to moisture.

D. Is durable and inexpensive.

E. Has prime functional properties of flexibility, softness, and diameter of the bristles or filaments, and of strength, rigidity, and lightness of the handle.

F. Has end-rounded filaments.

G. Is designed for utility, efficiency, and cleanliness.

II. GENERAL DESCRIPTION

A. Parts (Figure 27-1)

■ *Handle*: the part grasped in the hand during toothbrushing.

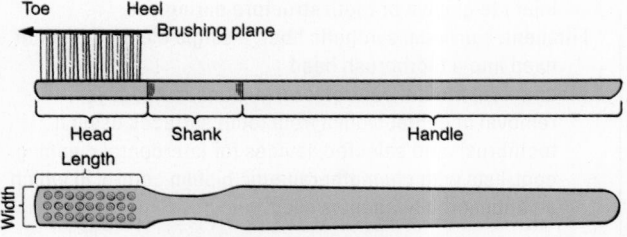

FIGURE 27-1 **Parts of a Toothbrush.**

- *Head*: the working end; consists of tufts of bristles or filaments and the stock where the tufts are secured.
- *Shank*: the section that connects the head and the handle.

B. Dimensions

- *Total Brush Length*: about 15–19 cm (6–7.5 inches); junior and child sizes may be shorter.
- *Head*: large enough to accommodate the tufts.
  - Length of brushing plane, 25.4–31.8 mm (1–1 1/4 inches); width, 7.9–9.5 mm (5/16–3/8 inch).
  - Bristle or filament height, 11 mm (7/16 inch).

III. HANDLE

A. Composition

- *Manufacturing specifications*. Most often a single type of plastic, or a combination of polymers.
- *Properties*. Combines durability, imperviousness to moisture, pleasing appearance, low cost, and sufficient maneuverability.

B. Shape

1. Preferred characteristics
   - Easy to grasp.
   - Does not slip or rotate during use.
   - No sharp corners or projections.
   - Light weight, consistent with strength.
2. Variations
   - A twist, curve, offset, or angle in the shank with or without thumb rests may assist the patient in the adaptation of the brush to difficult-to-reach areas.
   - A handle of larger diameter may be useful for patients with limited dexterity, such as children, aging patients, and those of any age with a disability.

IV. BRUSH HEAD

A. Design

- *Length*. May be 5–12 tufts long and 3–4 rows wide.
- *Spacing*. Tufts that are widely spaced allow for easy cleaning. Those closely spaced allow the filaments to support each other.
- *Arrangement*. Tufts may be of a consistent shape on the brush head or varied as shown in **Figure 27-2**.

B. Brushing Plane (Profile)

- *Trim*. Variously shaped filament profiles.
- *Length*. Range from filaments of equal lengths (flat planes) to those with variable lengths, such as rippled, tapered, bilevel, multilevel, and angled **(Figure 27-2)**.
- *Properties*. Soft and end-rounded for safety to oral soft tissues and tooth structure.

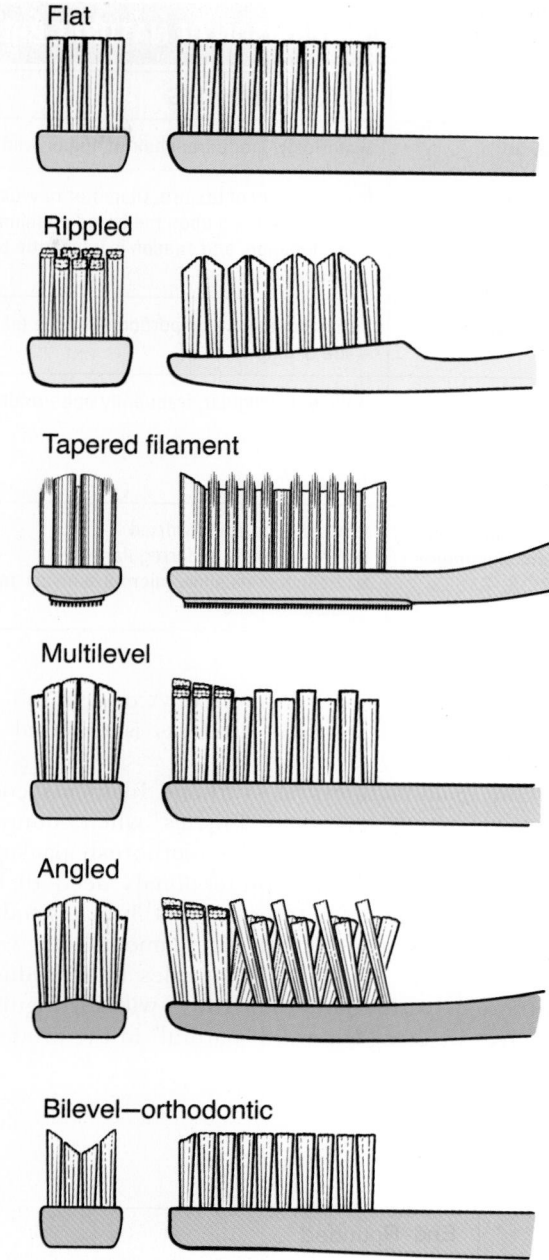

FIGURE 27-2 **Manual Brush Trim Profiles.** A variety of filament profiles are available. In addition to the classic flat planed brush, other trims include the rippled, tapered filaments, bilevel, multilevel, and angled. Brushes for use over orthodontic appliances are made with various bilevel shapes.

- *Efficiency in biofilm removal*. Efficiency for cleaning the hard-to-reach areas, such as extension onto proximal surfaces, malpositioned teeth, or exposed root surfaces, depends on individual patient abilities and understanding.

V. BRISTLES AND FILAMENTS

Most current toothbrushes have nylon filaments. Natural bristles are relatively unsanitary, and their physical

TABLE 27-1	COMPARISON OF NATURAL BRISTLES AND SYNTHETIC FILAMENTS	
	NATURAL BRISTLES	**FILAMENTS**
Source	Historically made from hair of hog or wild boar	Synthetic, plastic materials, primarily nylon
Uniformity	No uniformity of texture. Diameter or wearing properties depending upon the breed of animal, geographical location, and season in which the bristles were gathered	Uniformity controlled during manufacturing
Diameter	Varies depending on portion of bristle taken, age, and life of animal	Range from extra soft at 0.075 mm (0.003 inch) to hard at 0.3 mm (0.012 inch)
End shape	Deficient, irregular, frequently open-ended	End-rounded to ensure fewer traumas. There is a direct relation between gingival damage and the absence of end-rounding[8,9]; **Figure 27-3** shows examples of nonrounded and end-rounded filaments[10]
Advantages and disadvantages	■ Cannot be standardized ■ Wear rapidly and irregularly ■ Hollow ends allow microorganisms and debris to collect inside	■ Rinse clean, dry rapidly ■ Durable and maintain longer ■ End-rounded and closed, repel debris and water ■ More resistant to accumulation of microorganisms

qualifications cannot be standardized. A comparison of natural bristles and synthetic filaments is reviewed in **Table 27-1**.

Many manufacturers of synthetic filaments continue to refer to filaments as "bristles" when communicating with consumers on the toothbrush package and in advertising. Dental professionals need to be aware that most manufacturers of toothbrushes today produce brushes using "synthetic filaments" but will refer to these as "bristles." Companies that produce a toothbrush with "natural bristles" will distinguish themselves by using the word "natural" in the product description.

A. Factors Influencing Stiffness

The stiffness depends on the diameter and length of the filament. Brushes designated as soft, medium, or hard are not comparatively consistent between manufacturers.

- *Diameter.* Thinner filaments are softer and more resilient.
- *Length.* Shorter filaments are stiffer and have less flexibility.
- *Number of filaments in a tuft.* Increased density of filaments and tufts give added support to adjacent filaments, thus increasing the feel of stiffness.
- *Angle of filaments.* Angled filaments may be more flexible and less stiff than straight filaments of equal length and diameter; there is no straight end-line force applied as with the straight filament.

B. End-Rounding

- *Process of end-rounding.* Each nylon filament is sealed and rounded by heat treatment. The quality of end-rounding varies depending on manufacturers.[8] Natural bristles cannot be end-rounded.
- *Effect.* A direct relation exists between gingival damage and the absence of end-rounding.[9,10]
- *Examples.* **Figure 27-3** shows examples of nonrounded and end-rounded filaments.

TOOTHBRUSH SELECTION FOR THE PATIENT

I. INFLUENCING FACTORS

Factors that influence the selection of the proper manual or power toothbrush for an individual patient include the following:

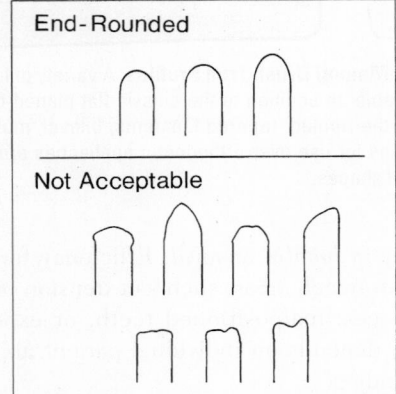

FIGURE 27-3 End-Rounded Filaments. Examples of the shape of acceptable end-rounding and of those that are not acceptable are shown. (Reprinted with permission from Silverstone LM, Featherstone MJ. A scanning electron microscope study of the end rounding of bristles in eight toothbrush types. Quintessence Int. 1988 Feb;19(2):87–107).

A. Patient

- Ability of the patient to use the brush and remove dental biofilm from all tooth surfaces without damage to the soft tissue or tooth structure.
- Manual dexterity of the patient.
- The age of the patient and the differences in the dentition and dexterity as related to age.

B. Gingiva

- Status of gingival or periodontal health
- Anatomic configurations of the gingiva

C. Position of Teeth

Displaced teeth require variations in brush placement.

- Crowded teeth
- Open contacts

D. Compliance

- Patient preference may dictate which method and which brush is recommended.
- Patient may have preferences and may resist change.
- Patient may lack motivation, ability, or willingness to follow the prescribed procedure.

E. Method Selected

Professional personnel may prefer to instruct patients in certain methods and with certain brushes.

II. TOOTHBRUSH SIZE AND SHAPE

- Brush head selection is dependent on the patient's ability to maneuver and adapt the brush correctly to all facial, lingual, palatal, and occlusal surfaces for dental biofilm removal.
- Multilevel brush heads have been shown to be beneficial and were developed on the basis of their ability to improve cleaning performance and to reach critical sites easier. (i.e., interproximal and at the gingival margin)[11]

III. SOFT NYLON BRUSH

The following are suggested as advantages for the use of a soft end-rounded brush that is applied appropriately.

- More effective in cleaning the cervical areas, both proximal and marginal.
- Less traumatic to the gingival tissue; therefore, patients can brush at the cervical areas without fear of discomfort or soft tissue laceration.
- Can be directed into the sulcus for sulcular brushing and into interproximal areas for cleaning the proximal surfaces.

- Applicable around fixed orthodontic appliances or fixation appliances used to treat a fractured jaw.
- Tooth abrasion and/or gingival recession can be prevented or may be less severe in an overvigorous brusher.
- More effective use for sensitive gingiva in such conditions as necrotizing ulcerative gingivitis or severe gingivitis, or during healing stages following scaling and debridement or periodontal surgery.
- Small size is ideal for a young child as a first brush on primary teeth.

GUIDELINES FOR MANUAL TOOTHBRUSHING

Complete toothbrushing instruction for a patient involves teaching what, when, where, and how. In addition to descriptions of specific toothbrushing methods, the succeeding sections consider the grasp of the brush, the sequence and amount of brushing, the areas of limited access, and supplementary brushing for the occlusal surfaces and the tongue. The possible detrimental effects from improper toothbrushing and variations for special conditions are described. The care of toothbrushes is outlined.

I. GRASP OF BRUSH

A. Objectives

- Grasp and manipulate the brush for successful removal of dental biofilm.
- Provide patients with specific instruction in how to hold and place the brush.
- Remove dental biofilm that has been colored with a disclosing agent to show the tenaciousness of the biofilm and the need for controlled pressure.
- Using a light, comfortable grasp, the following can be expected:
  - Control of the brush during all movements.
  - Effective positioning at the beginning of each brushing stroke, follow-through during the complete stroke, and repositioning for the next stroke.
  - Sensitivity to the amount of pressure applied.

B. Procedure

1. Grasp toothbrush handle in the palm of the hand with thumb against the shank.
   - Near enough to the head of the brush so that it can be controlled effectively.
   - Not so close to the head of the brush that manipulation of the brush is hindered or that fingers can touch the anterior teeth when reaching the brush head to molar regions.
2. Position filaments in the proper direction for placement on the teeth; direction depends on the brushing method to be used.

- Adapt grasp for the various positions of the brush head on the teeth throughout the procedure; adjust to permit unrestricted movement of the wrist and arm.
- Apply appropriate pressure for removal of the dental biofilm. Too much pressure, however, bends the filaments and curves them away from the area where brushing is needed.

II. SEQUENCE

- The procedure in brushing, for any method used, needs to ensure complete coverage for each tooth surface.
- Start brushing from a molar region of one arch around to the opposite side, then back around the lingual or facial. Repeat in the opposing arch.
- Each brush placement will overlap the previous one for thorough coverage **(Figure 27-4)**.
- Encourage the patient to begin by brushing one of the areas of greatest individual need as shown by disclosing agent.
  - Areas most frequently missed.
  - Areas most difficult for brush placement and/or manipulation, such as the right side for the right-handed brusher or the left side for the left-handed brusher.
- Suggest that the sequence be varied at least once each day so that the same areas are not always brushed last when time may be limited and biofilm removal may be less complete.

III. AMOUNT OF BRUSHING

The main consideration is the removal of the dental biofilm. For infection control, dental biofilm needs to be removed from all surfaces of all teeth as completely as possible. The number of strokes and length of time spent depend on the patient's ability and efficiency in accomplishing the task.

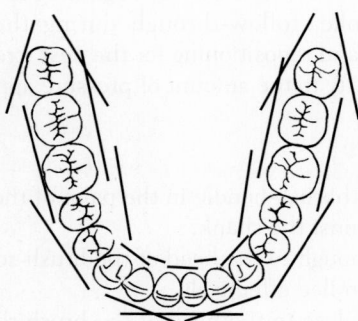

FIGURE 27-4 **Brushing Positions.** Each brush position, as represented by a black line, will overlap the previous position. Note placement at canines, where the distal aspect of the canine is brushed with the premolars and the mesial aspect is brushed with the incisors. Short lines on the lingual anterior aspect indicate brush placed vertically. The maxillary teeth require a similar number of brushing positions.

A. The Count System

To ensure thorough coverage with an even distribution of amount of brushing and to help the patient concentrate on the performance, a system of counting can be useful.

- Count 6 strokes in each area (or 5 or 10, whichever is most appropriate for the particular patient) for modified Stillman or other method in which a stroke is used.
- Count slowly to 10 for each brush position while brush is vibrated and filament ends are held in position for the Bass, Charters, or other vibratory method.

B. The Clock System

Some patients brush thoroughly while watching a clock or an egg timer for 3 or 4 minutes. Timed procedures cannot guarantee thorough coverage, because single areas that are most accessible may get more brushing time.

C. Combination

For many patients, use of the "count" system in combination with the "clock" system produces the most complete removal of dental biofilm.

D. Built-in Timers

- Many power toothbrushes have built-in timers that signal lapsed time.
- Signals may be set for 30 seconds, 1 or 2 minutes.
- Timers can motivate patients to increase the total time spent brushing.

IV. FREQUENCY OF BRUSHING

- Because of individual variations, one set rule for frequency cannot be applied. The emphasis in patient education is placed on complete biofilm removal daily rather than on the number of brushings.
- For the control of dental biofilm, and for oral sanitation and halitosis control, at least two brushings, accompanied by appropriate interdental care, are recommended as a minimum for each day.
- The longer the bacteria remain undisturbed, the greater the pathogenic potential of the biofilm bacteria.
- A clean mouth before going to sleep is encouraged. Bacteria thrive in the dark, warm, moist climate of the oral environment.
- Patients who use a chewable fluoride tablet, mouthrinse, or gel application before going to bed need to complete their biofilm removal before fluoride application.

METHODS FOR MANUAL TOOTHBRUSHING

Most toothbrushing methods can be classified based on the position and motion of the brush. Noted beside certain categories that follow are names of methods that utilize the designated motion as part or all of their particular procedure. Some of these methods are recorded for descriptive, comparative, or historic purposes only and are not currently recommended. A few may have been shown to be detrimental.

- Sulcular: Bass
- Roll: Rolling stroke, modified Stillman
- Vibratory: Stillman, Charters, Bass
- Circular: Fones
- Vertical: Leonard
- Horizontal
- Physiologic: Smith
- Scrub-brush

 THE BASS METHOD: SULCULAR BRUSHING

The Bass method is widely accepted as an effective method for dental biofilm removal adjacent to and directly beneath the gingival margin. The areas at the gingival margin and in the col are the most significant in the control of gingival and periodontal infections.

I. PURPOSES AND INDICATIONS

- For all patients for dental biofilm removal adjacent to and directly beneath the gingival margin.
- For open embrasures, cervical areas beneath the height of contour of the enamel, and exposed root surfaces.
- For the patient who has had periodontal surgery.
- For adaptation to abutment teeth, under the gingival border of a fixed partial denture, and orthodontic appliances (Figure 30-4, page 440).

II. PROCEDURE

A. Position the Brush

- Direct the filaments apically (up for maxillary, down for mandibular teeth).
- First position the sides of the filaments parallel with the long axis of the tooth (**Figure 27-6A**).
- From that position, turn the brush head toward the gingival margin to make approximately a 45° angle to the long axis of the tooth (**Figure 27-6B**).
- Direct the filament tips into the gingival sulcus (**Figure 27-5A,B**).

B. Strokes

- Press lightly so the filament tips enter the gingival sulci and embrasures and cover the gingival margin. Do not bend the filaments with excess pressure.
- Vibrate the brush back and forth with very short strokes without disengaging the tips of the filaments from the sulci.
- Count at least 10 vibrations.

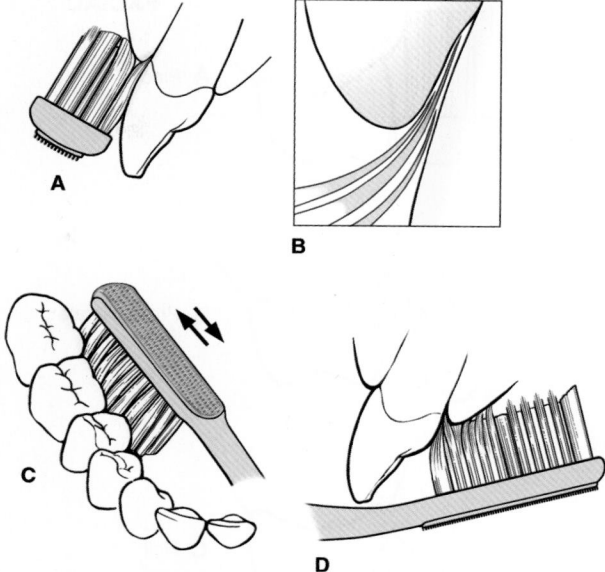

FIGURE 27-5 Sulcular Brushing. (A) Filament tips are directed into the gingival sulcus at approximately 45° to the long axis of the tooth. **(B)** Brushes designed with tapered filaments reach below the gingival margin with ease. **(C)** Brush in position for lingual surfaces of mandibular posterior teeth. **(D)** Position for palatal surface of maxillary anterior teeth.

C. Reposition the Brush

Apply the brush to the next group of two or three teeth. Take care to overlap placement, as shown in **Figure 27-4**.

D. Repeat Stroke

The entire stroke (steps A through C) is repeated at each position around the maxillary and mandibular arches, both facially and lingually.

E. Position Brush for Lingual and Palatal Anterior Surfaces (Figure 27-5D)

Hold the brush the long narrow way for the anterior components. The filaments are kept straight and directed into the sulci.[12]

III. LIMITATIONS

- An overeager brusher may convert the previously mentioned "very short strokes" into a vigorous scrub that can cause injury to the gingival margin.
- Dexterity requirement may be too high for certain patients. Because a 45° angle can be difficult to visualize, emphasis is on placing the tips of the filaments into the sulcus.
- Rolling stroke procedure may precede the sulcular brushing when a patient believes it helps to clean the teeth. The two methods are performed separately rather than trying to combine them in what has been referred to as a "modified Bass."

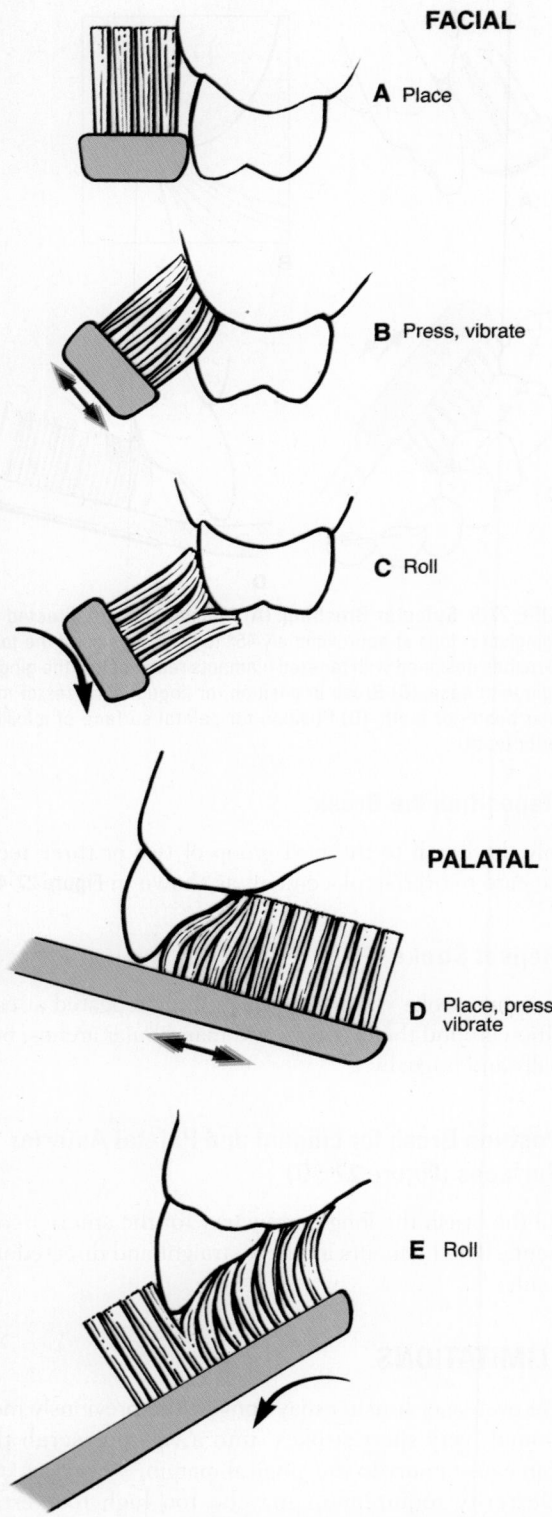

FACIAL

A Place

B Press, vibrate

C Roll

PALATAL

D Place, press vibrate

E Roll

FIGURE 27-6 **Modified Stillman Method of Brushing. (A)** Initial brush placement with sides of bristles or filaments against the attached gingiva. **(B)** The brush is pressed and angled, then vibrated. **(C)** Vibrating is continued as the brush is rolled slowly over the crown. **(D)** Maxillary anterior lingual placement with the brush applied the long way. **(E)** Vibrating continues as the brush is rolled over the crown and interdental areas. Placement is similar for the lingual surfaces of the mandibular anterior teeth. The roll or rolling stroke brushing method has the same brush positions.

■ The procedure of rolling the brush down over the crown after the vibratory part of the sulcular brush stroke has several disadvantages:
   A. Too often the brush is hastily and carelessly replaced into the sulcus position, or the opposite is true, and considerable time is consumed in the attempt to replace the brush carefully.
   B. Gingival margin injury by the constant replacement of the brush can result.
   C. The patient may tend to roll the brush down over the crown prematurely, thereby accomplishing very little sulcular brushing.

 THE ROLL OR ROLLING STROKE METHOD

I. PURPOSES AND INDICATIONS

■ Cleaning gingiva and removing biofilm, materia alba, and food debris from the teeth without emphasis on gingival sulcus.
   A. Meant for children with relatively healthy gingiva and normal tissue contour, when a sulcular technique may seem difficult for the patient of any age to master.
   B. Meant for general cleaning in conjunction with the use of a vibratory technique (Bass, Charters, Stillman).
■ Useful for preparatory instruction (first lesson) for modified Stillman method because the initial brush placement is the same. This can be particularly helpful when there is a question as to how complicated a technique the patient can master and practice.

II. PROCEDURE[4,13]

A. Position the Brush

■ *Filaments.* Direct filaments apically (up for maxillary, down for mandibular teeth).
■ *Place side of brush on the attached gingiva.* The filaments are directed apically. When the plastic portion of the brush head is level with the occlusal or incisal plane, generally the brush is at the proper height, as shown in **Figure 27-6A**.

B. Strokes

■ *Press to flex the filaments.* The sides of the filaments are pressed lightly against the gingiva. The gingiva will blanch.
■ *Roll the brush slowly over the teeth.* As the brush is rolled, the wrist is turned slightly. The filaments remain flexed and follow the contours of the teeth, thereby permitting cleaning of the cervical areas. Some filaments may reach interdentally.

C. Replace and Repeat Five Times or More

■ *Repeat the entire stroke.* The entire stroke (steps A and B) is repeated at least five times for each tooth or group of teeth.

- *Rotate the wrist.* When the brush is removed and repositioned, the wrist is rotated.
- *Stretch the cheek.* The brush is moved away from the teeth, and the cheek is stretched facially with the back of the brush head. Care is taken not to drag the filament tips over the gingival margin when the brush is returned to the initial position **(Figure 27-6A)**.

D. Overlap Strokes

When moving the brush to an adjacent position, overlap the brush position, as shown in **Figure 27-4**.

E. Position Brush for Anterior Lingual or Palatal Surfaces

- Use the brush the long, narrow way.
- Hook the heel of the brush on the incisal edge **(Figure 27-6D)**.
- Press (down for maxillary, up for mandibular) until the filaments lie flat against the teeth and gingiva.
- Press and roll (curve up for mandibular, down for maxillary teeth).
- Replace and repeat five times for each brush width.

III. LIMITATIONS

- Brushing too high during initial placement can lacerate the alveolar mucosa.
- Tendency to use quick, sweeping strokes results in no brushing for the cervical third of the tooth because the brush tips pass over rather than into the area; likewise for the interproximal areas.
- Replacing brush with filament tips directed into the gingiva can produce punctate lesions.

 # THE STILLMAN METHOD

- *Purpose.* As originally described by Stillman,[14] the method was designed for massage and stimulation, as well as for cleaning the cervical areas.
- *Brush position.* The brush ends were placed partly on the gingiva and partly on the cervical areas of the tooth and were directed slightly apically.
- *Pressure.* As the tips were pressed lightly, blanching of the tissue occurred.
- *Movement.* The handle was given a slight rotary motion, and the brush ends were maintained in position on the tooth surface.
- *Repeated.* After several applications, the brush was moved to the adjacent tooth.

THE MODIFIED STILLMAN METHOD

A modified Stillman, which incorporates a rolling stroke after the vibratory (rotary) phase, frequently is used. The

modifications minimize the possibility of gingival trauma and increase the biofilm removal effects.[15]

I. PURPOSES AND INDICATIONS

- Dental biofilm removal from cervical areas below the height of contour of the crown and from exposed proximal surfaces.
- General application for cleaning tooth surfaces and massage of the gingiva.

II. PROCEDURE (FIGURE 27-6)

A. Position the Brush

- *Filaments.* Direct filaments apically (up for maxillary, down for mandibular teeth).
- *Place side of brush on the attached gingiva.* The filaments are directed apically. When the plastic portion of the brush head is level with the occlusal or incisal plane, generally the brush is at the proper height, as shown in **Figure 27-6A**.

B. Strokes

- *Press to flex the filaments.* The sides of the filaments are pressed lightly against the gingiva. The gingiva will blanch.
- *Angle the filaments.* Turn the handle by rotating the wrist so that the filaments are directed at an angle of approximately 45° with the long axis of the tooth.
- *Activate the brush.* Use a slight rotary motion. Maintain light pressure on the filaments, and keep the tips of the filaments in position with constant contact. Count to 10 slowly as the brush is vibrated by a rotary motion of the handle.
- *Roll and vibrate the brush.* Turn the wrist and work the vibrating brush slowly down over the gingiva and tooth. Make some of the filaments reach interdentally.

C. Replace Brush for Repeat Stroke

Reposition the brush by rotating the wrist. Avoid dragging the filaments back over the free gingival margin by holding the brush out, slightly away from the tooth.

D. Repeat Stroke Five Times or More

The entire stroke (steps A through C) is repeated at least five times for each tooth or group of teeth. When moving the brush to an adjacent position, overlap the brush position, as shown in **Figure 27-4**.

E. Position Brush for Anterior Lingual and Palatal Surfaces

- Position the brush the long, narrow way for the anterior components, as described for the rolling stroke technique and shown in **Figure 27-6D** and **E**.
- Press and vibrate, roll, and repeat.

III. LIMITATIONS

A. Careful placement of a brush with end-rounded filaments can prevent tissue laceration. Light pressure is needed.

B. Patient may try to move the brush into the rolling stroke too quickly, and the vibratory aspect may be ineffective for biofilm removal at the gingival margin.

 THE CHARTERS METHOD

- *History.* During his long productive dental career, Dr. W. J. Charters emphasized the importance of prevention.

- *Purpose.* The interproximal toothbrushing method that he taught had as its objectives cleanliness through removal of the "film and mucin" from the proximal surfaces and gingival massage through mechanical stimulation.

- *Brush position.* Among his many published papers, Charters described two brush positions, one at a right angle to the long axis of the tooth[16] and another at a 45° angle with the tips of the bristles toward the occlusal plane. The right-angle position might have been intended primarily for patients with interdental periodontal tissue loss, where access permitted the bristles to enter the embrasure.

- *Method.* For either brush position, the instructions were to force the tips into the interproximal area.

- *Pressure.* "With the bristles between the teeth, as much pressure as possible is exerted, giving the brush several slight rotary or vibratory movements. This causes the sides of the bristles to come in contact with the gum margin, producing an ideal massage."[17]

- *Bristle position.* The classic periodontal textbooks[18] have described the Charters method with the bristles directed toward the occlusal plane at a 45° angle with the long axis.

I. PURPOSES AND INDICATIONS

- Loosen debris and dental biofilm.
- Massage and stimulate marginal and interdental gingiva.
- Aid in biofilm removal from proximal tooth surfaces when interproximal tissue is missing, for example, following periodontal surgery.
- Adapt to cervical areas below the height of contour of the crown and to exposed root surfaces.
- Remove dental biofilm from abutment teeth and under the gingival border of a fixed partial denture (bridge) or from the undersurface of a sanitary bridge.
- Cleansing orthodontic appliances (Figures 30-3 and 30-4, page 440).

II. PROCEDURE[16]

A. Apply Rolling Stroke Procedure

Instruct in a basic rolling stroke for general cleaning to be accomplished first.

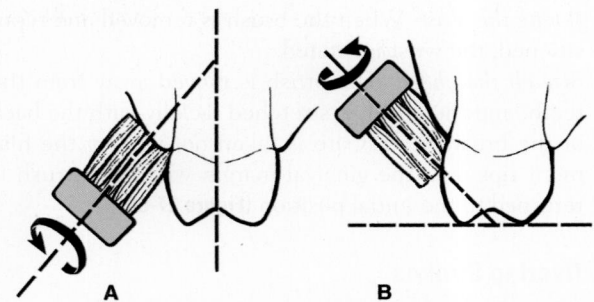

FIGURE 27-7 **Stillman and Charters Methods Compared.** **(A)** Stillman. The brush is angled at approximately 45° to the long axis of the tooth. **(B)** Charters. The brush is angled at approximately 45° to the occlusal plane, with brush tips directed toward the occlusal or incisal surfaces.

B. Position the Brush

- Hold brush (outside the oral cavity) with filaments directed toward the occlusal or incisal plane of the teeth that will be brushed.
- Point tips down for application to the maxillary and up for application to the mandibular arch.
- Insert the brush held in the direction it will be used.
- Place the sides of the filaments against the enamel with the brush tips toward the occlusal or incisal plane.
- Angle the filaments at approximately 45° to the occlusal or incisal plane.
- Slide the brush to a position at the junction of the free gingival margin and the tooth surface **(Figure 27-7B)**.
- Note contrast with position for the Stillman method **(Figure 27-7A)**.

C. Strokes

- Press lightly to flex the filaments and force the tips between the teeth.
- Press the sides of the filaments against the gingival margin.
- Vibrate the brush gently but firmly, keeping the tips of the filaments in contact with the tooth surface.
- Count to 10 slowly as the brush is vibrated with a rotary motion of the handle.

D. Reposition the Brush and Repeat

Repeat steps B and C, as described, several times in each position around the dental arches.

E. Overlap Strokes

When moving the brush to an adjacent position, overlap the brush position, as shown in **Figure 27-4**.

F. Position Brush for Anterior Lingual and Palatal Surfaces

Because the Charters brush position is difficult to accomplish on the lingual surfaces, a modified Stillman technique is frequently advised. When the Charters method is preferred, the positions are as follows:

- *Posterior*
  A. With brush tips pointed toward the occlusal surfaces, extend the brush handle across the incisal edge of the canine of the opposing side to be brushed.
  B. Place the sides of the toe-end filaments against the distal surface of the most posterior tooth and subsequently at each embrasure.
  C. Press and vibrate.
- *Anterior*
  A. With brush handle parallel with the long axis of the tooth, place the sides of the toe-end filaments over the interproximal embrasure.
  B. Press and vibrate.

G. Application of Brush for Fixed Partial Denture

When placing the brush, check that the filament tips are directed under the gingival border of the pontic.

III. LIMITATIONS

- Brush ends do not engage the gingival sulcus to remove subgingival bacterial accumulations.
- In some areas, the correct brush placement is limited or impossible; therefore, modifications become necessary, consequently adding to the complexity of the procedure.
- Requirements in digital dexterity are high.

OTHER TOOTHBRUSHING METHODS

The rolling stroke, modified Stillman, and Bass are the methods used most often for patient instruction either directly or as guidelines with variations. Other methods that have been used are included here. The technique and intent of some of the methods overlap. Assessment before special instruction may reveal that a mixture of techniques may be in use by a patient. The following other toothbrushing methods are described in this section.

I. HISTORICAL METHODS

- Circular: Fones method (**Table 27-2** and **Figure 27-8**)
- Vertical: Leonard method **(Table 27-2)**
- Physiologic: Smith's method **(Table 27-2)**

II. METHODS CONSIDERED DETRIMENTAL

A. Horizontal

- An unlimited sweep with a horizontal scrubbing motion bears pressure on teeth that are most facially inclined or prominent.
- With the use of an abrasive dentifrice, such brushing may produce tooth abrasion.

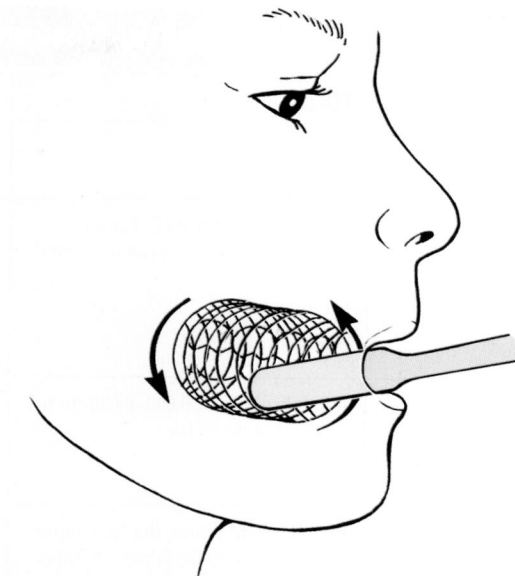

FIGURE 27-8 **Fones Method of Brushing.** With the teeth closed, a circular motion extends from the maxillary gingiva to the mandibular gingiva using a light pressure.

- Because the interdental areas are not touched by this method, dental biofilm can remain undisturbed on proximal surfaces.

B. Scrub-Brush

- A scrub-brush procedure consists of vigorously combined horizontal, vertical, and circular strokes, with some vibratory motions for certain areas.
- Without caution, vigorous scrubbing can encourage gingival recession and, with a dentifrice of sufficient abrasiveness, can create areas of tooth abrasion.

 POWER TOOTHBRUSHES

Power brushes are also known as power-assisted, automatic, mechanical, or electric brushes. The American Dental Association Council on Scientific Affairs evaluates power brushes for the reduction of dental biofilm and gingivitis (Figure 29-1, page 433).[24]

I. EFFECTIVENESS

A. Evolution

- Power toothbrushes have evolved through time due to improved designs and features.
- Power toothbrushes of the 1960–1980 era mimicked the motions of manual brushing.

B. Power Versus Manual

- Research showed equivalence for power and manual brushes in biofilm removal and reduction of gingivitis.[25,26]

TABLE 27-2	HISTORICAL TOOTHBRUSHING METHODS		
METHOD	**FONES**	**LEONARD**	**SMITH**
Alternate Description	Circular	Vertical	Physiologic
History	Advocated by Alfred C. Fones, founder of first course for dental hygienists	As described by Hirschfeld,[20] the up-and-down stroke was employed when teeth were cleaned with a primitive crude twig toothbrush.	Described by Smith[22] and advocated later by Bell.[23] Based on the principle that the toothbrush follows a physiologic pathway and traverses over the tissues in a "natural" masticating act.
Type of brush	A soft brush with 0.006–0.008-inch filament diameter	A soft brush with 0.006–0.008-inch filament diameter	A soft brush with "small tufts of fine bristles arranged in four parallel rows and trimmed to an even length"
Stroke	In abbreviated form, the technique described by Dr. Fones includes the following[19]: 1) With the teeth closed, place the brush inside the cheek over the last maxillary molar, lightly contacting the gingiva. 2) Use a fast, wide, circular motion with light pressure sweeping from the maxillary to the mandibular gingiva. 3) Bring anterior teeth in edge-to-edge contact holding lip out when necessary to make continuous circular strokes. 4) Lingual and palatal tooth surfaces require an in-and-out stroke. Brush sweeps across palate and back and forth to the molars on the mandibular arch. (See **Figure 27-8**)	Paraphrased, Leonard's method is described as follows[21]: 1) With the teeth edge-to-edge, place the brush filaments against the teeth at right angles to the long axes of the teeth. 2) Brush vigorously with light pressure and mostly up and down strokes with a slight rotation or circular motion after striking the gingival margin with force. 3) Use enough pressure to force the filaments into the embrasures, but not enough to damage the brush. 4) The upper and lower teeth are not brushed in the same series of strokes. The teeth are placed edge-to-edge to keep the brush from slipping over the occlusal or incisal surfaces.	Direct the brush down over the lower teeth onto the gingiva and upward over the teeth for the maxillary. It is also suggested that a few gentle horizontal strokes be used to clean the portion of the sulci directly over the bifurcations of the roots.
Recommendations	An easy-to-learn first technique for young children	Use when maxillary and mandibular teeth are to be brushed separately surfaces	
Limitations	Possibly detrimental for adults, particularly when used by a vigorous brusher		

- Current power brushes move in speeds and motions that cannot be duplicated by manual brushes.
- Research has shown consistently that power brushes are more effective than manual.[27–29]
- The safety of power brushes as compared to manual has been well established.[29–32]

II. PURPOSES AND INDICATIONS

A. General Application

- Recommended for physically able patients with ineffective manual biofilm removal techniques.

- To facilitate mechanical removal of dental biofilm and food debris from the teeth and the gingiva.
- Reduce calculus and stain buildup.[32]

B. Special Patients

Power brushes can be useful for many patients, including:

- Those with a history of failed attempts at more traditional biofilm removal methods.
- Those undergoing orthodontic treatment (page 438).
- Those undergoing complex restorative and prosthodontic treatment.

- Those with dental implants.
- Aggressive brushers: tendency to use less pressure when using a power brush than with a manual brush.[33–35]
- Patients with disabilities or limited dexterity.
- The large handles of power brushes can be of benefit.
- Handle weight needs to be considered for these patients.
- Patients unable to brush.
- A power brush may be readily used by a parent or caregiver.

III. DESCRIPTION

A. Motion

There is great variety in the manner in which power brushes move, for example:

- The entire brush head moves as a unit in one type of motion.
- Groups of tufts on the same brush head may move differently.
- The entire brush head moves as a unit, but in different, yet simultaneous motions.
- Different-shaped brush heads move separately, and in different, yet simultaneous motions.
- A synopsis of the types of motions of power brushes is seen in **Table 27-3**.

B. Speeds

- Vary from low to high.
- Generally, power brushes with replaceable batteries move slower than those with rechargeable batteries.

TABLE 27-3	POWER TOOTHBRUSH MOTIONS
MOTION	**DESCRIPTION**
Rotational	Moves in a 360° circular motion
Counter-rotational	Each tuft of filaments moves in a rotational motion; each tuft moves counter-directional to the adjacent tuft.
Oscillating	Rotates from center to the left, then to the right; degree of rotation varies from 25–55 degrees.
Pulsating	When brush head is on the tooth, direct pulsations toward the interproximal.
Cradle or twist	Side to side with an arc
Side-to-side	Side-to-side perpendicular to the long axis of the brush handle
Translating	Up-and-down parallel to the long axis of the brush handle.
Combination	Combination of simultaneous yet different type of movement.

- Movement varies from 3,800 to 40,000 movements per minute depending on the manufacturer and type.

C. Brush Head Design

- *Adult.* The variety of shapes is illustrated in **Figure 27-9**. They may be small and round, conical, or like traditional manual heads. Trim profiles include flat, bilevel, rippled, or angled.
- *Child.* A child's power brush head can be specially designed to accommodate a smaller mouth and the development of the dentition, as shown in **Figure 27-10**.
- *Interdental.* The interdental brush heads pictured in **Figure 27-11** are designed to fit a standard power brush handle and are similar in shape to manual interdental brushes, as shown in Figure 28-9, page 416.

D. Filaments

- Made of soft, end-rounded nylon.
- Diameters: from extra-soft, 0.075 mm (0.003 inch), to soft, 0.15 mm (0.006 inch).
- Some children's power brush heads feature specially manufactured filaments for extra softness.

E. Power Source

- *Direct*
  A. Connects to electrical outlet.
- *Replaceable batteries*
  A. Relatively inexpensive and convenient.
  B. As most batteries lose their power, brush speed is reduced.
  C. Advise patients to select a brush that has a watertight handle to avoid corrosion of batteries.
- *Rechargeable*
  A. Rechargeable, nonreplaceable battery.
  B. Recharges via a stand that is connected to the electrical outlet.
- *Disposable*
  A. Batteries can be neither replaced nor recharged.

IV. INSTRUCTION

A. Basis for Brush Selection

- Quality of clinical research that supports the efficacy and safety of the brush.
- Dental professional's experience with the product.
- Patient circumstances and preferences.
- Dexterity of the patient: detailed hand motion by patient is not a key requirement as it is with manual brushes.
- Brush head and batteries that can be replaced for maximum efficiency.
- Features that include a timer and pressure sensor.

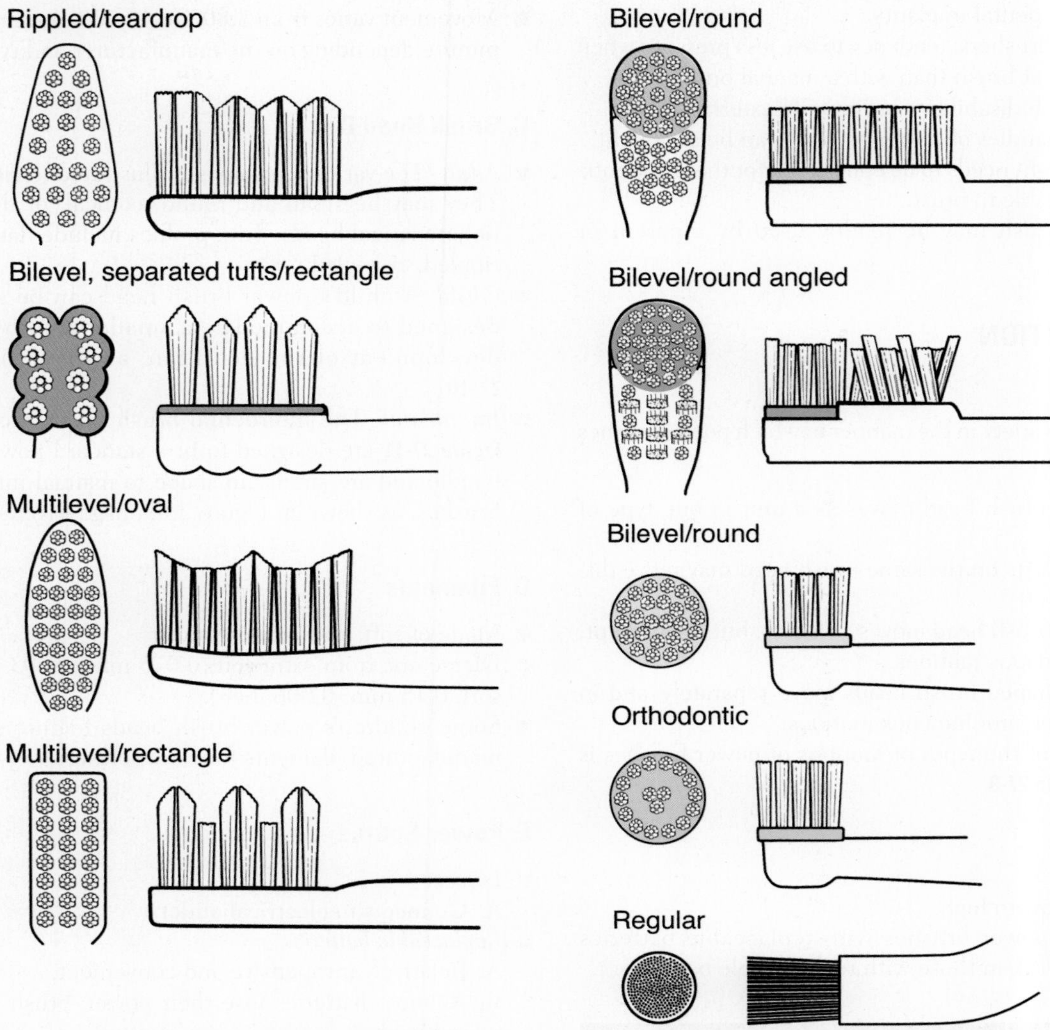

Rippled/teardrop

Bilevel, separated tufts/rectangle

Multilevel/oval

Multilevel/rectangle

Bilevel/round

Bilevel/round angled

Bilevel/round

Orthodontic

Regular

FIGURE 27-9 Power Brush Trim Profiles. Power brushes are made in a variety of brush head shapes, such as oval, teardrop, rectangular, and round. Some power brushes have two different-shaped heads on the same brush. In addition, there are a variety of brush head trims on power brushes, including, flat, bilevel, and multilevel.

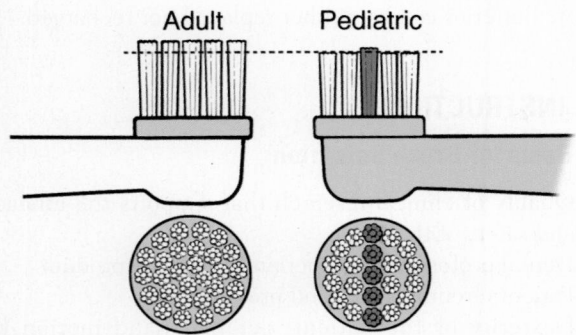

Adult   Pediatric

FIGURE 27-10 Child Power Brush Profile. Power brushes for children could necessitate smaller head sizes and shorter filaments to allow for distal reach in tight posterior areas. Raised blue filaments allow for better access to occlusal pits and fissures.

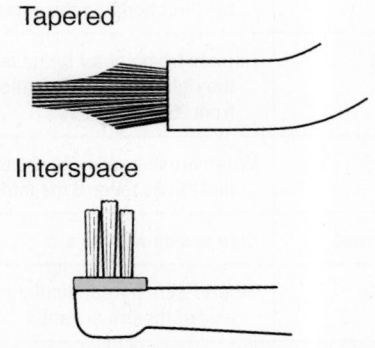

Tapered

Interspace

FIGURE 27-11 Interdental Power Brush Trim Profiles. Some power brushes offer brush heads especially for interdental and proximal surface dental biofilm removal and difficult-access areas such as around implants, orthodontic appliances, and exposed furcations.

B. Preparation for Instructing Patient

- Review manufacturer's instructions as they can differ.
- If possible, use the product before teaching a patient.

C. Hands-on Instruction

- Teach patients that use of power brushes does require practice.
- Provide a demonstration model of the brush and a video of the brushing instructions, if available.
- Show and tell the patient how to turn the handle to reach all areas of the mouth.

V. PROCEDURE

- Follow standard flossing procedure.
- Select brush with soft end-rounded filaments.
- Select dentifrice with minimum abrasivity.
- Place a small amount of dentifrice on the brush and spread the dentifrice over the teeth.
- Place brush in the mouth before turning power on to prevent splashing.
- Vary the brush position for each tooth surface. Brush each tooth and surrounding gingiva separately.
  - A. Apply the brush for sulcular brushing to the distal, facial, mesial, and lingual surfaces of each tooth as the brush is moved from the most posterior teeth toward the anterior, quadrant by quadrant.
  - B. Turn the brush to reach each proximal area.
  - C. Angulate for access to surfaces of rotated, crowded, or otherwise displaced teeth.
- Use light steady pressure. Pressure is not great enough at any time to bend the filaments.

SUPPLEMENTAL BRUSHING

I. PROBLEM AREAS

A. Adaptations

- Each surface of each tooth is brushed.
- Initial instruction necessarily may be limited to a basic procedure, particularly when it varies from the patient's present procedures.
- At succeeding lessons, the special hard-to-get areas can be reviewed.
- Suggestions are made and demonstrated for brush adaptation for areas that were missed.

B. Areas for Special Attention

- Facially displaced teeth, especially canines and premolars, where the zone of attached gingiva on the facial may be minimal and where toothbrush abrasion may occur.

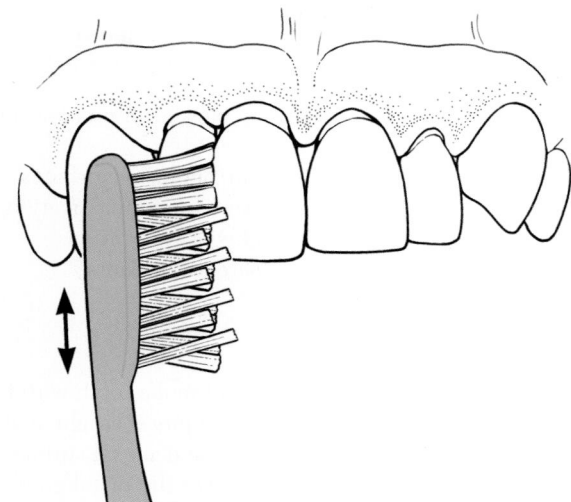

FIGURE 27-12 Brush in Vertical Position. For overlapped teeth, open embrasures, and selected areas of recession, the dental biofilm on proximal tooth surfaces can be removed with the brush held in a vertical position.

- Inclined teeth, for example, lingual surfaces of mandibular molars that are inclined lingually.
- Exposed root surfaces; cemental and dentinal surfaces.
- Overlapped teeth or wide embrasures, which require use of vertical brush position **(Figure 27-12)**.
- Surfaces of teeth next to edentulous areas.
- Exposed furcation areas.
- Right canine and lateral incisor, both maxillary and mandibular, which are commonly missed by right-handed brushers; the opposite is true for left-handed brushers.
- Distal surfaces of most posterior teeth **(Figure 27-13)**. At best, the brush may reach only the distal line angles. Supplementation with dental floss or textured dental floss is needed for the distal surface (Figures 28-3G and 28-6C; pages 412 and 414).

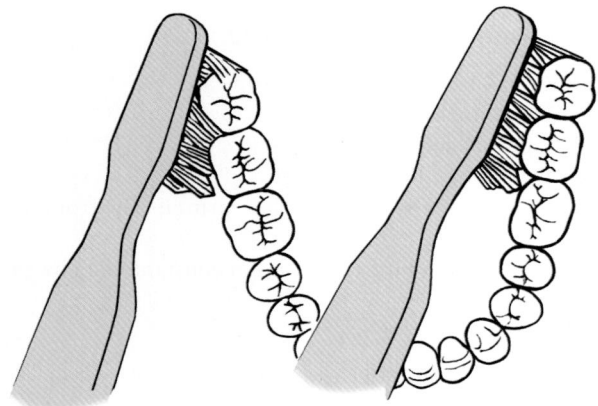

FIGURE 27-13 Brushing Problems. Brush placement to remove biofilm from the distal surfaces of the most posterior teeth. The distobuccal surface is approached by stretching the cheek; the distolingual surface is approached by directing the brush across from the canine of the opposite side.

II. OCCLUSAL BRUSHING

A. Objectives

■ Loosen biofilm microorganisms packed in pits and fissures.

■ Remove biofilm deposits from occlusal surfaces of teeth out of occlusion or not used during mastication.

■ Remove biofilm from the margins of restorations.

■ Clean pits and fissures to prepare for sealants.

B. Procedure

■ Place brush on occlusal surfaces of molar teeth with filament tips pointed into the occlusal pits at a right angle.

■ Position the handle parallel with the occlusal surface.

■ Extend the toe of the brush to cover the distal grooves of the most posterior tooth **(Figure 27-14A)**.

■ Strokes. Two acceptable strokes are suggested.
  A. Vibrate the brush in a slight circular movement while maintaining the filament tips on the occlusal surface throughout a count of 10. Press moderately so filaments do not bend but go straight into the pits and fissures **(Figure 27-14A)**.
  B. Force the filaments against the occlusal surface with sharp, quick strokes; lift the brush off each time to dislodge debris; repeat about 10 times.

■ Move brush to premolar area, overlapping previous brush position.

C. Precaution

Long scrubbing strokes from anterior to posterior on an occlusal surface may contact only the prominent parts of the cusps **(Figure 27-14B)**.

 ### III. TONGUE CLEANING

Total mouth cleanliness includes tongue care.

A. Microorganisms of the Tongue

■ Main foci for oral microorganisms are:
  A. Dorsum of tongue
  B. Gingival sulci and pockets
  C. Dental biofilm on all teeth

■ Microorganisms in saliva are principally from the tongue.

■ The microflora of the tongue is not constant, but changes frequently.[36]

B. Effects of Cleaning the Tongue

■ Slows dental biofilm formation and total biofilm accumulation.

■ Reduces number of microorganisms.

■ Reduces potential for halitosis.

■ Contributes to overall cleanliness.

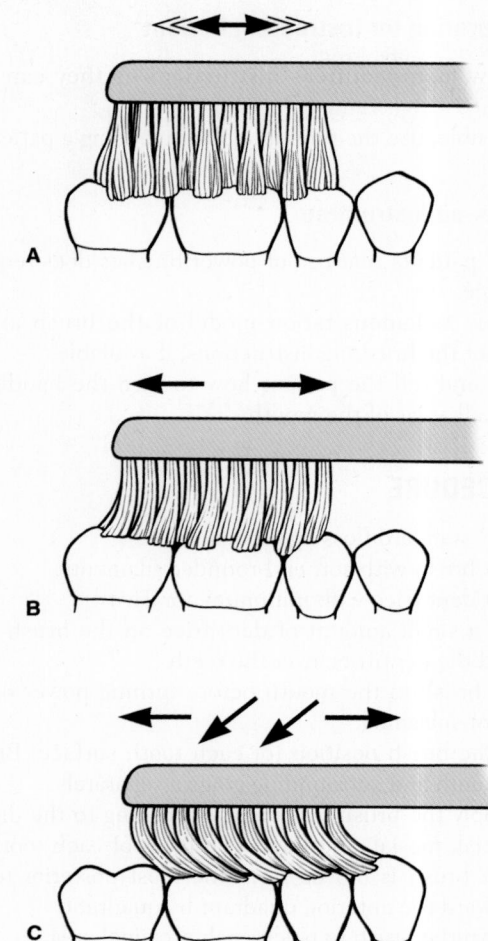

FIGURE 27-14 **Occlusal Brushing. (A)** Vibrating brush with light pressure while maintaining filament tips on the occlusal surface permits tips to work their way into pits and fissures. **(B)** Long horizontal strokes contact only the cusp tips. **(C)** Excess pressure curves the filaments so that tips cannot get into the pits and fissures.

C. Anatomic Features of Tongue Conducive to Debris Retention

■ *Surface papillae.* Numerous filiform papillae extend as minute projections, whereas fungiform papillae are not as high and create elevations and depressions that entrap debris and microorganisms (Figure 14-2, page 210).

■ *Fissured tongue.* Fissures may be several millimeters deep and retain debris.

D. Brushing Procedure

1. Hold the brush handle at a right angle to the midline of the tongue and direct the brush tips toward the throat.

2. With the tongue extruded, the sides of the filaments are placed on the posterior part of the tongue surface.

3. With light pressure, draw the brush forward and over the tip of the tongue. Repeat three or four times. Do not scrub the papillae.

4. A power brush should only be used for tongue cleaning when the switch is in the "off" position.

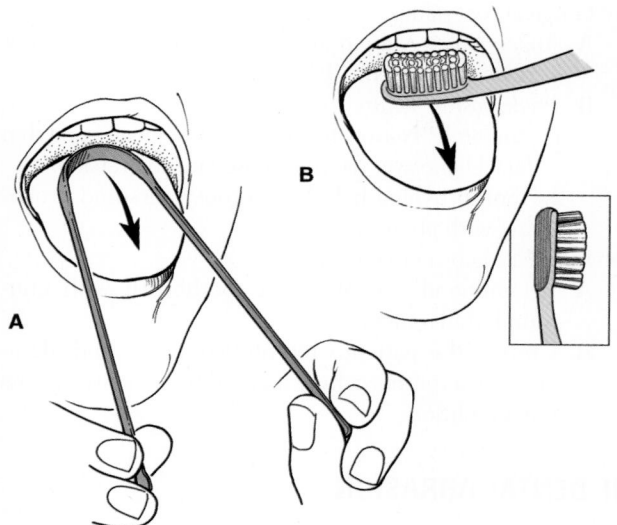

FIGURE 27-15 Tongue Cleaners. (A) A variety of plastic or flexible metal cleaners are available to clean the dorsal surface of the tongue. **(B)** An example of a toothbrush with a rubber tongue cleaner behind the brush head. The cleaner is pressed over the tongue with a light but firm stroke.

E. Tongue Cleaner

Tongue cleaners may be made of plastic, rubber, stainless steel, or other flexible metal. They are curved or raised, textured pads that are wide enough to fit over the tongue surface without hitting the teeth.

- *Types*
  A. Curved with a single handle
  B. Curved with two ends to hold **(Figure 27-15A)**
  C. Raised, textured rubber pad on the back side of the brush head **(Figure 27-15B)**
- *Purpose.* By removing debris and microorganisms, the patient can expect tongue cleaning to contribute to:
  A. overall mouth cleanliness
  B. reduction in the number of bacteria available for biofilm formation
  C. fewer mouth odors
  D. improvements for the patient who has xerostomia, a coated tongue, deep fissures, or who uses tobacco products.
- *Procedure*
  A. Place the cleaner toward the most posterior area of the dorsal surface **(Figure 27-15)**.
  B. Press with a light but firm stroke, and pull forward.
  C. Repeat several times, covering the entire surface of the tongue.
  D. Wash the tongue cleaner under running water.

TOOTHBRUSHING FOR SPECIAL CONDITIONS

Even when an unusual oral condition develops, a patient is encouraged to brush wherever possible to reduce the possibility of infection and promote healing. Prolonged omission of techniques of biofilm removal is never indicated. Examples of conditions that may require a temporary departure from personal care routines are included here.

I. ACUTE ORAL INFLAMMATORY OR TRAUMATIC LESIONS

When an acute oral condition precludes normal brushing, instruct the patient to:

- Brush all areas of the mouth that are not affected.
- Rinse with a warm, mild saline solution to encourage healing and debris removal.
- Resume regular biofilm control measures on the affected area as soon as possible.

II. FOLLOWING PERIODONTAL SURGERY

Provide specific instructions concerning brushing while sutures and/or a dressing are in place.

- Brush the occlusal surfaces of the teeth and use light strokes over the dressing.
- Avoid direct, vigorous brushing to prevent displacement of a dressing.
- Brush other teeth and gingiva, not involved in the surgery, as usual.
- Additional instructions appear in Table 42-2, page 671.

III. ACUTE STAGE OF NECROTIZING ULCERATIVE GINGIVITIS

- Lack of oral cleanliness can be a major contributing factor.
- Oral tissues are sensitive to any touch during the acute stage, and toothbrushing therefore is neglected.
- Careful brush placement and an extra soft brush are indicated to avoid trauma.

IV. FOLLOWING DENTAL EXTRACTION

- Brush all teeth and gingiva except the surgical wound area.
- Clean the teeth adjacent to the extraction site the day following surgery.
- Brush areas not involved in the surgery as usual to reduce biofilm collections and promote healing.
- Detailed instructions for pre- and postsurgery may be found in Chapter 54 on page 825.

V. FOLLOWING DENTAL RESTORATIONS

- Patients tend to avoid brushing a new crown, implant, newly placed fixed partial denture, or other prosthesis.
- Specific instructions are needed at the time of insertion.

EFFECTS OF TOOTHBRUSHING

I. THE GINGIVA

- Trauma occurs most frequently on the facial surfaces over prominent teeth in the dental arch.
- Lesions are frequently found over canines and premolars.
- Lesions occur most often immediately following initial instruction in the use of a new method of brushing; patient may be overzealous or may have misunderstood correct brush placement.
- Examination of patient's gingiva within a few days after instruction can be important.

A. Acute Alterations

Acute lesions are usually lacerations or ulcerations. The severity of the lesion may depend on the frequency and extent of brushing, as well as on the stiffness of the filaments and the force applied.

- Appearance
  A. Scuffed epithelial surface with denuded underlying connective tissue.
  B. Punctate lesions that appear as red pinpoint spots.
  C. Diffuse redness and denuded attached gingiva.
- Precipitating factors
  A. Horizontal or vertical scrub toothbrushing method.
  B. Excess pressure applied using firm palm grasp of handle.[37]
  C. Use of abrasive dentifrice.[38]
  D. Overvigorous placement and application of the toothbrush.
  E. Penetration of gingiva by filament ends.
  F. Use of a toothbrush with frayed, broken bristles or filaments.
  G. Application of filaments beyond attached gingiva.

B. Chronic Alterations

- Changes in gingival contour
  A. Appearance
    1. Rolled, bulbous, hard, firm marginal gingiva, in "piled up" or festoon shape ("McCall's festoon," Figure 14-10, page 219).
    2. Gingival cleft, which is a narrow groove or slit that extends from the crest of the gingiva to the attached gingiva ("Stillman's cleft," Figure 14-11, page 219).
  B. Location
    1. May appear only on the facial gingiva, because of the vigor with which toothbrush is used.
    2. Frequently inversely related to the right- or left-handedness of the patient.
    3. Areas most often involved are around canines or teeth in labioversion or buccoversion.

- Gingival recession
  A. *Appearance*. Margin has moved apically and root surface is exposed.
  B. *Predisposing factors*
    1. Anatomic: Narrow band of attached gingiva and thin facial bone over teeth malposed in labioversion.
    2. Toothbrushing habits: Vigorous pressured brushing with abrasive dentifrice.
- Suggested corrective measures
  A. Recommend use of a soft toothbrush with end-rounded filaments.
  B. Correct the patient's toothbrushing method; demonstrate a toothbrushing method better suited to the oral condition.

II. DENTAL ABRASION

Appearance. Wedge-shaped indentations with smooth, shiny surfaces, as seen in Figure 17-5, page 260.

A. Definition

- Abrasion is the wearing away of tooth structure that results from a repetitive mechanical habit.
- Incorrect toothbrushing, especially with an abrasive dentifrice is the most common cause.

B. Location

- Primarily on facial surfaces, especially of canines, premolars, and sometimes first molars, or, on any tooth in buccoversion or labioversion, those most available to the pressure of the toothbrush.
- The canines are susceptible because of their prominence on the curvature of the dental arches.
- Most abraded areas are on the cervical areas of exposed root surfaces, but occasionally they may occur on the enamel.
- When adjacent teeth are involved, the lesions appear in line with each other.

C. Contributing Factors

- Brushing with abrasive agent in the dentifrice.
- Horizontal brushing with excessive pressure.
- Form of filament ends: abrasion is less frequent when filaments are end-rounded.
- Prominence of the tooth surface labially or buccally.

D. Corrective Measures

- Explain the problem to the patient to ensure full cooperation.
- Advise use of a specific brush with end-rounded filaments.
- Change the toothbrushing procedure.
- Recommend a less abrasive dentifrice.

■ Use a smaller amount of dentifrice.
  A. Start brushing in the area of the dentition where the most biofilm and calculus are noted at a maintenance appointment.
  B. Avoid applying the dentifrice vigorously to the same tooth surfaces.

III. BACTEREMIA

Evidence suggests that toothbrushing and scaling can produce a detectable bacteremia.[39-41]

■ The incidence and magnitude of bacteremia after scaling is significantly higher in patients with periodontitis than in gingivitis and healthy patients.[40]
■ There is no definitive data on the relative risks of using manual or electric toothbrushes in patients who are predisposed to infective endocarditis.
■ The mere fact that bacterial endocarditis can be produced through toothbrushing makes the need for maintaining proper oral hygiene a priority.[41]

 ## CARE OF TOOTHBRUSHES

When discussing the type and features of the brush selected for an individual patient, the number of brushes needed and the frequency of replacement is included. Perhaps an ideal time to teach cleaning and daily care of brushes would be after a practice session.

The condition of a brush depends on many factors, including the amount and manner of use, the type of care, and the quality of the brush at the start.

I. SUPPLY OF BRUSHES

■ Advise at least two brushes for home use and a third in a portable container for use at work, school, or travel.
■ Purchase of brushes needs to be staggered so that all brushes are not new at the same time and, more important, so that they are all not old at the same time, thereby resulting in less than optimum maintenance of the gingival condition.

II. BRUSH REPLACEMENT

■ Frequent replacement recommended; at least every 2 to 3 months.
■ Brushes need to be replaced before filaments become splayed or frayed or lose resiliency. Duration of a brush is influenced by many factors, including frequency and method of use.
■ Brush contamination occurs with use.[42,43] Contamination has the potential for causing systemic or localized infection.
■ Patients who are debilitated, immunosuppressed, have a known infection, or are about to undergo surgery for any reason can be advised to disinfect their brushes or use disposable brushes.[43]

III. CLEANING TOOTHBRUSHES

■ Clean thoroughly after each use.
■ Hold brush head under strong stream of warm water from faucet to force particles, dentifrice, and bacteria from between the filaments.
■ Tap the handle on edge of sink to remove remaining particles.
■ Use one toothbrush to clean another brush; filaments can be worked between those of the other brush to remove resistant debris.
■ Rinse completely and tap out excess water.

IV. BRUSH STORAGE

■ Brushes need to be kept in open air with head in an upright position, apart from contact with other brushes, particularly those of another person.
■ Portable brush container needs sufficient holes to give air temporarily until the brush can be completely exposed for drying. A closed container encourages bacterial growth.

DOCUMENTATION

In the permanent record, the documentation for initial instruction will include the following:

■ Type of toothbrush patient has used to date: manual versus power.
■ Recommended changes in type of brush or method of use.
■ Identify needs or changes in the soft tissue and teeth from a "plaque score" using a disclosing agent.
■ Record areas patient has difficulty reaching with suggestions for follow-up.
■ Tongue cleaning method instructed.
■ **Box 27-3** shows a sample Progress Note.

BOX 27-3	**Example Progress Note: Toothbrushes and Toothbrushing**

Current brushing method: manual flat trim brush, combination of Fones method anterior teeth and rolling stroke posterior teeth. Recommend switch to manual brush, multilevel filaments, use 1×/day with Bass method (demonstrated). Suggested a power brush minimum 1×/day. Instructed to bring power brush next visit to adjust method if needed. Reminded to use tongue cleaner daily and suggested a manual brush with a tongue cleaner on the back of the brush head. **(Figure 27-15B)**

Signed: _____, RDH Date: _____.

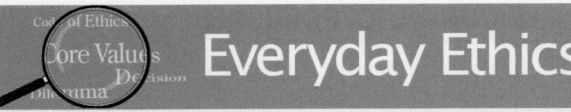

Everyday Ethics

Brandi greeted her new patient, Mr. Russell, who had recently moved to the area from across country. While completing the history, he told her about the dental hygienist in the other practice and how much he appreciated her telling him what a good job he was doing with his home care. "I went regularly every 6 months and she always spent a good half hour with me." When asked what type of brush, toothpaste, and other aids she had recommended for him to use, he said, "Oh, she never told me any special kinds; she always said I was doing OK."

The oral examination showed generalized moderate probing depths with a few up to 5 or 6 mm pockets with bleeding, generalized subgingival calculus and early furcation exposures in all first molars. There also was notable halitosis. When Brandi asked him to demonstrate homecare, it was obvious that more specific instruction would be needed. Mentally Brandi planned to start him on a power brush.

Questions for Consideration

1. Which core ethical values are represented in this scenario? Explain how each applies.
2. List factors that could have been in effect where Mr. Russell's former dental hygienist appears to have acted malevolently?
3. Take partners to role play an ethical approach Brandi can use to explain the following:
   a. The seriousness of his active periodontal disease even though he has had a history of regular dental hygiene care.
   b. Why she will need at least 4 hour-long appointments and use anesthesia for each quadrant to complete the initial scaling;
   c. How she will explain why she wants him to use a power brush and have more frequent appointments scheduled at 3–4 months rather than twice a year.

Factors To Teach The Patient

- How dental biofilm forms and its effects on the teeth and gingiva.
- Why it is necessary to remove dental biofilm from the teeth daily, especially before going to sleep.
- The type of brush: manual, power, or both, recommended to maintain optimal oral health for a particular patient.
- Individualized hands-on instruction using an appropriate manual or power brushing method.
- Proper care and maintenance of manual and power brushes.
- Indications for and use of a tongue cleaner.

References

1. Hirschfeld I. *The toothbrush: its use and abuse.* Brooklyn, NY: Dental Items of Interest; 1939. 1–27 pp.
2. McCauley HB. Toothbrushes, toothbrush materials and design. *J Am Dent Assoc.* 1946 Mar;33:283–93.
3. Weinberger BW. *An introduction to the history of dentistry.* St. Louis: Mosby; 1948. 140–44 pp.
4. American Academy of Periodontology. Committee report: the tooth brush and methods of cleaning the teeth. *Dent Items Interest.* 1920 Mar;42:193.
5. Menaker L, editor. *The biologic basis of dental caries.* Hagerstown, MD: Harper & Row; 1980, Chapter 22, Alexander JF: Toothbrushes and toothbrushing. 482–96 pp.
6. Koecker L. *Principles of dental surgery.* Baltimore: American Society of Dental Surgeons; 1842, Chapter III, *exhibiting a new method of treating the diseases of the teeth and gums.* 155–56 pp.
7. American Dental Association, Council on Dental Therapeutics. *Accepted dental therapeutics.* 40th ed. Chicago: American Dental Association; 1984. p. 386–87.
8. Checchi L, Minguzzi S, Franchi M, Forteleoni G. Toothbrush filaments end-rounding: stereomicroscope analysis. *J Clin Periodontol.* 2001 Apr;28(4):360–71.
9. Breitenmoser J, Mörmann W, Mühlemann HR. Damaging effects of toothbrush bristle end form on gingiva. *J Periodontol.* 1979 Apr;50(4):212–16.
10. Silverstone LM, Featherstone MJ. A scanning electron microscope study of the end rounding of bristles in eight toothbrush types. *Quintessence Int.* 1988 Feb;19(2):3–23.
11. Stiller S, Bosma MLP, Shi X, Spingel CM, Yankell SL. Interproximal access efficacy of three manual toothbrushes with extended, x-angled or flat multitufted bristles. *Int J Dent Hygiene.* 2010 Aug;8(3):244–48.
12. Bass CC. An effective method of personal oral hygiene. *J Louisiana State Med Soc.* 1954 Mar;106(3):57–73.
13. Bunting RW, editor. *Oral hygiene.* 3rd ed. Philadelphia: Lea & Febiger; 1957, Chapter 10, Hard D: Oral prophylaxis. 280–83 pp.
14. Stillman PR. A philosophy of the treatment of periodontal disease. *Dent Digest.* 1932 Sep;38(9):380.
15. Hirschfeld. op. cit., p. 380.
16. Charters WJ. Home care of the mouth. I. proper home care of the mouth. *J Periodontol.* 1948 Oct;19:136–39.
17. Charters WJ. Eliminating mouth infections with the toothbrush and other stimulating instruments. *Dent Digest.* 1932 April;38:130.
18. Miller SC. *Textbook of periodontia.* 3rd ed. Philadelphia: The Blakiston Co.; 1950. 327–28 pp.
19. Fones AC. *Mouth hygiene.* 4th ed. Philadelphia: Lea & Febiger; 1934. 299–306 pp.
20. Hirschfeld. op. cit., pp. 369–371.
21. Leonard HJ. Conservative treatment of periodontoclasia. *J Am Dent Assoc.* 1939 Aug;26:1308–15.
22. Smith TS. Anatomic and physiologic conditions governing the use of the toothbrush. *J Am Dent Assoc.* 1940 Jun;27:874.
23. Bell DG. Home care of the mouth. III. teaching home care to the patient. *J Periodontal Res.* 1948 Oct;19(4):140–3.
24. American Dental Association, Council on Scientific Affairs [Internet]. ADA acceptance program guidelines for toothbrushes. Chicago, American Dental Association; updated Nov 2009[Cited 2010 Aug 8]; [about 10 screens]. Available from: www.ada.org/sections/about/pdgs/guide_toothbrushes.pdf
25. McKendrick AJW, Barbenel LMH, McHugh WD. A two-year comparison of hand and electric toothbrushes. *J Periodontal Res.* 1968;3(3):224–31.

26. Loe H, Kleinman DV, editors. *Dental plaque control measures and oral hygiene practices*. Oxford: IRL Press; 1986, Frandsen A: Mechanical oral hygiene practices: state of the science review. 94 p.

27. Barnes CM, Russell CM, Weatherford TW. A comparison of the efficacy of 2 powered toothbrushes in affecting plaque accumulation, gingivitis, and gingival bleeding. *J Periodontol*. 1999 Aug;70:840–47.

28. Cronin M, Dembling W, Warren PR, King DW. A 3-month clinical investigation comparing the safety and efficacy of a novel electric toothbrush (Braun Oral-B 3D plaque remover) with a manual toothbrush. *Am J Dent*. 1998;11(Special Issue):S17.

29. Ho HP, Niederman R. Effectiveness of the Sonicare® sonic toothbrush on reduction of plaque, gingivitis, probing pocket depth, and subgingival bacteria in adolescent orthodontic clients. *J Clin Dent*. 1997;11(Special Issue):S17.

30. Warren PR, Ray TS, Cugini M, Chater BV. A practice-based study of a power toothbrush: assessment of effectiveness and acceptance. *J Am Dent Assoc*. 2000 Mar;131(3):389–94.

31. Danser MM, Timmerman MF, Ijzerman Y, van der Velden U, Warren PR, van der Weijden FA. A comparison of electric toothbrushes in their potential to cause gingival abrasion of oral soft tissues. *Am J Dent*. 1998 Sep;11:S35.

32. Sharma NC, Galustians HJ, Qaqish J, Cugini MA, Warren PR. The effect of two power toothbrushes on calculus and stain. *Am J Dent*. 2002 Apr;15(2):71–6.

33. van der Weijden GA, Timmerman MF, Reijerse E, Snoek CM, van der Velden U. Toothbrushing force in relation to plaque removal. *J Clin Periodontol*. 1996 Aug;23(8):724–9.

34. Heasman P, Wilson Z, Macgregor I, Kelly P. Comparative study of electric and manual toothbrushes in patients with fixed orthodontic appliances. *Am J Orthod Dentofacial Orthop*. 1998 Jul;114(1):45–9.

35. Boyd RL, McLey L, Zahradnik R. Clinical and laboratory evaluation of powered electric toothbrushes: *in vivo* determination of average force for use of manual and powered toothbrushes. *J Clin Dent*. 1997;8(Special Issue):72.

36. Van der Weijden GA, Van der Velden U. Fluctuation of the microbiota of the tongue in humans. *J Clin Periodontol*. 1991 Jan;18:26–9.

37. Niemi ML, Ainamo J, Etemadzadeh H. The effect of toothbrush grip on gingival abrasion and plaque removal during toothbrushing. *J Clin Periodontol*. 1987 Jan;14:19–21.

38. Niemi M, Sandholm L, Ainamo J. Frequency of gingival lesions after standardized brushing as related to stiffness of toothbrush and abrasiveness of dentifrice. *J Clin Periodontol*. 1984 Apr;11(4):254–61.

39. Kinane DF, Riggio MP, Walker KF, MacKenzie D, Shearer B. Bacteremia following periodontal procedures. *J Clin Periodontol*. 2005 Jul;32(7):708–13.

40. Forner L, Larsen T, Kilian M, Holmstrup P. Incidence of bacteremia after chewing, toothbrushing, and scaling in individuals with periodontal inflammation. *J Clin Periodontol*. 2006 Jun;33(6):401–7.

41. Hartzell JD, Torres D, Kim P, Wortmann G. Incidence of bacteremia after routine brushing. *Am J Med Sci*. 2005 Apr;329(4):178–80.

42. Glass RT. The infected toothbrush, the infected denture, and transmission of disease: a review. *Compend Contin Educ Dent*. 1992 Jul;13(7):592–8.

43. Müller HP, Lange DE, Müller RF. Actinobacillus actinomycetemcomitans contamination of toothbrushes from patients harbouring the organism. *J Clin Periodontol*. 1989 Jul;16(6):388–90.

Interdental Care and Irrigation

ESTHER M. WILKINS, BS, RDH, DMD
DEBORAH M. LYLE, RDH, BS, MS

Chapter Outline

Traditionally, toothbrushing has been considered to be first in line as the method for cleaning the teeth and removing dental biofilm for the prevention of gingival and periodontal infections. Toothbrushing cannot accomplish biofilm removal for the proximal tooth surfaces and adjacent gingiva to the same degree that it does for the facial, lingual, and palatal aspects. Interdental biofilm control, therefore, is essential to complete the patient's self-care program.

■ Objectives and procedures for removal of dental biofilm from proximal tooth surfaces are included in this chapter.

■ Key words are defined in **Box 28-1**.

■ When the preventive treatment plan is outlined for an individual, assessment is made of the oral condition, the problem areas, and the overall prognosis for improvement or maintenance of gingival health.

■ Measures for interdental biofilm control are selected to complement biofilm control by toothbrushing.

BOX 28-1	Key Words

Interdental Care

Col: the depression in the gingival tissue under a contact area between the lingual (palatal) papilla and the facial papilla.

Embrasure: V-shaped spillway space next to the contact area of adjacent teeth, narrowest at the contact and widening toward the facial, lingual (palatal), and occlusal contacts.

Floss cleft: a cleft in the gingival margin usually at a mesial or distal line angle of a tooth where dental floss was repeatedly applied incorrectly. The lining of the cleft can be completely lined with epithelium.

Floss cut: unintentional incision at the gingival margin due to incorrect positioning and placement of dental floss.

Hydrotherapy: the use of forced intermittent or steady stream of water for a cleansing or therapeutic purpose.

Interproximal space: the triangular region bounded by the proximal surfaces of contacting teeth and the alveolar bone between the teeth, which forms the base of the triangle; the space is normally filled with the interdental papilla; also called the interdental area.

Irrigant: substance used for irrigation.

Irrigation: flushing of a specific area or site with a stream of fluid; application of a continuous or pulsated stream of fluid to a part of the body for a cleansing or therapeutic purpose.

   Supragingival Irrigation: the point of delivery of the irrigation is at, or coronal to, the free gingival margin.

   Marginal Irrigation: the point of delivery of the irrigation is angled at, or placed apically to, the gingival margin.

   Subgingival Irrigation: the point of the delivery of the irrigation is placed in the sulcus or pocket and may reach the base of the pocket depending on its probing depth.

Keratinized epithelium: outer, protective surface of stratified squamous epithelium; covers the masticatory mucosa; interdental col area is not normally keratinized.

Proxabrush: another name for an interdental brush (Figure 28-9).

THE INTERDENTAL AREA

■ The three types of gingival embrasures are illustrated in **Figure 28-1**.

■ In health, the interdental gingiva fills the interproximal area and under the contact of the adjacent teeth in a Type I embrasure.

■ When the interdental papilla is missing or reduced in height, which is common as a result of periodontal infection, the shape of the interdental gingiva changes, and open Type II or Type III embrasures may be seen.

■ **Figure 28-2** shows a Type II embrasure from the proximal surface with the col and from the facial surface.

I. ANATOMY OF THE INTERDENTAL AREA

A review of the gingival and dental anatomy of the interdental area can give meaning to and clarify the role and purpose of the various devices available for interdental care.

A. Posterior Teeth

■ Between adjacent posterior teeth are two papillae, one facial and one lingual or palatal.

■ The papillae are connected by a col, a depressed concave area that follows the shape of the apical border of the contact area (Figure 14-8A, page 214).

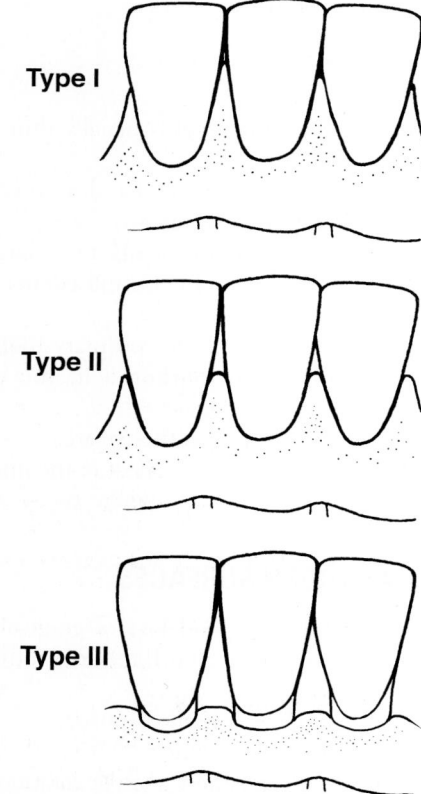

FIGURE 28-1 **Types of Gingival Embrasures.** Type I, interdental papilla fills the gingival embrasure. Type II, with slight to moderate recession of the interdental papilla. Type III, with extensive recession or complete loss of the interdental papilla.

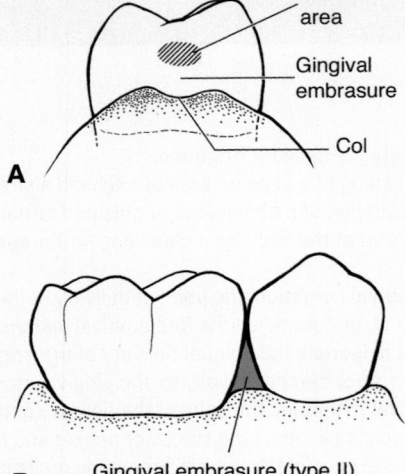

FIGURE 28-2 Type II Gingival Embrasure. (A) Embrasure shown from the proximal surface with the col. **(B)** Facial view, with gingival embrasure shown in blue.

B. Anterior Teeth

■ Between anterior teeth in contact is a single papilla with a pyramidal shape.
■ Tip of the papilla may form a small col under the contact area (Figure 14-8B, page 214).

C. Epithelium

■ The epithelium covering a col is usually thin and not keratinized.
■ Col epithelium is protected and is less resistant to infection than keratinized surfaces.
■ Inflammation in the papilla leads to enlargement, with increased inflammatory cells and edema; the col becomes deeper.
■ The col area is inaccessible for ordinary toothbrushing; microorganisms are harbored in the concave center.
■ Most gingival disease starts in the col area.
■ The incidence of gingivitis is greatest in the interdental tissues.[1]

II. PROXIMAL TOOTH SURFACES

■ With bacterial infection and loss of gingival attachment, the interdental papillae are reduced in height.
■ Proximal tooth surfaces become exposed.
■ Dental biofilm can accumulate.
■ Irregularities of tooth position, such as rotation or overlapping, and deviations related to malocclusion or tooth loss may be present.
■ Easy access for removal of bacterial deposits by the individual is prevented.

■ Root surface morphology of the proximal surfaces is typical for each tooth type.
■ Concavities and grooves are predisposed to bacterial accumulations.[2,3]
■ With advanced periodontitis, furcation areas of maxillary first premolars and molars open onto the proximal surfaces.

PLANNING INTERDENTAL CARE

I. PATIENT ASSESSMENT

A. History of Personal Oral Care

■ Type of toothbrush, dental floss, and other interdental devices currently used.
■ Frequency and personal time spent.
■ Estimate of the patient's apparent priorities on personal oral care.

B. Dental and Gingival Anatomy

■ Position of teeth.
■ Types and shapes of embrasures: variation throughout the dentition.
■ Probing depths: classification of the periodontal condition.
■ Prostheses present: special interdental care required for fixed and removable prostheses.
■ Areas where toothbrush cannot reach.

C. Extent and Location of Dental Biofilm

■ Preparation of a "plaque score" (in Chapter 22, pages 315 to 318) to show the patient the extent of biofilm needing removal on a daily basis.
■ Use of a disclosing agent to show specific sites where biofilms accumulate.
■ Evidence of the patient's ability to care for difficult access areas.

D. Personal Factors

■ Handicap or disability that limits ability to carry out needed personal oral hygiene.
■ Knowledge about and appreciation for interdental oral care.

II. DENTAL HYGIENE CARE PLAN

A. Objectives

■ Select appropriate interdental aids to help the patient reach optimum oral cleanliness and health.
■ Teach the patient correct system of oral care.
■ Motivate the patient to accept responsibility for daily personal care.

B. Initial Care Plan

- At first, the simplest procedures are selected for the patient's convenience and ease of learning based on the patient's current knowledge and oral care habits.
- Minimum frequency: thoroughly twice daily.
- Keep the daily oral care regimen at a realistic level with respect to the time the patient is able or willing to spend.
- As the values the patient places on oral health increase over time, and as the preventive maintenance program becomes a priority in the patient's slifelong self-care health goals, a more refined program can be introduced.

SELECTIVE INTERDENTAL BIOFILM REMOVAL

I. RELATION TO TOOTHBRUSHING

- Vibratory and sulcular toothbrushing, such as that performed with the Charters, Stillman, and Bass methods, can be successful to some degree in removing dental biofilm near the line angles of the facial and lingual or palatal embrasures.
- Brush in vertical position is effective for additional access around line angles onto the proximal surfaces (Figure 27-12, page 401).

II. SELECTION OF INTERDENTAL AIDS

- Dependent on oral health, disease status, and the risk for future recurrence.
- A patient working to control or arrest disease may need more frequent self-care than a patient practicing prevention.
- More than a toothbrush is needed for complete biofilm removal from exposed proximal tooth surfaces.
- With the judicious selection and use of the various methods for interdental care, disease control can be accomplished by the motivated patient.
- Dental floss, interdental brushes, and other aids are described in this chapter.

DENTAL FLOSS AND TAPE

- The effective use of dental floss contributes to gingival health by removing dental biofilm[4–7] and reducing interproximal bleeding.[8]
- Dental floss is most effective when interdental papillae are present and there has not been loss of attachment with root surface exposure.[9]
- As recession occurs, dental floss may still be used, but greater time, effort, and dexterity are required for complete removal of dental biofilm from the exposed proximal tooth surfaces.

I. TYPES OF FLOSS

- Research has shown no difference in the effectiveness of waxed or unwaxed floss for biofilm removal.[4,6,10–12]
- Biofilm removal depends on how floss is applied. For optimal patient compliance, the patient may use a preferred type.[4,13]

A. Materials

- *Silk:* Historically, floss was made of silk fibers loosely twisted together to form a strand and waxed for proximal surface cleaning.
- *Nylon:* Nylon multifilaments, waxed or unwaxed, have been widely used in circular (floss) or flat (tape) form for biofilm removal from proximal tooth surfaces.
- *Expanded PTFE:* Plastic monofilament polytetrafluoroethylene with wax is used for proximal tooth surface biofilm removal.

B. Features of Waxed or Expanded PTFE

- Smooth surface provided by the wax covering helps to prevent trauma to soft tissue.
- Slides through contact area with ease.
- Monofilament type resists breakage or shredding when passed over irregular tooth surface, restoration, or calculus deposit.
- Wax gives strength and durability during application; shredding or breakage is rare.

C. Features of Unwaxed

- Thinner floss may be helpful when contact areas are tight; however, forcing the floss through may break the floss.
- Pressure against a tooth surface spreads the nylon fibers and gives a wider surface for biofilm removal.
- Sharper thin edge requires special attention to prevent injury to the gingival tissue when guiding floss through a tight contact area or when moving floss on the tooth surface in an apical direction.
- Squeaking sound effect when floss moves over a clean tooth surface may provide a motivation for patient thoroughness.
- Unwaxed floss, which frays when rubbed over an irregular tooth surface, rough surface of a restoration, or calculus deposit, might cause the patient to become aggravated and discouraged, thereby resulting in lost motivation to floss regularly.
- Floss that is tightly wound around fingers tends to cut, hurt, and cause discomfort. This problem is not usually as evident with wide dental tape or with waxed floss or tape.

D. Enhancements

■ Color and flavor have been added to dental floss.
■ Therapeutic agents that have been added include fluoride and whitening agents. Limited research has been published relative to their effectiveness.

II. PROCEDURE

■ When dental floss is applied with firm pressure to a flat or convex proximal tooth surface, biofilm can be removed.
■ Older biofilm is tenacious and may require several strokes for removal.
■ When floss is placed over a concave surface, contact is not possible (**Figure 28-10A**), and supplementary devices are needed to remove a bacterial deposit completely.

A. When to Floss

For most patients, best results can be obtained by using dental floss before toothbrushing. The following reasons may apply:

■ When proximal tooth surfaces are flossed first and biofilm is removed, the fluoride from a dentifrice used while brushing reaches the proximal surfaces for prevention of dental caries.
■ When brushing is accomplished first, flossing may not be carried out.
  ■ The mouth feels clean; the need for flossing may not be appreciated.
  ■ Time may be short and flossing can be postponed.

B. Floss Preparation

■ **Figure 28-3** outlines the flossing steps that are described in detail here in this section.
■ Hold a 12- to 15-inch length of floss with the thumb and index finger of each hand; grasp firmly with only half inch of floss between the fingertips. The ends of the floss may be tucked into the palm and held by the ring and little finger, or the floss may be wrapped around the middle fingers (**Figure 28-3A, B,** and **C**).
■ A circle of floss may be made by tying the ends together; the circle may be rotated as the floss is used (**Figure 28-4**).[14]

C. Application

■ *Maxillary teeth:* Direct the floss up by holding the floss over two thumbs or a thumb and an index finger as shown in **Figure 28-3A** and **B**. Rest a side of a finger on teeth of the opposite side of the maxillary arch to provide balance and a fulcrum.
■ *Mandibular teeth:* Direct the floss down by holding the two index fingers on top of the strand. One index finger

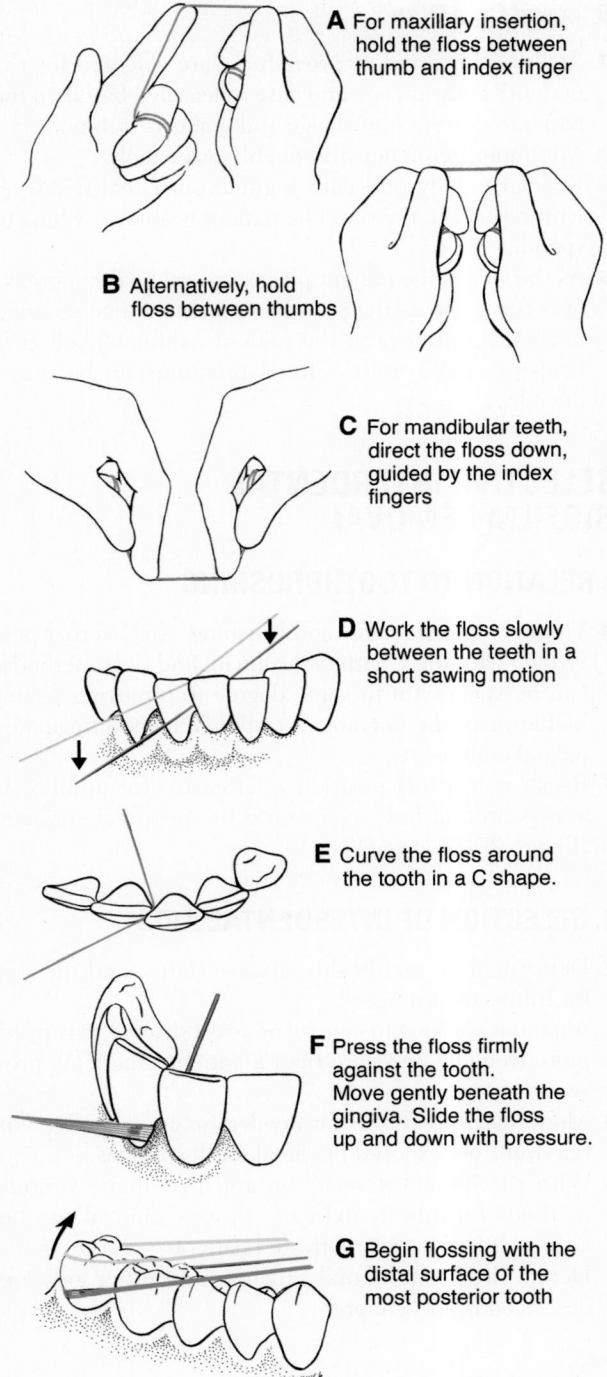

A For maxillary insertion, hold the floss between thumb and index finger

B Alternatively, hold floss between thumbs

C For mandibular teeth, direct the floss down, guided by the index fingers

D Work the floss slowly between the teeth in a short sawing motion

E Curve the floss around the tooth in a C shape.

F Press the floss firmly against the tooth. Move gently beneath the gingiva. Slide the floss up and down with pressure.

G Begin flossing with the distal surface of the most posterior tooth

FIGURE 28-3 Use of Dental Floss. For maxillary insertion, hold the floss between the thumb and index finger **(A)** or between thumbs **(B)**. Grasp the floss firmly. Allow only 1/2-inch length between fingers. **(C)** For the mandibular teeth, direct the floss down, guided by the index fingers. **(D)** Work the floss slowly between the teeth in a short sawing motion. Avoid snapping through the contact area. **(E)** Curve the floss around the tooth in a C-shape. Hold the floss toward the mesial for cleaning the distal surfaces and toward the distal for cleaning the mesial surfaces. **(F)** Press the floss firmly against the tooth. Move gently beneath the gingiva until tissue resistance is felt. Slide the floss horizontally and vertically with pressure to remove biofilm. **(G)** Begin flossing with the distal surface of the most posterior tooth, and work systematically around the arch.

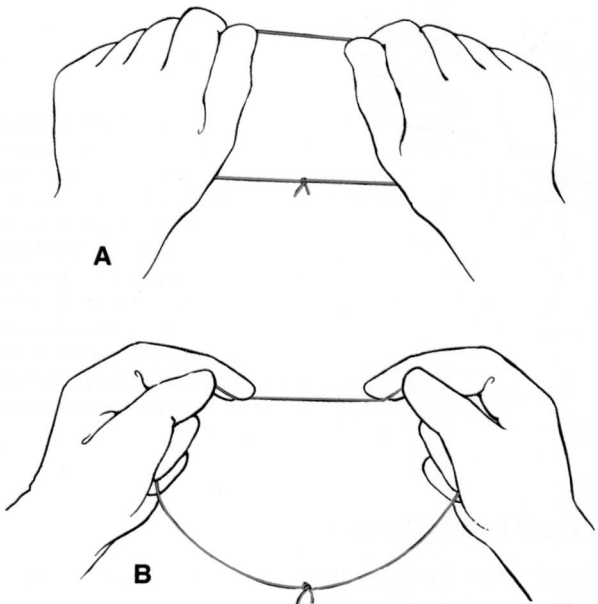

FIGURE 28-4 Circle of Floss. The ends of the floss are tied together for convenient holding. A child may be able to manage floss better with this technique. **(A)** Floss held for maxillary teeth. **(B)** Floss held for mandibular teeth.

holds the floss on the lingual aspect and the other on the facial aspect **(Figure 28-3C)**. The side of the finger on the lingual side is held on the teeth of the opposite side of the mouth to serve as a fulcrum or rest.

D. Insertion

- Hold floss firmly in a diagonal or oblique position **(Figure 28-5)**.
- Guide the floss past each contact area with a gentle sawing motion **(Figure 28-3D)**.
- Control floss to prevent snapping through the contact area onto the gingival tissue.

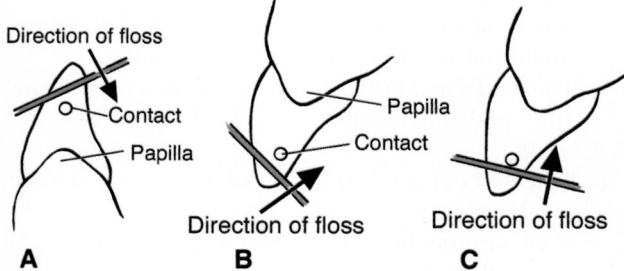

FIGURE 28-5 Insertion of Floss. Hold floss in a diagonal or oblique position over the teeth where the floss will be inserted. Arrows indicate the direction of movement of the floss. **(A)** Floss held for mandibular insertion. **(B)** Floss held for maxillary insertion. **(C)** Floss held incorrectly. When floss is held horizontally, the possibility for damage to the papilla is greater.

E. Cleaning Stroke

- Clean adjacent teeth separately; for the distal aspect, curve the floss mesially, and for the mesial aspect, curve the floss distally, around the tooth **(Figure 28-3E and F)**.
- Pass the floss below the gingival margin, curve to adapt the floss around the tooth, press, and slide up and down over the tooth surface. Repeat.
- Loop the floss over the distal surfaces of the most posterior teeth in each quadrant and the teeth next to edentulous areas **(Figure 28-3G)**. Hold firmly against the tooth and move the floss in both an up-and-down motion and a "shoe-shine" stroke.

F. Additional Suggestions

- Slide the floss to a new, unused portion for succeeding proximal tooth surfaces.
- Floss may be doubled to provide a wider rubbing surface.
- When a dentifrice is used with the floss, dental tape may be better than floss in retaining the dentifrice against the tooth.

III. PRECAUTIONS

A. Pressure in Col Area

- The col area is not keratinized and is vulnerable to bacterial invasion.
- Biofilm control of the area is of great importance because most gingival and periodontal infection begins in the col area.
- Too great a pressure with floss one or more times daily, particularly very fine floss that tends to cut more easily than thicker floss, can be destructive to the attachment.
- Excess pressure of the floss against the attachment is particularly significant in children in whom teeth are in the process of eruption and the junctional epithelium is less firmly attached.

B. Prevention of Floss Cuts and Floss Clefts

- *Location:* Floss cuts or clefts occur primarily on facial and lingual or palatal surfaces directly beside or in the middle of an interdental papilla. They appear as straight-line cuts from the gingival margin and may result in a floss cleft (Figure 14-11, page 219).
- *Causes*
  - Using too long a piece of floss between the fingers when held for insertion.
  - Snapping the floss through the contact area.
  - Not curving the floss about the teeth; holding floss straight across the papilla.
  - Not using a rest to prevent undue pressure.

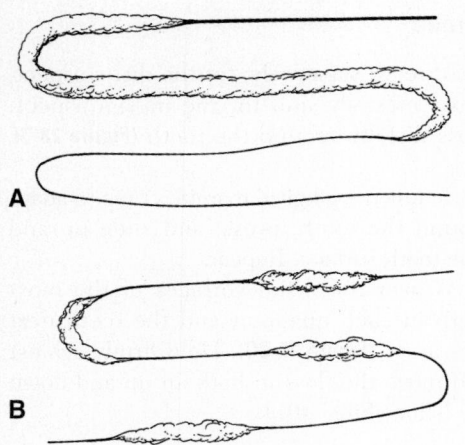

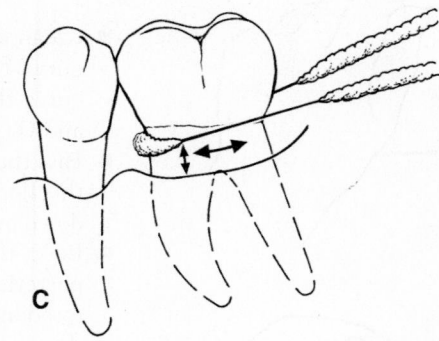

FIGURE 28-6 **Tufted Dental Floss.** The floss/yarn combination may be "Super Floss" **(A)** in a precut length with a tufted portion and a 3-inch stiffened end for insertion under a fixed prosthesis, or "NUFloss" **(B)** with tufted portions alternated with plain floss. A preferred length of "NUFloss" is obtained from the container. **(C)** "NUFloss" applied to the proximal surface of a molar. It may be used in an up-and-down and a shoe-shine stroke.

TUFTED DENTAL FLOSS

I. DESCRIPTION

Tufted dental floss is also called a floss/yarn combination. Regular dental floss is alternated with a thickened tufted portion. Two variations are available commercially.

A. Single, Precut Lengths

"Super Floss"[15] is available in a 2-foot length composed of a 5-inch tufted portion adjacent to a 3-inch stiffened end for inserting under a fixed appliance or orthodontic attachment **(Figure 28-6A)**.

B. Roll

"NUFloss"[16] is available in a roll that is similar to that of regular floss and has a cutting device to allow selection of a preferred length. The tufted portions (about 1 inch long) alternate with the plain floss (about 1½ inches long) **(Figure 28-6B)**.

II. INDICATIONS FOR USE

■ Biofilm removal from tooth surfaces adjacent to wide embrasures where interdental papillae have been lost.
■ Biofilm removal from mesial and distal abutments and under pontic of a fixed partial denture or orthodontic appliance. The stiff end of "Super Floss" is inserted; "NUFloss" is threaded using a floss threader (see Figures 31-2 and 31-3, page 451).

III. PROCEDURE

A. Individual Surface of Tooth or Implant

Curve floss and/or tufted portion around the tooth or implant in a "C" to remove dental biofilm. Move floss vertically and horizontally **(Figure 28-6C)**.

B. Fixed Partial Denture

Thread tufted floss over pontic and apply to distal surface of the mesial abutment and mesial surface of the distal abutment (Figure 31-3, page 451).

AIDS FOR FLOSSING

I. FLOSS HOLDER

A floss holder can be helpful for a person with a disability or for a parent or caregiver serving a child or patient. A floss holder is shown in Figure 56-11 (page 866) for use by a disabled person.

II. FLOSS THREADER

A floss threader is used for biofilm and debris removal around orthodontic appliances or under fixed partial dentures as shown in Figures 31-2 and 31-3 on page 451.

III. KNITTING YARN

■ *Indications for use*
  ■ For tooth surfaces adjacent to wide proximal spaces, dental floss may be too narrow and not remove biofilm efficiently.
  ■ For isolated teeth, teeth separated by a diastema, and distal surfaces of most posterior teeth.
  ■ For mesial and distal abutments of fixed partial dentures and under pontics, use a floss threader.
■ *Procedure*
  ■ Select about 8 to 10 inches of 3- or 4-ply smooth synthetic yarn.
  ■ Fold yarn double. Loop through about 8 inches of dental floss; tie floss with one overhand knot.
  ■ Insert floss through the contact area. Draw the yarn into the embrasure **(Figure 28-7)**.
  ■ Clean adjacent teeth separately with a facial-lingual, back-and-forth stroke. Hold the ends of the yarn distally and then around mesially.

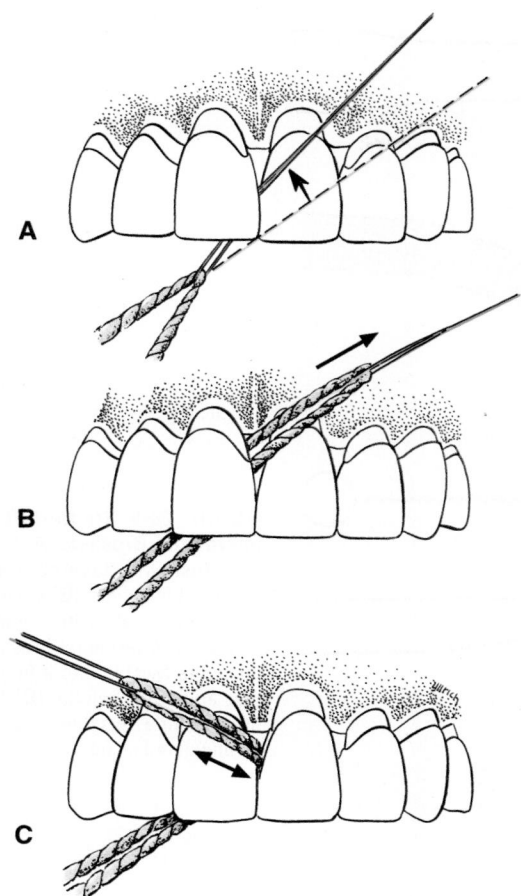

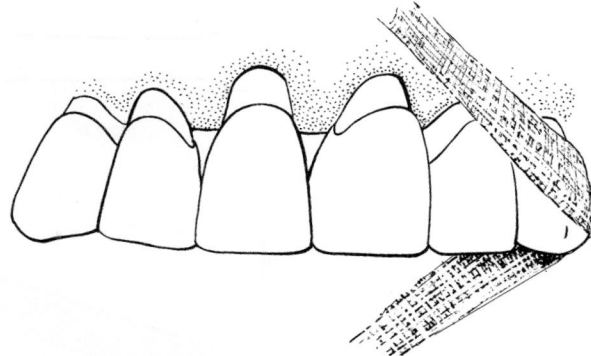

FIGURE 28-8 **Gauze Strip.** A 6- or 8-inch length of 1-inch bandage is folded in thirds and placed around a tooth adjacent to an edentulous area, a tooth with interdental spacing, or the distal surface of the most posterior tooth. A shoe-shine stroke is used to clean the dental biofilm from the surface.

- *Steps for procedure*
  - Cut 1-inch gauze bandage into a 6- to 8-inch length, and fold in thirds or down the center.
  - Position the fold of the gauze on the cervical area next to the gingival crest and work back and forth several times; hold ends in a distal direction to clean a mesial surface, and in a mesial direction to clean a distal surface **(Figure 28-8)**.

 ## INTERDENTAL BRUSHES

I. TYPES

A. Small Insert Brushes With Reusable Handle

- Soft nylon filaments are twisted into a fine stainless steel wire for insertion into a handle with an angulated shank **(Figure 28-9B)**. Select brush with plastic-coated wire.
- The small tapered or cylindric brush heads are of varying sizes approximately 12 to 15 mm (1/2 inch) in length, with a diameter of 3 to 5 mm (1/8 to 1/4 inch).

B. Brush with Plastic Handle

- Soft nylon filaments are twisted into a fine stainless steel wire. The wire is continuous with the handle, which is approximately 35 to 45 mm (1½ to 1¾ inches) in length **(Figure 28-9C)**.
- The very short, soft filaments form a narrow brush approximately 30 to 35 mm (1¼ to 1½ inches) in length and 5 to 8 mm (1/4 to 5/16 inches) in diameter **(Figure 28-9D)**.

II. INDICATIONS FOR USE

When sufficient space is available for the insertion of an interdental brush without excess force, the following applications are indicated:

FIGURE 28-7 **Knitting Yarn. (A)** Yarn is looped through dental floss, and the floss is drawn through the contact area in the usual manner, shown by the arrow. **(B)** Yarn is drawn through the embrasure. **(C)** Yarn is positioned against the surface of the tooth for biofilm removal. When tooth contact is missing and space permits, the yarn is used without floss.

- For specific areas where a papilla may be high or access is not otherwise sufficient for the wide yarn, use the dental floss end of the combination.
- Apply dentifrice and rub surface with the yarn back and forth, up and down.
- For closed contacts, use a floss threader (see Figure 31-2, page 451).

IV. GAUZE STRIP

- *Uses*
  - For proximal surfaces of widely spaced teeth. Gauze is too thick to pass through contact areas.
  - For surfaces of teeth next to edentulous areas.
  - For outer mesial and distal surfaces of abutment teeth of a fixed partial denture.
  - For areas under posterior cantilevered section of a fixed appliance, such as the distal portion of a denture supported by implants.

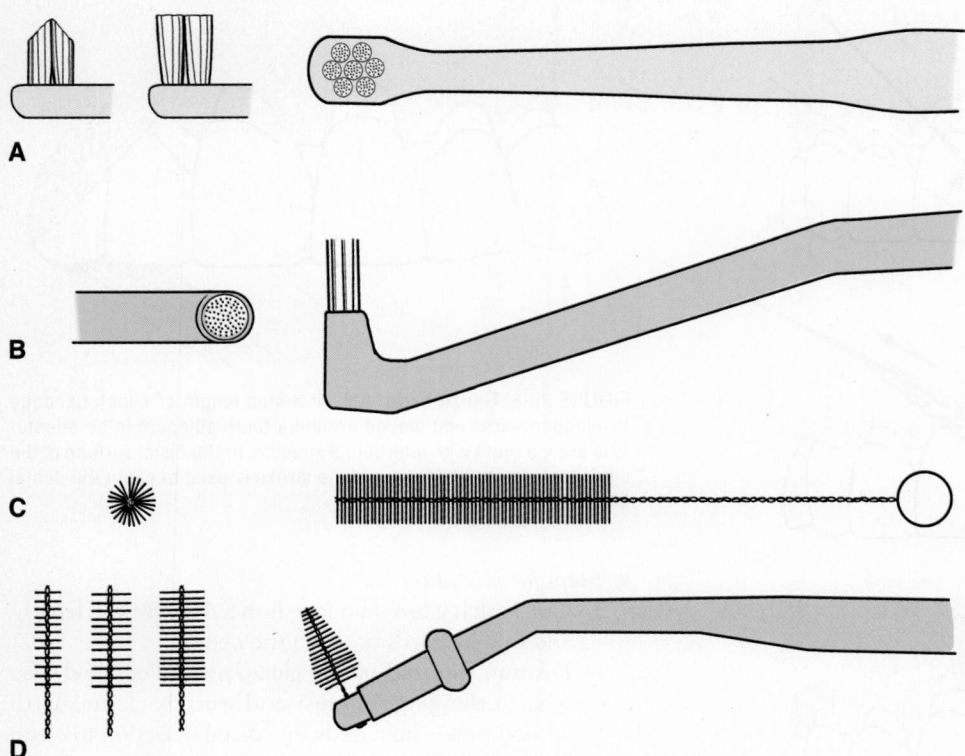

FIGURE 28-9 **Single-tuft and Interdental Brushes. (A)** Single-tuft brush with tapered and flat groups of filaments. **(B)** Single-tuft brush on handle with angulated shank. **(C)** Interdental brush with filaments twisted into a fine wire that ends in a handle. **(D)** Insert brushes for a reusable handle with an angulated shank.

A. For Removal of Dental Biofilm and Debris

■ Proximal tooth surfaces adjacent to open embrasures, orthodontic appliances, fixed prostheses, dental implants, periodontal splints, and space maintainers, and other areas that are hard to reach with a regular toothbrush.

■ Concave proximal surfaces where dental floss and other interdental aids cannot reach **(Figure 28-10A)**. Floss bridges over a concave surface, whereas the interproximal brush can reach and cleanse **(Figure 28-10B)**.[1,17]

■ Exposed Class IV furcations (Figure 16-3, page 250).

B. For Application of Chemotherapeutic Agents

■ Fluoride dentifrice, gel, and/or mouthrinse for prevention of dental caries, particularly root surface caries, and for surfaces adjacent to any prosthesis.

■ Antibacterial agents for control of dental biofilm and the prevention of gingivitis.

■ Desensitizing agents.

III. PROCEDURE

■ Select brush of appropriate diameter.

■ Moisten the brush and insert at an angle in keeping with gingival form; brush in and out.

IV. CARE OF BRUSHES

■ Clean brush during use to remove debris and biofilm by holding under actively running water.

■ Clean thoroughly after use and dry in open air.

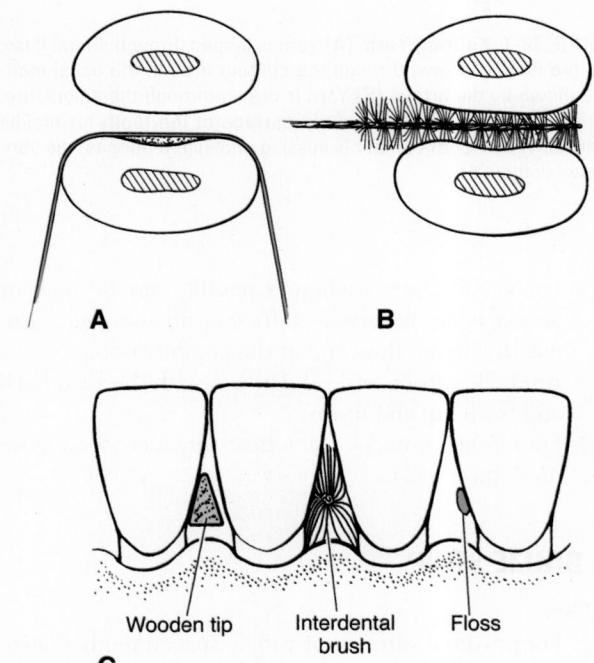

FIGURE 28-10 **Interdental Care. (A)** Floss positioned on the mesial surface of a maxillary first premolar shows the inability of the floss to remove dental biofilm on a concave proximal tooth surface. **(B)** Use of an interdental brush in the same interproximal area to show how the proximal surfaces can be cleaned free of dental biofilm. **(C)** Comparison of the access of a wooden tip, an interdental brush, and a piece of dental floss to an open interdental area.

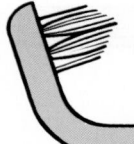

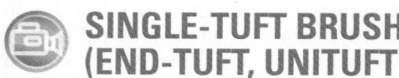

FIGURE 28-11 **Single-tuft Brush With Bent Shank.** Adaptation of brush with angulated handle permits easier access to lingual and palatal aspects of the natural teeth, as well as to orthodontic appliances, prostheses, and implant abutments.

■ Discard before the filaments become deformed or loosened.

 ## SINGLE-TUFT BRUSH (END-TUFT, UNITUFT)

I. DESCRIPTION

The single tuft, or group of small tufts, may be 3 to 6 mm in diameter and may be flat or tapered **(Figure 28-9A** and **B)**. The handle may be straight or contra-angled.

II. INDICATIONS FOR USE

A. For Open Interproximal Areas

B. For Fixed Dental Prostheses

The single-tuft brush may be adaptable around and under a fixed partial denture, pontic, orthodontic appliance, precision attachment, or implant abutment.

C. For Difficult-to-Reach Areas

The lingual surfaces of the mandibular molars, abutment teeth, the distal surfaces of the most posterior teeth, and teeth that are crowded are examples of areas where an end-tuft brush may be of value. The shank may be bent for easy adaptation **(Figure 28-11)**.

III. PROCEDURE

■ Direct the tip of the tuft into the interproximal area and along the gingival margin; go around the distal surfaces from lingual and facial of the most distal teeth in all 4 quadrants.
■ Combine a rotating motion with intermittent pressure especially in the interproximal areas to reach as much of the proximal surfaces as possible.
■ Use a sulcular brushing stroke.

 ## INTERDENTAL TIP

I. COMPOSITION AND DESIGN

Conical or pyramidal flexible rubber tip is attached to the end of the handle of a toothbrush or is on a special plastic

handle. The soft, pliable rubber tip is preferred because it can be adapted to the interdental area and below the gingival margin without causing damage to the epithelial lining.

II. INDICATIONS FOR USE

■ For cleaning debris from the interdental area and for removal of biofilm by rubbing the exposed tooth surfaces.
■ For biofilm removal at and just below the gingival margin.

III. PROCEDURE

■ Trace along the gingival margin with the tip positioned just beneath the margin (1 to 2 mm.). The adaptation is similar to the toothpick in holder **(Figure 28-12)**.
■ For additional cleaning of the proximal surfaces of the teeth, rub the tip against the teeth as it is moved in and out of an embrasure and under a contact area. Position tip with the gingival form; take care not to flatten the interdental tissue.
■ Rinse the tip as indicated during use to remove debris, and wash thoroughly at the finish.

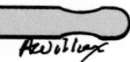 ## TOOTHPICK IN HOLDER

I. DESCRIPTION

A round toothpick is inserted into a plastic handle with contra-angled ends for adaptation to the tooth surface at

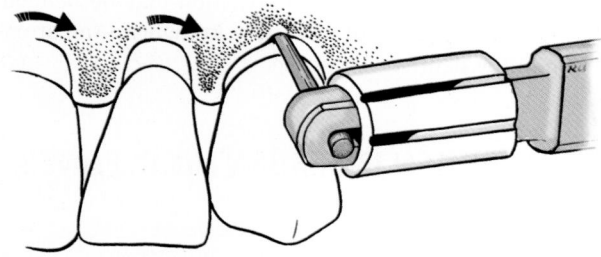

FIGURE 28-12 **Toothpick in Holder for Dental Biofilm at Gingival Margin.** The tip is placed at or just below the gingival margin. Trace the margin around each tooth.

the gingival margin for biofilm removal. The device also is called a "Perio-Aid."

II. INDICATIONS FOR USE

A. Patient With Periodontitis

For biofilm removal at and just under the gingival margin, for interdental cleaning, particularly for concave proximal tooth surfaces, and for exposed furcation area.

B. Orthodontic Patient

For biofilm removal at gingival margin above appliances.

III. PROCEDURE

A. Prepare Instrument

■ Insert round tapered toothpick into the end of the holder. One type of holder has angulated ends for use in various positions.

■ Twist the toothpick firmly into place. Break off the long end cleanly so that sharp edges cannot scratch the inner cheek or the tongue during use.

B. Application

■ Apply toothpick at the gingival margin. Apply just under the gingival margin at a slant, with moderate pressure: trace the gingival margin around each tooth to remove biofilm.

■ To remove biofilm just below the gingival margin, apply the end at less than 45°, maintain the tip on the tooth surface, and follow around the sulcus or pocket **(Figure 28-12)**.

■ Use a tip that has become soft and slightly frayed from use as a small cleaning "brush" to rub on tooth surfaces where biofilm has collected. Check for and remove loose bits of wood that could become deposited in the sulcus or gingiva.

■ For hypersensitive spots, usually at the cervical third of a tooth, the patient can use the tip daily to massage dentifrice for desensitization on the sensitive area.

■ When a contact is inadequate and the patient indicates that floss or toothpicks are required to relieve pressure from impacted food, dental attention may be needed. The area is charted or otherwise brought to the attention of the dentist.

WOODEN INTERDENTAL CLEANER

I. DESCRIPTION

The wooden cleaner is a 2-inch-long device made of basswood or birch wood. It is triangular in cross section, as shown in **Figure 28-13**.

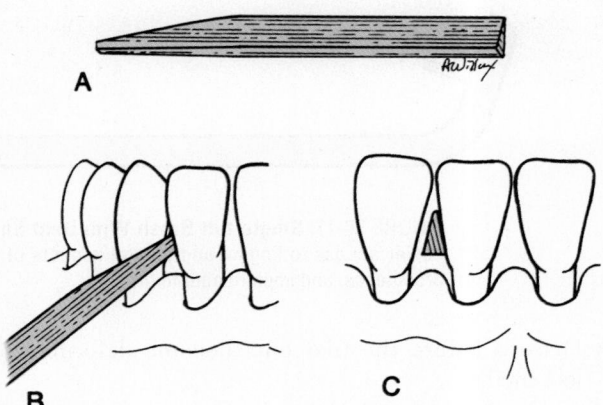

FIGURE 28-13 Wooden Interdental Cleaner. (A) The 2-inch wooden triangular cleaner. **(B)** Application on the proximal surface of a tooth with a Type III embrasure. The base of the triangle is on the gingival side. **(C)** The side of the triangle is rubbed in and out against the proximal surface to remove dental biofilm.

II. INDICATIONS FOR USE

A. Application

For cleaning proximal tooth surfaces where the tooth surfaces are exposed and interdental gingiva are missing. Space must be adequate otherwise the gingival tissue can be traumatized.

B. Limitation

■ As with most interdental devices, the wooden cleaner is advised only for the patient who follows instructions carefully.

■ A fresh cleaner may be advised for each arch or quadrant because the wood may become splayed.

III. PROCEDURE

A. Fulcrum (Rest)

First teach the patient to use a rest by placing the hand on the cheek or chin or by placing a finger on the gingiva convenient to the place where the tip will be applied. This precaution helps prevent insertion of the wedge with too much pressure.

B. Preparation

Soften the wood by placing the pointed end in the mouth and moistening with saliva.

C. Directions

■ Hold the base of the triangular wedge toward the gingival border of the interdental area and insert with the tip pointed slightly toward the occlusal or incisal surfaces to follow the contour of the embrasure **(Figure 28-13B and C)**. Do not hold the wedge horizontally because the interdental tissue can be flattened.

- When the surface feels rough, check for calculus and remove by scaling.
- Clean the tooth surfaces by moving the wedge in and out while applying a burnishing stroke with moderate pressure first to one side of the embrasure and then to the other, about four strokes each.
- Discard the cleaner as soon as the first signs of splaying are evident.

ORAL IRRIGATION

I. DESCRIPTION

- Irrigation is the targeted application of a pulsated or steady stream of water or other irrigant for preventive or therapeutic purposes.
  - The purpose of irrigation is to reduce the bacteria and inflammatory mediators that lead to the initiation or progression of periodontal infections.
  - For the patient, irrigation can be a part of routine self-care.
- Mechanical devices, including toothbrushes and interdental aids, can accomplish dental biofilm removal supragingivally and slightly below the gingival margin for the motivated patient.
  - Toothbrushes penetrate less than 1 mm into the gingival sulcus.[18]
- Benefits from removing loosely connected biofilm with the use of an oral irrigator include:
  - Reduction of gingivitis and bleeding.[19,20]
  - Reduction or alteration of subgingival dental biofilm.[21]
  - Subgingival access to pathogenic microorganisms.[22,23]
  - Subgingival delivery of antimicrobial agents.
- Supragingival and marginal irrigation are effective for removing loosely attached dental biofilm and reducing gingivitis.
- When an antimicrobial agent is used in the irrigator, reduction of the supragingival and subgingival biofilm and of gingivitis is enhanced.[20]

II. PENETRATION INTO POCKET: SUBGINGIVAL ACCESS

- The standard jet tip placed supragingivally can penetrate below the gingival margin 44 to 71% of the pocket depth.[22]
- Specialized tips used for marginal or subgingival delivery have shown penetration between 41 and 90% depending on tip use, technique, and presence of calculus.[23,24]

III. POWER-DRIVEN DEVICE

- Generates an intermittent or pulsating jet of fluid with an adjustable dial for regulation of pressure and flow.
- Delivers irrigant through a handheld interchangeable tip that rotates 360° for application at or below the gingival margin.

- Maintains steady flow or pulsations of irrigant from a reservoir.

DELIVERY METHODS

- When a standard delivery tip is directed perpendicularly to the long axis of the tooth, two zones of hydrokinetic activity are created.[25]
  - *Zone 1:* impact zone, where the irrigant makes initial contact.
  - *Zone 2:* flushing zone, where the irrigant is deflected from the tooth surface subgingivally.
- A pulsating stream has been shown to be superior to a steady stream, a fact to consider when recommending products.
- Patient-applied irrigation is divided into three categories based on tip placement and design:
  - Supragingival irrigation
  - Marginal irrigation
  - Subgingival irrigation

I. STANDARD JET TIP

A. Delivery Tips

- Monojet (single stream) **(Figure 28-14A)**
- Fractionated microjet **(Figure 28-14B)**
- Pulsating and nonpulsating

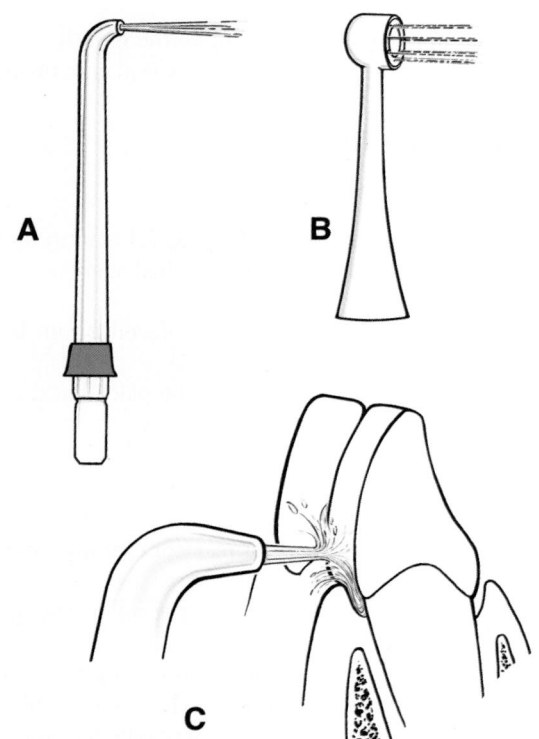

A   **B**

C

FIGURE 28-14 **Supragingival Irrigation Demonstrating Delivery of Irrigant. (A)** Monojet Tip (single stream). **(B)** Fractionated microjet tip (multiple streams). **(C)** Monojet delivery tip showing impact and flushing of subgingival area.

- Lean over the sink to allow the irrigant to flow from the oral cavity.
- Direct the jet tip toward the interdental area until almost touching the tooth surface.
- Hold tip at a right angle (90°) to the long axis of the tooth.
    This is generally referred to as supragingival irrigation **(Figure 28-14C)**.
- Increase pressure slightly over time depending on gingival inflammation and comfort.
- Follow a definite pattern around the teeth: maxillary arch first, then the mandibular, facial, palatal, and lingual.
- Pause briefly at each interproximal area.

B. Procedure

- Described in **Box 28-2**.
- Easy to do for most patients.

C. Special Instructions

- Always read and follow manufacturer's instructions regarding use of an irrigator.
- Irrigation imparts a clean feeling to the mouth.
- It is used as part of a comprehensive oral care regimen.

II. SPECIALIZED TIPS

A. Delivery Tips

- For application at or below the gingival margin for targeted delivery of water or antimicrobial agents.
- Types
    - Soft rubber tip designed to be placed 2 mm below the gingival margin **(Figure 28-15A)**.
    - Tapered plastic tip designed to be placed at the gingival margin **(Figure 28-15)**.

B. Procedure

- Identify appropriate areas for use (for example, specific pocket, furca, or implant).
- Set unit pressure on lowest setting or follow the manufacturer's instructions.
- Direct the tip at or below the gingival margin according to the manufacturer's directions. The use of a soft rubber tip or a tapered plastic tip is generally referred to as marginal irrigation **(Figure 28-15C)**.
- Activate flow of solution for a few seconds into designated area; stop flow and move to next designated area.

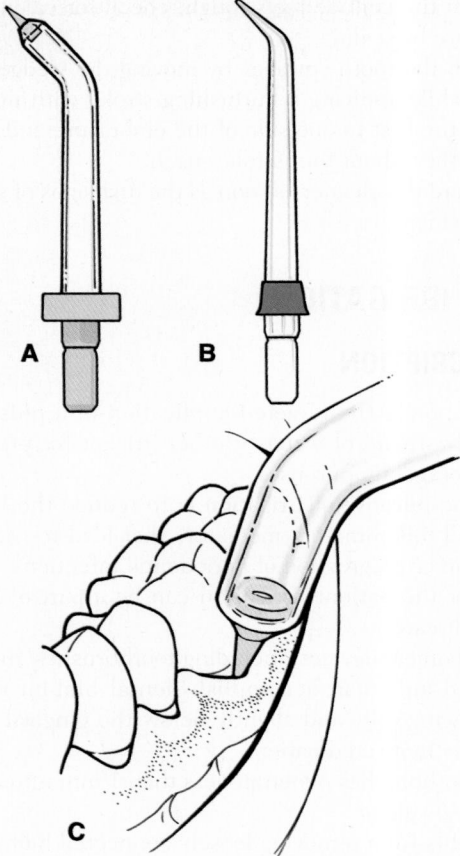

FIGURE 28-15 Patient-applied Marginal Irrigation. (A) and **(B)** Special tips for use by the patient. **(C)** Soft rubber tip designed to be placed 2 mm below gingival margin.

- When using a metal or plastic cannula, care must be given to ensure the patient can place the tip subgingivally and deliver the agent accurately and safely. Proper use of a cannula tip is considered subgingival irrigation.

APPLICATIONS FOR PRACTICE

Regular use of daily personal oral irrigation is beneficial. Even patients with good oral hygiene can benefit from the use of daily irrigation. Use a patient-centered approach to evaluate each patient individually to determine which techniques, products, or devices are appropriate.

I. ADVANTAGES OF PATIENT-APPLIED DAILY IRRIGATION

A. Reduction of Gingivitis

- The absence of bleeding is the best clinical measurement to predict minimal risk of periodontal breakdown.
- Irrigation consistently has shown a significant reduction of bleeding and gingivitis even with water as the irrigant.

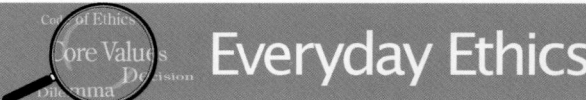

Everyday Ethics

Jane, here for a routine maintenance appointment, is excited about information she has just read on the internet about a new cleaning device for biofilm removal. She begins to ask Glenna, the dental hygienist, detailed questions about the product such as whether it really works, where it can be purchased, and how much it costs. Glenna is unfamiliar with the aid but doesn't want to be embarrassed in front of the patient so she tells Jane the product doesn't work and spends an extra 5 minutes at the end of the appointment going over manual flossing techniques.

Questions for Consideration
1. Which of the dental hygiene core values (Table II-1, page 38), have application in this scenario? Consider the relation to an ethical duty for lifelong learning.
2. From the patient's perspective, what is the role of the dental hygienist in this situation? Consider the roles of dental hygiene in Chapter 1, and Figure I-1 (page 1).
3. Is it unethical to mislead the patient about a product when the value is unknown or the dental hygienist prefers the benefits of another (perhaps rival) product? Why or why not?

B. Changes in Subgingival Biofilm[21]

- Quality of organisms, less viable or pathogenic
- Quantity of organisms, reduction in number

C. Problem Areas

- Areas that are difficult to access with traditional mechanical methods:
  - Open interdental areas
  - Malpositioned teeth
  - Exposed furcas
  - Periodontal pockets
  - Postperiodontal surgery problem areas

D. Special Needs Areas

- Prosthetic replacements and fixed partial dentures.
- Orthodontic appliances.
- Intermaxillary fixation appliances for orthognathic surgery and fractured jaw.
- Complex restorations and other extensive rehabilitation.
- Implant maintenance with soft rubber specialized tip.[26]
- Immunocompromised individuals who have an exaggerated inflammatory response.
- Ineffective interdental technique due to physical ability or lack of compliance.

II. SPECIAL CONSIDERATIONS

A. Premedication Requirement

A patient who requires antibiotic premedication for dental and dental hygiene treatment is evaluated before introducing the use of an oral irrigator or other mechanical device.

B. Incidence of Bacteremia

- The incidence of bacteremia from irrigation ranges from a low of 6% in patients with gingivitis to a high of 50% in patients with periodontitis.[27,28] This is consistent with bacteremia observed following toothbrushing and flossing.[29,30,31]
- The incidence and magnitude of bacteremia of oral origin have been shown to be proportional to the degree of oral inflammation and infection.[31] Therefore, it is imperative that patients at risk maintain optimal oral health.

C. Consultation

Contact with the patient's physician is needed when a question arises about the use of adjunctive oral hygiene aids that can create a bacteremia.

BOX 28-3	Example Progress Note

Regular 3 months maintenance. Jane came in with questions about her lower right area where she has had a lot of sensitivity since she has been using the interdental brushes that were recommended. She has had generalized recession ever since the periodontal surgery, and has perhaps been over-enthusiastic with her personal care.

    She already is using dentifrice with desensitizing agent. My main suggestion was to use the toothpaste on her interdental brush and leave some dentifrice on the teeth; not to rinse after brushing and waste the benefits especially before going to bed. Otherwise one other thing is to avoid real cold and real hot foods. Be patient, I told her, and let's see what nature will do. Your teeth and gingiva are just beautiful. I gave her a sample of another long thin interdental brush with very soft filaments to try out.

Signed: _____, RDH Date: _____

DOCUMENTATION

Documentation for a patient's interdental care progress notes need to include a minimum of the following:

■ Initially the complete health history including need or not for premedication to prevent bacteremia; extra- and intraoral examination, radiographs; and study casts if used for help in patient instruction.

■ Information for special needs concerning halitosis(with tests prescribed or given); xerostomia recommendations for oral care.

■ Notes on all personal oral care demonstrations and products recommended for use.

■ A sample progress note may be reviewed in **Box 28-3**.

 **Factors To Teach The Patient**

■ By demonstration with disclosing agent, how the toothbrush doesn't clean the interdental area thoroughly.
■ About dental biofilm and how it collects on the proximal tooth surfaces when left undisturbed.
■ How vulnerable the interdental area is to gingival infection.
■ How to use each recommended interdental aid to clean the proximal tooth surfaces.
■ To ask the dental hygienist and the dentist about new products they see advertised and whether the product should be tried.

References

1. Smukler H, Nager MC, Tolmie PC. Interproximal tooth morphology and its effect on plaque removal. *Quintessence Int.* 1989 April;20(4):249–55.

2. Gher ME, Vernino AR. Root morphology—clinical significance in pathogenesis and treatment of periodontal disease. *J Am Dent Assoc.* 1980 Oct;101(4):627–33.

3. Fox SC, Bosworth BL. A morphological survey of proximal root concavities: a consideration in periodontal therapy. *J Am Dent Assoc.* 1987 Jun;114(6):811–4.

4. Ciancio SG, Shibly O, Farber GA. Clinical evaluation of the effect of two types of dental floss on plaque and gingival health. *Clin Prev Dent.* 1992 May–Jun;14(3):14–8.

5. Abelson DC, Barton JE, Maietti GM, Cowherd MG. Evaluation of interproximal cleaning by two types of dental floss. *Clin Prev Dent.* 1981 Jul–Aug;3(4):19–21.

6. Lobene RR, Soparkar PM, Newman MB. Use of dental floss: effect on plaque and gingivitis. *Clin Prev Dent.* 1982 Jan–Feb;4(1):5–8.

7. Hanes PJ, O'Dell NL, Baker MR, Keagle JG, Davis HC. The effect of tensile strength on the clinical effectiveness and patient acceptance of dental floss. *J Clin Periodontol.* 1992 Jan;19(1):30–4.

8. Graves RC, Disney JA, Stamm JW. Comparative effectiveness of flossing and brushing in reducing interproximal bleeding. *J Periodontol.* 1989 May;60(5):243–7.

9. Killoy WJ. *American Academy of Periodontology. Proceedings of the world workshop in clinical periodontics.* Chicago: American Academy of Periodontology; 1989. p. II/11–II/15.

10. Hill HC, Levi PA, Glickman I. The effects of waxed and unwaxed dental floss on interdental plaque accumulation and interdental gingival health. *J Periodontol.* 1973 Jul;44(7):411–3.

11. Lamberts DM, Wunderlich RC, Caffesse RG. The effect of waxed and unwaxed dental floss on gingival health. Part I. Plaque removal and gingival response. *J Periodontol.* 1982 Jun;53(6):393–6.

12. Wunderlich RC, Lamberts DM, Caffesse RG. The effect of waxed and unwaxed dental floss on gingival health. Part II. Crevicular fluid flow and gingival bleeding. *J Periodontol.* 1982 Jun;53(6):397–400.

13. Beaumont RH. Patient preference for waxed or unwaxed dental floss. *J Periodontol.* 1990 Feb;61(2):123–5.

14. Masters DH. Oral hygiene procedure for the periodontal patient. *Dent Clin North Am.* 1969 Jan;13(1):3–17.

15. SUPER-FLOSS. Oral-B Laboratories, Inc., 600 Clipper Dr., Belmont, CA 94002-4199.

16. NU-FLOSS. 1311 W. Webster Ave., Winter Park, FL 32789.

17. Kiger RD, Nylund K, Feller RP. A comparison of proximal plaque removal using floss and interdental brushes. *J Clin Periodontol.* 1991 Oct;18(9):681–4.

18. Waerhaug J. Effect of toothbrushing on subgingival plaque formation. *J Periodontol.* 1981 Jan;52(1):30–4.

19. Barnes CM, Russell CM, Reinhardt RA, Payne JB, Lyle DM. Comparison of irrigation to floss as an adjunct to toothbrushing: effect on bleeding, gingivitis and supragingival plaque. *J Clin Dent.* 2005;16(3):71–7.

20. Flemmig TF, Newman MG, Doherty FM, Grossman E, Meckel AH, Bakdash MB. Supragingival irrigation with 0.06% chlorhexidine in naturally occurring gingivitis. I. 6 month clinical observations. *J Periodontol.* 1990 Feb;61(2):112–7.

21. Cobb CM, Rodgers RL, Killoy WJ. Ultrastructural examination of human periodontal pockets following the use of an oral irrigation device in vivo. *J Periodontol.* 1988 Mar;59(3):155–63.

22. Eakle WS, Ford C, Boyd RL. Depth of penetration in periodontal pockets with oral irrigation. *J Clin Periodontol.* 1986 Jan;13(1):39–44.

23. Braun RE, Ciancio SG. Subgingival delivery by an oral irrigation device. *J Periodontol.* 1992 May;63(5):469–72.

24. Boyd RL, Hollander BN, Eakle WS. Comparison of subgingivally placed cannula oral irrigator tip with a supragingivally placed standard irrigator tip. *J Clin Periodontol.* 1992 May;19(5):340–4.

25. Lugassy AA, Lautenschlager EP, Katrana D. Characterization of water spray devices. *J Dent Res.* 1971 Mar–Apr;50(2):466–73.

26. Felo A, Shibly O, Ciancio SG, Lauciello FR, Ho A. Effects of subgingival chlorhexidine irrigation on peri-implant maintenance. *Am J Dent.* 1997 Apr;10(2):107–10.

27. Romans AR, App GR. Bacteremia: a result from oral irrigation in subjects with gingivitis. *J Periodontol.* 1971 Dec;42(12):757–60.

28. Felix JE, Rosen S, App GR. Detection of bacteremia after the use of an oral irrigation device in subjects with periodontitis. *J Periodontol.* 1971 Dec;42(12):785–7.

29. Donley TG, Donley KB. Systemic bacteremia following toothbrushing: a protocol for the management of patients susceptible to infective endocarditis. *Gen Dent.* 1988 Nov–Dec;36(6):482–4.

30. Berger SA, Weitzman S, Edberg SC, Casey JI. Bacteremia after the use of an oral irrigation device: a controlled study in subjects with normal-appearing gingiva: comparisons with use of toothbrush. *Ann Intern Med.* 1974 Apr;80(4):510–1.

31. Pallasch TJ, Slots J. Antibiotic prophylaxis and the medically compromised patient. *Periodontol. 2000.* 1996 Feb;10:107–38.

CHAPTER 29

Dentifrices and Mouthrinses

TESSIE LAMADRID BLACK, RDH, BS

Chapter Outline

CHEMOTHERAPEUTICS

Recent advances in understanding the pathogenesis of periodontitis have led to alternative therapies that focus on reduction of inflammation in the oral cavity using both mechanical devices and chemotherapeutics.

- Inflammation of the periodontal tissues has an impact on the human body beyond the oral cavity, particularly in immunocompromised individuals.
- Oral inflammation has been linked to several conditions including stroke and heart disease.[1]
- Increased inflammation associated with diabetes can make a patient more susceptible to periodontal disease.[2-4]
- Oral pathogens can travel to the lungs to cause healthcare-associated pneumonias[5] as described on page xxx.
- Either the clinician or the patient can administer chemotherapeutics.
- Key words pertaining to chemotherapeutics are defined in **Box 29-1**.
- The benefits of using dentifrices and mouthrinses may be preventive, therapeutic, or cosmetic.

DENTIFRICES

A dentifrice is a substance applied with a toothbrush or other applicator for:

- Removal of biofilm, stain, and other soft deposits from the gingiva and tooth surfaces
- Application of therapeutic agents
- Superficial cosmetic effects

PREVENTIVE AND THERAPEUTIC BENEFITS OF DENTIFRICES

I. PREVENTION OF DENTAL CARIES

- Fluoride was recognized as an anticaries agent but the addition of stannous fluoride to a dentifrice was problematic owing to lack of compatibility with abrasive agents.[6]
- The first caries-preventive dentifrice containing stannous fluoride (0.4%) became available commercially in 1955.[7]
- More about fluoride dentifrices is in Chapter 35 on page 535.
- Xylitol, a flavoring agent in some dentifrices, has been shown to provide anticaries benefits.

II. REMINERALIZATION OF EARLY NONCAVITATED DENTAL CARIES

- Fluoride enhances remineralization (in Chapter 26, page 379)

III. REDUCTION OF BIOFILM FORMATION

- Agents used:
  - Triclosan
  - Zinc citrate
  - Stannous fluoride

BOX 29-1	Key Words

Dentifrice and Mouthrinses

Acidogenic: Acid-forming

Antimicrobial agent: chemical that is bacteriostatic or bactericidal.

Astringent: a substance that causes contraction or shrinkage and arrests discharges.

Chemotherapeutic agent: a chemical that is used for therapeutic reasons.

Chemotherapy: treatment of disease by means of chemical substances or pharmaceutical agents.

CHX: Chlorhexidine

Co-polymer: a substance with a high molecular weight that results from chemically combining two or more monomers

Efficacy: the benefits of a product or procedure that lead to intended results such as reduction in gingivitis.

Humectant: substance contained in a product (such as in a dentifrice) to retain moisture and prevent hardening upon exposure to air.

Hydrokinetic activity: activity relating to motions of fluids or the forces that produce or affect such motions; opposite of hydrostatic.

Inflammatory mediator: a chemical that impacts the immuno-inflammatory process causing either exacerbation (pro-) or reduction (anti-). Pro-inflammatory mediators include interleukin-1β and (IL-1β), prostaglandin E_2 (PGE_2), and tumor necrosis factor alpha (TNF-α). Interleukin-10 (IL-10) is an anti-inflammatory mediator.

Substantivity: the ability of an agent to bind to the pellicle, tooth surface, and soft tissue and be released over an extended period of time with the retention of its potency.

Synergism: process whereby the joint action of separate agents is greater than the sum of their effects taken separately.

Synergistic effect: coordinated action; acting jointly; for example, one drug might enhance the effect of another drug.

Therapeutic rinse: a chemical with therapeutic properties that is delivered by rinsing or irrigation device.

IV. REDUCTION OF GINGIVITIS/INFLAMMATION

- An antigingivitis dentifrice can contribute to the improved health of gingival tissue.
- Triclosan is the primary agent that has shown efficacy in reducing gingival inflammation.
- Triclosan combined with a copolymer of polyvinyl methoxyethylene and maleic acid (PVM/MA) increases the substantivity for 12 hours even after eating and drinking[8]
- Use of a dentifrice containing triclosan has demonstrated:[9,10,11]
  - Significant reductions in supragingival biofilm formation
  - Reduction in gingival inflammation *in vivo*.[10]
  - Inhibition of inflammatory mediators *in vitro* including interleukin-1β and prostaglandin E_2[11]

V. REDUCTION OF DENTIN HYPERSENSITIVITY

- The most effective agent in commercial dentifrices for the reduction of dentin hypersensitivity is 5% potassium nitrate.[12,13]
- Patients using a dentifrice for sensitivity are to be instructed to use the dentifrice for no longer than four weeks as it is important to determine the etiology of the sensitivity in the event it is more serious than exposed dentinal tubules.
- More information on reducing dentin hypersensitivity is located in Chapter 43 on page 683.

VI. REDUCTION OF SUPRAGINGIVAL CALCULUS FORMATION

- "Tartar-control" dentifrices have been researched with significant results.
- Dentifrices shown to help inhibit supragingival calculus may contain:
  - Pyrophosphate salts[14]
  - Zinc salts (zinc chloride and zinc citrate)[15,16]

- Sodium hexametaphosphate[17]
- Triclosan/copolymer[18]

COSMETIC EFFECTS OF DENTIFRICES

I. REMOVAL OF EXTRINSIC STAIN

- The pigments from foods, tobacco use, or chemical agents may become imbedded in the acquired pellicle and dental biofilm.
- Cosmetic results from dentifrice are based on:
  A. Mechanical removal of the stained biofilm
  B. Delivery of a bleaching agent
- Each commercially available product needs to be evaluated individually for efficacy and patient acceptance.
- More information on tooth staining is provided in Chapter 21 on page 305.

II. REDUCTION OF ORAL MALODOR (HALITOSIS)

- Delivery of active ingredients to reduce oral malodor on a temporary basis by inhibiting the production of volatile sulfur compounds (VSCs)
- Chlorine dioxide, essential oils and zinc chloride have a beneficial effect on reducing oral malodor via reduction of VSCs.[19]
- Triclosan/copolymer can control the bacteria associated with VSCs thereby reducing oral malodor.[20]
- Stannous fluoride combined with sodium hexametaphosphate can reduce VSC production.[21]

BASIC COMPONENTS OF DENTIFRICES: INACTIVES

Most dentifrices share a common composition of ingredients needed for a stable formulation. They are sold primarily as pastes and gels. The common ingredients and their function can be found in **Table 29-1**.

TABLE 29-1	INGREDIENTS AND FUNCTION OF COMMERCIALLY AVAILABLE DENTIFRICES	
INGREDIENT	**FUNCTION**	**AVERAGE FORMULATION PERCENTAGE**
Surfactant/Detergent	Foaming and cleansing	1–2%
Abrasive	Cleaning and polishing	20–40%
Binder	Thickening agent and stabilizes formula	1–2%
Humectant	Prevent water loss/hardening of dentifrice	20–40%
Preservative	Prevents microorganisms from destroying the dentifrice in storage	2–3%
Flavoring	Sweetener	1–1.5%
Water	Maintain the ingredient in formulation	20–40%

TABLE 29-2	THERAPEUTIC ACTIVE INGREDIENTS IN DENTIFRICES
BENEFIT	**ACTIVE INGREDIENTS**
Anti-Biofilm/ Anti-Gingivitis	Triclosan/copolymer, stannous fluoride, zinc citrate
Anti-Calculus	Tetra potassium pyrophosphate, tetra sodium pyrophosphate, sodium hexametaphosphate, triclosan/copolymer, zinc compounds
De-Sensitizer	Potassium nitrate, potassium citrate, potassium chloride, stannous fluoride, strontium chloride
Oral Malodor	Essential oils, chlorine dioxide, triclosan/copolymer, stannous fluoride/sodium hexametaphosphate

In addition to all of the ingredients included in **Table 29-1**, a therapeutic dentifrice will have a drug or chemical agent stated as an active ingredient for a specific preventive or therapeutic action. The active ingredient represents approximately 1.5–2% of the dentifrice's formulation. Therapeutic agents are outlined in **Table 29-2**.

I. DETERGENTS (FOAMING AGENTS OR SURFACTANTS)

A. Purposes

- Lower surface tension
- Penetrate and loosen surface deposits
- Suspend debris for easy removal by toothbrush
- Emulsify/disperse the flavor oils
- Contribute to foaming action

B. Substances Used

- Sodium lauryl sulfate USP
- Sodium N-lauryl sarcosinate

II. CLEANING AND POLISHING AGENTS (ABRASIVES)

A. Purposes

- Cleans well with no damage to tooth surface.
- A polishing agent is used to produce a smooth tooth surface.
- A smooth surface can prevent or delay the re-accumulation of stains and deposits.

B. Abrasives Used

- Calcium carbonate
- Phosphate salts
- Hydrated aluminum oxide
- Silica, silicates, and dehydrated silica gels

III. BINDERS (THICKENERS)

A. Purpose

- Stabilize the formulation
- Prevent separation of the solid and liquid ingredients during storage

B. Types Used

- Mineral colloids
- Natural gums
- Seaweed colloids
- Synthetic celluloses

IV. HUMECTANTS (MOISTURE STABILIZERS)

A. Purposes

- Retain moisture
- Prevent hardening on exposure to air

B. Substances Used

- Xylitol
- Glycerol
- Sorbitol

V. PRESERVATIVES

A. Purposes

- Prevent bacterial growth
- Prolong shelf life

B. Substances Used

- Alcohol
- Benzoates
- Dichlorinated phenols

VI. FLAVORING AGENTS (SWEETENERS)

A. Purposes

- Impart a pleasant flavor for patient acceptance
- Mask other ingredients that may have a less pleasant flavor

B. Substances Used

- Essential oils (peppermint, cinnamon, wintergreen, clove)
- Artificial noncariogenic sweeteners:
  A. Xylitol
  B. Glycerol
  C. Sorbital

ACTIVE COMPONENTS OF DENTIFRICES

Today's dentifrice selections offer a variety of active ingredients that may help prevent caries, sensitivity, biofilm, gingivitis, calculus formation, and oral malodor. The first active ingredient introduced in a dentifrice was fluoride. Since then, there have been major developments in this area. These actives provide benefits in the areas of:

- Anti-caries
- Anti-biofilm/Anti-gingivitis
- Anti-calculus
- Anti- oral malodor (Halitosis)
- Anti-sensitivity
- Specific active ingredients are summarized in **Table 29-2**.

SELECTION OF DENTIFRICES

I. PREVENTION OR REDUCTION OF ORAL DISEASE

- Dental caries
- Fluoride-containing dentifrice during remineralization program (page 383).
- Dentin hypersensitivity
- Inflammation
- Calculus formation
- Oral malodor/reduction of VSCs

II. CONSIDERATIONS FOR THE PEDIATRIC PATIENT

A. Birth to First Tooth Eruption

- Parents can clean the child's gums with a soft infant toothbrush or cloth and water.

B. Eruption of First Tooth

- Parents can begin to start brushing twice daily using fluoridated toothpaste and a soft, age-appropriate sized toothbrush.
- Use a very small "smear" of toothpaste to brush the teeth of a child less than 2 years of age. The small smear of fluoride paste is shown in Figure 49-7 on page 771.
- Children can be trained to spit out and not swallow excess toothpaste after brushing.

C. 2–5 Year old

- The parent can dispense a "pea-sized" amount of toothpaste (Figure 49-7, page 771), and perform or assist child's tooth brushing.
- Parents need to realize that young children do not have the ability to brush their teeth effectively without help and supervision.

- Parents can be role models for their child by brushing their teeth at the same time as the child.

III. PATIENT-SPECIFIC DENTIFRICE RECOMMENDATIONS

- Dentifrice recommendations are a key part of personal daily care planning and are patient specific.
- Considerations include:
  - Patient's current oral condition
  - Any patient complaint/concern
  - Sensitivities or allergies to a specific ingredient
  - Propensity of staining (stannous fluoride containing dentifrice)
  - Patient's nontherapeutic/cosmetic choices
  - Expectation of compliance. When a dentifrice does not appeal in either taste or texture, it will not be used no matter what its therapeutic benefits might be.
- Personal trial is needed before a recommendation is made. Dental hygienists need first-hand experience with each product they might recommend.

MOUTHRINSES

- Mechanical aids may not be sufficient to maintain optimum oral health for certain patients and may be supplemented with the use of a chemotherapeutic mouthrinse.
- Classification of mouthrinses: preventive, cosmetic, and therapeutic
- Chemotherapeutic rinses may have active ingredients to reduce inflammation.
- Cosmetic rinses can provide some extrinsic stain removal when it is superficial in unattached biofim.
- Delivery: rinsing can deliver an agent less than 2 mm into the sulcus or pocket and is not a delivery of choice for patients with moderate or deep pockets.[22]
- Functions: a list of general functions of chemotherapeutic agents is provided in **Box 29-2**.

BOX 29-2	Functions of Chemotherapeutic Agents

- Remineralization: Restore mineral elements
- Antimicrobial: Bactericidal or bacteriostatic
  - ☐ Biofilm control
  - ☐ Gingival health: Reduction/prevention of gingivitis
- Astringent: Shrink tissues
- Anodyne: Alleviate pain
- Buffering: Reduce oral acidity
- Deodorizing: Neutralize odor
- Oxygenating: Cleansing

PURPOSES AND USES OF MOUTHRINSES

I. BEFORE PROFESSIONAL TREATMENT

- To reduce the numbers of intraoral microorganisms available to aerosols.
- To reduce aerosol contamination during use of a hand-piece or ultrasonic scaler.

II. SELF-CARE

- As part of personal oral self-care for specific needs
- Biofilm control
- Dental caries prevention through remineralization of noncavitated early dental caries
- Prevention of gingivitis
- Contribute to malodor control
- Post-treatment therapy following scaling and root planing
  A. Periodontal surgery
  B. Removal of teeth

PREVENTIVE AND THERAPEUTIC AGENTS OF MOUTHRINSES

I. FLUORIDE

A. Mechanism of Action

- Stannous:
  - Deposit of fluoride ion on enamel
  - Tin ion from stannous fluoride interferes with cell metabolism for antimicrobial effect
- Sodium:
  - Deposit of fluoride ion on enamel
  - Cariostatic: inhibits demineralization and enhances remineralization

B. Availability and Use

- Available in varying concentrations in a dentifrice, gel, or rinse
- Uses:
  - Prevention of dental caries
  - Reduction of hypersensitivity
  - Reduction of gingivitis

C. Efficacy

- Reduction in biofilm or caries when dentifrice, gel, or rinse is used topically by the patient
- Modest reduction in gingivitis using stannous fluoride in a dentifrice[23,24]

D. Considerations

- Stannous: tooth staining; flavor
- Instruct patient to expectorate/not to swallow

II. CHLORHEXIDINE (CHX)

A. Mechanism of Action

- A cationic bisbiguanide with broad antibacterial activity
- Binds to oral hard and soft tissues
- Attaches to bacterial cell membrane, thereby damaging the cytoplasm causing lysis
- Binds to pellicle and salivary mucing to prevent biofilm accumulation
- Bactericidal and bacteriostatic depending on concentration
- Bactericidal concentrations cause cell lyses
- Bacteriostatic concentrations interfere with cell wall transport system
- The substantivity of chlorhexidine: 8–12 hours
- Antimicrobial and antigingivitis agent

B. Availability and Uses

- CHX is the most effective antimicrobial and antigingivitis agent available for clinical use.
  - Mouthrinse available by prescription in a 0.12% solution in the United States (higher concentrations are available in other countries); postsurgery for enhanced wound healing
- Recommend uses:
  - Preprocedural rinse to reduce bacterial load before instrumentation-producing aerosols
  - Before, during, and after periodontal debridement
  - Patients who are at a high risk for dental caries
  - Immunocompromised individuals who are more susceptible to infection
  - Postsurgery for enhanced wound healing

C. Efficacy

- CHX is safe and effective in:
- Preventing and controlling biofilm formation
- Reducing viability of existing biofilm
- Inhibiting and reducing the development of gingivitis[25]
- Reducing *Mutans streptocci*[25,26]
- CHX varnish is effective in:
  - Reduction of dental caries for children[27]
  - Reduction of dental caries in people with xerostomia[28]

D. Considerations

- Low level of toxicity due to poor absorption through mucous membranes
- Staining of teeth including pits and fissures, restorations, and soft tissues
- Increase in supragingival calculus formation
- Altered taste perception
- Minor irritation to soft tissues, lips, and tongue
- Chlorhexidine interacts with and is inactivated by sodium lauryl sulfate when rinsing is performed immediately after brushing. Wait 30 minutes after brushing before rinsing with chlorhexidine

III. TRICLOSAN

A. Mechanism of Action

- Bisphenol and nonionic antimicrobial agent
- A broad-spectrum agent effective against gram-negative and gram-positive bacteria
- Acts on the microbial cytoplasmic membrane, causing leakage of the cell contents, or bacteriolysis
- Antimicrobial and antigingivitis agent
- Low toxicity

B. Availability and Uses

- Triclosan-containing mouthrinse and dentifrice are available in other countries
- Available only in a dentifrice in the United States
- Recommended uses:
  - Reduction of biofilm and gingivitis
  - Reduced biofilm accumulation
  - Reduced supragingival calculus formation

C. Efficacy

- Reduction in biofilm and bleeding on probing[29]

D. Considerations

- Easily released from oral tissue binding sites such as tooth surface or soft tissue
- Combined with PVM/MA to increase substantivity and efficacy

IV. PHENOLIC-RELATED ESSENTIAL OILS

A. Mechanism of Action

- Phenolics disrupt cell walls and inhibit bacterial enzymes
- Poor substantivity
- Decreases pathogenicity of biofilm
- Antimicrobial and antigingivitis agent

B. Availability and Uses

- A combination of thymol, eucalyptol, menthol, and methyl salicylate is available as a brand name product and generic product.
- Recommended uses:
  - Individuals unable to perform adequate brushing and flossing
  - Initially or periodically to help improve oral hygiene
  - Adjunct for mechanical self-care routines that are not sufficient in reducing biofilm, bleeding, and gingivitis
  - Preprocedural rinse to reduce bacterial load before instrumentation producing aerosols

C. Efficacy

- Significant reduction in the levels of biofilm and gingivitis[30,31]

D. Considerations

- Burning sensation
- Bitter taste
- Efficacy of individual rinses based on following the manufacturer's instructions and not casual use of the rinse
- Contraindicated for current or recovering alcoholics due to alcohol content

V. QUATERNARY AMMONIUM COMPOUNDS

A. Mechanism of Action[32]

- Cationic agents that bind to oral tissues
- Rupture the cell wall and alter the cytoplasm
- Initial attachment to oral tissue is very strong, but released rapidly
- Decreases the ability for bacteria to attach to the pellicle
- Low substantivity

B. Availability and Uses

- The most commonly used agent is cetylpyridinium chloride (CPC), at 0.05–0.07%
- Recommended uses:
  A. Reduction in biofilm accumulation
  B. Adjunct for mechanical self-care routines

C. Efficacy

- Demonstrated reductions in biofilm.
- Reduction in gingivitis has been demonstrated in limited studies

D. Considerations

- Staining of teeth
- Increased supragingival calculus formation
- A burning sensation and occasional desquamation[33]

VI. OXYGENATING AGENTS

A. Mechanism of Action

- Alters bacterial cell membrane increasing permeability
- Release of oxygen acts to debride area
- Poor substantivity

B. Availability and Uses

- The common agents available in commercial rinses are:
- 10% carbamide peroxide

- 1.5% hydrogen peroxide
- Recommended for short-term use to reduce the symptoms of pericoronitis and necrotizing ulcerative gingivitis[34]

C. Efficacy

- Negligible antimicrobial effect
- Debriding agent

D. Consideration

- Prolonged use of 3% hydrogen peroxide rinses has resulted in gingival irritation and delayed tissue healing.[34]

VII. OXIDIZING AGENTS

A. Mechanism of Action

- Neutralization of volatile sulfur compounds (VSCs) that contribute to oral malodor
- Primarily a cosmetic claim

B. Availability and Uses

- The common agents available in commercial rinses are:
  - Chlorine dioxide
  - Chlorine dioxide/zinc combination
- Recommended short-term use to reduce volatile sulfur compounds in the control of oral malodor

C. Efficacy

- Mainly cosmetic

D. Consideration

- There is no clinical evidence to support the use of these products for reduction of biofilm or gingivitis.

COMMERCIAL MOUTHRINSE INGREDIENTS

Ingredients and their functions are listed in **Table 29-3**.

I. ACTIVE INGREDIENTS

- Commercial mouthrinses generally contain more than one active ingredient and, therefore, may advertise multiple claims for use.
- Factors that influence how effective an agent may be:
  - Dilution by the saliva
  - Length of time the agent is in contact with the tissue or bacteria
  - Evidence supporting the particular product
- General characteristics of an effective chemotherapeutic agent are shown in **Box 29-3**.

BOX 29-3	**Characteristics of an Effective Chemotherapeutic Agent**

- Nontoxic: The agent does not damage oral tissues or create systemic problems.
- No or Limited Absorption: The action is confined to the oral cavity.
- Substantivity: The ability of an agent to be bound to the pellicle and tooth surface and be released over a period of time with retention of potency.
- Bacterial Specificity: May be broad spectrum, but with an affinity for the pathogenic organisms of the oral cavity.
- Low Induced Drug Resistance: Low or no development of resistant organisms to agent.

II. INACTIVE INGREDIENTS

A. Water

- Makes up the largest percentage by volume

B. Alcohol

- Increases the solubility of some active ingredients
- Percentage varies from 0% to 26.9%
- Enhances flavor
- No link to oral cancer[35]

C. Flavoring

- Essential oils and their derivatives (eucalyptus oil, oil of wintergreen)
- Aromatic waters (peppermint, spearmint, wintergreen, or others)
- Artificial noncariogenic sweetener

III. PATIENT-SPECIFIC MOUTH RINSE RECOMMENDATIONS

Mouthrinses are formulated for a variety of oral benefits including mouth freshening, prevention of caries, biofilm control, control of oral malodor. Several factors are considered when making a mouthrinse recommendation including:

- Is the patient currently able to control biofilm through other methods?
- Does the patient consider rinsing a substitute for other mechanical procedures such as brushing and flossing?
- Does the patient's substance abuse history contraindicate recommending an alcohol-containing mouth rinse?
- Xerostomia could be worsened by the drying effect of an alcohol-containing mouthrinse.

TABLE 29-3	TYPICAL MOUTHRINSE FORMULATION
INGREDIENT	**FUNCTION**
Alcohol	Enhances flavor impact; contributes to cleansing
Flavor	Adds pleasantness/freshness; makes breath temporarily fresh;
Humectant	Adds "body"; inhibits crystallization around closure
Surfactant	Solubilizes the flavor; provides foaming action
Water	Major vehicle to carry other ingredients
Preservative	Preserves aqueous formulation
Dyes	Add color
Sweeteners	Contribute to overall flavor perception
Flavor	Make mouthrinse pleasant to use
Active or Functional Ingredient	Provide therapeutic and/or benefits

BOX 29-4	Steps: How to Rinse

1. Take a small amount of the fluid into the mouth.
2. Close lips; hold teeth slightly apart.
3. Force the fluid through the interdental areas with pressure.
4. Use the lips, cheeks, and tongue action to force the fluid back and forth between the teeth.
5. Balloon the cheeks, then suck them in, alternately several times.
6. Divide the mouth into three parts—front, right, and left.
7. Concentrate the rinsing first on the front, then on the right, and then on the left side.
8. Expectorate.
9. Follow manufacturer's directions on amount, length, and frequency of rinsing

IV. CONTRAINDICATIONS

- Use of a mouthrinse can enhance a patient's personal daily oral care regime. The patient needs to understand why rinsing is not a substitute for brushing or flossing.
- Some agents are contraindicated in children. Review manufacturer's instructions for age limits as they vary by product.
- Contraindicated in children younger than 6 years who have tendency to swallow instead of expectorate.
- Contraindicated in physically or mentally challenged patients who cannot follow rinsing instructions.

PROCEDURE FOR RINSING

- Many patients, particularly children, must be shown specifically how to rinse. The method can be practiced under supervision.
- **Box 29-4** suggests steps for teaching a patient how to rinse.

UNITED STATES FOOD AND DRUG ADMINISTRATION (FDA)[36]

The purpose of the United States Food and Drug Administration (FDA) is to ensure the safety and efficacy of medical and dental drugs, equipment, and devices that affect living tissue. All drugs require FDA approval. Rinses and dentifrices are classified by the FDA as either cosmetic, therapeutic, or a combination: cosmetic and therapeutic.[36]

I. BRIEF HISTORY OF THE FDA

- Oldest consumer protection agency in the US federal government.
- Officially began in 1906 with the passage of the Pure Food and Drug Act.

II. PURPOSES OF THE FDA

- Regulate drugs, equipment, and devices.
- Some devices and equipment are exempt (dental water jets, power and manual toothbrushes, dental floss) if they have existing or reasonably foreseeable characteristics of commercially distributed devices of the same type.

III. DENTAL PRODUCTS REGULATED

- Infection control products
- Dental equipment such as ultrasonic instruments
- Diagnostic test kits (i.e., dental caries detection devices)
- Prosthetic and restorative such as implants
- Surgical and periodontal such as guided tissue regeneration membranes, bone-filling material, and growth factors
- Prescription drugs, controlled and sustained-release devices, and chemotherapeutics
- In the case of dentifrice and mouthrinses, FDA has reviewed actives under over-the-counter (OTC) monographs, which are regulations that specify the active

TABLE 29-4	FDA CLEARANCE DOCUMENTATION PROCESS FOR ORAL CARE PRODUCTS	
PHASE	**STUDY TYPE**	**PURPOSE**
Pre-clinical	Animal studies	Safety/toxicity
I.	Clinical trial with small sample population (20–80)	Determine: 1. dosing/safety, 2. how drug is metabolized and excreted 3. identify side effects.
II.	Clinical trial with a larger sample population (100–200) who have disease or condition that the product is designed to treat. The test drug is compared to a standard treatment or placebo known as a control	Provides further safety data and preliminary evidence of efficacy.
III.	Clinical trial with a large sample population (1,000 to 3,000) who have a disease or condition to test efficacy, monitor side effects, and identify treatment parameters. The test drug is compared to a standard treatment or placebo known as a control	Identify possible less obvious side effects
IV.	Clinical trials on products that are already approved and on the market	Continue to measure long-term benefits, risks, and optimal protocol.

ingredients and permissible levels of those ingredients, as well as statements that the product labels must bear. However, the actual formulations of dentifrices excluding triclosan/copolymer have not been subject to any pre-market review by FDA.

IV. RESEARCH REQUIREMENTS AND DOCUMENTATION

■ **Table 29-4** outlines the documentation process for a product to receive FDA approval.[36]

AMERICAN DENTAL ASSOCIATION (ADA) SEAL OF ACCEPTANCE PROGRAM[37]

The ADA has promoted safety and effectiveness of dental products for over 125 years. The ADA Seal of Acceptance Program, which evaluates over-the-counter (OTC) products* offered to consumers, has been in place since 1930, and is internationally recognized. The program is voluntary, and products are awarded the ADA Seal only after the ADA Council on Scientific Affairs has thoroughly evaluated clinical and laboratory studies on a product, and determined that it meets the ADA criteria for safety and effectiveness, when used as directed.

For many years, the Seal Program website has provided a listing of all products that have the ADA Seal. Now there is a new Seal Program feature to help consumers and dental professionals choose OTC oral care prod-

ucts. The new feature provides detailed information on each of the approximately 300 Accepted products.

■ Each product has its ADA approved Seal Statement that lists the indications for which the product is accepted.
■ Information is included for each product on the basis for Acceptance (i.e., the data on which Acceptance is based), indications, directions for use, ingredients, label warnings and company contact information.
■ The Seal Web site also allows comparisons of the attributes of 2–6 products in a given product category.
■ This information is printable and can be used to help consumers make informed decisions about the oral care products they use.
■ It can also be useful to dental professionals in recommending OTC oral care products to their patients.
■ Visit http://www.ada.org/sealprogramproducts.aspx for more information on the ADA Seal Program and for access to product information on ADA Accepted products.

Following is information on some features of the ADA Seal of Acceptance Program:

I. PURPOSES OF THE SEAL PROGRAM

■ To help the public and dental professionals make informed decisions about consumer dental products.
■ To study and evaluate products for safety and efficacy, when used as directed.
■ To inform members of the dental team and the public about the safety and efficacy of each product that is accepted.

---

*In 2005 the ADA eliminated the Seal Program for professional products. These are now evaluated in the ADA'S Professional Product Review, which is distributed several times a year to ADA members.)

■ To maintain liaison with regulatory agencies and research and professional organizations.

II. PRODUCT SUBMISSION AND ACCEPTANCE PROCESS

■ Information required from the company
  A. Complete ingredient listing
  B. Objective data from clinical and laboratory studies that support the product's safety, and claimed effectiveness, when used as directed
  C. Compliance with specific product category; Acceptance guidelines if applicable (http://www.ada.org/3408.aspx)
  D. Evidence of good manufacturing processes.
■ Evaluation.
  A. Involves more than 125 expert consultants, members of the ADA Council on Scientific Affairs and Council staff scientists.
  B. Acceptance is for a 5-year period, after which the company can reapply for a new 5-year Acceptance.
  C. When composition, manufacturer, or owner of an Accepted product is changed, the company must resubmit for the Seal.

III. ACCEPTANCE AND USE OF THE SEAL

■ Claims of product effectiveness on labeling and in advertising and promotional materials must first be approved by the Council on Scientific Affairs.
■ The use of the ADA Seal **(Figure 29-1)** on labeling and in promotional materials must be accompanied by an ADA-approved Seal Statement.

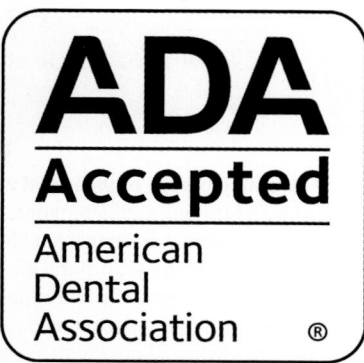

FIGURE 29-1 **ADA Seal of Acceptance, The American Dental Association, Council on Scientific Affairs.** The Seal is awarded to consumer products that meet ADA guidelines for safety and effectiveness. (Reprinted with permission of the ADA Council on Scientific Affairs.)

■ The Seal Statement tells the consumer what specific claims have been reviewed and approved, and indicates why the particular product was accepted.

DOCUMENTATION

■ Information to be documented in the patient's permanent record will include a minimum of the following:
  ▪ Recommended dentifrice and mouthrinse for personal oral care daily use: nonalcohol containing mouthrinse, antibacterial dentifrice.
  ▪ Patient instructed on proper usage including amount and frequency of use.
■ Summary of current oral findings showed need for additional demonstration.
■ Sample progress note may be found in **Box 29-5**.

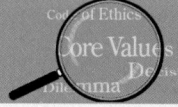 Everyday Ethics

Betty, a recent graduate, is just beginning her dental hygiene career in a private practice. Dr Dadaman, the dentist she practices with, has no particular opinions regarding dentifrices and considers one as good as the other. He requests that she simply hand out whatever sample-size products the office receives for free from visiting dental product reps. Betty has read up on the clinical support for many of the currently available products while in school and she is well versed on the differences. However, she is too shy and unsure of herself to challenge her employer and discuss the need to use an evidence-based approach to identifying the correct product for each patient.

　　When Betty gets home after at the end of the day, she reflects that maybe something that she learned in school might help her. She finds her Wilkins textbook and looks up the steps for ethical decision-making.

Questions for Consideration
1. By answering some of the questions listed in step three of the decision making steps (in Chapter 1, page 11), identify and develop a rationale to support at least three different choices or alternative actions that Betty could take to resolve this issue.
2. Discuss this scenario in the context of the legal and ethical concepts identified in Table IV-1 (page 339). Which of these concepts might help support Betty's choice of actions as she reflects on her own professionalism and determines her responsibilities in regard to making product recommendations for her patients?
3. Whatever course of action Betty takes now will likely set the course for future discussions with her employer regarding patient recommendations or the way Betty practices her profession. Which ADHA roles (Box 1-2, page 5) will Betty be filling when she determines the course of action she will take in this situation?

BOX 29-5	Sample Progress Note

Mr. Drew (just celebrated his 76th birthday last week) came on time as usual for routine maintenance using a cane for a strained ligament: "had 'small' accident 2 weeks ago." BP 117/72, extraoral/intraoral ok, nothing unusual. Perio exam: generalized firm, heavy keratinization attached gingiva and some 3–4 probing depths with no bleeding on probing. Asked about the heavy keratinization again (as I usually do) and he said he used to smoke: "stopped long time ago, and still miss it." Asked about diet he "eats lots of apples and other fruit." Checked toothpaste, and other possible oral products and he said "Mouthwash? I've used this great mouthwash every day for the past—oh—25 years—do you think that would toughen up my gums? My mouth is so dry I would think it could help."

(*Note added:* to check the alcohol content of that mouthwash (could contain high% alcohol to cause the drying.)

Signed: _____, RDH Date: _____.

Factors To Teach The Patient

- Significance of American Dental Association product acceptance seal, especially that it is a voluntary program and lack of a seal on a product does not signify it is unsafe or not effective.
- To ask dental hygienist and dentist about new mouthrinses, best way to use, and appropriateness for personal needs.
- How to avoid impulse buying with regard to dentifrices, oral rinses, and other chemical agents. To seek professional advice to avoid contraindications with oral condition and restorations.
- To understand that compliance with recommended chemical agent is directly related to expected outcomes (results or improvements).
- Why the use of chemotherapeutics is not a substitute for proper and daily mechanical biofilm removal.
- To check the ingredients of mouthrinses to prevent the purchase of high alcohol content if dry mouth is a problem.

References

1. Scannapieco FA, Bush RM, Paju S. Associations between periodontal disease and risk for atherosclerosis, cardiovascular disease, and stroke. A systematic review. *Ann Periodontol*. 2003 Dec;8(1):38–53.
2. Löe H. Periodontal Disease. The sixth complication of diabetes mellitus. *Diabetes Care*. 1993 Jan;16(1):329–34.
3. Nishimura F, Takahshi K, Kurihara M, Takashiba S, Murayama Y. Periodontal disease as a complication of diabetes mellitus. *Ann Periodontol*. 1998 Jul;3(1):20–9.
4. Ryan ME, Carnu O, Kamer A. The influence of diabetes on the periodontal tissues. *J Am Dent Assoc*. 2003 Oct;134 (Spec No):34S–40S. 8:38–53.
5. Scannapieco FA. Role of oral bacteria in respiratory infections. *J Periodontol*. 1999 Jul;70(7):793–802.
6. Mellburg JR. Fluoride dentifrices: current status and prospects. *Int Dent J*. 1991 Feb;41(1):9–16.
7. Fischman SL. The history of oral hygiene products: how far have we come in 6000 years? *Periodontol 2000*. 1997Oct;15:7–14.
8. Mariotti AJ, Burrell KH. Mouthrinses and dentifrices. In: American Dental Association. ADA/PDR guide to dental therapeutics. 5th ed. Chicago: ADA Publishing Division; 2009. Mouthrinses, pp. 213–23; Dentifrices, pp. 223–31.
9. Bolden TE, Zambon JJ, Sowinski J, Ayad F, McCool JJ, Volpe AR, DeVizio W. The clinical effect of a dentifrice containing triclosan and a copolymer in a sodium fluoride/silica base on plaque formation and gingivitis: a six-month clinical study. *J Clin Dent*. 1992;3(4):125–31.
10. Lindhe J, Rosling B, Socransky SS, Volpe AR. The effect of a triclosan-containing dentifrice on established plaque and gingivitis. *J Clin Periodontol*. 1993 May;20(5):327–34.
11. Gaffar A, Scherl D, Afflitto J, Coleman EJ. The effect of triclosan on mediators of gingival inflammation. *J Clin Periodontol*. 1995 Jun;22(6):480–4.
12. Schiff T, Zhang YP, DeVizio W, Stewart B, Chaknis P, Petrone ME, Volpe AR, Proskin HM. A randomized clinical trial of the desensitizing efficacy of three dentifrices. *Compend Contin Educ Dent Suppl*. 2000;(27):4–10.
13. Orchardson R, Gillam DG. The efficacy of potassium salts as agents for treating dentin hypersensitivity. *J Orofac Pain*. 2000 Winter;14(1):9–19.
14. Sowinski J, Petrone DM, Battista G, Petrone ME, Crawford R, Patel S, DeVizio W, Chaknis P, Volpe AR, Proskin HM. The clinical anticalculus efficacy of a tartar control whitening dentifrice for the prevention of supragingival calculus in a three-month study. *J Clin Dent*. 1999;10(3 Spec No):107–10.
15. Lobene RR, Soparkar PM, Newman MB, Kohut BE. Reduced formation of supragingival calculus with use of fluoride-zinc chloride dentifrice. *J Am Dent Assoc*. 1987 Mar;114(3):350–2.
16. Segreto VA, Collins EM, D'Agostino R, Cancro LP, Pfeifer HJ, Gilbert RJ. Anticalculus effect of a dentifrice containing 0.5% zinc citrate trihydrate. *Community Dent Oral Epidemiol*. 1991 Feb;19(1):29–31.
17. Schiff T, Saletta L, Baker RA, He T, Winston JL. Anticalculus efficacy and safety of a stablilized stannous fluoride/sodium hexametaphosphate dentifrice. *Compend Contin Educ Dent*. 2005 Sep;26(9 Suppl 1):29–34.
18. Volpe AR, Petrone ME, DeVizio W, Davies RM. A review of plaque, gingivitis, calculus and caries clinical efficacy studies with a dentifrice containing triclosan and PVM/MA Copolymer. *J Clin Dent*. 1993;4(Spec No):31–41.
19. Bosy A. A review of oral products for mouth odor. *ADHA In Touch*. 2004 Apr:4–6.
20. Pilch S, Williams MI, Cummins D. In vitro efficacy of Colgate Total advanced fresh. *Compend Contin Educ Dent*. 2003 Sep;24(9 Suppl):10–3.
21. Nachnani S. Oral malodor reduction with 3-week use of 0.454% SnF2 dentifrice [640]. *J Dent Res*. 2008;87(Spec Iss B):Abstract 2864.
22. Wunderlich RC, Singleton M, O'Brien WJ, Caffesse RG. Subgingival penetration of an applied solution. *Int J Periodontics Restorative Dent*. 1984;4(5):64–71.
23. Mankodi S, Bartizek RD, Winston JL, Biesbrock AR, McClanahan SF, He T. Anti-gingivitis efficacy of a stabilized 0.454% stannous fluoride/sodium hexametaphosphate dentifrice. *J Clin Periodontol*. 2005 Jan;32(1):75–80.
24. McClanahan SF, Beiswanger BB, Bartizek RD, Lanzalaco AC, Bacca L, White DJ. A comparison of stabilized stannous fluoride dentifrice and triclosan/copolymer dentifrice for efficacy in the reduction of gingivitis and gingival bleeding: six-month clinical results. *J Clin Dent*. 1997;8(2 Spec No):39–45.
25. Banting D, Bosma M, Bollmer B. Clinical effectiveness of a 0.12% chlorhexidine mouthrinse over two years. *J Dent Res*. 1989 Nov;68(Spec No):1716–18.

26. Grossman E, Reiter G, Sturzenberger OP, De La Rosa M, Dickinson TD, Ferretti GA, Ludlam GE, Meckel AH. Six-month study of the effects of a chlorhexidine mouthrinse on gingivitis in adults. *J Periodontol Res.* 1986;21(Suppl):33.

27. Baca P, Muñoz MJ, Bravo M, Junco P, Baca AP. Effectiveness of chlorhexidine-thymol varnish in preventing caries lesions in primary molars. *J Dent Child (Chic).* 2004 Jan–Apr;71(1):61–5.

28. Banting DW, Papas A, Clark DC, Proskin HM, Schultz M, Perry R. The effectiveness of 10% chlorhexidine varnish treatment on dental caries incidence in adults with dry mouth. *Gerodontol.* 2000 Dec;17(2):67–76.

29. Schaeken MJM, Van Der Hoeven JS, Saxton CA, Cummins D. The effect of mouthrinses containing zinc and triclosan on plaque accumulation, development of gingivitis and formation of calculus in a 28-week clinical test. *J Clin Periodontol.* 1996 May;23(5):465–70.

30. Overholser CD, Meiller TF, DePaola LG, Minah GE, Neihaus C. Comparative effects of 2 chemotherapeutic mouthrinses on the development of supragingival dental plaque and gingivitis. *J Clin Periodontol.* 1990 Sep;17(8):575–9.

31. Sharma N, Charles CH, Lynch MC, Qaqish J, McGuire JA, Galustians JG, Kumar LD. Adjunctive benefit of an essential oil-containing mouthrinse in reducing plaque and gingivitis in patients who brush and floss regularly: a six-month study. *J Am Dent Assoc.* 2004 Apr;135(4):496–504.

32. Mandel ID. Antimicrobial mouthrinses: overview and update. *J Am Dent Assoc.* 1994 Aug;125(Suppl 2):2S–10S.

33. Roberts WR, Addy M. Comparison of the *in vivo* and *in vitro* antibacterial properties of antiseptic mouthrinses containing chlorhexidine, alexidine, cetyl pyridinium chloride and hexetidine. Relevance to mode of action. *J Clin Periodontol.* 1981 Aug;8(4):295–310.

34. Weitzman SA, Weitberg AB, Niederman R, Stossel TP. Chronic treatment with hydrogen peroxide: is it safe? *J Periodontol.* 1984 Sep;55(9):510–1.

35. Cole P, Rodu B, Mathisen A. Alcohol-containing mouthwash and oropharyngeal cancer: a review of the epidemiology. *J Am Dent Assoc.* 2003 Aug;134(8):1079–87.

36. US Food and Drug Administration. FDA: Protecting and Promoting Your Health [Internet]. Silver Spring (MD): USFDA; [updated 2011 Jan 13]. Inside clinical trials testing medical products in people; [updated 2009 May 21; cited 2010 Oct 15]; [about 4 screens]. Available from: http://www.fda.gov/Drugs/ResourcesForYou/Consumers/ucm143531.htm

37. American Dental Association. ADA: America's leading advocate for health [Internet]. Chicago: ADA; c1995–2011. ADA seal and acceptance program and products; [cited 2011 Jan 14]; [about 1 screen]. Available from: www.ada.org/sealprogramproducts.aspx

The Patient With Orthodontic Appliances

ESTHER M. WILKINS, BS, RDH, DMD
MARYLOU E. GUTMANN, RDH, BS, MA

Chapter Outline

An individualized preventive program that includes a specific plan of instruction, motivation, and supervision is essential for the patient with orthodontic appliances. The patient needs to understand that much more effort is required while in treatment than was required before the appliances were placed. Terminology used in orthodontic therapy is defined in Box 30-1.

CEMENTED BANDS AND BONDED BRACKETS

Resin-bonded brackets have been used widely in orthodontic treatment. The brackets are usually placed on the facial surfaces of the teeth; however, sometimes brackets are bonded to the lingual surfaces. They aid in the application and control of applied forces necessary to accomplish tooth movement and bone remodeling for orthodontic therapy. Brackets can be metal or clear ceramic; their function is to retain the arch wire. Brackets are illustrated in Figure 30-1.

In some cases, circumferential molar bands used, for example for jaw stabilization following orthognathic surgery or when additional strength is needed to hold palatal bars, elastics, or other special devices.

I. ADVANTAGES OF BONDED BRACKETS[1]

A. Improved aesthetics.
B. Improved gingival condition due to better access for control of dental biofilm at the cervical third of the teeth.

BOX 30-1	Key Words

Orthodontics*

Aligner system: A series of customized transparent and removable aligners utilized in orthodontic therapy to align or straighten teeth.

Appliance: any device designed to influence the shape and/or function of the mouth/jaw system.

Fixed appliance: a bonded or banded appliance affixed to individual teeth or groups of teeth.

Orthodontic appliance: device used to influence growth and/or position of the teeth and jaws.

Orthopedic appliance: device used to influence growth and/or position of bones.

Arch wire: curved wire positioned in the brackets around the dental arch and held in place by elastomers or ligatures.

Band: preformed stainless steel ring fitted around a tooth and cemented in place; available in shapes for each tooth form; each band has a bracket attached on the facial side, which is the mode of attachment for the arch wire.

Bonding: process by which orthodontic brackets are affixed to the tooth surface; a fluoride-releasing, light-activated resin is frequently used.

Direct bonding: a single-step intraoral procedure in which orthodontic attachments are oriented and bonded individually.

Indirect bonding: a two-step process by which orthodontic attachments are affixed temporarily to the teeth of a study cast from which they are transferred to the mouth at one time by means of a template or tray that preserves the predetermined orientation and permits them to be bonded simultaneously.

Bracket: attachment that is bonded to the enamel for the purpose of holding the arch wire.

Ceramic: alumina ($Al_2 O_3$) used as a single-crystal material or as a polycrystalline material.

Debonding: removal of brackets and residual adhesive, after which the tooth surface is returned to its normal contour.

Elastomer: elastoplastic ring or latex elastic used to hold an arch wire in a bracket wing.

Fracture toughness: ability of bracket material to resist fracture.

Interceptive/preventive orthodontics: dental services intended to prevent the development of a malocclusion by maintaining the integrity of an otherwise normally developing dentition.

Ligature: cord, thread, elastic, or stainless steel wire used to secure the arch wire to the bracket.

Retainer: an orthodontic appliance, fixed or removable, used to maintain the position of the teeth following corrective treatment.

Hawley retainer: a removable plastic and wire appliance used to stabilize teeth; may be modified for special applications during or after orthodontic therapy.

Space maintainer: prosthetic replacement for prematurely lost primary teeth to prevent closure of the space before eruption of the permanent successors.

Space regainer: appliance used for correction of tooth displacement resulting from premature loss of one or more teeth without timely space maintenance.

Tensile: susceptible to extension; capable of being stretched.

Tensile strength: maximum stress that a material is capable of sustaining; usually expressed in pounds per square inch.

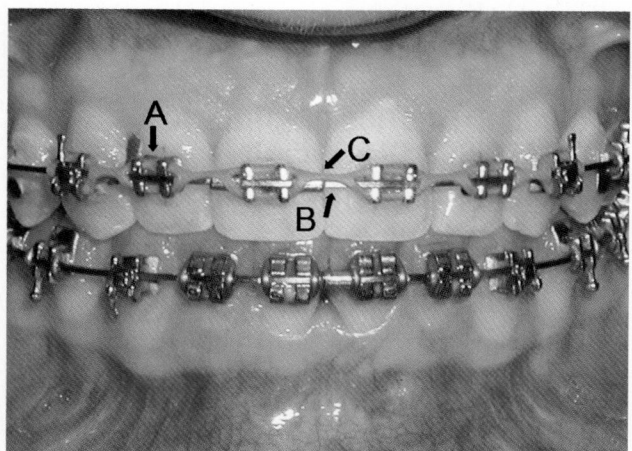

FIGURE 30-1 **Fixed Appliance System.** Bonded brackets **(A)** with arch wire **(B)** held in place by elastomers **(C)**.

C. Proximal surface dental caries can be detected and treated without bracket removal.

D. Patient can be aware immediately when a bracket loosens, whereas an unsecured band may go undetected.

E. Placement factors
- No need for tooth separation (as required for band placement); results in less patient discomfort and no band spaces to close at the end of treatment.
- Bonded appliances can be placed on partially erupted teeth, so waiting for tooth eruption is unnecessary before treatment can be started.
- Lingual brackets ("invisible braces") may be used for specially selected cases.
- Placement of brackets is faster and easier than placement of bands.

II. DISADVANTAGES OF BONDED BRACKETS[1]

A. Attachment may be weaker because less surface area is in contact with tooth. Bracket may detach more readily than a band. Bond strength is technique sensitive and also dependent on the adhesive resin selected for the bonding procedure.[2,3]

B. Rebonding a loose bracket is more time consuming and requires more tooth preparation than does recementing a loose band.

C. Debonding at the end of treatment is more time consuming than debanding, with more potential for damage to the tooth surface because of the higher bond strength.

D. Lower fracture toughness; enamel is subject to cracks.[4]

III. FIXED APPLIANCE SYSTEM

Figure 30-1 shows the bonded brackets with arch wire held in place by elastomers.

A. Brackets

- *Materials.*
  - Metal (stainless steel).
  - Plastic (polycarbonate).
  - Plastic with metal reinforcements.
  - Ceramic.
- *Forms.* Brackets are made in many styles, shapes, and sizes for different teeth, each designed to accomplish a specific objective of treatment. The basic forms are single or twin, as illustrated in **Figure 30-2**.
- *Base.* The base of the bracket is prepared with a mesh backing to assist in retaining the resin bonding agent. The mesh backing, or bonding pad as it is also called, is made to the exact size of the bracket so that no area of tooth is left uncovered where demineralization can occur. Mesh backings retain less dental biofilm than do other types of backings.[5,6]

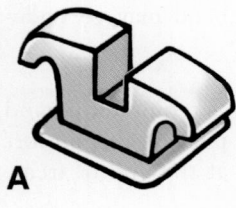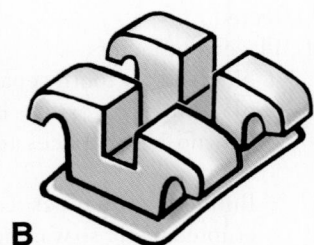

FIGURE 30-2 Orthodontic Brackets. (A) Single bracket with an incisal and a cervical wing. **(B)** Twin, or Siamese, bracket with two wings on each side of the central groove where the arch wire is held. The shape and style of each bracket vary with the tooth on which the bracket will be located.

B. Arch Wire

- The arch wire is used to generate and distribute forces that guide orthodontic tooth movement.
- Arch wires are made of stainless steel or an alloy of chromium or titanium, and they may be round, rectangular, or multistranded. The arch wire is illustrated in **Figure 30-1**.

C. Elastomers

An elastomer is used for the following:

- Hold wires in the brackets **(Figure 30-1)**.
- Apply force to close spaces between teeth.

CLINICAL PROCEDURES FOR BONDING[1,7,8]

I. ASSESSMENT EXAMINATION

Before bonding, documentation of any irregularities of the patient's teeth, such as white spots or cracks, is required to prevent misunderstanding by the patient after debonding.[9]

II. PROCEDURAL STEPS

A. The principles described in Chapter 36, page 545, for pit and fissure sealants apply for bonding orthodontic brackets.

B. Details are not included here, except to point out that calculus must be completely removed and the gingiva healed. Polishing the enamel surface before etching is unnecessary to achieve an acceptable bond.[10]

C. Follow procedures listed in Chapter 36, page 547, for sealant application. After bonding, the area around the bracket is cleaned of excess resin.

III. CHARACTERISTICS OF BONDING RELATING TO DEBONDING

A. Nature of the Bond

- The acid etch exposes the prism structure and creates microclefts, as illustrated in Figure 36-1 (page 544).
- The average depth of the microclefts ranges from 50 to 80 mm.[11–13]
- Some fine tag extensions have been observed to depths of 100 to 170 mm.[13]
- On the bracket side, the resin becomes locked into the mesh base.

B. Effect of Filler Particles

- Physical property values increase from unfilled to heavily filled resins. Fillers increase bond strength, hardness, and wear resistance.
- Heavily filled resins (composites) perform better for the posterior teeth because posterior attachments are subject to high forces of mastication.
- Ease of debonding can be related to the type of resin and length of etching time. Heavily filled composites are thicker and less viscous; they may be more difficult to remove.[2] When etching time is decreased from 60 seconds to 15 seconds, less adhesive resin remains on the teeth.[3] This shorter etching time makes the enamel surface less retentive, but it is adequate for orthodontic bonding.[3]
- The bond is stronger when a smaller (thinner) layer of resin is placed between the tooth surface and the bracket.
- In summary, anterior brackets may be bonded with a lightly filled resin, whereas posterior teeth may need a heavily filled resin to prevent detachment.

IV. USE OF FLUORIDE-RELEASING BONDING SYSTEM

- Demineralization around brackets can result in a serious caries problem for even the most conscientious patient.
- Use of fluoride-releasing bonding systems such as glass ionomers[14] have been shown to have positive preventive results.[15–17]

DENTAL HYGIENE CARE

- The patient may be under care with regular appointments for a long period, frequently over a few years.
- Periodic communication between the patient's referring dentist and dental hygienist is required to coordinate instruction along with other essential dental and dental hygiene care.

I. COMPLICATING FACTORS: RISK FACTORS

A. Age Groups

- Many orthodontic patients are in the preteen and teenage years, periods when the incidence of gingivitis is high. The incidence of periodontal infection increases from early childhood to late teenage years.
- There is a significant increase in the number of adult patients seeking orthodontic treatment. As with younger patients, the risk factors for caries and periodontal diseases increase.
- The adult orthodontic patient may be taking medications or have a systemic issue that can complicate therapy.

B. Gingivitis

- Dental biofilm retention by orthodontic appliances leads to gingivitis.
- The degree can vary from slight to severe with gingival enlargement, particularly of the interdental papillae.
- The tissue may greatly enlarge and cover the fixed appliance. The enlarged tissue with pockets provides additional biofilm-retentive areas.

C. Position of Teeth

- Teeth that are irregularly positioned are more susceptible to the retention of bacterial deposits and are more difficult to clean.
- With the severe malocclusions presented by orthodontic patients at the outset, this factor becomes even more significant.

D. Problems With Appliances

- Orthodontic appliances retain biofilm and debris.
- Accidents may cause a bracket to become detached.

E. Self-Care Is Difficult

- Even the patient who tries to maintain oral cleanliness has difficulty. The appliances are in the way and interfere with the application of the toothbrush and other devices used for dental biofilm control.
- Instruction needs to be very specific and reviewed at each appointment.

II. DISEASE CONTROL

A rigid program for dental caries and periodontal disease control is needed. The selection of biofilm control procedures for an individual patient is determined by the anatomic features of the gingiva, the position of the teeth, and the type and position of the orthodontic appliance.

A. General Instructions

- Give instructions before appliances are placed. Every attempt is made to have the oral tissues in health and the patient motivated to perform thorough daily biofilm removal before treatment starts.
- Perform brushing before a mirror so that brush application is accurate and brushing is thorough.
- Use a disclosing solution rinse to assist in self-evaluation. A patient wearing an orthodontic appliance may experience difficulty in chewing disclosing wafers without discomfort or pain. Also, it may be difficult to remove disclosing solution stains from the bonding resin.

■ Recommend an approved fluoride dentifrice to aid in dental caries control.

■ Recommend an approved mouthrinse to aid in dental caries control and periodontal inflammation control.

■ Place emphasis in brushing on sulcular brushing and cleaning the area between the orthodontic bands and brackets and the gingiva.

B. Toothbrushing: Brush Selection

■ *Power brush.* Used with soft filaments, a light stroke, and at a low speed, power brushes have been shown to be very effective for maintaining gingival health and cleaning around appliances.

■ Figure 27-9 (page 400) shows various designs of power brushes, including one designed especially for orthodontic use that has a pointed brush tip.

■ *Manual brush*

   ■ Soft brush. A soft brush with end-rounded filaments is recommended.

   ■ Bilevel. A special bilevel orthodontic brush designed with spaced rows of soft nylon filaments and a shorter middle row that can be applied directly over the appliance is shown in **Figure 30-3**. It is used with a short horizontal stroke.

C. Brushing Procedure

■ *Sulcular brushing.* A sulcular method is needed by most patients for cleaning the appliances and maintaining

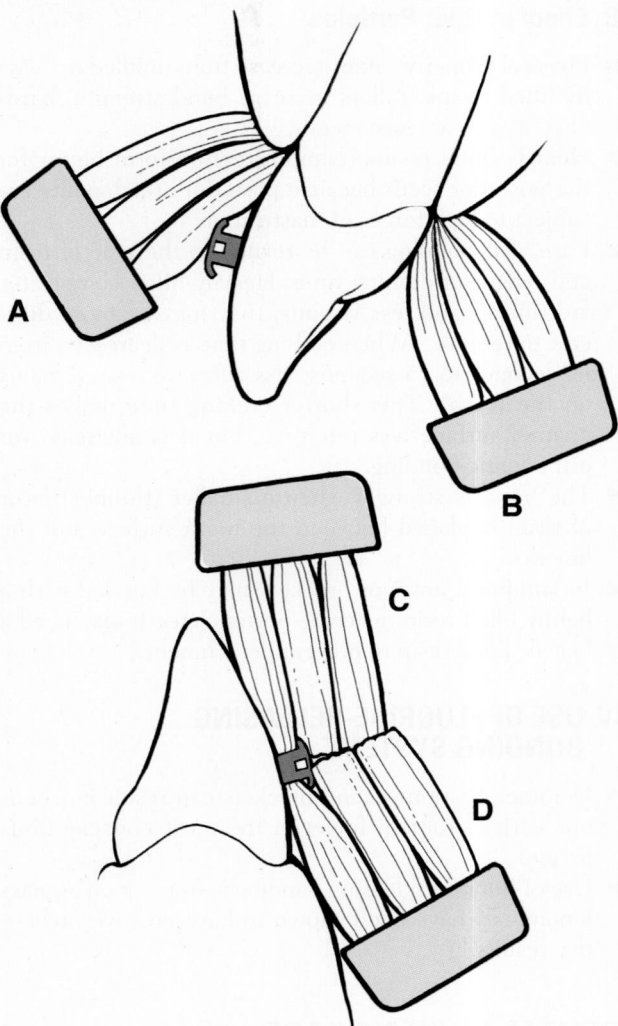

FIGURE 30-4 **Toothbrushing for Orthodontic Appliance. (A)** and **(B)** Sulcular brushing for periodontal tissues. **(C)** Brush in Stillman position for occlusal side of bracket and arch wire. **(D)** Cleaning the gingival side of bracket using brush in Charters brushing position.

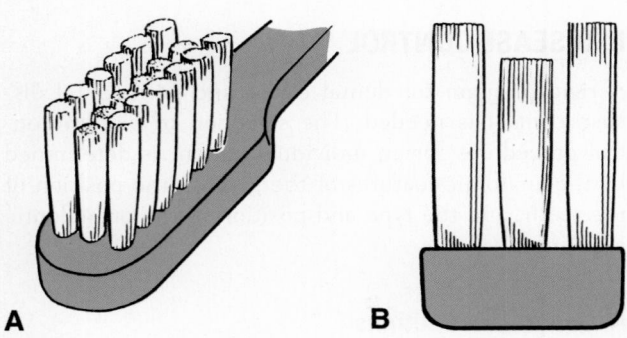

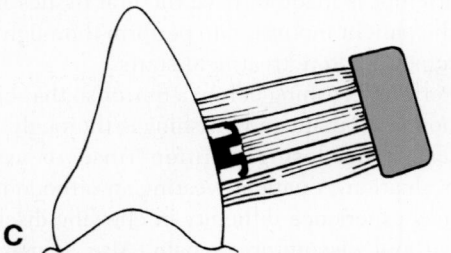

FIGURE 30-3 **Orthodontic Bilevel Toothbrush. (A)** Middle row of filaments trimmed shorter to fit over a fixed appliance. **(B)** Cross section. **(C)** Brush held over a bracket.

the gingiva. Power brushes are adapted for sulcular as well as any other brushing procedures.

■ *Adapt for appliance.* Special adaptation is required for facial surfaces. Place the brush with filament ends directed toward the occlusal surface (Charters' position, **Figure 30-4D**) to clean under the wire and bracket for mandibular arch) place in Stillman position for the opposite side **(Figure 30-4C)**.

■ *Clean all surfaces.* To ensure cleanliness, one needs to brush the appliances in any way that the filaments can be manipulated. Insert the brush from below, over, and above the arch wire; rotate and vibrate to remove biofilm and debris.

■ *Lingual and palatal.* Approach to brushing is similar to the basic strokes used on the facial surfaces.

D. Additional Measures

■ The entire system is kept as simple as possible; it is a challenge to find the most effective therapeutic aid that the patient will use.

■ When suggesting a new aid, be sure to eliminate one that did not work well for the patient.

■ Document changes to the oral care plan in the patient's chart.

■ *Interdental aids.* A floss threader is needed for biofilm removal from proximal tooth surfaces when the appliance prevents passage of floss from the occlusal aspect. Tufted dental floss used in the floss threader can remove the biofilm more efficiently than can regular dental floss.

■ An interdental brush and a single-tuft brush can be particularly beneficial around individual teeth. Premounted interdental brushes can provide access to areas around and under the arch wires and come in a container that is easy for patients to use away from home.

■ A rubber tip can be helpful in dislodging biofilm under brackets.

■ *Oral irrigation.* Most patients who wear orthodontic appliances can benefit from the regular use of water irrigation for removal of loose dental biofilm and food debris and prevention of gingival inflammation. Oral irrigation before brushing is recommended so that the debris is removed to provide access to enamel surfaces for the fluoride dentifrice.

E. Dental Hygiene Instrumentation

1. It is difficult to instrument manually around orthodontic bands and brackets. The use of an ultrasonic or sonic scaler can be helpful.

2. The use of an air polisher is indicated since the bands and brackets can tear polishing cups and the agent is less abrasive than polishing paste.

COMPLETION OF THERAPY

■ At the completion of therapy, patients are excited and are looking forward to the removal of the appliances. They may forget posttreatment instructions that are essential.

■ With this in mind, the dental hygienist provides written as well as verbal instructions on dental biofilm removal, the fluoride regimen, diet, care of the retainer, and follow-up appointments with the orthodontist and general practitioner.

■ In addition, a description and careful explanation of each step in the procedure for debanding and debonding will alleviate patient apprehension about the process.

■ Retained excess resin is biofilm retentive, irritating to oral tissues, unsightly and it must be removed.

CLINICAL PROCEDURES FOR DEBANDING

I. BAND REMOVAL

Bands are generally removed with orthodontic band-removing pliers.

II. CEMENT REMOVAL

Cement remaining on the teeth following band removal can be removed with an ultrasonic scaler.

CLINICAL PROCEDURES FOR DEBONDING

I. METHOD TYPES

■ Mechanical, electrothermal, laser, and ultrasonic methods have been studied in an attempt to determine which method is the most efficient and effective, provides the least discomfort for the patient, and causes the least damage to enamel.[18–22]

■ Debonding with a CO_2 or YAG laser has shown promise but is still in the experimental stage.[19,23]

II. REMOVAL OF RESIDUAL RESIN ADHESIVE

A. Procedure Objectives

■ Remove resin bulk.
■ Minimize damage to pulpal tissue.
■ Avoid damage to enamel surface.
■ Prevent excess enamel loss.

B. Examination

■ Varying amounts of resin remain after the bracket is removed, particularly in normal anatomic grooves, as shown in **Figure 30-5**.

■ During debonding, frequent examination is necessary using visual and tactile methods.

■ **Box 30-2** contains a summary of the steps necessary for complete removal of the orthodontic adhesive resin.

C. Identification of Residual Resin

■ Patient reports feeling roughness with the tongue.

■ Visual. When dry, the resin appears dull and opaque compared with clean, shiny enamel. Use of disclosing solution will also enhance the visibility of the adhesive resin remnant.[24]

■ Tactile. Application of an explorer reveals a rough surface, sometimes with catches along the margin of a resin tag. Filler particles from the resin may abrade the metal explorer tip, leaving a gray line on the resin surface.

■ *Use of loupes for magnification of the tooth surface.* A more accurate evaluation of the enamel surface can be made.

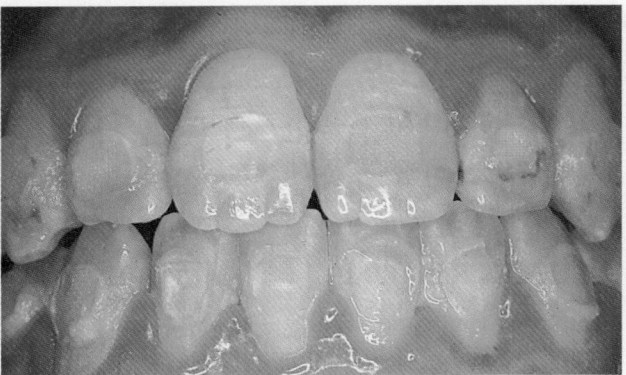

FIGURE 30-5 **Facial View of Anterior Teeth With Adhesive Resin Remaining Following Removal of Orthodontic Brackets.** (Reprinted with permission Gutmann ME. Composite adhesive resin removal following orthodontic treatment. *J Pract Hyg*. 1996 May-Jun;5:16.)

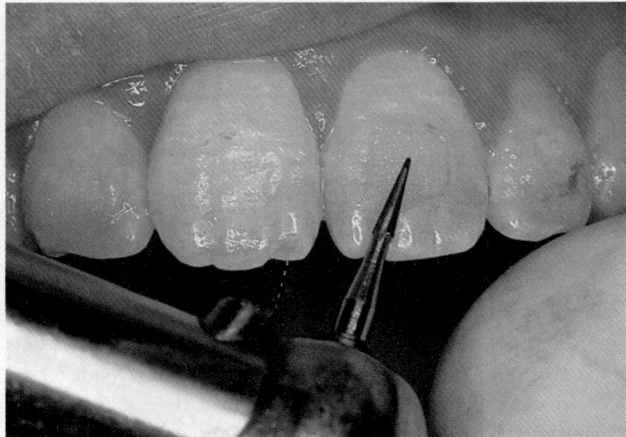

FIGURE 30-6 **Use of Tapered, Tungsten-Carbide Finishing Bur on Low-Speed Handpiece to Remove Bulk of Adhesive Resin.** (Reprinted with permission from *Journal of Practical Hygiene*. Gutmann ME. Composite adhesive resin removal following orthodontic treatment. *J Pract Hyg*. 1996 May-Jun;5:16.)

D. Removal of Resin from Tooth Surface[24,25]

- *Bur selection*. Use a tapered, plain-cut, tungsten-carbide finishing bur with a low-speed handpiece, as illustrated in **Figure 30-6**.
- *Speed*. Use low speed to control heat.
- *Stroke*. Use a smooth, evenly applied, light brush stroke in one direction to prevent faceting.
- *Direction*. Work systematically from cervical portion of the resin; move toward incisal or occlusal third. When removed, the resin resembles fine white shavings, as seen in **Figure 30-7**.
- *Evaluate frequently* to prevent overinstrumentation, rinse frequently, dry, and evaluate the surface. The resin will appear opaque in contrast to the glossy enamel. Reapply disclosing solution as necessary to visualize small remaining resin particles. Patients may also be helpful in identifying resin remnants with their tongues.

E. Final Finish

- *Objective*
  A. Restore pretreatment enamel surface finish.
- Examination
  - Perform visual and tactile examination to distinguish areas of normal enamel from irregularities.
  - Request patients to examine their teeth by slowly sliding the tongue over the enamel surfaces.

Box 30-2	**Steps for Orthodontic Adhesive Resin Removal Using Burs and Polishing Instruments**

1. Identify the location and extent of the resin with an explorer, disclosing solution, and patient feedback.
2. Using a tapered, tungsten-carbide finishing bur in a low-speed handpiece, move the bur from the cervical to incisal/occlusal portion of the resin in a light, brushlike stroke.
3. Evaluate progress frequently by rinsing and drying the tooth surfaces.
4. Polish each surface with aluminum oxide polishing points followed by aluminum oxide polishing cups.
5. Use a rubber cup in a slow-speed handpiece to polish each surface with a fine pumice slurry. Use intermittent strokes.
6. Use a brown polishing cup in a slow-speed handpiece to polish the enamel surfaces.
7. Use a green polishing cup in a slow-speed handpiece to provide the final finish to the enamel surfaces.

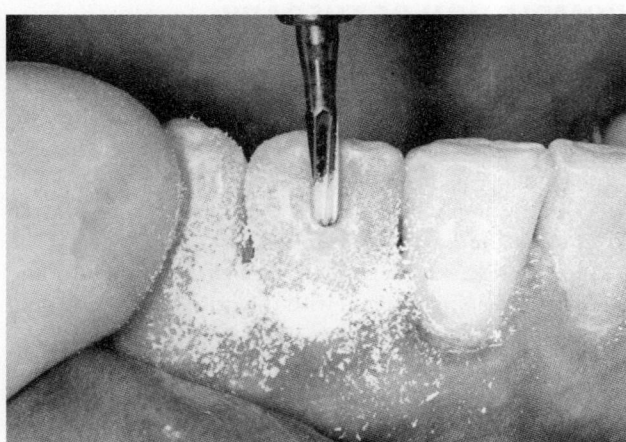

FIGURE 30-7 **Adhesive Shavings Following Use of Bur.** (Reprinted with permission from Gutmann ME. Debonding orthodontic adhesives. *J Dent Hyg*. 1985 Aug;59:369.)

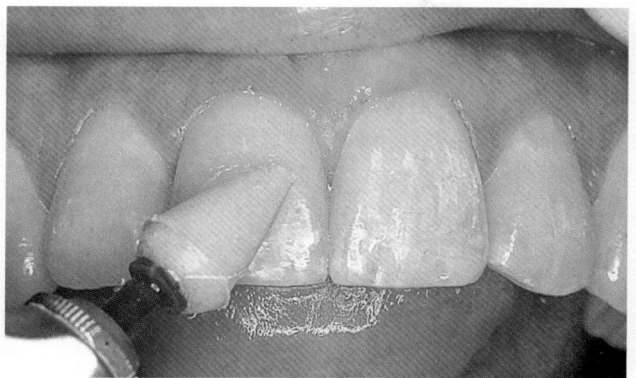
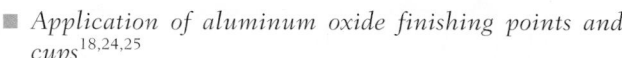

FIGURE 30-8 **Aluminum Oxide Finishing Point to Remove Any Enamel Scarring Resulting From Bur.** (Reprinted with permission from *Journal of Practical Hygiene.* Gutmann ME. Composite adhesive resin removal following orthodontic treatment. *J Pract Hyg.* 1996 May-Jun;5:16.)

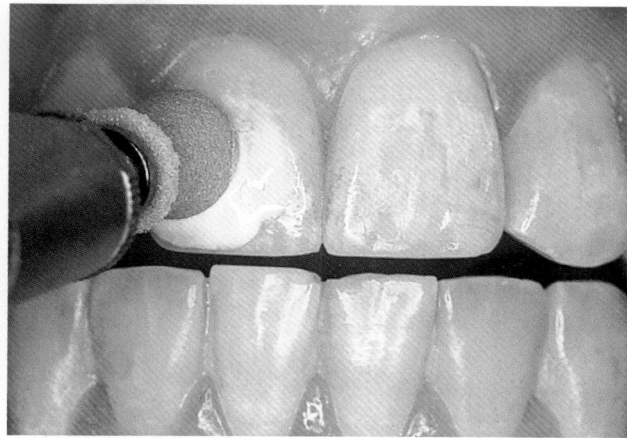

FIGURE 30-10 **Polishing With Fine Pumice Slurry and Rubber Cup.** (Reprinted with permission from *Journal of Practical Hygiene.* Gutmann ME. Composite adhesive resin removal following orthodontic treatment. *J Pract Hyg.* 1996 May-Jun;5:16.)

- *Application of aluminum oxide finishing points and cups*[18,24,25]
  - Use the finishing points first to remove any fine scarring resulting from the burs **(Figure 30-8)**.
  - Use a low-speed handpiece.
  - Follow with aluminum oxide cups and move from area to area in a cervical to incisal/occlusal direction **(Figure 30-9)**.
- *Application of the rubber cup*
  - Use a fine pumice water slurry, as seen in **Figure 30-10**.
  - Polish in a wet field to prevent overheating.
  - Use intermittent strokes to avoid overheating and move from tooth to tooth.
- *Final polish*
  - Use brown followed by green polishing cups to produce a natural-appearing, glossy enamel surface **(Figures 30-11 and 30-12)**.[25]

POST-DEBONDING EVALUATION

- Each step of bonding and debonding has a deleterious effect on the enamel surface.
- Realization that the enamel surface can be damaged can help the clinician avoid unnecessary trauma during the various procedures.

I. ENAMEL LOSS

- Total enamel loss from etching, bracket removal, residual resin removal, surface finishing, and application of pumice averages approximately 30–100 μm.[13,23,26,27] One laboratory study reported an average loss of enamel of only 7.4 μm with careful use of a tungsten-carbide finishing bur.[28]
- Enamel loss is greater when filled resins (composites) are used for bonding than when unfilled resins are

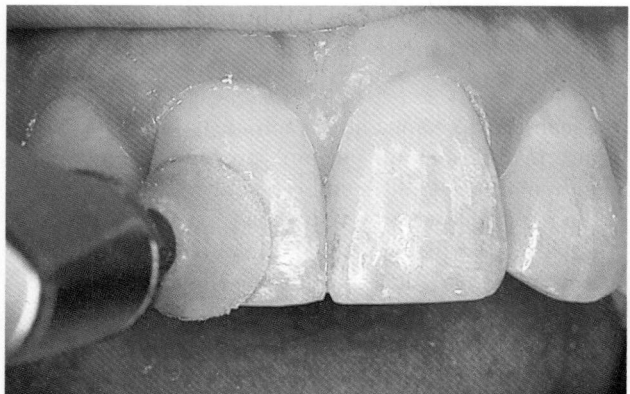

FIGURE 30-9 **Aluminum Oxide Finishing Cup to Remove Any Enamel Scarring Resulting From Bur.** (Reprinted with permission from *Journal of Practical Hygiene.* Gutmann ME. Composite adhesive resin removal following orthodontic treatment. *J Pract Hyg.* 1996 May-Jun;5:16.)

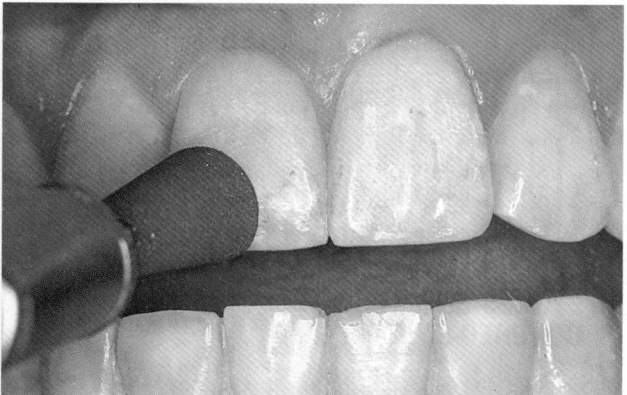

FIGURE 30-11 **Brown Polishing Cup Provides Maximum Gloss to Enamel Surface.** (Reprinted with permission from *Journal of Practical Hygiene.* Gutmann ME. Composite adhesive resin removal following orthodontic treatment. *J Pract Hyg.* 1996 May-Jun;5:16.)

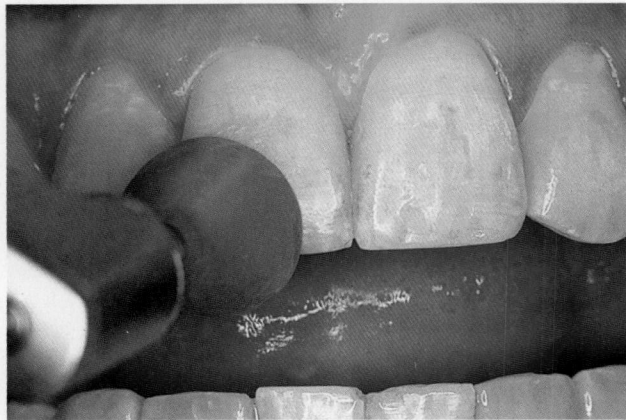

FIGURE 30-12 **Final Polishing With Green Polishing Cup.** (Reprinted with permission from *Journal of Practical Hygiene.* Gutmann ME. Composite adhesive resin removal following orthodontic treatment. *J Pract Hyg.* 1996 May-Jun;5:16.)

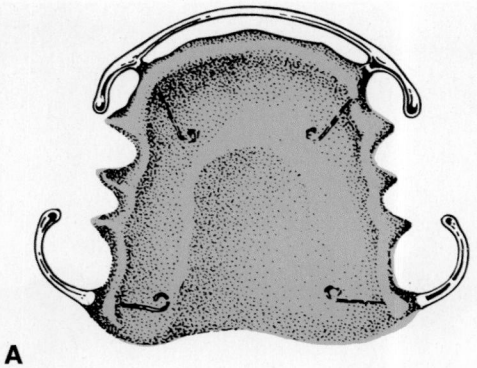

A

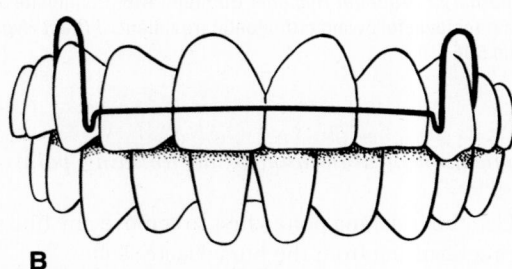

B

FIGURE 30-13 **Hawley Retainer. (A)** Removable acrylic retainer with facial retaining wire and clasps to be worn after removal of a fixed orthodontic appliance. **(B)** Anterior view shows a Hawley appliance in position. The method for cleaning the appliance is similar to that for cleaning a removable denture.

used. The loss is also greater when a rotating bristle brush rather than a rubber cup is used with the abrasive for finishing.

■ The outer layer of enamel is the most significant. The fluoride-rich surface enamel is approximately 50 μm deep. Without care during debonding, the entire protective layer can be removed.

■ When multiple bonding and debonding procedures are done, such as when a bracket becomes detached, the enamel loss is compounded. As much as 72 μm of enamel may be lost during a complete multiple procedure.[27]

■ The need for careful selection of instruments and abrasives, along with minimal instrumentation, to prevent unnecessary enamel loss is apparent.

II. DEMINERALIZATION (WHITE SPOTS)

■ White demineralization areas or dental caries have been relatively common findings after orthodontic treatment.

■ Patients with teeth that have been banded or bonded tend to develop these areas significantly more often than do patients who have not had orthodontic therapy.

■ Dental biofilm retention on the appliances and the resin, along with the difficulty of biofilm removal by the patient, contribute to demineralization and dental caries.

III. ETCHED ENAMEL NOT COVERED BY ADHESIVE

■ Surface areas etched but not covered with adhesive resin become remineralized when the fluoride contact is high through personal and professional applications.

■ Etched enamel has a high fluoride uptake.

RETENTION

After fixed appliances have been removed, a retainer is worn to give support to the teeth while the bone and other supporting tissues are stabilizing. One type of removable retainer is the Hawley appliance, shown in **Figure 30-13.** The use of a retainer provides another source for retention of dental biofilm. Special instruction for care and cleaning of a retainer is needed. General procedures are suggested here.

■ Clean the appliance after each meal and before retiring. Instructions for cleaning procedures and agents for removable appliances are described with the care of the removable denture (Chapter 31, page 453).

■ Brush and rinse teeth and gingival tissue under the appliance each time the appliance is removed. Unless necessary as directed by the orthodontist, the health of the underlying tissues is best maintained when the appliance is not kept in the mouth continuously.

■ Brush the mucosa under the appliance. Methods are described in Chapter 31 on page 453.

■ Keep appliance in a container with water when it is out of the mouth.

POST-DEBONDING PREVENTIVE CARE

I. PERIODONTAL EVALUATION

- A complete examination with careful probing and charting is necessary because many changes take place during treatment.
- Calculus removal is completed as needed.
- Clinical photographs assist the patient in comparing gingival tissue changes and teeth before and after treatment.
- Apply disclosing agent for documentation of biofilm and patient instruction.

II. DENTAL CARIES

- Examination for demineralization (white spots) and dental caries is essential.
- Dental biofilm retention by orthodontic appliances can be extensive. The configurations of the appliances make biofilm control efforts by the patient extremely difficult. Biofilm collects on brackets and some resins even when the patient's oral hygiene is generally good.[5]
- Composite resin may be left on the tooth surface around the bracket. The surface of resins is difficult to make smooth; thus, biofilm collects.

III. FLUORIDE THERAPY[29]

- A complete program of fluoride treatments, professionally applied at frequent maintenance appointments and used by the patient on a daily basis, is prerequisite both during and following orthodontic therapy.
- Application of a fluoride varnish immediately following bonding can help to reduce demineralization by up to 50%.[30] Varnish applications need to become a part of every maintenance appointment.
- With the loss of fluoride-rich enamel surface during bonding and debonding procedures, the need

Box 30-3	Example Progress Note

Maintenance appointment after completion of treatment.
  Patient first saw the orthodontist and then came for oral hygiene check.
  Gingiva normal color, except lingual mandibular molars with marginal redness with bleeding on probing. She said the soreness she had right after band removal has pretty much gone.
  Removed small calculus deposits mandibular anterior where she always had calculus during her treatment. Encouraged better flossing and positioning of her electric brush to get between those anterior teeth. She returns to her dental hygienist in general practice for next dental hygiene maintenance. I told her I would send a memo to her RDH to tell her about this appointment.

Signed: _____, RDH Date: _____

for remineralization and replenishment of fluoride is clear.

DOCUMENTATION

Over the long period of treatment, detailed recording of each step, the tissue reactions, and the outcomes are needed.

- Patient's personal hygiene, the implements used, and the biofilm observed at individual visits is a significant part of the records.
- At dental hygiene appointments, calculus occurrence and removal.
- Documentation by the orthodontist includes each step and the summaries of changes noted.
- A sample progress note may be found in **Box 30-3**.

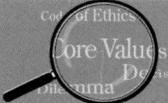

Everyday Ethics

Dorothy, a patient who had recently completed orthodontic therapy, presents for a maintenance appointment with Caroline, the dental hygienist in her general dentist's practice. The facial surfaces of tooth numbers 4–13 and 20–29 appear to harbor remnants of composite adhesive resin.

  Caroline, the dental hygienist, feels an obligation to remove these adhesive remnants but does not want to make any disparaging comments about the orthodontist, whose responsibility it was to remove the adhesive. There is not enough time to remove all of the resin and complete the examination, radiographs, and dental hygiene therapy at the current appointment.

Questions for Consideration

1. Which of the core values (Table II-1, page 38) have particular significance in this setting? How and why?
2. To maintain Dorothy's trust in her orthodontist, how can Caroline inform the patient of the accretions and explain the need for additional appointments?
3. Role play a conversation between Caroline and Dorothy as Caroline explains the problem.

Factors To Teach The Patient

- The significance of dental biofilm around orthodontic appliances and the teeth.
- How to apply the toothbrush (power or manual) and adjunctive devices to remove dental biofilm from the bracket, the arch wire, and the teeth.
- How, when, and why to use fluoride rinses, toothpaste, and brush-on gel.
- The frequency for professional follow-up during and after orthodontic therapy.

References

1. Zachrisson BU. Bonding in orthodontics. In: Graber TM, Vanarsdall RL. *Orthodontics, current principles and techniques.* 3rd ed. St. Louis: Mosby; 2000. p. 557–639.
2. David VA, Staley RN, Bigelow HF, Jakobsen JR. Remnant amount and cleanup for 3 adhesives after debracketing. *Am J Orthod Dentofacial Orthop.* 2002 Mar;121(3):291–6.
3. Osorio R, Toledano M, Garcia-Godoy F. Bracket bonding with 15- or 60-second etching and adhesive remaining on enamel after debonding. *Angle Orthod.* 1999 Feb;69(1):45–8.
4. American Dental Association, Council on Dental Materials, Instruments, and Equipment. Ceramic orthodontic brackets: how and when to use them. *J Am Dent Assoc.* 1992 Jul;123(7):243–4.
5. Gwinnett AJ, Ceen RF. Plaque distribution on bonded brackets: a scanning microscopic study. *Am J Orthod.* 1979 Jun;75(6):667–77.
6. Zachrisson BU, Brobakken BO. Clinical comparison of direct versus indirect bonding with different bracket types and adhesives. *Am J Orthod.* 1978 Jul;74(1):62–78.
7. Gwinnett AJ; American Dental Association, Council on Dental Materials, Instruments, and Equipment. State of the art and science of bonding in orthodontic treatment. *J Am Dent Assoc.* 1982 Nov;105(5):844–50.
8. Proffit WR. *Contemporary orthodontics.* 2nd ed. St. Louis: Mosby; 1993. Chapter 10, Mechanical principles in orthodontic force control; p. 353–7.
9. Zachrisson BU, Skogan O, Höymyhr S. Enamel cracks in debonded, debanded, and orthodontically untreated teeth. *Am J Orthod.* 1980 Mar;77(3):307–19.
10. Lindauer SJ, Browning H, Shroff B, Marshall F, Anderson RH, Moon PC. Effect of pumice prophylaxis on the bond strength of orthodontic brackets. *Am J Orthod Dentofacial Orthop.* 1997 Jun;111(6):599–605.
11. Buonocore MG, Matsui A, Gwinnett AJ. Penetration of resin dental materials into enamel surfaces with reference to bonding. *Arch Oral Biol.* 1968 Jan;13(1):61–70.
12. Retief DH. Effect of conditioning the enamel surface with phosphoric acid. *J Dent Res.* 1973 Mar-Apr;52(2):333–41.
13. Diedrich P. Enamel alterations from bracket bonding and debonding. A study with the scanning electron microscope. *Am J Orthod.* 1981 May;79(5):500–22.
14. Marcusson A, Norevall LI, Persson M. White spot reduction when using glass ionomer cement for bonding in orthodontics: a longitudinal and comparative study. *Eur J Orthod.* 1997 Jun;19(3):233–42.
15. Chan DC, Swift EJ, Bishara SE. In vitro evaluation of a fluoride-releasing orthodontic resin. *J Dent Res.* 1990 Sep;69(9):1576–9.
16. Bishara SE, Swift EJ Jr, Chan DC. Evaluation of fluoride release from an orthodontic bonding system. *Am J Orthod Dentofacial Orthop.* 1991 Aug;100(2):106–9.
17. Basdra EK, Huber H, Komposch G. Fluoride released from orthodontic bonding agents alters the enamel surface and inhibits enamel demineralization in vitro. *Am J Orthod Dentofacial Orthop.* 1996 May;109(5):466–72.
18. Osorio R, Toledano M, Garcia-Godoy F. Enamel surface morphology after bracket debonding. *J Dent Child.* 1998 Sep-Oct;65(5):313–7, 354.
19. Smith SC, Walsh LJ, Taverne AA. Removal of orthodontic bonding resin residues by CO_2 laser radiation: surface effects. *J Clin Laser Med Surg.* 1999 Feb;17(1):13–8.
20. Everett MS. Debonding orthodontic adhesives. *Dent Hyg.* 1985 Aug;59(8):364–70.
21. Bishara SE, Trulove TS. Comparisons of different debonding techniques for ceramic brackets: an in vitro study. Part I. Background and methods. *Am J Orthod Dentofacial Orthop.* 1990 Aug;98(2):145–53.
22. Bishara SE, Trulove TS. Comparisons of different debonding techniques for ceramic brackets: an in vitro study. Part II. Findings and clinical implications. *Am J Orthod Dentofacial Orthop.* 1990 Sep;98(3):263–73.
23. Bishara SE, Fehr DE. Ceramic brackets: something old, something new, a review. *Semin Orthod.* 1997 Sep;3(3):178–88.
24. Gutmann ME. Composite adhesive resin removal following orthodontic treatment. *J Pract Hyg.* 1996 May-Jun;5:16.
25. Campbell PM. Enamel surfaces after orthodontic bracket debonding. *Angle Orthod.* 1995 Nov;65(2):103–10.
26. Pus MD, Way DC. Enamel loss due to orthodontic bonding with filled and unfilled resins using various clean-up techniques. *Am J Orthod.* 1980 Mar;77(3):269–83.
27. Thompson RE, Way DC. Enamel loss due to prophylaxis and multiple bonding/debonding of orthodontic attachments. *Am J Orthod.* 1981 Mar;79(3):282–95.
28. van Waes H, Matter T, Krejci I. Three-dimensional measurement of enamel loss caused by bonding and debonding of orthodontic brackets. *Am J Orthod Dentofacial Orthop.* 1997 Dec;112(6):666–9.
29. Boyd RL. Comparison of three self-applied topical fluoride preparations for control of decalcification. *Angle Orthod.* 1993 Spring;63(1):25–30.
30. Todd MA, Staley RN, Kanellis MJ, Donly KJ, Wefel JS. Effect of a fluoride varnish on demineralization adjacent to orthodontic brackets. *Am J Orthod Dentofacial Orthop.* 1999 Aug;116(2):159–67.

CHAPTER 31

Care of Dental Prostheses

TAMMY K. SWECKER, BSDH, MED

Chapter Outline

Overall cleanliness of the oral cavity involves care of all natural teeth, soft tissues, and dental prostheses.

■ A *prosthesis* is an artificial replacement of a missing part of the body, and a dental prosthesis replaces one or more teeth and supporting structures. A prosthesis may be fixed or removable.

■ Awareness of the types and characteristics of prostheses, supporting tissues, and the common issues a patient may experience with prostheses is needed to provide information, comprehensive oral hygiene instruction, and treatment for the patient who has prostheses.

■ Common issues the patient may ask the dental hygienist about include the options to replace a missing tooth

BOX 31-1	Key Words

Dental Prostheses

Abutment: a tooth or implant used for the support or retention of a fixed or removable prosthesis.

Complete denture: dental prosthesis that replaces the entire dentition and associated structures; may be a complete maxillary denture or a complete mandibular, or both.

Coping: a thin covering or crown.

Denture: artificial substitute for missing natural teeth and adjacent tissues.

Denture adhesive: a soft material used to adhere a denture to the underlying mucosa; also referred to as an adherent.

Denture stomatitis: An inflammation of the oral mucosa that bears a complete or partial removable dental prosthesis, typically a denture.

Fixed partial denture: a replacement for one or more missing teeth that is securely retained to natural teeth and/or dental implant abutments that furnish the primary support for the prosthesis; also called a fixed prosthesis or bridge.

Immediate denture: any removable dental prosthesis fabricated for placement immediately following the removal of a natural tooth/teeth.

Interim prosthesis: a fixed or removable dental prosthesis designed to enhance esthetics, stabilization and/or function for a limited period, after which it is to be replaced by a definitive dental or maxillofacial prosthesis. Often such prostheses are used to assist in determination of the therapeutic effectiveness of a specific treatment plan or the form and function of the planned for definitive prosthesis. Also referred to as provisional prosthesis, provisional restoration.

Obturator: a prosthesis used to close a congenital or acquired opening, such as for a cleft palate, an area lost because of trauma, or after surgery for removal of a diseased area.

Occlusal vertical dimension: the distance measured between two points when the occluding members are in contact.

Pontic: an artificial tooth on a partial denture that replaces a missing natural tooth, restores its function, and usually occupies the space previously filled by the natural crown.

Precision attachment: a type of connector that consists of a metal receptacle and a close-fitting part; the metal receptacle usually is included within the restoration of an abutment tooth, and the close-fitting part is attached to a pontic or removable partial denture framework.

Prosthesis: artificial replacement of an absent part of the body; may be a therapeutic device to improve or alter function; may be a device employed to aid in accomplishing a desired surgical result.

Removable partial denture: a dental prosthesis that supplies teeth and/or associated structures in a partially edentulous jaw and can be removed and replaced at will.

Residual ridges: the portion of the residual bone and its soft tissue covering that remains after the removal of teeth.

Rest: a rigid, stabilizing extension of a fixed or removable partial denture that contacts a remaining tooth or teeth; prevents movement toward the mucosa and transmits functional forces to the teeth.

Ultrasonic cleaner: a device, in which a denture is placed in water or some type of solvent cleaner, that uses ultrasonic waves to dislodge debris on a denture.

or teeth, how to adjust to a new denture and relearn how to chew, or what to do if a denture feels loose.
- Definitions for this chapter may be studied in **Box 31-1**.
- Daily maintenance by the patient is a vital factor for success and longevity of a prostheses and the health of remaining teeth and oral tissues.
- Patients with prostheses may be at greater risk for dental caries and periodontal infections because of the biofilm-friendly margins of restorations, under clasps, and under fixed prostheses.
- A patient may have more than one prosthesis. A patient with a complete maxillary denture may have both fixed and removable partial dentures in the mandibular arch; an implant retained removable partial denture or an implant-retained mandibular overdenture.
- The customized regimen for personal care involves the natural teeth as well as the fixed and removable prostheses.
- A program of instruction is worked out for each patient specific to individual needs. Examples of fixed and removable prostheses and appliances are listed in **Box 31-2**.

BOX 31-2	Types of Oral Prostheses and Appliances

Fixed
Fixed partial denture
Periodontal splint
Implant-supported complete denture
Orthodontic appliance
Space maintainer

Removable
Removable partial denture
Natural tooth supported
Implant supported
Complete denture
Overdenture
Obturator
Removable orthodontic appliance
Removable space maintainer
Hawley appliance

MISSING TEETH

- A patient may have one or more missing teeth or may have tooth extractions planned.
- A patient is informed of the options to replace missing teeth as well as risk factors associated with a choice not to replace the missing teeth.
- A long history of poor oral hygiene, carious lesions, and periodontal infections may have lead to tooth loss; trauma is another common cause of tooth loss.

I. REPLACEMENT OPTIONS

A. Replacement options include the following:
- Fixed Prosthesis
- Removable prosthesis
- Dental Implants (page 465)

B. Dental hygienist's role
- Explain each possible choice for the patient.
- Clarify with questions from the patient.
- Prepare notes from the intraoral/extraoral examination to assist the dentist.
- Keep a neutral stand on the options until the dentist has studied the case and advised

II. NO REPLACEMENT

A. Replacement for a missing tooth may not be indicated for a patient who has sufficient remaining teeth for function, for example:
- Third molars are generally not replaced after extraction.
- Second molars that are extracted and have no opposing tooth.
- Teeth extracted for orthodontic reasons.

B. Risks of not replacing missing teeth include:
- *Migration of adjacent teeth.* Tilting and rotation of teeth may complicate future replacement options or lead to periodontal problems due to difficulty in biofilm control and misdirected occlusal forces when chewing.
- *Migration of opposing teeth.* An unopposed tooth may supererupt.
- *Remaining teeth may suffer from the added function and stress.* This may lead to fractures and tooth loss.
- *Loss of occlusal vertical dimension.* The bite may become overclosed due to many missing teeth and can lead to temporomandibular joint (TMJ) disorders.

FIXED PARTIAL DENTURE PROSTHESES

I. DESCRIPTION

A. Fixed partial dentures, commonly called dental *bridges*, are composed of the following, as shown in **Figure 31-1**:
- Abutments
- Connectors
- Pontics

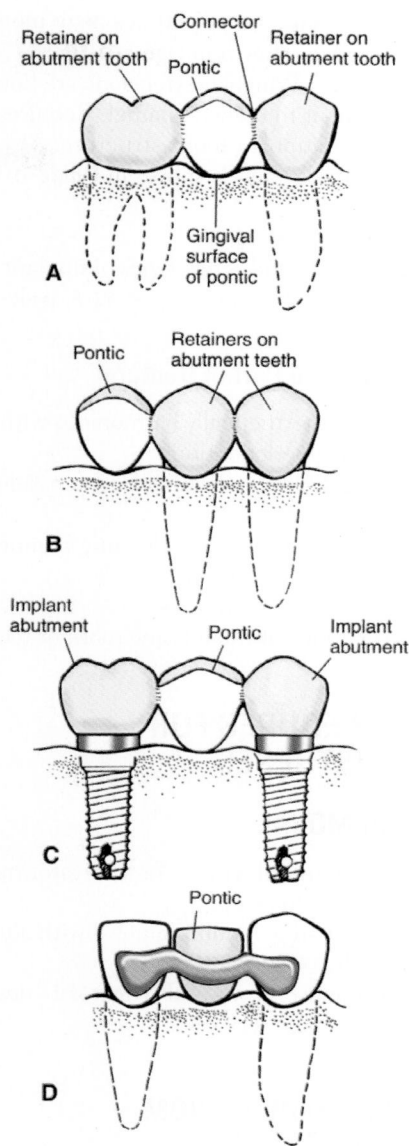

FIGURE 31-1 **Fixed Partial Dentures. (A)** Characteristic parts of a mandibular three-unit fixed partial denture. Cast gold crowns on the abutment teeth serve as the retainers for the bridge. **(B)** Cantilever bridge supported by a double abutment. **(C)** Fixed partial denture with implant abutments. **(D)** Fixed resin–retained partial prosthesis.

B. Bridges can be fabricated from various materials including:
- Metals
- Ceramics
- Combination of both

C. A fixed partial denture is affixed to the teeth or implants with a cement and is not removable.

II. CHARACTERISTICS

A. Types of Fixed Partial Dentures

1. *Natural tooth supported*
- *Traditional/bilateral.* Supported by one or more natural teeth at each end as shown in **Figure 31-1A**.

- *Cantilever.* Pontic supported by one or more teeth at one end only as shown in **Figure 31-1B**.
- *Resin retained.* Winglike extensions are bonded with a resin cement to etched enamel. Requires minimal or no preparation to tooth structure. Also called a Maryland Bridge and is shown in **Figure 31-1D**.
2. *Implant supported*
  - Shown in **Figure 31-1C**.
  - Blade, cylinder, and screw types of implants used for abutments are shown in Figure 32-3, page 466.

B. Criteria for Fixed Partial Denture[1]

- Biologically and aesthetically harmonious with the teeth and surrounding periodontium.
- All parts accessible for cleaning by the patient and the dental professional.
- Does not interfere with the cleaning regimen for the remaining natural dentition.
- Cannot traumatize oral tissues.
- Restores functions of the missing tooth or teeth.

CARE PROCEDURES FOR FIXED PROSTHESES

I. DEBRIS REMOVAL

- Loose debris removal with an oral irrigator may be recommended as a first step.
- Facilitates next step: biofilm removal with a toothbrush and other aids.
- Procedure for use of an oral irrigator is described in Chapter 28 on page 419.

II. BIOFILM REMOVAL FROM ABUTMENT TEETH

- Nearly all the methods proposed for dental biofilm control in Chapters 27 and 28 may be applicable to abutment teeth.
- The proximal surface of an abutment tooth and the gingiva adjacent to a pontic require special attention.

A. Toothbrushing

- Sulcular brushing is generally indicated.

B. Dentifrice Selection

- A *nonabrasive* dentifrice is indicated to prevent the abrasion of the prosthesis surfaces and any areas of exposed root on abutment teeth.
- A *fluoride-containing* dentifrice is selected for protection of remaining tooth surfaces, particularly exposed cementum. Acidulated fluoride preparations

are contraindicated for porcelain and composite restorations.[2]

C. Additional Interdental Care

- Removal of biofilm from proximal surfaces of tooth, abutment, and pontic is vital.
- The method is selected based on the abilities of each patient and the type of prosthesis.
- An interdental cleaning device is adapted specifically to the proximal surfaces of the abutments.
- The same interdental cleaning procedures can be applied to the gingival surface of the fixed partial denture.
- Interdental cleaning methods and devices are described on pages 412 and 413.

III. THE PROSTHESIS

A. Areas Requiring Emphasis

- Margins of the restorations may provide slightly irregular areas for retaining biofilm and require daily attention.
- The gingival surfaces of the pontics and beneath the connectors are particularly prone to biofilm retention.

B. Toothbrushing

- A toothbrush in the Charters position may be helpful for cleaning the gingival surface of the pontic from the facial aspect.
- The filaments can be directed under the pontic to clean the gingival surface.
- Charters brush position is described in Chapter 27 on page 396.

C. Dental Floss in Threader

Tufted dental floss is most efficient for cleaning a fixed partial denture. As shown in Figure 28-6, page 414, two types are available.

1. *Floss Threader*
  - Thread a 12- to 15-inch length into a floss threader. Several types are available and are shown in **Figure 31-2**.
  - Apply threader between abutment, pontic, and gingiva.
  - Draw the floss through, and using single or double thickness, remove loose debris, as in **Figure 31-3**.
  - Apply a new section of the floss with moderate pressure to the undersurface (gingival surface) of the pontic and then to the proximal surfaces of each abutment tooth to remove the biofilm.
2. *"Super Floss"*
  - Available in 2-foot lengths with a tufted segment.
  - Has a stiffened end for self-threading.

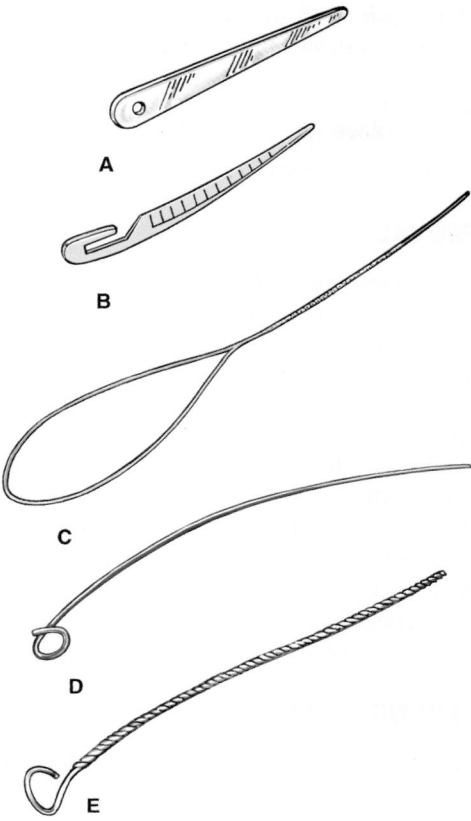

FIGURE 31-2 **Floss Threaders.** **(A)** Clear plastic with closed eye. **(B)** Tinted plastic with open eye. **(C)** Soft plastic loop. **(D)** Flexible wire. **(E)** Twisted wire.

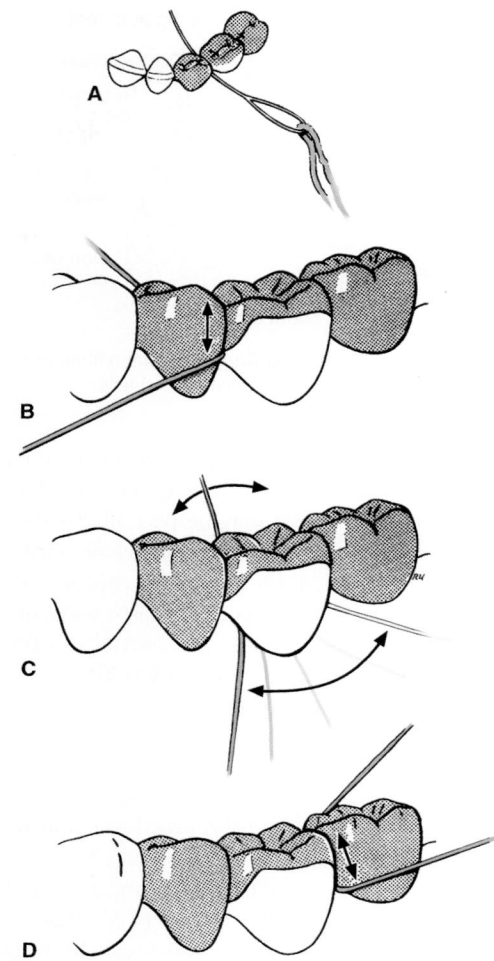

FIGURE 31-3 **Use of Floss Threader.** **(A)** Use floss threader to draw the floss or tufted floss between abutment and pontic. **(B)** Apply floss to the distal surface of the mesial abutment; pull through 1 or 2 inches. **(C)** Slide floss under pontic. Move back and forth several times, as shown by the arrows, to remove dental biofilm from the gingival surface of the pontic. **(D)** Apply new section of floss to the mesial surface of the distal abutment.

■ Use in same manner as described earlier for floss threader.

D. Other Interdental Devices

■ An interdental brush shown in Figure 28-9, page 416, and a single-tuft brush shown in Figure 28-11, page 417, can be recommended and demonstrated as indicated by the requirements of the individual prosthesis.
■ Interdental brushes may be used mesial and distal to the pontic when space allows easy entry.

E. Additional Factors

■ Margins of the restorations are evaluated for possible dental caries at every maintenance appointment.
■ One or more bridge abutments may become uncemented. Evidence of any movement is evaluated during dental appointments and by the patient while performing daily care.
■ Instruct the patient to inform the dental team when any problem or change with the fixed prosthesis become apparent.

REMOVABLE PARTIAL DENTURE PROSTHESES

I. DESCRIPTION

■ A removable partial denture replaces one or more, but less than all, of the natural teeth and associated structures.
■ The partial denture can be removed from the mouth and replaced at will.
■ The denture base rests on the oral mucosa and carries the artificial teeth.

II. TYPES

■ A typical partial denture consists of a stable metal framework made of chrome cobalt.
■ The framework engages abutment teeth or an abutment implant with a wide variety of clasp assemblies and rest seats or precision attachments.

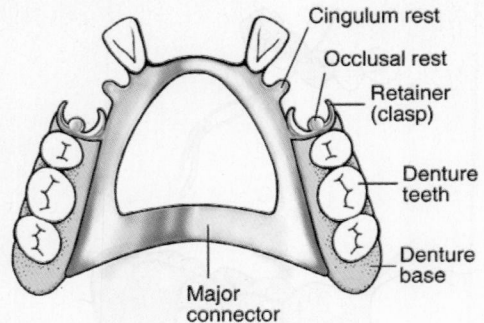

FIGURE 31-4 **Removable Partial Denture.** Components of a removable partial denture shown for a maxillary prosthesis.

- Depending on the location and number of remaining natural teeth, a partial denture may receive all its support from the teeth, or it may be partially tooth borne, partially implant borne, and partially tissue borne.
- The base is most frequently made of plastic acrylic resin.
- The teeth may be made of porcelain, plastic resin, or metal.
- The basic parts of a removable partial denture are shown in **Figure 31-4** and defined in **Box 31-1**.

III. CHARACTERISTICS

- Self-care procedures for the patient with a removable prosthesis involve cleaning the prosthesis and remaining natural teeth.
- The appliance is removed for cleaning the abutment teeth, gingival tissue, and the mucosa of edentulous areas.
- The health of the underlying tissues can be negatively affected by a removable partial denture because biofilm tends to accumulate more readily and in greater quantities.

- Biofilm control is a major factor in maintaining the long-term health of abutment teeth for a removable partial denture.
- All removable appliances are labeled for patient identification purposes. Methods of identification are described in Chapter 53 on pages 819 to 821.

IV. REMOVAL

A. It is most comfortable to have the patient remove the prosthesis because the patient is familiar with the path of insertion and removal.
B. If a patient is unable to remove the appliance, the dental hygienist proceeds as follows:
- Exert an even pressure on both sides of the denture simultaneously as the clasps slide up over their abutment teeth.
- The line of insertion and removal of a partial denture is designed and constructed for an even, vertical movement.
- Avoid grasping the clasp assemblies of the prostheses, which may damage or bend a clasp.

V. RECEIVING A DENTURE

A. Prevent cross-contamination when receiving a removable prosthesis from a patient by:
- Wearing personal protective mask, eyewear, and gloves.
- Offering a disposable cup in which the patient can place the prosthesis directly.
B. Rinse the prosthesis under slowing running water; take care not to splash.
C. Place in a cleaning solution in bag in an ultrasonic cleaner as shown in **Figure 31-5**.

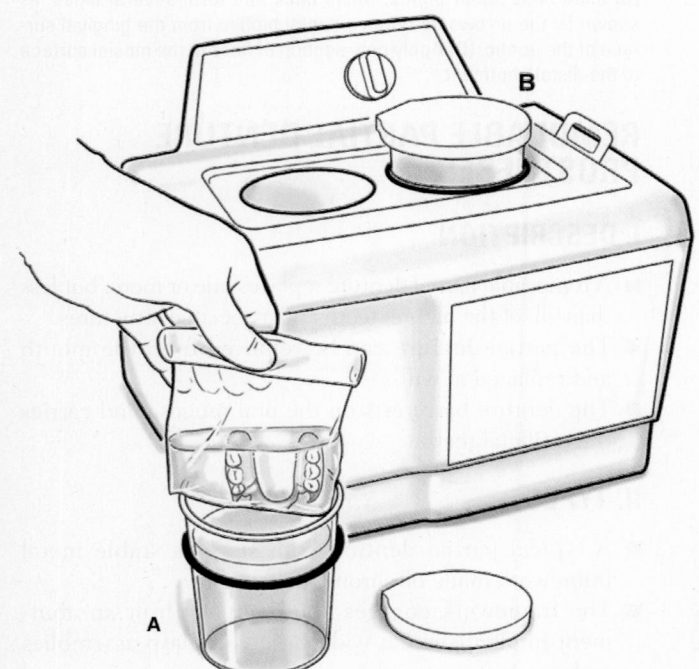

FIGURE 31-5 **Ultrasonic Denture Cleaner. (A)** First, the removable prosthesis is placed in a sealed bag with cleaning solution and placed in a beaker filled with water. **(B)** Beaker is then placed in an ultrasonic unit and set according to manufacturer directions.

SELF-CARE PROCEDURES FOR REMOVABLE PARTIAL PROSTHESES

- The selection of cleansing agents and the procedures for cleaning are complicated by the intricacy of the metallic parts and their relation to the natural teeth, as well as by the dental materials used in construction.
- Rinsing, immersing, and brushing methods, as well as the cleansing agents described for the complete denture on page 456, may apply to various other types of removable prostheses.
- After each meal, and at bedtime, the appliance is removed and both the appliance and the natural teeth are cleaned.
- Examples of other removable appliances are listed in **Box 31-2**.

I. OBJECTIVES FOR THE PATIENT

- Objective for all patients is to attain and maintain oral health and function.
- The objective for the natural teeth is to control biofilm for the prevention of dental caries and periodontal infection.
- Cleaning the prosthesis takes on added significance because it is adjacent to natural teeth and rests on soft tissue.
  A. The basic daily self-care objective is to:
   1. Remove all loose debris and attached biofilm.
   2. Disinfect the appliance to eliminate potential irritants to the teeth and oral tissues that may cause malodor.
  B. A professional cleaning for all removable prostheses is obtained on a routine scheduled maintenance appointment.

II. THE PROSTHESIS

A. Rinsing

- When regular cleaning facilities are not available, rinsing is beneficial for both the natural teeth and the removable prosthesis.
- Partial denture is removed, the mouth is rinsed with water, and the denture is rinsed under running water. The method for rinsing the mouth is outlined in Box 29-4, page 424.
- Rinsing does not remove biofilm, which is attached firmly, so it is not a substitute for complete care procedures.

B. Brushing

Precautions are taken during brushing a removable partial denture:

- Too tight a grasp of a partial prosthesis can result in bending or fracture of clasps or bars.
- Filaments of a brush can inadvertently catch the prosthesis and cause it to drop and break.

- Partially fill the sink with water or line the sink with a face cloth or towel to prevent breakage should the prosthesis be dropped.

C. Types of Brushes

1. *Toothbrush*
   - The use of a patient's regular toothbrush is not recommended for care of a removable prosthesis because brushing the clasps or other metal parts may deform the toothbrush filaments and make the brush ineffective for use on natural teeth.
   - When a patient chooses to use a regular toothbrush, a separate brush is indicated.
2. *Power brush*
   - A power brush is not used on a removable prosthesis because of the danger of catching the brush and damaging the prosthesis.
3. *Clasp brush*
   - A specially designed narrow, tapered brush about 2–3 inches long that can be adapted to the inner surfaces of clasps or precision attachments is recommended (**Figure 31-6**).
   - Difficult-to-clean clasp assemblies have protected internal surfaces prone to biofilm accumulation that can be carefully removed with a clasp brush.
4. *Denture brush*
   - A denture brush is described on page 457 and is available specifically for brushing dentures.
   - It is an excellent brush for cleaning all the surfaces and the metal bars of the partial removable denture.

D. Immersion

- Before immersion, the denture is cleaned by rinsing and brushing to remove all loose surface biofilm and debris.
- Avoid agents known to corrode or discolor.
- Procedures for immersion cleaning are described on page 457.

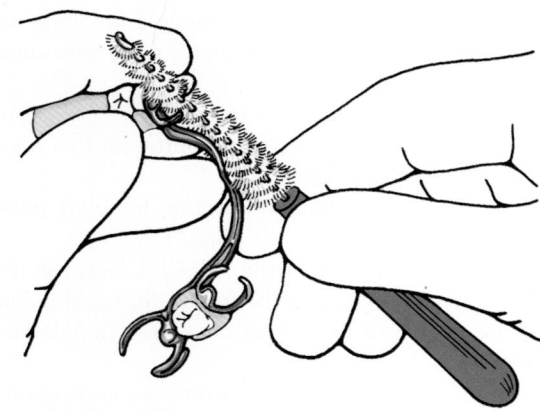

FIGURE 31-6 **Clasp Brush.** A brush specially designed to remove dental biofilm from the inside surfaces of clasps is available. The denture must be held carefully to avoid accidents.

III. THE NATURAL TEETH

A. Biofilm Control

- The removable prosthesis is taken out of the mouth before biofilm control of remaining teeth is performed.
- Toothbrushing and interdental cleaning methods selected for the particular needs of each patient are followed meticulously.
- The longevity of the removable appliance depends on the health of the supporting teeth, and the health of the natural teeth depends on the cleanliness of the prosthesis.

B. Dental Caries Prevention

- Abutment teeth are at increased risk for caries and periodontal disease. Protocol for caries prevention is found in Chapter 26 on page 383.
- Daily oral care, topical fluoride use, and diet may need modification to reduce caries risk.
- Caries and periodontal involvement involving any abutment tooth can lead to tooth loss and the patient may have more limited options for replacement.

OBTURATOR

I. DESCRIPTION

- Obturators present as a resin base with retainer clasps that provide stability for the appliance.
- Depending on the palatal defect, some obturators have anterior prosthetic teeth due to the nature of the defect.

II. PURPOSES AND USES

- Patients with previous cancers of the head involving the maxilla
- Cocaine abusers that snort the powder form of the drug develop necrosis of the nasal septum and surrounding tissues;[3]
- Patient with an area lost due to trauma
- Patients with cleft palate with an obturator that fits the dimensions of the palatal defect.[4]
- More information about obturators for cleft palates may be found in Chapter 50, page 780.
- Depending on the size of the palatal defect, the obturator may need to stay in the mouth during the dental hygiene treatment to prevent choking or inhalation of materials.
- Obturators need to be removed during the exposure of radiographic films. An appliance with metal clasps will interfere with the radiolucency of the teeth and surrounding tissues.

III. CARE OF OBTURATOR

- A minimum of semiannual visits to the dentist and dental hygienist are recommended as the palatal defect will change over time and the obturator will need to be adjusted.
- Treatment of natural dentition includes complete calculus and stains removal, oral hygiene instructions, and fluoride therapies based on caries risk assessment.
- Removal of an obturator during dental hygiene therapy is necessary to ensure access for complete calculus and biofilm removal and treatment of natural tooth surfaces.
- Daily cleaning and care of an obturator follows the care given for a removable partial denture.
- Patients may need to sleep with the obturator in place when the defect is severe; sleeping with an obturator in place increases the risk of demineralization and dental caries in the abutment teeth as well as the incidence of denture stomatitis.
- When the patient must sleep with the obturator in place, it is suggested that the patient remove the obturator for short periods during the day to allow the tissue to rest.

COMPLETE DENTURE PROSTHESES

- The initial adjustment to wearing a prosthesis is challenging to the patient, particularly with removable appliances.
- The entire dental team works together to assist the patient through the process of loosing teeth and adjusting to a new prosthesis.
- New dentures require several adjustment visits with the dentist.

I. TYPES OF DENTURES

A. *Immediate denture*. Delivered initially after teeth are extracted. Due to the amount of bone remodeling after extraction, the denture is relined or rebased about 6 months later.
B. *Interim denture*. A temporary denture used for diagnosis and treatment. A conventional denture is made later.
C. *Conventional denture*. The long-term complete denture prosthesis.

II. COMPONENTS OF A COMPLETE DENTURE (FIGURE 31-7)

A. Denture Base

- The part of a denture that rests on the oral mucosa and to which the teeth are attached.
- Most denture bases are made of plastic acrylic resin.
- Others may be metal such as chrome-cobalt or gold, in combination with a plastic resin.

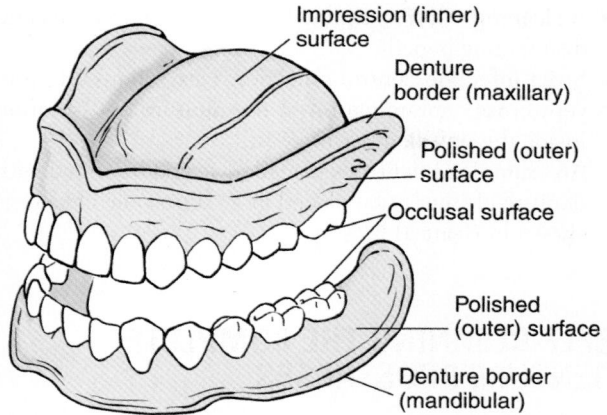

FIGURE 31-7 **Complete Denture.** The surfaces and borders of maxillary and mandibular dentures.

B. Surfaces

1. Impression surface. The tissue or inner surface of the denture.
   - Lies directly on the residual ridges and adjacent tissues.
   - The surface may be lined with a long-term material that is not to be removed by the patient such as a temporary soft liner, a tissue conditioner, or a permanent soft silicone liner.
   - A patient may place a denture adhesive material on the impression surface of the denture before inserting the denture.
   - The denture adhesive is removed from the denture during daily cleaning and from soft tissues to enable visual inspection.
     - A denture adhesive is a commercially available paste or powder preparation.
     - The adhesive is used to improve denture retention, stabilization, and comfort, as recommended by the dentist.
     - A patient may use an adhesive indefinitely in an attempt to get along with ill-fitting dentures that need to be adjusted or remade.
2. *Polished surface.* The external or outer surface is polished. The impression surfaces are not polished.
3. *Occlusal surface.* The surface of a denture that makes contact or near contact with the corresponding surface of the opposing denture or natural teeth.

C. Teeth

- The denture teeth may be made of plastic acrylic resin, composite resin, or porcelain.
- A patient may request to have decorative facings incorporated into certain teeth.
- Metal occlusal surfaces may be present, for example, to maintain a stable vertical dimension of occlusion when opposing teeth may cause excessive wear.

III. DENTURE DEPOSITS

Accumulation of stains and deposits on dentures varies between individuals in a manner similar to that on natural teeth. The phases of deposit formation may be divided as follows:

A. Mucin and Food Debris on the Denture Surface

Readily removed by rinsing and brushing.

B. Denture Pellicle and Denture Biofilm

- Denture pellicle forms readily after a denture is cleaned.
- Denture biofilm is composed predominantly of gram-positive cocci, rods, and filamentous forms of bacteria in an intermicrobial substance.
- Biofilm also includes varying accumulations of *Candida albicans,* the yeast that causes candidiasis, and gram negative microorganisms.[5]
- Biofilm serves as a matrix for calculus formation and stain accumulation when the denture is not cleaned.[6]
- Denture biofilm is associated with breath malodor and denture stomatitis.[7]

C. Denture Calculus

- Calculus is hard and fixed to the denture surface.
- Calculus can form anywhere on a denture, especially the facial surfaces of the maxillary molars and lingual surfaces of the mandibular anterior.

D. Stains

- Dentures can become stained similarly to natural teeth.
- Frequent causes of stain include tobacco, red wine, coffee, and tea.

IV. REMOVAL OF DENTURE

- Usually, it is most comfortable for the patient to remove the denture.
- The clinician may remove dentures for certain patients, particularly those with a physical limitation or in an emergency situation.
- Although denture removal may be complicated by anatomic features of an individual mouth, a general procedure is outlined in **Box 31-3**.

V. CARE OF DENTURES DURING INTRAORAL PROCEDURES

- Provide a cleansing tissue for the patient's use when requesting the patient to remove or insert the denture.
- Rinse in water to remove any unattached debris without splashing.

BOX 31-3	Method for Removal of a Complete Denture

The clinician follows standard procedures for infection control while removing and handling the denture from the patient's mouth.

The Complete Maxillary Denture
1. Clinician is positioned at 11–12 o'clock; left-handed clinician is at 12–1 o'clock.
2. Grasp the anterior portion of the denture firmly with the thumb on the facial surface at the height of the border of the denture under the lip and the index finger on the palatal surface.
3. With the other hand, elevate the lip to expose the border of the denture to break the seal.
4. Remove the denture gently in a downward and forward direction.
5. If the retention of the denture cannot be overcome by elevation of the lip, request the able patient to blow into the mouth with the lips closed to break the suction seal.

The Complete Mandibular Denture
1. Clinician is positioned at 8–9 o'clock; left-handed clinician is at 3–4 o'clock.
2. Grasp the denture firmly on the facial surface with the thumb and on the lingual surface with the index finger.
3. With the other hand, retract the lower lip forward and remove the denture gently.

■ Professionally clean the denture in an ultrasonic denture cleaner, following manufacturer's instructions, with appropriate cleaning solution (**Figure 31-5**).
■ Follow strict procedures to protect the denture from exposure to unclean areas during transportation and when in the ultrasonic cleaner.
■ Provide a disposable cup or sterile container with a fitted cover to hold the prosthesis after rinsing.
■ Immerse in antimicrobial solution to disinfect and prevent drying.
■ Place container in a safe place away from treatment area to prevent spilling or inadvertent discarding.
■ At the end of the appointment, remember to rinse and return the moist denture before the patient rises from the dental chair.
■ Do not allow denture to dry as it can cause distortion.

VI. PROFESSIONAL DENTURE CLEANING

■ Commercially available devices include ultrasonic, sonic, magnetic, and agitating mechanisms that can be combined with an immersion agent.
■ The action of the modern, well-functioning ultrasonic cleansing device is an effective method for cleaning a denture.

■ A cleaning solution is added for additional cleaning and disinfecting benefit.
■ Strict infection control procedures are followed to prevent cross contamination of the denture and solution inside the cleaning basin.
■ An example of dentures placed in sealed bag filled with denture cleaner to be placed in an ultrasonic cleaner is shown in **Figure 31-5**.

SELF-CLEANING THE COMPLETE DENTURE PROSTHESES

I. DESCRIPTION

■ Do not assume that the patient who is wearing a denture knows the proper methods for caring for the prostheses and intraoral tissue.
■ During questioning for the patient history, information about the method and frequency of oral care and care of the prostheses is recorded.
■ When the denture is removed, examine for deposits and stains.
■ Alternate cleansing agents, devices, or procedures are recommended and demonstrated as needed.
■ Instruction is individualized for each patient's need: for example, the patient receiving a maxillary and mandibular denture for the first time, the patient whose dentures have been remade or relined, or the patient with a single denture that opposes natural teeth.
■ Record all details of patient instructions and recommendations in the patient's permanent record.
■ Types of dentures and characteristics of the edentulous mouth are described in Chapter 53 on page 813.

II. PURPOSES FOR CLEANING

Inadequate oral tissue care and denture hygiene practices are major causes of oral lesions under dentures.

A. Prevent Irritation to the Oral Tissues

■ *Mechanical irritants.* Rough deposits of biofilm, calculus, thick stains.
■ *Chemical irritants.* Products of putrefaction of food debris and bacterial metabolic products.

B. Control Infection

Reactions to denture biofilm and/or secondary infections by way of traumatic lesions may occur.

■ Prevent mouth odors
■ Maintain appearance

III. WHEN TO CLEAN

- Several times each day, clean dentures manually after eating and at bedtime.
- Each day, clean dentures by chemical immersion, usually overnight.

IV. PROCEDURE FOR CLEANING

- Rinsing, immersion, followed by brushing, is recommended.
- When unable to clean, rinsing is advised.

V. PREPARATION FOR CLEANING

- Rinse the denture thoroughly when it taken from the mouth to remove saliva and loose debris.
- Remove denture-adhesive material with light brushing.
- Denture-bearing mucosa. Rinse and clean with a soft toothbrush two or more times daily.

VI. CLEANING BY IMMERSION

The denture is soaked in a solvent or detergent in which chemical action removes or loosens stains and deposits that can then be rinsed or brushed away

A. Advantages

- The solution reaches all areas of the denture for a complete cleaning.
- Minimizes the danger of dropping the appliance.
- Prevents need for handling, which is required during brushing.
- Offers safe storage when dentures are out of the mouth.
- Aids patients that have limited ability to manage a brush.
- When manual cleaning is not possible, immersion involves the least handling and observation. This advantage is particularly attractive to a caregiver who must clean the denture for a patient.

B. Procedure

- The procedure for cleaning a denture by immersion is found in **Box 31-4**.
- The solution needs to be changed and the container cleaned daily
- Mix fresh solution to prevent contamination and growth of microorganisms.[8]

C. Solutions

1. *Proprietary.* Available in powder or tablet form.
   - *Preparation.* Add measured warm water as directed by the manufacturer.
   - *Length of immersion.* Usually 10 to 15 minutes or as suggested by the manufacturer. Because the action depends on the mechanical bubbling effect

BOX 31-4	Procedure for Cleaning a Denture by Immersion

- Place denture in a plastic container with a fitted cover that is maintained specifically for this purpose.
- Use only warm water, which promotes the action of the cleanser, for rinsing and mixing the solution. Hot water is never used because it can distort plastic resin.
- Follow manufacturer's specifications to ensure correct dilution of cleanser and time length for immersion.
- Check that the denture is completely submerged in the solution; cover the container.
- When the denture is removed, rinse under running water and remove loosened debris and chemicals before proceeding to clean by brushing.
- Empty and clean container daily. Mix fresh solution to prevent contamination and growth of microorganisms.[8]

of released oxygen, the solution has little value after the available oxygen has been released.
   - *Effect.* The solutions are only effective against loose debris; denture cleanliness depends on regular daily immersion supplemented by brushing.
2. *Hypochlorite solution.* Household bleach (5% sodium hypochlorite) and Calgon. Calgon acts to improve the penetrating and detaching power of the bleach. This solution is not recommended for an appliance that consists of any metal.
   - *Proportions*
     1. 1 tablespoon (15 ml) sodium hypochlorite (household bleach).
     2. 2 tsp (8 ml) Calgon.
     3. 4 ounces (114 ml) water.
   - *Length of immersion*: Usually 10 to 15 minutes. When stains or calculus form, the patient needs instruction to soak the denture overnight provided there are no metal parts that can become corroded. Rinse thoroughly before insertion.

VII. CLEANING BY BRUSHING

Brush with water, soap, or other mild cleansing agent. Abrasive agents cause scratches, which promote biofilm accumulation.

A. Type of Brush

1. *Denture brush*
   - A good-quality denture brush with end-rounded filaments is recommended. The styles of denture brushes vary.
   - One type shown in **Figure 31-8** is designed with two arrangements of filaments: (1) round arrangement to access the inner, curved impression surface; (2) rectangular portion for convenient adaptation to the polished and occlusal denture surfaces.

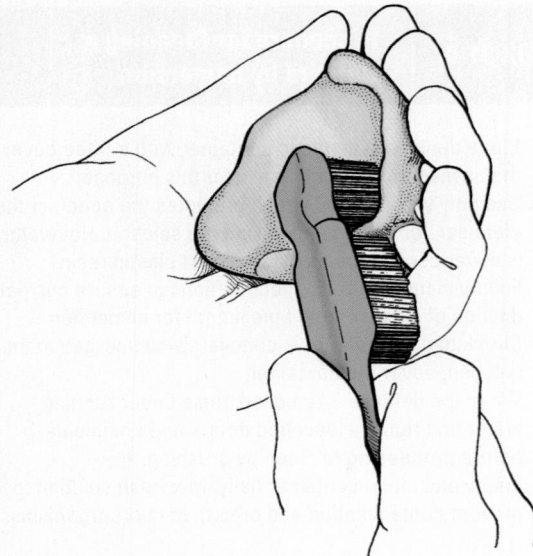

FIGURE 31-8 Denture Brush. The denture is held securely, but without squeezing, in the palm of the nonworking hand. Place a face cloth in the bottom of the sink and partially fill with water. The specially designed brush is preferred because one group of tufts is arranged to provide access to the inner impression surface of the denture, as shown.

■ Another brush designed for a patient with one hand or otherwise disabled, is shown in Figure 56-12, page 861.
2. *Other brushes*
   ■ A few patients prefer not to have a denture brush for personal reasons.
   ■ A hand brush can be used, provided the filaments are long enough to reach into the deeper portions of the impression surfaces.
   ■ Prerequisite is that each area of each surface of the denture be reached by the brush if denture biofilm formation is to be controlled.
   ■ If a patient prefers to use an ordinary toothbrush, a multitufted soft nylon brush with end-rounded filaments can be acceptable if access to all the inner curvatures is possible without applying undue pressure on certain parts in the attempt to clean others.
   ■ The patient who wears a single denture needs separate brushes for the natural teeth and the denture to maintain the brush for the natural teeth in the best condition possible.
   ■ Adjustments of brush technique may be needed to assist the disabled patient, as described in Chapter 56 on pages 864 to 866.

B. Procedure

Procedure for cleaning a denture is listed in **Box 31-5**.

C. Precautions Related to Brushing

■ Overzealous brushing and use of an abrasive cleansing agent on the impression surface could damage the fit of the denture.

BOX 31-5 | **Procedure for Cleaning Denture by Brushing**

1. Spread a towel, wash cloth, or rubber mat over the bottom of the sink to serve as a cushion should the denture be dropped; partially fill the sink with water.
2. Grasp denture in palm of hand securely (**Figure 29-8**) but without a squeezing pressure because dentures can be broken.
3. Apply warm water, nonabrasive cleanser, and brush to all areas of the denture. Pay particular attention to the impression surfaces where configurations of the surface correspond with those of the oral topography. The anterior areas of the inner surfaces of both the maxillary and mandibular dentures require special adaptations of the brush.
4. Rinse denture and brush under running water. Use the brush to remove denture cleanser that may be retained in the grooves.
5. Visually check each area carefully for biofilm.
6. Teach the patient to run a finger over the surfaces to find "slippery" biofilm areas.

■ Plastic resin can be abraded. Scratches make a rough surface; the denture may become more subject to the collection of biofilm, debris, and calculus.
■ Possibility of incomplete cleaning or cleaning with uneven pressure when the brush is applied more vigorously to accessible areas and misses difficult-to-access areas.
■ Danger of dropping and breaking the denture is increased when it is wet and slippery.
■ Advise patients to use their prescription eyewear when brushing to watch the procedure and to observe the cleanliness of the denture after brushing.

VIII. DENTURE CLEANSERS

A. Requirements for a Denture Cleanser[9]

■ Easy for a patient to use.
■ Bactericidal and fungicidal.
■ Effective removal of denture deposits (organic and inorganic) without abrasion of the denture surface.[10]
■ Nontoxic.
■ Harmless to the dental materials used for removable partial dentures, complete dentures, and obturators.
■ Reasonably priced.

B. Chemical Solution Cleansers (Immersion)

1. *Alkaline peroxide*
   ■ Active ingredient: alkaline detergent with an oxygen-liberating agent (sodium perborate or percarbonate).
   ■ Action: loosens debris and light stains by an oxygen-liberating mechanism. A preventive cleanser is used regularly from the day a denture has been cleaned

professionally to prevent accumulation of heavy deposits.
- ■ Examples: Most proprietary cleansers are in the form of a powder or tablet that is dropped into water to create the alkaline solution of hydrogen peroxide.
- ■ Disadvantages
  1. Does not remove heavy stains or calculus.
  2. Corrosion of metal parts of a denture.

2. *Dilute acids*
- ■ Active ingredient: inorganic acids.
- ■ Action: dissolves inorganic components of denture deposits.
- ■ Examples: 3% to 5% hydrochloric acid alone or with phosphoric acid, commercially prepared ultrasonic solutions. The strong acids (although in dilute forms) are not recommended for home use by the patient. The dental hygienist uses these agents during the dental hygiene appointment to cleanse and disinfect the appliance.
- ■ Disadvantage: corrosion of metal parts of a denture.

3. *Enzymes.* The enzymes act to break down biofilm proteins and polysaccharides. Enzyme agents have been incorporated into various immersion-type cleansers.

4. *Disinfectants*
- ■ A sanitary denture is necessary for the prevention of inflammation in the oral mucosa under the denture. Types of denture-induced lesions are described in Chapter 53 on page 815.
- ■ Regular daily maintenance procedures are necessary.
- ■ Patient instruction in disinfection of a denture is needed.
- ■ Commercially available sodium hypochlorite (household bleach) has been shown to be an effective antimicrobial. To disinfect, immerse the denture for 5 minutes with 5.25% sodium hypochlorite solution (1 tbsp household bleach/1 gallon of water). This concentration destroys most microorganisms.[11]
  - ■ Bleach can fade the color of the denture and is corrosive to metal parts of a denture.
  - ■ The denture needs to be rinsed completely.
- ■ Before disinfection, rinse the denture under running water, taking care not to splash and thus contaminate the area.

C. Abrasive Cleansers (Brushing)

1. *Denture pastes and powders, toothpastes and powders*
- ■ Active ingredient: an abrasive, such as calcium carbonate.
- ■ Action: mechanical removal of biofilm and stains by brushing.
- ■ Examples: various commercial products.
- ■ Disadvantages: can abrade the plastic resin denture base and acrylic teeth. Select a paste with low abrasiveness.

2. *Household agents*
- ■ Active ingredient: detergent and/or abrasive agent.
- ■ Examples: salt and bicarbonate of soda are mildly abrasive; hand soap is cleansing and not particularly

abrasive. Avoid scouring powders or other excessively abrasive cleansers.

IX. ADDITIONAL INSTRUCTIONS

A. Care of Plastic Resin

- ■ Immerse an appliance made with plastic resin in cool water or cleansing solution when it is not in the mouth.
- ■ Never place in hot or boiling water.

B. Prevention of Denture Deposits

- ■ When the denture is kept clean by regular procedures from the time of insertion, accumulation of stains and calculus can be prevented and the risk of tissue irritation can be reduced.
- ■ Home care includes a combination of mechanical and chemical methods to remove microorganisms associated with denture stomatitis.[10]

C. Professional Maintenance

- ■ Avoid scraping with a sharp instrument in the attempt to remove calculus deposits.
- ■ When the cleaning methods recommended in this chapter do not remove deposits, professional cleaning by the dental hygienist is needed.
- ■ A regular maintenance plan is arranged.

D. Paste Cleansers

- ■ Paste cleansers (dentifrices or denture pastes) may cling and be difficult to rinse from the denture.
- ■ Residual chemical agents, such as essential oils, may cause inflammatory or allergic reactions of the oral mucosa, and phenolic agents can have deleterious effects on plastic resin.

E. Soft Lining Materials

- ■ Temporary soft conditioning lining material may require proprietary cleansers to avoid harm to the material. Washing with cold water and a soft cloth, cotton, or soft brush (gently) can be suggested.
- ■ Denture biofilm needs to be removed several times each day. Brush outer, polished surfaces in the usual manner.
- ■ When the denture is placed in water overnight, the teeth are placed down so that the soft material at the denture border cannot become deformed.
- ■ Permanent silicone liners are softer and have a more porous surface to host biofilm accumulation; added diligence is required to remove biofilm and prevent build-up.

F. Denture Adhesives

- ■ Some patients prefer the added security of a denture adhesive to ensure stability and retention of a denture.

- An adhesive is not a solution for ill-fitting dentures; patient needs referral for evaluation and possible reline, rebase, or new denture.
- An adhesive may be necessary for the new denture patient as the immediate, interim denture begins to loosen with healing of the underlying tissues.
- Adhesive remaining attached to the tissue is removed to visualize the health status of the tissue underneath.

THE UNDERLYING MUCOSA

- The oral mucosa can be negatively affected by contact with a prosthesis, which results in the common condition called *denture stomatitis*.
- A strong association exists between *Candida albicans* biofilm on the denture, the constant wearing of a denture, amount of tissue covered by the denture, low vitamin A levels, cigarette smoking, and denture stomatitis.
- The residual biofilm may be laden with *Candida albicans* that could lead to regrowth and colonization on a patient's denture [11,12]
- Daily cleaning the denture, leaving the denture out for a period of time each day, and proper nutrition are factors in maintaining oral health.

I. EXAMINATION

- Soft tissue examination and oral cancer screening are recommended at least yearly for all patients by a dental professional, more frequently for patients with increased risk factors for oral cancer and pathology.
- Record and refer any changes and concerns for evaluation.
- Daily examination is performed by patient, taking notice of any oral changes and symptoms.
- Inform the patient to seek care when experiencing any oral change or when any concerns arise with the prosthesis.

II. RINSING

- Each time the denture is removed, the mouth is rinsed thoroughly with warm water or a mild salt solution, unless patient has dietary salt restrictions.
- The patient can learn to clean the mucosa by rubbing over the edentulous areas with the tongue.

III. CLEANING

- At least once daily a soft toothbrush with end-rounded filaments is applied lightly over the ridges and in the vestibules using long, straight strokes from posterior to anterior.
- Concurrently, the tongue is cleaned. Use a tongue cleaner as described in Chapter 27 on page 402.

IV. MASSAGE

For stimulation of circulation and increased resistance to trauma, frequent massage is recommended. Methods for massage that may be suggested to the patient are the following:

A. Digital

Place thumb and index finger over the ridge and apply massage with a press-and-release stroke. The palate may be rubbed with the ball of the thumb.

B. Soft Toothbrush

Apply sides of filaments and vibratory motion to each area. Prevent trauma to the tissue by placing the brush carefully and avoiding scrubbing with undue pressure.

C. Power Brush

Apply with no pressure to each area with smooth, even strokes.

V. SOFT TISSUE CONDITIONS

- Soft tissue changes are shown in Chapter 53 on page 817, particularly associated with patients who wear removable prostheses [13]
- Record and call to the dentist's attention lesions such as the following:
  A. Traumatic ulcerations
  B. Denture stomatitis
  C. Angular cheilitis
  D. Epulis formation

VI. DAILY REMOVAL OF PROSTHESES

- Generally, a removable appliance is left out of the mouth for a period of time each day to give the tissue underneath a rest from the constant contact.
- At night, the most convenient time to leave denture out of mouth may be while sleeping.
- In certain circumstances, a dentist may advise continual wear.
- Dentures are cleaned and kept moist while out of mouth.

COMPLETE OVERDENTURE PROSTHESES

An overdenture is a complete denture supported by both retained natural teeth or implants and the soft tissue of the residual alveolar ridge. Overdentures also have been called overlay dentures, coping dentures, and tooth-mucosa–supported dentures.

I. PURPOSES

The advantages of an overdenture compared with a denture in a completely edentulous mouth are that the natural teeth can provide the following:

- Help preserve bone, which may improve retention of denture.
- Allow the remaining teeth to bear occlusal pressures, thereby reducing the pressures placed on edentulous areas.
- Improve stability and retention of the denture. Improve the patient's tactile and proprioceptive senses by having the periodontal ligament present. Increase the patient's psychologic acceptance of the denture. The patient does not feel that all natural teeth have been lost.

II. NATURAL TOOTH–RETAINED OVERDENTURE

An overdenture may be possible for any patient whose treatment plan calls for extraction of teeth. Teeth frequently selected for overdenture abutments are the mandibular canines and premolars and the maxillary canines.

A. Periodontal Condition

Retained teeth must have a healthy periodontium, including healthy gingiva, bone level, and band of attached gingiva.

B. Endodontic Therapy

Most preserved teeth need endodontic therapy because the crowns will be reduced.

C. Restorative

- Tooth crowns are reduced to short rounded preparations or to the level and contour of the gingival margin.
- An amalgam or composite restoration may cover the root canal fillings.

III. IMPLANT-RETAINED OVERDENTURE

- Implants can be placed to help retain dentures and are becoming more common than natural tooth retained overdentures.
- Implants are generally placed in an area of each mandibular canine **(Figure 31-9B)**.
- Implants are not subject to dental caries, which is a factor with retained natural teeth.
- Peri-implant hygiene is described in Chapter 32 on page 469.

DENTAL HYGIENE CARE AND INSTRUCTION

I. GENERAL CARE

- The patient needs to be well informed concerning the care of the retained teeth, implants, the periodontium, and all intraoral and extraoral tissues.

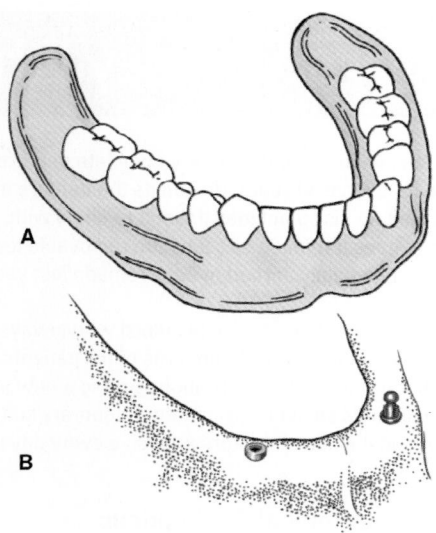

FIGURE 31-9 Overdenture. (A) Mandibular complete denture. **(B)** Examples of two different types of implant abutments. Generally, the same type of abutments are used in a denture.

- A high degree of motivation to save the remaining teeth is a primary concern.
- Patient is provided with the individualized instructions that are appropriate for the type of prosthesis or prostheses present.

II. FLUORIDE PROGRAM FOR CARIES PREVENTION

- A specific fluoride application plan is included for all natural tooth–retained overdentures and any patients with retained natural teeth.
- Fluoride application is not appropriate for use with implants.
- When the teeth have been extracted because of dental caries, caries control measures take on special significance, particularly if dietary habits remain the same.
- Current dietary habits are checked by asking the patient to keep a daily food diary; limitations on cariogenic food intake are recommended.

A. Fluoride Self-Application

- All patients need to use a fluoride dentifrice.
- In addition, a mouthrinse, prescription-strength toothpaste, and/or a gel tray are recommended daily.
- After cleaning, the patient's denture can be used for a custom tray, and the fluoride gel drops can be placed inside at the locations of the natural teeth.
- Pressure of the denture as it is seated forces the gel around the teeth.
- Higher concentrations of sodium fluoride (5000 ppm) have been shown to be more protective for overdenture abutments.[14]

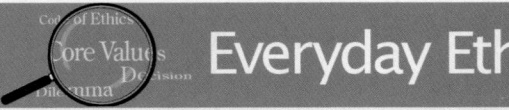

Everyday Ethics

Mr. Samuel wears an old maxillary complete denture that he has had for almost 30 years. He admits the denture moves around a bit and is sometimes difficult to chew with, but he refuses to have it remade because the removable lower partial denture he finally agreed to have remade last year was so expensive.

Bryce, a very caring dental hygienist who always tries to be sensitive to the financial concerns of his patients, decides to stop bothering Mr. Samuels about getting a new denture. He recommends an over-the-counter temporary soft reline material and the use of denture adhesive every day instead.

Questions for Consideration

1. What legal and ethical concepts (Table IV-I, page 339) are apparent in this scenario?
2. If he was asked, Bryce might say that his recommendations for this patient are supported by the core value of beneficence and that his personal values include helping Mr. Samuels keep the cost of his dental care low in any way he can. Do you agree or disagree? Explain why.
3. Explain how additional core values from Table II-1 on page 38 support a different approach to making recommendations.

B. Professional Topical Applications

■ Frequent maintenance appointments are needed to check the health of the gingival tissues; a fluoride varnish application can be made at each appointment.

■ Benefit is derived from fluoride in direct proportion to the frequency of application: the more frequent the application of fluoride, the greater the benefit.

III. SEALANTS

Application of sealants to overdenture abutment teeth has been shown effective in the prevention of dental caries.[15]

IV. MAINTENANCE APPOINTMENTS

■ Supervision by frequent maintenance appointments for scaling, biofilm debridement, topical fluoride applications, motivation, and instruction for biofilm control are essential.

■ Check for periodontal health, integrity of each restoration or sealant, and health of all oral tissues.

■ Check the condition of the removable prostheses by looking for fractures, cracks, chipped and worn teeth, and broken clasps.

■ More frequent maintenance appointments may be needed for patients at higher risk for periodontitis, dental caries, or other pathology.

DOCUMENTATION

The following items need to be included in the patient's permanent record of a patient with a fixed or removable prosthesis:

■ Description of the prosthesis.
■ Description of stability of the prosthesis.
■ Intraoral findings describing soft tissue, abutment teeth or placement of abutment implants.
■ Customized regimen for personal care.
■ Fluoride regimen of patient and recommendations.
■ Sample of Progress Note may be found in **Box 31-6**

BOX 31-6	**Example Progress Note: Partial Denture**

63-year-old male presents to clinic for an adult prophylaxis appointment with no chief complaint at this time. The patient does not take any medications. He presents with a removable partial denture on the mandibular arch. Patient states "the partial fits well." Underlying tissue is coral pink without lesions and salivary flow is normal. Abutment teeth are stable with pocket depths more 3 mm. Patient removes the partial nightly and soaks in water with an over the counter denture cleanser. Patient reports brushing denture twice a day and rinsing it after meals. Reappointed on a plan for three months' maintenance.

Signed: _____, RDH Date: _____.

Factors To Teach The Patient

■ How to perform a self-examination of the oral tissues.
■ How to evaluate the prosthesis.
■ Why all prostheses need cleaning more than once a day.
■ How to handle a removable prosthesis while it is cleaned.
■ The need to adapt toothbrushing, flossing, and use of other aids to the various configurations of abutment teeth whether natural tooth or implant.
■ How tongue cleaning contributes to complete oral health.
■ The significance of regular maintenance appointments: intraoral/extraoral screening for pathology, especially oral cancer screening; professional cleaning of remaining teeth and prostheses; and adjustments if needed.
■ Risks when missing teeth are not replaced.
■ The importance of seeking professional evaluation if any problems arise with existing prostheses; never attempt to repair or adjust a prosthesis.

References

1. Obreschkow C. Oral hygiene and periodontal considerations in restorative treatment with prefabricated attachments and precision-milled prosthetic devices. *Int J Periodontics Restorative Dent.* 1985;5(4):72–80.
2. American Dental Association, Council on Dental Materials, Instruments and Equipment; Council on Dental Therapeutics. Status report: effect of acidulated phosphate fluoride on porcelain and composite restorations. *J Am Dent Assoc.* 1988 Jan;116(1):115.
3. Brand HS, Gonggrijp S, Blanksma CJ. Cocaine and oral health. *Br Dent J.* 2008 Apr 12;204(7):365–9.
4. Reisburg DJ. Dental and prosthodontic care for patients with cleft or craniofacial conditions. *Cleft Palate Craniofac J.* 2000 Nov;37(6):534–7.
5. Yilmaz H, Aydin C, Bal BT, Qzcelik B. Effects of disinfectants on resilient denture-lining materials contaminated with *Staphylococcus aureus, Streptococcus sobrinus,* and *Candia albicans. Quintessence Int.* 2005 May;36(5):373–81.
6. Paranhos HF, Silva-Lovato CH, Souza RF. Effect of three methods for cleaning dentures on biofilms formed in vitro on acrylic resin. *J Prosthodont.* 2009 Jul;18(5):427–31.
7. Garrett NR. Poor oral hygiene, wearing dentures at night, perceptions of mouth dryness and burning, and lower educational level may be related to oral malodor in denture wearers. *J Evid Based Dent Pract.* 2010 Mar;10(1):67–9
8. DePaola LG, Minah GE. Isolation of pathogenic microorganims from dentures and denture-soaking containers of myelosuppressed cancer patients. *J Prosthet Dent.* 1983 Jan;49(1):20–4.
9. American Dental Association, Council on Dental Materials, Instruments, and Equipment. Denture cleansers. *J Am Dent Assoc.* 1983 Jan;106(1);77–9.
10. Budtz-Jörgensen E. Materials and methods for cleaning dentures. *J Prosthet Dent.* 1979 Dec;42(6)619–23.
11. Jose A, Coco B, Milligan S, Young B, Lappin D, Bagg J, Murray C, Ramage G. Reducing the incidence of denture stomatitis: are denture cleansers sufficient? *J Prosthodont.* 2010 Jun;19(4):252–7.
12. Ramage G, Tomsett K, Wickes BL, Lopez-Ribot JL, Redding SW. Denture stomatitis: a role for Candida biofilms. *Oral Surg Oral Med Oral Pathol Oral Radiol Endod.* 2004 Jul;98(1):53–9.
13. Shulman JD, Rivera-Hidalgo F, Beach MM. Risk factors associated with denture stomatitis in the United States. *J Oral Pathol Med.* 2005 Jul;34(6):340–6.
14. Ettinger RL, Olson, RJ, Wefel JS, Asmussen C. In vitro evaluation of topical fluorides for overdenture abutments. *J Prosthet Dent.* 1997 Sep;78(3):309–14.
15. Kurtz KS. Adjunctive caries control in overdenture abutment teeth: a new modality. *J Am Dent Assoc.* 1995 Feb;126(2):213–5.

The Patient With Dental Implants

STACY A. MATSUDA, RDH, BS, MS

Chapter Outline

Dental implants offer a means of tooth replacement that can preserve surrounding oral tissues normally compromised by a missing tooth by way of biomechanical force stimulation of the alveolar bone.

A dental implant simulates a natural tooth root. It may be used to replace one tooth or multiple teeth for a partially or completely edentulous patient. The various plates and parts used in the treatment of fractured bones or joint replacements are also implants.

Knowledge of dental implants is essential for all dental hygienists, especially the dental hygienist who is responsible for professional maintenance and monitoring of

peri-implant health. In addition, patients often will voice questions and/or concerns to the dental hygienist regarding their treatment options, which presents an opportune time for education to dispel confusion, alleviate fears, or reinforce a decision to proceed with needed treatment.

The success of an implant can depend on many factors, especially including patient understanding and skills for direct daily care of the prosthesis and the surrounding soft tissues. Frequent maintenance appointments for careful supervision and patient motivation are essential components for implant success. Key words and terminology are defined in **Box 32-1**.

BOX 32-1	Key Words

Dental Implants

Alloplast: an inert foreign body used for implantation within tissue.

Augment: to make greater, more numerous, larger, or more intense.

Augmentation: to increase the size beyond the existing size; in alveolar ridge or maxillary sinus augmentation: to increase the bone to accommodate a dental implant.

Biocompatible: capable of existing in harmony with the surrounding biologic environment.

Blade form dental implant: tooth root replacement with a wide, thin shape unlike that of a natural tooth.

Endosseous or root form dental implant: tooth root replacement with a cylindrical or conical shape similar to a natural tooth root.

Fibrous encapsulation: layer of fibrous connective tissue between the implant and surrounding bone. Also called fibrous integration; indicative of failed osseointegration.

Guided tissue regeneration: a procedure that attempts to regenerate lost periodontal structures, such as a barrier technique to exclude epithelial ingrowth.

Implant abutment: segment connecting the submerged implant body to the prosthetic component. The abutment enters the oral cavity providing a platform for attaching crowns or bridges.

Occlusal overload: masticatory force applied to an implant that exceeds the capacity of the bone implant interface or implant component to withstand it. Overload can compromise the integrity of an implant because no periodontal ligament is present to absorb the forces.

Osseointegration: the direct attachment or connection of osseous tissue to an inert alloplastic material without intervening connective tissue.

Peri-implantitis: inflammation of the periodontal tissues around an implant.

Provisional prosthesis or tooth crown: temporary or preliminary appliance or tooth used during healing or osseointegration for purposes of stability or appearance.

Root form dental implant: endosseous implant shaped in the approximate form of a tooth root.

Subperiosteal frame dental implant: framework placed under the periosteum that is tacked in place on the bone with a few small screws to support an overdenture; tooth root replacement with a cylindrical or conical shape.

Titanium: a uniquely biocompatible metal used for implants either in the commercially pure form or as an alloy.

Titanium alloy: a common titanium alloy (Ti-6A1–4V) used for dental implants that contains 6% aluminum to increase strength and decrease weight and 4% vanadium to prevent corrosion.

TYPES OF DENTAL IMPLANTS

Over the years, a variety of designs of dental implant systems have been tried clinically and studied with research. They are subperiosteal, transosseous, and endosseous. Currently, endosseous or "root form" implants are the most widely used.

I. SUBPERIOSTEAL

A. Definition

■ Custom-fabricated framework of metal that rests over the bone of the mandible or maxilla, under the periosteum: complete arch or unilateral.

B. Description[1,2]

■ Material: titanium or vitallium (cobalt-chromium-molybdenum).

■ *Two-step.* In the first step, a surgical flap is used to reflect mucosal tissues and to expose the underlying bone. An impression is made of the bony ridge. The metallic unit is cast and then placed in a second surgical step. Usually, four posts protrude into the oral cavity to hold the complete denture.

■ *One-step.* Computer-assisted tomography design and manufacturing have been applied, using a reformatted computed tomography scan from which approximate casts of the maxilla or mandible can be made. The implant is designed on this replica and is placed in one surgical procedure **(Figure 32-1)**.

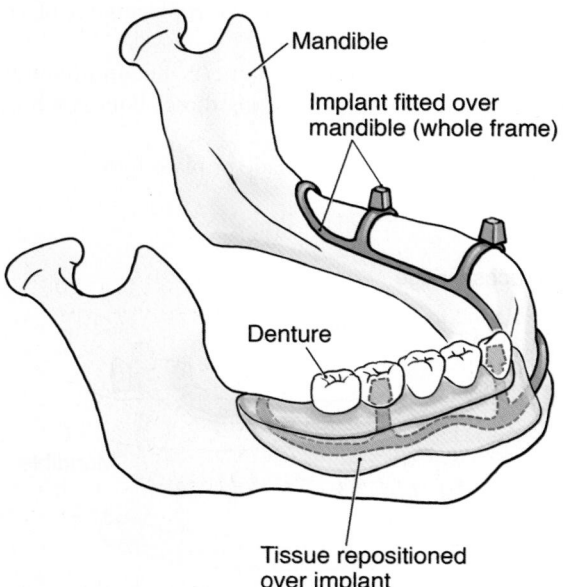

FIGURE 32-1 **Subperiosteal Implant.** The custom-fabricated framework is shown on the left side of the mandible; on the right side, the framework is shown by dotted lines under the denture.

II. TRANSOSSEOUS (TRANSOSTEAL)

A. Definition

- A dental implant that penetrates both cortical plates and passes through the full thickness of the alveolar bone.
- Also known as a *mandibular staple implant* or *staple bone implant*.

B. Description[3,4]

- Materials: stainless steel, ceramic-coated materials, and titanium alloy.
- A metal plate, fitted to the inferior border of the mandible, has five to seven pins extending toward the occlusal surface.
- Usually, two terminal pins protrude into the oral cavity to hold the overdenture. The pins are connected by a crossbar **(Figure 32-2)**.
- The transosteal implant can be used when the patient has an atrophic edentulous mandible or a congenital or traumatic deformity of the mandible.

III. ENDOSSEOUS (ENDOSTEAL)

Endosseous implants are placed fully within the bone and are the most widely used implants.

ENDOSSEOUS IMPLANT

I. DEFINITION

- An implant placed within the bone to replace a single tooth or provide support for the replacement of complete or partial loss of teeth.
- Successful tooth replacement is accomplished by osseointegration, which means direct bone anchorage to an implant body.
- Early forms (endosteal): blade or plate form.

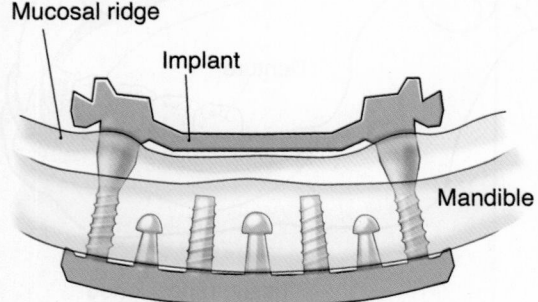

FIGURE 32-2 **Transosteal Implant.** Mandibular staple bone plate in the anterior region shows metal plate at the lower border of the mandible, with pins extending toward the occlusal surface. Terminal pins protrude into the oral cavity to hold the overdenture.

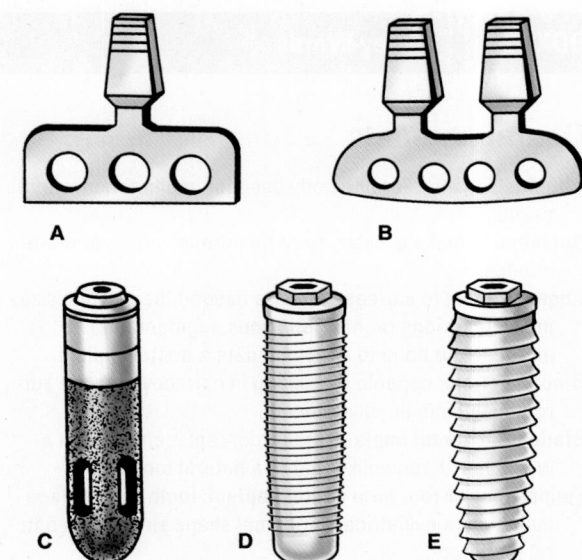

FIGURE 32-3 **Endosseous Implants.** (**A** and **B**) Blade types. (**C**) Cylinder type. (**D** and **E**) Screw types.

- Current forms (endosseous): "root form" or cylindrical; can be threaded, smooth, perforated or solid **(Figure 32-3)**.

II. DESCRIPTION

- Material: primarily plasma-sprayed titanium.
- May be placed in one or two phases.
- Immediate: the implant is placed immediately following extraction of the tooth it will replace.
- Two phase: the support, body, or fixture is placed in bone during the first surgical step and left covered by a periodontal flap for several months while the implant bonds with the bone. The abutment post is then exposed through the soft tissue at a second-stage surgical procedure. Placement of the crown or prosthesis follows.
- **Figure 32-4** illustrates the parts of an endosseous implant and the surrounding biologic tissues.

III. SURGICAL PREPARATION FOR IMPLANT PLACEMENT

- The surgical procedure requires a sterile placement of the implant into the bone.
- Whenever microorganisms are introduced during a surgical procedure, healing can be impaired.
- Manufacturers prepare implants in sterile packages.

IV. PROSTHODONTIC STEPS

- Attention to ideal requirements for acceptable prostheses is necessary.

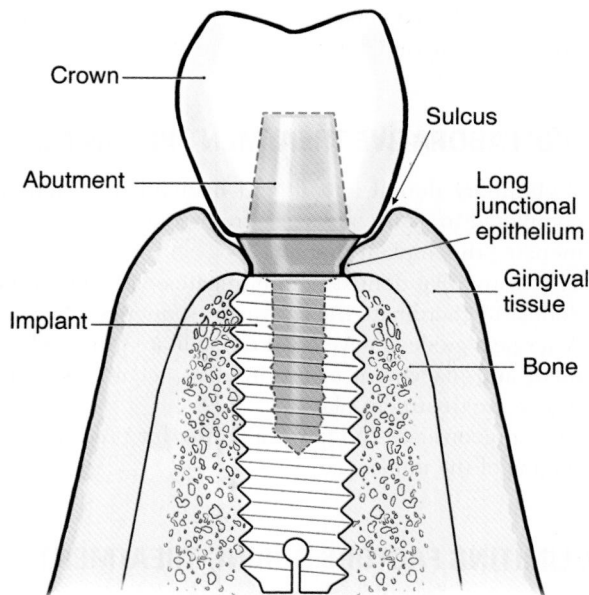

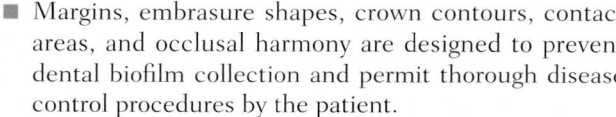

FIGURE 32-4 **Parts of an Endosseous Implant.** The crown, abutment, and implant are shown in relation to the surrounding bone and periodontal tissues.

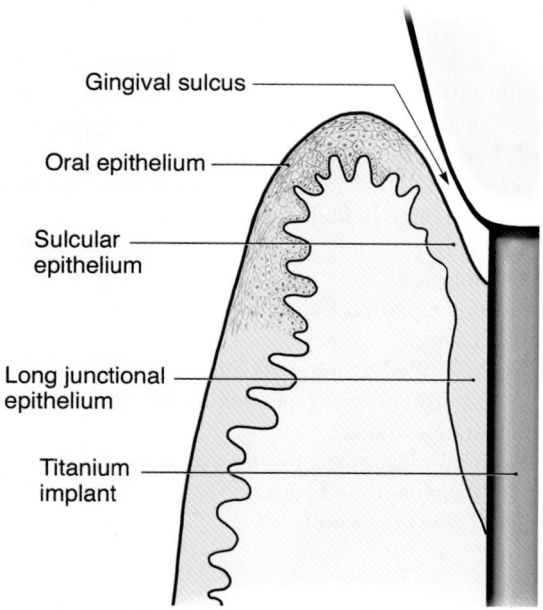

FIGURE 32-5 **The Implant/Soft Tissue Interface.** At the implant/soft tissue interface, there can be no connective tissue fiber attachment as when bone is present. The attachment resembles a long junctional epithelial attachment.

■ Margins, embrasure shapes, crown contours, contact areas, and occlusal harmony are designed to prevent dental biofilm collection and permit thorough disease control procedures by the patient.

IMPLANT INTERFACES

An implant has an inner interface with the *bone* and a *soft tissue* interface where the abutment, post, or other protruding portion of the implant is surrounded by the mucosal or gingival tissue.

I. IMPLANT/BONE INTERFACE

A. *Osseointegration*
   ■ Refers to direct structural and functional union between the implant and healthy living bone.
   ■ Indicates successful placement of the implant.
   ■ No mobility evident.
B. *Fibrous encapsulation (also called fibrous integration)*
   ■ Refers to the infusion of connective tissue cells between the implant body and surrounding bone.
   ■ Indicates failure of osseointegration.
   ■ Mobility of the implant is evident.

II. IMPLANT/SOFT TISSUE INTERFACE[5,6]

A. The external environment of an implant is the oral cavity, with saliva, dental biofilm, and debris.

B. Biologic seal (permucosal seal): between the implant and the soft tissue, a biologic seal exists to prevent microorganisms and inflammation-producing agents from entering the tissues.
C. Soft tissue connection: sulcular epithelium is in contact with the implant surface.
   ■ The attachment appears similar to the epithelial attachment of the junctional epithelium of a natural tooth. Hemidesmosomes and basal lamina have been identified.
   ■ The epithelium resembles a long junctional epithelium.
   ■ No connective tissue fibers (Sharpey's fibers) can exist to hold the attachment as with a natural tooth.
   ■ **Figure 32-5** illustrates the implant/soft tissue interface at the junctional epithelium.

PREPARATION AND PLACEMENT

I. PATIENT SELECTION

■ Careful screening is essential at the start.
■ Generally acceptable physical health.
■ Genuine desire to go through the required treatment.
   ■ Realistic expectations
   ■ Ability to manage oral self-care measures.
■ Diagnosis and treatment planning are based on a risk–benefit analysis and follow a detailed medical, dental, and behavioral history along with an oral and radiographic examination. Sometimes a psychologic examination is used.

A. Systemic Health

1. *Medical history.* The patient must be free of systemic conditions that can interfere with healing or acceptance of the implant. Biocompatibility of the implant with body tissues is essential.
2. *Contraindications.* Examples of conditions that make a patient a poor risk include:
   - Pregnancy
   - Debilitation
   - Recent radiation therapy to the affected part of the oral cavity
   - Uncontrolled diabetes mellitus
   - Alcoholism or heavy alcohol intake
   - Substance abuse
   - An immunosuppressive disease or medication
   - Anticoagulant medication
   - Psychosis or paranoia

B. Tobacco Use

- All forms of tobacco can increase the risk for implant failure.
- During implant placement, it has been recommended that the patient cease at least 1 week before surgery and continue to avoid tobacco at least until healing is completed.
- For high expectancy of best implant health, a tobacco cessation program is advised (Chapter 33, page 489).

C. Oral Examination

1. Evidence of adequate depth of alveolar bone:
   - Radiographic or other measurements for bone can be made
   - In the absence of adequate bone, or an intruding maxillary sinus, treatment planning may include bone grafting to augment the proposed treatment site.
2. Periodontal health
   - The presence of active periodontitis contraindicates implant placement until the disease is treated and under control.
   - The patient must demonstrate consistent and effective personal oral care.

II. INFORMATION FOR THE PATIENT

- The patient's role as a cotherapist in the long-term maintenance requirements for implant therapy.
- Explanation of procedures to be performed and the time frame for scheduling appointments.
- Review of possible complications.
- Understand the role of personal oral care and the need for daily dental biofilm control.
- Agreement to follow through with the recommendations for personal and professional care.

- Sign an informed consent statement and agreement of understanding (in Chapter 24, page 358).

III. COLLABORATIVE TREATMENT PLANNING

- Preliminary dental and dental hygiene treatment is completed to insure a disease-free mouth before commencing the implant therapy.
- The restorative dentist communicates with the periodontist to coordinate the treatment sequence.
- A surgical guide is developed to facilitate proper alignment and placement of the implant according to the prosthetic treatment plan.
- The surgeon uses the surgical guide for precise positioning of the implant.

IV. LIMITING FACTORS DURING TREATMENT

The success of implant therapy can be compromised by many factors. Problems can occur in any of the following ways:

- Tissue damage during surgery because of overheating of the bone
- Infection
- Premature biomechanical loading before osseointegration
- Bruxism and/or parafunction during healing
  - Excessive lateral forces with inflammation can result in bone loss. This is especially true in the maxillary posterior region where the bone is typically the poorest quality and occlusal forces are the highest.
  - The posterior maxillary region can be vulnerable to breakdown of the implant-to-bone interface.
  - Preventive measures include proper prosthetic design that compensates for biomechanical force and treatment planning the proper number of implants to distribute the occlusal load.
  - Corrective measures include splinting or fabrication of a bite appliance.

POSTRESTORATIVE EVALUATION

Once the implant or implants are fully integrated in the bone and restorative work is complete, a postrestorative evaluation is made. Using radiographs, clinical examination, and close visual inspection, evaluation, and documentation include the following:

- Radiographic: bone level; no space between implant and abutment; and no space between abutment and prosthesis
- Peri-implant tissue health: no inflammation, no calculus or biofilm, no suppuration
- Test for mobility: no movement
- Patient function and comfort

■ Sufficiency of patient's oral self-care; feedback provided and additional instruction as needed with hands-on practice.

PERI-IMPLANT HYGIENE

A key requirement for implant success is the disease control program for the tissue surrounding the implant. Meticulous daily personal hygiene is a necessity: repeated instruction may be needed.

I. CARE OF THE NATURAL TEETH

■ Transmission of microblmorganisms from the natural teeth and periodontal pockets to the peri-implant tissues can occur.
■ Periodontal pockets around the natural teeth act as natural reservoirs, and periodontal pathogens from the pockets colonize in the tissue around the implants.
■ Before placement of the implants, it is necessary for the periodontal condition to be treated and brought to a healthy state.
■ After the placement of the implants, the maintenance program emphasizes care of the natural teeth and tissues as well as the peri-implant tissues.

II. IMPLANT BIOFILM

■ Biofilm microorganisms around implants with healthy permucosal tissue have been shown to be similar to the flora around natural teeth. Gram-positive, nonmotile, coccoid, and other forms of bacteria predominate.[7,8]
■ The tissues around implant posts or abutments react to microorganisms and their toxic products in a manner similar to the gingiva surrounding natural teeth.
■ When inflammation and pocket depths increase, the total number of microorganisms including spirochetes and motile rods will increase.

III. PLANNING THE DISEASE CONTROL PROGRAM

A. Relation to Treatment

Supervision of a patient's oral hygiene begins before the surgical phase for implant placement and carries on throughout the treatment phases.

B. Types of Prostheses

1. Implant-supported prostheses may be partial, complete, fixed, removable, or single-tooth replacements. Instruction for their care is provided (pages 450 to 459).
2. *Examples*
   ■ Overdenture (Figure 31-9, page 461)
   ■ Screw-retained restoration
   ■ Cemented restoration

C. Monitoring Prostheses Fit

■ Instruct the patient to monitor the fit of the implant prosthesis on a regular basis by firmly wiggling the crown, bridge, or superstructure.
■ Components that have become loose need treatment and are considered true emergencies in the dental practice.

IV. SELECTION OF BIOFILM-REMOVAL METHODS

A. Each patient needs an individually planned program so that each type of abutment and prosthesis can be maintained in a biofilm-free environment.
   ■ Provide specific directions in a take-home printed form.
B. Abutments or posts are cleaned daily with meticulous care.
C. *Precautions*
   ■ Prevent damage to implant materials. Use implements, dentifrices, or other cleaning agents that will not scratch or abrade the titanium or other material.
   ■ Each device is checked and selected by the dental hygienist before recommended for use.
D. *Toothbrushes*
   ■ Select toothbrush filaments that are smooth, soft, and end-rounded to prevent damage to the titanium and the peri-implant tissue.
   ■ Power toothbrushes with soft, end-rounded filaments can be applied effectively.
E. *Dental floss*
   ■ Specialized spongy filament floss is available with a built-in threader (Figure 28-6, page 414).
   ■ Commercial floss products include corded varieties.
F. *Interdental care*
   ■ Use only smooth plastic coated wires for interdental brushes (Figure 28-9, page 416).
   ■ Avoid all metal core brushes.
   ■ Synthetic yarn or a folded section of gauze bandage can be used to clean abutments under overdentures.
   ■ A floss threader can be used to position yarn or dental floss around an abutment and under a fixed prosthesis (Figure 31-2, page 451).
   ■ The end-tuft brush with soft filaments is particularly useful in lingual and palatal embrasure spaces (Figure 28-11, page 417).
   ■ Round, wooden toothpicks used in plastic handles can be effective for cleaning exposed proximal tooth surfaces and "penciling" just under the crest of the gingiva (Figure 28-12, page 417).

V. RINSING AND IRRIGATION

A. General cleaning
   ■ Use of an irrigator can remove debris before specific cleaning with toothbrush and auxiliary aids.

B. Chemotherapy
- Rinsing or daily irrigation with an approved anti-microbial can be recommended to help minimize bacterial accumulation and inflammation. Specific directions for preparation of the solution and use of the irrigator are demonstrated and practiced with the patient.
- Example: Chlorhexidine, 0.12%, has been shown to be effective. A cotton swab, sponge tip, or interdental brush dipped in the solution can be applied directly to the gingival margins to help prevent staining of oral tissues or tooth-color restorations.

VI. FLUORIDE MEASURES FOR DENTAL CARIES CONTROL

- For the patient with natural teeth, daily fluoride self-application is incorporated into the regimen.
- Avoid acidic fluoride preparations.[9,10]
- Neutral sodium fluoride is recommended.

MAINTENANCE

Periodic care for professional maintenance and monitoring is scheduled according to the complexity of the restoration or prosthetic superstructure in addition to the patient's ability to perform adequate home self-care and their periodontal risk profile (susceptibility and present condition).

A. Continuing supervision of the patient with dental implants is essential.
B. Episodic nature of periodontal and peri-implant inflammation:
- A multitude of factors may affect the patient's ability to withstand the critical threshold beyond which pathogenic organisms can overwhelm the host response.
- Regular in-office periodontal maintenance care is a critical component of implant therapy success.
C. Patient expectations:
- The well-informed and conscientious patient who devotes much time each day on personal care procedures expects a maintenance appointment that thoroughly evaluates the health status of the periodontal tissues and the completeness of biofilm control efforts.

I. BASIC CRITERIA FOR IMPLANT SUCCESS

A. The long-term success of an implant is assessed during routine, frequent examinations.
B. Dental hygienists need to recognize the basic criteria by which an ailing/failing implant can be identified.
C. A healthy implant shows the following:
- No pain or discomfort reported by the patient.
- No mobility.
- Radiograph: no bone loss or peri-implant radiolucency; no space at the implant-abutment interface

or at abutment–prosthesis interface with confirmation of a tight fit.
- No clinical signs of peri-implantitis: close visual inspection shows healthy gingival tissue surrounding the abutment, firm in consistency with no edema.
- No bleeding or increased depths on gentle probing performed with a rounded, smooth plastic probe.
- No movement or loose components in the prosthesis; check for cracks, fractures, missing or non-secured screws by close visual inspection while applying coronally directed force to superstructure using a rigid instrument such as a carver or scaler.

II. FREQUENCY OF APPOINTMENTS

- The patient's daily oral biofilm removal with regular professional supervision and monitoring of maintenance appointments directly influence the long-term success of an implant.
- When teeth were lost originally because of lack of daily biofilm control by the patient, a more intense program of education and practice may be needed.
- Neglect may have been caused by lack of knowledge about, or appreciation for, preventive measures.
- Each patient needs a personalized appointment interval, depending on individual needs.
- The first series of appointments following placement of the implant(s) starts within a week and is scheduled weekly until healing is completed and the patient has demonstrated the ability to control the dental biofilm.
- Maintenance appointments during the first year may be at 1- or 2-month intervals.

III. THE MAINTENANCE APPOINTMENT

A. Health History Review; Vital Signs; Intraoral/Extraoral Examination

- Basic review questions can reveal the present state of health, recent illnesses, changes in medications, and other current information.
- Comparisons with previous records permit assessment of vital signs and extraoral/intraoral observations.

B. Selective Radiographs

- A standard procedure is used so that comparisons can be made for bone level to determine status of implant stability.
- Special film placement devices have been developed.[11,12]

C. Periodontal Assessment

1. *Peri-implant tissue.* Visual examination shows no signs of inflammation as evidenced by the usual criteria of changes in color, size, shape, and consistency.

2. *Probing*
   - A smooth plastic probe with rounded end is used.
   - Pressure-sensitive probes are available to guard against excess insertion pressure.
   - Sweep probe gently around the internal surface of the sulcus or pocket wall to determine bleeding tendency (Figure 22-11, page 326).
   - If bleeding occurs, the depth of attachment is carefully measured. Each millimeter of gingival sulcus is probed to detect incipient changes.
   - What could seem like a minute area of gingival bleeding on probing, whether the pocket is shallow or has started to deepen, can be a warning signal that an area may not be covered adequately by present self-care procedures or may need additional periodontal treatment.
3. *Mobility determination*
   - Implant mobility is always present in a failed implant.
   - Careful mobility testing is done with close visual inspection for fluid at the gingival margin; fluid emerging from the peri-implant area around an implant on mobility provocation can be a sign of ailment.
   - Inform the dentist and/or implant surgeon immediately of noticeable mobility.
4. *Dental biofilm*
   - Tested with a disclosing agent.
   - Examined for biofilm accumulation patterns for patient instruction, and documented.
5. *Calculus*
   - Mineralized deposits usually are not extensive, hard, or firmly attached to implant abutments or other protruding parts, provided the patient has been faithful with daily procedures and professional maintenance appointments.
   - Semi-soft, partially mineralized deposits can be effectively removed with variations of floss implements.
6. *Review of personal dental biofilm control procedures*
   - Bleeding points and/or probing depth increases are brought to the attention of the patient along with strategies to address oral self-care problem areas.
   - The patient demonstrates self-care methods, and the clinician provides feedback and recommendations for improvements.

D. Instrumentation

1. Care must be taken not to scratch or alter in any way the surfaces of titanium and other materials making up the implant superstructure.
2. *Biofilm removal.* Soft deposits are removed from the titanium abutment with gauze strips, sponge-filament dental floss, or yarn wrapped around the abutment 360°.
   - Floss alternatives such as textured cords are often sufficient to remove partially mineralized deposits that are loosely bound to the titanium abutment surface.
3. *Calculus removal.* Specialized implant-specific instruments are indicated for hard deposits that remain following soft deposit removal on titanium abutments.
   - Current implant-specific instruments mimic traditional universal curets and sickle scalers in design.
   - Titanium metal instruments safe for use on implants are available in addition to the more traditional nonmetal plastic instruments.
   - Gold-plated instruments are also available but must be monitored for wear to prevent inadvertent scratching of a titanium abutment from the metal beneath the gold.
   - Implant-specific ultrasonic tips and inserts are available for peri-implant debridement. Use *low* power when instrumenting implant abutments with an ultrasonic device.
4. *Prevention of damage to the implant surface*
   - Confine manual instrument strokes to the prosthesis and the supragingival area of the abutment.
   - Severe abrasion can result from application of an ultrasonic scaler without a specialized tip designed for implant use.
5. *Stain removal.* Unless it is necessary for esthetics, stain removal is not included routinely.
   - When selective stain removal with a rubber cup is indicated, only a nonabrasive agent is used and applied gently.
   - Tin oxide or nonabrasive toothpaste may be suitable for polishing agents.
6. *Professional subgingival irrigation.* The use of 0.12% chlorhexidine after professional instrumentation may be a treatment alternative when peri-implantitis has been present. Irrigation with chlorhexidine gluconate has been shown to be a safe procedure around implants.[13,14]

IMPLANT COMPLICATIONS

I. FACTORS THAT CONTRIBUTE TO IMPLANT FAILURE

A. Systemic Factors

- Not revealed or known in initial preparation of medical history
- Undiagnosed or uncontrolled diabetes
- Immunocompromised patient
- Poor vascularity
- Poor bone quality or quantity
- Unanticipated infection
- Cancer, osteoporosis

B. Surgical Phase of Treatment

- Traumatic insertion
- Break in sterile procedure

C. Restorative Phase of Treatment

■ Premature or excessive loading
■ Parafunctional forces
■ "Pericementitis:" iatrogenic peri-implantitis due to retained cement at implant–abutment interface.

D. Maintenance Phase

■ Patient neglect; noncompliance with self-care, instruction, and maintenance visits
■ Peri-implantitis: soft tissue reactions
■ Mechanical/structural complications:
  A. Fractured components
  B. Broken attachments
  C. Loose single tooth abutment (true emergency: instruct patient to call office immediately)

II. PERI-IMPLANT PROBLEMS

Two prominent contributing factors to breakdown of the peri-implant environment are occlusal overload (biomechanical stress) and bacterial infection.

■ *Initial stage: Peri-implant mucositis*
  A. Reversible bacterial infection in the soft tissue similar to gingivitis.
  B. Mild color change with accompanying bleeding may be present.
■ *Secondary stage: Peri-implantitis*
  A. Inflammation has reached the level of the bone.
  B. Edema or hemorrhage present in the surrounding tissues.
  C. Exudate may or may not be present.
  D. Increase in probing depth.

III. AILING IMPLANT

■ Inflammation present but no mobility.
■ Bone may appear normal in the radiograph or there may be incipient bone loss evident.
■ Review/reinforce patient's oral self-care practice.
■ Perform careful supragingival debridement.
■ Irrigate with an oral antimicrobial rinse (0.12% chlorhexidine gluconate); prescribe for daily home use.
■ Adjunctive therapy using local delivery antimicrobial placement may also be indicated.
■ Consultation with the surgeon may be needed if the tissue does not respond favorably to therapy within 2 weeks.

IV. FAILING IMPLANT

■ Inflammation present; may be accompanied by exudate on mobility testing.
■ Bone loss has occurred and continues.
■ Mobility is incipient, with movement faintly noticeable.
■ Consult the surgeon when an implant shows signs of failing.

V. FAILED IMPLANT

■ Evident mobility; signifies a serious problem.
■ Radiographic changes in bone level are apparent when compared with prior films; may show a vertical bony defect.
■ Implant mobility coupled with radiographic evidence of bone destruction are conclusive indications of a failed implant.
■ Patient is referred immediately back to the surgeon for evaluation and removal of the failed implant.

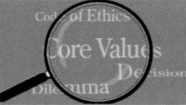 # Everyday Ethics

Karen reviewed the permanent record progress notes before receiving Ms. Halvee for her routine 4 months' continuing care. Dr. Richards had seen Ms. Halvee within the week for an examination and radiograph of tooth #10 where a root canal had been placed 2 years ago and was giving her trouble. The endodontic therapy had failed and Dr. Richards had recorded that the tooth was now indicated for extraction.

While Karen was updating blood pressure and medical history, she noticed that her patient did not seem to be her usual talkative self. "I guess I have to have a bridge put in and *I am not happy* about it," Ms. Halvee said.

Karen asked, "Have you discussed this with Dr. Richards?"

Ms. Halvee replied, "To tell the truth I'm really confused. My brother asked me why I'm not getting an implant. Dr. Richards just said we need to do a bridge."

Questions for Consideration

1. What obligation does Karen have, and what procedure does Karen need to follow, in terms of assuring that Ms. Halvee's treatment options have been fully presented and adequately explained and understood?

2. Is there an issue with societal trust in this incident? Which of the other dental hygiene core values are evident in this scenario? (Refer to Table II-I, page 38.)

3. With respect to core values and informed consent standards, role-play (1) additional conversation between Karen and Ms. Halvee, and (2) a dialogue that could ensue between Karen and Dr. Richards as Karen explains Ms. Halvee's concerns about the treatment he has indicated for her.

DOCUMENTATION

All members of the implant therapy team are kept informed and up to date on the status of the patient from initial consultation through the postrestorative evaluation. Reports and copies of progress notes are sent between surgical and restorative practices.

For documenting appointments concerning a dental implant, the following factors are recorded in the progress note:

- Consultation before implant treatment plan
  A. Patient advised of all options to replace missing tooth/teeth.
  B. Patient understands surgical, prosthetic and maintenance phases of dental implant therapy.
  C. Expected benefits, principal risks, and potential complications of dental implant therapy have been fully explained.
  D. Alternatives to suggested dental implant treatment have been outlined.
  E. Necessary follow-up care and home self-care with ongoing professional maintenance appointments have been fully explained to pt.
- Maintenance: examination

In addition to standard continuing care procedures, evaluate and document implant-specific assessments as follows:

A. Verify dental implant locations with chart and current radiographs.
B. Peri-implant tissue tone, color, and texture
C. Presence of inflammation: note erythema, edema, and/or exudate
D. Evidence of pathology: lightly probe peri-implant space if visual signs of inflammation present
E. Radiograph if pathology present, and/or every twelve months to look for changes in bone level

F. Implant mobility
G. Prosthesis stability
H. Biofilm and calculus accumulation: note quantity and location.
- An example of a Progress Note appears in **Box 32-2**.

Factors To Teach The Patient

- How to care for implants; special needs related to the titanium surfaces.
- How the health of the periodontal tissues and the duration of the implants and prostheses depend on meticulous daily self-care by the patient.
- The role of biofilm in periodontitis and peri-implantitis; vulnerability of the implant to infection from periodontal pathogens that may be present on adjacent natural teeth.
- How cleaning a mouth with complex restorations takes longer. Time must be allotted in the daily schedule for thorough biofilm removal each day, especially before going to bed.
- Why frequent, ongoing professional maintenance care and annual radiographs to document bone height around implants are necessary.

References

1. Harris BW. A new technique for the subperiosteal implant. *J Am Dent Assoc.* 1990 Sep;121(9):422–4.
2. Homoly PA. The restorative and surgical technique for the full maxillary subperiosteal implant. *J Am Dent Assoc.* 1990 Sep;121(9):404–7.
3. Cranin AN, Sher J, Schilb TP. The transosteal implant. A 17-year review and report. *J Prosthet Dent.* 1986 Jun;55(6):709–18.
4. Small IA. The fixed mandibular implant: Its use in reconstructive prosthetics. *J Am Dent Assoc.* 1990; Sept; 121(3):369, 372, 374.
5. Donley TG, Gillette WB. Titanium endosseous implant-soft tissue interface: a literature review. *J Periodontol.* 1991 Feb;62(2)153–60.
6. Cochran D. Implant therapy I. *Ann Periodontol.* 1996 Nov;1(11): 710–20.
7. Mombelli A, Lang NP. Microbial aspects of implant dentistry. *Periodontol 2000;1994;4:74–80.*
8. Mombelli A, Marxer M, Gaberthuel T, Grunder U, Lang NP. The microbiota of osseointegrated implants in patients with a history of periodontal disease. *J Clin Periodontol.* 1995 Feb;22(2):124–30.
9. Siirila HS, Kononen M. The effect of topical fluorides on the surface of commercially pure titanium. *Int J Oral Maxillofac Implants.* 1991; Spring: 6(1): 50–4.
10. Probster L, Lin W, Huttemann H. Effect of fluoride prophylactic agents on titanium surfaces. *Int J Oral Maxillofac Implants.* 1992 Fall; 7(4):390–4.
11. Cox JF, Pharoah M. An alternative holder for radiographic evaluation of tissue-integrated prostheses. *J Prosthet Dent.* 1986 Sep; 56(9):338–41.
12. Meijer HJA, Steen WHA, Bosman F. Standardized radiographs of the alveolar crest around implants in the mandible. *J Prosthet Dent.* 1992 Aug;68(8):318–21.
13. Lavigne SE, Krust-bray KS, Williams KB, Killoy WJ, Theisen F. Effects of subgingival irrigation with chlorhexidine on the periodontal status of patients with HA-coated integral dental implants. *Int J Oral Maxillofac Implants.* 1994 Number 2;9(2):156–62.
14. Felo A, Shibly O, Ciancio SG, Lauciello FR, Ho A. Effects of subgingival chlorhexidine irrigation on periimplant maintenance. *Am J Dent.* 1997 Apr;10(4):107–10.

BOX 32-2	Sample Progress Note

Patient presents for continuing care appointment following final seating of implant prosthesis #3. No patient chief concern/complaint. BP 132/84 Right arm; Pulse 79. Intraoral/extraoral exam within normal limits. Peri-implant soft tissue appears firm/healthy indicating apparent oral self-care; One periapical radiograph #3 implant: abutment-prosthesis interface within normal limits; no mobility evident on implant fixture or prosthesis; no biofilm or calculus accumulation #3; pt doing well overall. Treatment: reinforce personal care procedures, periodontal debridement with manual & ultrasonic scaling. Next: 3-month continuing care. Copy report to surgeon and general dentist.

Signed: _____, RDH Date: _____.

33 | CHAPTER

The Patient Who Uses Tobacco

ELAIN BENTON, RDH, BS, CTTS
JANE COTTER, RDH, MS

Chapter Outline

| BOX 33-1 | Key Words and Abbreviations |

Tobacco Use

Carcinogen: substance or chemical that has been known to cause cancer.

CDCP: Centers for Disease Control and Prevention

Chemical dependency: generic term relating to psychological or physical dependency, or both, on an exogenous substance.

COPD: chronic obstructive pulmonary disease

Cotinine: a by-product of nicotine found in body fluids; cotinine levels are used in behavioral research to determine recent use of nicotine-containing products or recent contact with passive smoke and in clinical research to determine correlations between cotinine levels and oral disease.

Drug abuse: any use of a drug that causes physical, psychological, economic, legal, and/or social harm to the person who uses or other persons affected by the user's behavior.

Drug addiction: a chronic disorder leading to negative physical, psychological, or social consequences from compulsive use of substance; characterized by continued use despite negative effects encountered by use.

Dysphoria: generalized feeling of ill being, malaise, restlessness, and discomfort.

FDA: Food and Drug Administration

Nicotine: a poisonous, addictive stimulant that is the chief psychoactive ingredient in tobacco.

Nicotine gum: polacrilex gum developed to aid in tobacco cessation; available as an over-the-counter product.

Nicotine lozenge: lozenge developed to aid in tobacco cessation; available as an over-the-counter product.

Nicotine nasal spray: a prescription nicotine withdrawal product used nasally by the patient to aid in tobacco cessation.

Nicotine patch: a transdermal form of nicotine withdrawal therapy; available as an over-the-counter product.

Nicotine inhaler: a prescription nicotine inhalation system used orally for tobacco cessation.

Nitrosamines: cancer-causing chemicals found in tobacco.

Oral cancer: in this chapter, the term "oral cancer" includes cancer of the lips, tongue, floor of the mouth, palate, gingiva, alveolar mucosa, buccal mucosa, and oropharynx.

Placenta abruptio: premature detachment of a normally situated placenta.

Placenta previa: placenta implanted in the lower segment of the uterus extending to the margin of the internal opening of the cervix; may obstruct opening partially or completely.

Psychoactive drug: possessing the ability to alter mood, behavior, cognitive processes, or mental tension.

Pyrolysis: chemical decomposition of a substance by heat.

Smoke: visible vapor and gases given off by a burning substance.

> **Environmental tobacco smoke (ETS) or passive smoke:** tobacco smoke present in room air resulting from ignited tobacco products burning in an ashtray or exhaled by a smoker (people who are currently smoking are also exposed to other smokers' sidestream smoke).
>
> **Mainstream smoke:** smoke that is inhaled directly into the user's lungs.
>
> **Sidestream smoke:** the aerosol emitted directly into the surrounding air from the lit end of a smoldering tobacco product; may be inhaled by the user; is a major component of environmental smoke.
>
> **Third-hand smoke:** tobacco smoke residue absorbed by furnishings.

Sudden infant death syndrome (SIDS): Sudden and unexpected death of an apparently healthy infant; typically occurring between the ages of 3 weeks and 5 months.

TSNAs: potent carcinogenic tobacco-specific nitrosamines.

Transdermal: method of drug delivery by patch on skin; a mode for slow release over extended time.

Transmucosal: type of drug delivery by infiltration of mucosal lining.

Use: using the substance of tobacco because of an individual's addiction to nicotine.

User: an individual who either smokes tobacco or places tobacco in the mouth.

Evidence began to accumulate many years ago that use of tobacco poses an enormous threat to human health.[1]

■ The Surgeon General's first report on tobacco, released in 1965, made an unqualified announcement of tobacco's harm.[2]

■ Subsequent reports further documented the health hazards and discussed the social, economic, and cultural aspects of tobacco use.[3]

■ Oral effects of tobacco use are well documented.

■ Advice from health professionals has been shown to be a powerful influence on patients' decisions to stop or not begin using tobacco.

■ Dental and dental hygiene professionals are in an ideal position and have a responsibility to provide patients who use tobacco with the opportunity to enter a tobacco cessation program to assist in stopping tobacco use.

■ Key words related to tobacco use and addiction are defined in **Box 33-1**. **Box 33-2** defines the various forms of tobacco.

HEALTH HAZARDS

■ Tobacco is toxic to humans. Tobacco use is the single most preventable cause of disease and premature death in the world. As detailed in **Figure 33-1** smoking has caused more preventable deaths in the United States

BOX 33-2	Key Words

Forms of Tobacco

Bidis: small, thin hand-rolled cigarettes consisting of tobacco wrapped in a tendu or temburni leaf (plants native to Asia), and may be secured with a colorful string at one or both ends.

Chaw: a golf-ball-sized portion of chewing tobacco held in the user's mouth usually inside the cheek or between the lower lip, gingiva, and mucosa.

Chewing tobacco: tobacco available in loose-leaf, twist, and plug forms manufactured by air-drying tobacco leaves; held inside cheek and/or chewed (chaw).

Cigar: 1 to 20 gm of air-cured fermented tobacco wrapped in paper that is smoked.

Cigarette: less than 1 gm of unfermented tobacco wrapped in a cylindrical paper-enclosed form that is smoked.

Hookah pipe: a water pipe used to smoke specially made flavored tobacco.

Kreteks: referred to as clove cigarettes—are imported from Indonesia and typically contain a mixture of tobacco, cloves, and other additives.

Pipe tobacco: ground leaf tobacco manufactured for smoking through a pipe.

Quid: a pinch of snuff held in the user's mouth for various periods of time.

Sachets: moist snuff in ready to use pouches that look like small tea bags.

Smokeless (spit) tobacco: term used to define all forms of tobacco that are not ignited or inhaled.

Smoking tobacco: any form of tobacco that is ignited and smoked by the user.

Snuff: fire-cured, finely ground or powdered tobacco sold in both dry and moist forms or baglike pouches; not chewed but a small amount ("pinch" or "quid") is placed and held between cheek and gingiva or lower lip, gingiva, and mucosa. Snuff can also be sniffed or inhaled into the nose.

Snus: moist powder tobacco product that is a smokeless, spitless pouch; originated from a variant of dry snuff used in the nineteenth century in Sweden.

Tobacco pipe: a tube with a bowl at one end used to smoke tobacco.

than AIDS, alcohol use, motor vehicle accidents, homicides, drug overdoses, and suicides combined.

- Nearly 21% of adult Americans smoke, and thousands of children and adolescents become regular users of tobacco every day.[4]
- Offspring of smokers are more likely to become smokers.[5]

- As years of tobacco use accumulate, so do the systemic and oral health effects of all forms of tobacco.
- Life expectancy is shortened.[6] The number of years lost depends on many factors.
- Women who smoke or are exposed to environmental tobacco smoke (ETS) are at risk for the same smoke-related health problems as men.[7]

Comparison of Causes of Preventable Deaths in the U.S.

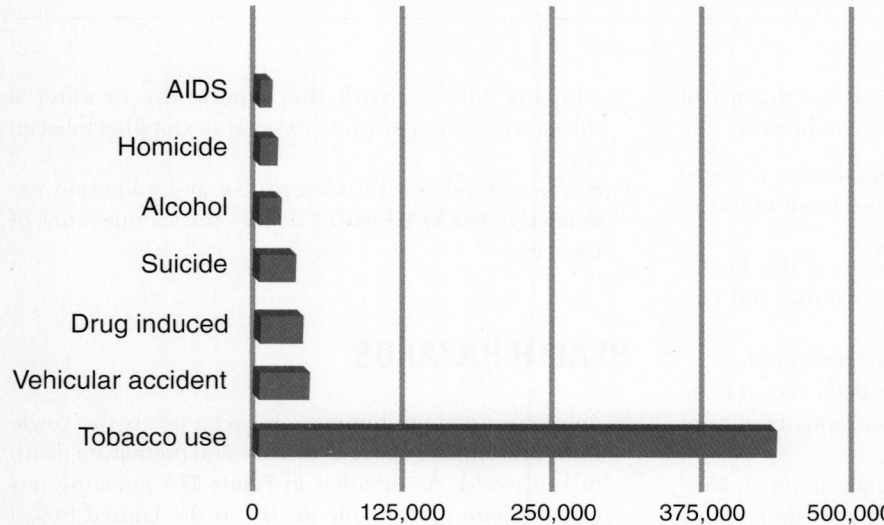

FIGURE 33-1 **Preventable Deaths in the United States in 2007.** (*Source:* Xu J, Kochanek KD, Murphy S, Tejada-Vera, B. Deaths: final data for 2007. National Vital Statistics Reports. 2010 May [cited 2010 Sept 29];58(19):1–135. Available from: http://www.cdc.gov/nchs/data/nvsr/nvsr58/nvsr58_19.pdf).

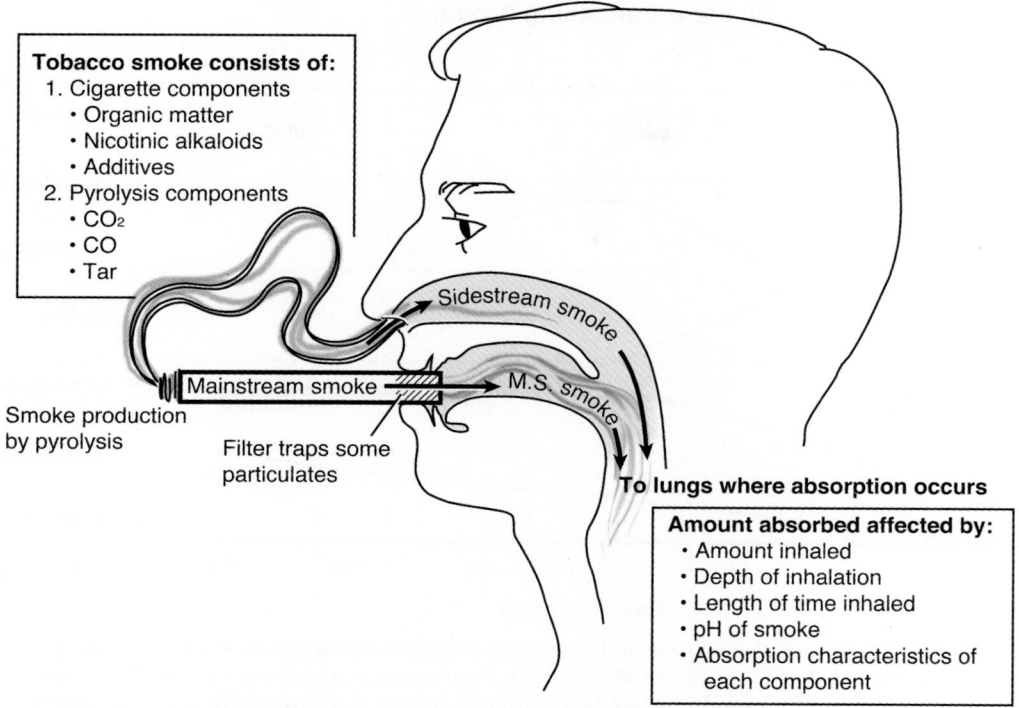

Tobacco smoke consists of:
1. Cigarette components
   • Organic matter
   • Nicotinic alkaloids
   • Additives
2. Pyrolysis components
   • CO_2
   • CO
   • Tar

Smoke production by pyrolysis

Filter traps some particulates

Mainstream smoke

Sidestream smoke

M.S. smoke

To lungs where absorption occurs

Amount absorbed affected by:
• Amount inhaled
• Depth of inhalation
• Length of time inhaled
• pH of smoke
• Absorption characteristics of each component

FIGURE 33-2 **Components of Mainstream Smoke and Factors Influencing Absorption by the Lungs.**

■ As much as 90% of lung cancer deaths in women are attributable to smoking; lung cancer has surpassed breast cancer to become the leading cause of cancer death among American women.

COMPONENTS OF TOBACCO PRODUCTS

■ The public mistakenly believes that nicotine is the harmful substance in tobacco. Instead nicotine is only the most addictive substance, it is the other chemicals, including pesticides, aldehydes, ketones, and amines, found in processed tobacco that are the most harmful.

■ Once tobacco is ignited, carcinogenic nitrosamines, polonium 210, carbon monoxide, and other substances become part of mainstream smoke and are emitted in ETS. **Figure 33-2** illustrates the smoking process.

■ **Table 33-1** lists differences in the quantity of nicotine delivered by tobacco products: the amount and rate at which a nicotine-containing product delivers nicotine to the bloodstream is a determinant of its addiction potential.[8]

METABOLISM OF NICOTINE

■ Absorption of nicotine occurs through the lungs, skin, and oral or nasal mucosa.[9]

■ Several factors influence absorption from smoked tobacco (cigarettes, pipes, and cigars), as identified in **Figure 33-2**. Regardless of the type of tobacco used, nicotine is primarily eliminated by liver metabolism and excreted through the kidneys in acid urine.

I. NICOTINE FROM SMOKING

A. Absorption: Lungs

Nicotine enters the lungs and quickly passes into arterial circulation by way of blood vessels lining the sacs of the bronchi.

TABLE 33-1	NICOTINE DELIVERY OF VARIOUS TOBACCO PRODUCTS
PRODUCTS	**AMOUNT OF NICOTINE DELIVERY**
Cigarettes	0.7–2.0 mg
Bidis	1.5–4.1 mg
Kreteks	1.9–2.6 mg
Moist Snuff	0.01–7.8 mg/g
Hookah Smoking (45 min–1 h)	Equivalent to inhaling 100–200 times the volume of smoke from one cigarette.[9,10,11,12,13,14]

Nicotine-Containing Products

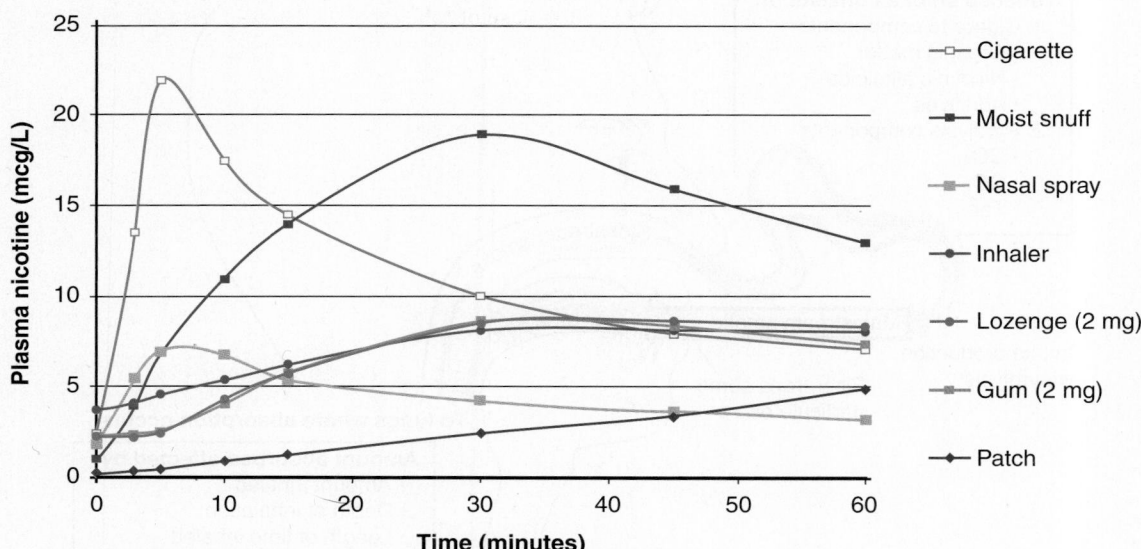

FIGURE 33-3 **Plasma Concentrations for Tobacco Products and Nicotine Pharmacotherapies.** (*Source:* Choi JH, Dresler CM, Norton MR, Strahs KR. Pharmacokinetics of a nicotine polacrilex lozenge. Nicotine Tob Res. 2003; 5:635–44; Fant RV, Henningfield JE, Nelson RA, Pickworth WB. Pharmacokinetics and pharmacodynamics of moist snuff in humans. *Tob Control.* 1999;8:387–92; and Schneider NG, Olmstead RE, Franzon MA, Lunell E. The nicotine inhaler: clinical pharmacokinetics and comparison with other nicotine treatments. *Clin Pharmacokinet.* 2001;40:661–84).

B. Distribution

1. *To the Brain.* Nicotine is delivered efficiently to the brain by the bloodstream in less than 20 seconds.
2. *Peak Plasma Concentration.* **Figure 33-3** illustrates the peak blood plasma concentrations from various tobacco products and nicotine replacement therapies (NRTs).
   - Following the onset of smoking, peak plasma concentration of nicotine occurs in approximately 4–5 minutes.
   - None of the NRTs can duplicate the speed or level of nicotine from cigarettes or snuff.
   - The objective of NRTs is to help prevent withdrawal symptoms.
   - NRTs are less likely to cause dependence when compared to tobacco products.
   - Dental hygienists are in an ideal position to discuss the immediate delivery of nicotine to the brain during smoking and to educate patients about the differences in nicotine delivery of various NRTs, particularly those that are available over-the-counter.
3. *Dissemination.* Nicotine is spread to all body tissues.
4. *Changes in the Liver.* Nicotine is metabolized in the liver into cotinine.
   - Cotinine concentrations in the blood, urine, and saliva are used to assess
     - Whether a person uses tobacco,
     - If so, to what extent,

- The level of exposure of nonsmokers to passive or environmental smoke.

II. SMOKELESS TOBACCO

Smokeless tobacco is the term applied to snuff and chewing tobacco products (defined in **Box 33-2**), which are not smoked but are placed in the mouth.[10]

- Of the 28 carcinogens found in chewing tobacco and snuff, the most harmful are the tobacco-specific N-nitrosamines (TSNAs). These chemical compounds are usually formed during the growing, curing, fermenting, and aging of tobacco.
- Other cancer-causing substances found in smokeless tobacco include benzo(a)pyrene, formaldehyde, acetaldehyde, arsenic, nickel, cadmium, and polonium–210.[11]

A. Absorption: Oral Cavity

- Nicotine is directly absorbed through the gingiva and oral mucous membranes.
- Once smokeless tobacco is placed in the mouth, the amount of nicotine absorbed is three to four times the amount delivered by a cigarette.[11]
- Nicotine concentration declines over 2 hours and is at a negligible level within 24 hours.
- Smokeless tobacco users experience nicotine blood plasma levels similar to the nicotine blood levels of smokers.

B. Absorption: Intestinal

- Most tobacco juice produced by smokeless tobacco is spit out.
- Juice that is intentionally and/or accidentally swallowed by the user is absorbed through the blood vessels lining the small intestine.

III. ELECTRONIC NICOTINE DELIVERY DEVICES

- An electronic cigarette or e-cigarette does not contain tobacco but delivers vaporized nicotine through a device that looks like a regular cigarette.
- The non-FDA approved item, the e-cigarette, consists of a battery, a heater, and a cartridge containing nicotine, water, propylene glycol and other chemicals and carcinogens.[12]
- The FDA has not approved e-cigarettes for use in the United States. Before they can be legally sold in the United States, they are required to have a FDA inspection and approval. The e-cigarettes do not have either, and there are no quality controls on the amount or potency of the substances, including nicotine, in them.[12,13]
- A serious concern is the different amounts of nicotine found in the cartridges. The nicotine amount in the cartridges would vary from the amount advertised leading to unpredictable nicotine dose delivery to the patient.[13]
- Puffing on the device activates the heating element and the solution is then vaporized and inhaled through a mouthpiece.
- The device is not approved for nicotine replacement therapy or for a method of smoking cessation.[14]

SYSTEMIC EFFECTS

- Use of tobacco products influences every system of the body. **Table 33-2** shows smoking-related conditions.
- The diseases that affect each system have consequences ranging from mild to deadly.

I. CARDIOVASCULAR DISEASES

- Smoking aggravates and accelerates the development of atherosclerosis and is a major risk factor for coronary heart disease, the leading cause of death for Americans.[15]
- Smokers who are over 50, who have used oral contraceptives, or who have a family history of coronary heart disease are at even greater risk.[16]

II. PULMONARY DISEASES

- Smoking is the major cause of chronic obstructive pulmonary disease (COPD), which includes emphysema and chronic bronchitis. More information on COPD is provided in Chapter 65 on page 1000.
- Emphysema slowly destroys a person's ability to breathe.
- Chronic bronchitis is a condition in which the airways produce excess mucus, which forces the smoker to cough frequently.[17]

III. CANCER

- Smoking is responsible for 87% of lung cancers in the United States and is the chief neoplastic cause of death in the United Kingdom.

TABLE 33-2	DISEASE CONSEQUENCES OF TOBACCO USE*			
CANCER	**RESPIRATORY DISEASES**	**CARDIOVASCULAR DISEASES**	**PREGNANCY INFANT HEALTH**	**OTHER CONDITIONS**
Oral cavity*	COPD	Atherosclerosis	Abortion	Osteoporosis
Lung	Emphysema	Coronary artery disease	Fetal neonatal death/ stillbirth	Alzheimer's
Larynx*	Bronchitis	Hypertension*	Placenta abruptio	Wrinkling
Pharynx*	Asthma	Aortic aneurysm	Placenta previa	Concomitant use of other drugs*
Esophagus	Bacterial Pneumonia	Arterial thrombosis	Premature/prolonged membrane rupture	Early menopause
Stomach* (peptic ulcer)*	Tuberculosis	Stroke	Preterm labor	
Bladder			Preeclampsia	
Uterine cervix			Growth retardation	
Breast			Sudden infant death syndrome	
Kidney			Low birth weight	
Pancreas*			Infertility	
Acute myeloid leukemia				
Colorectal				

*Associated with smoke and smokeless tobacco use.
Abbreviations: COPD, chronic obstructive pulmonary disease.

- Lung cancer is the leading cause of death for both black and white men and women.
- Approximately 75% of oral cancers are related to smoking and the use of smokeless tobacco.[18]

IV. TOBACCO AND USE OF OTHER DRUGS

- Smokers are more likely to consume alcohol. The combined use of alcohol and tobacco places the patient at greater risk for neoplasms and other oral problems.
- Heavy cigarette smoking is also highly correlated with cocaine and marijuana use.[19]

ENVIRONMENTAL TOBACCO SMOKE (ETS)

- A complex mixture of chemicals generated during the burning of tobacco products.
- The principal contributor is sidestream smoke, the material emitted from burning tobacco products between puffs.
- Other components include exhaled mainstream smoke and vaporized compounds diffused through a cigarette wrapper.
- Also called passive, secondary, or second-hand smoke.[20]
- In indoor areas, environmental smoke can last for many hours, depending on ventilation. Exposure for certain workers and family members can be extensive.
- **Third-hand smoke** is defined as tobacco smoke residue absorbed by furnishings.
  - Smoke reacts with a common pollutant on indoor surfaces, nitrous acid, which then forms TSNAs.
  - The TSNAs cling to the smoker's body, household dust, and every surface of the home, vehicle, or enclosed area where the smoking takes place. This process represents a health hazard.
  - The levels of the carcinogens increase with time and become higher if smoking is continued in enclosed areas.[21]
- Fortunately, many public areas, hospitals, and commercial work areas are now mandated smoke free.
- Individuals exposed to environmental tobacco smoke are at risk for the same health problems as are active smokers.
- A nonsmoker may be more sensitive to the toxic effects than the habitual smoker because the system of the smoker adapts to compensate for the deleterious effects of continued smoking.
- There is no risk-free level of exposure to ETS, as even brief exposure can be harmful.[22]

I. TOXICITY

- Many chemicals are contained in passive smoke, including the same carcinogenic compounds as those in mainstream smoke. Some toxic components are actually in higher concentrations in sidestream smoke than in mainstream smoke.
- Chemicals present in ETS include irritants and systemic toxicants (hydrogen cyanide and sulfur dioxide), mutagens and carcinogens (benzo[a]pyrene and formaldehyde), and reproductive toxicants (nicotine, cadmium, and carbon monoxide).
- Out of the 250 toxic chemicals in ETS, there are at least 50 that are associated with cancer.[22]

II. LUNG AND RESPIRATORY EFFECTS

- Exposure to cigarette smoke, whether active or passive, is the primary cause of lung cancer.[23]
- Eye and nasal irritation are the most commonly reported symptoms among adult nonsmokers.

III. CARDIOVASCULAR EFFECTS

- Both active and passive exposure to smoke have similar effects on the cardiovascular system.
- ETS is a major preventable cause of cardiovascular disease and death.[24]
- Nonsmokers exposed to ETS have 25 to 30% increased risk of developing heart disease.

PRENATAL AND CHILDREN

The fetus, infant, and growing children are exposed to ETS through the following:

- Homes and cars where smoking is permitted
- Daycare or preschool environments in which smoking is permitted
- Other enclosed environments that allow smoking, such as restaurants and sporting events
- Nonsmoking mother who is exposed to smoking environment.[25]

ETS exposure affects children's

- physical health,
- behavioral health,
- mental health.

I. IN UTERO

- Nicotine and carbon monoxide cross the placenta and enter the fetus.
- Adverse pregnancy risks include miscarriage, placenta previa, low birth weight, and increased perinatal mortality.
- Cleft lip, cleft palate, and delayed tooth formation have been associated with maternal smoking.[26]

II. INFANCY

- Chemicals are passed to the baby in the breast milk of mothers who smoke.

- Acute effects include increased incidence of upper respiratory tract illness.
- Postnatal ETS exposure is an independent cause of sudden infant death syndrome.[27]

III. YOUNG CHILDREN

- ETS affects lung development with symptoms of coughing, phlegm, and wheezing.
- Children are at higher risk for asthma; asthma sufferers have additional episodes and worsened condition.[28]
- Children have an increased incidence of middle ear infections.
- Behavioral problems and lower academic achievement in school may be related to missing school during illnesses.

ORAL MANIFESTATIONS OF TOBACCO USE

- The numerous oral conditions that are attributed to tobacco use vary with the type of tobacco used (smoking or smokeless) and the form in which it is used (cigarettes, pipes, cigars, chewing tobacco, moist snuff).[29]
- Pattern and severity of clinical presentation may vary with frequency and duration of use.
- **Table 33-3** lists examples of the wide variety of oral consequences of tobacco use; periodontal diseases and oral cancers provide the most serious destructive effects.[30]
- A systematic extraoral/intraoral examination is the most efficient and effective method for detecting tobacco-related conditions in and around the mouth.

- The extraoral/intraoral examination gives visual examples for use in encouraging the patient to start a tobacco cessation program.

TOBACCO AND PERIODONTAL INFECTIONS

Tobacco use is a major risk factor for periodontal diseases. Users are at a high risk for developing more severe periodontitis at younger ages than nonusers.[31]

I. EFFECTS ON THE PERIODONTAL TISSUES

A. Gingivitis

The degree of inflammatory response to dental biofilm accumulation is reduced compared with that in nonsmokers.

B. Periodontitis in Tobacco Users

- Increased rate and severity of periodontal destruction.[32]
- Increased bone loss, attachment loss, and pocket depths.[33]
- Pocketing is greater and gingival recession may be noted about anterior teeth especially maxillary linguals.[34]
- Gingival blood flow and gingival crevicular flow are diminished.[35]
- Increased tooth loss from periodontal causes.
- Increased prevalence with increased number of exposures to tobacco.[32]
- Prevalence and severity *lessen* with cessation.[35,36]

TABLE 33-3	ORAL CONSEQUENCES OF TOBACCO USE				
CANCER AND PRE-CANCER	**PERIODONTAL FACTORS**	**SOFT TISSUE PROBLEMS**	**HARD TISSUE PROBLEMS**	**ESTHETIC FACTORS**	**EXCERBATION—ORAL SIGNS IN SYSTEMIC DISEASES**
Squamous cell Leukoplakia (ST)* Homogeneous Nonhomogeneous Verrucous	ANUG & ANUP Relapse during maintenance Increased risk for periimplantitis and periimplant bone loss Localized recession and clinical attachment loss	Nicotine stomatitis (P) Smoker's melanosis Black hairy tongue Median rhomboid glossitis Median rhomboid glossitis Median rhomboid glossitis Leukodema (P) Hyperkeratosis (ST) Dry socket Delayed wound healing	Occlusal or incisal abrasion (P), (ST) Cervical abrasion (ST) Dehiscence of bone (ST) Tooth loss	Halitois Dental stains Prosthesis stains Orthodontic appliance stains Discoloration of restorations Impaired taste and smell	HIV/AIDS Type 1 and Type 2 diabetes

Abbreviations: mainly associated with P = pipe; ST = smokeless tobacco; no notation = smoked tobacco.

II. MECHANISMS OF PERIODONTAL DESTRUCTION

- No effect on the rate of dental biofilm accumulation.[36]
- Host response: lowered immune response.[37]
- Impaired neutrophils: decreased chemotaxis, phagocytosis, and adherence.[38]
- Altered antibody production; decreased serum IgG.[37]
- Impairment of revascularization; disruption of immune response; impact on healing; increased risk of periodontal disease.[37]
- Negative effect on bone metabolism; after menopause, women smokers have a deficit in bone density; smoking can influence osteoporosis.

III. RESPONSE TO TREATMENT

- Resistance to conventional therapy.[39]
- Ideal personal dental biofilm control can minimize the effect.
- Implants have greater risk for failure due to implantitis.[40]
- Delayed healing after surgical and nonsurgical procedures.[39]

NICOTINE ADDICTION

- Nicotine is tobacco's psychoactive agent (one that produces feelings of pleasure and well-being), and its use leads to tolerance, dependence, and addiction.[41]
- No one starts using tobacco to become addicted to it.
- Users seldom can explain why they use tobacco but often say that it helps their physical performance, mood, or ability to think. In fact, physical performance does not improve, mood is not better, and intellectual stimulation is minor.

I. TOLERANCE

A. Physiologic Adaptation

Tolerance refers to the user's need for more smoking or chewing the same amount of the same product over time as it becomes less and less effective in creating the desired feeling of well-being.

B. Amount of Use

To sustain the positive feelings associated with tobacco use, more and more has to be taken as time goes by.

II. DEPENDENCE

A. Characteristics

- As increased amounts are needed over time, the loss of control over the amount and frequency of tobacco use shows evidence of dependence.

BOX 33-3	Facts About Nicotine Dependency

- Nicotine addiction is similar to that produced by other substances such as alcohol, cocaine, and heroin.
- Tolerance to nicotine is demonstrated as the user experiences less nausea and dizziness following initial use.
- Tobacco abuse: Any use of tobacco products is considered a health hazard. Therefore, use of any amount is considered abuse.
- Nicotine addiction may be the most challenging of all addictions for complete recovery.
- 70% of smokers report that they would like to quit but only about one-third make a quit attempt each year; of these only about 2.5% are successful.
- Many tobacco users make many unsuccessful quit attempts before stopping use for indefinite or extended periods of time.
- Successfully quitting smokeless tobacco use may be equally or more difficult than stopping smoking. Smokeless tobacco is not considered a viable alternative for smokers who can quit.

Source: American Psychiatric Association. Diagnostic and statistical manual of mental disorders (DSM-IV), 4th ed. Washington, D.C.: American Psychiatric Association; 1994. pp. 243–7; Schmitz JM, Schneider NG, Jarvik ME. Nicotine, in Lowinson, JH, Ruiz P, Millman RB, Langrod JG. *Substance abuse: a comprehensive textbook,* 3rd ed. Baltimore, Williams & Wilkins; 1997. pp. 276–94.

- Facts about nicotine dependency are included in **Box 33-3**, and criteria for nicotine dependency are outlined in **Box 33-4**.

B. Reinforcing Effect

- Nicotine intensifies the release of dopamine by the brain, thereby increasing a feeling of pleasure and the compulsion to use tobacco.
- Positive reinforcement is produced with tobacco use, and abrupt stopping produces withdrawal symptoms.

III. ADDICTION

- Addiction is a chronic, progressive, relapsing disease characterized by compulsive use of a substance.
- The effects result in physical, psychological, and/or social harm to the user, but use continues despite that harm.
- Smoking is more addictive than alcohol and other drugs of abuse in terms of the proportion of those who are exposed and subsequently become dependent.
- The pattern of relapse is identical for tobacco, alcohol, and heroin.

BOX 33-4	Criteria for Nicotine Dependency

- Tolerance:
  - ☐ A need for markedly increased amounts of the substance to achieve intoxication or desired effect.
  - ☐ Markedly diminished effect with continued use of the same amount.*
- Withdrawal, as manifested by either:
  - ☐ Daily us of nicotine for several weeks.
  - ☐ Abrupt stopping or reducing nicotine will result in four or more of the following signs of nicotine withdrawal which is found in **Box 33-5** and they will occur within 24 hours.*
- Used in greater amounts over longer period of time than intended
- A persistent desire or unsuccessful efforts to cut down or quit
- A great deal of time spent using the substance
- Giving up important social, occupational, or recreational activities because of use of the substance
- Continued use despite knowledge of medical problems related to use and/or social and legal problems resulting from use.

*Preliminary draft revisions for the (DSM-V), 5th ed. is available for view. The above notations are from this edition, which will be published in May 2013.
Source: American Psychiatric Association. Diagnostic and statistical manual of mental disorders (DSM-IV), 4th ed. Washington, D.C.: American Psychiatric Association. 1994, pp. 243–7; Schmitz JM, Schneider NG, Jarvik ME. Nicotine, in Lowinson. JH, Ruiz P, Millman RB, Langrod JG. *Substance abuse: a comprehensive textbook,* 3rd ed. Baltimore: Williams & Wilkins; 1997. pp. 276–94.

BOX 33-5	Criteria for Nicotine Withdrawal Syndrome

- Dysphoric or depressed mood
- Insomnia
- Irritability, frustration, and anger
- Anxiety
- Difficulty concentrating
- Restlessness
- Decreased heart rate
- Increased appetite or weight gain
- Cravings for tobacco

Source: American Psychiatric Association. Diagnostic and statistical manual of mental disorders (DSM-IV), 4th ed. Washington, D.C.: American Psychiatric Association; 1994. pp. 243–7; Schmitz JM, Schneider NG, Jarvik ME. Nicotine, in Lowinson. JH, Ruiz P Millman RB, and Langrod JG. *Substance abuse: A comprehensive textbook,* 3rd ed. Baltimore: Williams & Wilkins; 1997. pp. 276–94.

- Most symptoms diminish over a few weeks when relapse does not occur.
- Cravings for tobacco, increased appetite, and weight gain may persist for months or years.

B. Alleviation of Symptoms

Table 33-4 lists activities that help to overcome withdrawal symptoms. The principle is to prevent relapse.

TREATMENT

Tobacco cessation methods or treatment for nicotine addiction fall into two categories: *self-help* and *assisted strategies.*[9,42]

I. REASONS FOR QUITTING

Success cannot be expected unless the individual makes a concentrated effort and believes in that effort's significance. Typical reasons include the following:

- General health awareness
- Specific health problem directly or indirectly related to tobacco use
- Effect on family
  - Need to act as a role model
  - Awareness of effects of ETS
- Effect of smoking and/or ETS on fetus during pregnancy
- Cost
- Social pressure and restrictions on smoking in many settings
- Personal recognition of the dangers of nicotine addiction and the desire to regain control of one's life.

- Factors affecting the development of addiction include:
  - Properties of psychoactive drug (dose).
  - Family, peer influences, and social acceptance.
  - Existing psychiatric disorders.
  - Cost and availability of the drug.
  - Influence of advertising.

IV. WITHDRAWAL

- Withdrawal refers to the effects of cessation of nicotine use by an individual in whom dependence is established.
- When users of nicotine products stop abruptly, within 24 hours they can experience maximal physical and/or psychological withdrawal symptoms.
- **Box 33-5** identifies typical nicotine withdrawal symptoms.

A. Duration

- Patients experience withdrawal symptoms almost immediately, and relapse within a week is not uncommon.

TABLE 33-4	ALLEVIATING NICOTINE WITHDRAWAL SYMPTOMS

SYMPTOMS	ACTIVITIES
Mood changes; anxiety, nervousness, stressed feelings	Breathe deeply; exhale through pursed lips. Take a walk or other relaxation exercise. Know your triggers, get more rest and take multivitamin. Make a list of things to do instead of smoking. Avoid places where you most commonly used tobacco.
Sleep disturbances	Avoid caffeine, drink a glass of warm milk instead. Avoid alcohol. Take a long walk hours before bed. Avoid naps, take a warm bath or meditate. Read a book, listen to soothing music.
Appetite increase	Eat only when you are hungry. Eat low-fat, low-calorie snacks. Chew sugarless gum or eat sugarless hard flavorful candy. Drink additional glasses of water. Exercise
Cravings	**Delay smoking or dipping:** Use tactics such as waiting 1 more minute; often cravings pass in 5 or 10 min. **Distract yourself:** Exercise; take a walk; call a friend. **Drink water:** to fight off cravings **Deep breaths:** Relax! Close your eyes and take 10 deep breaths; exhale through pursed lips. **Discuss your feelings:** with someone close to you or a support group*

*National Advisory Committee on Health and Disability. Guidelines for Smoking Cessation, Revised 2002. Wellington, New Zealand: National Advisory Committee on Health and Disability (National Health Committee); May 2002.
Adapted from Fiore MC, Jaén CR, and Baker TB, et al. Treating tobacco use and dependence: 2008 update. Quick reference guide for clinicians. Rockville (MD): U.S. Department of Health and Human Services. Public Health Service; 2008 [cited 2009 Apr].

II. SELF-HELP INTERVENTIONS

About one-third of adult smokers attempt to quit, but only 2 to 3% are able to achieve long-term abstinence on their own. The proportion of attempts and successes is similar among high-school students.

- Go cold turkey. Consider changing lifestyle, including exercise and diet modifications.
- Reduce number of daily tobacco exposures
- Select over-the-counter nicotine replacement patches, gum, or lozenges.
- Join a family member or friend in the tobacco cessation effort.

III. ASSISTED STRATEGIES

A. Counseling

- Provision of practical counseling, including problem solving and skills training.
- Provision of intra-treatment social support: "Our office staff and I are willing to assist you."

B. Pharmacotherapies[43]

Table 33-5 provides an overview of FDA-approved first-line pharmacotherapies.

C. Combination

Counseling combined with pharmacotherapy has been shown to be effective in helping patients to quit using tobacco.

PHARMACOTHERAPIES USED FOR TREATMENT OF NICOTINE ADDICTION

I. OBJECTIVES AND RATIONALE

- Make it easier to abstain from tobacco by partial replacement of nicotine or by counteracting nicotine's action.
- Reduce withdrawal symptoms.
- Fulfill, in part, the craving for tobacco by sustaining tolerance.
- Provide some effects (mood, cognitive changes) previously delivered from nicotine.

II. CONSIDERATIONS

- Discourage casual use of pharmacotherapies. Failure as a result of improper use can discourage future quit attempts.
- Inform patient of signs and symptoms of nicotine overdose: nausea, vomiting, dizziness, weakness, or rapid heartbeat.

TABLE 33-5	SUGGESTIONS FOR THE CLINICAL USE OF PHARMACOTHERAPIES FOR SMOKING CESSATION				
PHARMACOTHERAPY	**PRECAUTIONS/ CONTRA-INDICATIONS**	**SIDE EFFECTS**	**DOSAGE**	**DURATION**	**AVAILABILITY**
Bupropion SR	History of seizure History of eating disorder Using monoamine oxidase (MAO) inhibitor	Insomnia Dry mouth	Day 1–3: 150 mg each morning; Day 4-end: twice daily; take evening dose 8 hours before sleep	Start 1–2 wks before quit date; Use 2–6 mos	Zyban Wellbutrin SR Generic (Prescription only)
Varenicline**	Kidney problems or on dialysis Has not been studied In pregnant or nursing women; FDA warning re: potential for agitation, depressed mood, atypical behavior, or suicidal thoughts.	Nausea; Insomnia; Abnormal, vivid or strange dreams Constipation, gas and/or vomiting	Days 1–3: 0–5 mg 1 in morning; Days 4–7: 0.5 mg twice daily; Day 8 though end of treatment: 1 mg twice daily.	Use 3–6 mos; Start 1 wk before quit date	Chantix (Prescription only)
Nicotine gum	TMJ Disease Caution for denture wearers	Mouth soreness Dyspepsia Headaches	1–24 cigs/day 2 mg gum (up to 24 psc/day) 20+ cigs/day or smokeless tobacco-4 mg gum (up to 24 psc/day)*	Up to 12 wks Or as needed	Nicorette, -Mint (3 kinds) -Fruit -Cinnamon -Original (OTC only) Generic available
Nicotine inhaler	Asthma COPD	Local irritation of mouth and throat	6–16 cartridges/day*	Up to 6 mos; Taper at end	Nicotrol inhaler (Prescription only)
Nicotine nasal spray	Nasal polyps Rhinitis Sinusitis Asthma	Nasal and throat irritation Dependence potential	8–40 doses/day (No more than 48 sprays in 24 hrs)	3–6 mos; Taper at end	Nicotrol NS (Prescription only)
Nicotine transdermal patch	Allergy to patch adhesive; Do not use if have severe eczema or psoriasis DO NOT CUT PATCHES	Local skin reaction Insomnia Changes in dreams Headache	One patch per day If 10 cigs/day: 21 mg 4 wks, 14 mg 2–4 wks, 7 mg 2–4 wks If <10/day: 14 mg 4 wks, then 7 mg 4 wks One patch per day	8–12 wks	Nicoderm CQ (OTC only), Generic patches (prescription and OTC) Nicotrol (OTC only)
Nicotine lozenge	One lozenge at a time	Mouth soreness Dyspepsia Nausea Headache Cough Hiccups Heartburn Flatulence	2 mg if smoke/chew after 30 min of waking; 4 mg if smoke/chew within 30 min of waking. Maximum 20 lozenges in 24 hrs*	3–6 mos Wks 1–6: 1 every 1–2 hrs; Wks 7–9: 1 every 2–4 hrs; Wks 10–12: 1 every 4–8 hrs.	Commit -Mint -Cherry -Original (OTC only) Generic available
Nicotine Mini lozenge	Same as above	Same as above	2 mg if smoke/chew after 30 min of waking; 4 mg if smoke/chew within 30 min of waking. Maximum24 mini lozenges/day*	Same as above	Nicorette Mini -Mint (OTC only)

*Nothing to eat or drink 15 min prior to or during use.
Adapted from Fiore MC, Jaén CR, and Baker TB, et al. Treating tobacco use and dependence: 2008 update. Quick reference guide for clinicians. Rockville (MD): U.S. Department of Health and Human Services. Public Health Service; 2008 [cited 2009 Apr].
**Varenicline (Chantix) information. 2010 July 20. Available from: http://www.chantix.com.

- Consult physician before use if younger than 18 years or contraindications are present.

III. CONTRAINDICATIONS

- Self-medication without professional examination and advice.
- Pregnancy/breastfeeding: nicotine in the bloodstream, even in small amounts, can reach the fetus.
- Nicotine gum or lozenge: hypertension; using medication for asthma, depression, diabetes mellitus, cardiovascular disease, stomach ulcers.
- Nicotine patch: same as nicotine gum; in addition, some patients may be allergic to patch adhesives.
- Nicotine inhaler: same as nicotine gum; patients need to be cautious if allergy to menthol.
- Nicotine gum, lozenge, and inhaler: Avoid eating or drinking acidic beverages for 15 minutes before and during use due to decreased nicotine absorption.

IV. NICOTINE REPLACEMENT THERAPY (NRT)

A. Nicotine Gum

- *Transmucosal delivery:* Nicotine is released in the mouth during "chewing."
- *Description:* Nicotine gum is sweetened with xylitol and has either a mild mint, cinnamon or orange flavor.
- *Directions:* Chew one piece slowly until tingling or peppery taste is achieved; "park" gum in buccal vestibule; resume chewing when peppery taste or tingle fades; repeat chew/park activity.

B. Nicotine Patch

- *Transdermal delivery:* Nicotine is released through skin.
- *Directions:* Place a new patch on a hairless location upon rising; if sleep disruption occurs, remove 24-hour patch before bedtime or use 16-hour patch.

C. Nicotine Inhaler

- *Transmucosal delivery:* Nicotine is released in mouth during inhalation or puffing; hold vapor in oral cavity for absorption, do not inhale.
- *Requirements:* Store inhaler and cartridges in a warm place when temperatures drop below 40°F to prevent a decline in delivery of nicotine from the inhaler to the oral cavity.

D. Nicotine Nasal Spray

- *Nasal mucous membrane delivery:* Nicotine is released through lining of nose.
- *Dose delivery:* Avoid sniffing, swallowing, or inhaling while administering doses, as these increase irritating effects.

- *Directions:* Tilt head slightly back while delivering spray.
- Precaution for heavy smoker: increased dose.

E. Nicotine Lozenge

- *Transmucosal delivery:* Nicotine is released in mouth as lozenge dissolves.
- *Description:* the lozenge is sweetened with mannitol and aspartame and flavored with a mild mint or cherry.
- *Dose delivery:* **Table 33-5**
- *Directions:* do not bite or chew lozenge as it dissolves in the mouth: this can cause more nicotine to be swallowed quickly and may result in indigestion and/or heartburn.

NICOTINE-FREE THERAPY

A. Bupropion SR

- The first non-nicotine medication shown to be effective for tobacco cessation and approved by the FDA for that use.
- Mechanism of action is presumed to be mediated by its capacity to block neural uptake of dopamine and/or norepinephrine.
- Additional dosing information can be seen in **Table 33-5**.
- Take second dose 8 hours after first and with evening meal to reduce sleep disturbances.
- Bupropion SR can be used in combination with nicotine replacement therapies.

B. Varenicline Tartrate

- The second non-nicotine medication shown to be effective for smoking cessation and approved by the FDA for that use.
- Mechanism of action is: a partial nicotine agonist (blocks nicotine receptors in brain). It also causes reduction in dopamine release.
  - Always take after meals with full glass of water, to reduce nausea.
  - Take second dose 8 hours after first and with evening meal to reduce sleep disturbances.
  - Additional dosing information can be found in **Table 33-5**.
- Not currently recommended for use in combination with nicotine replacement therapies.

C. Combination Therapies

- Certain combinations of first-line medications have been shown to be effective smoking cessation treatments.

- Effective combination medications are:
  - Long-term (>14 weeks) nicotine patch + nicotine gum or spray
  - Nicotine patch + nicotine inhaler
  - Nicotine patch + bupropion SR

D. Second-Line Medications

- Second-line medications are pharmacotherapies for which there is evidence of efficacy for treating tobacco dependence, but they have a more limited role because of the following reasons:
  - The FDA has not approved them for a tobacco dependence treatment indication.
  - There are more concerns about potential side effects than exist with first-line medications.
  - Second-line treatments, clonidine and nortriptyline, can be considered for use on a case-by-case basis after first-line treatments have been used or considered and while under a physician's supervision.

DENTAL HYGIENE CARE FOR THE PATIENT WHO USES TOBACCO

- The tobacco-using patient presents a unique challenge to the oral health team. Specific treatment modifications are indicated.
- Helping the patient to quit using tobacco becomes an integral part of the dental hygiene care plan.

ASSESSMENT

I. PATIENT HISTORY

- Tobacco use status is assessed at each appointment.
- The basic history form in Chapter 9 (pages 119 to 120) used by all patients includes one or two questions to determine whether the patient currently uses tobacco and, if so, the types of tobacco (smoking and/or smokeless). A tobacco use assessment form from the National Cancer Institute is shown in **Figure 33-4**.

TOBACCO USE ASSESSMENT FORM

Name: _____   Date_____

1. Do you use tobacco in any form? ☐ Yes ☐ No
1A. If no, have you ever used tobacco in the past? ☐ Yes ☐ No
   How long did you use tobacco? Years____ Months____
   How long ago did you stop? Years____ Months____

If you are not currently a tobacco user, no other questions should be answered. Thank you for completing this form.
Question 2-10 are for current tobacco users only.

2. **If you smoke,** what type (check)   How many? (Number)
   ☐ Cigarettes   Cigarettes per day____
   ☐ Cigars   Cigars per day____
   ☐ Pipes   Bowls per day____
3. **If you chew/use snuff,** what type?   How much?
   ☐ Snuff   Days a can lasts____
   ☐ Chewing   Pouches per week____
   ☐ Other (describe)   Amount_____per_____
3A. **How long** do you keep a chew in your mouth? _____minutes
4. **How many days** of the week do you first use tobacco?   7 6 5 4 3 2 1
5. **How soon** after you wake do you first use tobacco?
   Within 30 minutes?____   More than 30 minutes?____
6. Does the person **closest to you** use tobacco?   ☐ Yes   ☐ No
7. **How interested are you** in stopping your use of tobacco?
   ☐ not at all   ☐ a little   ☐ somewhat   ☐ Yes   ☐ very much
8. Have you ever **tried to stop** using tobacco before?   ☐ Yes   ☐ No
9. Have you **discussed stopping** with your physician?   ☐ Yes   ☐ No
10. If you decided to stop using tobacco completely during the next two weeks, **how confident are you** that you would succeed?
   ☐ not at all   ☐ a little   ☐ somewhat   ☐ very confident

FIGURE 33-4 **Tobacco Use Assessment Form.** (Reprinted from Mecklenburg, RE, Greenspan D, Kleinman DV, Manley MW, Niessen LC, Robertson PB, Winn DE. Tobacco effects in the mouth: a national cancer institute and national institute of dental research guide for health professionals [Internet]. Washington, DC: U.S. Department of Health and Human Services, National Institutes of Health.; [NIH Publication No. 07-3330, reprinted Nov 2007; cited 2010 Nov]. Available from: https://cissecure.nci.nih.gov/ncipubs/searchres.aspx?sid=21MOElrJ2uYLRHKGNQNJzQ%3d%3d.

- Concomitant use of alcohol and other psychoactive drugs, with tobacco may necessitate modifications of clinical procedures.
- Figure 10-1 (page 136) illustrates tobacco use status as a vital sign along with temperature, pulse, respiratory rate, and blood pressure.[44]

II. EXTRAORAL EXAMINATION

A. Breath and Body Odor

- Halitosis
- Electropositive smoke: Smoke from cigars and other smoked tobacco products clings to skin, hair, and clothes and results in body odor.

B. Fingers

Smokers of nonfiltered cigarettes have a yellowish-brown discoloration of the fingers and fingernails.

C. Skin

Smokers experience premature and more extensive facial wrinkling.

D. Lips

Pipe and cigar smokers are at risk for development of precancerous and cancerous lip lesions.

III. INTRAORAL EXAMINATION

An excellent outline for conducting a thorough intraoral examination for the patient who uses tobacco is provided in Table 11-1 (page 148). Oral consequences of tobacco use are listed in **Table 33-3**.

A. Detection of an Intraoral Lesion or Problem

Upon detecting a problem or lesion that may or may not be tobacco-related, the clinician will:

- *Show the patient.* Provide a simple but thorough explanation related to the nature of the condition.
- *Explain.* Make certain that the patient understands the consequences of continuing tobacco use as it relates to the progress of the problem or lesion.
- *Record.* Provide a detailed description of the problem or lesion and note the information given to the patient in the dental record for the dentist's review.

B. Referral Indications

- If a lesion persists for more than 2 weeks, a biopsy is indicated (Chapter 11, page 154).
- *Refer* the patient for biopsy.

- *Ascertain.* Check to be certain that the patient undergoes the biopsy and receives results.
- *Consult.* Ensure the pathologist that reviews the biopsy provides the pertinent information.
- *Document.* Ensure that results are entered into the patient's treatment record.

C. Oral Self-Examination

- It is imperative to teach oral self-examination to all patients who use tobacco. The significance of oral self-examination in this high-risk group cannot be overstated.
- Teach patients to perform an oral self-examination by using the same techniques and components of the professional extraoral and intraoral examinations as shown in Table 11-1 (page 148).

D. Detect, Relate, Motivate

- Lesions that are a potential direct consequence of tobacco use are pointed out to the patient.
- The presence of tobacco-related problems/lesions can serve as a powerful motivational tool to encourage a quit attempt.
- The demonstration of the arrest or elimination of tobacco-related problems/lesions as the patient continues a nonuse status will aid in achieving permanent cessation.

IV. CONSULTATION

- Patients who do not seek routine medical care need referral to a physician for evaluation.
- Detection of underlying medical problems is essential so that necessary dental treatment modifications may be utilized.

CLINICAL TREATMENT PROCEDURES

Patients who use tobacco require longer and more frequent appointments due to the presence of increased risk of the following:

- dental stain,
- calculus,
- periodontal problems.

I. DENTAL BIOFILM CONTROL

- Self-care for daily dental biofilm control is the first priority in the care plan.
- Immaculate oral hygiene is required by this group of high-risk patients owing to their susceptibility to dental caries, periodontal infections, and other soft-tissue alterations.

II. SCALING AND ROOT PLANING

■ Inform the patient that healing will be jeopardized by continued tobacco use and that users cannot expect the same treatment results as nonusers.
■ When using power-driven instruments:
  ▨ Take precautions to prevent the patient from ingesting bacteria, water, and debris (smokers often have pulmonary and cardiovascular complications).
  ▨ Take other precautions (as described in Chapter 39 on page 624) when using power instrumentation.

III. OTHER PATIENT INSTRUCTION

A. Diet and Nutrition

■ Tobacco users may be poorly nourished because tobacco use decreases appetite. Conversely, the desire to control body weight through tobacco use may impede a patient's willingness to quit.
■ Suggestions about diet and exercise are included as a part of the cessation program.
■ Most smokeless tobacco products are sweetened with sugar or molasses, which increases their cariogenic potential. Appropriate instruction is needed.

B. Nonalcoholic Rinses

■ Tobacco users may be aware of halitosis and frequently use alcohol-containing mouthrinses to mask unpleasant odors.
■ Long-term use of alcohol-containing antibacterial agents, mouthrinses, and other oral hygiene products cannot be recommended owing to the synergistic effect of alcohol and tobacco in the initiation of head and neck cancers.

TOBACCO CESSATION PROGRAM

■ A program for tobacco cessation is an essential component of the dental hygiene care plan for all tobacco-using patients.[43,45]
■ The majority of users admit that they would like to quit or "know" that they need to, and about one-third of them are willing to try.
■ Interventions and their outcomes will vary depending on the motivation and experience of the clinician and the patient's acceptance of, and adherence to, the regimen.
■ Even a minimal intervention conducted by a clinician may help a patient become tobacco free.

MOTIVATIONAL INTERVIEWING

Motivational Interviewing techniques, described in Chapter 3 on page 29 are very useful in conversing with patients concerning behavior change.

THE "5 A's"

The "5 A's"—Ask, Advise, Assess, Assist, Arrange—provide the basis for a brief, simple, but effective tobacco dependence intervention.[40] A cessation program flow chart is presented in **Figure 33-5**.

I. ASK

A. Health History

■ Ask all patients about tobacco use.
■ Include questions about tobacco use on the health history (ADA Health History Form in Chapter 9 on pages 119 to 120) and document tobacco use at each maintenance appointment.

B. Present Questions Carefully

■ During review of the health history, present questions related to tobacco use nonjudgmentally.
■ Address tobacco use as a health issue, not as a moral and/or social issue.
■ Obtain facts without placing the patient on the defensive.

C. Obtain Patient's Confidence

■ Many minors use tobacco without their parents' knowledge or consent.
■ Social disapproval of tobacco use is increasing, and patients may hesitate to disclose their habit.

D. Children

■ By age 5, children are taking responsibility for themselves in many ways; therefore, it is recommended that this is the appropriate age to begin asking about tobacco use.
■ Children ages 3 to 6 can identify cartoon figures and relate them to a tobacco product. Children need to hear messages that counter those produced by the tobacco industry.
■ Ask parents about tobacco use in the home.
■ Discuss with the parents, the effects of ETS on health, developmental risks, and how tobacco use sets a bad example for children.

II. ADVISE

A. Never Users/Former Users

■ Advise every patient about tobacco use.
■ Praise "never users" and "former users" for their tobacco-free behavior.
■ Reinforcement counters the tobacco industry's message and other enticements to begin tobacco use and can help prevent relapse.

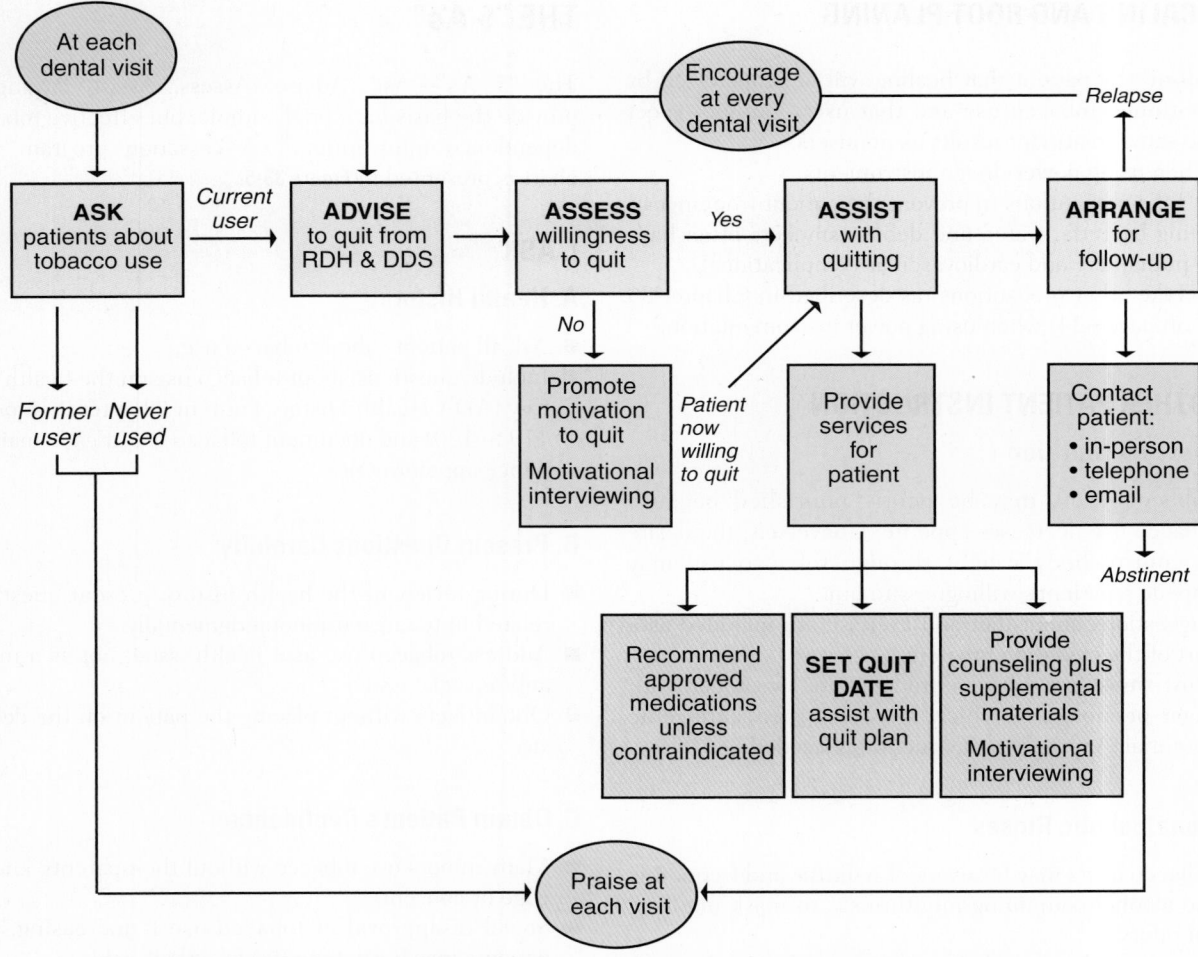

FIGURE 33-5 **Tobacco Cessation Flow Chart.** Flow chart to show how the 5 A's can be incorporated into the clinical setting. (Adapted from Fiore MC, Jaén CR, Baker TB, et al. Treating tobacco use and dependence: 2008 Update. Quick Reference Guide for Clinicians. Rockville (MD): U.S. Department of Health and Human Services. Public Health Service. April 2009.)

B. Current Users: Stop-Look-Listen Approach

1. *Stop now.* Clearly advise the patient about the importance of *stopping* now. Present the advice in a caring, compassionate manner so that patients realize that clinicians are interested in their health and well-being.
2. *Show.* Have patients *look* in their mouths during the initial oral examination to observe the clinical effects of tobacco use. Patients may or may not be impressed by a discussion of possible future health problems or of the effect of tobacco use on others. Advice needs to be relevant to existing conditions.

    Existing oral conditions that may serve as strong motivators to quit include,
    - extrinsic stain,
    - calculus,
    - halitosis,
    - gingival and/or periodontal infection,
    - soft-tissue lesions.

3. *Listen.*
    - Ask patients if they want to quit and their reasons. Most users want to quit. Their reasons may have little to do with health, but speaking out forces patients to focus and strengthen their reasons.
    - *Listening* to the patient allows the clinician to support the patient's thoughts and provide appropriate reinforcement.

C. Brief Advice to Patients

1. Significantly increases long-term abstinence rates.
2. Dentists and dental hygienists can and need to offer brief advice.

III. ASSESS

1. Ask the patient: "Are you ready to quit?"
2. If the patient is ready:
    - Determine if the patient could best be treated in your practice. (A patient may have multiple problems that might necessitate a referral.)

- If treatment is to be provided in your office, go to the *assist* step.
3. If the patient is not ready to quit, use the "5 R's":
   - *Relevance:* Patient indicates personal importance of quitting.
   - *Risks:* Patient identifies negative consequences of continued use.
   - *Rewards:* Patient identifies personal benefits of quitting.
   - *Roadblocks:* Patient identifies barriers to quitting and clinician helps address barriers.
   - *Repetition:* Reinforce the motivational message at every visit.

IV. ASSIST

A. Establish a Quit Plan

1. Set a quit date, preferably within 2 weeks.
2. Have the patient tell family, friends, and coworkers about quitting and request their understanding and support.
3. Warn the patient to anticipate challenges to the planned quit attempt, particularly during the first few weeks. This includes nicotine withdrawal symptoms.
4. Ask the patient to remove all tobacco-related products from home and work sites.

B. Provide Practical Counseling

1. Total abstinence is essential: "not even a single puff or dip after the quit date."
2. Review past quit attempts and identify what helped and what factors contributed to relapse.
3. Discuss challenges/triggers and how the patient will overcome them successfully.
4. Because alcohol can cause relapse, the patient needs to limit/abstain from alcohol use.
5. Quitting is more difficult when there is another smoker in the household. Tobacco-using housemates are encouraged to avoid use in the presence of the patient attempting to quit.

C. Pharmacotherapy

Suggest the use of approved over-the-counter (OTC) or prescription pharmacotherapy. Refer to **Table 33-5**.

D. Provide Educational Materials

1. Agencies that publish motivational materials are listed in **Table 33-6**.
2. Specific educational materials are available for
   - various cultures and ethnic groups,
   - different levels of education and literacy,
   - readers of all ages.

TABLE 33-6	SOURCES FOR TOBACCO CESSATION PATIENT EDUCATIONAL MATERIALS	
NAME OF SOURCE	**QUIT LINES**	**LINKS**
American Cancer Society	1–877-YES QUIT 1–877-937–7848	yesquit.com cancer.org
American Lung Association		lungusa.org
National Cancer Institute		cancer.gov
CDC Tobacco Information and Prevention Tips		cdc.gov/tobacco/
Nicotine Anonymous		nicotine-anonymous.org
QuitNet		quitnet.com
National Alliance for Tobacco Cessation		becomeanex.org
You Can Quit Smoking-Agency for Healthcare Research and Quality		ahrq.gov/consumer/tobacco
Smokefree.gov	National Quit Line 1–800-Quit-Now (1–800-784–8669)	smokefree.gov
American Dental Hygienists Association (Ask. Advice. Refer)		adha.org List of professional materials

3 Keep a supply of these materials in the office for distribution to patients.

V. ARRANGE

A. Follow-Up

1. Essential for successful quit rates.
2. Provide written documentation as a reminder, listing their quit date.
3. Suggest posting quit-date reminders in visible locations such as refrigerator door or bathroom mirror or placing index card with the quit date between cellophane and paper of the cigarette package.

B. Contact the Patient Before the Quit Date

1. Assure patient of care-provider's sincere interest in their tobacco cessation attempt via telephone call or email.
2. Inquire:
   - if information provided at initial contact has been helpful,
   - if there are any questions regarding the information received.

C. Follow-Up Contact

1. Follow-up, either in person or via telephone or e-mail, is essential.
2. Timely intervals would be once within the first week after the quit date when the patient's physical withdrawal symptoms are most intense, and again at the end of the first, second, and third months of their tobacco cessation.
3. More than four contacts help to increase long-term abstinence.

D. Actions During Follow-Up Contact

1. Congratulate and praise patients who have remained tobacco free.
2. Provide the opportunity for patients to ask questions. If they have none, encourage the patient to contact you if questions arise.
3. If relapse has occurred, ask the patient to recall and record the circumstances that led to reuse.
4. Encourage the patient to set another quit date, reminding the patient that a lapse can be a learning experience.
5. Review the use of pharmacotherapy.
6. Provide agencies and contact numbers for the patient who requests a more intensive cessation program.

THE TEAM APPROACH

I. ORGANIZE THE CLINIC TEAM

A. Select a Team Coordinator

The coordinator does not do everything, but sees that everything is done.

B. Responsibilities

1. Identify tobacco use status at patient's first visit.
2. Record appropriate documentation in patient's records.
3. Ensure that all tobacco-using patients are offered the opportunity to enter a cessation program.
4. Contact patients for follow-up.
5. Act as a coach for patients who relapse.
6. Maintain a supply of literature for patients.

C. Team Members

Tobacco users are interviewed to determine readiness to quit and are encouraged to enter a cessation program.

II. ORGANIZE A TOBACCO-FREE ENVIRONMENT

1. Remove ashtrays and post "Thank you for not smoking" signs.
2. Display tobacco use prevention and cessation materials prominently.
3. Eliminate magazines that contain tobacco advertising from reception area.

III. ORGANIZE A TOBACCO USER TRACKING SYSTEM

1. *Tobacco Use Assessment Form:* **Figure 33-4**.
2. *Patient Permanent Progress Report:* Records include dated case notes for all advice to quit, responses and interest in quitting, and progress.
3. *Tobacco status on records:* Clearly mark records so that status can be immediately seen by any clinic staff.

ADVOCACY

I. PUBLIC HEALTH POLICY

- The Surgeon General's Report on Oral Health[2] was the first report of a Surgeon General that focused on oral health and the report specifically identified tobacco use as a risk factor for oral cavity and pharyngeal cancer.
- Healthcare providers can help tobacco users quit and can become partners with one another and with community programs to prevent diseases and promote good health habits.
- The Centers for Disease Control and Prevention has been supporting state-based tobacco control coalitions

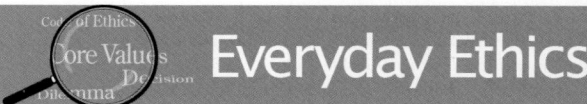

Everyday Ethics

Fifteen-year-old Jason comes with his mother for a regular maintenance appointment. During the oral examination, Edith, the dental hygienist who has been providing dental hygiene treatment for Jason and his family for many years, notices small red and white patches in the vestibular areas of the mandible adjacent to the molar teeth. She also records moderate brownish staining on the teeth and plans to use the air-powder polisher after scaling. She questions Jason about smoking and the use of smokeless tobacco, but he states that he has tried cigarettes only once or twice.

Questions for Consideration

1. What approach can Edith use to further assess and enhance Jason's understanding of the oral effects of tobacco use if she suspects he is not telling the truth?
2. What alternatives does Edith have in reporting her assessment findings that will maintain Jason's right to confidentiality but still inform his mother of the potentially serious oral tissue changes she has observed?
3. Which legal and ethical concepts, listed in Table VI-1 in Section VI Introduction on page 553, apply to this situation?

in all 50 states. Many local communities and municipalities are considering or have adopted smoke-free workplace ordinances.

- Oral health professionals can be valuable and welcome partners in these programs.

II. COMMUNITY ORAL HEALTH EDUCATIONAL PROGRAMS

No community oral health program can be considered complete without inclusion of tobacco prevention, control, and cessation education. Excellent materials are available from many nonprofit and professional organizations.

BOX 33-6	Example Progress Notes: Tobacco Use Assessment and Cessation Treatment

Patient presents for second quadrant scaling with anesthesia. Personal home care has improved; patient states he has noticed less bleeding. Cigarette smoker for 15 years; 1 to 2 packs a day. Patient presents with moderate periodontal disease (Type III), evidence of nicotine stomatitis, other oral cancer (OC) finding negative, and no cavitated caries lesions charted. DH diagnosis: Increased risk for oral and systemic disease due to tobacco dependence. Next step in care plan: basic ideas for smoking cessation introduced and explanation of oral and systemic effects of tobacco use provided. Patient motivated to quit because his wife is expecting new baby, but reports previous attempts to quit "Cold Turkey" were unsuccessful due to weight gain, mood swings and increased stress.

Discussed options for cessation support. Patient agreed to: 21 mg nicotine transdermal patch, transitioning to 14, then 7 mg patch over 8 to 10 weeks, combining patch therapy with nicotine gum to help prevent weight gain and provide relief for additional withdrawal symptoms and cravings. Follow up by telephone in 1 week and reevaluate at next visit scheduled in 2 weeks.

Signed: _____, RDH Date: _____

DOCUMENTATION

- Careful and complete documentation of tobacco use is a component of each patient assessment. It is part of the health history for new patients and part of the clinical (progress) notes for maintenance patients.
- Include tobacco history and/or current use, type of tobacco and amount typically used.
- Age, ethnicity, gender, periodontal and overall dental status as well as oral cancer screening findings
- Patient interest/confidence motivation/readiness to quit and previous quit attempts and techniques used.
- Options for cessation presented to patient and referrals to physician for examination/treatment.
- **Box 33-6** contains an example progress note for tobacco use assessment and cessation treatment.

Factors To Teach The Patient

- The most effective method to stop using tobacco is never to start.
- How to perform a regular self-examination of the oral cavity.
- Pregnant women who use tobacco products may harm the developing fetus and the newborn infant.
- Young children may experiment with or use tobacco products. Parents can be educated so they are prepared to provide guidance.
- All forms of social tobacco use can lead to addiction.
- Nonsmokers who breathe ETS can incur the same serious health problems as smokers. Children are especially susceptible.
- Smokeless tobacco use is *not* a safe alternative to smoking.
- Oral health team members can help patients become tobacco free.
- Learn about local or state tobacco legislation and public health policy to make informed choices related to a tobacco smoke-free society.

References

1. Pearl R. Tobacco smoking and longevity. *Science.* 1938 Mar; 87(2253):216–17.

2. Advisory Committee on Smoking and Health to the U.S. Surgeon General.Report. Washington, D.C., U.S. Department of Health, Education, and Welfare. 1965;31–40.

3. United States Department of Health and Human Services: Reducing tobacco use: a report of the surgeon general. Atlanta (GA):Centers for Disease Control and Prevention, National Center for Chronic Disease Prevention and Health Promotion, Office on Smoking and Health. 2000 Dec 22;49(RR-16):1–27.

4. Centers for Disease Control and Prevention. Cigarette smoking among adults and trends in smoking cessation: United States, 2008. MMWR [Serial Online]. 2008 [cited 2010 Apr 30] 58(44):1227–32.

5. Agrawal A, Scherrer JF, Grant JD, Sartor CE, Pergadia ML, Duncan AE, Madden PA, Haber JR, Jacob T, Bucholz KK, Xian H. The effects of maternal smoking during pregnancy on offspring outcomes. *Prev Med.* 2010 Jan–Feb;50(1–2):13–8.

6. Centers for Disease Control and Prevention. Smoking-attributable mortality, years of potential life lost, and productivity losses: United States, 2000–2004. *MMWR.* 2008;57(45):1226–8.

7. U.S. Department of Health and Human Services. Women and smoking: a report of the Surgeon General. U.S. Department of Health and Human Services, Centers for Disease Control and Prevention, National Center for Chronic Disease Prevention and Health Promotion, Office on Smoking and Health, 2001. [Updated 2001 March 27]. [cited 2010 June 16]. Available from: http://www.cdc.gov/tobacco/data_statistics/sgr/2001/complete_report/index.htm

8. Djordjevic MV, Doran KA. Part I: Nicotine content and delivery across tobacco products. *Handb Exp Pharmacol.* 2009;92:61–82.

9. Lowinson JH, Ruiz P, Millman RB, Langrod JG., eds. *Substance abuse: A comprehensive textbook.* 3rd ed. Baltimore: Williams & Wilkins; 1997. Chapter 25, Schmitz JM, Schneider NG, Jarvik ME. Nicotine. pp. 276–94.

10. Hatsukami D, Nelson R, Jensen J. Smokeless tobacco: current status and future directions. *Brit. J. Addict.* 1991 May;86(5):559–63.

11. National Cancer Institute. Smokeless tobacco or health, an international perspective. smoking and tobacco control monograph No. 2. Bethesda (MD): U.S. Department of Health and Human Services, National Cancer Institute, National Institutes of Health. NIH Pub. No. 93-3461. 1992: p 9. 91–126, 219–44. [cited 2010 Jun]. Available from: http://www.cancercontrol.cancer.gov/tcrb/monographs/index/html

12. FDA. Consumer updates: FDA warns of health risks posed by e-cigarettes [Internet]. Atlanta (GA): U.S. Food and Drug Administration, U.S. Department of Health and Human Services, 2009 July 23 [cited 2010 Jul 23] Available from: http://www.fda.gov/ForConsumers/ConsumerUpdates/ucm173401.htm

13. FDA. Summary of results: laboratory analysis of electronic cigarettes conducted by FDA [Internet]. Atlanta (GA): U.S. Food and Drug Administration, U.S. Department of Health and Human Services [updated 2009 July 22; cited 2010 July 23] Available from: http://www.fda.gov/NewsEvents/PublicHealthFocus/ucm173146.htm

14. Bullen C, McRobbie H, Thornley S, et al. Effect of an electronic nicotine delivery device (e cigarette) on desire to smoke and withdrawal, users preferences and nicotine delivery: randomized crossover trial. *Tob Control.* 2010 Apr;19(2):98–103.

15. United States Department of Health and Human Services: *The health consequences of smoking: a report of the Surgeon General [Internet].* Atlanta (GA): Department of Health and Human Services, Centers for Disease Control and Prevention, National Center for Chronic Disease Prevention and Health Promotion, Office on Smoking and Health; Washington, D.C. 2004 [updated 2009 May 29; cited 2010 May 10]:pp. 1–921 . Available from: http://www.cdc.gov/tobacco/data_statistics/sgr/2004/complete_report/index.htm

16. Farley TM, Meirik O, Chang CL, Poulter NR. Combined oral contraceptives, smoking, and cardiovascular risk. *J Epidemiol Community Health.* 1998 Dec;52(12):775–8.

17. Zielinski J, Bednarck M. Early detection of COPD in a high-risk population using spirometric screening. *Cardiopulmonary and Critical Care J.* 2001 Mar;119(3):731–6.

18. American Cancer Society. Cancer Facts and Figures 2002, Atlanta (GA): American Cancer Society. 2002;29–31.

19. Ford DE, Vu HT, Anthony JC. Marijuana use and cessation of tobacco smoking in adults from a community sample. *Drug and Alcohol Dependence.* 2002 Aug;67(3):243–8.

20. National Cancer Institute. Health effects of exposure to environmental tobacco smoke: the report of the California Environmental Protection Agency. Smoking and Tobacco Control Monograph No. 10. Bethesda (MD): U.S. Department of Health and Human Services, National Institutes of Health, National Cancer Institute, NIH Pub. No. 99-4645, 1999;ES-3–10.

21. Dreyfuss JH. Thirdhand smoke identified as potent, enduring carcinogen. *CA Cancer J Clin.* 2010 Jul–Aug;60(4):203–4. Epub 2010 Jun 8; [cited 2010 19 July].

22. U.S. Department of Health and Human Services. The health consequences of involuntary exposure to tobacco smoke: a report of the Surgeon General. Atlanta (GA): U.S. Dept. of Health and Human Services, Centers for Disease Control and Prevention, Coordinating Center for Health Promotion, National Center for Chronic Disease Prevention and Health Promotion, Office on Smoking and Health. 2006 [updated 2009 May 29; cited 2010 May]. Available from: http://www.surgeongeneral...gov/library/secondhandsmoke/report/

23. American Cancer Society. Cancer Facts and Figures 2010. Atlanta (GA): American Cancer Society 2002 [cited 2010 November];15–16.

24. Taylor AE, Johnson DC, Kazemi H. Environmental tobacco smoke and cardiovascular disease: A position paper from the council on cardiopulmonary and critical care. *American Heart Association, Circulation.* 1992 Aug;86(2):699–702.

25. Rosewich M, Adler S, Zielen S. Effects of active and passive smoking on the health of children and adolescents. *Pneumologie.* 2008 Jul;62(7):423–9. Epub 2008 Jul 3. [Cited 2010 June 20].

26. Kieser JA, Groeneveld HT, Da Silva P. Delayed tooth formation in children exposed to tobacco smoke. *J Clin Pediatr Dent.* 1996;20(2):97–100.

27. DiFranza JR, Aligne CA, Weitzman M. Prenatal and postnatal environmental tobacco smoke exposure and children's health. *Pediatrics.* 2004 Apr;113(4 Suppl):1007–15.

28. Metsios GS, Flouris AD, Koutedakis Y. Passive smoking, asthma and allergy in children. *Inflamm Allergy Drug Targets.* 2009 Dec; 8(5):348–52.

29. Mecklenburg RE, Greenspan D, Kleinman DV, Manley MW, Niessen LC, Robertson PB, Winn DE. Tobacco effects in the mouth: a National Cancer Institute and National Institute of Dental Research Guide for Health Professionals. U.S. Department of Health and Human Services. *Public Health Service.* 2000 Sep; NIH Publication No. 00-3330.27.

30. Tomar SL, Asma S. Smoking-attributable periodontitis in the United States: Findings from NHANES III. *J. Periodontol.* 2000 May;71(5):743–51.

31. Haber J, Wattles J, Crowley M, Mandell R, Joshipura K, Kent RL. Evidence for cigarette smoking as a major risk factor for periodontitis. *J. Periodontol.* 1993 Jan;64(1):16–23.

32. Bergstrom J, Eliasson S, Dock J. A 10-year prospective study of tobacco smoking and periodontal health. *J Perio.* 2000;71(8):1138–347.

33. Clasina G, Ramon CG, Echeverria JJ. Effects of smoking on periodontal tissues. *J Clin Periodontal.* 2002;29:771–6.

34. Haffajee AD, Socransky SS. Relationship of cigarette smoking to attachment level profiles. *J Clin Periodontol.* 2001;28:283–95.

35. Morozumi T, Kubota T, Sato T, Okuda K, Yoshie H. Smoking cessation increases gingival blood flow and gingival crevicular fluid. *J Clin Perio.* 2004;31:267–72.

36. Nair P, Sutherland G, Palmer RM, Wilson RF, Scott DA. Gingival bleeding on probing increases after quitting smoking. *J Clin Periodontol.* 2003;30:435–7.

37. Kibayashi M, Tanaka M, Nobuko N, et al. Longitudinal study of the association between smoking as a periodontitis risk and salivary bio-markers related to periodontitis. *J Periodontal.* 2007 May;78(5):859–67.

38. Apatzidou DA, Riggio MP, Kinane DF. Impact of smoking on the clinical, microbiological and immunological parameters of asdults patients with periodontitis. *J Clin Periodontol.* 2005;32:973–83.

39. Bergstrom J. Periodontitis and smoking: An evidence-based appraisal. *J Evid Base Dent Prac.* 2006;6:33–41.

40. Carcuac O, Jansson L. Peri-implantitis in a specialist clinic of periodontology. Clinical features and risk factors. *Swiss Dent J.* 2010;34(2):53–61.

41. Leshner AI. Understanding drug addiction: Implications for treatment. *Hospital Practice.* 1996 Oct;31(10):47–54, 57–9.

42. Mecklenburg RE, Christen AG, Gerbert B, Gift HC, et al. How to help your patients stop using tobacco: a National Cancer Institute Manual for the Oral Health Team, Smoking and Tobacco Control Program, National Cancer Institute, U.S. Department of Health and Human Services, Public Health Service. 1990 Dec; NIH Publication 91–3191.

43. Fiore MC, Jaen CR, Baker TB, et al. Treating Tobacco Use and Dependence:2008 Update. Clinical Practice Guideline. Rockville, MD, U.S. Department of Health and Human Services. Public Health Service. 2008 May [cited 2010 May 10]. Available from: http://www.ahrq.gov/clinic/tobacco/tobaqrg.pdf

44. Fiore MC. The new vital sign: Assessing and documenting smoking status. *JAMA.* 1991 Dec;266(22):3183–84.

45. Mecklenburg RE. How to help your patient be tobacco-free. National Cancer Institute, U.S. Department of Health and Human Services. *Public Health Service.* 2000 Jun;1–14.

Diet and Dietary Analysis

LUISA NAPPO-DATTOMA, RDH, RD, EDD

Chapter Outline

Nutrition is an integral part of an individual's general overall health as well as the health status of the oral cavity. The health of oral tissues can be affected by nutrition, diet, and food habits.

■ Box 34-1 defines relevant terms of standards, diet, nutrition, and oral health. Box 34-2 provides relevant abbreviations.

■ The interrelationship between nutritional status, systemic diseases, and oral conditions supports the need for timely and effective diet intervention.

■ Within the scope of practice, the dental hygienist has a responsibility to assess, screen, and deliver nutritional information and instruction as part of comprehensive education in health promotion and disease prevention and intervention.

■ Dietary and nutritional counseling, as part of a dental caries control program and periodontal maintenance, is an essential part of the dental hygiene treatment plan.

NUTRIENT STANDARDS FOR DIET ADEQUACY IN HEALTH PROMOTION

■ Education and instruction center around helping patients learn about selection of foods that make up an adequate diet.

■ To achieve an adequate balance in nutrition is a challenging task for all individuals.

■ To facilitate the learning process, multiple standards have been devised and are revised on a regular basis to reflect current research findings.

BOX 34-1	Key Words

Diet and Dietary Analysis

Anticariogenic: foods that do not lower the biofilm pH; encourage remineralization.

Antioxidant: a compound that stops the damaging effects of reactive substances seeking an electron (oxidizing agent).

Ariboflavinosis: a condition resulting from a lack of riboflavin.

Cariogenic: foods that lower the pH and are conducive to dental caries; the degree of cariogenicity depends on many factors, including physical form, texture, and consistency of the carbohydrate-containing food; its retention and clearance time from the oral cavity and the frequency of use.

Cariogenic exposure: individual ingestion of a cariogenic food that exposes tooth surfaces and lowers the pH in the dental biofilm.

Clearance time: the time from the cariogenic exposure until the food is cleared from the oral cavity; influenced by consistency and quantity of saliva; by the action of the tongue, lips, and cheeks; and by the consistency of food.

Diet: customary amount and kind of food and drink taken by an individual from day to day.

Dietary assessment: separation of a dietary food record into individual components of the Food Guide Pyramid; assessment of quality, of whether the individual is using an adequate diet, and of where modifications are needed.

Malnutrition: poor nourishment resulting from improper diet or some defect of metabolism that prevents the body from utilizing the intake of food properly.

Meal plan: a selectively planned or prescribed regimen of food to meet certain needs of the individual.

Noncariogenic food: does not support or promote bacterial growth responsible for caries formation.

Nutrient: a chemical substance in foods that is needed by the body for building and repair; the six classes of nutrients are proteins, fats, carbohydrates, minerals, vitamins, and water.

Macronutrients: energy-yielding nutrients that are needed in larger amounts in the diet; carbohydrate, protein, and fat.

Micronutrients: nutrients that are needed in small amounts in the diet and are not energy-yielding; vitamins and minerals.

Nutrient density: assessment of nutritional quality of a food by comparing the nutrient content with the amount of energy (kilocalories) it provides.

Nutrition: sum of processes involved in taking nutrients into the body and assimilating and utilizing them; includes ingestion, digestion, absorption, transport, utilization of nutrients, and excretion of waste products.

Nutritional deficiency: inadequacy of nutrients in the tissues; the result of inadequate dietary intake or impairment of digestion, absorption, transport, or metabolism.

Registered dietitian: a healthcare professional with a minimum of a bachelor's degree in nutrition or dietetics who has attended an internship program or equivalent and passed the registration examination, all under the approval of the American Dietetic Association (ADA). Continuing education is required to keep credentials current.

Synthesis: the process involved in the formation of a complex substance from simpler elements or compounds; the process of building up.

Vegan diet: A diet consisting of only plant foods. Other varieties of the vegan diet are: the fruitarian: fruits, nuts, honey, and vegetable oils; lacto-vegetarian: vegan based with the inclusion of dairy products; lacto-ovo-vegetarian: vegan based with the inclusion of dairy products and eggs.

BOX 34-2	Key Words

Abbreviations: Diet and Dietary Analysis

AIs: adequate intakes. The recommended nutrient intake utilized when there is not enough information to establish an EAR.

DRIs: dietary reference intakes. A comprehensive term for categories of reference values that concentrate on maintaining a healthy state for the healthy general population to avoid overeating and prevent chronic disease.

EARs: estimated average requirements. Estimates the nutrient requirements of the average individual.

RDAs: recommended dietary allowances; recommendations for the average amounts of nutrients recommended to be consumed daily by healthy people to achieve adequate nutrient intake to prevent deficiency.

ULs: tolerable upper intake levels, or upper levels; maximum intake by an individual that is unlikely to create risks of adverse health effects in almost all healthy individuals.

USDA: United States Department of Agriculture.

USDHHS: United States Department of Health and Human Services.

I. GOVERNMENT STANDARDS

A. Purposes of Standards

- Facilitate education for individuals about dietary needs and goals for health promotion.
- Help achieve diet adequacy for the public.
- Make recommendations relative to poor food habits such as missed meals, omission of essential foods and nutrients, and illogical dieting.
- Make specific recommendations for oral health.
- Motivate for behavioral modification.

B. Guidelines

- Provide guidelines through printed and Web-based educational materials.
- Guidelines reflect health concerns of the general public.

II. DIETARY STANDARDS

A. Dietary Reference Intakes (DRIs)[1]

- DRIs: a comprehensive term for categories of reference values that concentrate on maintaining a healthy state for the healthy general population to avoid overeating and prevent chronic disease.
- Encompasses the current nutrient recommendations made by the Food and Nutrition Board of the National Academy of Sciences.
- The categories include the RDAs, ALs, EARs, and ULs.
- Established for vitamins and minerals.
- Established by Institute of Medicine for the healthy general population to avoid overeating and to prevent chronic disease.

B. Estimated Average Requirements (EARs)[1]

- Estimates the nutritional requirements of the average individual.
- Categorized by age and gender.
- Provide the foundation for the RDAs.

C. Recommended Dietary Allowances (RDAs)[2]

- Recommendations for the average amounts of nutrients recommended to be consumed daily by healthy people to achieve adequate nutrient intake to prevent deficiency.
- Categorized by age and gender; do not include special needs such as illness.
- Reflect adequate nutrient intake of essential nutrients for healthy individuals to prevent deficiency.
- Based on gender and age; do not include special needs such as in illness.

D. Adequate Intakes (AIs)[3,4]

- The recommended nutrient intake utilized when there is not enough information to establish an EAR.

- AIs have been established for calcium, vitamin D, and fluoride for all age groups.

E. Tolerable Upper Intake Levels, or Upper Levels (ULs)[3,4]

- Maximum intake by an individual that is unlikely to create risks of adverse health effects in almost all healthy individuals.
- ULs were established to avoid toxicity due to excess intake of specific nutrients from food, fortified food, water, and nutrient supplements.

III. DIETARY GUIDELINES FOR AMERICANS

- Established by USDA and USDHHS as the basis for a federal nutrition policy based on the most recent scientific evidence review.
- Provides information and advice for choosing healthy eating patterns that focus on achieving and maintaining a healthy weight and embody food safety principles to avoid foodborne illness.
- Used as the basis for developing nutrition related programs, educational materials and consumer health messages.
- **Box 34-3** lists key recommendations in the 2010 Dietary Guidelines for Americans.

BOX 34-3	Key Recommendations: Dietary Guidelines for Americans, 2010

- Balance calories to manage weight
  - ☐ Prevent overweight and obesity
- Increase physical activity
- Foods and food components to reduce
  - ☐ Sodium
  - ☐ Saturated and trans fats
  - ☐ Added sugars
  - ☐ Refined grains
  - ☐ Alcohol
- Foods and nutrients to increase
  - ☐ Vegetables and fruits
  - ☐ Whole grains
  - ☐ Fat-free or low-fat milk and milk products
  - ☐ Protein foods, including seafood and vegetarian options
  - ☐ Oils instead of solid fats
  - ☐ Nutrients of concern, particularly potassium, dietary fiber, calcium, and vitamin D
- Build healthy eating patterns
  - ☐ Meet nutrients needs at appropriate caloric levels
  - ☐ Follow food safety to reduce foodborne illnesses

Source: U.S. Department of Agriculture and U.S. Department of Health and Human Services. *Dietary Guidelines for Americans, 2010.* 7th Edition, Washington, DC: U.S. Government Printing Office, December 2010. [cited 2011, April 25] Available from: http://health.gov/dietaryguidelines/.

IV. MYPLATE FOOD GUIDELINES

- Originally developed as a "Food Pyramid" by the United States Department of Agriculture (USDA) in 1991.
- Newest version established June 2011 using the graphic representation of a "dinner plate" icon as illustrated in **Figure 34-1**.
- Colorful graphic provides a visual reminder of the approximate proportions of five food groups necessary for a healthy diet.
- Educational materials accompanying the MyPlate food guidance system encourage consumers to:
- Build a healthy plate
  - Make half the plate vegetables and fruits
  - Switch to fat-free or low-fat milk
  - Choose whole grains.

- Vary protein choices (include seafood and beans) and keep meat portions small.
- Cut back on foods high in solid fat, added sugars, and salt
- Eat the right amount of calories
  - Enjoy food, but eat less and keep track what is consumed
  - Cook more often at home and choose lower calorie options when eating out
  - Limit alcoholic beverages
- Be physically active

V. RECOMMENDED FOOD INTAKE PATTERNS

- Food intake pattern recommendations, originally developed to accompany the MyPyramid food guidance system, have remained in place.

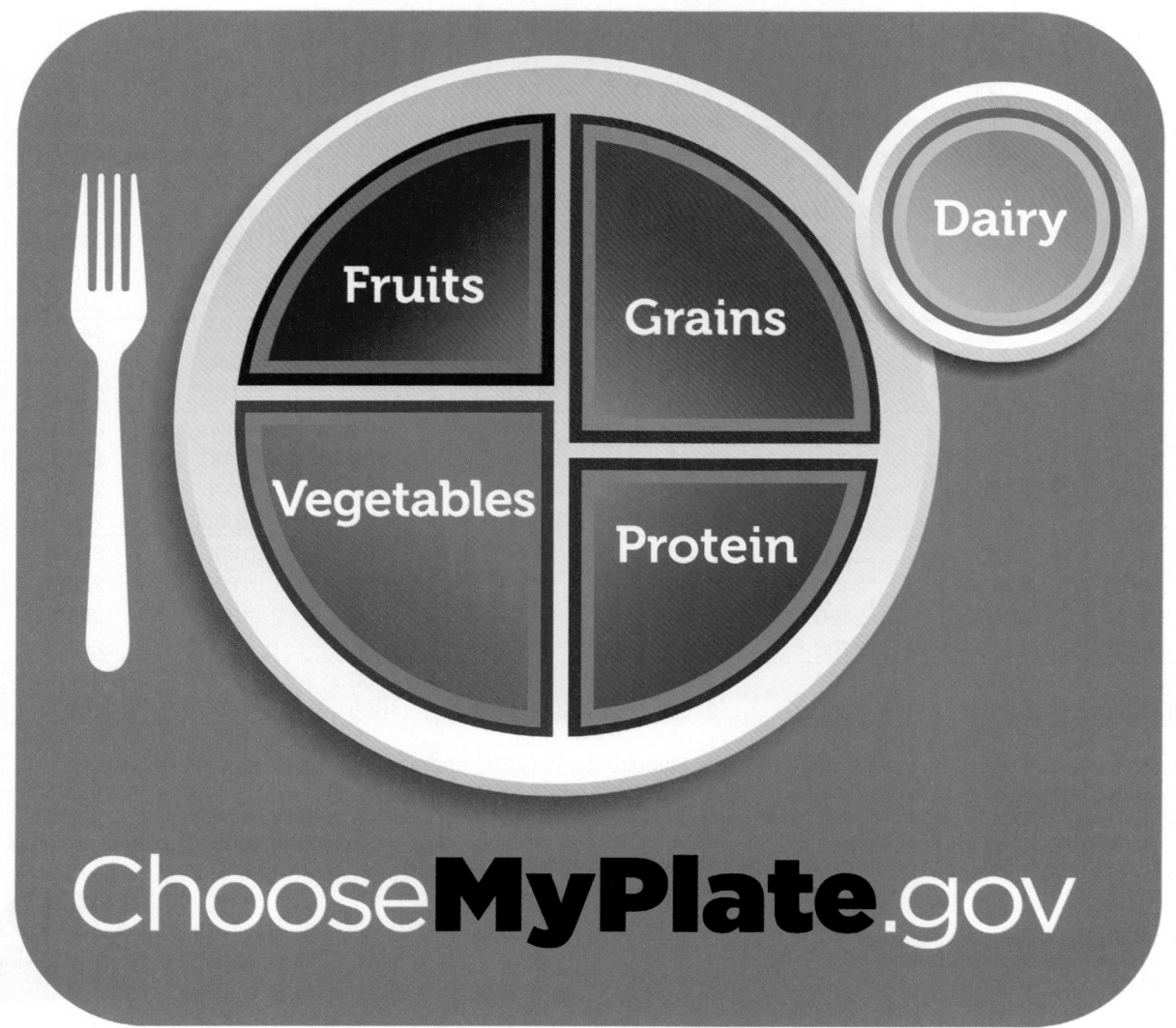

FIGURE 34-1 **ChooseMyPlate Guidelines Icon.** U.S. Department of Agriculture, Center for Nutrition Policy and Promotion, ChooseMyPlate Guidelines, June 2011. Available from http://www.choosemyplate.gov.

(Continued on page 502)

Food Intake Pattern Calorie Levels

Assigns individuals to a calorie level based on their sex, age, and activity level.

The chart below identifies the calorie levels for males and females by age and activity level. Calorie levels are provided for each year of childhood, from 2 to 18 years, and for adults in 5-year increments.

	MALES					FEMALES		
Activity level	Sedentary*	Mod. active*	Active*		**Activity level**	Sedentary*	Mod. active*	Active*
AGE					**AGE**			
2	1000	1000	1000		2	1000	1000	1000
3	1000	1400	1400		3	1000	1200	1400
4	1200	1400	1600		4	1200	1400	1400
5	1200	1400	1600		5	1200	1400	1600
6	1400	1600	1800		6	1200	1400	1600
7	1400	1600	1800		7	1200	1600	1800
8	1400	1600	2000		8	1400	1600	1800
9	1600	1800	2000		9	1400	1600	1800
10	1600	1800	2200		10	1400	1800	2000
11	1800	2000	2200		11	1600	1800	2000
12	1800	2200	2400		12	1600	2000	2200
13	2000	2200	2600		13	1600	2000	2200
14	2000	2400	2800		14	1800	2000	2400
15	2200	2600	3000		15	1800	2000	2400
16	2400	2800	3200		16	1800	2000	2400
17	2400	2800	3200		17	1800	2000	2400
18	2400	2800	3200		18	1800	2000	2400
19-20	2600	2800	3000		19-20	2000	2200	2400
21-25	2400	2800	3000		21-25	2000	2200	2400
26-30	2400	2600	3000		26-30	1800	2000	2400
31-35	2400	2600	3000		31-35	1800	2000	2200
36-40	2400	2600	2800		36-40	1800	2000	2200
41-45	2200	2600	2800		41-45	1800	2000	2200
46-50	2200	2400	2800		46-50	1800	2000	2200
51-55	2200	2400	2800		51-55	1600	1800	2200
56-60	2200	2400	2600		56-60	1600	1800	2200
61-65	2000	2400	2600		61-65	1600	1800	2000
66-70	2000	2200	2600		66-70	1600	1800	2000
71-75	2000	2200	2600		71-75	1600	1800	2000
76 and up	2000	2200	2400		76 and up	1600	1800	2000

*Calorie levels are based on the Estimated Energy Requirements (EER) and activity levels from the Institute of Medicine Dietary Reference Intakes Macronutrients Report, 2002.
SEDENTARY = less than 30 minutes a day of moderate physical activity in addition to daily activities.
MOD. ACTIVE = at least 30 minutes up to 60 minutes a day of moderate physical activity in addition to daily activities.
ACTIVE = 60 or more minutes a day of moderate physical activity in addition to daily activities.

United StatesDepartment of Agriculture
Center for Nutrition Policy and Promotion
April 2005
CNPP-XX

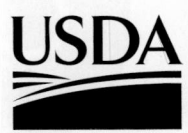

FIGURE 34-2 **MyPyramid Food Intake Pattern Calorie Levels.** U.S. Department of Agriculture, Center for Nutrition Policy and Promotion, MyPyramid Food Guidance System, April 2005. Available from http://www.choosemyplate.gov.

Food Intake Patterns

The suggested amounts of food to consume from the basic food groups, subgroups, and oils to meet recommended nutrient intakes at 12 different calorie levels. Nutrient and energy contributions from each group are calculated according to the nutrient-dense forms of foods in each group (e.g., lean meats and fat-free milk). The table also shows the discretionary calorie allowance that can be accommodated within each calorie level, in addition to the suggested amounts of nutrient-dense forms of foods in each group.

Daily Amount of Food From Each Group

Calorie Level[1]	1,000	1,200	1,400	1,600	1,800	2,000	2,200	2,400	2,600	2,800	3,000	3,200
Fruits[2]	1 cup	1 cup	1.5 cups	1.5 cups	1.5 cups	2 cups	2 cups	2 cups	2 cups	2.5 cups	2.5 cups	2.5 cups
Vegetables[3]	1 cup	1.5 cups	1.5 cups	2 cups	2.5 cups	2.5 cups	3 cups	3 cups	3.5 cups	3.5 cups	4 cups	4 cups
Grains[4]	3 oz-eq	4 oz-eq	5 oz-eq	5 oz-eq	6 oz-eq	6 oz-eq	7 oz-eq	8 oz-eq	9 oz-eq	10 oz-eq	10 oz-eq	10 oz-eq
Meat and Beans[5]	2 oz-eq	3 oz-eq	4 oz-eq	5 oz-eq	5 oz-eq	5.5 oz-eq	6 oz-eq	6.5oz-eq	6.5 oz-eq	7 oz-eq	7 oz-eq	7 oz-eq
Milk[6]	2 cups	2 cups	2 cups	3 cups	3 cups	3 cups	3 cups	3 cups	3 cups	3 cups	3 cups	3 cups
Oils[7]	3 tsp	4 tsp	4 tsp	5 tsp	5 tsp	6 tsp	6 tsp	7 tsp	8 tsp	8 tsp	10 tsp	11 tsp
Discretionary calorie allowance[8]	165	171	171	132	195	267	290	362	410	426	512	648

1 **Calorie Levels** are set across a wide range to accommodate the needs of different individuals. The attached table "Estimated Daily Calorie Needs" can be used to help assign individuals to the food intake pattern at a particular calorie level.

2 **Fruit Group** includes all fresh, frozen, canned, and dried fruits and fruit juices. In general, 1 cup of fruit or 100% fruit juice, or 1/2 cup of dried fruit can be considered as 1 cup from the fruit group.

3 **Vegetable Group** includes all fresh, frozen, canned, and dried vegetables and vegetable juices. In general, 1 cup of raw or cooked vegetables or vegetable juice, or 2 cups of raw leafy greens can be considered as 1 cup from the vegetable group.

Vegetable Subgroup Amounts are Per Week

Calorie Level	1,000	1,200	1,400	1,600	1,800	2,000	2,200	2,400	2,600	2,800	3,000	3,200
Dark green veg.	1 c/wk	1.5 c/wk	1.5 c/wk	2 c/wk	3 c/wk	3 c/wk	3 c/wk	3 c/wk	3 c/wk	3 c/wk	3 c/wk	3 c/wk
Orange veg.	.5 c/wk	1 c/wk	1 c/wk	1.5 c/wk	2 c/wk	2 c/wk	2 c/wk	2 c/wk	2.5 c/wk	2.5 c/wk	2.5 c/wk	2.5 c/wk
Legumes	.5 c/wk	1 c/wk	1 c/wk	2.5 c/wk	3 c/wk	3 c/wk	3 c/wk	3 c/wk	3.5 c/wk	3.5 c/wk	3.5 c/wk	3.5 c/wk
Starchy veg.	1.5 c/wk	2.5 c/wk	2.5 c/wk	2.5 c/wk	3 c/wk	3 c/wk	6 c/wk	6 c/wk	7 c/wk	7 c/wk	9 c/wk	9 c/wk
Other veg.	3.5 c/wk	4.5 c/wk	4.5 c/wk	5.5 c/wk	6.5 c/wk	6.5 c/wk	7 c/wk	7 c/wk	8.5 c/wk	8.5 c/wk	10 c/wk	10 c/wk

4 **Grains Group** includes all foods made from wheat, rice, oats, cornmeal, barley, such as bread, pasta, oatmeal, breakfast cereals, tortillas, and grits. In general, 1 slice of bread, 1 cup of ready-to-eat cereal, or 1/2 cup of cooked rice, pasta, or cooked cereal can be considered as 1 ounce equivalent from the grains group. **At least half of all grains consumed should be whole grains.**

5 **Meat & Beans Group** in general, 1 ounce of lean meat, poultry, or fish, 1 egg, 1 Tbsp. peanut butter, 1/4 cup cooked dry beans, or 1/2 ounce of nuts or seeds can be considered as 1 ounce equivalent from the meat and beans group.

FIGURE 34-3 **MyPyramid Food Intake Patterns.** U.S. Department of Agriculture, Center for Nutrition Policy and Promotion, MyPyramid Food Guidance System, April 2005. Available at http://www.choosemyplate.gov. (*continued*)

6 Milk Group includes all fluid milk products and foods made from milk that retain their calcium content, such as yogurt and cheese. Foods made from milk that have little to no calcium, such as cream cheese, cream, and butter, are not part of the group. Most milk group choices should be fat-free or low-fat. In general, 1 cup of milk or yogurt, 1 1/2 ounces of natural cheese, or 2 ounces of processed cheese can be considered as 1 cup from the milk group.

7 Oils include fats from many different plants and from fish that are liquid at room temperature, such as canola, corn, olive, soybean, and sunflower oil. Some foods are naturally high in oils, like nuts, olives, some fish, and avocados. Foods that are mainly oil include mayonnaise, certain salad dressings, and soft margarine.

8 Discretionary Calorie Allowance is the remaining amount of calories in a food intake pattern after accounting for the calories needed for all food groups—using forms of foods that are fat-free or low-fat and with no added sugars.

Estimated Daily Calorie Needs

To determine which food intake pattern to use for an individual, the following chart gives an estimate of individual calorie needs. The calorie range for each age/sex group is based on physical activity level, from sedentary to active.

	Calorie Range		
Children	Sedentary	⟶	Active
2–3 years	1,000	⟶	1,400
Females			
4–8 years	1,200	⟶	1,800
9–13	1,600	⟶	2,200
14–18	1,800	⟶	2,400
19–30	2,000	⟶	2,400
31–50	1,800	⟶	2,200
51+	1,600	⟶	2,200
Males			
4–8 years	1,400	⟶	2,000
9–13	1,800	⟶	2,600
14–18	2,200	⟶	3,200
19–30	2,400	⟶	3,000
31–50	2,200	⟶	3,000
51+	2,000	⟶	2,800

Sedentary means a lifestyle that includes only the light physical activity associated with typical day-to-day life.

Active means a lifestyle that includes physical activity equivalent to walking more than 3 miles per day at 3 to 4 miles per hour, in addition to the light physical activity associated with typical day-to-day life.

U.S. Department of Agriculture
Center for Nutrition Policy and Promotion
April 2005

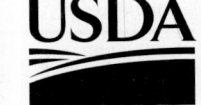

FIGURE 34-3 (*Continued*)

■ Caloric recommendations based on gender, age, and activity level are illustrated in **Figure 34-2**.

■ Twelve caloric patterns ranging from 1000 to 3200 kilocalories provide specific amounts of food consumption from the five food groups, oils, and discretionary kilocalories, as illustrated in **Figure 34-3**.

ORAL HEALTH RELATIONSHIPS

■ Nutrition, diet, and oral health are closely interrelated.
■ The oral cavity is the gateway to the health of the entire body.

■ Healthy masticatory function of the dentition contributes to proper dietary selection for maintenance of the nutritional status of the entire body.

■ Healthy diet selection provides essential nutrients for optimum health of oral tissues and prevention of manifestation of nutritional deficiencies.

I. SKIN AND MUCOUS MEMBRANE

■ Relevant vitamins: vitamin A, B complex, and ascorbic acid.
■ Relevant minerals: zinc and iron.
■ **Table 34-1** outlines the nutrients, their function and food sources.

(*Continued on page 505*)

TABLE 34-1	NUTRIENTS RELEVANT TO ORAL HEALTH		
NUTRIENT	**FUNCTION**	**DEFICIENCY DISEASE**	**FOOD SOURCE**
Vitamin A (Retinol, Provitamin A carotene)	• Fat soluble • Antioxidant • Bone and tooth development • Skin and mucous membrane integrity • Cell differentiation; essential for reproduction • Vision in dim light • Immune system integrity	• Night blindness • Xerophthalmia • Poor growth • Keratinization of epithelium • Dry, scaly skin • Toxic in large doses: (double vision, hair loss, dry mucous membranes, joint pain, liver damage)	Egg yolk, liver, fish liver oils, fortified milk, cream, cheeses; green leafy vegetables, orange, red, yellow pigmented fruits and vegetables
Vitamin D (Calciferol)	• Fat soluble • Aids in the absorption of calcium and phosphorus • Mineralization of bone	• Rickets in children • Osteomalacia in adults • Osteoporosis • Toxic in large doses: (calcification of soft tissues, growth retardation)	Exposure to UV sunlight, fortified milk, fish oils
Vitamin E (Tocopherol)	• Fat soluble • Antioxidant	• Low incidence of deficiency • Low toxicity	Whole grains, wheat germ, plant oils, margarines, legumes, seeds, nuts, greens
Vitamin K (Quinone)	• Fat soluble • Synthesis of prothrombin in blood clotting and bone proteins	• Prolonged clotting time • Hemorrhage • Toxic in large doses; (patients on blood thinners need to limit use in diet)	Synthesized by intestinal bacterial flora; dark green leafy vegetables, liver
Thiamin (B_1)	• Acts as coenzyme in carbohydrate and amino acid metabolism	• Essential for synthesis of acetylcholine for healthy nerves • Beriberi: weight loss, fatigue, edema, depression • Toxicity: not seen	Enriched whole grains and cereals, pork, meats, poultry, nuts, seeds, legumes
Riboflavin (Vitamin B_2)	• Coenzyme in energy metabolism of fat, carbohydrate, and protein	• Ariboflavinosis • Angular cheilosis • Growth failure • Eye disorders • Toxicity: not seen	Milk, cheese, enriched and whole grains and cereals, rice, mushrooms, liver
Niacin (Vitamin B_3)	• Coenzyme in energy metabolism of fat, carbohydrate, and protein	• Pellagra: diarrhea, dermatitis, dementia and death • Toxicity not seen in food sources • Toxicity with large doses of supplements for treatment of hypercholesterolemia: (skin redness and flushing, gastric ulcers)	Enriched whole grains and cereals, rice, meat, poultry, fish, green leafy vegetables
Pyridoxine (Vitamin B_6)	• Coenzyme in amino acid and lipid metabolism • Hemoglobin synthesis • Homocysteine metabolism	• Dermatitis • Depression • Convulsions • Peripheral neuritis • Toxicity not seen in food sources • Toxicity from supplements: neuropathy, irreversible nerve damage	Widespread food sources with exception of fat and sugar
Cobalamin (Vitamin B_{12})	• Maturation of RBC • Requires Intrinsic Factor from parietal cells for absorption • Cofactor in folate and homocysteine metabolism	• Pernicious anemia secondary to lack of intrinsic factor and total vegan diet • Toxicity: not seen	All animal foods, fortified cereals

(*continued*)

TABLE 34-1	NUTRIENTS RELEVANT TO ORAL HEALTH (*Continued*)		
NUTRIENT	**FUNCTION**	**DEFICIENCY DISEASE**	**FOOD SOURCE**
Folate (Folic Acid)	• Maturation of RBC • DNA synthesis • Homocysteine metabolism	• Megaloblastic anemia, • Neural tube defects: Spina bifida • Masks B12 deficiency • Toxicity not seen	Green leafy vegetables, fruits, legumes, fortified grains
Ascorbic Acid (Vitamin C)	• Antioxidant • Collagen synthesis • Wound healing • Aids in absorption of iron	• Scurvy • Poor wound healing • Petechial hemorrhages • Increased periodontal symptoms • Toxicity: potential for rebound scurvy	Citrus fruits, broccoli, strawberries, peppers, tomatoes, cantaloupe
Calcium	• Muscle contraction • Blood clotting • Nerve impulse transmission • Calcification of bone and tooth structure	• Osteoporosis • Incomplete calcification of hard tissues • Toxicity: not seen	Dairy products, tofu, fortified orange juice, and soy milk, green leafy vegetables, canned salmon and sardine bones
Phosphorus	• Required for bone and teeth strength • Acid-base balance • Muscle contraction	• Poor bone maintenance • Incomplete calcification of teeth • Compromised alveolar integrity • Toxicity: skeletal porosity	Dairy products, meat, poultry, processed foods, soft drinks, nuts, legumes, whole grain cereals
Magnesium	• Bone strength and rigidity • Hydroxyapatite crystal formation • Nerve impulse • Muscle contraction	• Muscle weakness • Alveolar bone fragility • Toxicity seen in medications containing magnesium	Wheat bran, whole grains, green leafy vegetables, legumes, nuts, chocolate
Fluoride	• Prevention of dental caries • Remineralization	• Increased incidence of caries • Toxicity: tooth mottling; enamel hypoplasia	Fluoridated water, tea, seaweed, toothpaste
Iron	• Component of hemoglobin • Carries oxygen to cells • Immune function • Cognitive development	• Anemia: pallor of face, conjunctiva, lips, mucosa and gingiva • Shortness of breath • Fatigue • Decreased immunity • Toxicity: GI upset; pigmentation; seen in persons with hemochromatosis	Meat, poultry, fish, whole grains, dried fruit, enriched grains
Zinc	• Required for over 100 enzymes • Normal growth and development • Taste and smell sensitivity • Sexual development and reproduction • Immune integrity • Wound healing	• Altered taste • Growth retardation • Decreased wound healing • Impaired immunity • Toxicity: rare (stomach irritation; cramps; diarrhea; vomiting)	Seafood, meats, whole grains, greens
Copper	• Aids in iron metabolism • Collagen formation	• Anemia • Poor growth • Low WBC • Bone demineralization • Tissue fragility • Decreased trabeculae of alveolar bone • Toxicity: vomiting; diarrhea	Whole grains, nuts, dried fruits, meats legumes, shell fish, organ

Source: Palmer CA, editor. *Diet and nutrition in oral health.* 2nd ed. Upper Saddle River: Pearson Prentice Hall; 2007. Chapter 8, Palmer, CA Papas, AS: The minerals and mineralization; Chapter 9, Palmer, CA: Vitamins today; pp. 163, 169–71, 204–5, 222–5.

TABLE 34-2	ORAL MANIFESTATIONS OF NUTRIENT DEFICIENCIES
ORAL SYMPTOM ASSOCIATED WITH THE TONGUE	**NUTRIENT DEFICIENCY**
Altered taste sensations	Riboflavin, thiamin, zinc, vitamin A, vitamin B_{12}
Glossitis	Folate, niacin, riboflavin, vitamin B_6, vitamin B_{12}
Glossodynia	Niacin, vitamin B_6, vitamin B_{12}
Sore or burning tongue	Iron, niacin, riboflavin, thiamin, vitamin B_6, vitamin B_{12}
ORAL SYMPTOMS ASSOCIATED WITH MUCOSAL TISSUE	
Angular cheilosis	Folate, iron, riboflavin, vitamin B_6, vitamin B_{12}
Candidiasis	Folate, iron, zinc, vitamin A, vitamin C
Delayed wound healing	Riboflavin, zinc, vitamin A, vitamin C
Mucositis/Stomatitis	Folate, niacin, thiamin, vitamin B_{12}

Source: Palmer CA, editor. Diet and nutrition in oral health. 2nd ed. Upper Saddle River: Pearson Prentice Hall; 2007. Chapter 8, Palmer, CA Papas, AS: The minerals and mineralization; Chapter 9, Palmer, CA: Vitamins today; pp. 163, 169 –71, 204–5, 222–5.

II. PERIODONTAL TISSUES

Periodontal diseases are not caused by nutritional deficiencies, but malnutrition may contribute to the progression of periodontal disease symptoms and influence how treatment can succeed in bringing the tissues back to health.

- *Nutritional deficiencies do not cause periodontal diseases.* Without local factors, including the periodontal pathogens in biofilm, biofilm-retentive factors (such as calculus and defective restorations), and lack of the patient's personal daily care to remove biofilm, periodontal infections cannot occur.
- *Severe deficiencies are rare in developed countries.* Symptoms of deficiencies such as listed in **Table 34-2** may be seen in cases of severe deprivation, starvation, and long-term patients with alcoholism or other drug addictions.
- *RDAs are essential to the health of the periodontal tissues.* As part of total body health, the daily diet nourishes the oral tissues.
- *The physical character of the diet contributes.* A soft sticky diet that stays on the tooth surfaces, especially cervical third and proximal areas, encourages biofilm buildup and proliferation of bacteria, including the periodontal pathogens.
- *Malnutrition suppresses the immune system and so impairs the host's reaction to infections.* Increased activity of pathogenic microorganisms may result in increased periodontal disease.

- *Nutrients contribute to healing and tissue repair.*[5] The elements strongly associated with wound healing include the vitamin B complex, vitamin C (ascorbic acid), and dietary calcium.
  - *B complex* refers to all the water-soluble vitamins except vitamin C. They are thiamin (vitamin B_1), riboflavin (vitamin B_2), niacin (vitamin B_3), pyridoxine (vitamin B_6), cobalamin (vitamin B_{12}), biotin, folic acid, and pantothenic acid. Each member of the B complex has individual functions.
  - *Vitamin C* is needed for collagen formation and intercellular material, and healing tissues after procedures including scaling and root planing.
  - *Dietary calcium.* 99% of the calcium in the body is in the bones and teeth; 1% is in the body tissues and fluids; essential for cell metabolism, muscle contraction, and nerve impulse transmission. Vitamin D is necessary for the continuous exchange of calcium between the blood, skeletal bones, and other cells.
  - *Low dietary intake of calcium can be a risk factor for periodontal disease.* Loss of alveolar bone and soft tissue attachment are typical of periodontal disease symptoms.[6]
  - *Current and former smokers show increased severity of periodontal disease. When smokers have low dietary vitamin C intake, their periodontal disease is more severe.*[7] There is no research to show whether intake of vitamin C can improve periodontal health.[7]

- *Obesity and periodontal disease*
  - Obesity is a significant predictor of periodontal disease.[8]
  - A younger population with overall and abdominal obesity shows increased periodontal disease. Underweight individuals have decreased periodontal disease.[9]
  - Promotion of healthy nutrition, adequate physical exercise, and weight control may be factors in the prevention of periodontal disease and slowing its rate of progression.[9]
- *Dietary assessment for periodontal conditions*
  - Periodontal therapy patients need specific instruction in diet selection.
  - Recommendation of firm fibrous foods, such as raw carrots or apples, may stimulate the tissues and improve circulation.
  - Chewing firm foods increases salivary flow. Saliva acts as a buffer, and increased saliva aids in oral clearance.
  - Surgical intervention patients may need to alter diet consistency following treatment during the healing period.
  - A soft diet of high-quality protein is indicated for adequate wound healing. Puddings, scrambled eggs, milkshakes, yogurt, and cottage cheese have high-quality protein to promote healing.

III. TOOTH STRUCTURE AND INTEGRITY

A. Nutrients and Health of Tooth Structure

- Adequate nutrition during tooth development is essential for mineralization.
- Relevant minerals: calcium, phosphorus, magnesium, and fluoride.
- Relevant vitamin: vitamin A.
- **Table 34-1** outlines nutrients, their function, and food sources.

B. Dietary Assessment

- Diet assessment during early tooth development is essential to assist parents.
- Anticipatory guidance for the parents has special significance (page 755).
- Prevention of early childhood caries is described in Chapter 49 on pages 768.

IV. DENTAL CARIES

A. Prevention[10]

- Fluoride is the essential mineral for dental caries prevention.
- The complexity of dental caries formation is illustrated in **Figure 34-4**.

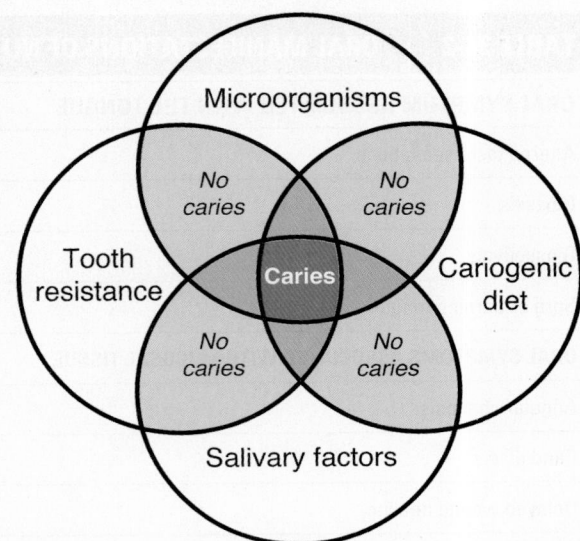

FIGURE 34-4 Dental Caries Process. Four overlapping circles illustrate the factors involved in the development of dental caries. All four act together, and as shown by the center, dental caries results. (Adapted from United States Department of Health and Human Services, Public Health Service, National Institute of Dental Research: Broadening the scope. Long-range research plan for the 1990s. NIH Publication No. 90-1188, Washington DC: United States Government Printing Office; 1990.)

B. Role of Cariogenic Foods[11]

- Caries is a result of excess cariogenic foods, not a nutrient deficiency.
- Fermentable carbohydrates produce acids when acted on by specific biofilm microorganisms.
- *Streptococcus mutans*, *Lactobacilli*, and other acid-forming organisms use fermentable carbohydrate from the diet to produce acids.

C. Consistency of Food

- Soft sticky foods cling to the teeth and gingiva and encourage biofilm accumulation.
- Microorganisms are protected and nourished in dental biofilm on the tooth leading to increased acid formation.

D. Dietary Assessment and Counseling

- Use of dietary assessment and patient instruction relative to dental caries control.
- Personal recommendations foster behavioral modification in disease prevention.

COUNSELING FOR DENTAL CARIES CONTROL

A. Risk Factors

- Control of dental biofilm.
- Modification of intake of sugars and cariogenic food.

- Strengthening the tooth surface to resist caries activity.
- Presence of saliva is essential; xerostomia increases the risk for demineralization.
- **Figure 34-4** illustrates the intricate relationship of all four factors in the development of dental caries.

B. Other Preventive Measures That Support Dietary Control

- Pit and fissure sealants.
- Restoration of existing carious lesions.
- Implementation of fluoride therapy.

THE DIETARY ASSESSMENT

- The dietary assessment is an integral part of disease prevention and health promotion in the scope of dental hygiene care.
- The patient and dental hygienist have the opportunity to collaborate in the evaluation of diet adequacy and in diet intervention.

I. PURPOSES OF A DIETARY ASSESSMENT

- Identify the patient who may be at nutritional and oral health risk.
- Refer to a registered dietitian when intervention beyond the scope of dental hygiene practice is indicated.
- Provide an opportunity for a patient to study personal dietary habits objectively.
- Obtain an overall picture of the types of food in the patient's diet, food preferences, and quantity of food eaten.
- Study the food habits and snacking patterns.
- Record frequency of use and consumption of cariogenic food.
- Determine the overall consistency of the diet.
  A. Identify fibrous foods regularly consumed.
  B. Identify soft sticky foods regularly consumed.
- Identify the nutritional status of an individual with regard to overall requirements, and then collaborate with the patient to make suggestions for modification in nutritional adequacy of the diet in health promotion.
- Plan with the patient for necessary changes to improve the health of the oral mucosa and periodontium, and prevent dental caries.

II. PRELIMINARY PREPARATION FOR DIETARY ASSESSMENT[11]

A. Patient History

1. Information obtained from medical, dental, and social histories is essential in assessing oral health and nutritional status.
   - Disease states
   - Medications
   - Disabilities
   - Learning limitations
   - Significant unintentional change in body weight
   - Factors influencing food use and food intake
2. Dietary influences can be identified by intra- and extra-oral examination, which may reveal oral tissue that is suggestive of nutritional deficiencies.

B. Clinical Evaluation

- Evaluation detects high-risk patients by noting factors suggestive of a dietary problem.
- Clinical examination and charting of cavitated carious lesions and demineralizing areas.
- Identification of any abnormalities in the patient's overall appearance; weight, skin, nails, and hair.
- **Table 34-2** lists oral manifestations of severe deficiencies.

III. FORMS USED FOR ASSESSMENT

A. *Food Diary* (Figure 34-5)

- A diary of the patient's dietary intake over the previous 24 hours.
- Obtained by interview with patient.
- Assesses nutrients, food groups, diet adequacy, form and frequency of the carbohydrate intake, and snacking patterns.
- Results are reviewed and appropriate instruction given at appointment or a follow-up appointment.
- It is quick and easy to administer and can be done chairside in one visit.
- Is limited to one day's intake, therefore, it is not necessarily representative of a patient's normal diet.

B. *Dietary Analysis Recording Form* 3–7 Days (Figure 34-6)

- A more accurate account of a patient's intake.
- Patient completes food diary for 3, 5 or 7 days, inclusive of one weekend day.
- Affords the patient a more active role in the dietary assessment and a chance to observe areas that require modification.
- Provide patient with three to seven copies of the *Food Diary* (Figure 34-5). Request patient to return the forms at follow-up visit.
- At follow-up visit the patient's diary is evaluated for:
  - Eating patterns
  - Consumption and frequency of fermentable carbohydrates
  - Nutritional adequacy

IV. PRESENTATION OF THE *FOOD DIARY* TO THE PATIENT

A. Explain the Purpose

- Briefly describe how diet relates to the dental situation.

FOOD DIARY

NAME_____TEL_____

AGE_____SEX_____Height _____Weight_____BMI____

Type of Foods/Beverages		Quantity Eaten (cup, oz, tbsp, tsp, etc.)	Preparation Method
BREAKFAST			
7:30 AM:	Orange juice	½ cup	Bagel Shop
	Bagel	Whole	
	Cream cheese	2 tablespoons	
	Coffee	2 cups	
	Milk and sugar	½ cup , 2 packets	
SNACK			
10:00 AM	Chocolate cookies	2	
	Orange soda	12 oz can	
LUNCH			
1:00 PM	Mushroom Pizza	2 slices	School Cafeteria
	Orange soda	12 oz can	
	Cheese cake	1 slice	
SNACK			
4:00 PM	Whole wheat pretzels	1 bag	Vending machine
DINNER			
7:00 PM	Turkey	6 oz	Roasted
	Potato	1 medium	Baked
	Sour Cream	2 Tablespoons	
	Broccoli	1 cup	Sauteed
	Oil	2 Tablespoons	
	Gravy	½ cup	Canned
SNACK			
9:30 PM	Popcorn	3 cups	Microwave

FIGURE 34-5 **Food Diary.** Sample of a form for patients to use to record the daily intake of foods. Can be used for the 24-hour recall or multiple forms used in the 3–7 day food diary.

- Provide a foundation for the education to follow.
- Avoid mention of specific foods not to bias patient.

B. Explain the Form

- Provide written and oral instructions for use of the *Food Diary*.
- Provide suggestions for listing various foods and use of household measurements for indicating quantity **(Box 34-4)**.

- Instruction for completing the food diary encourages the patient to provide a more accurate portrayal of eating behaviors.

C. Complete the Current Day's Food Diary With the Patient

- Helps to illustrate how to itemize and list foods eaten.
- Provides an example while completing the patient's own daily diary.

Name _____

Date _____ Age _____

Dietary Analysis

Food Groups	Day 1	2	3	4	5	6	7	Daily Average	"MyPyramid" Food Guidance System Recommendations for Six Most Used Caloric Levels (12 Total Levels)						
									1000 kcals	1600 kcals	1800 kcals	2200 kcals	2800 kcals	Adequate	
														Yes	No
Grains									3 oz-eq	5 oz-eq	6 oz-eq	7 oz-eq	10 oz-eq*		
Vegetables									1 cup	2 cups	2.5 cup	3 cups	3.5 cups		
Fruits									1 cup	1.5 cups	1.5 cups	2 cups	2.5 cups		
Milk									2 cups	3 cups	3 cups	3 cups	3 cups		
Meat & Beans									2 oz-eq	5 oz-eq	5 oz-eq	6 oz-eq	7 oz-eq		
Oils									3 tsp	5 tsp	5 tsp	6 tsp	8 tsp		
Discretionary Calories									165 kcals	132 kcals	195 kcals	290 kcals	426 kcals **		

* eq is the abbreviation for the word equivalents. See MyPyramid Food Intake Patterns (Figure 32-3) for more details on equivalents.

**kcals = kilocalories

Sweets									Total	
Liquid	With Meal									Total all liquid exposures and multiply by 20 minutes and divide by total number of days to equal daily acid attack from liquids. **Total Liquid Minutes_____**
	End of Meal									
	Between Meal									
Soft/Solid Sticky/ Retentive	With Meal									Total all soft and hard solid exposures and multiply by 40 minutes and divide by total number of days to equal daily acid attack from solids. **Total Solid Minutes_____**
	End of Meal									
	Between Meal									
Hard/Solid Slowly Dissolving	With Meal									Add both liquid and solid totals to determine number of minutes per day teeth are under acid attack. **Total Daily Minutes of Acid Attack _____**
	End of Meal									
	Between Meal									

FIGURE 34-6 **Dietary Analysis Recording Form.** From the food diary kept by the patient (**Figure 34-5**), each serving is entered as a check in the space beside the appropriate food group. Each category is totaled, averaged, and compared with the recommendation on the right.

D. General Directions

1. Emphasize importance of completing the diary for each meal as soon after eating as possible to avoid forgetting.
2. Encourage use of typical days, uncomplicated by illness, dieting, holidays, or other unusual events.
3. Review details of recording the component parts of a combination dish, such as a sandwich:
   - 2 slices of whole wheat bread
   - 4 oz of turkey
   - 1 teaspoon of mustard or light mayonnaise
   - 2 slices tomato with lettuce
   - 1 slice of cheddar cheese
4. Indicate need for recording nutritional supplements and all fluids consumed, including alcoholic beverages.
5. Request that meals eaten other than at home be identified:
   - Restaurant
   - Guest at friend's home
   - Party

BOX 34-4	*Food Diary* Instructions

- Write down everything eaten on the food diary form provided on page 508.
- Record each meal as soon after eating as possible to avoid forgetting.
- Do not choose days when dieting, fasting, or ill.
- Be accurate in determining the amounts eaten, using household measurements (e.g., 1/2 cup cereal, 1 tsp margarine, 3 oz fish). A 3-oz serving size can be compared to the size of a deck of cards.
- Use brand names whenever possible.
- Record added sauces, gravies, condiments, and all extras (e.g., sugar or cream in coffee, mayonnaise, chewing gum, cough drops).
- Record food preparation methods (e.g., baked, fried, boiled, grilled).
- Record all fluids; include water and alcoholic beverages.

6. Instruct patient to select consecutive days and at least one weekend day for a realistic representation of diet pattern.

V. RECEIVING THE COMPLETED *FOOD DIARY*

A. Obtain Supplemental Data

- Receive the *Food Diary* soon after its completion.
- Question the patient to clarify presented information.
- Does food diary represent a typical day or week?
- Identify influences on appetite such as illness or stress.
- Identify food likes and dislikes; food preferences; intolerances; food allergies.
- Frequency of dining out.
- Identify special diets being followed in the home.
- Average alcohol intake.
- Which family member is doing the cooking and food shopping?

B. Review Patient's *Food Diary*

1. Common omissions
   - Garnishes: frosting, whipped cream, butter or margarine on vegetables, salad dressings, oil.
   - Beverages: quantity, sweetened, decaffeinated.
   - Snacks: type, brand, quantity.
   - Chewing gum or mints: sugarless, nonsucrose sweetener such as xylitol, quantity.
   - Canned fruit: packed in water, heavy or light syrup, own juices, or nonsucrose sweetened, quantity.
   - Fruit and vegetables: canned, fresh, or frozen.
   - Cereal: sugar-treated or low sugar brand, type of milk and/or sugar added, quantity.

- Potato: baked, mashed, fried.
- Seasonings or sauces: quantity, type.
2. Determine common food habits, such as snacking at night or fast food choices at lunch.

VI. ANALYSIS OF DIETARY INTAKE

Three principal parts of the food diary to analyze are the number of servings in each food group, the frequency of cariogenic foods, and the consistency of the diet.

A. Nutritional Analysis for Adequacy of 24-Hour Recall Intake

- When time is a factor a 24-hour analysis is appropriate.
- Compare food groups represented in the patient's 24-hour food diary with that of the pyramid.
- Determine nutritional adequacy.
- Calculate the patient's "sweet score" as outlined in **Figure 34-7** *Scoring the Sweets*.
- Cariogenic foods are listed and categorized as solid, liquid, or slowly dissolving (**Figure 34-7**).
- Totals for the one day are multiplied by respective time factors and a score determines patient's caries risk.

B. Nutritional Analysis for Adequacy of Food Intake From the *Food Diary*

- Use the *Dietary Analysis Recording Form* to summarize adequacy of daily portions of each food group (**Figure 34-6**).
- Each food eaten is entered into a food group with number of servings.
- Comparison of patient's food diary with the *MyPyramid Food Guidance System* (**Figures 34-1, 34-2, 34-3**).
- Totals for the week are added and the average per day calculated.
- The average is compared to the recommended servings for each food group.
- Web-based nutrition analysis program available at *www.mypyramidtracker.gov* to analyze a 3-, 5-, or 7-day diary:
  - Charts comparing patient's averages to the RDA.
  - Tables comparing patient to *MyPyramid* recommendations.
- Assist patient while deficiencies are identified.
- Analysis of cariogenic foods.[11]
- Identify physical form of carbohydrate.
  - Liquids: sweetened or unsweetened soft drinks; fruit juice with added sugars.
  - Soft solid/sticky and retentive: retentive cakes, cookies, chips, pretzels, jellybeans, and chewy, sticky candies.
  - Hard solid/slowly dissolving: hard candies, mints, and cough drops.
- Identify frequency of meals and snacks.
  - When snacks are consumed.
  - Number of between-meal snacks consumed daily.

SCORING THE SWEETS (Caries-Promoting Potential)				
Food Items (from patients 24 hour recall)	**Reference Foods Considered Cariogenic**	**Frequency** (Place a check for each exposure to cariogenic food)	**Weighted Score**	**Total Points Each Category**
1. 2. 3. 4.	**Liquid** Soft drinks, fruit drinks, cocoa, sugar, and honey in beverages, nondairy creamers, ice cream, sherbet, flavored or frozen yogurt, pudding, custard, jello	___ ___ ___ ___	X 1	
1. 2. 3. 4. 5. 6.	**Solid & Sticky** Cakes, cupcakes, doughnuts, sweet rolls, potato chips, pretzels, pastry, canned fruit in syrup, bananas, cookies, chocolate candy, caramel, toffee, jelly beans, other chewy candy, chewing gum, dried fruit, marshmallows, jelly, jam	___ ___ ___ ___	X 2	
1. 2. 3.	**Slowly Dissolving** Hard candies, breath mints, antacid tablets, cough drops	___ ___ ___	X 3	

TOTAL SCORE _____

Using the 24-hour recall diary:
- Classify each sweet into liquid, solid and sticky, or slowly dissolving. (Use reference food list)
- For each time a sweet was eaten, either at a meal or between meals (at least 20 minutes apart) place a check in the frequency column.
- In each category tally the number of sweets eaten and multiply by the weighted score. Record the category points in the respective column.
- Tally all the category points to determine the total score.

Sweet score: (Risk for dental caries)	How to lower your risk for caries:
0-1 **low risk** 2-4 5-7 **moderate risk** 8-9 >10 **high risk**	1. Cut down on the frequency of between-meal sweets 2. Don't sip constantly on sweetened beverage 3. Avoid using slowly dissolving items like hard candy, cough drops etc. 4. Eat more nondecay promoting foods such as: (low fat cheese, raw (vegetables, crunchy fruits, nuts, popcorn.)

FIGURE 34-7 **Scoring the Sweets.** Form to be used to determine patient's caries risk when doing a 24-hour recall at chairside. (Adapted with permission from Carole A. Palmer Ed.D., R.D., Division of Nutrition and Oral Health Promotion, Department of General Dentistry, Tufts University School of Dental Medicine.)

- Circle in red and tally the number of cariogenic foods; both solid and liquids.
- Frequency more relevant than quantity in caries incidence.
- High frequency of eating events decreases ability of calcium and phosphate to remineralize teeth between episodes.
- During counseling appointment, show the patient how to:
  - Select and circle in red the cariogenic foods on the *Scoring the Sweets* form **(Figure 34-7)**.
  - Select liquid, soft solid, hard solid, and time of eating.
- Total the number of sweets for liquid and solids and multiply total by 20 minutes (liquids) and 40 minutes (solids).
- Divide by number of days (3, 5, or 7 day diary).
- Add the liquid and solid score for total minutes teeth are exposed to sweets and acid attack **(Figure 34-6)**.

C. Analysis of Diet Consistency

- Help patient to identify the types of firm and fibrous foods from the *Food Diary* such as:
  - Uncooked fruits and vegetables.
  - Cooked; crisp-tender vegetables.

- Help patient to identify the frequency of use:
  - Daily or occasionally.
  - During meal, end of meal, or between meals.

D. Benefits of *Food Diary* Analysis

- Patient can identify appropriate and inappropriate practices for dental caries control.
- Corroborate findings with clinical findings and patient's oral health problems in preparation for counseling session.

PREPARATION FOR ADDITIONAL COUNSELING

I. DEFINE OBJECTIVES

- To help patient understand the individual oral problems and appreciate the need for changing habits.
- To explain specific alterations in the diet necessary for improved general and oral health.
- For dental caries control.
  - To promote the minimal consumption of cariogenic foods, particularly between meals.
  - To substitute noncariogenic foods into diet.

II. PLANNING FACTORS

A. Patient Attitude

- Consider patient's willingness and ability to cooperate as evidenced by keeping appointments and following personal oral care procedures.
- Consider patient's health care beliefs and nutrition and dental knowledge.

B. Possible Barriers

- Difficulty and resistance to change of normal habits.
- Patient dissatisfaction with loss of usual or customary foods.
- Patients may not attempt to make modifications if recommendations are numerous or overwhelming.
- Lack of appreciation of need for change due to limited knowledge of diet, nutrition, and oral health relationship.
- Common misconception about concentrated sugar as an indispensable energy source.
- Social prejudices.
- Cultural and religious patterns significant to food selection and preparation.
- Financial considerations in food purchasing.
- Emotional eating patterns and cravings for sweets.
- Parental attitude toward sweets in the diet.
  - Elimination of all sugars would deprive a child of normal childhood pleasures.
  - All sugars are viewed as "bad" foods for children to have.

III. APPROPRIATE TEACHING MATERIALS

- Patient's radiographs, charting, and food diary.
- Diagrams, food models, food labels, or charts of dietary standards and requirements.
- Educational leaflets to illustrate patient's special dietary or oral health needs.
- An outline of a realistic diet plan with specific suggestions for food substitutes.
- A list of snack suggestions.

COUNSELING PROCEDURES

I. SETTING

- An environment free from interruptions and distracting background sounds.
- Apart from the clinical treatment room.
- Patient comfort promotes environment conducive to learning.
- Provide limited but pertinent educational information.
  - Posters and pamphlets.
  - Food labels and food models of portion sizes.
  - Avoid overloading with too much new information to minimize confusion.
- Persons involved in promoting change.
  - For a younger patient, the primary caregiver is present since this individual supervises the child's eating and oral care.
  - Person preparing meals and grocery shopping needs to be present to learn about appropriate food choices.

II. POINTERS FOR SUCCESS OF A CONFERENCE

- Be prepared and on time.
- Plan for only a few simple visual aids.
- Concentrate on the factors related to the patient's diet-based dental problem.
- Encourage parents to exclude small children (other than patient) from the conference; they may create distractions.
- Develop a permissive, friendly atmosphere; establish eye contact with a warm, nonthreatening environment.
- Take care not to follow a written outline of recommendations so rigidly that the conference lacks spontaneity.
- Use question format that provides a response filled with information.[12]
  - Use open-ended questions that elicit information. Example: "Tell me what was the first thing you ate today," "How was the omelet prepared?" and "What did you put on the bagel?"
  - Limit closed-ended questions; they provide "yes" or "no" responses and limited information. Example: "Did you eat breakfast today?"
  - Avoid using "why." It might put the patient on the defensive.

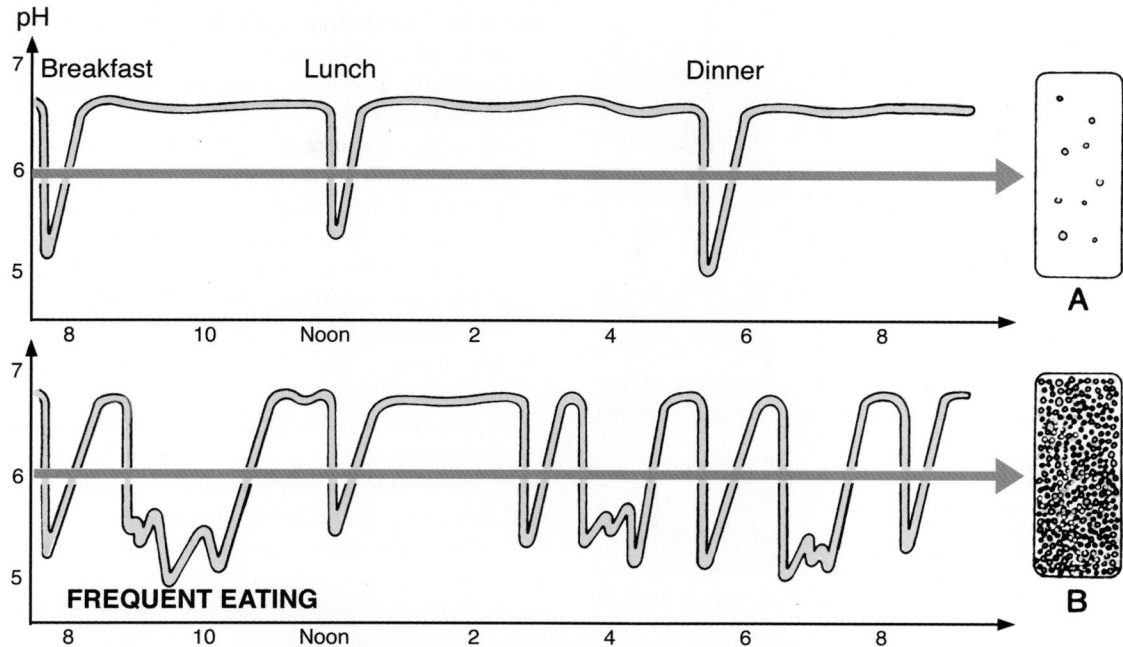

FIGURE 34-8 **Cariogenic Foods and Biofilm pH.** The range of pH in dental biofilm from 5 to 7 is shown on the left. Time intervals are shown across the bottom of each graph. The double-line curve represents the variations in biofilm pH throughout a day. Each time sugar or a cariogenic food is taken in, the pH of the dental biofilm drops to or below the critical pH (5.2 to 5.5). As shown in the lower graph, frequent eating keeps the pH at the critical level below which enamel demineralization can occur. On the right, (A) shows that bacterial counts are lower, whereas in (B), aciduric microorganisms are greatly increased in numbers. The critical pH for the root surfaces is 6.0 to 6.7. (Adapted with permission from Larmas, M.: *Int Dent J.* June 1985;35:109).

Example: "Why do you put sugar in your coffee?"

■ Guide patients to develop their own behavioral changes.
　▨ Use a patient-centered approach to the counseling session.
　▨ Foster greater patient compliance.
　▨ Empower the patient to get involved in making the suggestions and recommendations for change.
　▨ Put the responsibility for change on the patient.
　▨ Keep goals simple, small, and realistic.
■ Adequately discuss all questions from patient or parent using a conversational tone without lecturing.
■ Keep session brief, informative, and engaging for the patient without taking notes.

III. PRESENTATION

A. Review Purposes of the Meeting

■ Provide explanation of the relevance between diet and patient's particular problem.
■ Emphasize health promotion and disease prevention.

B. Clarification of "Cariogenic" Foods

■ Calculate the sugar score from the *Scoring the Sweets* or *Dietary Analysis Recording Form* to emphasize caries risk.
■ Clarify confusion of hidden sugars, added sugars, and natural sugars.

■ Clarify the moderation of sugar intake and select substitutions.

C. Review of Dental Caries Initiation

■ The sucrose from cariogenic food on the tooth surface can be changed to acid in minutes.
■ The pH drops to below 5.5, which is the critical level for demineralization of enamel.
■ Acid left undisturbed will be cleared from the mouth from 40 minutes to up to 2 hours, depending primarily on salivary flow. For a patient with xerostomia, clearance takes much longer.
■ **Figure 34-8** illustrates how the frequent intake of sucrose lowers the pH for several hours in the course of the day.

D. Frequency and Time of Exposure

■ Each exposure of the tooth surface to sucrose or other cariogenic food in a meal or snack increases the amount of acid on the tooth.
■ The quantity of a cariogenic food is not as significant as when and how often the tooth is exposed.
■ Prolonged intake of a cariogenic liquid or solid, such as continuous sipping of a sucrose-containing beverage while working at a desk, does not allow for a remineralization period to occur in which the pH can rise above the critical level.

E. Retention

- Vigorous rinsing with (fluoridated) water immediately after eating a cariogenic food can help remove the sucrose before it is metabolized by the acid-forming bacteria and reaches the tooth surface.
- Cariogenic foods taken after brushing and flossing before retiring are not cleared readily because salivary flow decreases during sleep.
- Cariogenic liquids are removed from the teeth in relatively less time than are solids.
- Oral retentiveness of cariogenic foods is related to length of time food debris with fermentable carbohydrate remains on the teeth and exposure to decreased biofilm pH.[13,14,15]
    - Sticky foods are retained for longer periods of time and have a longer oral clearance.[13,14]
    - Highly retentive fermentable carbohydrates have a delayed rate of oral clearance increasing exposure of teeth to a decreased pH and higher potential for demineralization.[13,14]
- Sequence of food consumption within a meal pattern is related to caries incidence.[15,16,17,18]
    - Eating fermentable carbohydrates at the beginning of a meal or between other noncariogenic foods (protein and fat) is less cumulative in cariogenic potential.
    - Protein and fat are not metabolized by bacteria and are recommended to be eaten at the end of a meal.
    - Cheese eaten after sweets or at the end of a meal prevents the decrease in pH and production of acids in the oral cavity.[18]
- Water aids in rinsing sugars from tooth surfaces and decreases cariogenic activity.
- Noncariogenic sweeteners contribute to caries prevention.[19]
- Sugar-free gums decrease lactic acid production and increase salivary flow potentially buffering acids.
    - Chewing a gum with xylitol immediately after each meal reduces the levels of *Streptococcus mutans* and promotes remineralization.
    - Xylitol is the sugar substitute of choice because it is not fermentable by caries promoting bacteria. Sorbitol can be fermented by *Streptococcus mutans* at a very slow rate.[20]

IV. SPECIFIC DIETARY RECOMMENDATIONS

A. Examination of the Patient's Food Diary

- After analyzing the diet, the patient can identify the deficiencies and excesses and suggest alternate choices.
- Try to retain as many as possible of the patient's present food habits.
- Make recommendations that can be adapted to the patient's pattern of living.

- Discuss foods from each food group that the patient likes and can be added to the diet.
- Guide the patient to identify foods in the diary that need changing.
- Assist patient in finding acceptable substitutions for the cariogenic food choices.
    - Patients may accept light yogurt as an alternative to ice cream for a snack.
    - Fruit may be an appealing suggestion.
    - Patients need to be involved in making changes in their own diets.
- To enhance compliance, help patients create their own meal plans for one day.
    - Incorporate the principles discussed during the counseling.
    - Collaborate on modifications the patient can achieve realistically and is willing to try.
    - Avoid too many changes that may be overwhelming.
    - Determine patient comprehension of information presented and patient's motivational level.
    - Include morning, afternoon, and evening snacks as well as breakfast lunch and dinner in a meal plan for a day.

B. Basic Principles for Dietary Changes

- Directions for the patient are simple and specific because interpretation of new ideas can be difficult.
- Incorporate foods from the food groups to complete the patient's diet to ensure adequacy and balance of nutrients.
- Limit the use of cariogenic foods to mealtimes.
    - Evaluate the final food in a meal because it may remain on the teeth if rinsing is not possible.
    - Recommend chewing a gum containing xylitol at the end of each meal especially for a caries-susceptible person.
    - Recommend specific stores within the area where patients can purchase xylitol gums.
- Foods that require chewing increase salivary flow.
    - Saliva provides buffering effect.
    - Saliva helps remove cariogenic foods.
- Limit between-meal snacking and select snacks from noncariogenic foods.
    - Nonflavored milk.
    - Cheese.
    - Peanut butter on sliced apples.
    - Cream cheese on celery.
    - Sugar-free gelatin or pudding.
- Use as little concentrated sweetener in the preparation of foods as possible.
    - Decrease the amount of granulated or brown sugar by half when baking.
    - Consider substituting non-sucrose sweeteners such as xylitol

- Observe care in the purchase of prepared foods and include more foods such as unsweetened fruit juice and canned fruits with no sugar added.
  - Natural sugars are just as detrimental as refined sugars (e.g., honey, maple syrup).
- Encourage daily use of fluoride through water, foods, dentifrices, and rinses.
- Encourage rinsing with water if toothbrushing and flossing is not available.

EVALUATION OF PROGRESS

The success of the dental caries control guidelines and meal plan depends on learning by the patient. Learning implies a change of behavior and progress toward goals that are clearly understood by the learner.

I. IMMEDIATE EVALUATION

- The patient's verbal and nonverbal expressed interest, comprehension, and demonstration of cooperation in the dietary analysis and counseling session.
- Patient motivation level of caries control plan.

II. THREE-MONTH FOLLOW-UP

- Request patient to keep a 3-, 5- or 7-day food diary for assessment and evaluation.
- Review personal oral care procedures and provide suggestions as needed.
- Scaling as needed; fluoride varnish application.
- Collaborate on ideas for further modifications when indicated. Smaller goals may need to be established for greater compliance.
- Document progress, additional material reviewed, and plan for continued behavior modification.

III. SIX-MONTH FOLLOW-UP

- Perform examination and clinical procedures.
  - Charting of carious lesions and demineralized areas.
  - Disclose and check biofilm score and reteach as needed with new biofilm removal brush, interdental and tongue cleaning devices.
  - Scaling as needed; fluoride varnish application.
- Compare dental caries incidence with previous chartings and completed restorative dentistry.
- Make collaborative dietary recommendations with patient in accord with new assessment.
- Document progress, education provided, and plan.

IV. OVERALL EVALUATION

- Consistent reduction in dental caries rate in the years following the initial counseling shows sustained change in habits.
- Patient's and parents' attitudes toward maintaining adequate oral health habits.
- Attempts to maintain a diet containing minimum cariogenic foods.
- Compliance with keeping regular appointments for professional dental care.

DOCUMENTATION

The following factors are included when documenting patient care that includes diet analysis and patient counseling:

- Rationale for dietary analysis
- The type of dietary intake utilized for dietary assessment
- The results of the dietary analysis

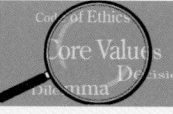

Everyday Ethics

Ms. Carlson presents with Type I diabetes and several significant changes in her oral cavity since her last dental hygiene appointment including angular cheilosis, glossitis, and several proximal carious lesions. The hygienist, Bettina, believes that Ms. Carlson has advanced dietary needs beyond the scope of practice of a dental hygienist and therefore, avoids any chairside dietary assessment with the patient. Routine personal daily oral care instructions are given. On completion of the examination, Bettina mentions her concerns about Ms. Carlson's dietary status to the dentist but does not record any recommendations in the patient's permanent record.

Questions for Consideration
1. What professional protocol for referrals can be followed by the dental hygienist since she believes giving dietary advice to a patient with diabetes is beyond the scope of practice for a dental hygienist?
2. By eliminating the chairside dietary assessment for dental caries prevention did Bettina act nonmaleficently toward the patient? Explain your response.
3. Which ethical principles would be ignored if Bettina does not educate the patient about the preventive measures for her dental caries or document this information in the patient's record?

Patient presented with two new carious lesions since last dental hygiene maintenance visit 1 year ago. Patient has been informed of the need to assess caries risk with an evaluation of dietary habits. A 24-hour recall was performed chair side. Dietary analysis revealed a sweet score of 9 indicating a moderate caries risk. Evaluation of diet for nutritional adequacy revealed an inadequate representation of fruits and vegetables and overconsumption of fat intake. As a result of the 24-hour recall, the patient requested a more extensive evaluation. A 7-day food diary was given to the patent with instructions on proper recording of food quantity and preparation. A follow-up appointment was made in 2 weeks.

Signed: _____, RDH Date: _____.

Factors To Teach The Patient

Medications With Sucrose
- The need to avoid liquid or chewable forms containing sucrose.
- Reasons to avoid frequent daily use of medications with sucrose.
- Reasons for rinsing with water after a medication contained in a syrupy sucrose mixture.

Medications With Side Effect of Xerostomia
- Drugs the patient is using that cause xerostomia (dry mouth).
- How xerostomia increases the risk of dental caries development.
- Why it is necessary to use saliva substitutes, chew gum containing xylitol, and avoid slowly dissolving in the mouth candies containing sucrose.
- Effect of xerostomia on chewing and swallowing and how it compromises nutrient intake.

Facts About Dental Caries
- How dental caries on the tooth surface starts and progresses.
- How the interaction of cariogenic foods, tooth surface, saliva, and microorganisms act together contributing as factors in the dental caries process **(Figure 34-4)**.
- How repeated, frequent acid production and the pH in the dental biofilm adversely affect the teeth.
- Why there is a need to avoid frequent episodes of eating or drinking food or beverages that contain sucrose **(Figure 34-8)**.

- The results of the sugar score and the level of caries risk
- Instructions given on completing the food diary
- **Box 34-5** contains an example progress note for a patient receiving dietary analysis and counseling.

References

1. Dietary reference intakes: Application in dietary planning. Washintong, DC: The National Academies Press; 2003. Available from: http://www.nap.edu/openbook.php?record_id=10609&page=156
2. National Research Council, Committee on Dietary Allowances, Food and Nutrition Board. Recommended dietary allowances, 10th ed. Washington DC: National Academy of Sciences, Office of Publications; 1989.
3. Institute of Medicine. Dietary reference intakes: the essential reference to nutrient requirements. Washington DC: National Academies Press; 2006.
4. Institute of Medicine. DRIs for thiamin, riboflavin, niacin, vitamin B6, folate, pantothenic acid, biotin, and choline. Washington DC: National Academies Press; 1999.
5. Neiva RF, Steigenga J, Al-Shammari KF, Wang HL. Effects of specific nutrients on periodontal disease onset, progression and treatment. *J Clin Periodontol.* 2003 Jul;30(7):579–89.
6. Nishida M, Grossi SG, Dunford RG, Ho AW, Trevisan M, Genco RJ. Calcium and the risk for periodontal disease. *J Periodontol.* 2000 Jul;71(7):1057–66.
7. Nishida M, Grossi SG, Dunford RG, Ho AW, Trevisan M, Genco RJ. Dietary vitamin C and the risk for periodontal disease. *J Periodontol.* 2000 Aug;71(8):1215–23.
8. Genco RJ, Grossi SG, Ho A, Nishimura F, Murayama Y. A proposed model linking inflammation to obesity, diabetes, and periodontal infections. *J Periodontol.* 2005 Nov;76(11 Suppl):2075–84.
9. Al-Zahrani MS, Bissada NF, Borawskit EA. Obesity and periodontal disease in young, middle-aged, and older adults. *J Periodontol.* 2003 May;74(5):610–15.
10. Featherstone JD. The science and practice of caries prevention. *J Am Dent Assoc.* 2000 Jul;131(7):887–99.
11. Boyd LD, Dwyer JT. Guidelines for nutrition screening, assessment, and intervention in the dental office. *J Dent Hyg.* 1998 Fall; 72(4):31–43.
12. Rosal MC, Ebbeling CB, Lofgren I, Ockene JK, Ockene IS, Hebert JR. Facilitating dietary change: the patient-centered counseling model. *J Am Diet Assoc.* 2001 March;101(3):332–41.
13. Kashket S, Van Houte J, Lopez LR, Stocks S. Lack of correlation between food retention on the human dentition and consumer perception of food stickiness. *J Dent Res.* 1991 Oct;70(10):1314–19.
14. Kashket S, Zhang J, Van Houte J. Accumulation of fermentable sugars and metabolic acids in food particles that become entrapped on the dentition. *J Dent Res.* 1996 Nov;75(11):1885–91.
15. Lingström P, Birkhed D, Ruben J, Arends J. Effect of frequent consumption of starchy food items on enamel and dentin demineralization and on plaque pH in situ. *J Dent Res.* 1994 Mar;73(3):652–60.
16. Linke HA, Birkenfeld LH. Clearance and metabolism of starch foods in the oral cavity. *Ann Nutr Metab.* 1999;43(3):131–9.
17. Rugg-Gunn AJ, Edgar WM, Geddes DA, Jenkins GN. The effect of different meal patterns upon plaque pH in human subjects. *Br Dent J.* 1975 Nov 4;139(9):351–6.
18. Linke HA, Riba HK. Oral clearance and acid production of dairy products during interaction with sweet foods. *Ann Nutr Metab.* 2001; 45(5):202–8.
19. Hayes C, The effect of non-cariogenic sweeteners on the prevention of dental caries: a review of the evidence. *J Dent Educ.* 2001 Oct; 65(10):1106–9.
20. Hildebrandt GH, Sparks BS. Maintaining mutans streptococci suppression with xylitol chewing gum. *J Am Dent Assoc.* 2000 Jul; 131(7):909–16.

CHAPTER 35

Fluorides

DURINDA J. MATTANA, RDH, MS

Chapter Outline

The use of fluorides provides the most effective method for dental caries prevention and control.

Fluoride is necessary for optimum oral health at all ages and is made available at the tooth surface by two general means:

- *Systemically,* by way of the circulation to developing teeth (preeruptive exposure).
- *Topically,* directly to the exposed surfaces of erupted teeth (posteruptive exposure).

Topically applied sources of fluoride can be swallowed during tooth development to provide both preeruptive exposure to developing teeth of young children and posteruptive exposure to teeth currently erupted in the oral cavity. The beneficial effects of fluoride are due primarily to its topical effect after the teeth have erupted into the oral cavity.[1] However, epidemiologic evidence shows maximum caries inhibiting effect when there is systemic exposure before tooth eruption and frequent topical fluoride exposure throughout life.[2]

Key words associated with fluoride and fluoride therapy are defined in **Box 35-1**.

FLUORIDE METABOLISM[1,3]

I. FLUORIDE INTAKE

- Fluoride is a systemic nutrient taken into the body by way of water that contains fluoride naturally or has been fluoridated, from prescribed dietary supplements, and, in small amounts, from foods.
- Foods and beverages prepared at home or processed commercially using water containing fluoride are also sources of fluoride.
- Varying amounts are ingested from dentifrices, mouthrinses, supplements, and other fluoride products used by the individual.

II. ABSORPTION

A. Gastrointestinal Tract

- Fluoride is rapidly absorbed by passive diffusion in the stomach as hydrogen fluoride (HF): the rate and amount of absorption depends on the solubility of the fluoride compound and the gastric acidity.
- Most is absorbed within 60 minutes.
- Most of the fluoride that is not absorbed in the stomach will be absorbed by the small intestine.
- There is less absorption when the fluoride is taken with milk and other food.

B. Blood Stream

- Plasma carries the fluoride for its distribution and elimination throughout the body.

- Maximum blood levels are reached within 30 minutes of intake.
- Normal plasma levels are low and rise and fall according to intake.

III. DISTRIBUTION AND RETENTION

- Fluoride is distributed by the plasma to all tissues and organs.
- There is a strong affinity for calcified tissues. Approximately 99% of fluoride in the body is located in the mineralized tissues.
- Concentrations of fluoride are highest at the surfaces next to the tissue fluid supplying the fluoride.
- The fluoride ion (F) is stored as an integral part of the crystal lattice of teeth and bones. The amount stored varies with the intake, the time of exposure, and the age and stage of the development of the individual. The teeth store small amounts, with highest levels on the tooth surface.
- Fluoride that accumulates in bone can be mobilized slowly from the skeleton over time due to the constant resorption or remodeling of bone. In contrast, once tooth enamel is fully matured the fluoride deposited during development can only be altered by cavitated dental caries, erosion, or mechanical abrasion.[1]

IV. EXCRETION

- Most fluoride is excreted through the kidneys in the urine, with a small amount excreted by the sweat glands and in the feces.
- There is limited transfer from plasma to breast milk for excretion by that route.[1]

FLUORIDE AND TOOTH DEVELOPMENT

Fluoride is a nutrient essential to the formation of sound teeth and bones, as are calcium, phosphorus, and other elements obtained from food and water. A more comprehensive review of the histology of tooth development and mineralization can be a helpful supplement to the information included here.[4,5]

I. PREERUPTIVE: MINERALIZATION STAGE

- Fluoride is deposited during the formation of the enamel, starting at the dentinoenamel junction, after the enamel matrix has been laid down by the ameloblasts. **Figure 35-1A** shows the distribution of fluoride in parts of the tooth during mineralization.
- Fluoride is incorporated directly into the hydroxyapatite crystalline structure during mineralization of all of the parts of the teeth to become fluorapatite which

BOX 35-1	Key Words

Fluorides

Abrasive system: substances with cleaning and polishing properties utilized in the formulation of a dentifrice; to be compatible with fluoride compounds and other ingredients and not alter the tooth structure unfavorably.

Acidogenic: producing acid or acidity.

Apatite: a group of minerals of the general formula Ca_{10} $(PO_4)_{6\times 2}$ wherein the X might include hydroxyl (OH), carbonate (CO), fluoride (F), or oxygen (O); crystalline mineral component of hard tissues (bones and teeth).

Hydroxyapatite: $Ca_{10}(PO_4)_6(OH)_2$; the form of apatite that is the principal mineral component of teeth, bones, and calculus.

Fluorapatite: the form of hydroxyapatite in which fluoride ions have replaced some of the hydroxyl ions; with fluoride, the apatite is less soluble and therefore more resistant to the acids formed from carbohydrate intake.

Fluorhydroxyapatite: apatite formed when low concentrations of fluoride react with tooth mineral; at higher concentrations, calcium fluoride is formed.

Cariogenic challenge: exposure of a tooth surface to an acid attack; acid is from the action of dental biofilm and cariogenic food ingested.

Cariostatic: exerting an inhibitory action on the progress of dental caries.

Defluoridation: lowering the amount of fluoride in fluoridated water to an optimum level for the prevention of dental caries and dental fluorosis.

Demineralization: breakdown of the tooth structure with a loss of mineral content, primarily calcium and phosphorus.

Dilution: the reduction in the absolute measurable benefits of the effectiveness of an intervention.

Efficacy: with reference to a product: an efficacious product produces a statistically and clinically significant benefit under ideal testing conditions in carefully controlled clinical trials.

Fluoride: a salt of hydrofluoric acid; the ionized form of fluorine that occurs in many tissues and is stored primarily in bones and teeth.

Fluorosis: form of enamel hypomineralization due to excessive ingestion of fluoride during the development and mineralization of the teeth; depending on the length of exposure and the ppm of the fluoride, the fluorosed area may appear as a small white spot or as severe brown staining with pitting.

Gel: semisolid or solid phase of a colloidal solution.

Glycolysis: process by which sugar is metabolized by bacteria to produce acid.

Hypocalcification: deficient calcification.

Enamel hypocalcification: defect of enamel maturation caused by hereditary or systemic irregularities.

Halo or diffusion effect: occurs when foods and beverages processed in a fluoridated community are imported and consumed in a nonfluoridated community.

Maturation: stage or process of becoming mature or attaining maximal development; with respect to tooth development, maturation results from the continuous dynamic exchange of ions into the surface of the enamel from pellicle, dental biofilm, and oral fluids.

O.T.C.: over the counter.

Prevented Fraction: the proportion of disease occurrence in a population that is averted due to an intervention.

ppm: parts per million; measure used to designate the amount of fluoride used for optimum level in fluoridated water, dentifrice, and other fluoride-containing preparations (1 ppm is equivalent to 1 mg/L).

Remineralization: restoration of mineral elements in a tooth surface; enhanced by presence of fluoride; remineralized lesions are more resistant to initiation of dental caries than is normal tooth structure.

Rx: prescription

Subsurface lesion: demineralized area below the surface of the enamel created by acid that has passed through micropores between enamel rods; subject to remineralization by action of fluoride.

Thixotropic: type of gel that sets in a gel-like state but becomes fluid under stress; the fluid form permits the solution to flow into interdental areas.

"White spot": term used to describe a small area on the surface of enamel that contrasts in appearance with the rest of the surface and may be visible only when the tooth is dried; two types of white spots can be differentiated: an area of demineralization and an area of fluorosis (also referred to as an "enamel opacity").

produces a less soluble apatite crystal.[2] Preeruptive fluoride also results in the development of shallower occlusal grooves, reducing the risk of fissure caries.[2]

■ Table 49-10, page 766 shows the weeks *in utero* when the hard tissue formation begins for the primary teeth.

■ The first permanent molars begin to mineralize at birth as shown in Table 17-1, page 258.

■ Fluoride is available to the developing teeth by way of the blood plasma to the tissues surrounding the tooth buds.

■ Effect of excess fluoride (fluorosis)[6,7]

■ Dental fluorosis is a form of hypomineralization that results from systemic ingestion of an excess amount of fluoride during tooth development.

■ The effects of fluoride on enamel formation that cause dental fluorosis are cumulative rather than a threshold amount.

■ During mineralization the enamel is highly receptive to free fluoride ions.

■ The normal activity of the ameloblasts may be inhibited, and the defective enamel matrix that can form results in discontinuity of crystal growth.

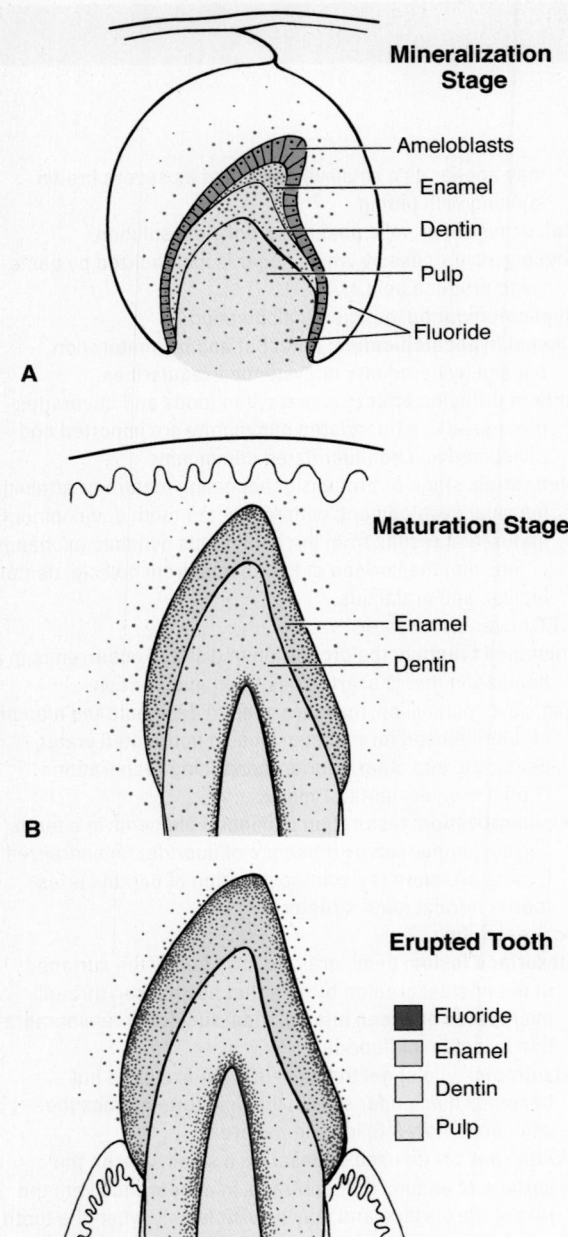

FIGURE 35-1 Systemic Fluoride. Green dots represent fluoride ions in the tissues and distributed throughout the tooth. **(A)** Developing tooth during mineralization shows fluoride from water and other systemic sources deposited in the enamel and dentin. **(B)** Maturation stage before eruption, when fluoride is taken up from tissue fluids around the crown. **(C)** Erupted tooth continues to take up fluoride on the surface from external sources. Note concentrated fluoride deposition on the enamel surface and on the pulpal surface of the dentin.

■ Dental fluorosis can appear clinically in varying degrees from white flecks or striations to cosmetically objectionable stained pitting as outlined in Tables 22-2 and 22-3, pages 331 and 332.

II. PREERUPTIVE: MATURATION STAGE

■ After mineralization is complete and before eruption, fluoride deposition continues in the surface of the enamel. **Figure 35-1B** shows fluoride around the crown during maturation.

■ Fluoride is taken up from the nutrient tissue fluids surrounding the tooth crown.

　■ Much more fluoride is acquired by the outer surface during this period than in the underlying layers of enamel during mineralization.

　■ Children who are exposed to fluoride for the first time within the two years before eruption have the greatest amount of fluoride acquired during this preeruptive stage.

III. POSTERUPTIVE

■ After eruption and throughout the life span of the teeth

　■ The concentration of fluoride on the outermost surface of the enamel is dependent upon topical sources of fluoride from fluoridated drinking water, dentifrices, mouthrinses, and other surface exposures. The fluoride on the outermost surface is available to inhibit demineralization and enhance remineralization as needed on a daily basis. **Figure 35-2** depicts the areas on the tooth that acquire fluoride after eruption.

　■ The continuous presence of fluoride on the tooth surfaces can inhibit the initiation and progression of dental caries.

■ Uptake is most rapid on the enamel surface during the first years after eruption.

　■ Continuing intake of drinking water with fluoride provides a topical source as it washes over the teeth throughout life.

TOOTH SURFACE FLUORIDE

Fluoride concentration is greatest on the surface next to the source of fluoride. For the enamel of the erupted tooth, that is the outer surface exposed to the oral cavity. For the dentin, the highest concentration is at the pulpal surface until after recession of the periodontal attachment when the root surface is exposed to the oral cavity.

I. FLUORIDE IN ENAMEL

A. Uptake

■ Uptake of fluoride depends on the level of fluoride in the oral environment and the length of time of exposure.

■ Hypomineralized enamel absorbs fluoride in greater quantities than sound enamel, becoming incorporated into the hydroxyapatite crystalline structure to become fluorapatite.[6]

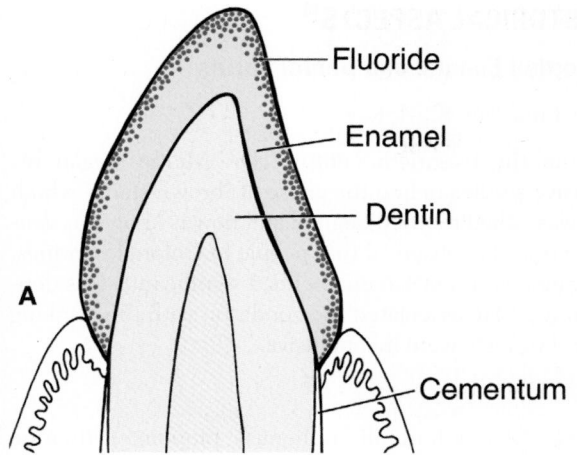

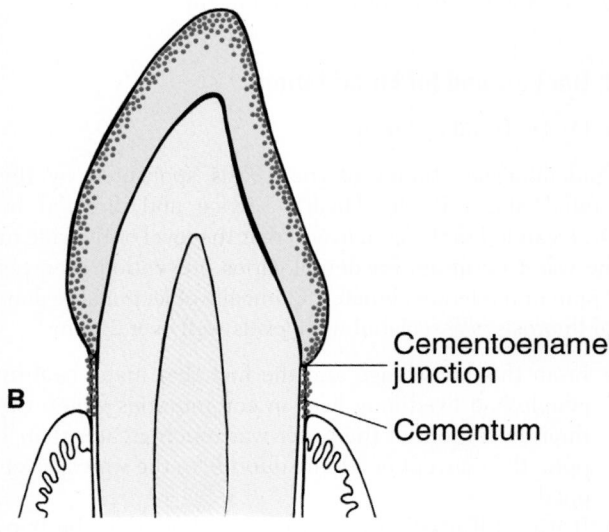

FIGURE 35-2 **Fluoride Acquisition after Eruption. (A)** Fluoride represented by green dots on the enamel surface is taken up from external sources, including dentifrice, rinse, topical application, and fluoridated drinking water passing over the teeth. **(B)** Gingival recession exposes the cementum to external sources of fluoride for the prevention of root caries and the alleviation of sensitivity.

■ Therefore, demineralized enamel that has been remineralized in the presence of fluoride will have a greater concentration of fluoride than sound enamel.

B. Fluoride in the Enamel Surface

■ Fluoride is a natural constituent of enamel.
■ The intact outer surface may have the highest concentration, for example, 1,000–2,000 parts per million, which falls sharply toward the interior of the tooth which may have 20–100 ppm.[8]

II. FLUORIDE IN DENTIN[9]

■ The fluoride level may be greater in exposed dentin than in enamel.

■ A higher concentration is at the pulpal or inner surface, where exchanges take place.
■ Newly formed dentin absorbs fluoride rapidly.

III. FLUORIDE IN CEMENTUM[9]

■ The level of fluoride in cementum is high and increases with age.
■ With recession of the clinical attachment level in periodontal infection, the root surface is exposed to the fluids of the oral cavity. **Figure 35-2B** shows fluoride acquisition to exposed cementum. Fluoride is then available to the cementum from the saliva and all the sources used by the patient, including drinking water, dentifrice, and mouthrinse.

DEMINERALIZATION– REMINERALIZATION[8]

Figure 35-3 illustrates the comparative levels of fluoride that may be found in the tooth surface and the sublevel lesion in early dental caries.

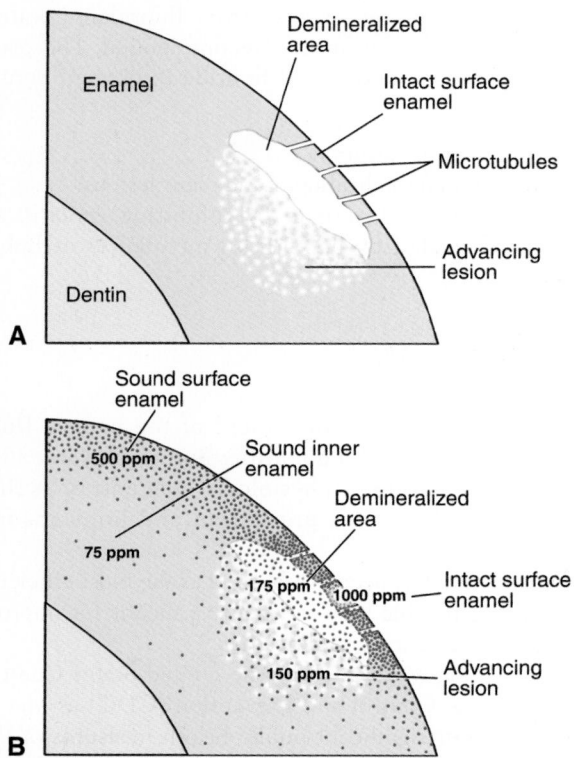

FIGURE 35-3 **Examples of Enamel Fluoride Content. (A)** Early stage of dental caries with an intact surface enamel and subsurface demineralized area. **(B)** A demineralized area readily takes up available fluoride. As shown, the fluoride content (1000 ppm) of the relatively intact surface over a subsurface demineralized white spot is higher than that of the sound surface enamel (500 ppm). The body of the advancing lesion has a higher fluoride content (150 ppm) than does the sound inner enamel (75 ppm). (Source: Melberg JR, Ripa LW, Leske GS. Fluoride in preventive dentistry: theory and clinical applications. Chicago: Quintessence; 1983. p. 31.)

I. FLUORIDE IN BIOFILM AND SALIVA

- Saliva and biofilm are reservoirs for fluoride so it is available for remineralization when needed.
- Fluoride aids to inhibit demineralization when it is present at the crystal surface during an acid challenge.
- Fluoride enhances remineralization by adsorbing to the crystal surface and attracting calcium and phosphate ions.
- At high concentrations, fluoride interferes with the growth and metabolism of bacteria.
- Dental biofilm may contain 5–50 ppm fluoride. The content varies greatly and is constantly changing.
- Brought by the saliva from the same sources, or from an exchange with the fluoride in biofilm, fluoride may be acquired directly from fluoridated water, dentifrice, and other topical sources, and the demineralizing tooth surface under the biofilm.

II. SUMMARY OF FLUORIDE ACTION

Having fluoride available topically to the tooth posteruptively is key to its effectiveness. Frequent exposure to fluoride, such as from fluoridated water, dentifrice, and mouthrinse, is recommended. There are three basic topical effects of fluoride to prevent dental caries.[8]

- Inhibit demineralization.
- Enhance remineralization of incipient lesions.
- Inhibit bacterial activity by inhibiting *enolase*, an enzyme needed by bacteria to metabolize carbohydrates.

FLUORIDATION

- Fluoridation is the adjustment of the natural fluoride ion content of a domestic municipal water supply to the optimum physiologic concentration that will maximize caries prevention and limit enamel fluorosis.[10]
- Fluoridation has been established as the most efficient, effective, reliable, and inexpensive means for improving and maintaining oral health
- Fluoridation was named by the United States Centers for Disease Control and Prevention (CDC) as one of the 10 most significant public health measures of the twentieth century.[10]
- The estimated annual cost per person per year is approximately $0.54–3.44, with lower cost per person for communities of more than 20,000 people.[11]
- In 2008, 64.3% of the total U.S. population received fluoridated water whereas 72.4% of the population served by public (municipal) water systems received fluoridated water. These percentages vary greatly from state to state.[12]

I. HISTORICAL ASPECTS[13]

A. Mottled Enamel and Dental Caries

- Dr. Frederick S. McKay

Early in the twentieth century, Dr. McKay began his extensive studies to find the cause of "brown stain," which later was called mottled enamel and now is known as *dental fluorosis*. He observed that people in Colorado Springs, Colorado, with mottled enamel had significantly less dental caries.[14] He associated the condition with the drinking water, but tests were inconclusive.

- H.V. Churchill

In 1931, H.V. Churchill, a chemist, pinpointed fluorine as the specific element related to the tooth changes that Dr. McKay had been observing clinically.[15]

B. Background for Fluoridation

- Dr. H. Trendley Dean

Epidemiologic studies of the 1930s sponsored by the United States Public Health Service and directed by Dr. Dean led to the conclusion that the level of fluoride in the water optimum for dental caries prevention averages 1 ppm in moderate climates. Clinically objectionable dental fluorosis is associated with levels well over 2 ppm.[16]

- From this knowledge and the fact that many healthy people had lived long lives in communities where the fluoride content of the water was much greater than 1 ppm, the concept of adding fluoride to the water developed.
- It was still necessary, however, to show that the benefits from controlled fluoridation could parallel those of natural fluoride.

C. Fluoridation—1945

- The first communities were fluoridated in 1945.
- Research in the communities began before fluoridation was started to obtain baseline information and it continued over the years with detailed examinations and reports.

D. Control Cities

- Aurora, Illinois, where the natural fluoride level is optimum (1.2 ppm), was used to compare the benefits of natural fluoride in the water supply with those of fluoridation, as well as with a fluoride-free city, Rockford, Illinois.
- Original cities with fluoridation and their control cities in the research are shown in **Box 35-2**.
- The research conducted in these cities, as well as throughout the world, has documented the influence of fluoride on oral health.

BOX 35-2	First Fluoridation Research Cities

Research City	Control City
Grand Rapids, Michigan (January, 1945)	Muskegon, Michigan
Newburgh, New York (May, 1945)	Kingston, New York
Brantford, Ontario (June, 1945)	Sarnia, Ontario
Evanston, Illinois (February, 1947)	Oak Park, Illinois

■ The documented effects and benefits are predominantly due to the topical, posteruptive exposure of the surfaces of the teeth to fluoride of all sources, particularly the fluoride in fluoridated water, throughout life.

II. WATER SUPPLY ADJUSTMENT

A. Fluoride Level

■ Since 1962, the United States Public Health Service has recommended the optimal fluoride concentration of 0.7 ppm (for warmer climates) to 1.2 ppm (for colder climates) to prevent dental caries and minimize fluorosis.[17]

■ The range in fluoride concentration was based on the assumption that people in warmer climates drink more water and therefore receive more fluoride.

■ In 2011, the United States Department of Health and Human Services updated their recommendation for the optimal concentration of water fluoridation to a single number to 0.7 ppm for all communities rather than the range. The decision is based on the fact that Americans have access to many more sources of fluoride today than they did when water fluoridation was introduced in the United States.[18]

■ The change still provides an effective level of fluoride to reduce the incidence of dental caries while minimizing the rate of fluorosis.

B. Chemicals Used

All fluoride chemicals must conform to the appropriate American Water Works Association (AWWA) standards to ensure that the drinking water will be safe.[17]

1. Sources

Compounds from which the fluoride ion is derived are naturally occurring and are mined in various parts of the world. Examples of common sources are fluorspar, cryolite, and apatite.

2. Criteria for acceptance of a fluoride compound for fluoridation include:

■ Solubility to permit its regular use in a water plant.

■ Relatively inexpensive.

■ Readily available to prevent interruptions in maintaining the proper fluoride level.

3. Compounds used:

■ Dry compounds: sodium fluoride and sodium silicofluoride.

■ Liquid solution: hydrofluorosilicic acid.

EFFECTS AND BENEFITS OF FLUORIDATION

Fluoridated water is not only a systemic source of fluoride to developing teeth, but most importantly a topical source of fluoride on the surfaces of erupted teeth throughout life.[19] Even in the presence of multiple sources of topical fluoride available from dentrifices and other consumer products today, fluoridation continues to play a dominant role in the decline in the prevalence and severity of dental caries rates.

I. APPEARANCE OF TEETH

■ Teeth exposed to an optimum or slightly higher level of fluoride appear white, shining, opaque, and without blemishes.

■ When the level is slightly more than optimum, exposed developing teeth may exhibit mild enamel fluorosis seen as white areas in bands or flecks. These areas can be seen by drying the teeth and observing them under a dental light. Without such close scrutiny, such spots may blend with the overall appearance.

■ The majority of fluorosis today is mild and not considered an esthetic problem.[10,20]

■ Dental fluorosis, associated with higher than optimum fluoride levels during tooth development, has been classified according to several epidemiological indexes for assessing severity, including Dean's Fluorosis Index as shown in Table 22-2, page 331 and the Tooth Surface Index of Fluorosis (TSIF) as shown in Table 22-3, page 332.

II. DENTAL CARIES: PERMANENT TEETH

A. Overall Benefits

■ Maximum benefit is seen with continuous use of fluoridated water from birth.

■ It is estimated that the reduction in caries due to water fluoridation alone (factoring out other sources of topical fluoride) among adults of all ages is 27%.[19]

■ The effects are similar to communities with optimum levels of natural fluoride in the water.

■ Many more individuals are completely caries-free when fluoride is in the water.

B. Distribution

■ Anterior teeth, particularly maxillary, receive more protection from fluoride than do posterior teeth[16] because the anterior teeth are contacted by the drinking water as it passes into the mouth.
■ Fluoride is added to the surface of the enamel after eruption.

C. Progression

■ Not only are the numbers of carious lesions reduced, but the caries rate is slowed.
■ Caries progression is also reduced in the surfaces that receive fluoride for the first time after eruption.[21]

III. ROOT CARIES

■ Root caries experience in lifelong residents of a naturally fluoridated community is in direct proportion to the fluoride concentration in the water compared with the experience of residents of a fluoride-free community.[22]
■ The incidence of root caries is approximately 50% less in lifelong residents of a fluoridated community.[23]

IV. DENTAL CARIES: PRIMARY TEETH

■ With fluoridation from birth, the caries incidence is reduced up to 40% in the primary teeth.[10]
■ The introduction of fluoridation into a community significantly increases the proportion of caries-free children and reduces the dmft/DMFT scores when compared to areas that are nonfluoridated over the same time period.[20]
■ For example, children aged 6–9 years in Newburgh, New York, had five times as many caries-free primary teeth present as did the children of Kingston, where fluoride was not present in the community drinking water.[24]

V. TOOTH LOSS

Tooth loss due to dental caries is much greater in both primary and permanent teeth without fluoride[24] because of increased dental caries, which progresses more rapidly.

VI. ADULTS

■ When a person resides in a community with fluoride in the drinking water throughout life, benefits continue.
■ In Colorado Springs, adults aged 20–44 years who had used water with natural fluoride showed 60% less caries experience than did adults in fluoride-deficient Boulder, Colorado. In Boulder, adults also had had three to four times as many permanent teeth extracted.[25]

■ In a survey of adults in Rockford, Illinois (no fluoride), there were about seven times as many edentulous persons as there were in a comparable group in Aurora, Illinois (natural fluoride).[26]

VII. PERIODONTAL DISEASES

■ Indirect favorable effects of fluoride on periodontal health can be shown. Improved bone density resulting from fluoride can affect the alveolar bone, along with all bones, and may provide beneficial resistance against bone resorption.
■ Dental carious lesions favor dental biofilm retention and, therefore, contribute to the development of periodontal diseases, particularly lesions adjacent to the gingival margin and proximal surface lesions, which favor food impaction.
■ The incidence of periodontal diseases increases with age because of the cumulative effects of etiologic factors and the disease processes. With the use of fluorides, particularly fluoridation, fewer teeth are lost because of dental caries at younger ages. Therefore, periodontal disease prevention and control is to be emphasized in communities with fluoride in the drinking water.

PARTIAL DEFLUORIDATION

■ Water with excess fluoride does not meet the requirements of the United States Public Health Service.
■ Several hundred communities in the United States have water supplies that contain more than twice the optimal level of fluoride.
■ Defluoridation can be accomplished by one of several chemical systems.[27] The efficacy of the methods has been shown.
■ The water supply in Britton, South Dakota, has been reduced from almost 7 ppm to 1.5 ppm since 1948, and in Bartlett, Texas, from 8 ppm to 1.8 ppm since 1952. Examinations have shown a dramatic reduction in the incidence of objectionable fluorosis in children born since defluoridation.[27,28]

SCHOOL FLUORIDATION

■ To bring the benefits of fluoridation to children living in rural areas without the possibility for community fluoridation, adding fluoride to a school water supply has been an alternative.
■ Because of the intermittent use of the school water (5 days each week during the 9-month school year), the amount of fluoride added is increased over the usual 1 ppm.
■ Example: After 12 years of fluoride at 5 ppm in the school drinking water of Elk Lake, Pennsylvania, children who had attended that school regularly had 39% fewer decayed, missing, and filled teeth than did those

in the control group. The greatest benefits were found on proximal tooth surfaces.[29]

- Example: In the schools of Seagrove, North Carolina, after 12 years with the fluoride level at 6.3 ppm, the children experienced a 47.5% decrease in decayed, missing, and filled surfaces compared with those in the control group.[29]
- Such systems have significance in the long history of efforts for fluoridation for all people in the United States.
- School fluoridation has been phased out in several states, and the current extent of this practice is unknown. Operations and maintenance of small fluoridation systems are problematic.[10]

DISCONTINUED FLUORIDATION

- When fluoride is removed from a community water supply that had dental caries control by fluoridation, the effects can be clearly shown.
- Example: In Antigo, Wisconsin, the action of anti-fluoridationists in 1960 brought about the discontinuance of fluoridation, which had been installed in 1949. Examinations in the years following 1960 revealed the marked drop in the number of children who were caries-free and the steep increases in caries rates. From 1960 to 1966, the number of caries-free children in the second grade decreased by 67%.[30] Fluoridation was reinstated in 1966 by popular demand.

FLUORIDES IN FOODS

I. FOODS[31]

- Certain foods contain fluoride, but not enough to constitute a significant part of the day's need for caries prevention.
- Meat, eggs, vegetables, cereals, and fruits have very small but measurable amounts, whereas tea and fish have larger amounts.
- Foods cooked in fluoridated water retain fluoride from the cooking water.

II. SALT[32,33,34]

- Fluoridated salt has not been promoted in the United States, but is widely used in Germany, France, and Switzerland where 30–80% of the domestic marketed salt is fluoridated. Another 30 countries or more use fluoridated salt worldwide for its effectiveness as a community health program.
- Fluoridated salt results in a reduced incidence of dental caries, but there is insufficient evidence for its overall effectiveness.

- Fluoridated salts currently available supply about one third to one half of the amount of fluoride ingested daily from 1 ppm fluoridated water.
- Fluoridated salt is recommended by the World Health Organization as one alternative to fluoridated water to target underprivileged groups.

III. HALO/DIFFUSION EFFECT

- Foods and beverages that are commercially processed (cooked or reconstituted) in optimally fluoridated cities can be distributed and consumed in nonfluoridated communities.
- This halo or diffusion effect can result in increased fluoride intake by individuals living in nonfluoridated communities, providing them some protection against dental caries.[31]

IV. BOTTLED WATER

Bottled water usually does not contain optimal fluoride unless it has a label indicating that it is fluoridated. Patients need to be advised to fill their water bottles from a fluoridated water supply.

V. WATER FILTERS[35]

- Reverse osmosis and water distillation systems remove fluoride from the water, but water softeners do not.
- Carbon filters (on the end of the faucet or in pitchers) vary in their removal of fluoride.
- Carbon filters with activated alumina remove fluoride.
- Patients need to be warned that water filters have the ability to remove fluoride from their drinking water and it is best to check with the manufacturer.

VI. INFANT FORMULA[36,37,38]

- Even though there has been an increase in breast-feeding in the United States, infant formula remains a major source of nutrition for many infants.
- Ready-to-feed formulas do not need to be reconstituted, but water is added to powdered and liquid concentrate formulas.
- Breast milk may contain 0.02 ppm fluoride and all types of infant formula themselves contain a low amount of fluoride (0.11–0.57 ppm).[37]
- The level of fluoride in the water supply used to reconstitute powdered or liquid concentrate formulas determines the total fluoride intake.
- The American Dental Association (ADA) recommends continuing to use optimally fluoridated water to reconstitute infant formula while being aware of the possible risk of mild enamel fluorosis in the primary teeth.[38]

DIETARY FLUORIDE SUPPLEMENTS[10,39,40]

- Prescribed dietary supplements were introduced in the late 1940s and are intended to compensate for fluoride-deficient drinking water.
- The current supplementation dosage schedule developed by the ADA and the American Academy of Pediatric Dentistry, revised in 1994, includes children aged 6 months through 16 years that consume drinking water that contains <0.6 ppm of fluoride. **Table 35-1** contains the daily dosage amounts based on the age of the child and the amount of fluoride that is in the primary water supply.
- Clinical recommendations from the American Dental Association Council on Scientific Affairs include the use of fluoride supplements for children: 1) at a high risk of developing dental caries and 2) those whose primary source of drinking water is deficient in fluoride.[41]

I. ASSESS POSSIBLE NEED

- Review the history to be certain the child is not receiving other fluoride in such preparations as vitamin-fluoride supplements.
- Determine that the fluoride level of all sources of drinking water is below 0.6 ppm.
- Refer to the list of fluoridated communities available from state or local health departments.
- Request water analysis when the fluoride level has not been determined.
- Determine the child's risk for dental caries as high before considering the use of fluoride supplements.[39]
- Reassess the caries risk at frequent intervals as the status may be affected by the child's development, personal and family situations, and behavioral factors such as oral hygiene practices.[33,41]

II. AVAILABLE FORMS OF SUPPLEMENTS

- Sodium fluoride supplements are available as tablets, lozenges, and oral drops.

- Prescribed on an individual patient basis for daily use at home.

A. Tablets and Lozenges

- Tablets are chewed before swallowing, lozenges are dissolved for one or two minutes in the mouth to provide both preeruptive and posteruptive benefits.[41]
- Tablets, lozenges, and drops are available in 0.25 mg, 0.50 mg, and 1.0 mg dosages.
- Chewable tablets, and lozenges, are best taken at bedtime, after the teeth have been brushed. Instruct parent and patient not to eat, drink, or rinse for at least 15 minutes after chewing a tablet or dissolving a lozenge for a topical effect.
- Maximum topical effect occurs on newly erupted teeth.

B. Drops

- A liquid concentrate with directions that specify the number of drops for the prescription dose.
- Oral solutions may be dropped directly in the mouth or mixed with cereal, fruit juice, or other food. If mixed with foods or beverages containing calcium, the amount of sodium fluoride absorbed may be reduced.
- Primary use: for the child from 6 months to 3 years and those unable to use other forms that require chewing and/or swallowing.

III. PRESCRIPTION

- *Prescription guidelines*
  - No more than 264 mg NaF (120 mg of fluoride ion) are to be dispensed per household at one time.
  - Take supplements with juice or water. Taking fluoride supplements with dairy products is not recommended because the fluoride can combine with the calcium and be poorly absorbed.

TABLE 35-1	FLUORIDE SUPPLEMENTS DOSE SCHEDULE (mg NaF/day)*		
	WATER FLUORIDE ION CONCENTRATION (ppm)		
AGE OF CHILD	**LESS THAN 0.3**	**BETWEEN 0.3 AND 0.6**	**GREATER THAN 0.6**
Birth–6 months	0	0	0
6 months – 3 years	0.25 mg	0	0
3–6 years	0.50 mg	0.25 mg	0
6–16 years	1.0 mg	0.50 mg	0

*2.2 mg of sodium fluoride provides 1 mg of fluoride ion.
Source: American Dental Association and the American Academy of Pediatrics.

- *Storage:* Keep tablets out of the reach of children, in the original container, away from heat and direct light, and away from damp places such as the bathroom or kitchen sink.
- *Missed dose:* Take as soon as remembered, however if it is almost time for the next dose, skip the missed dose and go back to the regular dosing schedule.

IV. BENEFITS AND LIMITATIONS

- Administration of prenatal dietary fluoride supplements is not recommended despite evidence that fluoride crosses the placenta during the fifth and sixth months of pregnancy and enters the prenatal deciduous enamel.[42] Use of fluoride supplements by pregnant women has not been shown to benefit their offspring and furthermore, cannot effect the permanent teeth because they do not develop *in utero*.
- Overall, there is weak evidence to support the use of fluoride supplements to prevent dental caries in primary teeth.
- Daily fluoride supplements can offer caries preventive benefits in permanent teeth. School aged children who chewed and swallowed 1 mg fluoride tablets daily on school days had significantly lower caries than children who did not use fluoride supplements.
- Consider the child's age, caries risk, and all sources of fluoride exposure before recommending the use of fluoride supplements.[33,41]

PROFESSIONAL TOPICAL FLUORIDE APPLICATIONS

Topical fluorides are an essential part of a total preventive program for patients of all ages.

- Fluoridated water and fluoride toothpaste are the primary sources of topical fluoride for patients of all ages and levels of caries risk.
- Additional topical fluoride sources can be professionally applied and self-applied by the patient, primarily for those at moderate or high caries risk.
- For children age 6 years or younger, fluoride varnish is the only topical application recommended.
- Professionally applied fluorides may be gels or foams delivered in trays (not to be used for children under age 6 years) or varnish that is applied with a very soft brush on the teeth.

I. INDICATIONS[43]

The professional application of a high-concentration fluoride preventive agent is:

- Based on caries risk assessment for the individual patient.
- *Low caries risk:* use professional judgment; application may not provide additional benefit.

BOX 35-3 | **Indications for Professional Topical Fluoride Application: Individual Risk Factors for Developing Dental Caries[43]**

- Primary teeth (varnish only)
  Suboptimal fluoride exposure
  Low socio-economic status
- Posteruptive period
  Rapid uptake of fluoride for newly exposed enamel
- Active caries (new carious lesions at regular maintenance)
- Secondary/recurrent caries adjacent to previous restorations
- Wearing orthodontic appliances: bands, bonded brackets
- Compromised salivary flow
  Radiation therapy to head and neck
  Sjögren's syndrome or another condition that limits salivary secretion by the glands
  Medication with side effect of xerostomia
- High titers of cariogenic bacteria
- Chemo/radiation therapy
- Eating disorders
- Drug/alcohol abuse
- Cariogenic diet
- Exposed root surfaces
- Irregular Dental Care
- Poor oral hygiene
- Natural teeth supporting an overdenture
- Exposed root surfaces following periodontal recession
- Lack of compliance and conscientious efforts for daily dental biofilm removal
- Low or no fluoride in drinking water
- Early carious lesions
  Pit and fissure: restore caries; sealant for all others
  Proximal surfaces: need fluoride application

Source: American Dental Association Council on Scientific Affairs. Professionally applied topical fluoride: evidence-based clinical recommendations. *J Am Dent Assoc.* 2006 Aug;137(8):1151–9.

- *Moderate caries risk* (presence of at least one risk factor): application at 6-month intervals or more frequent.
- *High caries risk* (multiple risk factors, xerostomia, or suboptimal fluoride exposure): application at 6-month or 3-month intervals.
- Factors contributing to moderate or high caries risk are listed in **Box 35-3**.

II. HISTORICAL PERSPECTIVE

- Professionally applied fluoride has been instrumental in the reduction of dental caries in the United States and other industrialized countries since the early 1940s.
- Dr. Basil G. Bibby conducted the initial topical sodium fluoride study using Brockton, Massachusetts, schoolchildren.[44]

- More than one-third fewer new carious lesions resulted from a 0.1% aqueous solution applied at 4-month intervals for 2 years.
- The research led to extensive studies by Dr. John W. Knutson and others sponsored by the United States Public Health Service. The aim was to determine the most effective concentration of sodium fluoride, the minimum time required for application, and procedural details.[45,46] Their results still provide the basis for the applications currently used and described in the following sections.

III. COMPOUNDS

Table 35-2 provides a summary of the generally available professional fluoride applications that include the following:

- 2.0% sodium fluoride as gel or foam delivered in trays.
- 1.23% acidulated phosphate fluoride as a gel or foam delivered in trays.
- 5% sodium fluoride as a varnish brushed on the teeth.

A. 2.0% Sodium Fluoride (NaF) Gel

- Sodium fluoride, also called neutral sodium fluoride due to its neutral pH of 7.0, contains 9,050 ppm fluoride ion.
- Clinical trials demonstrating the efficacy of neutral NaF are based on a series of four or five applications on a weekly basis.[47]
- Quarterly or semiannual applications are most common in clinical practice.

B. 2.0% Sodium Fluoride (NaF) Foam

- There is limited clinical evidence to demonstrate foam's effectiveness in caries prevention.

C. 1.23% Acidulated Phosphate Fluoride (APF) Gel

- Contains 12,300 ppm fluoride ion.
- A 4-minute tray application is recommended four times per year for individuals at a high risk for dental caries.[48]

- Widely used because of its storage stability, acceptable taste, and tissue compatibility.
- Low pH of 3.5 enhances fluoride uptake, which is greatest during the first four minutes.[48]
- APF may etch porcelain and composite restorative materials so it is not indicated for patients with porcelain, composite restorations, and sealants.
- The hydrofluoride component of APF dissolves the filler particles of the composite resin restorations.
- Macroinorganic filler particles of composite materials demonstrate noticeable etched patterns generated by APF, whereas more recent micro-filled materials are not sensitive to the APF agent.[49]
- The prevented fraction of dental caries ranged from 18–41% with the use of APF or NaF gels.[50]

D. 1.23% Acidulated Phosphate Fluoride (APF) Foam

- There is limited clinical evidence to for the effectiveness of foam in caries prevention.

E. 5% Neutral Sodium (NaF) Varnish

- Fluoride varnishes were developed during the late 1960s and early 1970s to prolong contact time of the fluoride with the tooth surface.[51]
- Varnishes are safe and effective, fast and easy to apply, and patient acceptance is good.
- The prevented fraction of dental caries ranged from 34–57% with the use of fluoride varnish.[50]
- Varnishes have been widely used in Western Europe, Scandinavia, and Canada since the 1980s.[51]
- Varnish received approval from the United States Food and Drug Administration (FDA) in 1994 for use as a cavity liner and for treatment of hypersensitive teeth. Its use in the United States as a caries preventive agent is considered off-label, but has become a standard of care in practice.[52]
- Varnish has a higher concentration of fluoride than gel or foam (22,600 ppm fluoride ion), but an overall less amount of fluoride is used per application (<7 mg

TABLE 35-2	PROFESSIONALLY APPLIED TOPICAL FLUORIDES			
AGENT	**FORM**	**CONCENTRATION**	**APPLICATION MODE**	**NOTES**
Sodium Fluoride (NaF) Neutral or 7 pH	2% Gel or *Foam	9,050 ppm 0.90% F ion	Tray (4 minutes)	Do not overfill: see **Figure 35-5**
Acidulated phosphate 3.5 pH	1.23% Gel or *Foam	12,300 ppm 1.23% F ion	Tray (4 minutes)	Do not overfill: see **Figure 35-5**
Sodium fluoride (NaF) Neutral or 7 pH	5% Varnish	22,600 ppm 2.6% F ion	Apply thin layer with brush (1–2 minutes)	Sets up to a hard film

*There is limited published clinical evidence supporting the effectiveness of foam.[30]

varnish versus 30 mg of gel for a child) because it is applied with a very soft brush in a thin layer.

■ Varnish sets quickly and remains on the teeth for a number of hours releasing fluoride into the pits and fissures, proximal surfaces, and cervical areas of the tooth where it is needed the most.[52]

■ Clinical studies regarding caries reduction are based on applications every 3–6 months.

■ Varnish is effective in reversing active pit and fissure enamel lesions in the primary dentition[53] and remineralizing enamel lesions regardless of whether the varnish is applied over or around the lesion.[54]

■ Varnish is also effective in reducing demineralization white areas around orthodontic brackets.[55]

■ Varnish is the fluoride application of choice for those with dentin hypersensitivity and the only professional topical fluoride to be used for children under the age of 6 years.

CLINICAL PROCEDURES: PROFESSIONAL TOPICAL FLUORIDE

I. OBJECTIVES

A. Prevention of Dental Caries

■ Identify special problems, including areas adjacent to restorations, orthodontic appliances, xerostomia, and other risk factors. **Box 35-3** contains indications for the application of a professional fluoride.

■ Examples: Active or secondary caries, exposed root surfaces, current orthodontic treatment, low or no fluoride exposure, or compromised salivary flow.

B. Remineralization of Demineralized Areas

■ Demineralized white areas on the cervical third, especially under dental biofilm.

C. Desensitization

■ Fluoride aids in blocking dentinal tubules, as explained in Chapter 43, page 683.

■ Varnish covers and protects a sensitive area, and fluoride is slowly released for uptake.

II. PREPARATION OF THE TEETH FOR TOPICAL APPLICATION

■ *General preparation for tray and varnish applications*

■ Instruct patients about all methods of caries prevention and how they work together.

■ Most patients will receive the professional topical application following their routine maintenance appointment with complete dental hygiene procedures of personal oral hygiene care instruction, scaling, and stain removal.

■ When the fluoride application is to be applied at a time other than following scaling and debridement, rubber cup polishing is not routinely necessary because fluoride will penetrate biofilm and provide the same benefits with or without prior polishing.[56]

■ Calculus and stain removal are to be completed.

■ After calculus removal apply principles of selective polishing for stain removal. Select an appropriate cleaning or polishing agent that will not harm the tooth surface or the restorative material present (Chapter 44, page 694).

■ A fluoride-containing polishing paste is not effective as a fluoride application.[57]

■ Preparation and procedure for gel or foam tray application is included in **Table 35-3**; preparation and procedure for varnish application is found in **Table 35-4**.

III. PATIENT AND/OR PARENT COUNSELING

■ Help patients understand the purposes and benefits as well as the limitations of topical applications.

■ Fluoride is one part of the total prevention program that includes daily biofilm control and limitation of cariogenic foods.

IV. APPOINTMENT SEQUENCE

A. *Tray application*
 1. Schedule the appointment to end at least 30 minutes before the patient's eating time.
 2. Prepare the patient for any discomfort, for example, the 4-minute timing when tray application is to be used.
 3. Explain the need not to swallow but to expectorate immediately after the tray is removed.

B. *Varnish application*
 1. Schedule the appointment when the patient can refrain from consuming hard foods and hot liquids and
 2. Avoid toothbrushing and flossing for 4–6 hours after the application or until the next morning.
 3. Remove the next morning.

V. TRAY TECHNIQUE: GEL OR FOAM

■ **Figure 35-4** shows tray selection for coverage of all exposed root surfaces.

■ Design of trays: maxillary and mandibular trays may be hinged together or separated, are of a natural rounded arch shape to hold the gel or foam and prevent ingestion, and are available in various sizes and brands.

■ **Figure 35-5** shows the amount of gel to be placed in each tray.

■ Most gels are thixotropic to offer better physical and handling characteristics for use in trays.

■ Procedures for a professional gel or foam tray fluoride application are listed in **Table 35-3**.

TABLE 35-3	PROCEDURE FOR TOPICAL GEL OR FOAM PROFESSIONAL TRAY
Patient	■ Determine need based on caries risk assessment (not to be used for children under age 6 years) ■ Choose the type of fluoride (APF or NaF and Gel or Foam); Data support use of Gel ■ Seat upright ■ Explain procedure including length: 4 min ■ Instruct not to swallow ■ Tilt head forward slightly
Tray Coverage	■ Choose appropriate size for full coverage ■ Complete dentition must be covered, including anterior and posterior vertical coverage, distal dam depth, and close fit to teeth ■ Check for coverage of areas of recession (if unable to cover exposed root surfaces use varnish application) ■ Proper and improper tray coverage is shown in **Figure 35-4**
Place Gel or Foam	■ Use minimum amount of gel or foam in the trays, as shown in **Figure 35-5** ■ Fill tray 1/3 full with gel; completely fill, but do not over-fill with foam
Dry the Teeth	■ Place a saliva ejector in the mouth during the drying procedure ■ Dry the teeth before insertion of trays starting with the maxillary teeth; facial, occlusal, and palatal surfaces and then the mandibular teeth; lingual, occlusal, and facial surfaces
Insert Trays	■ Place both filled trays in mouth ■ A two-step procedure (one tray at a time) may be required; if so, patient may not rinse but must expectorate after the removal of each tray to prevent swallowing.
Isolation	■ Use a saliva ejector with maximum efficiency suction
Attention	■ Do not leave patient unattended
Timing	■ Use a timer; do not estimate (4 min) ■ Procedure will take 8 minutes when a two-step procedure is used
Completion	■ Tilt head forward for removal of tray ■ Request patient to expectorate for several minutes; do not allow swallowing ■ Wipe excess gel or foam from teeth with gauze sponge ■ Use high-power suction to draw out saliva and gel ■ Instruct patient that nothing is to be placed in the mouth for 30 min; do not rinse, eat, drink, or brush teeth

Source: American Academy of Pediatric Dentistry. *Oral health policies for children: protocol for fluoride therapy.* Chicago: AAPD; 1967, rev. 2008.

VI. VARNISH TECHNIQUE[52]

■ Dispense varnish: If dispensed from a tube (rather than a single-dose packet), discard any clear varnish because the ingredients have separated and will contain only a fraction of the intended amount of fluoride.[58]

■ Unit-dosed 5% NaF varnish is available in premeasured wells or individual packets of different dosages with an applicator brush to mix the varnish and then apply.

■ Unit dosages are generally 0.25 ml, 0.4 ml, or 0.5 ml for the primary, mixed and permanent dentitions, respectively.

■ Procedures for a professional varnish fluoride application are listed in **Table 35-4**.

VII. AFTER APPLICATION

■ *Tray application*
  ■ Instruct patients not to rinse, eat, drink, brush, or floss for at least 30 minutes after gel or foam applications.

  ■ Rinsing immediately after a tray application has been shown to significantly lessen the benefits.[59]

■ *Varnish application*
  ■ Instruct patients to avoid hot drinks and alcoholic beverages, eating hard foods, and brushing or flossing the teeth for 4–6 hours or if possible until the next day to allow fluoride uptake to continue undisturbed.
  ■ Inform the patient that the treated teeth will feel as if they have a coating or film, but the product dries clear and is not visible.
  ■ Varnish is removed by the patient via toothbrushing and flossing the next day.

SELF-APPLIED FLUORIDES

■ Self-applied fluorides (prescription and over-the-counter products) are available as dentifrices, mouthrinses, and gels.
■ Concentrations of 1500 ppm fluoride or less can be sold over the counter.[39] Some products containing less than 1500 ppm of fluoride are available only by prescription.

(continued on page 532)

TABLE 35-4	PROCEDURE FOR VARNISH APPLICATION (5% NaF)
Patient	■ Determine need based on caries risk assessment (only professional fluoride for children under age 6 years) ■ Explain procedure ■ Seat supine ■ For the infant and toddler the parent and clinician can sit knee to knee with the child held across the knees (Figure 49-5, page 767) ■ Instruct not to swallow during the procedure
Prepare Product	■ Dispense from a tube or open a single-dose packet ■ Have applicator brush available
Dry Teeth	■ Varnish sets up in the presence of saliva, but it is recommended to remove excess saliva by wiping the teeth with a gauze square
Apply Varnish	■ Dip applicator brush in varnish and mix well ■ Systematically brush a thin layer over all tooth surfaces ■ For prevention of early childhood caries in the infant, toddler, or very young child, apply to the maxillary anterior teeth first and then proceed to other areas of the dentition if patient is cooperative ■ For all other patients, use a systematic approach. Begin with mandibular teeth; facial, occlusal, and lingual surfaces and then the maxillary teeth; palatal, occlusal, and facial surfaces ■ Provide full coverage to all areas of the teeth including areas of recession and the cervical third of facial, lingual, and palatal surfaces and occlusal surfaces ■ Application time is approximately 1 to 3 minutes
Completion	■ Instruct patient that the teeth will feel like they have a coating or film, but this is not visible ■ Ask the patient to avoid hard foods, drinking hot or alcoholic beverages, brushing, and flossing the teeth until the next day or at least 4–6 hours after application ■ It is advisable to drink through a straw for the first few hours after application ■ Patient is to remove the varnish the next day with toothbrushing and flossing

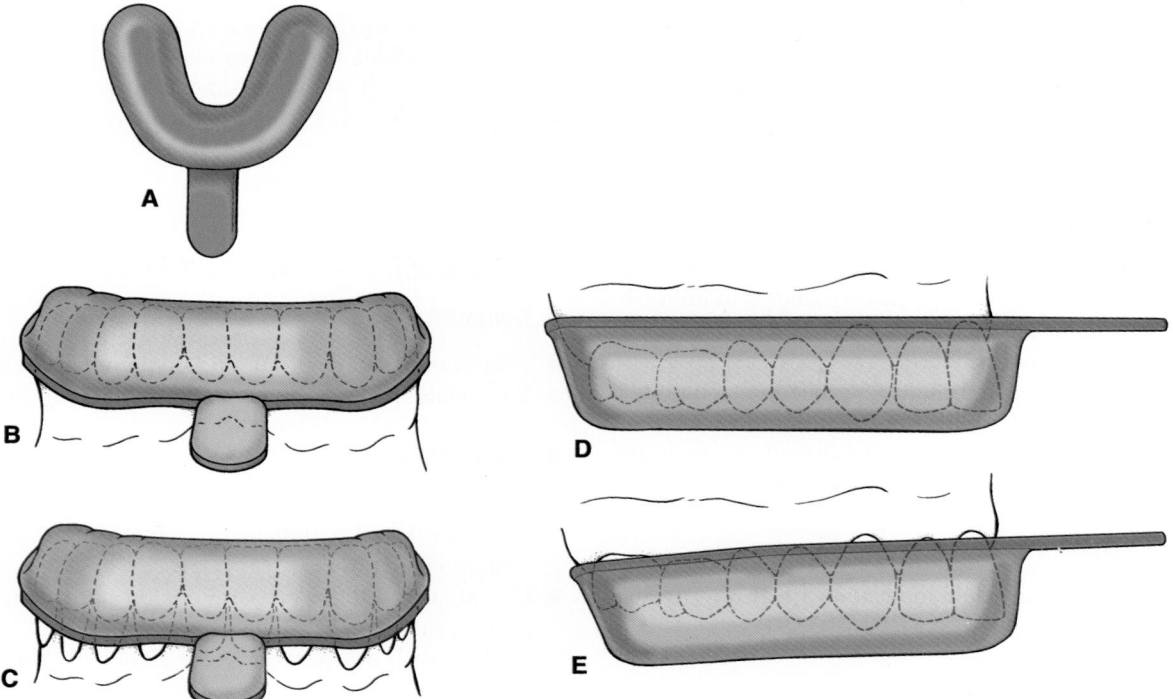

FIGURE 35-4 **Tray Selection. (A)** Mandibular tray held for try-in. **(B)** Tray over teeth is deep enough to cover the entire exposed enamel above the gingiva. **(C)** In the patient with recession and areas of root surfaces exposed, the same tray is not deep enough to cover the root surfaces where fluoride is needed for prevention of root caries or hypersensitivity. A custom-made tray is needed. **(D)** Tray adequately covers the distal surface of the most posterior tooth. **(E)** The tray does not cover the distal surface of the most posterior tooth or the cervical third of canine and central incisor adequately. The tray may need to be repositioned to cover the distal surface, or a larger stock or custom tray is needed.

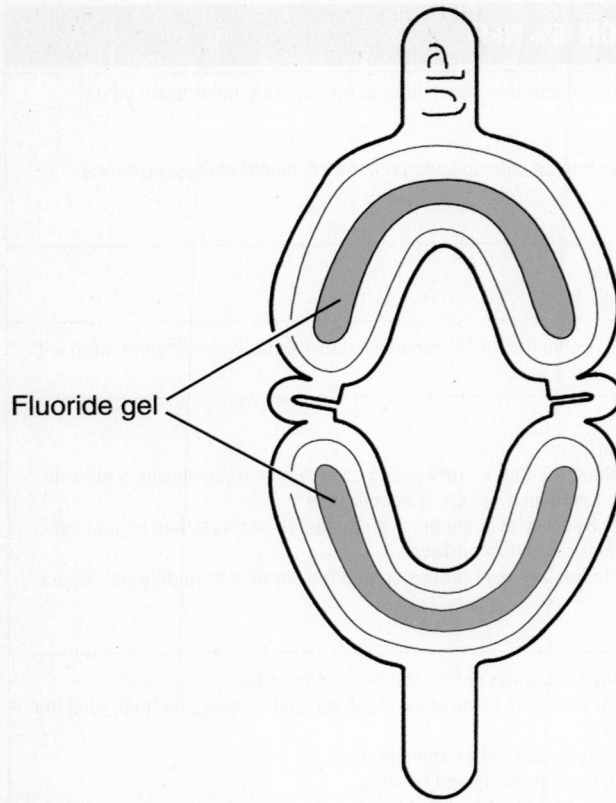

Fluoride gel

FIGURE 35-5 Measured Gel in Tray. No more than 2 ml of gel is placed in each tray for children, and no more than 5 ml is placed in each tray for adults. This amount fills each tray size 1/3 full.

■ May be applied by toothbrushing, rinsing, or trays that are custom made or disposable.

I. INDICATIONS

■ Patient needs are determined as part of total care planning.
■ Indications for use of tray, rinsing, and/or toothbrushing depend on the individual patient prevention needs and caries risk assessment.
■ Certain patients need multiple procedures combined with professional applications at the regular maintenance appointments. Special indications are suggested as each method is described in the following sections.

II. METHODS

The three methods for self-application are by tray, rinsing, and toothbrushing.

A. Tray

■ Custom-made or disposable tray. The tray is selected to fit the individual mouth and completely cover the teeth being treated.
■ **Figure 35-4** shows adequate and inadequate tray coverage on the teeth.
■ Instruction is provided not to overfill the tray.

B. Rinsing

■ The patient swishes for 1 minute with a measured amount of a fluoride rinse and expectorates.
■ Certain patients will need to learn how to rinse properly to force the solution between the teeth. Box 29-4, page 431, lists steps for teaching how to rinse.

C. Toothbrushing

■ A fluoride-containing dentifrice is used for regular brushing after breakfast and before going to bed and not eating again.
■ Brush-on gel is used after regular brushing to provide additional benefits.
■ Use an interdental brush to apply fluoride to proximal surfaces or open furcations.

TRAY TECHNIQUE: HOME APPLICATION

The original gel tray studies using custom-fitted polyvinyl mouthpieces compared the use of 1.1% acidulated NaF with plain NaF gel.

The gel was applied daily over a 2-year period by schoolchildren aged 11–14 years during the school years. Dental caries incidence was reduced up to 80%.[60]

I. INDICATIONS FOR USE

■ Rampant enamel or root caries in persons of any age to prevent additional new carious lesions and promote remineralization around existing lesions.
■ Xerostomia from any cause, particularly loss of salivary gland function.
■ Exposure to radiation therapy.
■ Root surface hypersensitivity.

II. GELS USED (AVAILABLE BY PRESCRIPTION)

A. Concentrations[39]

■ 1.1% neutral sodium (NaF); 5,000 ppm fluoride.
■ 1.1% acidulated phosphate (APF); 5,000 ppm fluoride.

B. Precautions[39]

■ Dispense small quantities. Maximum adult dose is 16 drops per day (4–8 drops on the inner surface of each custom-made tray).
■ Use neutral sodium preparations on porcelain, composites, titanium, or sealants.
■ Patients with mucositis may experience irritation with the APF.

C. Patient Instructions

■ Use the gel tray once each day, preferably just before going to bed.
■ **Box 35-4** outlines the procedures for the patient to follow for a home tray application.

BOX 35-4	Instructions for Home Tray Application

1. One daily application: recommended after tooth-brushing just before bedtime; do not eat or drink again. If applied at other time of day, do not eat or drink for at least 30 minutes.
2. Brush and floss before applying tray to remove biofilm and food debris.
3. Use prepared custom-made polyvinyl trays. Disposable trays can be used if the appropriate fit can be obtained.
4. Distribute no more than 4–8 drops—or a thin ribbon—of the gel on the inner surface of each tray. Each drop is equivalent to 0.1 mL.
5. Expectorate to dry out the mouth.
6. Apply one tray at a time. Hold head upright.
7. Apply the mandibular tray first; close gently to hold the tray in place.
8. Time by a clock for 4 minutes. Do not swallow.
9. Expectorate several times when the tray is removed to prevent swallowing gel, and prepare the mouth for the other tray.
10. Apply the maxillary tray and follow steps 7, 8 and 9 as for the other tray.
11. After tray removal, do not eat, drink or brush teeth for at least 30 minutes.
12. After both trays are removed, rinse the trays under running water and brush them clean.
13. Keep in open air for drying.

■ A copy of the instructions needs to be given to the patient.

FLUORIDE MOUTHRINSES

■ Mouthrinsing is a practical and effective means for self-application of fluoride for individuals at moderate or high caries risk. Do not use for patients age 6 or younger, or for patients unable to rinse for a physical or other reason.[61]

■ Rinsing can be part of an individual care plan or can be included in a group program conducted during school attendance.

I. INDICATIONS

Mouthrinsing with a fluoride preparation may be an additional benefit for the following:

■ General prevention of dental caries in:
  ■ Young persons during the high-risk preteen and adolescent years.
  ■ Patients with areas of demineralization.
  ■ Patients with root exposure following recession and periodontal therapy.
  ■ Participants in a school health group program for all grades except grade 1.

■ Patients with moderate to rampant caries risk who live in a fluoridated or nonfluoridated community.
■ Patients whose oral health care is complicated by biofilm-retentive appliances, including orthodontics, partial dentures, or space maintainers.
■ Patients with xerostomia from any cause, including head and neck radiation and saliva-depressing drug therapy.
■ Patients with hypersensitivity of exposed root surfaces.

II. LIMITATIONS

■ Children under 6 years of age and those of any age who cannot rinse because of oral and/or facial musculature problems or other disability are excluded from the practice of this method.
■ Alcohol content
  ■ Use of alcohol-based mouthrinses is not recommended; aqueous solutions are available.
  ■ Alcohol content of commercial preparations is not advisable for children.
  ■ Alcohol-containing preparations are never to be recommended for a recovering alcoholic person.
■ Compliance is greater with a daily rinse than with a weekly rinse when practiced on an individual basis at home.

III. PREPARATIONS[39]

■ Oral rinses are categorized as low-potency/high-frequency rinses or high-potency/low-frequency rinses.
■ Most low-potency rinses may be purchased directly over-the-counter (OTC); whereas most high potency rinses are provided by prescription.
■ **Table 35-5** contains the compounds, concentration, and recommended frequency of use for currently available self-applied fluoride rinses.

TABLE 35-5	SELF-APPLIED FLUORIDE MOUTHRINSES	
TYPE/ PERCENTAGE (RX OR OTC)	**CONCENTRATION IN PPM**	**FREQUENCY OF USE (10 ML OR 2 TEASPOONS SWISHED FOR 1 MIN)**
0.2% NaF (Rx)	905	Once daily or once weekly
0.044% NaF and APF (Rx and OTC)	200	Once daily
0.05 NaF (OTC)	230	Once daily
0.0221% NaF (OTC)	100	Twice daily

A. Low-Potency/High-Frequency (Available OTC)

1. *Preparations*
   - 0.05% NaF; 230 ppm.
   - 0.044% NaF and APF; 200 ppm. (available by prescription or OTC depending on the brand)
   - 0.0221% NaF; 100 ppm.
2. *Specifications*
   - No more than 264 mg NaF (120 mg of fluoride) can be dispensed at one time.
   - A 500-mL bottle of 0.05% NaF rinse contains 100 mg of fluoride.
   - Bottle is required to have a child-proof cap.
   - Rinses are not to be used by children under 6 years of age or by children or adults with a disability involving oral and/or facial musculature. Young children do not have sufficient control to expectorate, and they tend to swallow quickly.
   - The rinse is to be fully expectorated without swallowing.
3. *Procedure for use*
   - Low-potency rinses are used once or twice daily with 2 teaspoonfuls (10 mL) after brushing and before retiring. The adult and pediatric maximum dose is 10 mL of solution.
   - Swish between teeth with lips tightly closed for 60 seconds; spit out.
   - See Directions for Rinsing (29–4) and have the patient practice rinsing at the dental chair.
   - Do not eat or drink 30 minutes after rinsing.

B. High-Potency/Low-Frequency (Available by Prescription)

- 0.20% NaF; 905 ppm
  - Originally recommended as a weekly rinse, but can be used up to once per day.
  - Procedure for use is the same as for high frequency/low potency rinses.
  - The prevented fraction of dental caries ranges from 30–59% with the use of 0.2% fluoride rinse on various rinsing schedules.[50]

IV. BENEFITS

Benefits from fluoride mouthrinsing have been documented many times since the original research using various percentages of various fluoride preparations.[62,63] Frequent rinsing with low concentrations of fluoride has the following effects:

- A 26% to 29% average reduction in the dental caries incidence.[64]
- Greater benefit for smooth surfaces, but some benefit to pits and fissures.
- Greatest benefit to newly erupted teeth (thus, the program needs to be continued through the teenage years to benefit the second and third permanent molars).

- Added benefits for a community with fluoridation.[64]
- Effective in preventing and reversing root caries.[65]
- Primary teeth present in school-aged children benefit by as much as a 42.5% average reduction in dental caries incidence.[66]

BRUSH-ON GEL

- Brush-on gel has been used as an adjunct to the daily application of fluoride in a dentifrice and as a supplement to periodic professional applications.
- Regular use has been shown to help control demineralization about orthodontic appliances[67] and to provide protection against postirradiation caries in conjunction with other fluoride applications.[68]

I. PREPARATIONS

Table 35-6 contains the type, concentration, and daily usage guidelines for currently available self-applied fluoride gels.

A. 1.1% Sodium Fluoride (Neutral pH) or 1.1% Acidulated Sodium Fluoride (3.5 pH); 5000 ppm

- Available as a gel to be used separate from toothbrushing.
- Also available as a dentifrice: 1.1% neutral NaF with an abrasive system added.
- The rationale for the dentifrice product is to increase compliance with one step (brushing only) rather than brushing followed by application of the high-concentration gel with a toothbrush.
- Requires a prescription.

TABLE 35-6	SELF-APPLIED FLUORIDE GELS: BRUSH-ON OR USE IN CUSTOM TRAYS	
TYPE/ PERCENTAGE (RX OR OTC)	**CONCENTRATION IN PPM**	**DAILY USAGE GUIDELINES**
1.1% NaF (Rx)	5,000	4–8 drops on inner surface of custom tray or brush-on teeth, preferably at night
1.1% APF (Rx)	5,000	4–8 drops on inner surface of custom tray or brush-on teeth, preferably at night
0.4% SnF (OTC)	1,000	Brush-on teeth, preferably at night

B. Stannous Fluoride (SnF₂) 0.4% in Glycerin Base (1,000 ppm)

- Available as a gel to be used separate from toothbrushing.
- Available OTC.

II. PROCEDURE

- Teeth are cleaned first with thorough brushing and flossing before gel application with a separate toothbrush.
- Use once a day or more as recommended, preferably at night after toothbrushing and flossing.
- Place about 2 mg of the gel over the brush head and spread over all teeth.
- Brush 1 minute, then swish to force the fluid between the teeth several times before expectorating.
- Do not rinse.

FLUORIDE DENTIFRICES

I. DEVELOPMENT

- Historically tried with various compounds, including stannous fluoride, sodium fluoride, sodium monofluorophosphate, and amine fluoride.
- Early research objectives: to find compatible fluoride, abrasive systems, and formulations containing available fluoride for uptake by the tooth surface.
- In 1960 the first fluoride dentifrice gained approval by the American Dental Association, Council on Dental Therapeutics: 0.4% stannous fluoride.[69]

II. INDICATIONS

A. Dental Caries Prevention

A fluoride dentifrice approved by the ADA is an integral part of a complete preventive program and is a basic caries prevention intervention for all patients.[34]

B. All Patients Regardless of Their Caries Risk

- Toothbrushing at least twice per day with a fluoridated toothpaste is the foundation to all patients' fluoride regime.
- Patients with moderate to rampant dental caries are advised to brush three or four times each day with a fluoride-containing dentifrice and to chew xylitol gum after a meal when they cannot brush.
- Expectorate, but do not rinse after toothbrushing, to give the fluoride a longer time to be effective.

III. PREPARATIONS

Fluoride dentifrices are available as gels or pastes. Amine fluorides have not been developed and promoted in the United States.

A. Current Fluoride Constituents[70]

- Sodium fluoride (NaF) 0.24% (1100 ppm).
- Sodium monofluorophosphate (Na₂PO₃ F) 0.76% (1000 ppm).
- Stannous fluoride (SnF₂) 0.45% (1000 ppm).

B. Guidelines for Acceptance

The requirements for acceptance of a fluoridated toothpaste by the ADA are described in Chapter 29, on page 433. The Seal of Acceptance is illustrated in Figure 29-1, page 433.

IV. PATIENT INSTRUCTION: RECOMMENDED PROCEDURES

Advise the patient in the selection of a dentifrice, the need for frequent use, the method for application to the tooth surfaces, and the importance of using a fluoride dentifrice to promote oral health.

- Select an accepted fluoride-containing dentifrice.
- Place a small amount of dentifrice on the toothbrush.
- *Children (age less than 2 years):* Twice daily brushing with a "smear" of fluoridated dentifrice (about one-half the size of a small pea or a tiny touch) is used and spread along the brushing plane as shown in Figure 49-7, page 771.[71] The paste is then spread over all the teeth before starting to brush so that all teeth benefit and large amounts are not available for swallowing.
- *Older child (ages 3 to 5 years):* Twice daily brushing with the size of a small pea. Demonstrate spreading this amount over the ends of the filaments, and explain that the child is not to swallow excess amounts of dentifrice.[71]
- *Adults:* Use 1/2 inch or less twice daily.
- Spread dentifrice over the teeth with a light touch of the brush.
- Proceed with correct brushing positions for sulcular removal of dental biofilm (in Chapter 27, page 393).
- Keep dentifrice container out of reach of children.
- Rinsing after brushing is to be kept to a minimal amount of water to retain fluoride in the oral fluids.[71,72]

V. BENEFITS

- Twice daily use has greater benefits than once daily use.[61]
- Moderate and high caries-risk patients and patients that live in a nonfluoridated community benefit from using a dentifrice several times per day to maintain salivary fluoride levels.
- The dentifrice is a continuing source of fluoride for the tooth surface in the control of demineralization and the promotion of remineralization.
- The use of a dentifrice with a fluoride concentration of 1000 ppm and above compared to a nonfluoridated dentifrice prevents dental caries up to 23%.[73]

COMBINED FLUORIDE PROGRAM

- All adult patients, regardless of caries risk, benefit from twice daily use of a fluoridated dentifrice and consumption of fluoridated water multiple times during each day. Patients at moderate to high caries risk benefit from additional methods of fluoride exposure.
- Additional caries reduction can be expected when another topical fluoride such as a mouthrinse or gel tray is combined with a fluoride dentifrice.[74]
- When self-administered methods are chosen, patient cooperation is a significant factor.
- Age and eruption pattern influence the method selected.
- Newly erupted teeth need frequent fluoride exposure as soon after eruption as possible and continued indefinitely to control demineralization.
- Maintenance appointments can be scheduled for frequent professional topical applications for those at moderate and high caries risk and for continuing instruction and motivation regarding daily fluoride use for all patients.
- All methods are supplements to the daily use of fluoridated water and a dentifrice with fluoride.

FLUORIDE SAFETY

- Fluoride preparations and fluoridated water have wide margins of safety.
- Fluoride is beneficial in small amounts, but it can be injurious if used without attention to correct dosage and frequency.
- All dental personnel need to be familiar with the following:
    - Recommended approved procedures.
    - Potential toxic effects of fluoride.
    - How to administer general emergency measures should accidental overdoses occur as shown in Table 69-4, page 1076. Internal poisoning is described on page 1081, in Table 69-5.

I. SUMMARY OF FLUORIDE MANAGEMENT

- Use professionally and recommend only approved fluoride preparations for patient use. Products have approval from the Food and Drug Administration and the ADA in the United States. Read about the programs of the ADA Council on Scientific Affairs and the Seal of Approval of Products on page 433.
- Use only researched, recommended amounts and methods for delivery.
- Know potential toxicity of the various products, and be prepared to administer emergency measures for treating an accidental toxic response.

- Instruct patients in proper care of fluoride products.
    A. Dentist prescribes no more than 120 mg of fluoride at one time (no more than 480 of the 0.25 mg tablets or 240 of the 0.5 mg tablets).[39] Do not store large quantities in the home.
    B. Request parental supervision of a child's brushing or other fluoride administration. Rinses, for example, are not to be used by children under 6 years of age.
    C. Fluoride products have child-proof covers and are to be kept out of reach of small children and other persons, such as the mentally challenged, who may not understand limitations.
    D. In school health programs, dispensing of the fluoride product is to be supervised by responsible adults. Containers are to be stored under lock and key when not in active use.

II. TOXICITY

- *Acute toxicity* refers to rapid intake of an excess dose over a short time.
- *Chronic toxicity* applies to long-term ingestion of fluoride in amounts that exceed the approved therapeutic levels.
- *Accidental ingestion* of a concentrated fluoride preparation can lead to a toxic reaction.
- Acute fluoride poisoning is rare.[75]

A. Certainly Lethal Dose (CLD)[76]

A lethal dose is the amount of a drug likely to cause death if not intercepted by antidotal therapy.

- *Adult CLD:* 5–10 g of sodium fluoride taken at one time. The fluoride ion equivalent is 32 to 64 mg of fluoride per kilogram body weight (mg F/kg; **Box 35-5**).
- *Child:* Approximately 0.5 to 1.0 g, variable with size and weight of the child.

B. Safely Tolerated Dose (STD): One-Fourth of the CLD

- *Adult STD:* 1.25 to 2.5 g of sodium fluoride (8 to 16 mg F/kg).
- *Child:* **Box 35-5B** shows STDs and CLDs for children.
    A. Weights given for each selected age are minimal, and calculations for the doses are conservative.
    B. As can be noted in **Box 35-5B**, less than 1 g (1000 mg) may be fatal for children 12 years old and younger, and 0.5 g (500 mg) exceeds the STD for all ages shown.
    C. For children under 6 years of age, however, 500 mg would be lethal.[76]

III. SIGNS AND SYMPTOMS OF ACUTE TOXIC DOSE

Symptoms begin within 30 minutes of ingestion and may persist for as long as 24 hours.

BOX 35-5	Lethal and Safe Doses of Fluoride

A. LETHAL AND SAFE DOSES OF FLUORIDE FOR A 70-KG ADULT

Certainly Lethal Dose (CLD)
5–10 g NaF
or
32–64 mg F/kg

Safely Tolerated Dose (STD) = 1/4 CLD
1.25–2.5 g NaF
or
8–16 mg F/kg

B. CLDS AND STDS OF FLUORIDE FOR SELECTED AGES

Age (years)	Weight (lbs)	CLD (mg)	STD (mg)
2	22	320	80
4	29	422	106
6	37	538	135
8	45	655	164
10	53	771	193
12	64	931	233
14	83	1,206	301
16	92	1,338	334
18	95	1,382	346

Reprinted with permission from Heifetz SB, Horowitz HS. The amounts of fluoride in current fluoride therapies: safety considerations for children. *ASDC J Dent Child*. 1984 Jul-Aug;51(4):257–69.

A. Gastrointestinal Tract

Fluoride in the stomach is acted on by the hydrochloric acid to form hydrofluoric acid, an irritant to the stomach lining. Symptoms include:

- Nausea, vomiting, diarrhea.
- Abdominal pain.
- Increased salivation, thirst.

B. Systemic Involvements

- *Blood.* Calcium may be bound by the circulating fluoride, thus causing symptoms of hypocalcemia.
- *Central nervous system.* Hyperreflexia, convulsions, paresthesias.
- *Cardiovascular and respiratory depression.* If not treated, may lead to death in a few hours from cardiac failure or respiratory paralysis.

IV. EMERGENCY TREATMENT

A. Induce Vomiting

- *Mechanical.* Digital stimulation at back of tongue or in throat.
- *Drug.* Ipecac syrup.

B. Second Person

Call emergency service; transport to hospital.

C. Administer Fluoride-Binding Liquid When Patient Is Not Vomiting

- Milk.
- Milk of Magnesium.
- Lime water ($CaOH_2$ solution 0.15%).

D. Support Respiration and Circulation

E. Additional Therapy Indicated at Emergency Room

- Calcium gluconate for muscle tremors or tetany.
- Gastric lavage.
- Cardiac monitoring.
- Endotracheal intubation.
- Blood monitoring (calcium, magnesium, potassium, pH).
- Intravenous feeding to restore blood volume, calcium.

V. CHRONIC TOXICITY

A. Skeletal Fluorosis[75]

- Isolated instances of osteosclerosis, an elevation in bone density, can result from chronic toxicity after long-term (10 or more years) ingestion of water with 8 to 10 ppm fluoride or from inhalation of industrial fumes or dust.
- Skeletal fluorosis in its early stages is characterized by stiff and painful joints and becomes crippling in its later stages.
- It has never been a public health concern in the United States, even in communities that have had high levels of fluoride in the water for generations, but is endemic in certain countries such as China and India. Predisposing factors, dietary deficiencies, and population differences in regard to fluoride metabolism may play a role in its development in addition to exposure.
- Methods for defluoridation have been developed, as described in this chapter on page 524.

B. Dental Fluorosis

- Ingestion of naturally occurring excess fluoride in the drinking water and/or fluoridated dental products can produce visible fluorosis only when used during the years of development of the crowns of the teeth, namely, from birth until age 12 or 16 years or when the crowns of the third permanent molars are completed.
- No systemic symptoms result from the fluoride, and the individual has protection against dental caries. Indices used to describe dental fluorosis are found in Chapter 22, on page 332.

C. Mild Fluorosis

1. *Clinical evaluation*
   - Mild and very mild forms, dental fluorosis appears as white opacities in the enamel surface.
   - No esthetic or health problem is involved. Many such white spots are not visible except when scrutinized under a dental light and the surface is dried.

■ All white spots in the enamel are not related to fluoride intake; distinction is to be made by reviewing the patient's dental and fluoride-intake history, by noting the location and distribution of the white spots, and by considering the sequence of tooth development.

2. *Relation to fluoride sources*

■ Mild fluorosis may result from inadvertent ingestion of excess fluoride by young children during topical procedures both self-applied and professional. No problem exists when care is taken to follow basic steps, such as those listed in **Tables 35-3** and **35-4** for professional applications and those shown in Figure 49-7, page 771 for daily use of dentifrice the size of a smear or small pea (depending on the age of the child). Mouthrinses are not indicated for children less than 6 years of age.

■ Small amounts of dentifrice may be swallowed incidentally at each brushing. A child of 4 years who lives in a nonfluoridated community, uses a daily supplement (0.5 mg), and swallows two or three small amounts of dentifrice ingests far less than the STD of 106 mg shown in **Box 35-5B**.

VI. HOW TO CALCULATE AMOUNTS OF FLUORIDE[76,77]

Figure 35-6 is a flowchart that shows the steps necessary to determine the amount of fluoride in a fluoride compound. By doing so, one can then calculate the amount ingested by the patient.

■ Multiply the percentage of fluoride ion in the compound by the molecular weight conversion ratio, as shown in **Figure 35-6**.

■ Obtain the ratio by dividing the molecular weight of the compound by the atomic weight of fluoride.

■ Example: The molecular weight of sodium fluoride is 42 (Na = 23, F = 19). When divided by 19, a 1 to 2.2 ratio results, as used in the example in **Figure 35-6**.

BOX 35-6	Example Progress Note

(Patient is a 26-year-old male)
Patient presents with high caries risk as shown by the presence of two proximal cavitated lesions and frequent daily consumption of soda pop. States that he uses a fluoride toothpaste twice daily and consumes fluoridated water. Applied 5% NaF varnish to the entire dentition and provided postoperative instructions. Prescribed 1.1% NaF gel (2 refills) to apply with a separate toothbrush at night. Discussed the need for an additional varnish application in three months.

Signed: _____, RDH Date: _____.

DOCUMENTATION

A patient receiving a topical fluoride application and/or counseling regarding fluoride needs the following documented in the permanent record:

■ Caries risk level (document as low, moderate, high, or extreme)

■ Current use of fluoride toothpaste and exposure to fluoridated water

■ Type, concentration, mode of delivery, and postoperative instructions if a professional fluoride application is provided

■ Type, amount, and instructions for the use of any prescription or OTC patient-applied fluoride products recommended

■ A sample progress note is provided in **Box 35-6**.

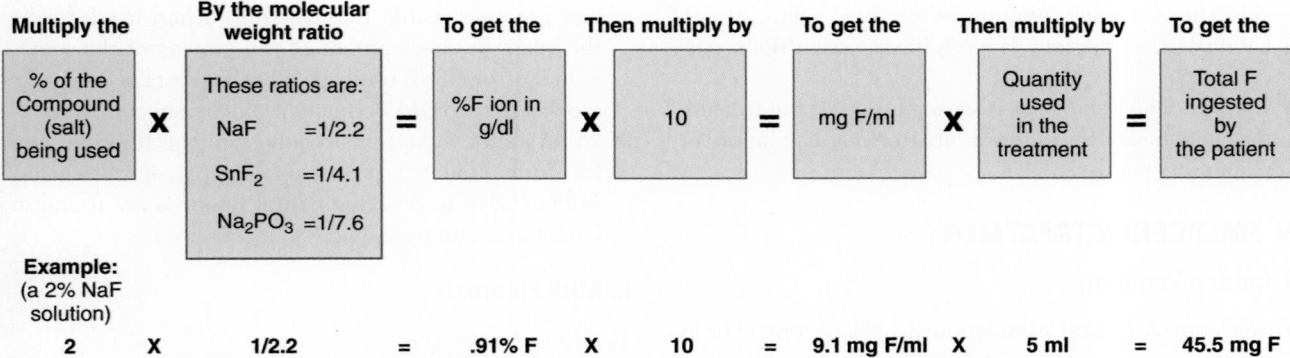

FIGURE 35-6 **Fluoride Calculation.** Flowchart shows steps in the calculation of the amount of fluoride in a compound used in treatment. The example shows that 5 mL of a 2% solution of NaF contains 45.5 mg F, an amount slightly greater than half of the safely tolerated dose (STD) for a 2-year-old child (**Box 35-5B**). (Data from Heifetz SB, Horowitz HS. The amounts of fluoride in current fluoride therapies: safety considerations for children. *Source: ASDC J Dent Child.* 1984 Jul–Aug;51(4):257–69.)

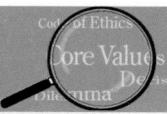

Everyday Ethics

Daniel was an extremely well-behaved and cooperative 4 1/2-year-old boy at a moderate to severe risk for dental caries due to having one carious lesion and living in a nonfluoridated area. When it came time for the fluoride treatment the dental hygienist, Nina, spent a few extra minutes explaining to Daniel how she will brush a coating on his teeth to make them stronger. Although Daniel's parents did not have insurance coverage, the hygienist decided it would be important for him to receive a fluoride application regardless of the fee. Daniel tolerated the procedure well. After the appointment Nina explained to Daniel's mother the varnish postoperative instructions. Daniel's mother became upset and said, "Why did you give my son a fluoride treatment without my permission? My husband just lost his job and I cannot afford this added cost."

Questions for Consideration

1. Because Daniel's mother brought him to the clinic for a scheduled appointment, Nina assumed *implied consent* for Daniel to receive dental hygiene treatment. Was it appropriate for Nina to have assumed that consent for the fluoride application was also implied? Why or why not?
2. Discuss ways in which the legal/ethical concepts of professional liability, scope of practice, standard of care, and informed consent are related to this scenario.
3. Answer the questions in the steps for resolving ethical issues or dilemmas found in Chapter 1, on page 10. Use the answers to determine at least one course of action Nina can take now to resolve the issue. Make sure to consider all individuals who might be affected by the decision.

Factors To Teach The Patient

I. Personal Use of Fluorides
- Purposes, action, and expected benefits relative to the specific forms of fluoride treatment the patient will receive.
- Specific instruction concerning self-applied techniques that will be performed at home. Prepared printed instruction materials can be especially useful.

II. Need for Parental Supervision
- Supervise daily care of child's teeth and mouth, including brushing of teeth using a smear (2 years of age or younger) or small, pea-sized (2–5 years of age) quantity of dentifrice to prevent excess ingestion of fluoride.
- Keep fluoride products out of reach of small children.
- Brush teeth before using chewable or lozenge dietary supplements. Avoid eating and drinking after use. Preferred time for use is just before going to bed.

III. Determine Need for Fluoride Supplements
- Recommendations for use are limited.
- Must determine child is at high caries risk and consumes fluoride-deficient drinking water.
- Reference a list of communities with fluoride in the drinking water at optimum level.
- Where to send private water source sample for fluoride analysis.

IV. Fluorides Are Part of the Total Preventive Program
- Emphasize fluoride toothpaste and fluoridated water as the cornerstone for prevention of dental caries.
- Control of cariogenic foods in the diet, particularly between meals.
- Regular professional supervision and care.

V. Fluoridation
- In a nonfluoridated community, information concerning the significance of fluoridation.
- How drinking fluoridated water helps people of all ages.
- How to access the Department of Health and Human Services Centers for Disease Control and Prevention website to obtain reliable information about fluoridation in the United States.

VI. Bottled Drinking Water/Water Filters
- Use fluoridated water.
- When bottled water does not have a label indicating that it is fluoridated, how the water bottle can best be filled from a water supply that is fluoridated.
- Inform that water filters can remove fluoride from drinking water so it is best to check with the manufacturer to be certain the fluoride will not be removed.
- Distillation and reverse osmosis systems remove fluoride from drinking water, but water softeners do not.

VII. Infant Formula
- Educate parents that powdered or liquid concentrate infant formula and the water to reconstitute this formula may contain fluoride.

References

1. Ellwood R, Fejerskov O, Cury JA, Clarkson, B. Chapter 18: Fluorides in caries control. In: Fejerskov O, Kidd E. *Dental caries The disease and its clinical management*. 2nd ed. Oxford UK: Blackwell Munksgaard Ltd.; 2008. pp. 293–4.

2. Newbrun E. Systemic benefits of fluoride and fluoridation. *J Public Health Dent*. 2004 Sept;64(S1):35–9.

3. Ekstrand J. Chapter 4: Fluoride metabolism. In: Fejerskov O, Ekstrand J, Burt BA. *Fluoride in dentistry*. 2nd ed. Copenhagen: Munksgaard; 1996. pp. 55–67.

4. Bath-Balough M, Fehrenbach M. *Dental embryology, histology, and anatomy*. 2nd ed. St. Louis:. Saunders; 2006. pp. 179–189.

5. Melfi RC, Alley KE. *Permar's oral embryology and microscopic anatomy*. 10th ed. Philadelphia: Lippincott Williams & Wilkins; 2000. pp. 43–87.

6. Levy S. An update on fluorides and fluorosis. *J Can Dent Assoc*. 2003 May;69(5):286–91.

7. Aoba T, Fejerskov O. Dental fluorosis: chemistry and biology. *Crit Rev Oral Bio Med*. 2002;13(2):155–70.

8. Featherstone JD. The science and practice of caries prevention. *J Am Dent Assoc*. 2000 Jul;131(7):887–99.

9. Yoon SH, Brudevold F, Gardner DE, Smith FA. Distribution of fluoride in teeth from areas with different levels of fluoride in the water supply. *J Dent Res*. 1960 Jul–Aug;39:845–56.

10. Centers for Disease Control and Prevention. Recommendations for using fluoride to prevent and control dental caries in the United States. *MMWR Recomm Rep*. 2001 Aug 17;50(RR-14):1–42.

11. Centers for Disease Control and Prevention. Populations receiving optimally fluoridated public drinking water–United States, 1992–1996. *MWWR Morb Mortal Wkly Rep*. 2008 Jul;57(27):737–41.

12. Department of Health and Human Services, Centers for Disease Control and Prevention: Community Fluoridation [Internet]. Atlanta (GA): 2008 Water Fluoridation Statistics. [updated 2010 Oct 22; cited 2011 Jan 3.] [about 4 screens] Available from: http://www.cdc.gov/fluoridation/index.htm

13. Herschfeld JJ. Classics in dental history: Frederick S. McKay and the "Colorado brown stain," *Bull Hist Dent*. 1978 Oct;26(2):118–26.

14. McKay FS. The relation of mottled enamel to caries. *J Am Dent Assoc*. 1928 Aug;15:1429.

15. Churchill HV. Occurrence of fluorides in some waters of United States. *J Indust Engin Chem*. 1931; 23:996.

16. Dean HT, Arnold FA Jr, Elvove E. Domestic water and dental caries. V. Additional studies of the relation of fluoride domestic waters to dental caries experience in 4425 white children, aged 12 to 14 years, of 13 cities in 4 states. *Public Health Rep*. 1942 Aug;57:1155.

17. Centers for Disease Control and Prevention. Engineering and administrative recommendations for water fluoridation, 1995. *MMWR Recomm Rep*. 1995 Sep;44(RR-13):1–40.

18. Department of Health and Human Services, Centers for Disease Control and Prevention: Division of Oral Health [Internet]. Atlanta (GA): Changes Proposed to National Fluoridation Level. [updated 2011 Jan 14; cited 2011 Jan 3.] [about 2 screens] Available from: http://www.cdc.gov/oralhealth

19. Griffin SO, Regnier E, Griffin PM, Huntley VN. Effectiveness of fluoride in preventing caries in adults. *J Dent Res*. 2007 May;86(5):410–15.

20. Yeung CA. A systematic review of the efficacy and safety of fluoridation. *Evid Based Dent*. 2008;9(2):39–43.

21. Dirks OB, Houwink B, Kwant GW. Some special features of the caries preventive effect of water fluoridation. *Arch Oral Biol*. 1961 August;4:187–92.

22. Burt BA, Ismail AI, Eklund SA. Root caries in an optimally fluoridated and a high-fluoride community. *J Dent Res*. 1986 Sep;6(9):1154–8.

23. Stamm JW, Banting DW, Imrey PB. Adult root caries survey of two similar communities with contrasting natural water fluoride levels. *J Am Dent Assoc*. 1990 Feb;120(2):143–9.

24. Ast DB, Fitzgerald B. Effectiveness of water fluoridation. *J Am Dent Assoc*. 1962 Nov;65:581–7.

25. Russell AL, Elvove E. Domestic water and dental caries. VII. A study of the fluoride-dental caries relationship in an adult population. *Public Health Rep*. 1951 Oct;66(43):1389–1401.

26. Englander HR, Wallace DA. Effects of naturally fluoridated water on dental caries in adults: Aurora-Rockford, Illinois, Study III. *Public Health Rep*. 1962 Oct;77(10):887–93.

27. Horowitz HS, Maier FJ, Law FE. Partial defluoridation of a community water supply and dental fluorosis. *Public Health Rep*. 1967 Nov;82(11):965–72.

28. Horowitz HS, Heifetz SB. The effect of partial defluoridation of a water supply on dental fluorosis—final results in Bartlett, Texas, after 17 Years. *Am J Public Health*. 1972 Jun;62(6):767–9.

29. Horowitz HS. Effectiveness of school water fluoridation and dietary fluoride supplements in school-aged children. *J Public Health Dent*. 1989;49(5 Spec No):290–6.

30. Lemke CW, Doherty JM, Arra MC. Controlled fluoridation: The dental effects of discontinuation in Antigo, Wisconsin. *J Am Dent Assoc*. 1979 Apr;80(4):782–6.

31. Jackson RD, Brizendine EJ, Kelly SA, Hinesley R, Stookey GK, Dunipace AJ. The fluoride content of foods and beverages from negligibly and optimally fluoridated communities. *Community Dent Oral Epidemiol*. 2002 Oct;30(5):382–91.

32. Burt BA, Marthaler TM. Chapter 16: Fluoride Tablets, Salt Fluoridation, and Milk Fluoridation. In: Fejerskov O, Ekstrand J, Burt BA. *Fluoride in Dentistry*. 2nd ed. Copenhagen: Munksgaard; 1996. pp. 291–310.

33. Espelid I. Caries preventive effect of fluoride in milk, salt and tablets: a literature review. *Eur Arch Paediatr Dent*. 2009 Sep;10(3):149–56.

34. European Academy of Paediatric Dentistry. Guidelines on the use of fluoride in children: an EAPD policy document. *Eur Arch Paediatr Dent*. 2009 Sep;10(3):129–35.

35. American Dental Association. *Fluoridation facts*. Chicago: ADA; 2005.

36. Hujoel PP, Zina LG, Moimaz SA, Cunha-Cruz J. Infant formula and enamel fluorosis: a systematic review. *J Am Dent Assoc*. 2009 Jul;140(7):841–54.

37. Siew C, Strock S, Ristic H, Kang P, Chou HN, Chen JW, Frantsve-Hawley J, Meyer DM. Assessing the potential risk factor for enamel fluorosis: a preliminary evaluation of fluoride content in infant formulas. *J Am Dent Assoc*. 2009 Oct;140(10):1228–36.

38. Berg J, Gerweck C, Hujoel P, King R, Krol D, Kumar J, Levy S, Pollick H, Whitford G, Strock S, Aravamudhan K, Frantsve-Hawley J, Meyer D. Evidence-Based clinical recommendations regarding fluoride intake from reconstituted infant formula and enamel fluorosis. *J Am Dent Assoc*. 2011 Jan;142(1):79–87.

39. Burrell KH. Chapter 10: Fluorides. In: Mariotti AJ, Burrell KH. *American Dental Association, Council on Scientific Affairs: ADA/PDR guide to dental therapeutics*. 5th ed. Chicago: ADA and Thomson PDR Publishing Co; 2009. pp. 323–37.

40. Ismail AI, Hasson H. Fluoride supplements, dental caries, and fluorosis: a systematic review. *J Am Dent Assoc*. 2008 Nov;139(11):1457–68.

41. Rozier RG, Adair S, Graham F, Iafolla T, Kingman A, Krol D, Levy S, Pollick H, Whitford G, Strock S, Frantsve-Hawley J, Aravamudhan K, Meyer DM. Evidence-based clinical recommendations on the prescription of dietary fluoride supplements for caries prevention. *J Am Dent Assoc*. 2010 Dec;141(12):1480–9.

42. Toyama Y, Nakagaki H, Kato S, Huang S, Mizutani Y, Kojima S, Toyama A, Ohno N, Tsuchiya T, Kirkham J, Robinson C. Fluoride concentrations at and near the neonatal line in human deciduous tooth enamel obtained from a naturally fluoridated and a non-fluoridated area. *Arch Oral Biol*. 2001 Feb;46(2):147–53.

43. American Dental Association Council on Scientific Affairs. Professionally applied topical fluoride: evidence-based clinical recommendations. *J Am Dent Assoc*. 2006 Aug;137(8):1151–9.

44. Bibby BG. Use of fluorine in the prevention of dental caries. II. The effects of sodium fluoride applications. *J Am Dent Assoc*. 1944 March;31:317.

45. Knutson JW. Sodium fluoride solutions: technique for application to the teeth. *J Am Dent Assoc*. 1948 Jan;36(1):37–9.

46. Galagan DJ, Knutson JW. The effect of topically applied fluorides on dental caries experience; experiments with sodium fluoride and calcium chloride; widely spaced applications; use of different solution concentrations. *Public Health Rep.* 1948 Sep;63(38):1215–21.

47. Warren DP, Chan JT. Topical fluorides: efficacy, administration, and safety. *Gen Dent.* 1997 Mar–Apr;45(2):134–40, 142.

48. Ripa LW. An evaluation of the use of professionally (operator applied) topical fluorides. *J Dent Res.* 1990 Feb;69 Spec No:786–96.

49. Soeno K, Matsumura H, Atsuta M, Kawasaki K. Influence of acidulated fluoride agents and effectiveness of subsequent polishing on composite material surfaces. *Oper Dent.* 2002 May-Jun;27(3):305–10.

50. Paulson S. Fluoride-containing gels, mouthrinses and varnishes: an update of evidence of efficacy. *(Report) Eur Arch Paediatr Dent.* 2009 Sep;10(3):157–62.

51. Beltrán-Aguilar ED, Goldstein JW, Lockwood SA. Fluoride varnishes: a review of their clinical use, cariostatic mechanism, efficacy and safety. *J Am Dent Assoc.* 2000 May;131(5):589–96.

52. Bawden JW. Fluoride varnish: a useful new tool for public health dentistry. *J Public Health Dent.* 1998 Fall;58(4):266–9.

53. Autio-Gold JT, Courts F. Assessing the effect of fluoride varnish on early enamel carious lesions in the primary dentition. *J Amer Dent Assoc.* 2001 Sep;132(9):1247–53.

54. Castellano JB, Donly KJ. Potential remineralization of demineralized enamel after application of fluoride varnish. *Am J Dent.* 2004 Dec;17(6):462–4.

55. Demito CF, Vivaldi-Rodrigues G, Ramos AL, Bowman SJ. The efficacy of fluoride varnish in reducing enamel demineralization adjacent to orthodontic brackets: an in vitro study. *Orthod Craniofacial Res.* 2004 Nov;7(4):205–10.

56. Ripa LW. Need for prior toothcleaning when performing a professional topical fluoride application: review and recommendations for change. *J Am Dent Assoc.* 1984 Aug;109(2):281–5.

57. Vrbic V, Brudevold F, McCann HG. Acquisition of fluoride by enamel from fluoride pumice pastes. *Helv Odontol Acta.* 1967 Apr;11(1):21–6.

58. Shen C, Autio-Gold J. Assessing fluoride concentration uniformity and fluoride release from three varnishes. *J Am Dent Assoc.* 2002 Feb;133(2):176–82.

59. Stookey GK, Schemehorn BR, Drook CA, Cheetham BL. The effect of rinsing with water immediately after a professional fluoride gel application on fluoride uptake in demineralized enamel: an in vivo study. *Pediatr Dent.* 1986 Jun;8(3):153–7.

60. Englander HR, Keyes PH, Gestwicki M, Sultz HA. Clinical anticaries effect of repeated topical sodium fluoride applications by mouthpieces. *J Am Dent Assoc.* 1967 Sep;75(3):638–44.

61. Adair SM. Evidence-based use of fluoride in contemporary pediatric dental practice. *Pediatr Dent.* 2006 Mar–Apr;28(2):133–42.

62. Torell P, Ericsson Y. The potential benefits derived from fluoride mouth rinses. In: Forrester DJ, Schulz EM, eds. *International workshop on fluorides and dental caries reductions.* Baltimore: University of Maryland School of Dentistry; 1974. pp. 114–76.

63. Birkeland JM, Torell P. Caries-preventive fluoride mouthrinses. *Caries Res.* 1978;12(Suppl 1):38–51.

64. Driscoll WS, Swango PA, Horowitz AM, Kingman A. Caries-preventive effects of daily and weekly fluoride mouthrinsing in a fluoridated community: final results after 30 months. *J Am Dent Assoc.* 1982 Dec;105(6):1010–13.

65. Heijnsbroek M, Paraskevas S, Vav der Weijden GA. Fluoride interventions for root caries: a review. *Oral Health Prev Dent.* 2007;5(2):145–52.

66. Ripa LW, Leske GS, Varma A. Effect of mouthrinsing with a 0.2 percent neutral NaF solution on the deciduous dentition of first to third grade school children. *Pediatr Dent.* 1984 Jun;6(2):93–7.

67. Stratemann MW, Shannon IL. Control of decalcification in orthodontic patients by daily self-administrated application of a water-free 0.4 percent stannous fluoride gel. *Am J Orthod.* 1974 Sept;66(3):273–9.

68. Wescott WB, Starcke EN, Shannon IL. Chemical protection against postirradiation dental caries. *Oral Surg Oral Med Oral Pathol.* 1975 Dec;40(6):709–19.

69. American Dental Association, Council on Dental Therapeutics. Evaluation of Crest toothpaste. *J Am Dent Assoc.* 1960 Aug;61:272.

70. Mariotti MJ, Burrell K. Mouthrinses and dentifrices. In: *American Dental Association, Council on Scientific Affairs: ADA/PDR guide to dental therapeutics.* 5th ed. Chicago: ADA and Thompson PDR Publishing Co; 2009. pp. 305–21.

71. American Academy of Pediatric Dentistry Liaison with Other Groups Committee; American Academy on Pediatric Dentistry Council on Scientific Affairs. Guideline on fluoride therapy. *Pediatr Dent.* 2008–2009;30(7 Suppl):121–4.

72. Sjogren K, Melin NH. The influence of rinsing routines on fluoride retention after toothbrushing. *Gerodontology.* 2001 Jul;18(1):15–20.

73. Walsh T, Worthington HV, Glenny AM, Appelbe P, Marinho VCC, Shi X. Fluoride toothpastes of different concentrations for preventing dental caries in children and adolescents. *Cochrane Database Syst Rev.* 2010 Jan 20;(1):CD007868.

74. Marinho VC. Cochrane reviews of randomized trials of fluoride therapies for preventing dental caries. *Eur Arch Paediatr Dent.* 2009 Sep;10(3):183–91.

75. Whitford GM. Acute and chronic fluoride toxicity. *J Dent Res.* 1992 May;71(5):1249–54.

76. Heifetz SB, Horowitz HS. The amounts of fluoride in current fluoride therapies: safety considerations for children. *ASDC J Dent Child.* 1984 Jul–Aug;51(4):257–69.

77. Bayless JM, Tinanoff N. Diagnosis and treatment of acute fluoride toxicity. *J Am Dent Assoc.* 1985 Feb;110(2):209–11.

Sealants

ESTHER M. WILKINS, BS, RDH, DMD

Chapter Outline

As part of a complete preventive program, pit and fissure sealants are indicated for selected patients. Because topically applied fluorides protect smooth tooth surfaces more than occlusal surfaces, a method to reduce the incidence of occlusal dental caries is needed.

- The incidence of new pit and fissure caries can be lowered significantly by the application of adhesive sealants.
- Sealant application is a part of a complete prevention program, not an isolated procedure.
- As an isolated procedure, patient (and parent) may misunderstand the selected area of prevention that sealants represent. Other surfaces and other teeth still need other methods of preventive protection.

- Box 36-1 provides definitions and terminology relative to sealants and their application.

DEVELOPMENT OF SEALANTS

Sealants were developed by Dr. Michael Buonocore and the group of dental scientists at the Eastman Dental Center in Rochester, New York.

- The focus of the early research was on the need to prepare the enamel surface so that a dental material would adhere.
- They demonstrated that by using an acid etch process, the enamel could be altered to increase retention.

BOX 36-1	Key Words

Pit and Fissure Sealants

Acid etchant: in sealant placement, the enamel surface is prepared by the application of phosphoric acid, which etches the surface to provide mechanical retention for the sealant.

Articulating paper: an inked ribbon held between teeth to determine tooth contacts.

Bibulous: absorbent; a flat bibulous pad, placed in the cheek over the opening of Stensen's duct, is used to aid in maintaining a dry field while placing sealants.

Biocompatibility: the ability of things to exist together without harm.

Bis-GMA: bisphenol A-glycidyl methylacrylate; plastic material used for dental sealants.

Bonding (mechanical): physical adherence of one substance to another; the adherence of a sealant to the enamel surface is accomplished by an acid-etching technique that leaves microspaces between the enamel rods; the sealant becomes mechanically locked (bonded) in these microspaces.

Bond strength: expression of the degree of adherence between the tooth surface and the sealant.

Conditioner: a substance added to another substance to increase its usability; in sealant placement, the acid etchant is added to the enamel to prepare it for bonding with the sealant.

Curing: the process by which plastic becomes rigid.

Incipient caries: beginning caries, caries limited to the enamel.

In vitro: under laboratory conditions.

In vivo: within the living body.

Micropores: tiny openings.

Polymer: a compound of high molecular weight formed by a combination of a chain of simpler molecules (monomers).

Polymerization: a reaction in which a high-molecular-weight product is produced by successive additions of a simpler compound.

   Photopolymerization: polymerization with the use of an external light source.

   Autopolymerization: self-curing; a reaction in which a high-molecular-weight product is produced by successive additions of a simpler compound; hardening process of pit and fissure sealants.

Sealant: organic polymer that bonds to an enamel surface by mechanical retention accommodated by projections of the sealant into micropores created in the enamel by etching; the two types of sealants, filled and unfilled, both are composed of Bis-GMA.

   Filled sealant: contains, in addition to Bis-GMA, microparticles of glass, quartz, silica, and other fillers used in composite restorations; fillers make the sealant more resistant to abrasion.

Viscosity: in general, the resistance to flow or alteration of shape by any substance as a result of molecular cohesion.

■ The research proved to be a major breakthrough, particularly in esthetic and preventive dentistry.[1,2]

HOW SEALANTS WORK

I. DEFINITION

A pit and fissure sealant is an organic polymer (resin) that flows into the pit or fissure and bonds to the enamel surface mainly by mechanical retention when the acid etch process precedes the application of the sealant material.

II. ACTION

A. Purpose of the Sealant

■ To provide a physical barrier to "seal off" the pit or fissure.

■ To prevent oral bacteria and their nutrients from collecting within the pit or fissure to create the acid environment necessary for the initiation of dental caries.

■ To fill the pit or fissure as deep as possible and provide tight smooth margins at the junction with the enamel surface.

■ When sealant material is worn or cracked away on the surface around the pit or fissure, the sealant in the depth of the micropore can remain and provide continued protection while sealant material is added for repair and to reseal the enamel/sealant junction.

B. Purpose of the Acid Etch

■ To produce irregularities or micropores in the enamel.

■ To allow the liquid resin to penetrate into the micropores and create a bond or mechanical locking.

■ **Figure 36-1** illustrates the sealant placed on a smooth enamel surface in contrast with placement on an etched surface with retention.

SEALANT MATERIALS

I. CRITERIA FOR THE IDEAL SEALANT[1]

1. Achieve prolonged bonding to enamel.
2. Be biocompatible with oral tissues.

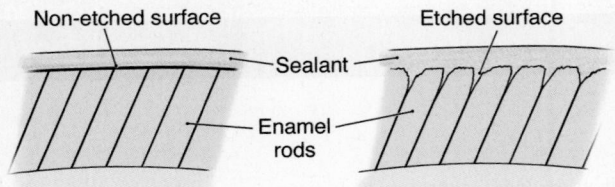

FIGURE 36-1 **Enamel–Sealant Interface.** Diagram of enamel–sealant interface to compare nonetched with etched surface. Etching produces microscopic porosities in the enamel to increase the area of retention. The unpolymerized resin flows into the porosities and hardens in taglike projections, as shown on the right. (Adapted with permission from Buonocore MG, Matsui A, Gwinnett AJ. Penetration of resin dental materials into enamel surfaces with reference to bonding. *Arch Oral Biol.* 1968 Jan;13(1):61–70.)

3. Offer a simple application procedure.
4. Be a free-flowing, low-viscosity material capable of entering narrow fissures.
5. Have low solubility in the oral environment.

II. CLASSIFICATION OF TYPES OF SEALANT MATERIALS

- A majority of sealants in clinical use are made of Bis-GMA (bisphenol A–glycidyl methylacrylate). The techniques of application vary slightly among available products.
- The three types of sealants currently available are filled, unfilled, and fluoride-releasing filled.
- Sealants are also identified by the method required for polymerization.

A. Classification by Method of Polymerization

1. *Self-cured or autopolymerized*
   - Preparation: material supplied in two parts. When the two are mixed they quickly polymerize (harden).
   - Advantages: no special equipment required.
   - Disadvantages: mixing required; working time limited because polymerization begins when the material is mixed.
2. *Visible Light–cured or photopolymerized*
   - Preparation: material hardens when exposed to a special curing light.
   - Advantages: no mixing required; increased working time due to control over start of polymerization.
   - Disadvantages: extra costs and disinfection time required for curing light, protective shields, and/or glasses.

B. Classification by Filler Content

1. *Filled*
   - Purpose of filler: To increase bond strength and increase resistance to abrasion and wear.

- Fillers: Glass and quartz particles give hardness and strength to resist occlusal forces.
- Effect: Viscosity of the sealant is increased. Flow into the depth of a fissure varies.
2. *Unfilled*
   - Clear, does not contain particles.
   - Less resistant to abrasion and wear.
   - May not require occlusal adjustment when placed, so at an advantage during school and community health programs where sealants are placed.
3. *Fluoride releasing*
   - Purpose: enhance caries resistance.
   - Action: remineralization of incipient caries at base of pit or fissure.

C. Classification by Color

- Available: clear, tinted, and opaque.
- Purpose: quick identification for evaluation during maintenance assessment.
- Effect: clear, tinted, or opaque sealants do not differ in retention.

INDICATIONS FOR SEALANT PLACEMENT

I. PATIENTS WITH RISK FOR DENTAL CARIES (ANY AGE)

- Xerostomia: from medications or other reasons.
- Patient undergoing orthodontics.
- Incipient caries (limited to enamel) and there is no radiographic evidence of caries on adjacent proximal surface.

II. TEETH

- Newly erupted: place sealant as soon after eruption as possible.
- Occlusal contour: when pit or fissure is deep and irregular.
- Caries history: other teeth restored or have carious lesions.

III. CONTRAINDICATIONS

- Radiographic evidence of adjacent proximal dental caries.
- Pit and fissures are well coalesced and self-cleansing; low caries risk.

IV. SELECTION OF TEETH

Figure 36-2 is a flowchart to assist in decision making.

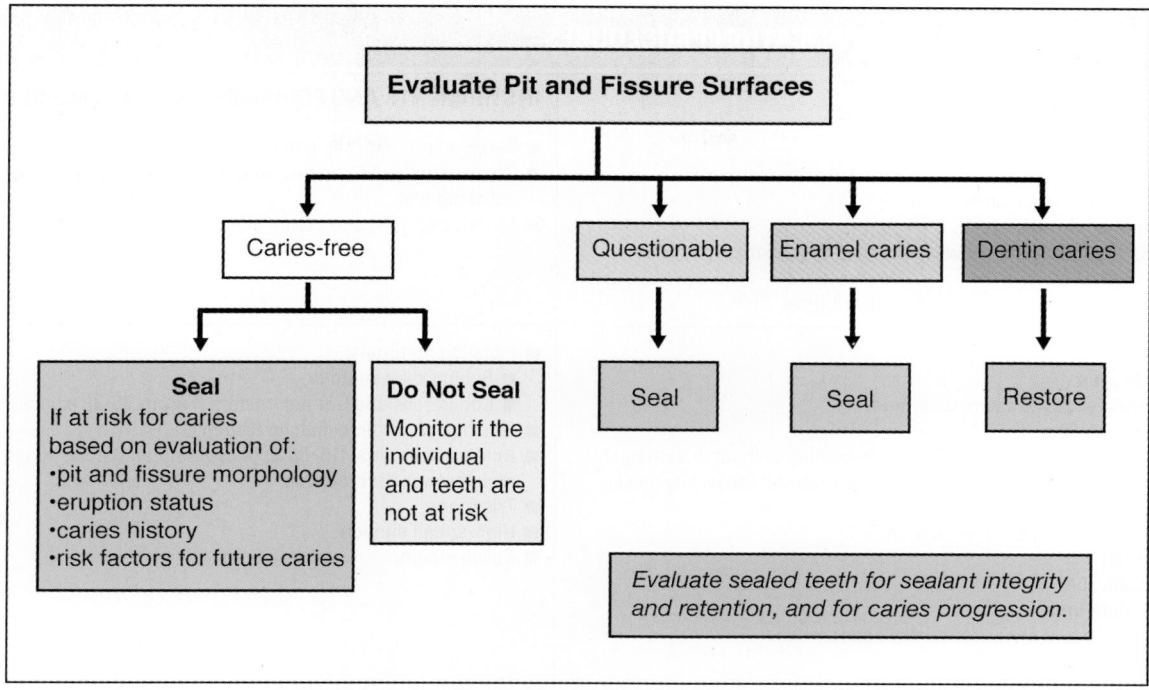

FIGURE 36-2 **Tooth Selection for Sealant Placement.** Flow chart to assist in decision making for placement of sealants. (Adapted with permission from Workshop on guidelines for sealant use: recommendations. The Association of State and Territorial Dental Directors, the New York State Health Department, the Ohio Department of Health and the School of Public Health, University of Albany, State University of New York. *J Public Health Dent.* 1995;55(5 Spec):263–73.)

 CLINICAL PROCEDURES

I. GENERAL RULES

- Treat each quadrant separately.
- Use four-handed method with assistant
  A. To ensure moisture control.
  B. To work efficiently and save time.
- Follow manufacturer's directions for each product.
- Success of treatment (retention) depends on the precision in each step of the application.
- Retention of sealant depends on maintaining a dry field during etching and sealant placement.
- Steps in procedure: follow the outline in **Table 36-1**.

II. PATIENT PREPARATION

- Explain the procedure and steps to be performed.
- The patient must wear safety eyewear for both protection from the chemicals of etching and sealant, and also from the light of the curing lamp.

III. PREPARATION OF TOOTH

A. Purposes

1. Remove deposits and debris.
2. Permit maximum contact of the etch and the sealant with the enamel surface.
3. Encourage sealant penetration into the pit or fissure.

B. Examine the Surfaces: Remove Calculus and Stains

C. Patient With No Stain or Calculus

1. Request patient to brush; apply filaments straight into occlusal pits and fissures (Figure 27-14A).
2. Suction the pits and fissures with high-velocity evacuator.
3. Use explorer tip to dig out debris and bacteria from the pit or fissure.
4. Suction again to remove loosened material.
5. Evaluate for additional cleaning; the brushing may be sufficient.

D. Cleansing Procedure: Choices

1. Polishing cup and brush with pumice; low-speed handpiece.
   - Disadvantage: pumice particles become lodged in the pits and not rinsed out.
   - Alternative: use bristle brush with clear water.
2. Air-powder polisher.[3,4]
3. Rinse out thoroughly.

IV. ISOLATION

A. Purposes of Isolation

- Keep the tooth clean and dry for optimal action and bonding of the sealant.

TABLE 36-1	SEALANT APPLICATION PROCEDURES

PROCEDURE: WHAT TO DO	INSTRUMENTS AND EQUIPMENT: WHAT IS NEEDED
Preparation ■ Set up tray. ■ Seat patient comfortably. ■ **Debride** occlusal surface. ■ Use toothbrush, air-powder polisher device or prophy brush. ■ **Rinse** for 20–30 s. ■ **Evaluate** teeth to be sealed clinically **(Figure 36-2)**.	■ Safety glasses for the patient ■ Prophy angle and brushes, toothbrush, or an air-powder polishing unit ■ Mirror, explorer, and cotton pliers

Etching
■ **Isolate area.**
■ **Dry** area for 20–30 s with trisyringe.
■ **Etch** for 30–60 s.
  ■ Gel: brush on surface and leave in contact without disturbing it.
  ■ Liquid: cover surface and continue to keep surface wet by adding.
  ■ Do not rub.
■ **Rinse** until surface is free of etch.
  ■ Gel: 60 s
  ■ Liquid: 30 s
■ **Re-isolate area**
■ **Dry** for 20 s and check for chalky appearance.
■ *If not chalky, re-etch.*
	■ Isolation materials:
	  ■ Rubber dam setup or
	  ■ Cotton rolls and Garmer holders **(Figure 36-3)**, bibulous pads
	■ Brushes or cotton pellets to dispense
	■ Acid etch material (15–50%) phosphoric etch acid, additional etch throughout etch time
	■ Trisyringe
	■ High-speed suction
	■ Saliva ejector

Application
■ **Apply** sealant material.
  ■ Mix autopolymerized sealant material prior.
  ■ Light-cured needs no mixing.
■ **Cure** while maintaining a dry field.
	■ Sealant material
	■ Brushes or flow tubes or cannulas for placement to dispense sealant material
	■ Mixing sticks (if using self-cured)
	■ Material tray or waxed paper pad
	■ Ultraviolet safety glasses or shield for clinician
	■ Timer or watch with a second hand

Evaluation ■ Evaluate the placed sealant for voids and air bubbles ■ Add additional sealant if necessary. ■ Re-etch before placement of material if salivary contamination occurs. ■ Check occlusion with articulating paper, adjust if sealant interferes with occlusion. ■ Floss contact areas.	■ Articulation paper ■ Dental floss ■ Fluoride gel and trays
Follow-Up ■ Educate the patient. ■ Administer fluoride treatment. ■ Re-evaluate at each subsequent appointment.	

■ Eliminate possible contamination by saliva and moisture from the breath.
■ Keep the materials from contacting the oral tissues, being swallowed accidentally, or being unpleasant to the patient because of flavor.

B. Rubber Dam

■ Rubber dam application is the method of choice because the most complete isolation is obtained. This method is especially helpful when more than one tooth in the same quadrant is to be sealed.
■ Rubber dam is essential when profuse saliva flow and overactive tongue and oral muscles make retraction and consistent maintenance of a dry, clean field impossible.

■ Combined treatment is planned. When a quadrant has a rubber dam and anesthesia for restoration of other teeth, teeth indicated for sealant can be treated.
■ Use anesthesia when application of the clamp cannot be tolerated by the patient.
■ Rubber dam may not be possible when a tooth that is essential for holding the clamp is not fully erupted.

C. Cotton-Roll Isolation

■ Patient position: tilt head to allow saliva to pool on the opposite side of the mouth.
■ Position cotton-roll holder (Garmer holder, **Figure 36-3**).
■ Place saliva ejector.

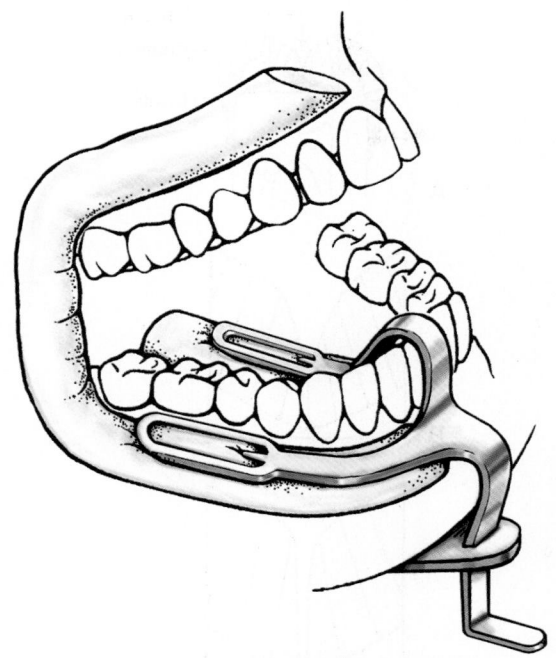

FIGURE 36-3 **Isolation Using Cotton-Roll Holders.** Two quadrants can be treated simultaneously. A continuous cotton roll extends from the mandibular anterior vestibule to the maxillary anterior vestibule. Bevel end of cotton rolls to facilitate retention. Lingual prong holds cotton roll adjacent to tongue over floor of the mouth.

- Apply triangular saliva absorber over the opening of the parotid duct in the cheek (bibulous pad).
- Take great care to prevent contamination from entering the area to be etched.

V. DRY THE TOOTH

A. Purposes

- Prepare the tooth for acid etch.
- Eliminate moisture and contamination.

B. Use Clean Air

- Clear the air by releasing the spray into a sink.
- Test for absence of moisture by blowing on a mouth mirror or other dry surface.

C. Time

- Air dry the tooth for at least 10 seconds.

VI. ACID ETCHING

A. Action

- Create micropores to increase the surface area and provide retention for the sealant **(Figure 36-1)**.
- Remove contamination from enamel surface.
- Provide antibacterial action.

B. Etch Forms

- *Phosphoric acid:* 15 to 50%, depends on product and manufacturer.
- *Liquid:* Low viscosity allows good flow into pit or fissure but may be difficult to control.
- *Gel:* Tinted gel with thick consistency allows increased visibility and control but may be difficult to rinse off the tooth surface.
- *Semi-gel:* Tinted, with viscosity between the gel form and the liquid allows good visibility, control, and rinsing ease.

C. Etch Timing

- Varies from 15 to 60 seconds. Follow manufacturer's instructions for each product.

D. Etch Delivery

- *Liquid etch:* Use a small brush, sponge, or cotton pellet; apply continuously throughout the etch time to keep the surface moist; do not rub, pat.
- *Gel and semi-gel:* use a syringe, brush, or manufacturer-supplied single-use cannula.

E. Completion of Etching

- Rinse thoroughly; apply suction to prevent saliva from reaching the etched surface.
- Dry, and examine the etched surface.
- Repeat etching process if the surface does not appear white and chalky.
- Dry for 15 to 20 seconds; maintain dry isolation ready for sealant application.

VII. SEALANT APPLICATION

A. Follow Manufacturer's Instructions

B. General Instructions

- Avoid overmanipulation to prevent producing air bubbles.
- Use disposable implement supplied for application.
- Cover all pits and fissures but do not overfill to a high, flat surface.
- After placement: leave in place for 10 seconds to allow for optimum penetration.

C. Curing

- *Timing:* 20 to 30 seconds in accord with manufacturer's instructions. Longer curing time is related to increased retention.
- *Apply curing light:* Use eye protection. Cover entire tooth surface to allow complete polymerization.
- *Check for voids:* Material can be added if surface has not been contaminated or wet.

VIII. OCCLUSION[5,6]

- Use articulating paper to locate high spots; adjust as required.
- Occlusal wear: unfilled sealants wear down to correct height; filled sealants require occlusal adjustment.

PENETRATION OF SEALANT

The penetration of a sealant depends on the following:

- The configuration of the pit or fissure
- The presence of deposits and debris within the pit or fissure
- The properties of the sealant itself

I. PIT AND FISSURE ANATOMY

A review of the anatomy of pits and fissures may be helpful in understanding the effects of sealants in the prevention of dental caries. The shape and depth of pits and fissures vary considerably even within one tooth.

- *Wide V-shaped* (**Figure 36-4B**) or *narrow V-shaped*.
- *Long narrow pits* and grooves reach to, or nearly to, the dentinoenamel junction (**Figure 36-4C**).
- *Long constricted form with a bulbous terminal portion* (**Figure 34-4D**). The pit or fissure may take a wavy course; it may not lead directly from the outer surface to the dentinoenamel junction.

II. CONTENTS OF A PIT OR FISSURE

A pit or fissure contains the following:

- Dental biofilm, pellicle, debris
- Rarely but possibly intact remnants of tooth development

III. EFFECT OF CLEANING

- The narrow, long fissures are difficult to clean completely.
- Retained cleaning material can block the sealant from filling the fissure and can also become mixed with the sealant.
- Removal of pumice used for cleaning and thorough washing are necessary for the success of the sealant.

IV. AMOUNT OF PENETRATION

- Wide V-shaped and shallow fissures are more apt to be filled by sealant (**Figure 36-5B**).
- Although ideally the sealant penetrates to the bottom of a pit or fissure, such penetration is frequently impossible.
- Microscopic examination of pits and fissures after sealant application has shown that the sealant does not penetrate to the bottom because residual debris,

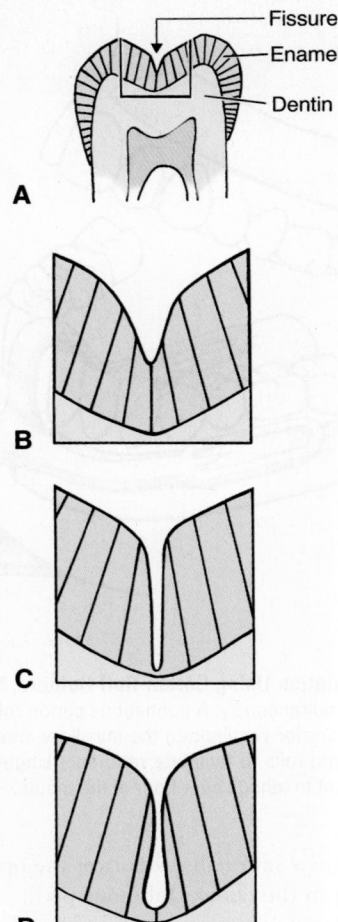

FIGURE 36-4 Occlusal Fissures. Drawings made from microscopic slides show variations in shape and depth of fissures. **(A)** Tooth with section enlarged for B, C, and D. **(B)** Wide V-shaped fissure. **(C)** Long narrow groove that reaches nearly to the dentinoenamel junction. **(D)** Long constricted form with a bulbous terminal portion.

cleansing agents, and trapped air prevent passage of the material (**Figure 34-5C** and **D**).

- Incipient dental caries at the base of a well-sealed pit or fissure has no access to nutrients required for survival.

MAINTENANCE

I. REEXAMINATION

At each maintenance appointment, or at least every 6 months, each sealant needs to be examined for deficiencies that may have developed.

II. RETENTION

A. Retention Time

- Sealants can be retained for many years.[7]
- Although surface sealant may be lost, sealant in the pits and fissures and sealant that penetrated into the microspaces of the enamel can still remain and provide some protection.[8]

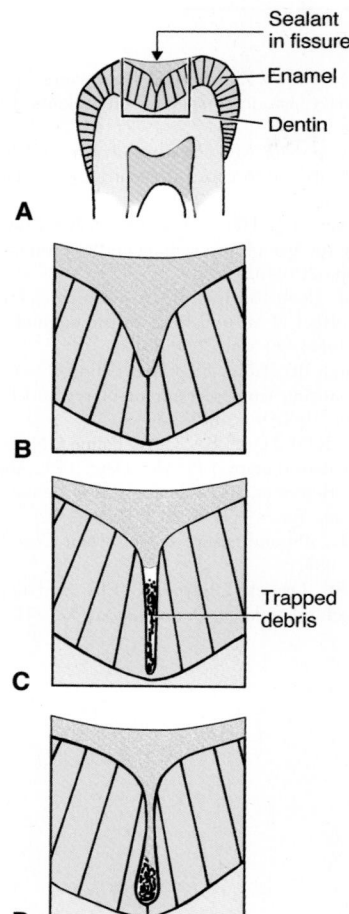

A

B

C

Trapped debris

D

FIGURE 36-5 **Pit and Fissure Sealant in Fissures.** Drawings made from microscopic slides show extent to which sealant may fill a fissure. **(A)** Tooth with section enlarged for B, C, and D. **(B)** Sealant fills wide V-shaped fissure and extends a short way up the slopes of surrounding cusps. **(C)** and **(D)** Fissures partially filled as a result of narrow constriction of the groove and blockage by trapped debris.

Labels in figure A: Sealant in fissure; Enamel; Dentin

B. Factors Affecting Retention

■ *During placement:* precision of technique with exclusion of moisture and contamination.
■ *Care of existing sealants.* Avoid using an air-powder polisher on intact existing sealants during maintenance appointments. Sealant wear increases with time of exposure to air-powder polisher abrasion.[9]

III. REPLACEMENT

A. Consult the manufacturer's instructions.
B. Tooth preparation: same as for original application.
C. Removal of firmly attached sections of retained sealant is not usually necessary.
D. Re-etching of the tooth surface is always essential.

DOCUMENTATION

Documentation in the record of a patient receiving a sealant needs to contain a minimum of the following:

■ Reason for selection of certain teeth for sealants; informed consent of patient, parent or other caregiver.
■ Type of sealant used, preparation of tooth, manner of isolation, patient cooperation during administration; post-insertion instructions given.
■ A sample progress note may be reviewed in **Box 36-2**.

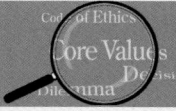

Everyday Ethics

Lillian had always enjoyed doing sealants when she was in dental hygiene school. They had been required to do quite a few, and as students they got to participate in "Sealant Day," a volunteer program carried out by the local dental hygienists every spring.

Now, when she came back from the state dental hygiene meeting, she was all excited about the new interpretation of the practice act by the Dental Board and greeted her employer, Dr. Fine, with the news the first thing Monday morning. The Board had voted that the dental hygienist who had been in practice for 2 years full-time (or part-time equivalent) could make the decision whether a pit or fissure needed a sealant. There was a continuing education course and an examination required.

Lillian added: "Remember Jack—that teenager that was here last week? He had some really deep fissures that I was sure would benefit from sealants. Can I go ahead and schedule him? I told him he needed them. He has an appointment with you to have a few cavities filled, but that wouldn't fit in

your book until nearly the end of the month. They are giving the exam and CE next week."

Dr. Fine continued quietly to tie on his gown for the first patient, and then he smiled and said, "Well, Lil, let's wait until he comes in for his appointment with me and I'll look at them."

Questions for Consideration
1. Professionally, what action(s) can Lillian take to initiate a system of calibration between her and Dr. Fine to pursue the new practice protocols?
2. What ethical issues may be involved here? How can they be resolved?
3. Which of the core values describe the friendly relationship between Lillian and Dr. Fine? And which core values describe Lillian's wishes to extend the services for Jack's (the patient's) benefit?

BOX 36-2	Example Progress Note

Clara (age 9) scheduled for two sealants in occlusals of 3 and 30, very inquisitive and interested in what was going on. As I was getting ready she said "how long will these last? I answered they would last a very long time, at least until she is 25. She said 'this one down here (pointing to #30, "wasn't in very long—that's why Mom wants you to do it over." Shocked, I asked if the other person did it same as I am—she said "I dunno it didn't hurt anyway." *Told her* I was doing it a real special way, nice and dry—it should be perfect. (So I made a double effort to clean the pit and keep it dry with a cotton roll holder and saliva ejector.) Scheduled in a week for the other side.

Signed:_____, RDH Date:_____

Factors To Teach The Patient

- Sealants are part of a total preventive program. Sealants are not substitutes for other preventive measures. Limitations of dietary sucrose, use of fluorides, and dental biofilm control are major factors with sealants for prevention of dental caries.
- What a sealant is and why such a meticulous application procedure is required.
- What can be expected from a sealant; how long it lasts, how it prevents dental caries.
- Need for examination of the sealant at frequent, scheduled appointments, and need for replacement when indicated.

References

1. Handleman SL, Shey Z. Michael Buonocore and the Eastman Dental Center. A historic perspective on sealants. *J Dent Res.* 1996 Jan;75(1):529–34.
2. Cueto EI, Buonocore MG. Sealing of pits and fissures with an adhesive resin: its use in caries prevention. *J Am Dent Assoc.* 1967 Jul;75(1):121–8.
3. Scott L, Brockmann S, Houston G, Tira D. Retention of dental sealants following the use of airpolishing and traditional cleaning. *Dent Hyg.* 1977 Sep;62(8):402–6.
4. Brockmann SL, Scott RL, Eick JD. A scanning electron microscopic study of the effect of air polishing on the enamel-sealant surface. *Quintessence Int.* 1990 Mar;21(3):201–6.
5. Stach DJ, Hatch RA, Tilliss TS, Cross-Poline GN. Change in occlusal height resulting from placement of pit and fissure sealants. *J Prosthet Dent.* 1992 Nov;68(5):750–3.
6. Tilliss TS, Stach DJ, Hatch RA, Cross-Poline GN. Occlusal discrepancies after sealant therapy. *J Prosthet Dent.* 1992 Aug;68(2):223–8.
7. Simonsen RJ. Retention and effectiveness of dental sealant after 15 years. *J Am Dent Assoc.* 1991 Oct;122(10):34–42.
8. Buonocore MG. Pit and fissure sealing. *Dent Clin North Am.* 1975 Apr;19(2):367–83.
9. Huennekens SC, Daniel SJ, Bayne SC. Effects of air polishing on the abrasion of occlusal sealants. *Quintessence Int.* 1991 Jul;22(7):581–5.

Implementation: Treatment

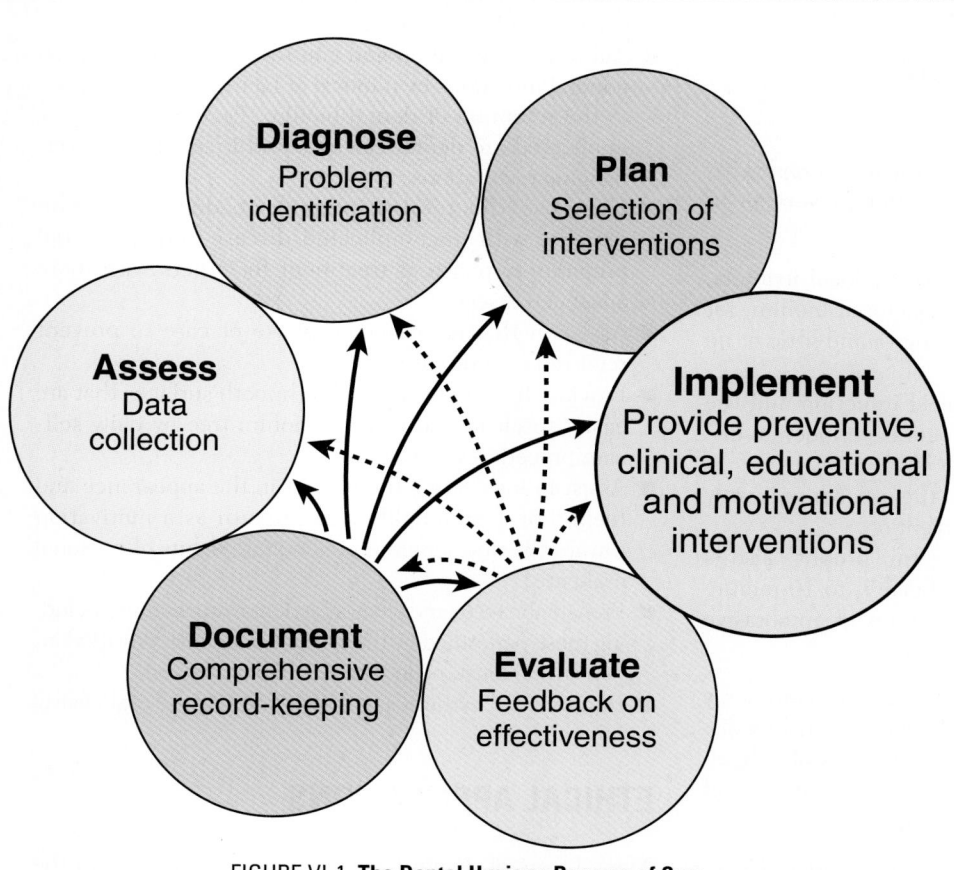

FIGURE VI-1 **The Dental Hygiene Process of Care.**

INTRODUCTION

Instrumentation for scaling, root planing, extrinsic stain removal, care of dental restorations, and postcare procedures are included in Section VI. Placement and removal of dressings, removal of sutures, and treatment of hypersensitive teeth are described. Immediate evaluation of techniques and their effects, short-term follow-up, and maintenance assessment follow instrumentation. These procedures are all part of dental hygiene implementation of treatment using nonsurgical periodontal therapy and preventive care as a part of the Dental Hygiene Process of Care (**Figure VI-1**, page 551).

The first objective of treatment is to create an environment in which the tissues can return to health.

- In the sequence of patient treatment, introduction to preventive measures occurs first, before professional instrumentation.
- After health has been attained, the patient's self-care on a daily basis is essential to keep the teeth and gingival tissues free from new or recurrent inflammatory disease caused by the microorganisms of dental biofilm.
- Professional instrumentation makes a limited contribution to arresting the progression of disease without daily biofilm control measures performed by the patient.

ORAL PROPHYLAXIS VERSUS PERIODONTAL THERAPY

As defined in any medical dictionary, the term *prophylaxis* refers to actions that are undertaken for prevention of disease.

- *Oral prophylaxis* is aimed at removing local irritants, including all calculus as well as bacterial biofilm, for a patient with relatively healthy gingiva and little or no attachment loss.
- The purpose is to prevent gingival infection and the loss of attachment that can happen as periodontal disease progresses.
- Performed with these objectives, the procedure is truly a preventive dental hygiene intervention.
- Unfortunately, the abbreviated term "prophy" also is sometimes used to mean a superficial 5- to 10-minute application of a rubber polishing cup with an abrasive paste to the enamel surfaces.

The term *therapy,* on the other hand, most commonly refers to treatment that is aimed at healing an existing disease or condition. *Periodontal therapy* consists of subgingival instrumentation that is applied in the presence of diagnosed periodontal or gingival disease.

- *Periodontal therapy* takes the form of subgingival scaling, root planing, and overall debridement. All calculus, biofilm, and toxins clinging to the tooth and root surface are removed with the express goal of eliminating active disease and creating clean, smooth, toxin-free tooth and root surfaces.
- Thorough periodontal instrumentation enhances reattachment and allows healing of gingival tissues.
- Continuing care, provided following periodontal therapy intervention, is referred to as *periodontal maintenance.*

The professional dental hygienist has a responsibility to assess each patient's oral health status thoroughly, determine any disease state, and select appropriate dental hygiene interventions based on the patient's individual needs. Appropriate terminology to discuss and document dental hygiene interventions will enhance understanding and help patients and health professions' colleagues develop a meaningful concept of dental hygiene practice.

OBJECTIVES OF TREATMENT

For each type of instrumentation, specific objectives are included that describe the details of the technique. General objectives of dental hygiene instrumentation are as follows:

- Create an environment in which the tissues can return to health and then be maintained in health.
- Eliminate or suppress periodontal pathogenic microorganisms and control reinfection.
- Aid in the prevention and control of gingival and periodontal infections by removal of factors that predispose to the retention of dental biofilm. Factors particularly implicated are dental calculus and irregular and overhanging restorations.
- Compose the total treatment needed for certain patients with uncomplicated disease and the initial preparatory phase of treatment for others with more advanced disease.
- Assist in the maintenance phase of care to prevent recurrence of disease.
- Provide the patient with smooth tooth surfaces that are easier to clean and to keep biofilm-free by daily self-care procedures.
- Assist in instructing the patient in the appearance and feeling of a thoroughly clean mouth as a motivation toward the development of adequate habits of personal oral care.
- Prepare the teeth and gingiva for dental procedures, including those performed by the restorative dentist, prosthodontist, orthodontist, pedodontist, and oral surgeon.
- Improve oral esthetics and sanitation of the oral cavity.

ETHICAL APPLICATIONS

Many facets of dental hygiene care relate directly to the provider-patient relationship and surrounding professional issues.

TABLE VI-1	ETHICAL AND PROFESSIONAL ISSUES	
PROFESSIONAL ISSUES	**EXPLANATION**	**APPLICATION EXAMPLES**
Expressed or Implied Contracts	An agreement to perform tasks that can be written (third-party payment) or oral (between provider and patient) for a course of treatment.	(1) Coding of dental hygiene services based on current edition of Current Dental Terminology (CDT) guidelines. (2) Documenting a code for a gingivitis diagnosis versus periodontal maintenance.
Whistle-Blowing	The disclosure of illegal or immoral wrongs that are under the control of the individual practitioner. May involve negligent acts.	(1) Reporting the lack of infection control procedures. (2) Reporting the actions of an impaired colleague to a state dental board.
Privacy Rights	Involves the reform of health information through protection of privacy, insurance access, preventing fraud and abuse, and standardization within the healthcare industry.	Health Insurance Portability & Accountability the confidentiality of dental records, especially where computers are used to document patient data.
Supervision	The ethical and legal working relationship between the dentist, dental hygienist, and other dental personnel.	A dental hygienist rendering treatment to patients of record that now reside in a nursing home

■ Concerns such as insurance contracts, whistle-blowing, and maintaining privacy rights of patients affect the overall delivery of dental services.

■ The dental hygienist acknowledges the ethical implications of providing care beyond the treatment alone.

■ Thus, the conduct of the professional dental hygienist prior to, during, and following the dental hygiene appointment is subject to moral assessment.

Both rights and duties are significant in the ongoing relationship between the patient and the dental hygienist.

■ A responsibility exists to treat patients equitably, aware of their best interest at all times.

■ Practicing a consistent and professional demeanor with all patients and all members of the dental team can be achieved and will uphold high standards and quality of care. Several ethical and professional issues to be considered are found in **Table VI-1**.

Anxiety and Pain Control

DONNA J. STACH, BS, RDH, MEd

Chapter Outline

Concern for patient anxiety and pain is an integral part of a dental hygiene appointment. Recognizing and managing a patient's anxiety and pain is an essential part of dental hygiene care planning. The decision to use a pharmacologic agent for management of anxiety and pain is dependent on a number of factors. Periodontal health status, the treatment being rendered, and the patient's pain threshold must all be considered. Pain threshold is highly individual and variable. **Box 37-1** provides terminology and definitions relative to anxiety and pain and to their management.

COMPONENTS OF PAIN

There are two components of pain. *Pain perception* is primarily a neurologic experience of pain; *pain reaction* is the personal interpretation and response to the pain message. Pain may occur during or following treatment.

I. PAIN PERCEPTION

- Relates to the physical process of receiving a painful stimulus and transmitting the information through the nervous system to the brain.
- In the brain, it is interpreted as pain.
- There is little variability in pain perception between individuals with intact nervous systems.

II. PAIN REACTION

- The reaction is a combination of the interpretation and the response to the pain message.
- The reaction is highly variable between individuals and even in the same individual at different times.
- Accounts for much of the variability seen between patients in personal pain management needs.
- Many factors influence pain reaction. Factors included are age, fatigue, emotional state, and both cultural and ethnic learned behaviors.
- The presence of anxiety has special significance because with anxiety the patient is predisposed to feel pain.
- People with a strong or rapid reaction to pain are said to have a low pain threshold.

PAIN CONTROL MECHANISMS

Five pain control mechanisms are available. They are often combined for optimum effect. Decisions about anxiety and pain management are included during dental hygiene care planning and written into the care plan. It is important to match the pain control method to the patient's treatment needs and medical status. All pain management techniques are more effective if utilized before the patient experiences pain.

The five categories of pain control mechanisms are the following:

I. REMOVE THE PAINFUL STIMULUS

- Affects pain perception.
- Examples: patient avoids dental appointment; clinician corrects faulty, pain-causing instrument technique.

II. BLOCK THE PATHWAY OF THE PAIN MESSAGE

- Affects pain perception.
- Examples: use of local anesthetic, topical anesthetic.

III. PREVENT PAIN REACTION BY RAISING PAIN REACTION THRESHOLD

- Affects pain reaction.
- Examples: use of nitrous oxide–oxygen conscious sedation; nonopioid analgesics such as nonsteroidal anti-inflammatory drugs (NSAIDs).

IV. DEPRESS CENTRAL NERVOUS SYSTEM

- Affects pain reaction.
- Example: general anesthesia.

V. USE PSYCHOSEDATION METHODS (ALSO CALLED IATROSEDATION)

- Affects both pain perception and pain reaction.
- Includes any nonpharmacologic technique that reduces patient anxiety, builds a trust relationship, or lets the patient feel more in control.
- May be used alone or may be combined with pharmacologic pain management.
- Examples: Explain procedures carefully; allow patient to express concerns; use relaxation or distraction techniques.

BOX 37-1	Key Words

Anxiety and Pain Control

Ambient air: surrounding atmosphere.

Analgesia: diminution or elimination of pain in the conscious patient.

Anesthesia: loss of feeling or sensation, especially loss of tactile sensitivity, with or without loss of consciousness.

Block anesthesia: induced by injecting the anesthetic close to a nerve trunk; may be at some distance from the area to be treated.

General anesthesia: the elimination of all sensations, accompanied by the loss of consciousness.

Infiltration anesthesia: induced by injecting the anesthetic directly into or around the tissues to be anesthetized.

Local anesthesia: loss of sensation, especially pain, in a circumscribed area without loss of consciousness; also called regional anesthesia.

Noninjectable local anesthesia: a thermosetting anesthetic gel extruded into the periodontal pocket results in loss of sensation to the adjacent soft tissue and typically partial dental/pulpal anesthesia.

Topical anesthesia: a form of local anesthesia whereby free nerve endings in accessible structures are rendered incapable of stimulation by the application of an anesthetic drug directly to the surface of the area.

Anxiety: a negative, emotional response to an anticipated event, the outcome of which is unknown. This is a learned response from personal experience or the stories of others.

Aspiration: recommended technique for preventing injection of local anesthetic directly into circulatory system. Negative pressure is created in anesthetic cartridge. If needle tip is in artery or vein, blood will be visible in cartridge.

Conscious: state in which patient is capable of rational response to commands and protective reflexes are intact, including the ability to maintain a patent airway independently and continuously.

Conscious sedation: the calming or allaying of nervous excitement while maintaining a conscious state by pharmacologic, nonpharmacologic, or combined methods.

Epinephrine: a hormone secreted by the adrenal medulla that, among many functions, causes vasodilation of blood vessels of skeletal muscles, vasoconstriction of arterioles of skin and mucous membranes, and stimulation of heart action; used in local anesthetics for its vasoconstrictive action.

Hypoxia: diminished availability of oxygen to body tissues.

Diffusion hypoxia: lack of adequate amounts of oxygen that can result from the rapid diffusion of nitrous oxide molecules from the blood stream into the lungs. Occurs if 100% oxygen is not administered at the conclusion of a nitrous oxide–oxygen sedation procedure.

Iatrosedation: reduction of anxiety as a result of the clinician's behavior or actions. A psychosomatic method of pain control.

Metered spray: a method for dispensing topical anesthetic that administers a fixed volume of drug and then stops automatically.

Occupational exposure: subject to an action or influence, usually negative, as a result of one's occupation or work environment.

Pain: a sensation in which a person experiences discomfort, distress, or suffering; may vary in intensity from mild discomfort to intolerable agony.

Pain threshold: point at which a sensation starts to be painful and a response results. Varies between individuals based on interpretation of sensation. May be altered by some drugs.

High pain threshold: a greater than average tolerance to a painful stimulus.

Low pain threshold: a strong or rapid reaction to a painful stimulus.

Potency: strength of a drug. Amount of a medication or drug necessary to achieve a desired effect.

Psychosomatic method: any nonpharmacologic technique that reduces anxiety and improves pain control. Effective because the mind influences the body's perception and interpretation of pain.

Scavenging device: that part of the nitrous oxide equipment that collects exhaled nitrous oxide and removes it. The main component is the scavenging nasal hood. Since 1980, the American Dental Association has recommended that effective scavenging devices be installed whenever nitrous oxide is used to reduce occupational exposure.

Sedation: one of the stages of anesthesia in which the patient is still conscious but is under the influence of a central nervous system depressant drug.

Titration: a technique for individualization of drug dose. Administration of small, incremental dose of a drug until the desired clinical action is observed.

Vasoconstrictor: a drug that constricts blood vessels. An additive to most local anesthetic solutions to offset the vasodilating actions of the local anesthetic.

NONOPIOID ANALGESICS

Over-the-counter (OTC) analgesics are an effective adjunct for preventing or reducing the mild to moderate discomfort that patients experience during dental hygiene therapy or postoperatively.

I. DRUGS

■ Nonsteroidal anti-inflammatory drugs (NSAIDs).
  ■ The drugs of choice for dental pain.[1]
  ■ Ibuprofen: Details are shown in **Box 37-2**.
■ Acetaminophen.

BOX 37-2	Ibuprofen*

Analgesic Activity
Onset: 30 minutes after administration.
Peak analgesic: 2–3 hours after administration.
Maintenance analgesia: Administer second dose 4 hours after initial dose.

Suggestions for Time of Administration
For treatment pain: Take 2 hours before.
For postoperative pain without local anesthetic: Take immediately before treatment.
For postoperative pain with local anesthetic: Take at completion of treatment.

*Ibuprofen is considered the drug of choice for dental pain.

II. ACTION OF NSAIDs

- Blocks prostaglandin synthesis at peripheral nerve endings to inhibit generation of pain message.[2]
- Suppresses onset of pain.
- Decreases pain severity.

III. INDICATIONS

- Mild to moderate pain during treatment.
- Mild to moderate pain postoperatively.

NITROUS OXIDE–OXYGEN SEDATION

The gases nitrous oxide and oxygen, in combination, are widely used in dental and dental hygiene practice settings. A state of conscious sedation is produced with the patient awake, relaxed, responsive to commands, able to cooperate with treatment, and having intact protective reflexes. The patient has some degree of analgesia and a higher pain reaction threshold.

CHARACTERISTICS OF NITROUS OXIDE

I. ANESTHETIC AND ANALGESIC PROPERTIES

- Produces analgesia.
- Achieves optimum analgesia and patient cooperation at 30 to 40% nitrous oxide for most patients. The need for higher or lower concentrations depends on individual biologic variability.
- Reduces the intensity of pain but does not block it; only mildly potent as an anesthetic gas.
- Combines with local anesthetic when the patient experiences significant discomfort.

II. CHEMICAL AND PHYSICAL PROPERTIES

- Gas at room temperature and pressure.
- Heavier than air.
- Colorless; sweet smelling.
- Nonirritating and nonallergenic.
- Nonflammable but will support the combustion of flammable substances.

III. BLOOD SOLUBILITY

- Relatively insoluble in blood; primary saturation of blood occurs in 3 to 5 minutes.[3]
- The gas molecules at the alveoli-blood interface and blood-brain interface pass readily to the tissue with the lowest concentration of nitrous oxide.
  - Results in rapid onset and recovery.
  - Results in potential diffusion hypoxia at completion of sedation procedure if 100% oxygen is not administered.

IV. PHARMACOLOGY OF NITROUS OXIDE

- Is not metabolized in the body; remains unchanged in blood and tissues.
- Enters and exits almost entirely through the lungs.

EQUIPMENT FOR NITROUS OXIDE–OXYGEN

- The equipment for nitrous oxide–oxygen conscious sedation is available as a portable unit or a central storage system with gas piped to individual treatment rooms.
- Currently available units have several built-in safety features to ensure that a minimal level of oxygen is always delivered and that the two gases could not be reversed inadvertently in delivery.
- The equipment can be divided into three basic parts: gas storage cylinders, a gas delivery system, and a scavenger system with the nasal hood (mask) having components of both the gas delivery and scavenger portions.

I. COMPRESSED GAS CYLINDERS

A. Nitrous Oxide

- *Color code:* Light blue.
- *Physical state:* Gas and liquid.
- *Pressure:* Constant at 750 pounds per square inch (psi) until almost empty.

B. Oxygen

- *Color code:* Green (international = white).
- *Physical state:* Gas.
- *Pressure:* Falls at a uniform rate with use from a full pressure of 2,000 psi or 2,200 psi for size E or H cylinders, respectively.

- *Use ratio:* About 2.5 cylinders of oxygen are used for each comparably sized cylinder of nitrous oxide.

C. Handle Carefully

- Use no grease, oil, lubricant, or hand cream around the cylinder valves or any fittings that come in contact with the gases.
- Store vertically on a rack or in another stable and secure manner.
- Open cylinder valves slowly in a counterclockwise direction.

II. GAS DELIVERY SYSTEM

A. Regulator or Reducing Valve

1. Converts high pressure of gas in the cylinders to a usable, lower level.
2. Subject to extreme high temperature if compressed gas cylinders are opened quickly.

B. Flow Meter

1. Visual indicator of liters per minute (l/min) flow of oxygen and nitrous oxide.
2. Flow meter comes in two designs:
   - Gas flow rates of nitrous oxide and oxygen are adjusted independently. The sum of the two is the total gas flow rate.
   - A total combined gas flow rate is established and the respective concentrations of the two gases are adjusted concurrently.

C. Reservoir Bag

1. Reservoir of gases to accommodate an exceptionally deep breath.
2. Allows for visualization of respirations for monitoring.
3. Degree of inflation can be used to help establish total flow rate of gas needed by the patient for comfortable respirations.
4. May be used to provide oxygen in assisted ventilation if attached to a full-face mask with relief valve.

D. Conducting or Breathing Tubes

III. NASAL HOOD, NOSE PIECE, MASK

- Deliver gas for patient inhalation.
- Collect exhaled gas and direct it into scavenger system.
- Good fit and seal around patient's nose are essential in size selection.
- Ideally, use a disposable item, or sterilize before each use.

IV. SCAVENGER SYSTEM

- Removes exhaled gas to keep nitrous oxide levels low in the ambient air of the treatment room.
- Connects to the office central evacuation system.
- Vents to outside of building and away from windows and air intakes.

V. SAFETY FEATURES

- *Universal color coding* of cylinders, hoses, flow controls for each gas.
- *Pin index* and *diameter index* safety systems physically prevent gas cylinders or hoses from being mistakenly interchanged between the gases due to incompatible placement of pins (projections) and diameter differences in the couplings.
- *Minimum oxygen flow,* 30% or 3 l/min.
- *Oxygen fail-safe system* automatically shuts off nitrous oxide if the oxygen falls below a minimum level.
- *Emergency air inlet* to provide room air if system shuts down.
- *Oxygen flush button* to supply 100% oxygen quickly.

VI. EQUIPMENT MAINTENANCE

A. Function Checks

- Maintain working order and safe practice by periodic checking of equipment.

B. Gas Leaks

- All equipment connections and rubber goods are subject to leaking. **Figure 37-1** shows the places that should be examined for tight connections, defects, and wear. Apply soapy water to connections; bubbles will form if leaks are present.

PATIENT SELECTION

I. INDICATIONS

- Patient with mild to moderate anxiety.
- Medically compromised patient who would benefit from additional oxygen and/or anxiety reduction. Examples: patient with a cardiovascular or cerebrovascular disease, or with stress-induced bronchial asthma.
- Procedures that are short in duration and cause a low level of pain. The analgesic effect is most pronounced on the soft tissues, making it especially useful during dental hygiene procedures.
- Patient with strong gag reflex.

II. CONTRAINDICATIONS

The gas is nonirritating to the respiratory system and does not interact chemically or biotransform within the body. There are no known allergies.

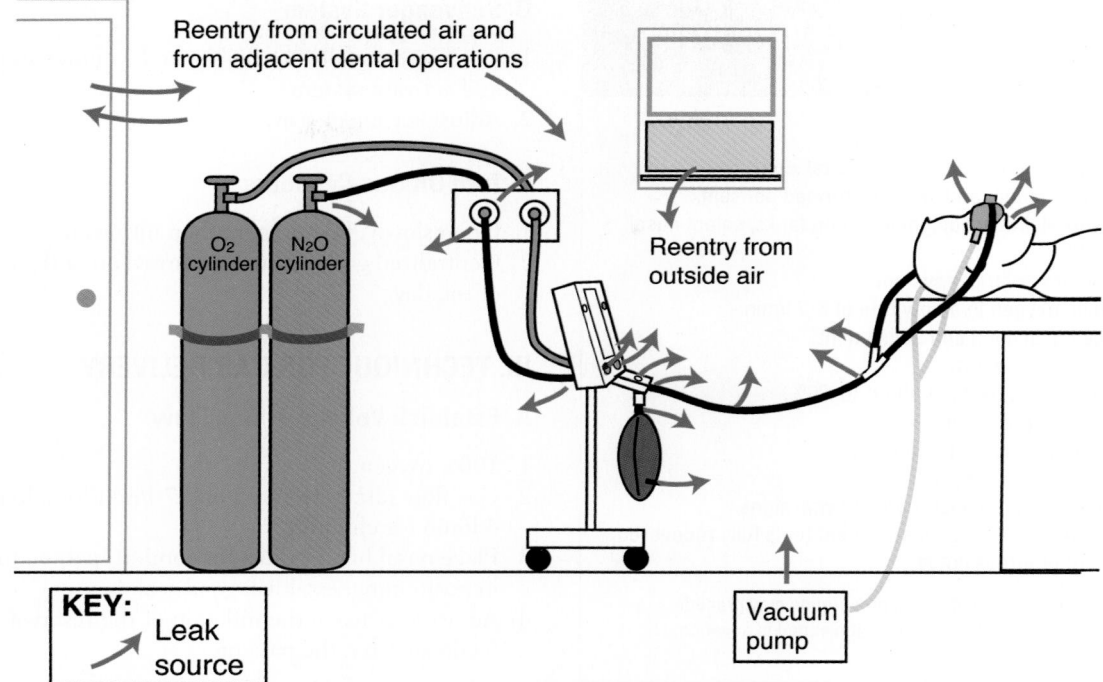

FIGURE 37-1 Potential Sources of Leaks from Nitrous Oxide/Oxygen Delivery Systems. Arrows show locations where regular inspection and testing is necessary. The most common sites of leakage are: *High-pressure connections:* from the gas delivery cylinders, the wall connectors, the hoses connecting to the anesthetic machine, and the anesthesia machine itself (especially the on-demand valve). *Low-pressure connections:* from the anesthetic flow meter and the scavenging mask. Look for loose-fitting connections, loosely assembled or deformed slip joints and threaded connections, defective or worn seals, and gaskets. *Rubber goods:* hoses and reservoir bag. Look for cracks and tears. (Adapted from National Institute for Occupational Safety and Health (US). Alert: controlling exposures to nitrous oxide during anesthetic administration. Cincinnati: US Department of Health, Education, and Welfare; 1994. p. 5. Publication No. 94–100. Joint publication of Public Health Service, Centers for Disease Control, National Institute for Occupational Safety and Health).

Individuals with the following conditions should be evaluated carefully before nitrous oxide–oxygen sedation:

■ Recent ophthalmic surgery using intraocular gases.
 ▪ Absolute contraindication following surgery with:
  1. Perfluoropropane for 8 weeks.
  2. Sulfur hexafluoride for 2 weeks.
 ▪ Vision damage could result from increased pressure on the eye during healing.[4]
■ Unable to cooperate and/or communicate.
 ▪ Unwilling to breathe through nose and/or leave nasal hood in place.
 ▪ Claustrophobia.
■ Moderate to severe chronic obstructive pulmonary disease (COPD). Examples: emphysema, chronic bronchitis.
■ Upper respiratory tract obstruction or infection if nose breathing would be difficult or breathing apparatus cannot be sterilized or replaced.
■ Conditions of confined air spaces within the body that would be adversely affected by increased pressure, such as middle ear or tympanic membrane problems, blockage of Eustachian tube or sinuses, bowel obstruction.

■ Severe personality disorders characterized by a tenuous grasp on reality.
■ Compulsive personalities who do not like the feeling of "losing control."
■ Patients who do not want nitrous oxide–oxygen sedation for any of a variety of personal reasons.
■ Severe vitamin B_{12} deficiency, as may result from gastric bypass surgery (more research needed).
■ Pregnancy
 ▪ Prudent practice would suggest that no elective drugs be administered during pregnancy, especially during the first trimester.
 ▪ Consultation with the patient's obstetrician is advisable.
 ▪ Second and third trimester: Dose and exposure should be kept to a minimum.
 ▪ May be sedation method of choice because of lack of effect in most organ systems, rapid removal from body, and lack of metabolism in the body.[5]

BOX 37-3	Steps in Nitrous Oxide/Oxygen Administration

1. Assess patient's medical status.
2. Take and record pretreatment vital signs.
3. Educate patient and secure informed consent.
4. Prepare delivery equipment (open tanks, select nasal hood).*
5. Activate scavenger system.
6. Turn on oxygen to a flow rate of 5–7 l/min.
7. Place nasal hood and adjust to fit.
8. Adjust gas flow rate.
9. Begin nitrous oxide at about 10–20%.
10. Titrate to optimum level.
11. Monitor throughout treatment.
12. Return to 100% oxygen.
13. Take and record posttreatment vital signs.
14. Remove nasal hood when patient feels fully recovered.
15. Record progress notes.

*Sequence may vary. Equipment preparation may precede patient assessment steps if treatment planned in advance.

CLINICAL PROCEDURES FOR NITROUS OXIDE–OXYGEN ADMINISTRATION

Box 37-3 lists the sequence of steps for nitrous oxide–oxygen administration.

I. PATIENT PREPARATION

A. Inform

- Before appointment
  - No specific food limitations but generally avoid fasting or heavy meals just before the appointment.
  - Wear comfortable clothing and loosen tight collars.
- At time of appointment
  - Explain procedure in positive terms. Stress the pleasant sense of relaxation; the patient will be aware and in control at all times.
  - Establish informed consent.

B. Assess

1. Evaluate patient's medical status.
2. Take and record vital signs.

II. EQUIPMENT PREPARATION

A. Nasal Hood

1. Select the appropriate size for optimum comfort and minimum gas leakage.
2. Attach to tubing.

B. Scavenger System

1. Connect, usually to high-speed volume evacuation, and activate system.
2. Adjust setting of scavenger system.

C. Turn On Gas Cylinders

1. Open slowly, first oxygen, then nitrous oxide.
2. Centralized gas systems are turned on at the beginning of the day.

III. TECHNIQUE FOR GAS DELIVERY

A. Establish Volume of Gas Flow

1. 100% oxygen.
2. Gas flow rate between 5 and 7 l/min for adults, 3 and 4 l/min for children.
3. Place nasal hood, adjust for comfort; patient may assist in positioning; establish good seal.
4. Adjust flow using the inflation of the reservoir bag and feedback from the patient.

B. Titration

Individualized drug dose is determined by increasing the percentage of nitrous oxide in small increments until the optimum sedation level is achieved based on clinical signs and symptoms.

1. *Initial concentration.* Start titration at about 10 to 15% concentration of nitrous oxide. Because of the rapid uptake of nitrous oxide in the lungs and distribution through the body, the effect of each dose can be assessed after 1 to 2 minutes.
2. *Patient response.* Observe the patient for signs of relaxation or other changes. Ask the patient what is felt. Use the patient's signs and symptoms to determine when the optimum level of sedation has been reached. **Table 37-1** lists signs and symptoms for various levels of nitrous oxide–oxygen sedation.
3. *Adjust dose.* Increase or decrease the nitrous oxide by 5 to 10% when the optimum individual dose has not been achieved. Wait 1 to 2 minutes and reassess. Repeat as needed.
   - Distribution of optimum sedation dose for different individuals follows a bell curve. For about 70% of patients, the ideal is in the 30 to 40% nitrous oxide range.[6]
   - At high altitudes, greater nitrous oxide concentrations will be needed because of the change in the partial pressure of the gases.
4. *Time.* Allow approximately 5 minutes for titration.
5. *Monitor.* Continue to monitor and adjust the concentration throughout the appointment. As the appointment proceeds or during less anxiety-producing parts of the appointment, a lower dose may be more comfortable. Avoid excessive fluctuations.

TABLE 37-1	CORRELATION OF SIGNS AND SYMPTOMS TO LEVELS OF NITROUS OXIDE/OXYGEN SEDATION	
LEVELS	**SYMPTOMS**	**SIGNS**
1. Early to ideal sedation	Light-headedness (dizziness) Tingling of hands and feet Body warmth Feeling of vibration throughout body Numbness of hands and feet Numbness of soft tissues of oral cavity Feeling of euphoria Feeling of lightness or heaviness in extremities Analgesia	Blood pressure, heart rate slightly elevated early in procedure, then return to baseline values Respirations are normal Peripheral vasodilation Flushing of extremities, face Decreased muscle tone as anxiety decreases (arms and legs relax)
2. Heavier sedation/slight oversedation	Hearing, especially of distant sounds, becomes more acute Visual images become confused (patterns on ceiling begin to move) Sleepiness Laughing, crying Dreaming Nausea	Movement increases Heart rate, blood pressure increase Rate of respiration increases Sweating increases Possible tearing
3. Oversedation	Nausea	Vomiting Loss of consciousness

Adapted with permission from Malamed SF. Sedation, a guide to patient management. 4th ed. St. Louis: Mosby; 2003. 245 p.

6. *Attend patient.* Never leave a sedated patient unattended; sedation can become deeper without some stimulation or interaction.
7. *Outcome.* Titration increases clinical success rate of nitrous oxide–oxygen conscious sedation and decreases adverse responses.

IV. COMPLETION OF SEDATION

A. Recovery

1. *Procedure.* At the completion of sedation, return the patient to 100% oxygen for at least 3 to 5 minutes or longer if needed for full recovery.
2. *Factors affecting recovery time.* Biologic variation, duration of sedation procedure, and concentration of nitrous oxide administration. Generally, the more nitrous oxide administered, the longer the recovery time.
3. *Signs of recovery.* Patient's report of feeling "back to normal," comparable presedation and postsedation vital signs.

B. Diffusion Hypoxia

If patient is returned directly to room air rather than 100% oxygen, diffusion hypoxia can result.

1. Nitrous oxide diffuses into an area of lower concentration more rapidly than oxygen, causing inadequate

oxygen in the alveoli if the patient is not given supplemental oxygen at the completion of sedation.
2. Hypoxia can result in patient discomfort or syncope.
3. Inadequate postsedation oxygen may result in a feeling of lethargy or headache.

C. Dismissal Follows Full Recovery

Usually the patient is able to return to all normal activities, including driving.

D. Record Keeping

The following items need to be included in the patient's record:

1. Presedation and postsedation vital signs.
2. Concentrations of both nitrous oxide and oxygen administered.
3. Total gas flow rate (l/min).
4. Length of time for sedation procedure.
5. Length of time on recovery oxygen.
6. Statement of patient's recovery status and any postcare instructions given.
7. Summary of patient's response to nitrous oxide can be helpful for subsequent appointments.
8. An example of progress notes is shown in **Box 37-4.**
9. Signature and date.

BOX 37-4   **Example Progress Notes: Nitrous Oxide/Oxygen Conscious Sedation**

Patient presented with a pronounced gag reflex that caused anxiety about dental treatment. Medical history is nonsignificant. Total gas flow rate: 5 l/min; 35% nitrous oxide and 65% oxygen (OR 2 l/min nitrous oxide and 4 l/min oxygen) for 40 min. Patient reported tingling in extremities and a relaxed feeling. Full-mouth debridement completed without incident. After treatment, 100% oxygen was administered for 5 min; patient said he felt fully recovered.

VITAL SIGNS	PRETREATMENT	POSTTREATMENT
Blood pressure	124/84	120/82
Pulse	75	70
Respirations	12	12

Signed: _____, RDH Date: _____.

POTENTIAL HAZARDS OF OCCUPATIONAL EXPOSURE

Chronic occupational exposure to nitrous oxide may have deleterious effects on health. Overexposure must be prevented.[7,8]

I. ISSUES OF OCCUPATIONAL EXPOSURE

A. Potential Health Problems

- Reduced fertility with as little as 3 to 5 hours of unscavenged nitrous oxide exposure per week.[9]
- Spontaneous abortion.[10]
- Increased rate of neurologic, renal, and liver disease.[10]
- Decreased mental performance, audiovisual ability, and manual dexterity.[11]

B. Recommended Exposure Levels

- Consensus has not been reached on occupational exposure limits; there is currently no exposure standard.
- National Institute of Occupational Safety and Health (NIOSH) recommends no more than 25 parts per million (ppm) during administration.

II. METHODS FOR MINIMIZING OCCUPATIONAL EXPOSURE

- Use an effective scavenging system that can move 45 l/min of air.
- Maintain equipment and inspect regularly for gas leaks, especially at the locations shown in **Figure 37-1**.

- Shut off and secure equipment at the end of each day's use.
- Improve general air quality: introduce fresh air, use a nonrecycling air-conditioning system, or open a window. Vent the scavenger system gases outside the building and away from windows and air intakes.
- Use an air sweep fan to direct nitrous oxide away from the clinician's breathing zone; periodically monitor air quality in the clinicians' breathing zone.
- Minimize patient conversations and mouth breathing; fit the nasal hood carefully to avoid leaks.
- Set conservative limits on the duration and concentration of nitrous oxide use per patient.

ADVANTAGES AND DISADVANTAGES OF NITROUS OXIDE/OXYGEN SEDATION ANESTHESIA

I. ADVANTAGES

- Both a mild analgesic and sedative: reduces patient's reaction to pain by raising pain threshold.
- Increases relaxation and cooperation during treatment.
- Reduces the gag reflex.
- Very safe with few side effects and few medical contraindications.
- Excellent for management of many medically compromised patients:
  - Provides oxygen enrichment as well as stress reduction.
  - Helps prevent emergencies because of anxiety and pain management.
- Readily absorbed and excreted from the body; rapid onset and recovery from drug effect.
  - Able to titrate to optimum level.
  - Recovery complete so patient can be dismissed to return to normal activities.
- Appointments less stressful for clinician because of relaxed, conscious, cooperative patient.

II. DISADVANTAGES

- A low-potency analgesic drug.
  - Not effective with all patients because of low potency; does not block all perception.
  - Severely distressed or phobic patient may need a more potent drug or combination of drugs.
- Patient must be able and willing to breathe through the nose.
- Equipment and gases are expensive.
- Use of poor techniques such as failure to titrate or use a scavenger system results in undesirable patient experiences and potential staff health risks.
- Potential for recreational abuse by health professionals.
- May stimulate sexual fantasies in some patients, and any resulting accusations can result in embarrassment, loss of reputation, and/or license.

LOCAL ANESTHESIA

Local anesthesia is the main modality for the management of dental pain. It blocks sensations, especially of pain, from teeth, soft tissues, and bone in the anesthetized area. Root instrumentation without discomfort requires a profound pulpal and periodontal tissue level of anesthesia.

Dental hygiene treatment provided with the use of local anesthesia is a more comfortable and satisfying treatment for both the patient and clinician. Instrumentation can be comprehensive and definitive, and patient compliance can increase.

PHARMACOLOGY OF LOCAL ANESTHETICS

Local anesthetics are the most frequently used drugs for dental and dental hygiene treatment. They are safe when administered in the recommended manner and amounts.

I. CONTENTS OF A LOCAL ANESTHETIC CARTRIDGE

A dental cartridge is prefilled by the manufacturer to include the following:

1. *Amide anesthetic:* Blocks the transfer of ions across the nerve membrane, which stops the transmission of pain messages.
2. *Vasoconstrictor:* Constricts local blood vessels to offset the vasodilation caused by the amide anesthetic. Cartridges without vasoconstrictor are available.
3. *Antioxidant:* Preservative for the vasoconstrictor, usually sodium metabisulfite or sodium bisulfite.
4. *Sterile water:* Diluent.
5. *Sodium chloride:* Creates an isotonic match with the body.

II. ESTER AND AMIDE ANESTHETIC DRUGS

Dental local anesthetic drugs can be divided chemically into two major groups: esters and amides. The first dental anesthetic was procaine (Novocain), an ester, which has not been available in dental cartridges in the United States since 1996. Except for topicals, all currently used local anesthetic agents are amides. There are a number of available drugs in this group that are similar for safety and effectiveness.[12,13]

A. General Characteristics of Ester Anesthetics

- Widely used in topical anesthetic agents.
- Have a higher incidence of allergic reactions; are less effective and shorter acting compared with amides.

- Metabolized in the blood plasma by the enzyme cholinesterase. The medical condition atypical plasma cholinesterase may result in the slow removal of the drug from the body.

B. General Characteristics of Amide Anesthetics

- Extremely low incidence of allergic reactions.
- Potential for toxicity or drug overdose make attention to detail in technique of administration and total drug dose critical.
- Metabolized by the liver (see specific medical considerations, page 566).
- Cause vasodilation of local blood vessels.

III. CHARACTERISTICS OF SPECIFIC SHORT- AND MEDIUM-ACTING AMIDE DRUGS

A. Lidocaine

- Proprietary names include Xylocaine, Octocaine, Lignospan.
- First amide and still most widely used dental anesthetic; also available as a topical.
- Used with vasoconstrictor to give adequate working time.
- FDA pregnancy category B; generally considered drug of choice for pregnant patient

B. Mepivacaine

- Proprietary names include Carbocaine, Polocaine, Isocaine.
- Causes less vasodilation than lidocaine; therefore, can be used without vasoconstrictor for short procedures.
- Mepivacaine 3%, also called Mepivacaine Plain, is often the drug of choice when vasoconstrictors or their sulfite antioxidants are contraindicated.
- FDA pregnancy category C

C. Prilocaine

- Proprietary names are Citanest Plain and Citanest Forte.
- May cause increased risk of paresthesia.[14]
- Metabolic by-products can cause transient methemoglobinemia, a condition that reduces the blood's oxygen-carrying capacity (see specific medical considerations, page 566).
- Can be used without vasoconstrictor because it causes limited vasodilation.
- When injected into tissues with limited vascularity, the duration of action is similar with and without vasoconstrictor. Example: inferior alveolar nerve block injection.
- FDA pregnancy category: B.

D. Articaine

- Proprietary names are Septocaine, Septanest, and Ultracaine.

■ Reported to diffuse through soft and hard tissues better than other amides.
■ May cause increased risk of paresthesia.[14]
■ Metabolic by-products can cause transient methemoglobinemia.
■ Metabolized primarily in plasma; has shorter half-life so reinjection may occur sooner.
■ FDA pregnancy category: C.

IV. CHARACTERISTICS OF SPECIFIC LONG-ACTING AMIDE DRUGS

A. Bupivacaine

■ Proprietary name: Marcaine, Vivacaine.
■ Long-lasting anesthetic with an extended period of analgesia for postcare pain management.
■ May have delayed onset of action.
■ FDA pregnancy category: C.

V. VASOCONSTRICTORS

A. Reasons for Use

1. *Safety.* Potential for toxic reaction (overdose) to anesthetic is reduced by slowing the rate at which it enters circulation.
2. *Longevity.* Duration of anesthetic effect is increased.
3. *Effectiveness.* Depth and profoundness of anesthetic is increased.
4. *Hemostasis.* Only if drug is locally injected directly into the area.

B. Potential Risks With Use of Vasoconstrictors

1. Hypersensitivity to the drugs.
2. Medical problems (see specific medical considerations, page 566).

3. Drug interactions (see potential drug interactions, page 567).
4. Degree of risk to medically compromised patients, including those with heart disease, varies. Use of vasoconstrictors in low doses is considered safe.[15]

C. Drugs Used

1. *Epinephrine*
   ■ Potent sympathomimetic amine.
   ■ Used in low concentrations, usually 1:100,000 or 1:200,000.
   ■ Maximum recommended doses (MRDs) for healthy patients and for medically compromised, especially those with cardiac disease, are given in **Table 37-2**.
2. *Levonordefrin* (Neo-Cobefrin)
   ■ Half as potent as equal doses of epinephrine and with less cardiac effect.
   ■ Used at higher concentration (1:20,000) to accomplish adequate vasoconstriction.
   ■ Higher doses may result in greater increase in blood pressure than epinephrine.
   ■ MRDs for healthy patients and for medically compromised, especially those with cardiac disease, are given in **Table 37-2**.

VI. CRITERIA FOR DRUG SELECTION

Amide local anesthetics are safe and effective when employed properly.

1. Length of time pain control is needed is a primary criterion for drug selection. **Table 37-3** shows the typical duration of action for common local anesthetics.
2. Medical status of the patient.
3. Potential for prolonged discomfort after treatment.

TABLE 37-2	VASOCONSTRICTORS: CONCENTRATIONS AND MAXIMUM RECOMMENDED DOSE (MRD)			
VASOCONSTRICTORS AND CONCENTRATIONS	**MRD IN HEALTHY PATIENTS**		**MRD IN MEDICALLY COMPROMISED PATIENTS**	
	MG/APPT	**CARTRIDGES/APPT**	**MG/APPT**	**CARTRIDGES/APPT**
Epinephrine				
1:50,000	Use not recommended		Use not recommended	
1:100,000 (0.018 mg/cart.)	0.2	10	0.04	2
1:200,000 (0.009 mg/cart.)	0.2	*	0.04	4
Levonordefrin				
1:20,000 (0.09 mg/cart.)	1.0	10	0.2	2

*Local anesthesia is the limiting drug.

TABLE 37-3	DURATION OF ACTION OF COMMON LOCAL ANESTHETICS	

DRUG NAME GENERIC NAME	DURATION OF ACTION	
	SOFT TISSUE	PULPAL
Short Acting		
3% mepivacaine	2–3 h	Infiltration: 20 min Block: 40 min
4% prilocaine	Infiltration: 1½–2 h	Infiltration: 10–15 min
Medium Acting		
2% lidocaine w/epinephrine 1:100,000	3–5 h	60 min
2% mepivacaine w/levonordefrin 1:20,000×	3–5 h	60–90 min
4% prilocaine	Block: 2–4 hr	Block: 60 min
4% prilocaine w/epinephrine 1:200,000	3–8 h	60–90 min
4% articaine w/epinephrine 1:100,000	3–6 h	60–75 min
Long Acting		
0.5% bupivacaine w/epinephrine 1:200,000	4–9 + h	90–180 min

Source: Malamed SF. Handbook of local anesthesia. 5th ed. St. Louis: Mosby; 2004. pp. 62–75.

4. Potential for self-inflicted injury before anesthetic wears off.

VII. DRUG FOR REVERSAL OF LOCAL ANESTHESIA

1. Phentolamine mesylate
   - Proprietary name: OraVerse™.
   - Indication: rapid reversal of soft-tissue anesthesia and associated effects of local anesthetic.
   - Drug action: vasodilation.
   - Cartridge contains: 0.4 mg drug in 1.7 ml solution.
   - Label: green
   - FDA pregnancy category: C.
2. Technique
   - Administered by injection in same location and with same technique as the local anesthesia being reversed.
   - Dose determined by amount of local anesthetic given in a 1:1 relationship or 1 cartridge of Phentolamine mesylate per cartridge of anesthetic.

INDICATIONS FOR LOCAL ANESTHESIA

Local anesthesia is indicated for treatment that has the potential to cause discomfort or pain. Anesthesia prevents both the patient and the clinician from the anticipation of discomfort, thus allowing both to relax and to make treatment comfortable.

I. DENTAL HYGIENE PROCEDURES

1. Scaling and root planing in areas with probing depths of 4 mm or greater.
2. Extensive instrumentation with either manual or power-driven instruments.
3. Treatment in areas of challenging pocket topography, furcations, or other difficult root anatomy.
4. Instrumentation of sensitive root surfaces.
5. Instrumentation in areas of painful, inflamed soft tissue.
6. Treatments that involve soft tissue manipulation.
   - Gingival curettage.
   - Suture removal.
   - Removal of subgingival overhang.
7. Treatment in areas of excessive hemorrhage.

II. PATIENT FACTORS

- Extent of patient's disease and deposits directly influence the extent or rigor of the needed treatment.
- Patient's pain reaction or pain threshold.

PATIENT ASSESSMENT

The goal of patient assessment is to ensure an effective and safe local anesthesia experience. Pretreatment evaluation is the first and most important step for avoiding a medical emergency.

I. SOURCES OF INFORMATION FOR COMPLETE PREANESTHETIC ASSESSMENT

1. Vital signs.
2. Medical history; ASA status (Table 23-1, in Chapter 23, page 342).
3. Current medications.
4. Emotional status/anxiety level.
5. Dental history related to local anesthesia.
6. Chief complaint and presence of inflammation.

II. TREATMENT OPTIONS BASED ON ASSESSMENT FINDINGS

Amide local anesthetics and the small amount of vasoconstrictor normally incorporated into the dental anesthetic cartridge can be administered safely to almost all patients. Options for treatment include:

1. Use local anesthetic without special precaution.
2. Avoid use of local anesthetic or of a specific local anesthetic because of high medical risk.
3. Select an alternative drug that will minimize or avoid risk.
4. Limit the dose of drug given at any specific appointment.
5. Use local anesthesia combined with maximum stress management; use in combination with nitrous oxide–oxygen conscious sedation.
6. Seek medical intervention, consult, or additional testing before proceeding.
7. Increase drug dose for an infiltration or give block or regional injections rather than infiltration in inflamed tissue as low pH inhibits drug distribution and effectiveness.

III. GENERAL MEDICAL CONSIDERATIONS

1. ASA IV patients and some ASA III patients (especially those who are anxious about injections) may not have the functional reserve to tolerate the injection procedure and the subsequent treatment (ASA, Table 23-1, in Chapter 23, page 342).
2. Patients who are too medically compromised for local anesthesia may not be appropriate for any elective dental therapy.
3. When performing a risk-benefit analysis for use of local anesthesia, consider the potential for medical distress that can result from inadequate pain control.
4. Seek a medical consult when there is doubt about the safety of a local anesthetic choice.
5. Calculate the safe total drug dose for children or small adults based on patient's weight. Every drug has a maximum recommended dose (MRD) in mg/lb and mg/kg that is used for the calculation.

IV. SPECIFIC MEDICAL CONSIDERATIONS

Most contraindications are relative, meaning that a case-specific evaluation needs to focus on the severity of the condition and treatment needs.

A. Allergy

- *Amide anesthetics:* True allergy is rare. If confirmed, avoid all amide anesthetics.
- *Ester anesthetics:* Allergy is fairly common. If confirmed, avoid all ester anesthetics, including topical anesthetics; and para-aminobenzoic acid (PABA) preservatives, such as methylparaben.
- *Bisulfites:* Sodium metabisulfite, acetone sodium bisulfite, and sodium or potassium bisulfite are used as the preservatives for the vasoconstrictor. If allergy is known, avoid anesthetics containing vasoconstrictors.

B. Hyperthyroidism

- *Uncontrolled:* Avoid vasoconstrictor.
- *Controlled:* Normal local anesthesia.

C. Impaired Liver or Kidney Function

- Only severe impairment is clinically relevant.
- Half-life of amide anesthetic could be prolonged, which could result in overdose.

D. Malignant Hyperthermia

- Trend is to consider amide anesthetics used in dentistry as safe.
- Medical consult is indicated as this could be a life-threatening condition.

E. Methemoglobinemia

- A congenital or acquired condition; hemoglobin molecule is converted to methemoglobin, which has less oxygen-carrying capacity. A cyanosis-like state may develop if a high percentage of molecules convert.
- Prilocaine and articaine cause a dose-related methemoglobinemia. Avoid their use in patients with a preexisting condition.

F. Heart Failure

- Reduced circulation resulting from heart failure slows elimination of amide anesthetic, which increases potential for anesthetic overdose.
- Patient is stress intolerant: pain and anxiety must be carefully managed. Consider use of nitrous oxide–oxygen sedation alone or in combination with local anesthesia.

G. Coronary Disease, Heart Attack, Recent Heart Surgery, Angina Pectoris, Hypertension, and Stroke

- Concern is for use and amount of vasoconstrictor.
- Decision based on patient ASA category, treatment, and treatment time needs; possible medical consultation.
- Usual treatment decision is to limit total amount of vasoconstrictor or, in some cases, to eliminate its use.

H. Hemophilia

- Excessive bleeding may result from needle contact with blood vessel.
- Decision, based on severity of condition, can range from treatment in hospital to avoiding injections into highly vascularized areas (example: the posterior superior alveolar [PSA]).

I. Pregnancy

■ Local anesthetics and vasoconstrictors are not terato-gens and may be safely administered.
■ Select a drug in the FDA pregnancy risk category B, usually lidocaine with vasoconstrictor. The FDA classifies drugs according to their safety for the fetus. Drugs are placed in category A, B, C, D, X from least to most risk for harm based on the best study evidence.[16]
■ It is prudent practice to limit any elective drug administration, especially during the first trimester.

J. Potential Drug Interactions

All medications reported in a patient's medical history need to be checked for potential drug interactions before selecting the pain control plan. Following are examples of frequently prescribed or otherwise used drugs that interact with an anesthetic or a vasoconstrictor. Precaution is needed.

1. Cimetidine and amide anesthetic. Probably not clinically significant.
2. Nonselective beta blockers and amide anesthetic or vasoconstrictors.
3. Tricyclic antidepressants and vasoconstrictors.
4. Phenothiazines and vasoconstrictors. Probably not clinically significant.
5. Cocaine and local anesthetics or vasoconstrictors.

ARMAMENTARIUM FOR LOCAL ANESTHESIA

I. SYRINGE

A. Design Features

1. Durable metal or plastic can be sterilized and reused with the addition of a new needle and cartridge.
2. Single-use, disposable syringes have safety features to prevent inadvertent needle stick after use.
3. Provide good visibility of the cartridge.

B. Promote Easy Aspiration

1. Manual aspiration is the traditional design.
2. Self-aspirating syringe works well for small hands.

II. NEEDLE

A. Disposable

Intended for single patient use.

B. Parts and Lengths of the Needle (Figure 37-2)

1. *Long needle:* approximately $1^1/_2$ inches or 40 mm.
2. *Short needle:* approximately 1 inch or 25 mm. Used for most injections.
3. *Ultra-short needle:* approximately $^1/_2$ inch or 12 mm.

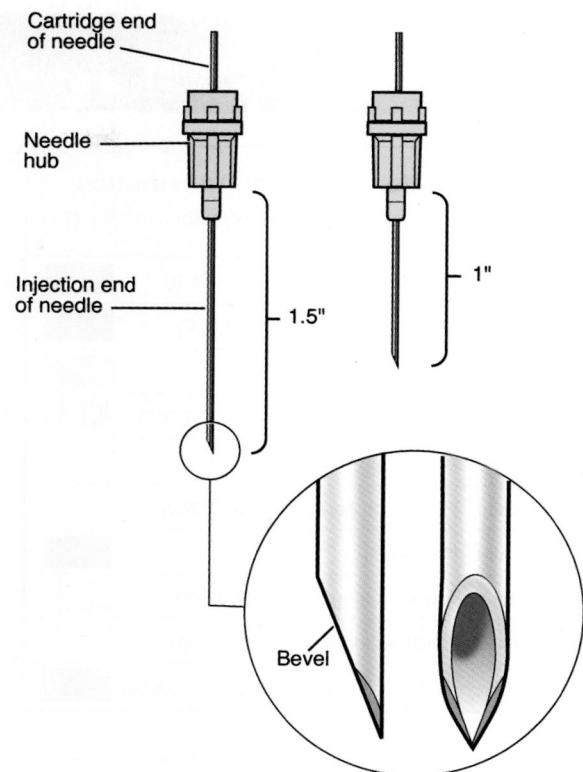

FIGURE 37-2 The Dental Anesthetic Needle. Dental needles are available in two lengths, *long* and *short.* Lengths vary slightly between manufacturers. The components of the needle are *cartridge end,* which penetrates the rubber diaphragm of the dental cartridge; *hub,* which attaches the needle to the syringe (made of plastic or metal); *injection end* or shank or shaft, which penetrates the oral tissue so that anesthetic solution is deposited at the desired site. INSERT: Shows an enlargement of the tip of the needle with sharp terminus and bevel. When giving an injection, the needle is oriented so that the bevel is parallel to the bone to help prevent the needle from catching the periosteum, the sensitive covering over the bone.

C. Gauge or Needle Diameter

1. *Size:* Ranked from largest to smallest, 25-, 27-, and 30-gauge needles are used in dentistry.
2. *Rigidity:* Because they penetrate the tissue, 25-gauge needles are stiffer and deflect less. They are preferred for accuracy when a long needle is needed.
3. *Aspiration:* Larger-gauge needles provide easier and more accurate aspiration.

III. CARTRIDGE OR CARPULE

1. Volume: 1.8 ml of solution in the United States.
2. Storage
   ■ Store at cool room temperature and away from the light.
   ■ Do not store in an alcohol or disinfectant solution.
3. Label on each cartridge: drugs, manufacturer, and expiration date.
4. Color coding: local anesthetic drug is identified by color on cartridge. Color codes are shown in **Box 37-5.**

BOX 37-5 Anesthesia Color Code

Color Codes for Local Anesthetics
A uniform system for easy recognition and safety

Lidocaine 2% with epinephrine (1:100,000)	
Lidocaine 2% with epinephrine (1:50,000)	
Lidocaine plain	
Mepivacaine 2% with levonordefrin (1:20,000)	
Mepivacaine 3% plain	
Prilocaine 4% with epinephrine (1:200,000)	
Prilocaine 4% plain	
Articaine 4% with epinephrine (1:100,000)	
Articaine 4% with epinephrine (1:200,000)	
Bupivacaine 0.5% with epinephrine (1:200,000)	

IV. ADDITIONAL ARMAMENTARIUM

1. Topical antiseptic to prevent postinjection infections.
2. Topical anesthetic to increase patient comfort.
3. Cotton gauze to wipe the injection site to clean, dry, and remove the topical anesthetic. May also be used to improve grasp for lip or cheek retraction.
4. Needle recapping device, if self-recapping needle is not used.
5. Sharps disposal system to meet safe practice standards for used needle disposal.

V. SEQUENCE OF SYRINGE ASSEMBLY

Figure 37-3 illustrates the assembly of the conventional anesthetic syringe; sequence makes the attachment between the harpoon and rubber stopper easier without applying excess force to the glass cartridge.

VI. COMPUTER-CONTROLLED ANESTHESIA DELIVERY SYSTEM

A. Pressure, volume, and rate of speed of local anesthetic delivery are precisely regulated by a computer.
B. Device includes a light, penlike hand piece attached to a computer-controlled, 2-speed motor that is activated by a foot or finger control. Any gauge Luer-lock needle and standard anesthetic cartridge may be used.
C. Slow, controlled delivery of anesthesia solution promotes more comfortable injections, especially palatal and periodontal ligament (PDL) injections; allows unique injections, the anterior middle superior alveolar (AMSA) and the palatal anterior superior alveolar (P-ASA), as well as all traditional dental injections.

CLINICAL PROCEDURES FOR LOCAL ANESTHETIC ADMINISTRATION

Administer the most comfortable injections possible by using gentle tissue manipulation, careful needle penetration, slow deposition of solution, and good patient communication. An example progress note for a patient receiving local anesthesia is found in **Box 37-7**.

I. INJECTION(S) SELECTION

A. Basic Injections

Table 37-4 lists injections with hard and soft tissues anesthetized, and the branches of the trigeminal nerve involved.

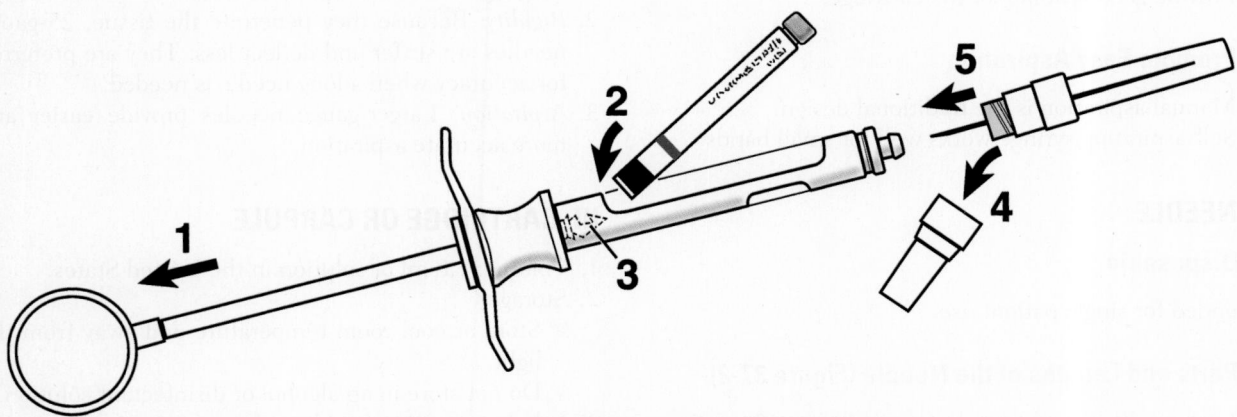

FIGURE 37-3 **Sequence for Assembling a Breech-Loading Aspirating Syringe.** 1. Pull back on thumb ring. 2. Insert anesthetic cartridge, rubber stopper end first, toward the thumb ring, then the diaphragm end toward the needle opening. 3. Set harpoon and test for lock into rubber stopper. 4. Remove safety cap from needle. 5. Screw needle onto the syringe.

TABLE 37-4	COMMON LOCAL ANESTHETIC INJECTIONS FOR DENTAL HYGIENE PROCEDURES	
INJECTION	**TISSUES ANESTHETIZED**	**BRANCH OF THE TRIGEMINAL NERVE**
Maxillary Arch		**Maxillary Division**
Posterior superior alveolar (PSA)	*Hard tissue:* second and third molars; first molar excluding mesiobuccal root; associated supporting structures *Soft tissue:* overlying facial tissues	Posterior superior alveolar
Middle superior alveolar (MSA)	*Hard tissue:* first and second premolars, mesiobuccal root of first molar, and associated supporting structures *Soft tissue:* overlying facial tissues	Middle superior alveolar
Anterior superior alveolar (ASA)	*Hard tissue:* canine and incisors and associated supporting structures *Soft tissue:* overlying facial tissues and lip	Anterior superior alveolar
Infraorbital (IO)	*Hard tissue:* premolars, canine, incisors, and associated supporting structures *Soft tissue:* overlying facial tissues, cheek, and lip	Infraorbital (includes both anterior and middle superior alveolar)
Greater palatine (GP)	*Hard tissue:* none *Soft tissue:* palatal tissue from teeth to midline from distal of third molar to canine	Greater palatine
Nasopalatine (NP)	*Hard tissue:* none *Soft tissue:* palatal tissues from left canine to right canine	Nasopalatine
Infiltration (Inf)	*Hard tissue:* individual teeth associated supporting structures *Soft tissue:* facial tissue overlying individual teeth	Individual terminal branches
Mandibular Arch		**Mandibular Division**
Long buccal (LB)	*Hard tissue:* none	Buccal (long buccal)
Inferior alveolar with lingual (mandibular block) (IA)	*Soft tissue:* facial tissue of molars *Hard tissue:* molars, premolars, canine, and incisors to midline, as well as associated supporting structures *Soft tissue:* facial tissue anterior to mental foramen, including lip *Hard tissue:* none *Soft tissue:* lingual tissue from molar to midline, including anterior two thirds of tongue; floor of mouth	Inferior alveolar (includes dental, mental, and incisive branches) Lingual
Gow–Gates technique (GG)	*Hard tissue:* mandibular teeth to midline; body of mandible; inferior portion of ramus *Soft tissue:* facial and lingual tissue; anterior two thirds of tongue and floor of mouth; skin over the zygoma; posterior portion of the cheek and temporal regions	Third division nerve block (includes inferior alveolar, mental, incisive, lingual, mylohyoid, auriculotemporal, and buccal nerves)
Mental and incisive (M/I)	*Hard tissue:* premolars, canine, incisors, and associated supporting structures *Soft tissue:* facial tissue and lip anterior to mental foramen	Mental and incisive branch of inferior alveolar
Either Arch		
Interpapillary	*Hard tissue:* none *Soft tissue:* individual papilla	Free nerve endings
Periodontal ligament (PDL)	*Hard tissue:* individual tooth *Soft tissue:* adjacent	Terminal nerve endings

Adapted with permission from Woodall IR. Comprehensive Dental Hygiene Care, 4th ed. St. Louis: Mosby; c1993. Stach DJ. Pain and pain control: topical and local anesthesia; p. 688.

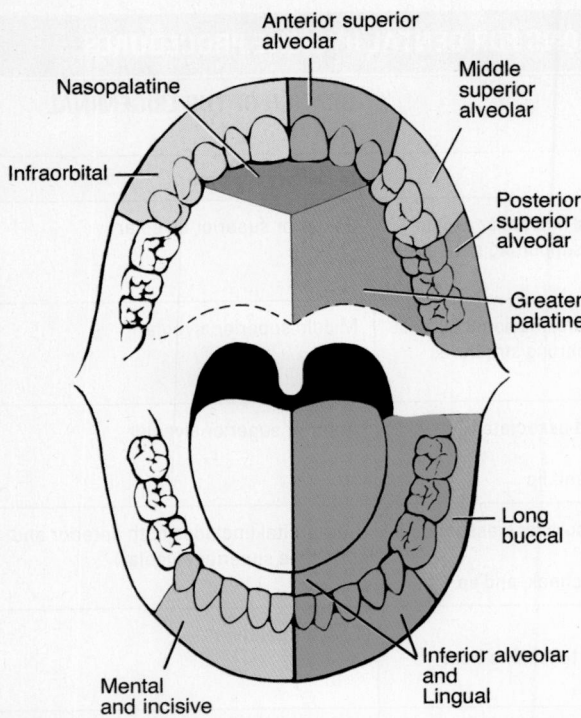

FIGURE 37-4 **Diagrammatic Representation of Teeth and Soft Tissues Anesthetized by Common Dental Injections.**

B. Areas Anesthetized

Figure 37-4 shows the areas to be anesthetized.

C. Steps and Procedures

Box 37-6 outlines the sequence and procedures for the administration of local anesthesia.

II. ASPIRATION

A. Purpose

To determine that the tip of the needle is not within a blood vessel. An anesthetic solution must be deposited extravascularly to be effective and to prevent toxicity.

B. When to Aspirate

- Before depositing anesthetic solution.
- Periodically throughout injection.

C. Procedure

1. Hold the needle steady so that the tip does not change position.
2. Create negative pressure within the dental cartridge.
   - *Standard harpoon-style syringe:* Pull back gently on the thumb ring. Movement is small, if any.

BOX 37-6	Steps in the Administration of Local Anesthesia

1. Assess patient medical status, treatment, and pain control needs in order to select injection(s) and anesthetic drug.
2. Assemble and test the syringe set-up **(Figure 37-3)**.
   a. Orient the needle so that the bevel will be toward the bone during the injection.
   b. Test the assembled syringe.
3. Position patient for good visibility and to prevent syncope with head level with or lower than heart.
4. Use topical anesthetic.
   a. Apply topical to dry tissue at the injection site for the appropriate time. For benzocaine, 1 to 2 minutes is optimal.
   b. Remove residual topical anesthetic.
5. Wipe injection site with gauze to dry and clean surface bacteria, saliva, and topical anesthetic from the area before injection.
6. Retract the lip or cheek for good visibility; stretch the tissue for easier needle penetration.
7. Keep the syringe out of the patient's sight.
8. Establish a fulcrum or hand rest for stability during the injection.
9. Insert the needle into the tissue and gently advance to desired site for administration of anesthetic.
10. Aspirate before depositing solution; reaspirate as needed throughout procedure.
11. Deposit the anesthetic solution slowly (1 to 2 minutes for full cartridge) to prevent patient discomfort and to reduce potential for a toxic reaction.
12. Withdraw the needle carefully at the completion of the injection, and recap the needle using a safe technique.
13. Remain with and observe the patient. Adverse drug reactions are most likely to occur during or shortly after the injection.
14. Record injection information in patient chart.
15. Use positive, supportive communication with the patient throughout the procedure.

- *Self-aspirating syringe:* Stop applying positive pressure to the thumb ring.
3. Rotate the syringe by a quarter turn and repeat aspiration (prevent a false negative).

D. Interpretation

1. Any fluid at the tip of the needle will be drawn into the cartridge. If the tip of the needle is in an artery or vein, blood will become visible; it may only be a small amount at the needle end of the cartridge.
2. *Negative aspiration:* No blood in cartridge; proceed with injection.

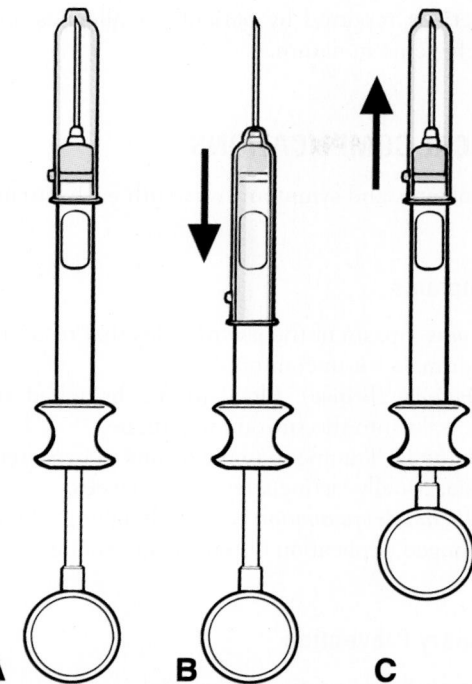

FIGURE 37-5 **Prevention of Percutaneous Injury: Self-sheathing Safety Needle.** **(A)** Syringe with protective sheath over the needle. **(B)** As the injection is made, the sheath slides back. **(C)** After injection, the sheath returns to cover the needle and protect the clinician during disposal.

3. *Positive aspiration:* Blood in the cartridge.
   - A small amount of blood with most of the cartridge clear: move to a new location and reaspirate.
   - Cartridge generally bloody: withdraw needle, replace cartridge, and repeat injection.

III. SHARPS MANAGEMENT[17,18]

A. Needle Recapping

- Needles with engineered sharps injury protection are preferred, such as a self-sheathing safety needle or safety syringe. An example of a device that meets these requirements is shown in **Figure 37-5**.
- Also acceptable:
   A. One-handed "scoop" technique **(Figure 37-6A)**.
   B. Mechanical device to hold the needle sheath **(Figure 37-6B)**.

B. No Manipulation

Do not manipulate needles; do not bend, break, or shear.

C. Needle Removal

Disposal containers for contaminated sharps should be readily accessible and located as close as possible to the area of use.

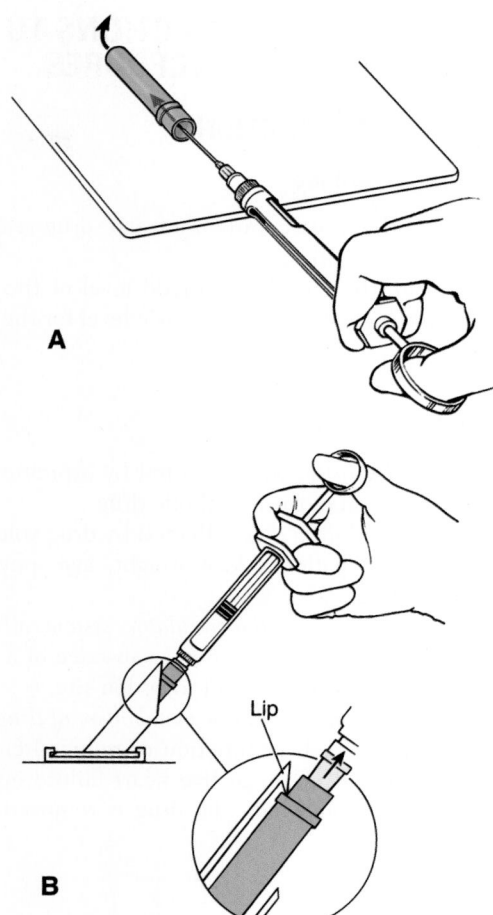

FIGURE 37-6 **Prevention of Percutaneous Injury: Alternative Needle Recapping Methods.** One-handed recapping or recapping with a safety mechanical device to hold the needle sheath is acceptable. **(A)** "Scoop" technique. Cap is placed on the tray and the needle is guided into it. **(B)** Example of commercially available holder for cap. Device is fastened to the tray, and cap is removed and recapped by directing the needle into the cap holder. Needles must be discarded in a puncture-resistant container.

BOX 37-7	Example Progress Notes: Local Anesthesia

Nonsignificant medical history, BP 120/80, pulse 68. Patient reported general root sensitivity. For periodontal debridement of max. and mand. right quadrants, administered 3.6 ml 2% lidocaine (lido) with epinephrine (epi) 1:100,000 for right anterior superior alveolar (ASA), middle superior alveolar (MSA), posterior superior alveolar (PSA), inferior alveolar (IA) long buccal (LB). Benzocaine topical. Anesthesia profound; procedure well tolerated.

Signed: _____, RDH Date: _____.

POTENTIAL ADVERSE REACTIONS TO LOCAL ANESTHESIA PROCEDURES

I. ADVERSE DRUG REACTIONS

A. Toxic Drug Overdose

- Overdose is the most common adverse drug reaction with amide anesthetics.
- Occurs when the circulating blood level of the drug becomes too high and reaches a toxic level for the individual.

B. Typical Causes of Overdose

1. *Intravascular injection:* prevented by aspiration before deposition of the anesthetic drug.
2. *Excessive total drug dose:* affected by drug volumes; drug choice; patient's lean weight, age, physical/medical status.
3. *Rapid absorption into the circulatory system:* affected by rate of injection, presence or absence of a vasoconstrictor, or vascularity of injection site.
4. *Reduced elimination and/or metabolism of drug:* Reduced kidney or liver function or reduced circulation as a result of congestive heart failure may reduce the rate at which the drug is removed from circulation.

C. Allergy

1. *Incidence:* Although often reported, incidence is rare with amide drugs. (Review allergy under specific medical considerations [page 566].)
2. *Definition:* Allergy is a hypersensitive state where a subsequent exposure to an allergen results in an exaggerated response. In local anesthesia, the most common allergens are the bisulfite antioxidant or ester topical anesthetic.
3. *Symptoms:* Response may range from mild, such as localized erythema or itching, to life threatening, such as generalized anaphylaxis or laryngeal edema.
4. *Onset:* May range from a few seconds to many hours.
5. *Management:* Table 69-4 (page 1079) presents procedures for managing an allergic reaction.

II. PSYCHOGENIC REACTIONS

A. Cause

Anxiety response to the injection procedure.

B. Symptoms

1. Vasodepressor syncope (fainting) and hyperventilation are most common.
2. Symptoms can be highly varied and may mimic drug reactions or other medical conditions.

3. Reactions reported by patients as allergies are often psychogenic in nature.

III. LOCAL COMPLICATIONS

The problems and symptoms vary with each situation.

A. Symptoms

1. *Trismus:* Spasm of the jaw muscles that restricts opening or makes it uncomfortable.
2. *Hematoma* (bruise): Blood from a breached artery or vein leaks into the surrounding tissue.
3. *Paresthesia:* Trauma to nerve results in persistent anesthesia, usually lasting a few days to weeks.
4. *Epithelial desquamation* (tissue sloughing): May follow prolonged application of topical anesthetic.

B. Primary Prevention

Use of excellent injection technique.

ADVANTAGES AND DISADVANTAGES OF LOCAL ANESTHESIA

I. ADVANTAGES

- Patient experiences no pain or discomfort during treatment procedure.
- Clinician has increased confidence to provide complete treatment when the patient is pain free.
- Local effect results in loss of sensation in area of treatment without a change in level of consciousness or patient cooperation.
- Completely reversible without residual side effects.
- Rapid onset of action.
- Adequate duration of clinical action that is reasonably predictable and that can be varied by choice of commercially available drugs.
- Relatively free of allergic reactions.
- Hemostasis if injected directly into area of desired hemorrhage control.

II. DISADVANTAGES

- Anticipating and receiving dental injections may cause high anxiety for patient. Effects may include:
  - Need for special anxiety reduction technique.
  - Undesirable psychogenic reactions.
  - Avoidance of needed care.
- Significant potential exists for toxicity (overdose) with amide drugs.
- There are systemic side effects from both the local anesthetic drug and vasoconstrictor.

- Where state law or skill levels preclude the dental hygienist from administering local anesthesia, it may be inconvenient or time consuming for the dentist to provide the injections.

NONINJECTABLE ANESTHESIA

Noninjectable anesthesia is a relatively new drug delivery modality. The anesthetic drugs are applied to the surface of the pocket lining tissue making this a topical application for legal and practical purposes. It provides adjacent soft tissue anesthesia and in varying degrees dental anesthesia. The anesthesia is available under the brand name Oraqix™.[19]

I. INDICATIONS FOR USE

- Adults; has not been studied in children.
- Initial or maintenance treatment of periodontal pockets where profound pulpal anesthesia is not needed.
- Management of mild to moderate discomfort during scaling especially over multiple quadrants in the same appointment; treatment where full dentition local anesthesia would be inappropriate.
- Needle phobic adults.

II. CONTRAINDICATIONS

- Allergy to amide anesthetic or other components of the anesthetic cartridge.
- Methemoglobinemia.

III. ARMAMENTARIUM AND PHARMACOLOGY

A unique dispenser with a blunt-tipped applicator delivers a gel containing both lidocaine and prilocaine into the periodontal pocket. Both the dispenser and the anesthetic gel are contraindicated for injections.

A. Cartridge and Blunt-Tipped Applicator

- Packaged together; for single-patient use.
- For use only with special dispenser and not for injection.
- Blunt-tipped applicator is individually bent by clinician with either a single or double bend.
- Cartridge contains 1.7 g anesthetic gel.
- Store at room temperature.

B. Anesthetic Gel

- Gel contents
  1. *Anesthetics:* 2.5% lidocaine and 2.5% prilocaine amide anesthetics (see amide anesthetic drugs, page 563).

  2. *Poloxamers:* thermosetting agents.
  3. *pH adjuster:* hydrochloric acid.
  4. *Purified water.*
- Gel characteristics
  1. Low viscosity fluid at room temperature.
  2. Gel at oral temperature.

C. Dispenser

IV. TECHNIQUE

A. Administration

1. Dispense a thin layer of the anesthetic gel at the gingival margin; wait 30 seconds.
2. Insert blunt-tipped applicator into the subgingival pocket, dispense product until pocket begins to overflow, then repeat in adjacent area.

B. Treatment Time[20]

1. *Onset:* 30 seconds.
2. *Duration:* 20 minutes with a range of 14–31 minutes.

C. Maximum Dose

- 5 cartridges per appointment.

TOPICAL ANESTHESIA

- A topical anesthetic is a drug applied directly to the surface of the mucous membrane to produce a loss of sensation.
- A topical anesthetic is used with varying degrees of success for short-duration desensitization of the gingiva, but it does not influence sensations in the teeth.
- The topical anesthetic is not a substitute for local anesthetic administered by injection.

I. INDICATIONS FOR USE

A topical anesthetic can be used conservatively for selected dental hygiene and dental services, including the following:

A. Preparation for local anesthesia injection.
B. Prevention of gagging in radiographic techniques and impression taking.
C. Temporary relief of pain from localized diseased areas, such as oral ulcers, wounds, or inflammation.
D. During instrumentation for probing and scaling. When discomfort involves the teeth as well as gingiva, a local anesthetic usually is indicated.
E. Suture removal.

II. ACTION OF A TOPICAL ANESTHETIC

A. Purpose

1. The purpose of a topical anesthetic is to desensitize the mucous membrane by anesthetizing the terminal nerve endings.
2. The superficial anesthesia produced is related to the amount of absorption of the drug by the tissue.

B. Absorption of Drug

1. Varies with:
   - Thickness of stratified squamous epithelial covering.
   - Degree of keratinization.
2. Tissue absorption
   - Highly resistant: skin, lips, palatal mucosa.
   - Absorb slowly: attached gingiva, buccal mucosa.
   - Prompt absorption: tissue without keratinization, such as vestibular mucosa or over the pterygomandibular space.

III. AGENTS USED IN SURFACE ANESTHETIC PREPARATIONS

Table 37-5 provides onset and duration of topical anesthetics.

A. Benzocaine or Ethyl Aminobenzoate (Ester Type)

1. Used in 20% formulation; most widely used topical agent.
2. Available as liquid, gel, ointment, and spray.
3. Not readily absorbed into circulation; potential for toxicity is minimal.
4. May cause allergic reaction, especially with prolonged or repeated application.

B. Tetracaine Hydrochloride (Ester Type)

1. Typically available as part of a combination of drugs in liquid, gel, and controlled-dose spray.
2. Readily absorbed causing deeper penetration, longer effect, and more potential for toxicity. Not to be used over a large area.

C. Lidocaine and Lidocaine Hydrochloride (Amide Type)

1. The only amide used alone as a topical.
2. Available in ointment, spray, transoral patch, and in combination with prilocaine.
3. Toxicity unlikely from topical alone but would be additive with other amide anesthetics. Greatest risk from sprays.

D. Lidocaine: Transoral Patch[21]

1. A delivery system that uses a bioadhesive patch to improve the duration of contact between the topical and oral soft tissue.
2. Provides profound soft tissue anesthesia as well as minimal pulpal anesthesia in some cases.
3. **Figure 37-7** shows relation of the position of a patch to the gingival margin.

E. Dyclone or Dyclonine Hydrochloride (Ketone Type)

1. Available in 0.5 or 1% formulation from a compounding pharmacy.
2. Available as a liquid.
3. As a gargle is good for gag reflex suppression.
4. Slow onset, up to 10 minutes; long duration, up to 1 hour.

TABLE 37-5	NONINJECTABLE AND TOPICAL ANESTHETIC APPLICATION TIMES			
	DRUG	**INITIAL ONSET**	**OPTIMUM APPLICATION (FOR DEPTH AND INTENSITY)**	**DURATION**
NONINJECTABLE LOCAL ANESTHESIC	2.5% Lidocaine and 2.5% prilocaine	30 s		14–31 min 20 min average
TOPICAL ANESTHETIC	Benzocaine	30 s	1–2 min	5–15 min
	Tetracaine (combined with other drugs)	2 min		20–60 min
	Lidocaine ointment	1–2 min	3–5 min	15 min
	Lidocaine transoral patch	$2^{1}/_{2}$–5 min	Varies by procedure (maximum 15 min after application)*	45 min (after 15-min application)
	Dyclonine	2–10 min	10 min	30–60 min

*See application technique transoral patch, page 575.

APPLICATION OF TOPICAL ANESTHETIC

I. PATIENT PREPARATION

- Consult history and other records for pertinent information concerning a patient's previous experiences with anesthetics. A patient with an allergy to a local anesthetic may also be allergic to a topical anesthetic.
- Determine the most appropriate anesthetic agent and method of application.
- Explain purpose and anticipated effect to the patient.

II. APPLICATION TECHNIQUES

Several application techniques are available. Not all methods are applicable to all products. Select the most appropriate method from the following:

A. Surface Application

1. May be used with liquid, gel, or ointment formulations of any of the available topical agents.
2. Topical is applied with a cotton-tipped swab or cotton roll.
3. Time before becoming effective varies with the drug used.
4. After application, excess topical is removed by rinsing or gentle wiping.

B. Aerosol Spray

1. Prevent inhalation by avoiding spray preparations when another method would be as effective. A spray must never be directed toward the throat.
2. Use metered- or controlled-dose spray dispensers to prevent inadvertent overdose.

C. Transoral Patch[21]

Topical anesthetic applied to the tissue using the transoral patch method provides a profound level of anesthesia to the soft tissues. It may provide slight loss of sensation to the teeth as well.
1. Air-dry the tissue for 30 seconds, apply the patch, and hold in place with firm finger pressure for an additional 30 seconds.
2. Apply for 5 to 10 minutes before most procedures; may be left in place for up to 15 minutes. Suggested application times for typical procedures are:
   - 5 minutes for most injections.
   - 8 to 10 minutes for palatal injections.
   - 15 minutes for most instrumentation (may be able to begin after 5 minutes).
3. Test tissue to confirm level of anesthesia after an appropriate application time. If adequate, remove the patch.

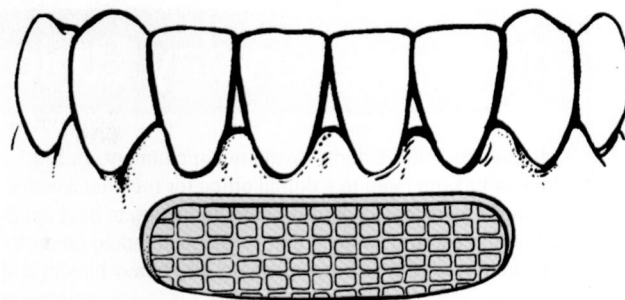

FIGURE 37-7 Transoral Lidocaine Patch Placement. In this example, for topical anesthesia to the mandibular incisors and facial tissues, patch is placed over the roots of the incisors with the upper edge 2 to 4 mm apical to the free gingival margin. Patch may be left in place during scaling and root planing for up to 15 minutes.

- Periodontal instrumentation may be started while the patch is in place if anesthesia is adequate; remove after 15 minutes.
- Injections are not to be given through a patch.
- Typical patch placement for scaling of the mandibular incisors is shown in **Figure 37-7**.

III. COMPLETION OF TOPICAL ANESTHETIC APPLICATION

1. Wait appropriate length of time for anesthetic to take effect before proceeding.
2. Limit drug exposure.
   - Apply only to the area of need.
   - Use the smallest effective amount.
   - Remove residual drug after application time.
3. Apply to a limited area at a time when using a drug with a short duration of action for a long procedure such as scaling.
4. Record topical anesthetic drug information in the patient's record.

DOCUMENTATION

Documentation in the permanent record for each appointment when a pain control drug or technique is used includes a minimum of the following factors:

- Medical status and vital signs.
- Rational for pain control use.
- Location or type of injection; topical anesthetic surfaces or teeth treated.
- Recovery time on 100% oxygen following nitrous oxide conscious sedation.
- Signature and date.
- An example progress note documenting an appointment for a patient receiving nitrous oxide oxygen conscious sedation is located in **Box 37-4** on page 562 and for a patient receiving local anesthesia is located in **Box 37-7** on page 571.

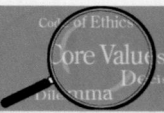

Everyday Ethics

Mr. Denver, in for a dental hygiene appointment, stated that he has not been to a dental office for the past 5 years because he is fearful of oral treatment owing to past painful experiences. Oral examination revealed bleeding on probing, generalized 5- to 6-mm pockets, and heavy biofilm and calculus deposits. Proposed treatment is four appointments for scaling and root debriding with anesthesia and patient instruction, followed by a reevaluation.

Questions for Consideration

1. What anxiety and pain management methods could be used for this patient? Refer to pain control mechanisms (page 38) to make your list as complete as possible. Which of these methods are legal for a dental hygienist to utilize in your state or province?
2. In the past, this patient has had painful treatment, you plan to provide comfortable treatment, how do the core values of dental hygiene (Table II-I in Section II Introduction, page 38) relate to these two approaches for patient care?
3. Thinking of ethics as expressed by the core values is the patient's expectation for pain management different if a dentist or a dental hygienist provides the deep scaling? Explain.

Factors To Teach The Patient

I. NITROUS OXIDE–OXYGEN CONSCIOUS SEDATION

■ Inform the clinician if the sedation becomes too strong or is too weak so that adjustments can be made. The level of sedation should be adjusted individually for optimum relaxation and comfort.

■ The gas will not result in unusual or undesirable behavior; the patient will maintain control of all personal actions.

■ Eat normally before treatment; avoid fasting or heavy meals.

II. LOCAL AND TOPICAL ANESTHESIA

■ Be careful not to bite lip, cheek, or tongue while tissues are without normal sensations. Warn and watch children to prevent injury. Do not test anesthesia by biting the lip.

■ Avoid chewing hard foods and avoid hot food and drinks until normal sensation has returned.

References

1. Jeske A, Zahrowski J. Good evidence supports ibuprofen as an effective and safe analgesic for postoperative pain. *J Am Dent Assoc.* 2010 May;141(5):567–8.
2. Dionne RA, Phero JC, Becker DE. *Management of pain and anxiety in the dental office.* Philadelphia: W.B. Saunders Co.; 2002. Chapter 2, Mechanisms of orofacial pain and analgesia; pp. 14–33.
3. Clark MS, Brunick AL. *Handbook of nitrous oxide and oxygen sedation.* 3rd ed. St. Louis: Mosby; 2008. Chapter 5, Physical properties and pharmacokinetics of nitrous oxide; pp. 33–40.
4. American Dental Association. Nitrous oxide use dangerous after intraocular gas injection: FDA. *J Am Dent Assoc.* 2002 Nov;133(11):1476.
5. Malamed SF. *Sedation: a guide to patient management.* 4th ed. St. Louis: Mosby; 2003. Chapter 12, Pharmacosedation: rationale; pp. 185–95.
6. Malamed SF. *Sedation: a guide to patient management.* 4th ed. St. Louis: Mosby; 2003. Chapter 15, Inhalation sedation: techniques of administration; pp. 237–56.
7. National Institute for Occupational Safety and Health. Control of Nitrous Oxide in Dental Operatories [Internet]. Washington: NIOSH; [updated 1998 March 2; cited 2010 Sept 21]. Available from: http://www.cdc.gov/niosh/nitoxide.html
8. ADA Council on Scientific Affairs. ADA Council on Dental Practice: nitrous oxide in the dental office. *J Am Dent Assoc.* 1997 March;128(3):364–5.
9. Rowland AS, Baird, DD, Weinberg CR, Shore DL, Shy CM, Wilcox AJ. Reduced fertility among women employed as dental assistants exposed to high levels of nitrous oxide. *N Engl J Med.* 1992 Oct 1;327(14):993–7.
10. Cohen EN, Gift HC, Brown BW, Greenfield W, Wu ML, Jones TW, Whitcher CE, Driscoll EJ, Brodsky JB. Occupational disease in dentistry and chronic exposure to trace anesthetic gases. *J Am Dent Assoc.* 1980 July;101(1):21–31.
11. National Institute for Occupational Safety and Health (US). Alert: controlling exposures to nitrous oxide during anesthetic administration. Cincinnati: US Department of Health, Education, and Welfare; 1994. p. 1. Publication No. 94–100. Joint publication of Public Health Service, Centers for Disease Control, National Institute for Occupational Safety and Health.
12. Malamed SF. *Handbook of local anesthesia.* 5th ed. St. Louis: Mosby; 2004. Chapter 4, Clinical action of specific agents; pp. 55–83.
13. Haveles EB. *Applied pharmacology for the dental hygienist.* 5th ed. St. Louis: Mosby; 2007. Chapter 15, Cardiovascular drugs; pp. 186–212.
14. Garisto GA, Gaffen AS, Lawrence HP, Tenenbaum HC, Haas DA. Occurrence of paresthesia after dental local anesthetic administration in the United States. *J Am Dent Assoc.* 2010 July;141(7):836–44.
15. Jastak JT, Yagiela JA, Donaldson D. *Local anesthesia of the oral cavity.* Philadelphia: Saunders; 1995. Chapter 3, Pharmacology of vasoconstrictors; pp. 61–85.
16. National Women's Health Information Center (US). womenshealth.gov: The Federal Government Source for Women's Health Information [Internet]. Washington: Office on Women's Health, Dept of Health and Human Services; [cited 2010 Nov 1]. Frequently asked questions: pregnancy and medicines [updated 2010 April 14, cited 2010 Nov 1]; [about 7 screens]. Available from: http://www.womenshealth.gov/faq/pregnancy-medicines.cfm

17. Occupational Safety and Health Administration (US). Occupational exposure to bloodborne pathogens; needlestick and other sharps injuries. Final Rule. *Fed Regist*. 2001 Jan 18;66(12):5317–25.

18. Organization for Safety and Asepsis Procedures. Infection control in practice. Annapolis (MD): 2002 Nov; Devices with sharps safety features; p. 1.

19. Dentsply Pharmaceutical. Oraqix: The Only FDA-Approved Needle-Free Anesthetic [Internet]. York (PA): Dentsply Pharmaceutical; c2010 [cited 2010 Sept 22]. Available from: http://www.oraqix.com/

20. Nilsson FJ, Isacsson G. The anesthetic onset and duration of a new Lidocaine/Prilocaine gel intra-pocket anesthetic (Oraqix) for periodontal scaling/root planing. *J Clin Periodontol*. 2001 May;28(5):453–8.

21. Hersh EV, Houpt MT, Cooper SA, Feldman RS, Wolff MS, Levin LM. Analgesic efficacy and safety of an intraoral lidocaine patch. *J Am Dent Assoc*. 1996 Nov;127(11):1626–34.

Instruments and Principles for Instrumentation

ESTHER M. WILKINS, BS, RDH, DMD

Chapter Outline

Instrumentation begins with the identification of the various types of instruments for specific dental hygiene assessment and treatment services to be performed and knowledge of the parts of those instruments. The requirements for putting the instruments into action to accomplish a particular task are *stabilization* by means of a correct *grasp* and *rest, adaptation, angulation, lateral pressure,* and *stroke.* Key words related to basic instrumentation are defined in **Box 38-1**.

■ A study of oral and dental anatomy and histology accompanies learning instrumentation procedures and skills.

■ Development of a thorough, efficient, and safe procedure for treatment depends on an understanding of the normal, healthy, and diseased characteristics of the dental and periodontal tissues being treated.
■ A high degree of skill in the care and use of the fine instruments is required.
■ Skill depends on knowledge and understanding of the goals of therapy and of how the goals can be reached through application of the fundamental principles of instrumentation.

BOX 38-1	Key Words

Principles for Instrumentation

Adaptation: relationship between the working end of an instrument and the tooth surface being treated.
Angulation: the angle formed by the working end of an instrument with the surface to which the instrument is applied for treatment.
Blade: working end of an instrument with special design for a particular clinical treatment.
Curet: a curved, rounded dental instrument utilized for scaling, root planing, and gingival curettage.
   Area-specific curet: a specialized instrument designed with specific angles in the shank for adaptation to a certain group of tooth surfaces.
   Universal curet: a curet designed for use on any tooth surface where the adaptation, angulation, and other principles of instrument used can be correctly and effectively accomplished.
Curettage: removal of inflamed soft tissue lining of a pocket wall.
Dominant hand: the hand generally used for performing fine tasks such as writing and holding instruments for scaling.
Finger rest: for an intraoral rest, the place on a tooth or teeth where the third or ring finger of the hand holding the instrument is placed to provide stabilization and control during activation of the instrument.

Fulcrum: the support upon which a lever rests while force intended to produce motion is exerted.
Indirect vision: use of a dental mouth mirror to view the area of instrumentation. Indirect lighting is provided by the mirror.
Instrumentation zone: section of the tooth where treatment is indicated and instrumentation is performed.
Lateral pressure: the minimal pressure that is required of an instrument against the tooth or soft tissue to accomplish the objective of the designated assessment or treatment.
Offset blade: the blade of an area-specific Gracey curet in which the lower shank is at a 70° angle to the face of the blade; contrasts with a universal curet blade, which is at a 90° angle with the lower shank **(Figure 38-6)**.
Scaler: instrument designed for initial removal of calculus, prior to finishing with a curet.
Scaling: instrumentation of a tooth surface to remove calculus and biofilm.
Shank: the part of the instrument between the handle and the working end.
   Lower or terminal shank: the part of the shank next to the blade.
Stroke: a single unbroken movement made by an instrument against a tooth surface during an examination or treatment procedure to accomplish a particular objective; the motion made for activation of an instrument.

INSTRUMENT IDENTIFICATION

The instruments needed for assessment and evaluation were described in Chapter 15 on pages 226 to 238. Instruments for scaling and related procedures are described in this chapter.

I. RECOGNITION OF INSTRUMENTS

■ Each instrument is recognized by sight and distinguished at a glance by the profile of the instrument.
■ The clinician is able to designate the names and numbers, and to associate each instrument promptly with the various phases of instrumentation.
■ Such spot identification contributes to organization of tray arrangement and efficiency of service rendered through prompt selection of the appropriate instrument for the service to be performed.

II. CLASSIFICATION BY PURPOSE AND USE

■ *Examination Instruments:* Probes, explorers.
■ *Treatment Instruments:* Curets, scalers (sickle, Jacquette, file, hoe, chisel).

III. DESCRIPTION ON THE INSTRUMENT HANDLE

■ *Design Name:* The school or individual responsible for the design or development.
■ *Design Number:* The traditional number used to identify the specific instrument. The same instrument may be made by various manufacturers using the same number.

INSTRUMENT PARTS AND BALANCE

The three major parts are the *working end,* the *shank,* and the *handle.* The relationship of these parts is illustrated by the curet in **Figure 38-1**.

I. WORKING END

■ The working end refers to that part used to carry out the purpose and function of the instrument. Each working end is unique to the particular instrument.
■ The working end of a scaler or curet is called a blade.

■ The parts of a sharp blade are:
  ■ *Cutting Edge:* A very fine line where two surfaces meet. For example, the *face* and the *lateral surface* meet to form the sharp cutting edge of a curet (Example: **Figure 38-4**).
  ■ *Lateral Surfaces:* The lateral surfaces meet or are continuous (as in the round back of a curet) to form the *back* of the instrument.

II. SHANK

■ The shank connects the working end with the handle, as shown in **Figure 38-1**.
■ The shape, length, and rigidity of the shank govern the access of the working end to accomplish the intended purpose for which the instrument was designed.
■ The section of the shank adjacent to the blade is called the *lower or terminal shank* as labeled in **Figure 38-1**.

A. Shape

■ *Straight (flat):* for adaptation to tooth surfaces with unrestricted access, such as for anterior teeth. With many instruments, the straight lower shank can provide the line-up for correct positioning for treatment.
■ *Angled:* For adaptation to tooth surfaces with restricted access, such as proximal surfaces of posterior teeth, deep periodontal pockets on narrow roots, and furcation areas. In general, the more restricted the access, the more angulated a shank needs to be and the sharper the bends of the angles.
  ■ Examples are the Gracey curets 11/12, 13/14, and 15/16, each of which has three bends.
  ■ Because the *distal* surfaces of molars and premolars are much less accessible than are the mesial surfaces, the angles in the shanks of 13/14 and 17/18 are designed with deeper bends to make access possible.

B. Effect of Shank Length

■ The distance from the cutting edge (working end) of the blade to the junction of the shank and handle in most all instruments is 35 to 40 mm (1½ inches).
■ Too short a distance limits action.
■ Extended lower shank length (for example adding on 3 mm.) permits accessing the blade into deep pockets along narrow roots, and into furcation areas. Examples are the mini-bladed and the micro-mini-bladed curets, which are described in this chapter.

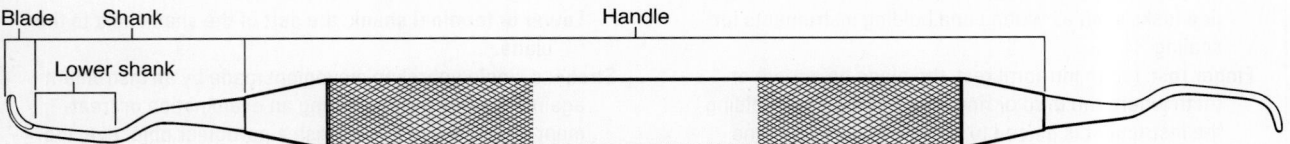

FIGURE 38-1 Parts of an Instrument. Curet shows the relationship of the working end (blade), shank, and handle. The section of the shank next to the blade is referred to as the terminal or lower shank.

C. Shank Flexibility

Instruments are made with shanks of varying degrees of thickness and rigidity that relate to the purpose for which the instrument is used.

1. *Rigid, Thick Shank.* A heavier shank is stronger and is able to withstand greater pressure without flexing when applied during instrumentation. Strong instruments are needed for removal of heavy calculus deposits.
2. *Less Rigid, More Flexible Shank.* A thinner shank may provide more tactile sensitivity and is used, for example, for removal of fine deposits of calculus and for maintenance root debridement.

III. HANDLE

The position and grasp of the handle in conjunction with the finger or hand rest are significant in the tactile sensitivity and the activation of the working end.

A. Overall Design

1. *Single-Ended Instrument:* Handle has one working end.
2. *Double-Ended Instrument:* May have paired (mirror image) or complementary working ends.
   - Paired working ends may be an instrument with its mirror image on the opposite end. One is used for access to proximal surfaces from the facial and the other for a lingual or palatal approach.
   - Complementary working ends may be composed for use during examination with a probe on one end and an explorer at the other end.
3. *Cone Socket Handles:* These are separable from the shank and working end. They permit screw-in instrument exchanges and replacements.

B. Weight

Handles with lighter weight enhance tactile sensitivity and lessen fatigue related to a tighter grasp. They are sometimes referred to as ergonomic handles.

C. Diameter

- In general, four diameters of instrument handles are available. As shown in **Figure 38-2**, the most common diameters available from manufacturers are 3/8, 5/16, 1/4, and 3/16 inch.
- The ideal instrument for comfort and best tactile sensitivity has for example, a lightweight, serrated, handle with a 3/8- or 5/16-inch diameter.

D. Surface Texture: Serrations

- Instrument handles may be smooth, ribbed, or knurled. A thinner, smooth handle may require a tighter grasp to prevent slipping, which can lessen tactile sensitivity and increase clinician's fatigue.

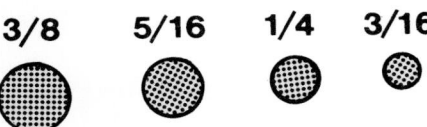

FIGURE 38-2 **Diameters of Instrument Handles.** The most common diameters are 3/8, 5/16, 1/4, and 3/16 inch. For comfort and tactile sensitivity, the widest diameter with a lightweight handle is recommended.

- The ribbed or knurled handle with a wider diameter can provide better control with a firm, but lighter grasp without lessening tactile sensitivity.

IV. INSTRUMENT BALANCE

- The working end of a balanced instrument is centered in line with the long axis of the handle **(Figure 38-3)**
- The design of the balance of each instrument provides the ability for its adaptation, angulation, and activation that can accomplish the objectives of the treatment plan.

THE TREATMENT INSTRUMENTS

Each instrument is designed for a specific type of application during treatment procedures. An instrument may be categorized first by whether it is intended primarily for supragingival or for subgingival treatment procedures. Scalers and curets are then designed for the blade size and anatomy of the cutting edges to meet the need of the purpose during treatment.

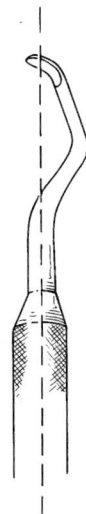

FIGURE 38-3 **Instrument Balance.** The working end of a balanced instrument is centered in line with the long axis of the instrument handle.

I. CATEGORIES

A. Curets

1. *Universal*
2. *Area Specific*
3. *Minibladed and Micro minibladed*

B. Scalers

1. *Scaler*
   - Curved scaler/sickle scaler
   - Straight scaler/Jacquette
2. *File Scaler*
3. *Hoe Scaler*
4. *Chisel Scaler*

II. INSTRUMENT BLADE ANATOMY

The parts of the blade of a scaler or a curet are the

1. *face* (inner surface)
2. *lateral surface*
3. *back*
4. *tip* (scaler) or *toe* (curet)
5. *cutting edges*

A cutting edge is formed by the junction of the face and the lateral surface.

Figure 38-4 shows a curet with each part labeled. The parts of a scaler are named the same. The differences are the pointed tip and the V-shaped back of the scaler shown in Figure 38-9. Each type of instrument is described in the next section.

 # UNIVERSAL CURET

A universal curet can be adapted for instrumentation on any tooth surface.[1] The working ends are paired mirror images on a single handle.

I. DESCRIPTION

A. Blade

1. *Face*
   - Perpendicular (at a 90° angle) to the lower shank **(Figure 38-6A)**.
   - Flat in cross section **(Figure 38-4B)** and curved lengthwise.
2. *Cutting Edges*
   - Two parallel cutting edges on a curved blade **(Figure 38-4A)**.
   - Continuous around the face; used and therefore sharpened, on both sides and around the toe.
3. *Back or Undersurface:* Rounded.
4. *Cross Section of the Blade:* Shaped like a half circle **(Figure 38-4B)**.
5. *Internal Angles*
   - Angles of 70° to 80° are formed where the lateral surfaces meet the face.
   - **Figure 38-5** shows the cross section of a curet with the internal angles marked.

B. Shank

- Angles or curves in the shank are specific for each of the many different universal curets available.[1]

II. PURPOSES AND USES

- Removal of calculus and root debridement for patients of all ages.
- Standard instrument for subgingival scaling to be followed by root planing with Gracey curets.
- After ultrasonic or sonic scaling to complete the procedure to remove residual calculus, to be followed by Gracey curets to plane the tooth surface as needed.

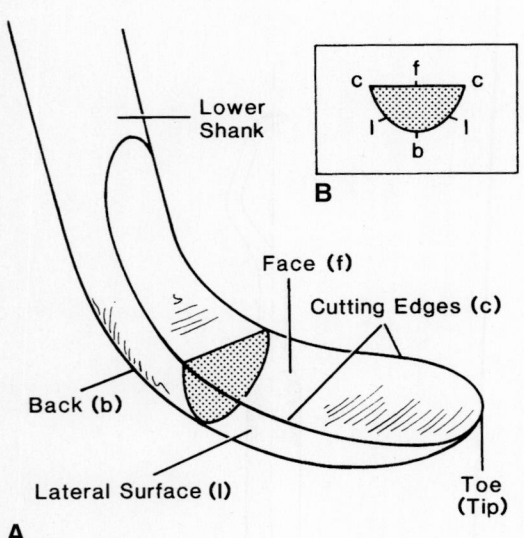

FIGURE 38-4 **Parts of a Curet. (A)** Curet with parts labeled. Lower shank is also called the terminal shank. The curet has a round toe, whereas the scaler has a pointed tip. **(B)** Cross section of a curet labeled f (face), c (cutting edges), l (lateral surfaces), and b (back).

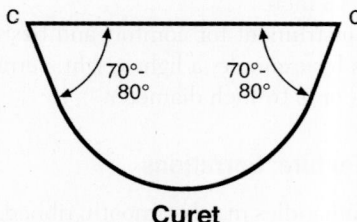

FIGURE 38-5 **Internal Angles of a Curet.** Cross section of a curet shows the 70° to 80° internal angles at the cutting edges. These angles are restored by sharpening techniques.

- Removal of supragingival calculus: especially the fine supragingival calculus close to the gingival margin.
  - Supragingival calculus commonly seen in pediatric patients.
  - The rounded instrument is best adapted to the cervical area.
  - Round back does not traumatize the gingival margin or base of sulcus or pocket when placed subgingivally.
- Useful for obtaining a sample of subgingival biofilm to place on a glass slide for the phase microscope or for microbiologic tests.

 AREA-SPECIFIC CURETS

The Gracey curets are area specific, which means that each curet is designed for adaptation to specific surfaces.

I. DESCRIPTION

A. Gracey Curets

1. *Working Ends:* Paired mirror-image, usually placed on a single handle. The original seven pairs are numbers 1–2, 3–4, 5–6, 7–8, 9–10, 11–12, and 13–14.
2. *Face:* "Offset" (at an angle of approximately 70°) in relation to the lower shank **(Figure 38-6B)**.
3. *Cutting Edge:* Each Gracey has one long sharpened cutting edge and the curved toe, which is also sharpened and used for treatmemt.
4. Only the longer, outer cutting edge that is lower when the handle is held down vertically is sharpened and used during instrumentation.

B. Miniblade and Micro Miniblade

Variations of area-specific curets provide clinicians with greater opportunities to complete deep subgingival

instrumentation on narrow roots and in furcations with improved skills.

1. *Objectives*
   - To facilitate access to the base of deep pockets.
   - To conform to the curvatures of roots on multirooted teeth and single-rooted teeth with moderate to severe loss of attachment.
2. *Shank:* Terminal (lower) shank elongated by 3 mm to adapt in deep pockets. The total length of the shank from blade to handle not changed.
3. *Miniblade*
   - Blade is one-half as long as a traditional Gracey curet.
   - Reduced length facilitates adaptation to the curved features of root morphology including concavities; longitudinal depressions on proximal surfaces; root surfaces within furcations; and interradicular convexities.
4. *Micro Miniblade*
   - Blade is one-half the length of the traditional Gracey curet.
   - It is narrower and 20% thinner with increase in rigidity of the shank to allow pressure when very deep calculus deposit is firmly attached.

II. PURPOSES AND USES

- Standard instruments for subgingival scaling and root planing.
- Necessary after ultrasonic or sonic scaling to complete the procedure as needed.
- A universal curet or a rigid Gracey curet is used for scaling for removal of as much of the calculus as possible.
- Area-specific curets follow for fine scaling and root planing.
- The design of the curet with a slender shank allows entrance into the sulcus or pocket with minimal trauma to the gingival margin.
- The curved blade with rounded end permits access to the base of the sulcus or pocket.
- The rounded back minimizes possible trauma at the base of the sulcus or pocket.

III. APPLICATION

A. Angulation

Blade is applied to the tooth so that the face forms a 70° angle with the tooth surface to be treated.

B. Adaptation

Principles of adaptation are described on page 590 in this chapter.

- Toe third or lower third of the cutting edge is maintained on the tooth surface at all times.
- Minimize soft tissue trauma caused by toe extending away from the tooth in the narrow pocket.

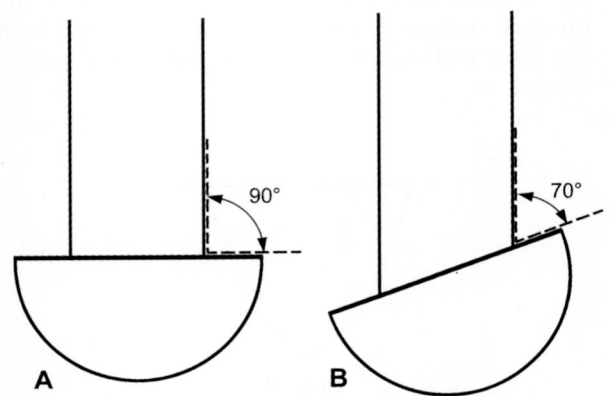

FIGURE 38-6 **Curet Design. (A)** A universal curet with the blade at a 90° angle to the lower shank. **(B)** Offset blade of an area-specific curet at a 70° angle to the lower shank.

- Changes in tooth surface contour require constant attention so that safe contact is maintained.
- On line angles, only 1 or 2 mm near the toe may be used (see Figure 39-5, page 618, Instrument Adaptation).

C. Curet Selection

- Universal curets are used for scaling for removal of as much of the calculus as possible.
- Area-specific curets follow for fine scaling and root planing.

D. Design

- The design of the curet with a slender shank allows entrance into the sulcus or pocket with minimal trauma to the gingival margin.
- The curved blade with rounded end permits access to the base of the sulcus or pocket.
- The rounded back minimizes possible trauma at the base of the sulcus or pocket.

E. Stroke

- *Stroke:* Pull stroke is applied in vertical, horizontal, or oblique directions **(Figure 38-18)**.
- Cutting edge is prepared when the instrument is sharpened for use at 70°. When the instrument is applied at a different angle, a bevel will be created, and the instrument will no longer be sharp.

SCALERS

I. TYPES OF SCALERS: SICKLES AND JACQUETTES

The "sickle" scaler **(Figure 38-7)** and the "Jacquette" scaler **(Figure 38-9)** may be referred to simply as "scalers," either curved or straight, respectively. Scalers may have a straight, curved, or contra-angled shank. The blades and cutting edges may be straight or curved.

A. Curved Scaler/Sickle Scaler

- Two cutting edges on a curved blade **(Figure 38-7)**.
- Face is flat in cross section and curved lengthwise.
- The face converges with the two lateral surfaces to form the *tip* of the scaler, which is a sharp point.
- In cross section, the blade is triangular **(Figure 38-7B)**.
- Internal angles of 70° to 80° are formed where the lateral surfaces meet the face at the cutting edges. **Figure 38-8** shows the cross section of a scaler with the internal angles marked.

B. Straight Scaler/Jacquette

- Two cutting edges on a straight blade **(Figure 38-9)**.
- Face (between the cutting edges) is flat.

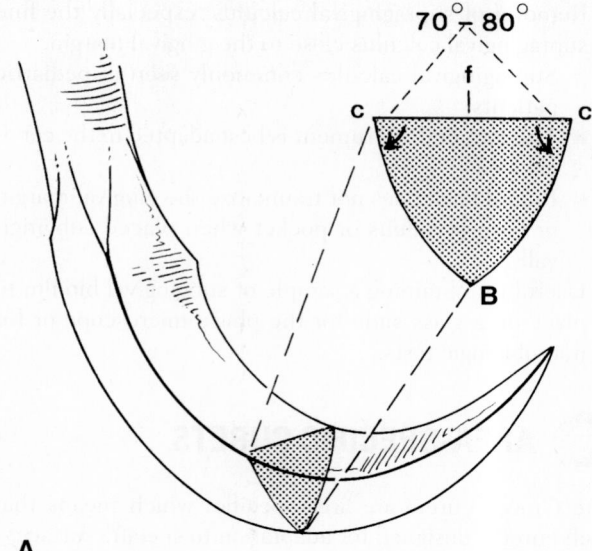

FIGURE 38-7 Curved Scaler (Sickle scaler). (A) The curved blade terminates in a point. **(B)** Cross section shows the face (f) and the two cutting edges (c) formed where the lateral surfaces meet the face at 70° to 80° angles. This type of scaler is also called a sickle scaler.

- The face converges with the two lateral surfaces to form the tip of the scaler, which is a sharp point.
- Cross section of the blade is triangular **(Figure 38-9B)**.
- Internal angles of 70° to 80° are formed where the lateral surfaces meet the face at the cutting edges **(Figure 38-8)**.

C. Angulation of the Shank

- *Straight:* Single instrument in which the relationships of the shank, blade, and handle are in a flat plane; adaptable primarily for anterior teeth, although may be used for scaling premolars when the lips and cheeks permit retraction for correct angulation.
- *Modified or Contra-Angle:* Paired instruments that are mirror images of each other to provide access to the proximal surfaces of posterior teeth; one adapts from the facial and the other from the lingual and palatal aspects.

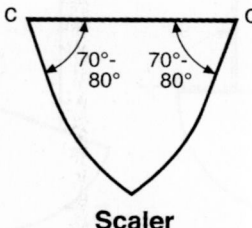

FIGURE 38-8 Internal Angles of a Scaler. Cross section of a scaler shows the 70° to 80° internal angles. These angles are restored by sharpening techniques.

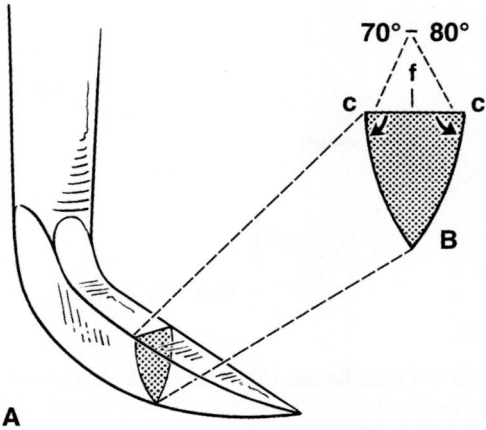

FIGURE 38-9 **Straight Scaler (Jacquette). (A)** The straight blade converges to a point where the two cutting edges meet at the tip. **(B)** Cross section of the scaler shows the face (f), the two cutting edges (c), and the 70° to 80° internal angles. This type of scaler is also known as the Jacquette scaler.

D. Purposes and Uses of Scaler

- Principally for the removal of supragingival calculus.
- May be useful for removal of gross calculus that is slightly below the gingival margin when the calculus is continuous with the supragingival calculus, and when the gingival tissue is spongy and flexible to permit easy insertion of the instrument.

E. Contraindications for Use of Scalers Subgingivally

- Cause undue trauma to the gingival tissue because of the large size, thickness, and length of the blade.
- Pointed tip and straight cutting edges cannot be adapted to the curved root surfaces. Risk of grooving or scratching the cemental surface is greater.
- Tactile sensitivity decreased with larger, heavier blades.

F. Application

- *Angulation:* The face of the blade is adapted to the tooth surface at an angle of approximately 70°.
- *Stroke:* Pull stroke only for this type of blade.
- Small scalers can be useful for removal of fine supragingival deposits directly under contact areas and between overlapping teeth.

II. FILE SCALER

A. Characteristics

- May be metal or diamond.
- Multiple cutting edges lined up as a series of miniature hoes on a round, oval, or rectangular base **(Figure 38-10A)**.
- The metal multiple blades are at a 90° angle with the shank **(Figure 38-10B)**.

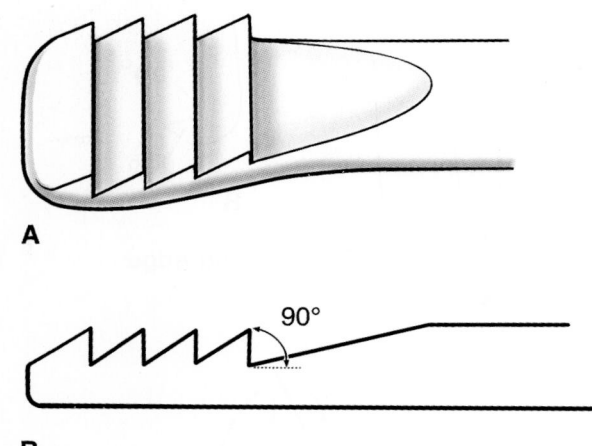

FIGURE 38-10 **File Scaler. (A)** A file has multiple cutting edges. **(B)** Each blade is at a 90° angle with the shank.

- Shanks are variously angulated: most are paired instruments.
- Reduced tactile sensitivity because of the series of blades.

B. Purposes and Uses of a File Scaler

- Removal of calculus
  - Crushes and fractures calculus into fragments prior to use of curets.
  - Burnished calculus that is impervious to removal with other bladed instruments can be removed with the file scaler.
  - Gross deposits of calculus on patients for whom ultrasonic use is contraindicated.
- Smoothing of the tooth at the cementoenamel junction.
- Smoothing down of overextended or rough amalgam restorations, particularly on proximal surfaces or in the cervical areas.

C. Application

- *Adaptation*
  Entire working surface is placed flat against the area to be treated. Flat blade adapted to the curved tooth surfaces is difficult. In certain relationships, such as on a line angle, the file has only a tangential contact.
- Pressure applied permits the cutting edges to grasp the surface.
- *Stroke:* pull only, using a linear motion.
- *File Use:* must always be followed with curet(s) to leave a smooth surface on roots.

III. HOE SCALER

A. Characteristics

- Single straight cutting edge **(Figure 38-11)**.
- *Blade:* Turned at a 99° angle to the shank.

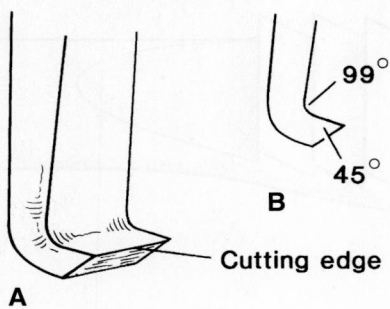

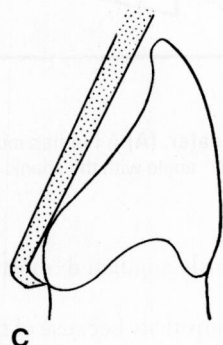

FIGURE 38-11 **Hoe Scaler. (A)** The hoe has a single cutting edge. **(B)** The blade is turned at an angle of 99° to the shank, and the cutting edge is beveled at a 45° angle. **(C)** Adaptation to a tooth for removal of calculus is with a two-point contact where possible.

■ *Cutting Edge:* Beveled at a 45° angle to the end of the blade **(Figure 38-11B)**.
■ *Shank:* Variously angulated for adaptation of cutting edges to accessible tooth surfaces; some are paired.

B. Purposes and Uses of a Hoe Scaler

■ Removes supragingival calculus, particularly large, accessible, tenacious pieces.
■ *Contraindications for use subgingivally:*
  A. Insertion of the thick-bladed instrument into the sulcus can cause unnecessary distention of the pocket wall.
  B. Lack of adaptability of the wide straight cutting edge to the curved root surface.
  C. Difficulty of use without gouging the cemental surface. The sharp "corners" need to be rounded with sharpening, as shown on page 605 later in this chapter.
  D. Lack of sensitivity because of the bulk of the instrument and the marked angulation of the shanks of some hoes.

C. Application

■ Full width of the cutting edge may be in contact with the calculus.
■ Two-point contact is maintained with the tooth to stabilize the instrument during the positioning and activation. Two-point contact means contact of the cutting edge and the side of the shank with the tooth **(Figure 38-11C)**.

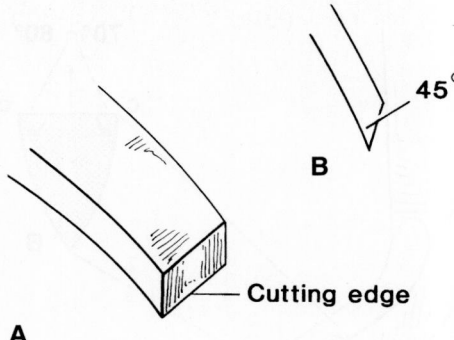

FIGURE 38-12 **Chisel Scaler. (A)** A chisel scaler has a single cutting edge, and the blade is continuous with a slightly curved shank. **(B)** A 45° bevel is at the cutting edge.

■ Hoes are not generally applied to proximal surfaces except the surface adjacent to an edentulous area.
■ *Pull stroke* is used in a coronal direction.

IV. CHISEL SCALER

A. Characteristics

■ Single straight cutting edge **(Figure 38-12)**.
■ Blade is continuous with a slightly curved shank.
■ End of blade is flat and beveled at 45° **(Figure 38-12B)**.

B. Purposes and Uses of a Chisel Scaler

■ Removal of supragingival calculus from exposed proximal surfaces of anterior teeth where interdental gingiva is missing.
■ Dislodgement of heavy calculus from the proximal areas of mandibular anterior teeth. When the calculus on the lingual surfaces may form a continuous bridge across several teeth, the chisel can be pushed horizontally from the facial aspect to break up the large masses of calculus.
■ Proximal surfaces of premolars when flexibility of the lips and cheeks permits retraction for proper positioning of the cutting edge.

C. Application

■ *Apply full width of cutting edge:* Sharp corners can nick and groove the tooth surface. Round the sharp "corners" during sharpening (page 581).
■ *Stroke:* Horizontal only, from facial to lingual on proximal surfaces of anterior, particularly mandibular, teeth.

PRINCIPLES FOR INSTRUMENT USE

Understanding the purpose of each instrument and developing dexterity in the effective use of the instruments are basic to clinical dental hygiene practice. The clinical results obtained for the patient depend on the proficiency and thoroughness with which the instrumentation is accomplished.

Stability is essential for effective, controlled action of an instrument. The correct use depends on maintaining *control* of the movement of the instrument through use of an effective *grasp* and the establishment and maintenance of an appropriate, firm, fulcrum *finger rest*.

INSTRUMENT GRASP

I. FUNCTIONS OF THE INSTRUMENT GRASP

A. Dominant Hand

■ The right hand is the dominant hand for the right-handed clinician.
■ A few rare people are completely ambidextrous, and others are partially dexterous with the nondominant hand, a useful capability when carrying out dental and dental hygiene procedures.
■ Exercises for developing dexterity are provided on pages 594 to 596 in this chapter.
■ The dominant hand is used to hold and activate the treatment instrument. The manner in which the instrument is held influences the entire procedure.

B. Nondominant Hand

■ The right-handed clinician uses the left hand and the left-handed clinician uses the right hand for essential supplementary functions to assist the dominant hand.
■ **Figure 38-13** shows the recommended modified pen grasp for each hand.
■ The mouth mirror is held by the nondominant hand.
■ With the appropriate grasp and finger rest, the following effects can be provided:
   A. Control of the position of the mirror for indirect vision, indirect lighting, and retraction.
   B. Assistance in providing the dominant hand with an auxiliary finger rest.

C. Grasp Dynamics

■ A rigid grasp, in which the instrument is gripped tightly, lessens the tactile sensitivity and, hence, the effectiveness of instrumentation.
■ The appropriate grasp is controlled, displays the confidence of the clinician in the work being done, and provides the following effects:
   ▪ Increased fingertip tactile sensitivity.
   ▪ Positive control of the instrument with balance and flexibility during motion.
   ▪ Decreased hazard of trauma to the dental and periodontal tissues, which in turn results in less postcare discomfort for the patient.
   ▪ Prevention of fatigue to clinician's fingers, hand, and arm.

II. TYPES OF GRASPS

A. Modified Pen Grasp for Internal Finger Rests

1. *Description:* The modified pen grasp is a three-finger grasp with specific target points of the thumb, index finger, and middle (second) finger all in contact with the instrument.
   ▪ *Thumb:* the center of the upper aspect of the pad.
   ▪ *Index finger:* the center of the upper aspect of the pad.
   ▪ *Middle finger:* the inside upper corner of the pad, behind the upper corner of the nail.
2. *Location on Handle*
   ▪ The instrument is held by the thumb and index finger on the handle.
   ▪ The upper corner of the middle finger is placed on the upper portion of the shank to hold and guide the movement **(Figure 38-13)**.
3. *Role of Middle Finger*
   ▪ The shank of the instrument is held against the inside upper corner of the pad of the middle finger.
   ▪ The instrument *is not* held across the nail or the side of the middle finger, as in a pen grasp usually used for writing.

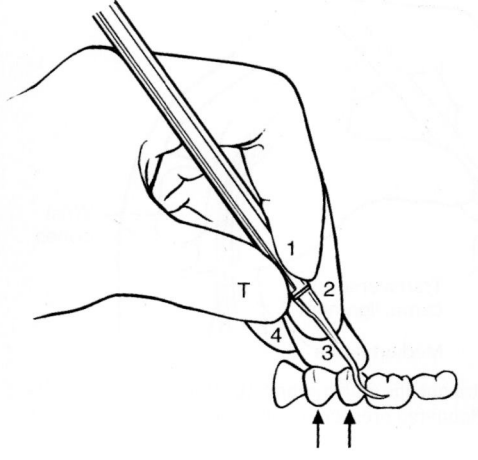
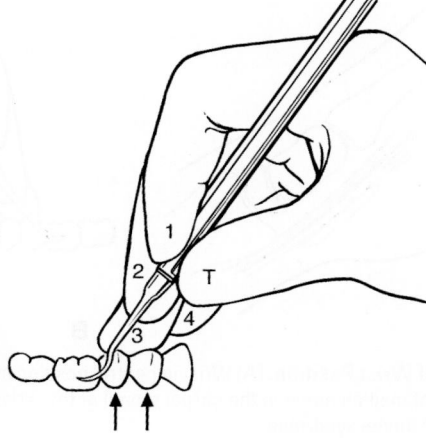

FIGURE 38-13 **Modified Pen Grasp for Left and Right Hands.** An instrument is held by the thumb (T), index finger (1), and the second, or "middle," finger (2), which also provides support. The third, or "ring," finger (3) serves as the finger rest, and the fourth, or "little," finger (4) is positioned beside the ring finger to supplement the finger rest.

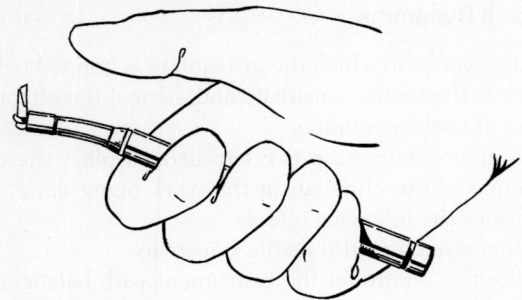

FIGURE 38-14 Palm Grasp of Instrument. The instrument handle is held in the palm by cupped index, middle, ring, and little fingers. Thumb is free and serves as the finger rest.

■ The specific position of the middle finger is essential to instrument control to prevent the instrument from slipping during adaptation and activation and to optimize application of lateral pressure.

4. *Role of Ring Finger:* The ring finger is used to establish a finger rest/fulcrum.

5. *Additional Support:* The side-to-side contact of index, middle, and ring fingers allows for greater stability, strength, and control during instrumentation.

B. Palm Grasp

1. *Description:* The handle of the instrument is held in the palm by cupped index, middle, ring, and little fingers. The thumb is free to serve as the fulcrum **(Figure 38-14)**.

2. *Limitations of Use:* Instruments for calculus removal, root planing, and maintenance root debridement are not used with a palm grasp. The possible exception is a chisel scaler when it is used to remove gross calculus by a push stroke.

3. *Examples of Uses for Palm Grasp*
   ■ Air syringe
   ■ Rubber dam clamp holder

■ Chisel for restorative work
■ Nondominant hand stabilizing the instrument for sharpening **(Figure 38-25A)**

NEUTRAL POSITIONS

Neutral positions for the wrist, forearm, elbow, and shoulder are basic to the following:

■ Efficient performance directed at the prevention of occupational pain risks, particularly those risks related to cumulative trauma disorders.
■ Clinical activities to prevent cumulative trauma disorders, particularly prevention of carpal tunnel syndrome described in Chapter 7, Figure 7-5 (page 95) and Table 7-1 (page 95).
■ General clinician and dental chair positioning and neutral body positioning are described in Chapter 7 on pages 90 to 92.

I. WRIST

■ The wrist is straight, and the forearm and the hand are in the same horizontal plane when in the neutral position.
■ **Figure 38-15** illustrates the straight wrist and the effect of a bent wrist.
■ Carpal tunnel syndrome, brought on by pressure on the median nerve in the carpal tunnel, is one of the nerve entrapment conditions that results from inappropriate work habits, such as working with a bent wrist.

II. ELBOW

The neutral elbow is 90° or greater, with the forearm positioned horizontally or slightly oblique. The hand is in straight alignment with the forearm.

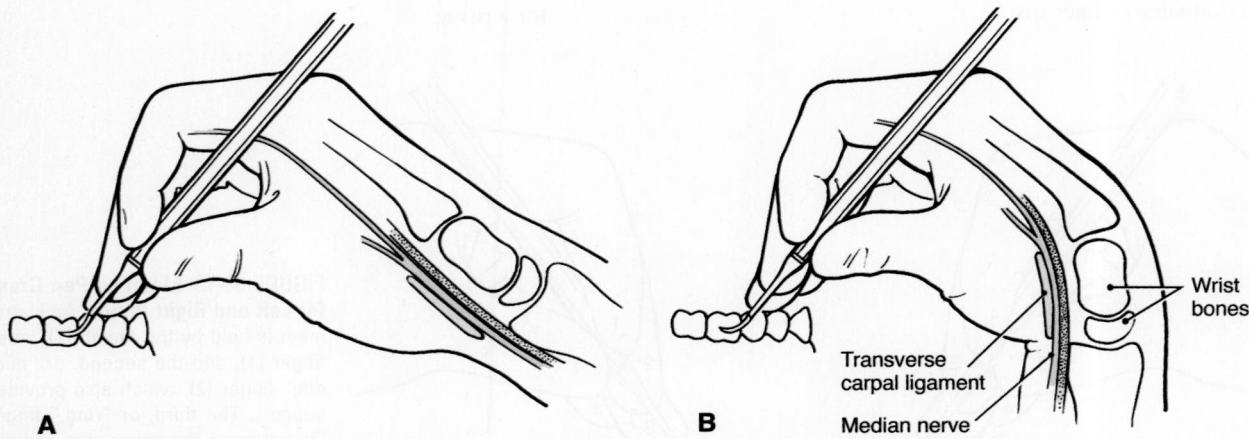

A

B

Wrist bones

Transverse carpal ligament

Median nerve

FIGURE 38-15 Effect of Wrist Position. (A) Wrist in neutral position in straight line with forearm. **(B)** Bent wrist shows cramping of median nerve in the carpal tunnel of the wrist. Repeated pressure on the median nerve can cause carpal tunnel syndrome.

III. SHOULDER

In neutral, both shoulders are level and relaxed to their lowest position. From a lateral position, each is vertically in line with, and beneath, each ear. The upper arms are straight down to the elbow.

FULCRUM: FINGER REST

A finger rest is always be used when instruments are applied to the teeth and gingiva.

I. DEFINITION

A. Fulcrum

The support, or point of rest, on which a lever turns in moving a body.

B. Finger Rest

The support, or point of finger rest on the tooth surface, on which the hand turns in moving an instrument.

II. OBJECTIVES

An effective, well-established finger rest is essential to the following:

A. Stability

For controlled action of the instrument.

B. Unit Control

Provides a focal point from which the whole hand can move as a unit.

C. Prevention of Injury

Injury to the patient's oral tissues can result from irregular pressure and uncontrolled movement.

D. Comfort for the Patient

Confidence in the clinician's ability, which results from the feeling of securely applied instruments.

E. Control of Length of Stroke

With instrument grasp, the finger rest limits the instrumentation to where it is needed.

III. INTRAORAL RESTS

The intraoral finger rest is essentially a total hand-coordinated effort to provide stabilization. **Figure 38-13** (page 587) shows the fingers grouped together with the fulcrum where the ring finger (no. 3 in **Figure 38-13**) maintains its position on a tooth near the tooth being treated.

A. Digits Used for Finger Rest

1. *Modified Pen Grasp*
   - *Ring finger:* Little finger is held close beside ring finger (finger nos. 3 and 4 in **Figure 38-13**).
   - *Supplementary:* Middle finger is held beside ring finger to provide total hand unity; ring finger maintains regular fulcrum position, and middle finger maintains its grasp on the instrument.
2. *Palm Grasp:* Thumb.

B. Location of Finger Rest

1. *Purposes:* The location of a finger rest is selected for the following reasons:
   - Convenience to area of instrumentation
   - Ease in instrument adaptation
   - Maintenance of an effective grasp
   - Application of the appropriate angulation
   - Stability and control of instrument during the activation (strokes)
   - Safety of the clinician. A finger rest is not placed in line of the stroke direction to prevent a rubber glove puncture and/or a finger stab if the patient moved suddenly or the instrument slipped for any reason.
2. *Principles*
   - The first choice for an intraoral finger rest is the tooth or teeth adjacent to the tooth being treated.
   - Maintain the rest on firm stable tooth or teeth. The patient's chin, lips, and cheeks are mobile and flexible and therefore less reliable for stability.
   - Where possible, the rest is placed in the same arch, maxillary or mandibular, as the instrumentation; also, where possible, the rest is placed in the same quadrant.

IV. VARIATIONS OF FINGER REST[2,3]

A basic fulcrum location cannot always be used or may require supplementation.

A. Problems

1. Limitations of oral anatomic features:
   - Patient's facial musculature
   - Mouth opening (microstomia)
   - Size of tongue
   - Arrangement of the teeth or malocclusions of individual teeth
   - Physical disability affecting the oral cavity indirectly may interfere with customary positioning for instrumentation.

2. Tenacious calculus in difficult-access areas may not be removed and root surfaces may not be planed by the usual procedures. Greater support and pressure to the instrument are required.

3. When the problem in instrumentation seems to be related to space and accessibility, the height and position of the patient's oral cavity needs to be checked. Also, a change in the clinician's working position may be necessary.

B. General Categories of Variations[3]

When a variation in finger rest is used, basic rules for stability and control are applied, and rests on movable tissues are avoided. Three types of variations are suggested here: *substitute, supplementary,* and *reinforced* finger rests. Any of these variations may require an external position.

1. *Substitute*
   ■ Missing teeth where finger rest is usually applied.
      ■ For an edentulous area, a cotton roll or gauze sponge may be packed into the area to provide a dry finger rest.
      ■ Otherwise, a rest across the dental arch or in the opposite arch may be required to provide stability.
   ■ Mobile teeth, or teeth with inadequate bony support.
      ■ Avoid mobile teeth for finger rests or use only with minimal pressure for brief periods.
      ■ Not only would the rest on a mobile tooth be unstable, but also pressure, movement, and undue stress on the tooth could traumatize and tear the periodontal ligament fibers.
   ■ Index finger of nondominant hand may be placed in the vestibule over a cotton roll or a dry gauze square.
      ■ The usual finger rest can be placed on the index finger to aid retraction and visibility, particularly in the mouth of a small child.

2. *Supplementary*
   Place the index finger of the nondominant hand on the occlusal surfaces of teeth adjacent to the working area. The finger rest can then be applied to the nondominant index finger.
   ■ This is known as a "finger-on-finger" rest.
   ■ Such supplements are helpful for achieving a parallel orientation of the terminal shank to proximal surfaces.
   ■ Supplemental rests are not useful for certain distal surfaces where the mouth mirror is essential for vision.

3. *Reinforced*
   In this type, a support is placed between the instrument handle and the working end to provide additional strength and force, particularly for hard, tenacious calculus in pockets.
   ■ Index finger of nondominant hand can be rested on the tooth adjacent to the one being scaled, while the thumb is placed on the instrument shank (or handle) for a reinforcement.
   ■ Greater control of the instrument can result and, when applied correctly, the danger of instrument breakage is reduced.
   ■ A definite rest for both hands is needed to distribute the pressure.

V. TOUCH OR PRESSURE APPLIED TO FINGER REST

A. Balance

■ The fulcrum finger rest maintains a secure hold with variable pressure to balance the action of the instrument being applied.
■ A balance is needed between the pressure exerted against the tooth and the pressure into the finger rest. These pressures will be described under "Activation: Stroke."

B. Effects of Excess Pressure

■ Decreased stability
■ Diminished control
■ Overtightened grasp to accommodate
■ Fatigue of patient caused by use of mandibular fulcrums; heavy pressure on the movable mandible can cause fatigue in the temporomandibular joint and related muscles and, thus, discomfort for the patient
■ Fatigue in clinician's fingers and hand

ADAPTATION

With an appropriate grasp and finger rest, the instrument is next ready for application. The working end of the instrument is adapted to the surface of the tooth where instrumentation is to take place.

I. RELATION TO TOOTH SURFACE

■ Select the correct end of a double-ended paired instrument.
■ The side of the tip or toe is maintained in close approximation to the surface being examined or treated.
■ The blade of an instrument is divided into thirds referred to as the shank third, the middle third, and the toe (or tip) third, as shown in Figure 39-4 (page 618).

II. CHARACTERISTICS OF A WELL-ADAPTED INSTRUMENT

A. Working End

■ The working end of the instrument is positioned correctly for the task to be accomplished. Example: when scaling, the angle formed by the face of the instrument and the tooth surface is crucial for effective calculus removal. ("Angulation" is described in a following section.)

■ The instrument is adapted for maximum usefulness of the working end. Example: 2 to 3 mm of the toe third of a curet may be adaptable when on a "flat" surface, whereas at a line angle or convex surface of a narrow root, less than 2 mm may be adaptable.

■ The working end is applied to conform to the contour of the tooth surface.

■ As the instrument is activated, it is adjusted to changes required by variations in the surface topography.

B. Soft Tissue

A properly adapted instrument harms neither the tissue being treated nor the surrounding or adjacent tissues.

III. PROBLEM AREAS

Areas where instrument adaptation is most difficult and requires more attention, time, and careful application of skill include the following:

A. Line Angles

All line angles require that the instrument be rolled between the fingers to turn the working end as the instrument is activated. At each change of direction around a line angle, the instrument must be rolled to keep it adapted to the surface. **Figure 38-16** shows the adaptation of an explorer tip to a line angle.

B. Convex and Rounded Surfaces

Particularly of narrow roots.

C. Cervical Area

Where the root is constricted.

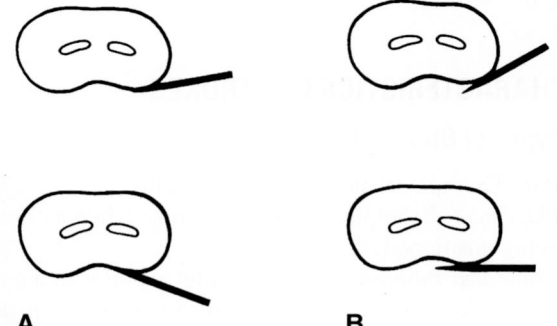

FIGURE 38-16 Instrument Adaptation. Cross section of maxillary first permanent premolar to show adaptation of the tip of an explorer. **(A)** Appropriate adaptation in which the tip of the explorer is maintained on the tooth surface in a series of strokes to explore around a line angle. **(B)** Incorrect adaptation with the tip of the explorer extended away from the tooth surface.

D. Proximal Root Surface

Root surfaces may be concave, have longitudinal grooves, or have narrow furcation openings.

ANGULATION

A factor closely related to and directly influencing instrument adaptation is angulation. Angulation refers to the angle formed at the cutting edge of an instrument between the tooth surface and the face of the instrument. Each instrument is applied to a surface in a specific manner for optimum adaptation and angulation.

I. PROBE

■ The usual adaptation of a probe is to maintain the side of the working tip on the tooth, with the long axis of the working end nearly parallel with the tooth surface.

■ As used for a bleeding index, the tip is placed inside the pocket wall and pressed lightly on the wall as the probe is moved horizontally around the tooth (see Figure 22-11, page 326).

II. EXPLORER

■ An explorer is held with the tip at a right angle to the occlusal surface when detecting occlusal pit or fissure caries.

■ On other surfaces, the side of the tip is kept on the tooth at all times.

■ The angle is 5° or less. Figure 15-14 (page 238) illustrates the use of the subgingival explorer.

III. SCALERS AND CURETS

Angulation for a scaler or a curet means the angle formed by the face at the cutting edge of the instrument with the surface to which the instrument is applied. **Figure 38-17** shows the various angles for curet adaptation. At zero angulation the curet face is flat against the tooth surface **(Figure 38-17A)**.

A. Scaling and Root Planing

■ For curets and scalers, an angle of 70° between the face of the instrument and the tooth surface permits effective calculus removal **(Figure 38-17B)**.

■ Markedly closed angulation uses only the side of a sharp cutting edge and can result in burnishing.

■ Burnishing produces a smooth veneer, making the calculus difficult or impossible to detect with an explorer.

B. Gingival Curettage

The face is turned toward the soft tissue wall of the pocket. The angle formed by the face of the curet blade

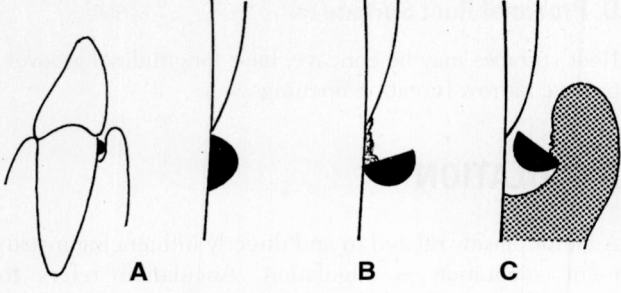

FIGURE 38-17 Instrument Angulation. Enlargement of pocket area from the tooth on the left shows cross section of a curet blade in black. **(A)** The curet is angulated at 0° with the tooth surface when used in an exploratory or insertion stroke. At 0° the face of the blade is flat against the tooth surface. **(B)** Blade angulated at approximately 70° with the tooth surface for scaling and root planing. **(C)** Open blade angulated toward the pocket wall in position for gingival curettage. The face of the blade forms an angle of approximately 70° with the soft tissue pocket wall.

and the soft tissue pocket wall being treated is approximately 70° **(Figure 38-17C)**.

LATERAL PRESSURE

Lateral pressure means the pressure of the instrument against the tooth surface during activation. It is described as light, moderate, or heavy pressure.

I. DETECTION INSTRUMENTS

Explorers and probes are used with a light pressure to maximize the sense of touch in detecting irregularities.

II. TREATMENT INSTRUMENTS

A. Assessment Stroke

A light pressure equal to that used by an explorer is applied as the curet blade is moved across the tooth surface. The purpose of the assessment stroke is to do the following:

- Assess the surface texture of the root.
- Confirm the positioning of the back of the curet at the soft tissue attachment.
- Rehearse an intended movement of the curet before activating a working stroke to confirm correct adaptation.

B. Scaling Stroke or Working Stroke

A definite, well-controlled, firm stroke of moderate to heavy pressure is used for calculus removal.

C. Root Planing Stroke

- A varying amount of pressure is applied, dependent upon the surface textures of the root surface.

- Lateral pressure begins as moderately firm if deposits are present.
- As strokes continue, a lighter pressure is applied progressively as the root surface becomes smooth and all the calculus has been removed.

D. Root Debridement Stroke

A lighter pressure is applied as a curet disrupts and removes dental biofilm from the root surface of a previously root planed tooth.

III. ERRORS IN TECHNIQUE

A. Effects of Insufficient Pressure

- Burnishing of calculus.
- Loss of control when both fulcrum and lateral pressure are insufficient.

B. Effects of Excessive Pressure

- Excess removal of tooth structure; gouging of root surfaces
- Loss of instrument control
- Potential damage to soft tissue, pocket lining; bleeding
- Patient discomfort; discomfort during healing later
- Clinician fatigue

ACTIVATION: STROKE

A stroke is an unbroken movement made by an instrument; it is the action of an instrument in the performance of the task for which it was designed.

Strokes may be identified by the instrumentation being performed. Examples are the "probing stroke," "scaling stroke," or "root planing stroke." Technique for each type is described in the chapters covering the specific procedures.

I. CHARACTERISTICS OF STROKES

A. Types of Strokes by Action

- *Pull.* Example: scaler removing calculus.
- *Placement.* Example: exploratory stroke when a curet is being positioned.
- *Combined Push and Pull:* Example: explorer in a walking stroke, which is moving the instrument up and down with equal pressure on the surface (see Figure 15-14, page 238).
- *Walking Stroke.* Example: probe is moved up and down, gently touching the coronal border of the periodontal attachment with each down stroke (see Figure 15-6, page 231).

B. Types of Strokes by Function

■ *Assessment Stroke*

A. Used to detect irregularities of the tooth surface such as the presence of calculus, a carious lesion, or a rough overhanging margin.

B. The assessment stroke is also called an exploratory stroke. The grasp pressure is light so that tactile sense is magnified.

C. Examples:

1. Probe is used to locate the attachment at the bottom of the periodontal pocket (page 231 in Chapter 15) and to estimate the amount of deposit present on the root surfaces while probing.

2. Explorer is used to evaluate for surface smoothness following treatment.

3. Ultrasonic tip is used with the power turned off only to confirm the soft tissue attachment for adequate access to the base of the pocket.

■ *Working Stroke*

The stroke applied to accomplish a task such as calculus removal or reshaping an overhanging margin.

C. Types of Strokes by Direction (Figure 38-18)

1. *Diagonal or Oblique:* Stroke that is diagonal across the surface being treated (**Figure 38-18A**).

2. *Vertical:* Strokes parallel with the long axis of the tooth being treated (**Figure 38-18B**).

3. *Horizontal:* Strokes parallel with the occlusal surface of the tooth being treated (**Figure 38-18C**). They are sometimes called circumferential, which should not be interpreted to mean that a stroke can be made to go around a tooth or large segment of a tooth. A horizontal stroke necessarily must be a short stroke because of the constant changes in the topography of the tooth surface.

4. *Curvilinear or Circular*

■ Stroke used with a handpiece. A small circular stroke is used with varying pressure to:

■ Apply polishing agent with a rubber cup (page 700).

■ Polish amalgam restorations using stones, burs, rubber cups, and points.

■ Assessment stroke with an explorer, to check a surface for residual calculus.

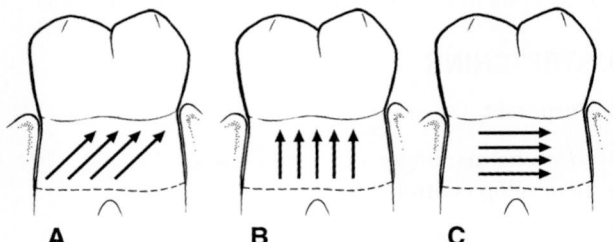

FIGURE 38-18 Directions of Instrument Strokes. Arrows on root surface represent (**A**) diagonal or oblique strokes, (**B**) vertical strokes, and (**C**) horizontal strokes.

II. FACTORS THAT INFLUENCE SELECTION OF STROKE

■ Size, contour, and position of gingiva

■ Surface and section of surface where the instrument is used

■ Probing depth

■ Size and shape of instrument used

■ Procedure objective, for example, nature of the deposit to be removed

III. NATURE OF STROKE

A. Grasp

■ The grasp of a scaler or curet is light while the working end is positioned for the stroke, and then the instrument is held more firmly during movement.

■ An explorer and a probe are held lightly for tactile sensitivity at all times.

B. Hand Stability

■ During a stroke, the whole hand pivots or rotates on the fulcrum.

C. Motion

■ The motion for a stroke is generated by a unified action of the shoulder, arm, wrist, and hand.

D. Length

■ The length of the scaling stroke is limited by the extent of calculus deposit and by the anatomic features of the area where the deposit is located.

■ The stroke is short, controlled, decisive, and directed to protect the tissues from trauma.

■ Instrumentation is applied to the section of the tooth where treatment is indicated. This section is called the *instrumentation zone.*

■ Avoid strokes long enough to pass over the whole crown when the calculus represents only a small area at the cervical third of the tooth.

■ The length of a stroke varies with each instrument and purpose. A description of strokes for each instrument is included in the respective chapters. In Chapter 15, the probe is described on page 226 and the explorer on page 234. **Figure 38-18** shows direction of strokes for various instruments.

IV. BALANCE OF PRESSURE

For control, a balance or equalization of pressure exists between the instrument blade against the tooth surface and the pressure on the fulcrum. Keeping the two forces equal will facilitate a stable, intentional control of the instrument as it is activated.

A. Assessment

- When exploring the tooth surface, the pressure of the instrument on the tooth is light.
- The grasp pressure of the fingers holding the instrument is also light, in order to achieve tactile sensitivity.
- The pressure of the rest, whether a fulcrum finger or hand, is light but secure and stable.

B. Calculus Removal

- When moving from assessment to activation of a working stroke, the pressure on the tooth and on the fulcrum increases dramatically.
- The lateral pressure on the handle of the instrument engages the blade for the working stroke. This is equal to the pressure of the instrument against the tooth.
- As the working stroke is initiated to remove calculus on a tooth surface, the pressure of the instrument against the tooth is firm. It may vary from medium heavy to heavy depending on the age of the calculus and the strength of its attachment to the tooth.
- The pressure of the finger or hand rest (fulcrum) must be equally firm to achieve stability and control of the instrument as it is activated.

C. Maintenance Root Debridement

- When removing dental biofilm from a tooth surface with minimal deposit, the pressure of the instrument on the tooth is light to moderate.
- The pressure of the specific grasp fingers supplying lateral pressure to the handle of the instrument equals the pressure of the blade on the tooth.
- The pressure of the finger/hand rest is similarly moderate.
- Pressures vary with the textures encountered.
  - When the texture changes from grainy to rough, the pressure of both finger/hand rest and blade against the tooth surface will increase in order to remove the deposit on the tooth surface.
  - Pressure is, therefore, responsive to the tactile information transmitted as the instrument progresses along the tooth surface.

VISIBILITY AND ACCESSIBILITY

I. EFFECTS OF ADEQUATE VISION AND ACCESSIBILITY

- Instrumentation is more thorough.
- Trauma to the oral tissues is minimized.
- Length of time required may be lessened, thereby lessening fatigue for patient and clinician.
- Patient cooperation can be increased because of shortened treatment time and less discomfort.

II. CONTRIBUTING FACTORS

- Patient and clinician positions.
- Efficient use of direct or reflected illumination by mouth mirror for each tooth surface.
- Adequate, yet gentle, retraction of lips, cheeks, and tongue with consideration for the patient's comfort and clinician's convenience.
- Magnification: use of loupes.

DEXTERITY DEVELOPMENT

- The dental hygiene student and the dental hygienist returning to practice after a temporary leave of absence can appreciate the need for exercises to develop dexterity and strength for the efficient and effective use of instruments.
- In addition, all students, returning retirees, and dental hygienists continuing in practice need an understanding of preventive measures that can preserve the health of their hands, arms, shoulders, and all muscles and joints involved when undertaking patient care.
- However generally dexterous a person may be, the use of new or unusual instruments requires different procedures for coordination. Control is essential, and guided strength contributes to control.
- Proficiency during procedures comes from repeated correct use of the instruments. Exercises for the fingers, hands, and arms supplement experience. Directed exercises are needed for both hands, separately and together. During the training period, a regular period of time each day can be set aside for exercises.

I. SQUEEZING THERAPY PUTTY OR A SOFT BALL

A. Purpose

To develop strength and control.

B. Procedure

- Hold putty in palm of hand; grip with thumb and all fingers (**Figure 38-19A**).
- Tighten and release grip at regular intervals.
- One hand rests while other is exercising.
- Use a ball in each hand to exercise at the same time.

II. STRETCHING

A. Purposes

- To strengthen finger and hand muscles.
- To develop control of finger movements.

B. Rubber Band on Finger Joints

- Place band at joint between first phalanx and second phalanx.

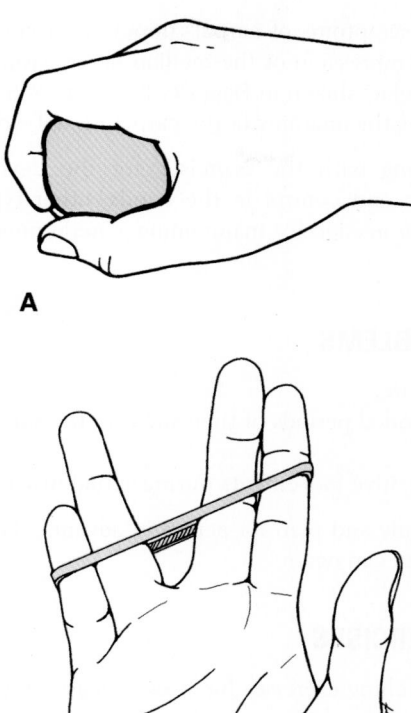

FIGURE 38-19 Exercises for Dexterity Development. (A) Squeezing therapy putty can aid in developing strength and control. **(B)** A rubber band can be applied at each group of finger and thumb joints and stretched.

■ Stretch band by separating middle and ring fingers **(Figure 38-19B)**.
■ Place band at joint between second phalanx and third phalanx and proceed as before.
■ Place bands on both hands and do exercises together.

C. Rubber Band on Finger Joints With Use of Fulcrum

■ Place band on joint between first phalanx and second phalanx.
■ Establish fulcrum (ring finger) on tabletop with little finger closely adjacent to it; elbow and forearm are free, as they are during instrumentation. Keep wrist straight, in same horizontal line as the forearm, and hold elbow at 90°. Stretch band by separating middle and ring fingers.
■ Touch thumb and index and middle fingers to simulate a modified pen grasp for holding an instrument. Stretch band by separating middle and ring fingers.
■ Variations
  ▪ Hold instrument in modified pen grasp while doing the exercise.
  ▪ Do writing exercise with rubber band in place.
■ Rest one hand while other is being exercised.

III. WRITING

A. Purposes

■ To develop correct modified pen grasp.
■ To propel instrument by activation from wrist and arm, without moving fingers.
■ To practice use of instruments when mouth mirror is required.
■ To develop control and precision.

B. Circles and Vertical Lines

■ Hold long, well-sharpened pencil with modified pen grasp.
■ Establish fulcrum (ring finger) on a piece of paper on tabletop. Keep wrist straight in line with forearm; elbow is at 90°, and shoulder is in neutral position. Forearm and elbow are free.
■ Inscribe counterclockwise small circles and vertical lines on paper, rapidly and lightly at first, slowly and with more pressure later.
■ Accomplish writing by activation of the hand by the upper arm, without flexing or extending the thumb and fingers holding the pencil.
■ Practice with each hand separately at first; then use a pencil in each hand at the same time, alternating writing action to simulate adaptation of the mirror first and then the explorer or scaler.

C. Using Mouth Mirror

■ Hold mouth mirror with modified pen grasp in non-dominant hand close to pencil while practicing writing exercises (previous section) through the mirror. Reverse hands.
■ Using engineer's graph paper and modified pen grasp with fulcrum as described earlier, follow the lines of the small squares while looking in mirror held with opposite hand.

D. Everyday Penmanship

■ Use modified pen grasp whenever possible for writing.
■ Practice word writing with the left hand (with the right hand for left-handed person) to increase dexterity for handling instruments.

IV. MOUTH MIRROR, COTTON PLIERS, AND EXPLORER

A. Purposes

■ To develop ability to turn mouth mirror at various angles.
■ To develop dexterity in holding objects with cotton pliers.
■ To establish desired grasp of explorer to ensure maximum touch sensitivity.

B. Mouth Mirror

- Hold mouth mirror with modified pen grasp, ring finger on tabletop as fulcrum finger with little finger closely adjacent to it; elbow and forearm are free. The mirror is used most frequently in the nondominant hand.
- Practice turning mirror with fingers, adjusting as to the several surfaces of the tooth.
- Hold a small object in the dominant hand for viewing in mirror held in nondominant hand.
- Practice crossing the mirror over fulcrum finger as in position for retracting lower lip while viewing lingual surfaces of mandibular anterior teeth in mouth mirror.

C. Cotton Pliers

- Make small, tight cotton pellets with thumb and index and middle fingers of each hand; then make one in each hand simultaneously.
- Hold cotton pliers with modified pen grasp and establish fulcrum finger on tabletop; elbow and forearm are free.
- Practice picking up cotton pellets using mirror vision (right hand, then left).
  - Use in wiping motion on tabletop or other object.
  - Move to different area to release pellet as if to a waste-receiving cup.

V. TACTILE SENSITIVITY

A. Explorer

- Mount small pieces of various grades of fine-grain sandpaper on a card.
- Hold explorer with modified pen grasp, and establish fulcrum finger on tabletop, with upper arm and forearm free. With eyes closed, compare roughness of the various grades of sandpaper. Use a light, exploring stroke.
- Use extracted teeth to feel with explorer tip until a light grasp permits maximum security of grasp and maximum sense of touch. Extracted teeth can be used to provide a contrast between exploring enamel, cementum, calculus, or other rough area of tooth surface.

B. Probe

- Repeat exercises described for explorer.
- Compare with explorer.

PREVENTION OF CUMULATIVE TRAUMA

Hand in hand with learning the instruments and attaining dexterity in their use for the treatment of patients is the well-being of the dental hygienist.

- Primary occupational hazards are related to personal everyday habits during chairside practice.

- The symptoms of carpal tunnel syndrome are caused by compression of the median nerve within the carpal tunnel as shown in **Figure 38-15B** (page 588). Figure 7-5 shows the anatomy of the carpel tunnel wrist area.

Along with the exercises for the development of strength and control in the hands, other types of exercises are needed for maintaining general musculoskeletal health.

I. PROBLEMS

- Posture.
- Extended periods of time spent in the same work position.
- Repetitive movements during actual instrumentation.

Study and plan for action in advance, before serious disability can occur.

II. EXERCISES

- Stretching exercises for stress release, improvement of posture, and counteracting repetitive movements used during instrumentation are suggested in **Figure 38-20**.
- Other exercises are shown in Figure 7-6 (page 98).

III. CLINICAL APPLICATION

- Exercises performed chairside, between appointments, can contribute greatly to long-range prevention.
- One idea for an exercise during patient treatment is shown in **Figure 38-21**. Each time an instrument is returned to the tray, fingers and wrists can be stretched before picking up the next instrument needed.

INSTRUMENT SHARPENING

Objectives for techniques of sharpening emphasize the **preservation of the original shape of the blade** *while restoring a sharp cutting edge.* Instruments designed for a particular purpose need to continue to be used in the manner for which they were designed. Inaccurate sharpening techniques can distort the blade and render the instrument useless for its intended purpose.

- Sharpening procedures are not easy to learn and require skill and patience to accomplish. While the process may seem tedious and time consuming, sharpening is an essential and integral part of instrumentation.
- Successful clinical outcomes using bladed instruments are dependent upon correctly contoured and sharpened instruments.
- Frequent (daily) sharpening prevents loss of blade structure to the stage when the need for recontouring becomes necessary to restore the original shape.

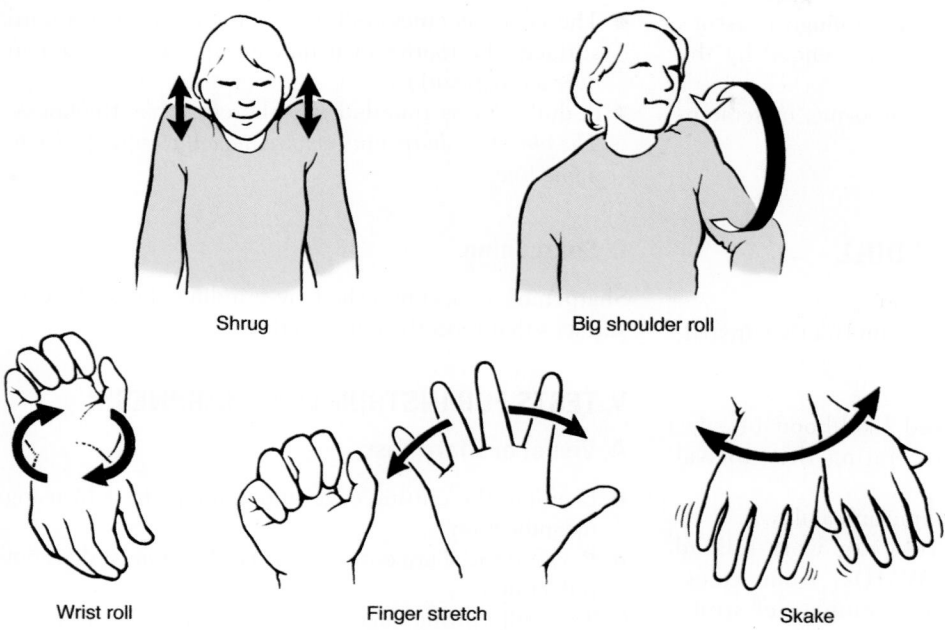

Shrug

Big shoulder roll

Wrist roll

Finger stretch

Skake

FIGURE 38-20 **Chairside Stretching Exercises.** Stretching exercises to relax the back, shoulders, and neck are shown with the shrug and rolling the head around with the big shoulder roll. Hand and finger rolls, stretches, and shaking can be performed anytime, even while attending a patient.

■ Terms related to instrument sharpening are defined in Box 38-2.

I. BENEFITS FROM USE OF SHARP MANUAL INSTRUMENTS

Instruments must be sharp if scaling, root planing, and maintenance root debridement are to be completed efficiently with minimal trauma to the tissues. When the instrument blade is maintained with its original contour and sharp cutting edges, the following may be expected:

■ Greater precision of treatment, improved quality of results, and less working time involved.

■ Increased tactile sensitivity during instrumentation. A sharp instrument does not have to be gripped as firmly as a dull one.

■ Greater control of the instrument because of the lighter grasp needed; less pressure on the tooth being scaled or planed and decreased pressure on the finger rest are required.

■ Fewer strokes required.

■ Less possibility of burnishing rather than removing the calculus.

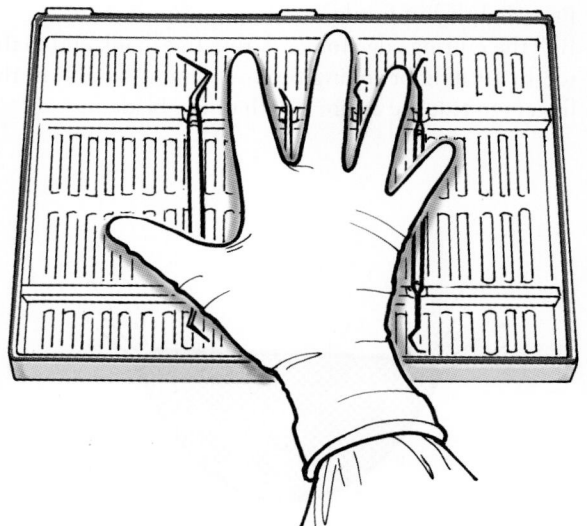

FIGURE 38-21 **Stretching Fingers Prior to Instrument Retrieval.** One of the exercises that can be used during actual clinical practice.

BOX 38-2	Key Words

Sharpening

Arkansas stone: fine-grained sharpening stone quarried from natural mineral deposits.

Burnish: to smooth and polish; an effect that can result when a dull scaler or curet is passed over tenacious calculus in an attempt to remove the deposit.

Cutting edge: the fine line formed where the face and lateral surfaces of a scaler or curet meet when the instrument is sharp; when the instrument is dull, the line has thickness and may even reflect light.

Hone: a sharpening stone (noun).

Honing: sharpening (verb).

Sharpness: when a scaler or curet is sharp, the cutting edge is a fine line that does not reflect light.

Testing stick: plastic 1/4-inch rod, 3 inches long, used to test the sharpness of a scaler or a curet.

- Prevention of unnecessary trauma to gingival tissues and, therefore, less discomfort experienced by the patient.
- Decreased possibility of nicking, grooving, or scratching the tooth surfaces.
- Less fatigue for the clinician.

II. CONSEQUENCES OF USING DULL MANUAL INSTRUMENTS

- Stress and frustration of using ineffective instruments.
- Wasted time, effort, and energy.
- Loss of control and increased likelihood of slipping with instrument and lacerating the gingival tissue.
- Loss of patient confidence in clinician's ability.
- Increased likelihood of developing work-related musculoskeletal disorders (WMDs) from excessive muscle strain and increased number of stroke repetitions.

III. SHARPENING STONES: MATERIALS

- *Natural Abrasive Stones:* Quarried from mineral deposits, the hard Arkansas stone is used for dental instruments because of its fine abrasive particle size.
- *Artificial Materials*
  - Hard, nonmetallic substances impregnated with aluminum oxide, silicon carbide, or diamond particles. Examples: ruby stone, carborundum stones, and the diamond hone.
  - Ceramic aluminum oxide.
  - Steel alloys are metals that are harder than most dental instrument steel and, therefore, are capable of sharpening the instrument.

IV. DYNAMICS OF SHARPENING[4]

A. Sharpening Stone Surface

- A sharpening stone acts as an abrasive to reshape a dulled blade by grinding the surface until the cutting edge is restored.
- The surface of the stone is made up of masses of minute crystals, which are the abrasive particles that accomplish the grinding of the instrument.
- A smaller particle size or a finer grain, as it is generally called, abrades or reduces more slowly and produces a finer cutting edge.

B. Cutting Edge

- The cutting edge is a very fine *line* formed where the face and lateral surface meet at an angle.
- The edge is a line and, therefore, has length but no thickness.

- The edge becomes dull when pressed against a hard surface (the tooth), or it may be nicked when drawn over a rough surface.
- A dull edge is rounded and therefore has thickness. *The object in sharpening is to reshape the cutting edge to a fine line.*

C. Sharpening

Sharpening is accomplished by grinding the surface or surfaces that form the cutting edge.

V. TESTS FOR INSTRUMENT SHARPNESS[5]

A. Visual or Glare Test

- Examine the cutting edge under adequate light using magnification.
- Because the sharp cutting edge is a fine *line*, it does not reflect light.
- The dull cutting edge presents a rounded, shiny *surface,* which reflects light.
  - **Figure 38-22** shows the cross section of a dull universal curet.
  - The dull cutting edges are tiny surfaces that reflect light.
  - Compare the cutting edges in **Figure 38-22** with **Figure 38-5**, which shows the sharp cutting edges, at the points labeled "c," on a universal curet.

B. Plastic Testing Stick

- Use a sterile plastic or acrylic 1/4-inch rod, 3 inches long.
- Place the fulcrum finger on the end of the stick.
- Apply the heel (shank end) of the cutting edge to the plastic stick, first at 90°, then closed to the correct angle for scaling (70°).
- Press lightly but firmly.
- Roll the cutting edge forward from the shank end to the toe by turning or rolling the instrument handle in the fingers to test the entire length of the blade.

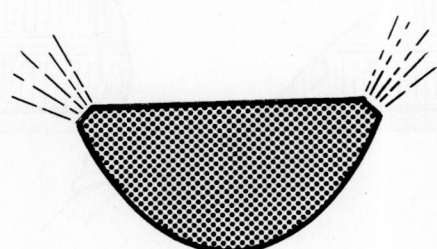

FIGURE 38-22 **Cross Section of a Dull Curet.** A sharp curet has a fine line at the cutting edge that will not reflect light. A dull cutting edge is like a small surface and reflects light as shown.

C. Confirming Sharpness Using the Plastic Testing Stick

- The **sharp** cutting edge engages or grips the plastic as the length of the blade is tested. Each portion of the cutting edge will engage the plastic uniformly as the blade advances.
- The **dull** cutting edge does not catch without undue pressure and slides easily over the surface of the stick.
- Because the edge is not uniformly dulled during use, there will be portions of a blade that exhibit varying degrees of sharpness or dullness.
- As the instrument blade is rolled along the testing stick, the degree of slipping vs. engagement will indicate the degree of sharpness or dullness. If only limited portions of the blade exhibit dullness, attempt to note the segments that slip as the blade is rolled along the testing stick.
  - The entire length of the cutting edge is always sharpened to maintain the original form.
  - Awareness of the portion(s) exhibiting dullness can guide pressure and the number of strokes.
  - This helps to minimize oversharpening.
  - Careful evaluation will increase efficiency and raise the likelihood that dull portions of the blade are restored to sharpness.

VI. EVALUATION OF TECHNIQUE

- Observe closely the stabilization of both the instrument and stone, each kept aligned in a single plane, to evaluate sharpening technique.
  - *Self-check:* As the stone is activated for sharpening, observe the top of the instrument to ensure it is secure and not moving.
  - *Self-check:* Observe stone to ensure it remains in a single plane of movement back and forth as it is activated.
- Evaluate by turning the instrument over to examine the back of the lateral surfaces under well-lit magnification.
- A solid, consistent bevel results from
  - instrument and stone positioned at the correct angle,
  - movement occurring in a single plane.
- Irregular bevel is revealed by
  - breaks in the fine line of the blade edge,
  - varying facets indicating the improper stone placement/movement.

SOME BASIC SHARPENING PRINCIPLES

I. STERILIZATION OF THE SHARPENING STONE

- A sterile sharpening stone and testing stick are parts of a basic clinical setup for a scaling appointment.
- Instruments then may be sharpened throughout the procedure as they show signs of dullness.

- Efficiency increases, and the patient benefits from receiving a more thorough treatment in less time.
- Sterilization of stones may be accomplished using any of the acceptable sterilization methods described on page 77, in accord with specific manufacturer's recommendations.
- Over time, the steam autoclave may dry out an Arkansas stone and lead to chipping or breakage.

II. INSTRUMENT HANDLING

All instruments must be handled with care to preserve sharpness and prevent accidental damage to the cutting edges.

III. PREPARATION OF STONE FOR SHARPENING

A. Dry Stone

- *Advantage:* The problems related to maintaining a sterile stone and preventing contamination when oil, tap water, or a lubricant is applied, the use of a dry stone provides a particular advantage.
- A dry stone contributes to the following effects:
  - Sharpens the cutting edge without nicks in the blade; nicks can be created from particles of metal suspended in a lubricant.
  - Allows the stone to be completely sterilized without the problem of interference by the oil left in and on the stone.

B. Water on Stone

Ceramic stones may be used dry or with water.

C. Lubricated Stone

- Certain quarried stones need lubrication to prevent drying out.
- Instruments are autoclaved before sharpening, and the stone and instruments are sterilized again after nonsterile lubricant is used.
- The lubricant can facilitate the movement of the instrument blade over the stone and prevent scratching of the stone, and suspend the metallic particles removed during sharpening help to prevent clogging of the pores of the stone (glazing).

IV. SHARPENING

A. Objectives

The objectives during sharpening are twofold:

- To produce a sharp cutting edge.
- To preserve the original shape of the instrument.
  A. Instrument shape is also known as contour.
  B. The contour of a curet toe is a smooth, continuous curvature with no points or flat edges.

B. When to Sharpen

- Sharpen at the first sign of dullness during an appointment.
- When instruments become grossly dulled, recontouring wastes the instrument.
- Restoring original contour to a grossly dull instrument often leaves a blade that is not functional and therefore useless.

C. Angulation

- Before starting to sharpen, analyze the cutting edge and establish the proper angle between the stone and the blade surface.
- Maintain the angle through the firm grasp, secure hand rest, moderate pressure, short stroke, and other features of the technique appropriate to the individual instrument.

D. Maintain Control

- Maintain control so that the entire surface is reduced evenly.
- Care must be taken not to create a new bevel at the cutting edge.

E. Care of Sharpening Stone

- Prevent grooving of the sharpening stone by varying the areas for instrument placement.
- Cleaning and stain removal procedures are described on page 606.

V. AFTER SHARPENING

A. Finishing the Instrument

Newly sharpened instruments are finished by carefully inspecting the edges for a clean consistent bevel with no particles or "wire edge" remaining.

B. How the Wire Edge Is Produced

- During sharpening, some of the metal particles removed during grinding remain attached to the edge of the instrument and create the wire edge.
- If allowed to remain, the tiny particles may be removed when the instrument is applied to the tooth surface during treatment.
- By sharpening into, toward, or against the cutting edge, the production of a wire edge is minimized.

C. Removal of Wire Edge

- Wipe the instrument carefully with a dry gauze square or an alcohol wipe to remove particles.

VI. INSTRUMENT WEAR

- As curets are used, the cutting edge wears down, leaving a narrower face and shorter length over a period of time.
- Sharpening also contributes to the size reduction.
- After sufficient reduction, instruments must be retired and discarded.
    - Blades will no longer access or adapt to the tooth surface.
    - Thinner blades are more susceptible to breakage with lateral pressure.
- Used instruments that have become excessively narrow are reserved for patients with minimal deposit and require biofilm debridement.
- Exert care when using overly thinned curets. If strong lateral pressure is applied, they may break off at the tip, leaving the last few millimeters embedded in the sulcus or pocket.
- Protocol for retrieving a broken instrument tip is included in Box 39-5, page 636.
- Evaluation during sharpening procedures provides the opportunity for proper attention to instrument maintenance.
    - Consider usefulness and suitability of instruments for various procedures as they are sharpened and assigned to tray setups.
    - Assign thinner-bladed instruments to procedures that do not require moderate or heavy calculus removal, such as maintenance appointments.
    - Discard or recycle instruments that have outlived their usefulness with shortened blades that cannot access proximal surfaces sufficiently.

SHARPENING CURETS AND SCALERS

In the sections following, procedures for a variety of sharpening techniques are outlined. In general, manual sharpening procedures are the methods of choice so that the blade is not reduced unnecessarily by a rapid-cutting mounted stone.

I. TECHNIQUE OBJECTIVES

- Preserve the original contour of the blade.
- Sharpen frequently to prevent need for excessive recontouring of the blade.

II. SELECTION OF CUTTING EDGES TO SHARPEN

A. Scalers/Sickles

- Most scalers are universal instruments.
- Cutting edges on both sides of the face are sharpened **(Figure 38-23)**.
- A two-step sharpening procedure is used

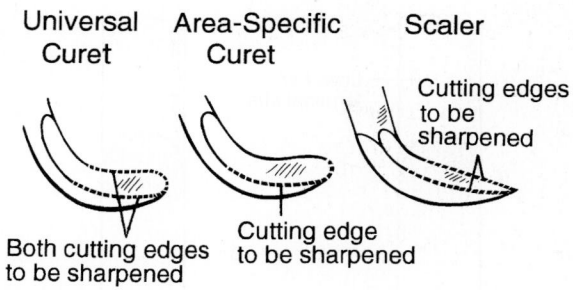

Universal Curet   Area-Specific Curet   Scaler

Cutting edges to be sharpened

Both cutting edges to be sharpened

Cutting edge to be sharpened

FIGURE 38-23 **Selection of Cutting Edge to Sharpen.** Both cutting edges and the rounded toe are sharpened for a universal curet. An area-specific curet is sharpened on the longer cutting edge and the rounded toe. A scaler is sharpened on the two sides, and the tip is brought to a point.

B. Curets: Universal

- Cutting edges on both sides of the face and the toe are sharpened (**Figure 38-23**).
- A three-step sharpening procedure is used.

C. Curets: Area Specific

- Cutting edge on one side of the face and the toe are sharpened.
- Sharpen the longer cutting edge, generally it will be the one farthest from the handle. In **Figure 38-23**, it is shown with a dotted line.
- A two-step sharpening procedure is used: one side of the face and the toe.

 MOVING FLAT STONE: STATIONARY INSTRUMENT

The side of the cutting edge formed by the lateral surface is reduced by this method. The technique described applies to both curets and scalers. Because the scaler has a pointed tip and the curet has a round toe end, a variation is necessary in the adaptation of the sharpening stone to that portion of the blade.

I. EXAMINE THE CUTTING EDGE TO BE SHARPENED

Test for sharpness to determine specific areas that are dull, but plan to sharpen the whole cutting edge(s) to maintain original contour.

II. REVIEW THE ANGULATION TO BE RESTORED AT THE DULL CUTTING EDGE

- Internal angle of the blade at the cutting edge(s) is 70° to 80° (**Figures 38-5** and **38-8**).
- Visible angle at which the stone will be placed will be 110°, as shown in **Figure 38-24**.

III. STABILIZE AND POSITION THE INSTRUMENT[6]

- Grasp the instrument in the nondominant hand in a palm grasp.
- Lean the hand against the edge of an immovable workbench or table under bright light (**Figure 38-25A**).
- The instrument should be low enough to allow the clinician to see the cutting edges clearly.
- Turn the face of the instrument up and parallel with the floor. Point the curet toe (or scaler tip) toward the clinician to provide better access for moving the stone.
- Note the shape of the face from above as outlined in **Figure 38-26**.
- The cutting edges begin at the lower shank.
- The cutting edges are parallel, until they converge.
- For the curet, they curve to form the toe.
- For the scaler, they taper to make the pointed tip.

IV. APPLY THE SHARPENING STONE

- Hold the stone perpendicular to the floor, at the shank third of the cutting edge.
- From the 90° angle with the face of the instrument, open the stone to make an angle of 110° (**Figure 38-24**).

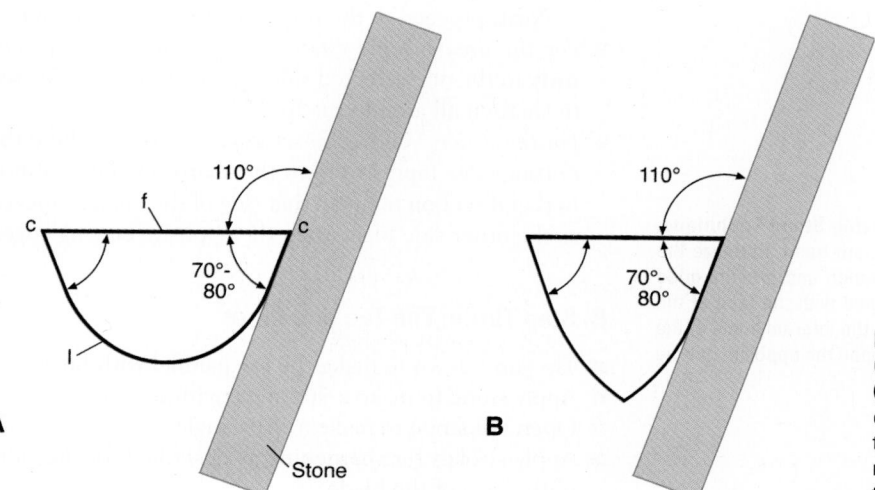

A   B

FIGURE 38-24 **Angulation for Sharpening.** Cross sections of a curet (**A**) and a scaler (**B**) show correct angulation of the face (f) of the blade with the flat sharpening stone to reproduce the internal angle of the instrument at 70°. Note the cutting edges (c) and the lateral surfaces (l).

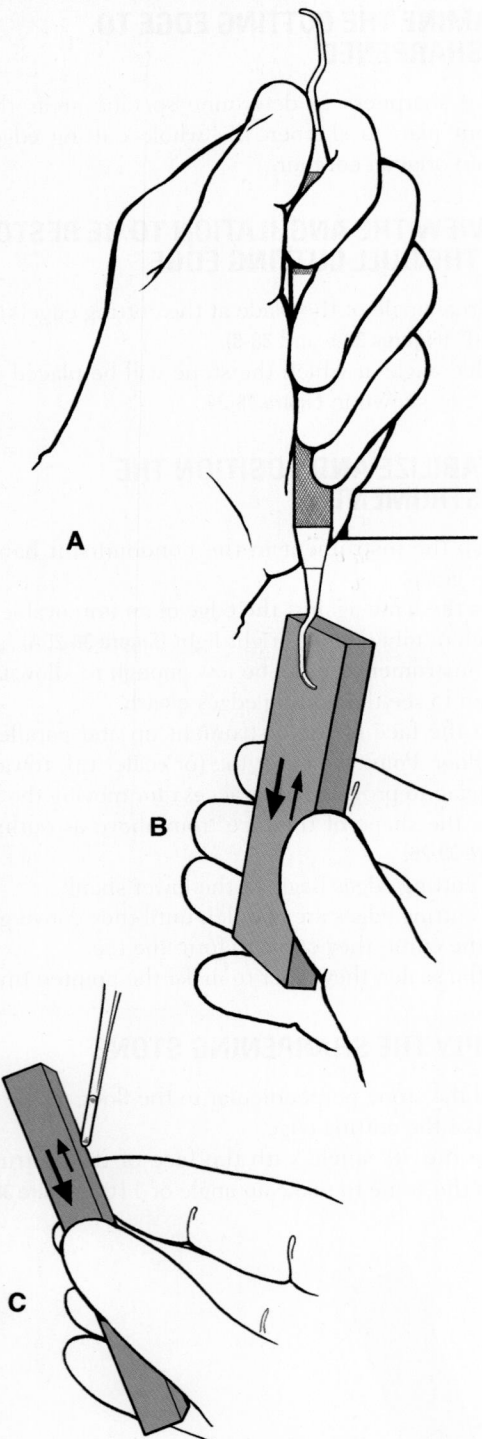

FIGURE 38-25 Stationary Instrument—Moving Stone Technique. (A) Grasp the instrument with the nondominant hand. Stabilize the hand on the edge of a stationary table or bench and provide good light on the instrument. **(B)** The stone is angled with the face of the instrument at 110° **(Figure 38-24)** to maintain the internal angle of the blade at 70° to 80°. **(C)** Stone reversed to sharpen the opposite cutting edge of a universal curet.

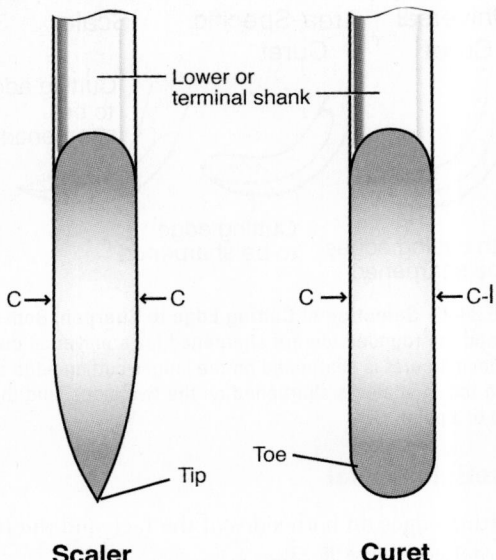

FIGURE 38-26 View of a Scaler and a Curet Looking Into the Face. The cutting edges (*c* and *c-1*) are parallel until they curve in to form the pointed tip (scaler) or the round toe (curet).

V. ACTIVATE THE SHARPENING STONE

A. Steps One and Two

- Maintain the stone in contact with the blade and at the proper angle throughout the procedure.
- Tighten the grasp on the instrument (nondominant hand) while applying a smooth even pressure to the cutting edge to keep the instrument stable and motionless.
- Move the stone up and down with short rhythmical strokes about ½-inch high. Place more pressure on the down stroke. Maintain the 110° angle precisely. Finish each area with a down stroke.
- *For the universal curet:*
  - Follow the cutting edge to where the curvature for the toe begins, applying 3 or 4 down strokes overlapping at each millimeter of the cutting edge.
  - Proceed to the opposite side to sharpen, repeating the steps just described **(Figure 38-25)**.
  - Next, proceed to the third step to sharpen the toe.
- *For the area-specific curet:* Apply sharpening strokes **only** to the one selected side: proceed to the third step to sharpen all around the toe.
- *For the scaler:* Follow the same procedure to where the cutting edge tapers to form the sharp tip and continue in that direction to finish that side of the blade. Proceed to the other side to sharpen the opposite cutting edge.

B. Step Three: The Toe of a Curet[6]

- Tip curet down to make the toe parallel with floor.
- Apply stone to make a 90° angle with the toe.
- Open the stone to make a 110° angle.
- Apply strokes for sharpening as described for the sides of the face of the blade.

VI. TEST FOR SHARPNESS

- Apply testing stick along the entire cutting edges.
- Repeat sharpening procedures as necessary to retain clean sharp cutting edges.

STATIONARY FLAT STONE: MOVING INSTRUMENT

I. CURET

- Place the stone flat on a steady surface.
- Examine the cutting edges to be sharpened. Test for sharpness.
- Hold the instrument in a modified pen grasp, and establish a secure finger rest **(Figure 38-27A)**.
- Apply the cutting edge to the stone. An angle of 110° is formed by the stone and face.
  - Because the curet is curved, only a small section of the cutting edge can be applied at one time.
  - Sharpening is performed in a *series* of applications of the cutting edge to the stone, each overlapping the previous, as the instrument is turned and drawn steadily along the stone.
  - The portion of the cutting edge nearest the shank is applied first **(Figure 38-27B, a)**.
- Apply moderate to light but firm pressure while the instrument is activated.
- Use a slow, steady stroke to maintain control and to ensure that each portion of the cutting edge receives equal treatment.
- Move the blade forward into the cutting edge. Turn the instrument continuously until the center of the round end of the blade is reached **(Figure 38-27B, b)**.
- Test for sharpness along the entire cutting edge; reapply to stone as necessary for ideal sharpness.
- Turn the instrument to sharpen the second cutting edge. Overlap at the center of the round toe. Universal curets are sharpened on both sides and around the toe. Gracey curets are sharpened on one side only and around the toe (see **Figure 38-23**).
- Carefully wipe the instrument with a gauze square or an alcohol wipe to remove the wire edge.

II. SCALER: SICKLE OR JACQUETTE

- Place the stone flat on a firm table or bench top under adequate light. Do not tilt the stone while sharpening.
- Examine cutting edges to be sharpened. Test for sharpness.
- Hold the instrument with a firm pen grasp, using thumb, index, and middle (second) fingers to prevent the instrument from rotating or changing angles during sharpening **(Figure 38-28A)**.
- Establish finger rest on side of stone using ring and little fingers.

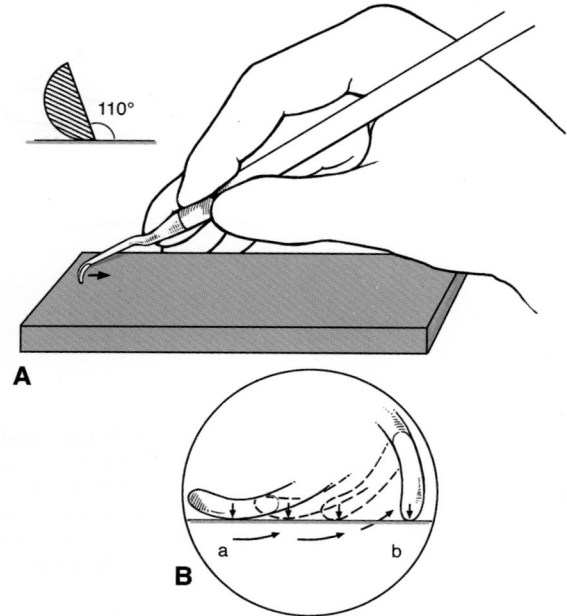

FIGURE 38-27 Stationary Stone—Moving Instrument Technique for a Curet. (A) Stone placed flat with blade in position at the beginning of the sharpening stroke. With the finger rest stabilized on the edge of the stone, the cutting edge is maintained at the proper angulation (110°) as the instrument is drawn along the stone with an even, moderate pressure. **(B)** The movement of the blade is shown by the arrows, which indicate each portion of the cutting edge as the blade is turned on the stone from the beginning (a) to the completion (b) of the stroke at the center of the round toe of the curet. For a universal curet, the instrument is turned over and the opposite cutting edge is sharpened.

- Stabilize stone with fingers of opposite hand.
- Apply cutting edge to be sharpened to the stone. Maintain 70° to 80° internal angle of the instrument **(Figure 38-28B)**. The portion of the cutting edge nearest the shank is applied first.
- Apply moderate to light but firm pressure while instrument is in motion. Heavy pressure can reduce control of instrument, cause scratching of the stone, and produce an unfavorable bevel at the cutting edge.
- Use a short, slow stroke to maintain the exact relation of the cutting edge to the stone.
  - Pull blade forward, toward the cutting edge.
  - All fingers move with the arm as a unit.
  - Use a slow, steady stroke to maintain control and to ensure that each portion of the cutting edge receives equal treatment.
  - Turn the instrument continually to follow the shape of the blade to the pointed tip.
- Test for sharpness after one or two strokes. Repeat as needed for ideal sharpness.
- Turn instrument and proceed to sharpen other lateral surface. When instrument placement is awkward for a modified contra-angle scaler, use a narrow side of the stone.

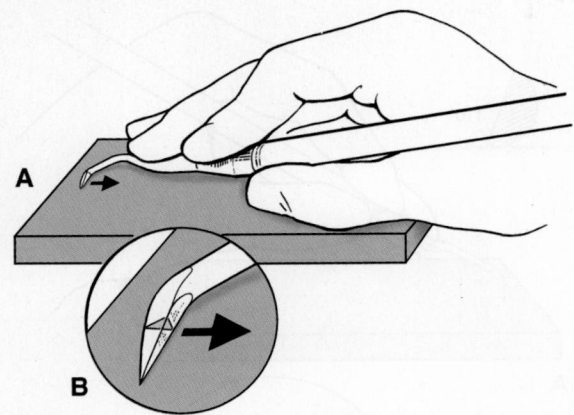

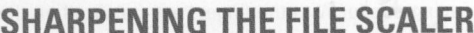

FIGURE 38-28 Stationary Stone Technique for a Straight Scaler. **(A)** With a modified pen grasp and a finger rest established on the side of the stone, the scaler is positioned for sharpening. **(B)** The portion of the cutting edge nearest the lower shank is applied first with an angle of 110° between the face and the stone. The instrument is turned continuously to follow the arc-like shape of the blade. The cutting edges are sharpened to the pointed tip.

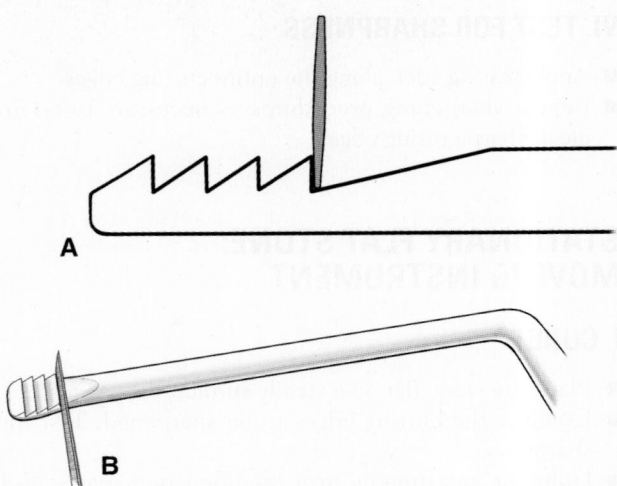

FIGURE 38-29 Sharpening a File Scaler. (A) Tanged file in position against one of the several surfaces to be ground. **(B)** With the file scaler stabilized to prevent movement, the Tanged file is pulled through the channel using a moderate, steady pressure against the surface to be ground.

SHARPENING THE FILE SCALER

Files are sharpened with a flat sharpening instrument called a *tanged file*. Use of magnification and good illumination are necessary when sharpening files to ensure correct placement of the tanged file.

- Use a testing stick to check for the degree of sharpness to determine whether the file will need to be sharpened.
- If the file blades do not grasp the plastic testing stick when adapted lightly, they will need to be sharpened.

I. SURFACE TO BE GROUND

- Examine the file closely with the head of the working end positioned outward (**Figure 38-10A**, page 585).
- Note the two angular surfaces that meet to form a "V" shape (**Figure 38-10B**).
- The surface to be contacted with the tanged file and ground during sharpening is the surface of the "V" that is farthest away.

II. SHARPENING PROCEDURE

- Prepare a workplace with good illumination and some means of magnification such as loupes or a magnified light ring.
- Place the sterile file on a clean surface. Secure it with the series of teeth facing up.
- Position the right end of the tanged file in the channel as shown in the illustration (**Figure 38-29A**). (Left-handed clinicians reverse the process, positioning the left end of the tanged file in the channel.)

- With light to moderate steady pressure, pull the tanged file through the channel, moving in a straight line from one end to the other in one direction only.
- Release pressure and reposition the tanged file back at the starting point. Repeat the process. Two or three passes with the tanged file are usually sufficient to bring each edge back to sharpness.
- Sharpen the remaining blades using the same technique.
- Test for sharpness and repeat the sharpening stroke as needed for ideal edge sharpness.

SHARPENING THE HOE SCALER

The hoe has only one surface to be ground. Because placement of the small surface on the flat stone is difficult to visualize, magnification is needed.

I. SURFACE TO BE GROUND

Examine surface to be ground (**Figure 38-30A**). Test for sharpness.

II. SHARPENING PROCEDURE

- Use stationary flat stone.
- Hold instrument in modified pen grasp. Establish finger rest on the side of the stone.
- Apply the surface to be ground to the stone in correct relationship to maintain the 45° bevel (**Figure 38-30B**).
- With moderate, steady pressure, pull the instrument toward the cutting edge a short distance. Allow the whole hand to move with the arm as a unit to aid in maintaining the correct angulation.

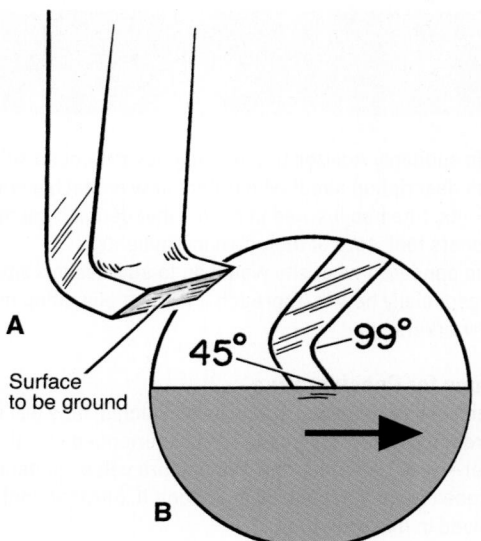

FIGURE 38-30 **Sharpening a Hoe Scaler. (A)** Surface to be ground. **(B)** Hoe adapted to the surface of a stationary flat stone at the proper angle to maintain the original bevel of 45°. Arrow indicates direction of the sharpening stroke leading into the cutting edge.

■ Release pressure and slide the instrument back. Repeat.
■ Test for sharpness and reapply as needed for ideal sharpness.
■ Wipe the instrument carefully with a dry gauze square or an alcohol wipe to remove particles.

III. ROUND CORNERS

Corners need to be rounded at each end of the cutting edge.

■ Rounded corners help to prevent laceration of soft tissue or grooving of tooth surface.
■ Hold instrument in nondominant hand with corners of cutting edge directed inward.
■ Rub the surface of the sharpening stone across each corner with a gentle rolling motion **(Figure 38-31)**. Two or three applications are usually sufficient.

SHARPENING THE CHISEL SCALER

Sharpening procedures for the chisel are similar to those for ~~hoe~~. Again, the surface is small, the angulation is dif-~~ficult to vis~~ualize, and the use of magnification is needed.

~~GROUND~~

~~ground~~ **(Figure 38-32A)**. Test for

~~PROCEDU~~RE

~~ied~~ pen grasp, establish ~~surface~~ to be ground to the ~~t~~ip to maintain the 45°

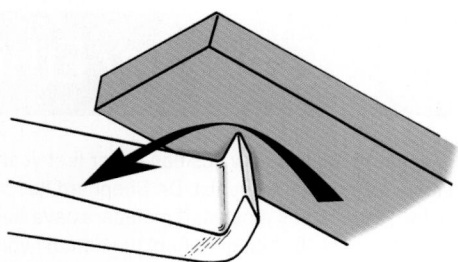

FIGURE 38-31 **Rounding a Hoe Scaler.** To round the sharp corners of the hoe scaler, a flat stone is rubbed over the instrument with a gentle rolling motion.

■ With moderate, steady pressure, push the instrument forward, toward the cutting edge, without changing the relationship with the stone.
■ After two or three applications, test for sharpness and reapply as necessary for an ideal cutting edge.
■ Wipe the instrument carefully with a dry gauze square or an alcohol wipe to remove particles.

III. ROUND CORNERS

Round the corners at each end of the cutting edge. In a manner similar to that shown in **Figure 38-31** for the hoe scaler, rub the surface of the flat stone across each corner of the chisel with a gentle, even, rolling motion. Two or three applications are usually sufficient.

SHARPENING EXPLORERS

I. TESTS FOR SHARPNESS

A. Visual

When examined under concentrated light, a dull explorer tip appears rounded.

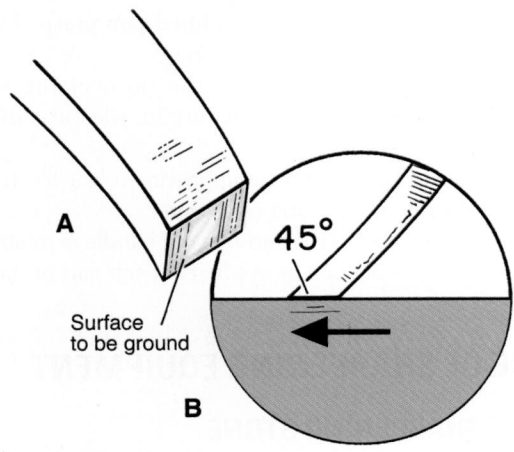

FIGURE 38-32 **Sharpening a Chisel Scaler. (A)** Surface to be ground. **(B)** Chisel is adapted to the surface of a stationary flat stone at the proper angle to maintain the original bevel of 45°. Arrow indicates direction of the sharpening stroke leading into the cutting edge.

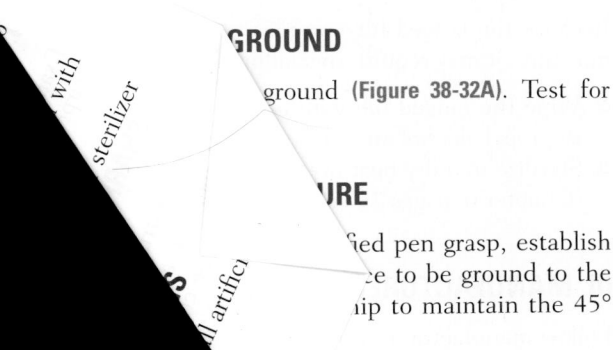

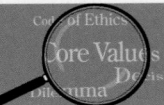

Everyday Ethics

Leslie is eager to begin a new position in her first year of clinical practice as a dental hygienist. Dr. Shepherd has been in practice for 15 years and most staff members have been with him at least the past 10, including Ann, the dental hygienist with whom she will be practicing. Leslie is glad to have someone with experience take her under her wing.

A dental assistant takes care of instrument sterilization and tray setups for the dental hygienists. As she sat down to her first patient, she noticed the instruments on her tray were all sickle scalers and she wanted curets. On closer inspection, however, she discovered that all but one instrument were indeed curets; they had just been mis-sharpened, leaving them with no contour (curvature) at the toe.

She excused herself to go into the instrument supply room only to find that all of the curets had sharp, pointed toes. Going back to the clinical area, she peeked in to ask Ann if the assistant did the sharpening for her, (as she glanced at Ann's tray she noted the curets were equally sharpened to a distinct point). Ann answered, "No, I do all the sharpening myself because I am very picky."

Leslie suddenly realizes that nothing has ever been said in a work description about who orders new dental hygiene instruments. She had learned in school that dental hygiene practitioners took care of their own instruments.

Leslie pondered what she would do to address this situation—especially how to approach it without alienating her new co-workers.

Questions for Consideration

1. Given Leslie's neophyte status as a clinician, how will she approach her new colleague—an experienced practitioner—with her concerns? Which core values of dental hygiene (Table II-1, page 38 in Section II, Introduction) are involved in this scenario?
2. What harm, if any, is affecting Dr. Shepherd's patients? Discuss whether or not the dentist needs to be notified about the condition of the instruments.
3. Utilizing an ethical decision framework (page 10 in Chapter 1), describe realistic alternatives for Leslie's course of action in this situation.

B. Plastic Testing Stick

A sharp explorer grips the plastic tester on light pressure and moves with resistance when pulled over the surface. A dull explorer does not catch and will slide.

II. RECONTOUR

Small-nosed pliers can be used to straighten a bent tip.

III. SHARPENING PROCEDURE

- Use flat stone.
- Instrument is held with a modified pen grasp. Finger rest is established on side of stone.
- Placement and movement of the tip over the stone resemble somewhat the procedure for the curet on the stone (see **Figure 38-27B**).
- Place side of tip on stone at approximately a 15° to 20° angle of stone with shank of explorer.
- As tip is moved over the surface, the handle is rotated so that even pressure can be applied to each part of the tip.

CARE OF SHARPENING EQUIPMENT

I. FLAT SHARPENING STONE

A. Prepare for Sterilization

Submerge in ultrasonic cleaner or scrub with soap and water to remove metal particles left from sharpening.

B. Stain Removal

- Check manufacturer's recommendation
- Alternate cleaning suggestions: Use ammonia, gasoline, or kerosene when stone becomes discolored. If the stone becomes "glazed" by metal particles ground into the surface, rub the stone over emery paper placed on a flat, solid surface.

C. Storage

- Keep in sealed, sterilized packages for sharpening at instrument preparation area.
- A stone and testing stick are stored with each instrument setup in the cassette for use during the treatment appointment.

II. CARE OF THE TANGED FILE

Because the tanged file corrodes easily when exposed to moisture, it may require special handling.

- Wipe the tanged file with a sterile gauze soaked isopropyl alcohol after use.
- Sterilize in a dry heat oven or chemical vapor (Chapter 6, pages 79 and 80).

III. MANUFACTURER'S DIRECTION

Follow manufacturer's directions for a

BOX 38-3	**Example Progress Note Related to Instrument Selection**

Patient presents for third in a series of scaling and root planing appointments (maxillary left quadrant). Complete debridement accomplished with universal and standard Gracy curets in all areas except the distal of tooth #15, where mini curets were used to access a deep pocket with furcation involvement and the mesial of tooth # 13, where use of a mini curet and careful adaptation was necessary to access a deep mesial concavity.

Signed: _____, RDH Date: _____

Factors To Teach The Patient

- Why it is necessary to use a variety of instruments for treatment.
- When and why there is a need for several appointments.
- Benefits of using a finely sharpened instrument for calculus removal.
- Harmful effects of using dull instruments.
- The relationship of personal daily care using dental floss and a toothbrush to the need for frequent appointments with the dental hygienist.

DOCUMENTATION

Documentation of instrument selection and instrumentation techniques in a patient chart can provide guidance during subsequent dental hygiene care. For example, notes made in the patient chart may include the following:

- Identification of specific instruments used in specific areas, such as mini-curets used to access a particularly deep pocket area.
- Areas in the patient's dentition that require more careful attention or careful application of skill.
- An example progress note is found in **Box 38-3**.

References

1. Scaramucci MK. The versatility of the universal curet: a review of a hand instrumentation staple. *Dimens Dent Hyg.* 2010 Feb;8(2):32,36,38.
2. Pattison AM, Matsuda S, Pattison GL. Extraoral Fulcrums. *Dimens Dent Hyg.* 2004 Oct;2(10):20–3.
3. Pattison AM, Pattison GL. *Periodontal instrumentation.* 2nd ed. Upper Saddle River (NJ): Prentice Hall; 1991. p. 166, 232, 371.
4. Scaramucci MK. A primer on instrument sharpening. *Dimens Dent Hyg.* 2009 Sep;7(9):32–5.
5. Hodges K. On the cutting edge. *Dimens Dent Hyg.* 2004 Apr;2(4):16–20,36.
6. Matsuda SA. Troubleshooting technique—sharpening. *Dimens Dent Hyg.* 2005 Jun;3(6):32,34.

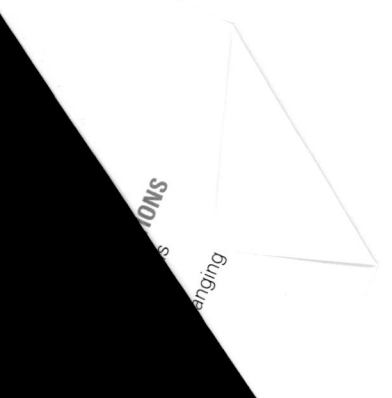

Nonsurgical Periodontal Instrumentation

STACY A. MATSUDA, RDH, BS, MS
ESTHER M. WILKINS, BS, RDH, DMD

Chapter Outline

Basic treatment for inflammatory gingival and periodontal infections is the removal of dental biofilm, bacterial toxic materials (endotoxins), and supragingival and subgingival calculus. The term *debridement* has been applied to the group of procedures involved and includes professional intervention by the clinician as well as the procedures carried out by the patient daily, when using a toothbrush and proximal biofilm-removal devices.

Periodontal debridement includes all of the following therapeutic interventions:

■ Scaling (manual and power-driven) to remove calculus and all soft deposits.
■ Root planing to eliminate subgingival calculus and smooth the tooth surface.
■ Root debridement to eliminate subgingival biofilm and mineralized deposits.

Periodontal debridement can provide the definitive or complete treatment for many patients with less advanced infections. For those with more advanced disease, debridement is the preparatory or initial therapy. The progress and success of treatment can be influenced by innate or acquired host factors.

Dental hygiene care aims to prevent, arrest, control, or eliminate the infection in the gingiva (page 245). The ultimate goals of the instrumentation are to eliminate pathogenic microorganisms that initiate the infection and to promote continuing health in the periodontal tissues. **Box 39-1** contains key words related to nonsurgical therapy.

The long-range success of treatment depends on the *control* of the dental biofilm by the patient on a daily basis. Therefore, instruction and monitoring biofilm-control ~~cedures precedes, continues simultaneously with, and~~ ~~professional instrumentation.~~

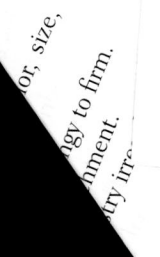

~~NONSURGICAL THERAPY~~

~~techniques for the removal of~~
~~al deposits using manual and~~
~~res. Chapter 40, following~~
~~f adjunctive interventions~~
~~of nonsurgical periodon-~~
~~ach procedure is assessed~~
~~s that includes periodontal~~

risk assessment. Nonsurgical therapy may include a combination of the following procedures:

■ Removal of dental biofilm, endotoxins, other bacterial products, and calculus.
■ Root planing to remove residual calculus and create a smoother tooth surface.
■ Irrigation using an antimicrobial agent.
■ Sustained-release antibiotic or antimicrobial agent particularly for refractory infections.
■ Removal of iatrogenic biofilm retainers.
   ▪ Overhanging margins of restorations.
   ▪ Unfinished, poorly contoured, or unpolished restorations.
■ Concurrent dental therapeutic interventions. Examples include:
   ▪ Restoration to arrest advanced carious lesions to aid gingival healing by preventing food impaction and making personal biofilm removal possible.
   ▪ Analysis of occlusal irregularities.

PREPARATION OF THE CLINICIAN

■ Skill in procedures for disease control for a patient requires more than the development of manual procedures for applying instruments to the tooth surfaces.
■ In these refined and exacting techniques, knowledge of the anatomic, histopathologic, and physiologic characteristics of the teeth and supporting tissues is necessary.
■ Such knowledge is tied together with recognition of the clinical manifestations of the tissues in disease and then in health as the effects of treatment become apparent.

FOCUS OF TREATMENT

■ The focus of clinical treatment is on the education and motivation of the patient.
■ The patient needs to understand how the disease is produced and how to contribute daily to the elimination of the risk factors of the infection.
■ Dental biofilm, endotoxin and other bacterial products, cementum, and calculus are all involved, but the sources of the inflammation are periodontal pathogenic microorganisms in the biofilm.

BOX 39-1	Key Words

Nonsurgical Instrumentation

Bactermia: presence of bacteria in the blood.
Endotoxin: lipopolysaccharide (LPS) complex found in the cell wall of many gram-negative microorganisms; contained superficially within periodontally involved cementum.
Furcation: anatomic area between the roots of a multi-rooted tooth.
Furcation invasion: pathologic resorption of bone within a furcation.
Instrumentation zone: area on tooth where instrumentation is confined; area where calculus and altered cementum are located and treatment is required.
Nonsurgical periodontal therapy: dental biofilm removal and control, supragingival and subgingival scaling,

root planing, and adjunctive treatments such as the use of chemotherapy; the basic objectives are to restore periodontal health; arrest or slow the progression of early periodontal disease; or, for more advanced disease, to prepare the tissues for more complex periodontal therapy.
Root planing: a definitive treatment procedure designed to remove altered cementum or surface dentin that is rough, impregnated with calculus, or contaminated with toxins or microorganisms. Also termed **debridement** or **root preparation.**
Scaling: instrumentation of the crown or root surfaces to remove dental biofilm and calculus.

I. DENTAL BIOFILM

- Gingival inflammation and periodontal destruction result from the action of pathogenic microorganisms in dental biofilm.
- Dental biofilm attaches to the surfaces of the gingiva and the teeth. Dental calculus is mineralized dental biofilm.

II. ENDOTOXIN

- Lipopolysaccharides or endotoxins, derived from the cell walls of gram-negative pathogenic microorganisms, are toxic to human tissue and lead to inflammation and destruction of the periodontal attachment.
- Endotoxins exist in the biofilm and can be removed readily from the parts of the teeth and tissues that the patient can reach with toothbrush, dental floss, interdental brushes, and whatever system works best for the individual patient.[1-4]

III. CEMENTUM

- The cementum is thin at the cervical third of the root. Some or even complete removal of the cementum during instrumentation for calculus removal is inevitable.
- Excess removal of the cementum and dentin beyond the point of tactile smoothness is not necessary.[5,6] However, a smooth surface is significant, since the microorganisms collect and colonize on a rough surface much more rapidly than on a smooth surface.[7,8]

IV. CALCULUS

- Calculus is not directly a cause of gingival inflammation, but the irregular surface provides a nidus for bacteria of the biofilm to collect and multiply.
- Calculus must be removed to provide a healing environment for the periodontal tissues.

V. RESTORATIVE BIOFILM-RETENTIVE FACTORS

- Overhanging margins and rough surfaces of restorations create a niche for microorganisms to collect, multiply, and mature into gram-negative strains.
- Personal oral self-care efforts by the patient are impeded by overhanging margins, irregular margins that are breaking down, and poorly contoured restorations.

AIMS AND EXPECTED OUTCOMES

The effects and benefits of complete, carefully performed nonsurgical periodontal therapy are summarized here.

I. INTERRUPT OR STOP THE PROGRESS OF DISEASE

- Reduce formation of dental biofilm.
- Delay repopulation of pathogenic microorganisms.
- Change behavioral and lifestyle habits of the patient to reduce risk factors for periodontal infections.

II. CREATE AN ENVIRONMENT THAT ENCOURAGES THE TISSUE TO HEAL AND THE INFLAMMATION TO BE RESOLVED

- Convert pocket (disease) to sulcus (health).
- Shrink previously enlarged spongy tissue.
- Reduce probing depths.
- Eliminate bleeding on probing.
- Regenerate the gingival tissues to normal co[lor] and contour.
- Change the quality of the tissues from spo[ngy]
- Improve the integrity of the clinical attac[hment]
- Remove calculus and restorative denti[stry] to reduce biofilm retention.

TABLE 39-1	EFFECT OF INSTRUMENTATION ON POCKET MICROFLORA
PERIODONTAL INFECTION BEFORE TREATMENT	**PERIODONTAL HEALTH AFTER TREATMENT**
Predominant flora is: Anaerobic Gram-negative Motile Spirochetes, motile rods; pathogenic	**Predominant flora is:** Aerobic Gram-positive Nonmotile Coccoid forms; nonpathogenic
Total count microorganisms: Very high total count of all types of microorganisms	**Total count microorganisms:** Much lower total counts of all types of microorganisms
Leukocyte count: Many leukocytes	**Leukocyte count:** Lower leukocyte counts

III. INDUCE POSITIVE CHANGES IN THE QUALITY AND QUANTITY OF THE SUBGINGIVAL BACTERIAL FLORA

■ Before instrumentation, the predominant microorganisms are anaerobic, gram-negative, motile forms with many spirochetes and rods, high counts of all types of microorganisms, and many leukocytes.

■ After instrumentation, the composition of the bacterial flora shifts to a predominance of aerobic, gram-positive, nonmotile, coccoid forms with lowered total counts and fewer leukocytes **(Table 39-1)**.

IV. PROVIDE INITIAL PREPARATION (TISSUE CONDITIONING) FOR PERIODONTAL THERAPY REQUIRED FOR ADVANCED DISEASE

■ Reduce or eliminate etiologic and predisposing factors.
■ Permit reevaluation. Surgical procedures may be lessened in extent.

V. EDUCATE AND MOTIVATE THE PATIENT

...reciate the values of a healthy mouth.
...o-therapist role in maintaining the health
... treatment phase.
...ment to perform daily personal bio-
...s.
...iodic maintenance appointments
...terval for ongoing monitoring of

Pati...

...RUMENTATION

...t are identified through
... treatment is defined by

the dental hygiene diagnosis and care plan. Included in the care plan are the following:

■ The special management required for the individual patient.
■ The distribution and severity of the periodontal infection.
■ The treatment sequence needed for the individual.
■ The length and number of appointments required to fulfill the need.
■ A plan for reevaluation and continuing care (described in Chapter 46 on pages 725 to 729).

OVERALL APPOINTMENT SYSTEMS

■ Whether a single or multiple appointment plan is required, the initial step is patient instruction.
■ The overall care plan is described and the informed consent of the patient, parent, or guardian obtained.
■ Treatment begins with the patient's own treatment through daily removal of biofilm.
■ In this chapter, the segment of the appointments devoted to instrumentation to include the removal of calculus, subgingival dental biofilm, and overhanging restorations is described.

I. WHEN A SINGLE APPOINTMENT MAY BE ADEQUATE

■ The diagnosis may be gingivitis or early periodontis (Tables 16-1 and 16-2, pages 245 and 246) with small areas of deposits readily accessible; anesthesia may not be needed.
■ Only a few teeth present; limited areas of anesthesia may be needed.
■ Patient presents with an acceptable biofilm score, and evidence of reasonable personal care without need for time for extended instruction and motivation.
■ Patient acts responsibly in keeping appointments for maintenance and continued monitoring for disease control.

II. PLANNED MULTIPLE APPOINTMENTS

The extent of periodontal involvement as shown by probing measurements, distribution and extent of calculus deposits, and oral cleanliness that shows evidence of the patient's personal care or lack of it are major determinants in the number of appointments needed. The patient is never promised that the treatment will be completed in a given number of appointments.

A. Quadrant Scaling Appointments

■ One efficient system for appointment planning is by quadrants or sextants for a more severely diseased mouth, anesthesia, at 1-week intervals to permit patient learning and progressive healing.

- With less severe periodontitis and a compliant patient, two quadrants of the same side (maxillary and mandibular arches) may be completed at an appointment.
- The patient is informed that after the scaling is completed, an appointment for evaluation will be needed.
- The concept of periodic maintenance care that will be needed is introduced.

B. Tissue Conditioning

- At the initial appointment, basic personal daily dental biofilm removal is introduced.
- Interdental devices to complement the use of a toothbrush can be added as the patient demonstrates readiness.
- At each successive appointment, a biofilm score is shown to the patient, and procedures are reviewed.
- With a motivated patient, the tissues will show changes toward a healthy state each week.
- The patient is self-treating and at the same time is *conditioning* the tissue for the clinician. As a result, there is less debris and less bleeding during instrumentation and fewer bacteria for the aerosol contamination created during instrumentation.
- The effect is a cleaner environment in which the clinician can carry out the professional treatment procedures and the patient can appreciate the feeling of a healthy mouth.

C. Evaluation

- At each appointment, the quadrants previously treated are examined for evidence of healing.
- Calculus left inadvertently can be removed by remedial scaling procedures.
- Evaluation: at least 2 weeks after the scaling series, healing of the tissues is expected to be well under way. Restoration of the clinical attachment permits probing.

III. "FULL-MOUTH DISINFECTION"

A. Definition

- System of scaling in two long appointments completed within a 24-hour period.
- The procedures are best accomplished under anesthesia practicing with a chairside assistant.
- Original research combined the concentrated deposit removal with professional and personal multiple treatments with chlorhexidine for additional oral disinfection.[9,10] Follow-up research showed no significant difference with or without the intense disinfection using chlorhexidine.[11,12]

B. Rationale

- Periodontal diseases are infections: ridding the mouth of as many of the pathogens as possible at one time can encourage healing.

- In the quadrant system, it is potentially possible for a scaled quadrant to become reinfected from pathogens left in untreated quadrants.

C. Limitations

- Case selection: Many patients would not be able to withstand such intense treatment.
- Patient instruction: Opportunities for review and repeated instruction at the patient's learning pace are not available without a series of extra appointments.
- Reevaluation by the clinician has advantages after a period of time. Completed increments can be evaluated and tissue response can be monitored.

IV. PRELIMINARY PARTIAL SCALING

One system used by some clinicians involved an initial or full-mouth debridement or "gross scaling," usually with an ultrasonic scaling device.

- A series of appointments was then planned for deep scaling by quadrants to complete the instrumentation.
- This approach was abandoned many years ago due to the potential for problems related to incomplete scaling.
- These problems could ultimately compromise the patient's health and interfere with favorable outcomes.

V. PROBLEMS OF INCOMPLETE SCALING

Removing the coronal-most portion of the deposit while leaving pathogenic bacteria beneath the soft tissues is not recommended for a number of reasons. Before using such a plan, the following needs to be considered:

A. Healing at the Gingival Margin: Limited Access

- When the irritants are removed around the opening of the pocket, the tissue heals and the gingival margin can close tight around the tooth.
- The marginal tissue may take on a color and shape that appears normal to the patient, but deep calculus and adherent biofilm remain undisturbed on the root surfaces.
- Despite the appearance of improvement, the probing depth and bleeding on probing have not changed.
- With tightening of the opening of the pocket, insertion of curets for additional deep instrumentation at subsequent appointments can be difficult. This acce limitation compromises the thoroughness of ins mentation that is necessary for healing and res of infection.

B. Potential for Abscess Formation[13]

- *Predisposing factors:*
  - Deep suppurating pockets; adva infection.
  - Pockets extending into furcati defects.

- ■ Patient susceptible to infection, such as with uncontrolled diabetes, with an immunodeficiency disease, or being treated with an immunosuppressive drug.
- ■ *Sequence: With partial scaling.*
  - ■ Healing can begin.
  - ■ The tissue at the gingival margin tightens.
  - ■ The pocket closes.
  - ■ Microorganisms multiply within.
  - ■ An abscess develops.

C. Patient Instruction

- ■ When supragingival calculus and dental biofilm are removed from the crowns of the teeth, the "visible lesson" is taken away.
- ■ As gingival swelling, sensitivity, and bleeding subside at the margin, the patient may be less motivated to return for the completion of treatment.
- ■ When treatment is carried out quadrant by quadrant, the patient has unscaled areas with which to compare the healing quadrants. The patient can see and feel changes and improvements that contrast with untreated areas.

D. Roughened Calculus

- ■ Calculus roughened by partial removal can be a source of increased subgingival biofilm collections. The surface of calculus is highly porous microscopically, allowing bacteria to collect and colonize.
- ■ The rough surface thus provides more sources for infection by holding pathogenic microorganisms and their inflammatory byproducts in intimate contact with the surrounding gingival tissues.[7,8]

E. Patient Misunderstanding

- ■ For the patient with limited understanding of the seriousness and extent of periodontal infection, the mouth may feel good and look good after a gross "cleaning."
- ■ As a result, the patient may not appreciate the need to return for the continuing appointments to complete the deep scaling. The personal objective of "clean teeth" had been fulfilled.
- ■ Later, when severe periodontitis develops, the patient may claim that incomplete treatment was provided originally.
- ■ By receiving repeated information at each successive quadrant treatment and by seeing the changes, the patient can gain a better understanding of the seriousness of the disease in the periodontal tissues.

VI. SCALING TO COMPLETION

A. Segmental Approach

- ■ Quadrant or sextant treatments to completion are recommended to prevent the aforementioned problems associated with incomplete scaling.

- ■ Decisions are made according to what can reasonably be completed by the individual clinician within the time frame of a given appointment. Reevaluations as the quadrants continue provide opportunities for removal of residual calculus not detectable at a first, or even a second reexamination.
- ■ Treatment appointments are scheduled accordingly.

B. Care Planning Factors to Consider

- ■ *Access:* the relative ease of insertion to base of the soft tissue pocket.
  - ■ Fibrosity and tissue tone of the free gingiva.
  - ■ Probing depths: attachment pattern around the full circumference of each tooth.
- ■ *Deposit on tooth surfaces*
  - ■ Extent and distribution of calculus.
  - ■ Age of calculus/degree of mineralization.
  - ■ Strength of attachment of calculus to the tooth.
- ■ *Root anatomy*
  - ■ Multirooted teeth with furcation involvement.
  - ■ Deep concavities.
- ■ *Patient factors*
  - ■ Need for local anesthetic or nitrous oxide/oxygen sedation.
  - ■ Limited capacity for opening mouth.
  - ■ Behavioral factors such as apprehension.

PREPARATION FOR INSTRUMENTATION

I. REVIEW THE PATIENT'S ASSESSMENT RECORD

- ■ *Note special needs:* from medical history and previous appointment experiences.
- ■ *Identify:* systemic or physical problems with potential for emergency.

II. REVIEW RADIOGRAPHIC FINDINGS

A. Findings Applicable During Instrumentation

- ■ Anatomic features of roots, furcations, and bone level, which may need special adaptations of curets.
- ■ Overhanging restorations to be removed or scheduled for replacement.

B. Use Radiographs as Guide

Keep radiographs on lighted viewbox throughout the treatment for reference to observe bone level and root anatomy for each area.

III. REVIEW CARE PLAN AND TREATMENT RECORDS

- ■ Note flow and sequence of planned appointments.
- ■ Note findings that apply to the instrumentation process.
  - ■ Examine periodontal probings to review attachment topography and access limitations.
  - ■ Assemble procedure tray setup to include appropriate instruments.

- Review previous appointment progress notes.
  - Read details of prior treatment, noting segments completed, which will be reassessed for healing.
  - Ascertain how previous treatment appointments have been tolerated by the patient.
  - Anticipate anesthesia requirements.
- Keep periodontal probing chart prominently displayed throughout the treatment for reference.

IV. PATIENT PREPARATION

A. Premedication Requirements for Patient at Risk

- Transient bacteremia can occur during and immediately after scaling procedures.
- Frequency and duration of bacteremia depends on severity of periodontal infection and inflammation and the degree of trauma during the instrumentation.[14,15]
- Check that the patient has taken the antibiotic premedication as prescribed.

B. Provide Preprocedural Bactericidal Rinse

C. Prepare for Anesthesia as Indicated

V. SUPRAGINGIVAL EXAMINATION

A. Visual

- Gross deposits and tooth surface irregularities can be seen by direct vision. Fine, unstained, white or yellowish calculus is frequently invisible when wet with saliva.
- Observe tooth surfaces closely while a gentle stream of compressed air is applied. Dry calculus is more visible than wet calculus.

B. Tactile

- Without deposits or anatomical irregularities, the enamel surface is smooth.
- An explorer tip passed over the surface slides freely, smoothly, and quietly.
- When rough calculus deposits are present, the explorer tip does not slide freely but meets with resistance over varying textures.
- Deposits can produce a scratchy sound or an audible click as the explorer passes over them.

VI. SUBGINGIVAL EXAMINATION

A. Visual

- *Gingiva.* The clinical appearance suggestive of underlying calculus may be the following:
  - Soft, spongy, bluish-red gingiva, with enlargement of the interdental papillae over proximal surface calculus
  - Dark-colored area beneath relatively translucent marginal gingiva

- *Calculus*
  - A loose, resilient pocket wall can be deflected from the tooth surface with a gentle stream of compressed air.
  - Dark, subgingival calculus can be seen within the pocket on the root.

B. Tactile

1. *Periodontal charting*
   - Use probing depth recordings as a basic guide.
   - Confirm recorded probing depths of segment to be instrumented.
   - Study the soft tissue attachment pattern to select effective procedures.
2. *Identify shallow pockets (sulci)*
   - Scaling in shallow pockets of fewer than 3 mm can lead to loss of periodontal attachment.[16–18]
   - Research has shown that repeated use of a curet when no calculus is present can result in detachment of periodontal ligament fibers and that healing does not bring them back.[18]
   - Root surfaces free of calculus may require biofilm removal.
   - Confine instrumentation to light-pressured but comprehensive biofilm debridement.
3. *Determine distribution and extent of deposits*
   - **Figure 39-1** illustrates probing. As the probe passes over the surface it may be intercepted by calculus **(Figure 39-1B)**.
   - Use an explorer for distinction of fine hard deposits.
4. *Evaluate tooth topography*
   - Detect grooves and furcations using a horizontal stroke **(Figure 39-1C)**.
   - Use a furcation probe to examine furcations.
   - Note root and furcation variations **(Figure 39-2)**.

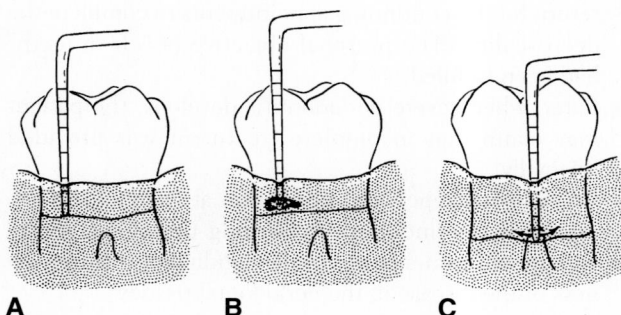

A   **B**   **C**

FIGURE 39-1 **Subgingival Examination Using a Probe. (A)** Probe inserted to the bottom of a pocket for complete examination prior to subgingival scaling. **(B)** As the probe passes over the root surface, it may be intercepted by a hard mass of calculus. **(C)** Using a horizontal probe stroke to examine the topography of a furcation area. Keep the side of the tip of the probe on the tooth surface and slide over one root, into the furcation, and across to the other root.

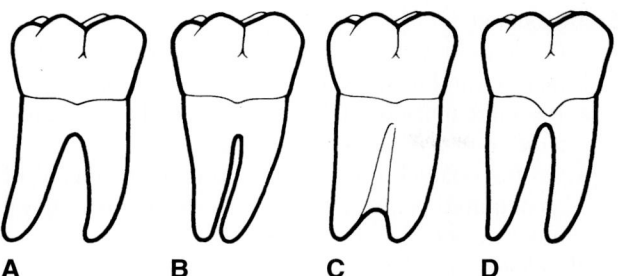

FIGURE 39-2 **Anatomic Variations of Furcations. (A)** Widely separated. **(B)** Separated but close together. **(C)** Fused roots separated only in the apical portion. **(D)** Presence of an enamel projection that may be conducive to an early furcation involvement. (Source: Carranza FA, Newman MG. *Clinical periodontology*. 8th ed. Philadelphia: Saunders; 1996. p. 641.)

5. *Evaluate restorative margins*
   ■ Detect overhanging restorations that need to be evaluated and treatment planned.
   ■ Detect marginal irregularities that retain biofilm.

VII. FORMULATE STRATEGY FOR INSTRUMENTATION

■ Combine clinical findings with information documented in the patient's record.
■ Check overall treatment objectives for the patient.
■ Determine a strategy for instrumentation.

CALCULUS REMOVAL

I. PREREQUISITES

■ Position of clinician to prevent cumulative trauma.
■ Clear visibility with excellent lighting.
■ Sharp instruments with proper contour.

II. LOCATION OF INSTRUMENTATION

Figure 39-3 illustrates the location of instrumentation. Instrumentation and the selection of the correct instrument depend on the following:

■ Type of pocket (gingival or periodontal)
■ Location of calculus (on crown or root surface)
■ Position of gingival margin (recession or covering cementoenamel junction)
■ Level of clinical attachment (normal or clinical attachment loss)

III. THE SCALING PROCESS

The process is the series of procedures and events that lead to achievement of a specific result.

A. Definitions

■ *Scaling:* removal of calculus and dental biofilm from the supragingival and subgingival exposed tooth surfaces(clinical crown).
■ *Periodontal debridement:* removal of all residual calculus and toxic materials from the root to produce a clean, smooth tooth surface. Other terms include *root planing, root detoxification,* and *root preparation.*

B. Instrumentation Zone[19]

■ Area of the tooth where instrumentation is performed for scaling and root planing.
■ *Location:* above the clinical attachment of the periodontal fibers; extends the height and width of the hard and soft deposits of calculus and biofilm to be removed.
■ Scaling and root planing strokes for deposit removal are limited to the instrumentation zone. Extending the strokes to clean areas where no deposits exist can be harmful to the tooth, allow the clinician to lose control, dull the instrument, and waste time.

C. Systematic Deposit Removal

1. Tooth to tooth
2. Section to section of deposit on each tooth surface
3. Strokes overlap in channels
4. The instrument is positioned progressively along the area of the deposit, within the *instrumentation zone.*

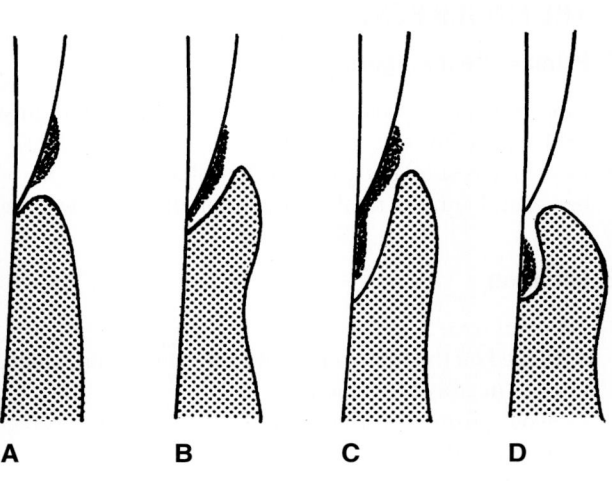
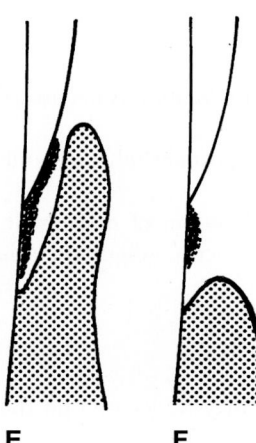

FIGURE 39-3 **Location of Instrumentation.** The location of calculus deposits, level of periodontal attachment, depth of pocket, and position of the gingival margin determine the site of instrumentation. **(A)** Supragingival calculus on the enamel. **(B)** Gingival pocket with both supragingival and subgingival calculus on enamel. **(C)** Periodontal pocket with both supragingival and subgingival calculus. **(D)** Periodontal pocket with subgingival calculus only on root surface. **(E)** Periodontal pocket with subgingival calculus on both enamel and root surface. **(F)** Calculus on root surface exposed by gingival recession.

5. *Nature of the deposit*
   - The oldest calculus, located next to the tooth surface, is the hardest.
   - The outermost calculus is covered with a layer of dental biofilm that has not yet started to mineralize.

IV. SPECIAL SUBGINGIVAL CONSIDERATIONS

Although the basic steps described for calculus removal apply to both supragingival and subgingival deposits, subgingival techniques are unique and complicated by several significant factors. The instrumentation is more complex and difficult than supragingival calculus removal. Some of the variables are included here.

A. Subgingival Anatomy

1. *Tooth surface pocket wall*
   - As shown in **Figure 39-3C**, and **E**, some subgingival instrumentation is on the crown (enamel), and some on the root (cementum or dentin).
   - In the cervical third of the root, the cementum is thin (0.03 to 0.06 mm) and may have been removed during previous instrumentation.
2. *Soft tissue pocket wall*
   - The pocket wall hugs closely to the tooth surface covered with rough calculus, which in turn is covered with bacterial biofilm.
   - Only a narrow area is available for manipulation of instruments.
   - The pocket narrows in the deeper area next to the clinical attachment.
   - Bleeding during instrumentation is inevitable because of the inflammation in the wall of the pocket.
3. *Variations in probing depths*
   - The periodontal charting is a primary guide to subgingival instrumentation and will serve as a road map to guide instrument depth of insertion.
   - Probing depths are recorded around each tooth because the depths can vary on a single surface.

B. Accessibility and Visibility

1. Pocket is a confined area; instrumentation is necessary in areas where access is difficult.
2. Instrumentation is dependent almost entirely on tactile sensitivity.
3. Soft tissue pocket wall limits freedom of movement. Careful adaptation to tooth surface configurations is essential.

C. Subgingival Calculus

1. *Location:* Subgingival calculus may be located on the enamel, the root, or both **(Figure 39-3B, C, D, E)**.

2. *Attachment*
   - Calculus attaches to the cementum in minute irregularities and in areas of cemental resorption.
   - It is more tenacious than on the enamel and requires a different technique for removal.
   - On the enamel it is attached primarily by means of an acquired pellicle, which makes calculus removal much easier.
3. *Morphology of calculus*
   - Subgingival calculus is irregularly deposited. It occurs in nodular, ledge, smooth veneer, and other forms (Table 20-1, page 301).
   - Previously scaled or burnished calculus: Subgingival calculus that has been partially scaled and left after incomplete instrumentation may be smooth and may not be detected when an explorer is used to check the area.

MANUAL SUBGINGIVAL SCALING STEPS

Types of instruments and the basic principles for their use are included in Chapter 38. This chapter continues from Chapter 38 to describe the use of the instruments for deposit removal. **Box 39-2** summarizes the steps.

I. INSTRUMENT GRASP

A. *Apply a modified pen grasp* (Figure 38-13).
   - Thumb and index and middle fingers make up the grasp points.
B. *Use a light grasp for:*
   - Instrument insertion and positioning.
   - Assessment strokes.
   - Root debridement strokes to remove biofilm.
C. *Keep the grasp firm and secure* during calculus removal.
D. *Apply a light grasp with light lateral pressure after calculus removal.*
   - To remove small irregularities.
   - To leave the treated area smooth.

II. STABILIZATION: ESTABLISH THE FINGER REST

A. Primary Rest Fingers

- Ring and little fingers (numbers 3 and 4 in Figure 38-13, page 587).
- Rest fingers are kept close to the middle finger (number 2) and join the total hand motion during activation.

B. Location

1. *Intraoral rests:*
   - Placed on the tooth adjacent to the one being scaled, or as near as convenient.
   - Avoid position in the path of the strokes to protect from accidental glove and finger cut.

BOX 39-2	Steps for Calculus Removal Using Manual Instruments

Assessment
- Probe to determine pocket/sulcus characteristics and confirm soft tissue attachment topography.
- Explore to determine location and extent of deposits and tooth surface irregularities.
- Select correct instruments that will adapt and conform to concavities and other root morphology characteristics for areas being treated.

Preparation: Instrument Control
- Hold instrument with a modified pen grasp.
- Identify correct cutting edge of blade for surface being scaled.
  - A. For area-specific curets: terminal shank parallel with surface being scaled.
  - B. For universal curets: terminal shank *less* than parallel with surface being scaled (approximately 20°).
- Establish a light hand rest for instrument placement to allow for adjustment and repositioning.
- Insert: use placement or exploratory stroke to locate apical edge of deposit.
- Adjust working angulation (average at 70°).

Action: Strokes
- Secure a stable, functional extraoral hand rest or intraoral finger rest that can support instrument placement and activation at correct working stroke angulation.
  - A. Pressure into the fulcrum equals the pressure against the tooth.
  - B. Balance fulcrum pressure with lateral pressure of the strokes.
- Activate for working stroke.
  - A. Apply firm lateral pressure for calculus removal.
  - B. Apply moderate lateral pressure to smooth the surface.
  - C. Apply light lateral pressure for biofilm debridement.
  - D. Control length and direction of stroke: respect the Instrumentation Zone.
  - E. Maintain continuous adaptation throughout the stroke.

Channels: Overlap to Completion
- Continue channel scaling with overlapping multidirectional strokes.
  - A. Apply placement stroke to reposition blade for next stroke.
  - B. Activate instrument circumferentially around tooth.
  - C. Keep toe adapted around line angles by rolling handle.
  - D. Cover all surfaces comprehensively to remove all traces of calculus and biofilm.

Evaluation
- Use explorer to determine end point of treatment.

2. *Distance rests:* a long span between the rest and the point of instrument application.
   - Requires an extended grasp.
   - Requires a secure finger rest.
3. *Variations:* Substitute, supplementary, and reinforced rests are described on pages 589 to 590.
4. *Dry the rest position:*
   - Biofilm and saliva make tooth surfaces slippery.
   - Use compressed air or dry with gauze sponge.

III. SELECT CORRECT CUTTING EDGE

A. Universal Curets

- Curets are paired and usually mounted on double-ended handles. Single-ended handles may be selected for certain patients or procedures.

- Correct cutting edge for scaling: when positioned on the tooth surface, only the back of the blade can be seen.
- Incorrect blade adaptation: the open face of the blade will be seen.
  - It would be impossible to angulate at 70° for scaling.
  - The *open* blade is in the correct position for gingival curettage to remove the inner soft tissue lining of the pocket wall.

B. Gracey Curets

- Hold instrument with the terminal shank perpendicular to the floor.
- Look into face.
- Select longer, lower cutting edge.

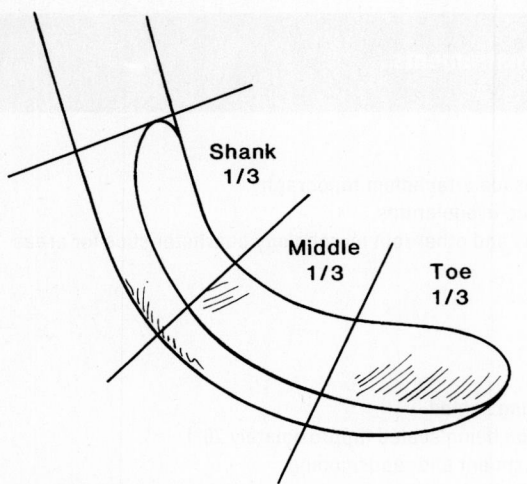

FIGURE 39-4 **Curet Divided Into Thirds.** The toe third is kept in contact with the tooth surface during instrumentation. Because of tooth contours, most strokes for scaling and root planing are accomplished using the toe third. Adaptation of the toe third is shown in **Figure 39-5.**

IV. ADAPTATION OF CUTTING EDGE

A. Apply Blade to Conform to Tooth Surface Being Treated

- Because of tooth contours, only a portion of a blade can be adapted.
- The toe and middle thirds of a curet blade are used most frequently **(Figure 39-4)**.

B. Maintain Adaptation

- Roll the handle around line angles and other tooth convexities.

- Maintain close adaptation of the cutting edge to prevent trauma of the adjacent soft tissue **(Figure 39-5B)**.
- At the same time maintain the 70° angulation.

V. ANGULATION

A. Insertion

Close the angle to nearly flat against the tooth surface (0°) as the instrument is inserted to the base of a pocket **(Figure 39-6A and B)**.

B. Establish Optimal Angle for Scaling

A 70° angle is effective for deposit removal using a scaler or a curet.

VI. LATERAL PRESSURE

A. Degree of Pressure of Blade against Tooth

Whether a light, moderate, or heavy pressure is needed will depend on the nature of the deposit and the type of therapy being performed.

1. *Light pressure*
   - Assessment.
   - Instrument insertion.
   - Confirmation of the soft tissue attachment.
2. *Moderate to heavy pressure*
   - Calculus removal.
   - Working strokes require heavy to moderate lateral pressure depending on the degree of mineralization of the calculus.
   - Recently formed calculus can be removed more readily than established calculus.

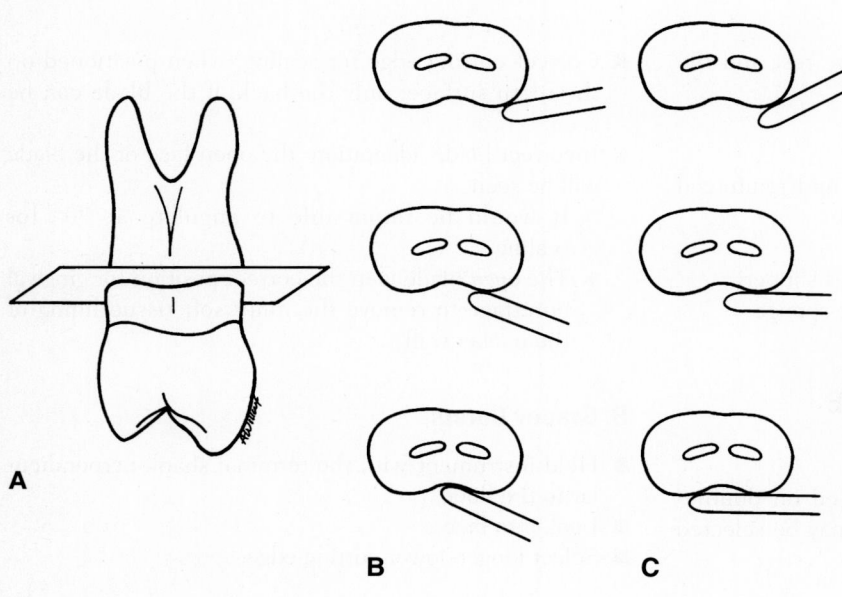

FIGURE 39-5 **Instrument Adaptation.** **(A)** Maxillary first premolar shows cross section of root drawn for **(B)** and **(C)**. **(B)** Diagram of three positions of a curet shows correct adaptation at a line angle and on the concave mesial surface with toe third of the instrument maintained on the tooth as the instrument is adapted. **(C)** Diagram shows incorrect adaptation with toe of curet extended away from the tooth surface.

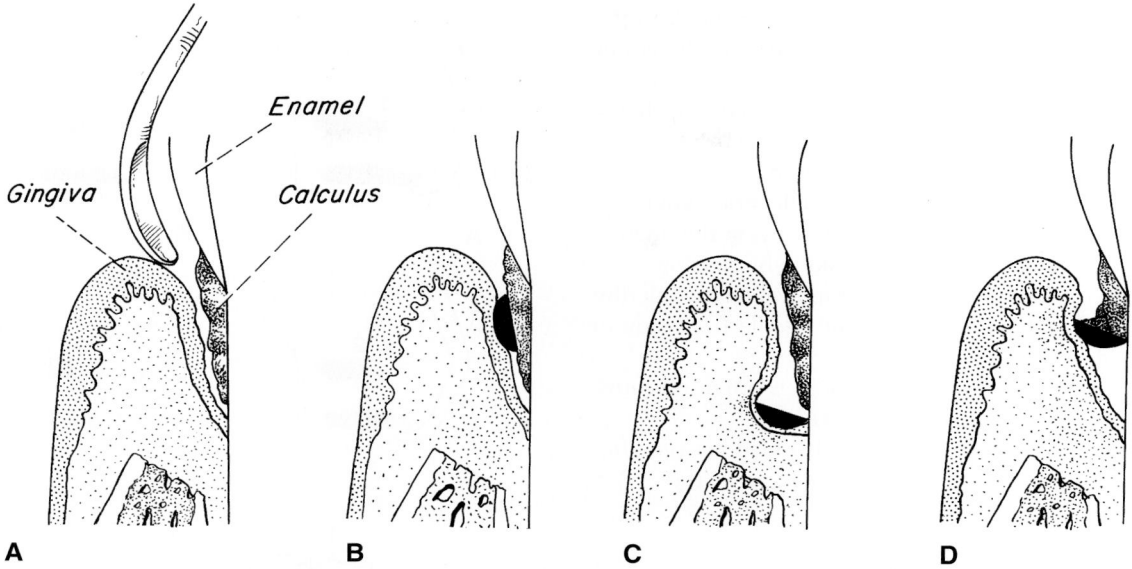

A   B   C   D

FIGURE 39-6 **Subgingival Scaling and Root Planing. (A)** The curet is inserted gently under the gingival margin. **(B)** With a placement stroke, the blade is passed over the surface of the tooth or calculus. Note 0° angle of the face of the curet with the calculus. **(C)** The curet is lowered to the base of the pocket until the tension of the soft tissue is felt with the rounded back of the curet. The curet then is positioned at an angle of 70° to 80° with the tooth surface beneath the calculus deposit. **(D)** The blade is moved along the root surface in a scaling stroke to remove the calculus.

3. *Biofilm debridement*
   - When the root surface is free of calculus, confine instrumentation to light-pressured debridement over the entire subgingival surface.
   - The tactile sense transmits vibrations felt from any irregularities present.
   - Lateral pressure against the tooth can be increased for removal.
   - Unnecessary and unwarranted tooth structure removal can be minimized.

B. Balance of Pressure During Stroke

Careful control is accomplished by a balance of pressure between

- the grasp of the instrument,
- the pressure on the finger rest,
- the lateral pressure against the tooth.

C. Factors Affecting Lateral Pressure

1. *Sharp instrument*
   - A minimum degree of pressure allows the cutting edge to "grab" the calculus.
   - Engaging the deposit provides strong leverage for effective, clean removal.
   - Less time, with fewer strokes, is required.
   - Fatigue is kept to a minimum.
2. *Dull instrument*
   - When dull, the blade cannot engage the deposit and will slide over it, burnishing it on the surface.

- The more the deposit is burnished with repeated strokes, the more difficult it becomes to remove.
- More strokes are taken, causing increased fatigue.
- Inefficiency increases treatment time.
- Grasp and lateral pressures increase to compensate for the sliding effect.
- Stroke control is reduced with the heavier pressure needed to activate a dull blade; this can lead to instrument slippage and trauma to the patient's gingival tissues.
- Loss of confidence by the clinician.
- Loss of patient confidence in the clinician.

VII. ACTIVATION: STROKE

A. Tighten the Grasp

- Renew the stability of the rest position.
  - Whether an intraoral finger rest or an extraoral hand rest, the pressure of the rest will equal the pressure against the tooth.
- Move the instrument firmly and deliberately, making each stroke intentional.
- Wrist and arm bear the weight during the stroke, rather than flexing the fingers in the grasp.

B. Maintain Cutting Edge Evenly During the Stroke

1. *Adaptation:* Keep blade closely aligned with the surface of the tooth.
2. *Angulation:* Maintain blade position by observing lower shank from beginning to end of each stroke.

- Relationship of the angle of the lower shank to the tooth surface stays consistent for the full length of the stroke.
- Orientation of lower, terminal shank to surface being scaled:
  - *Gracey curets:* parallel orientation.
  - *Universal curets:* less than parallel orientation.
- Guard against blade closure. Changing the angulation at the cutting edge can lead to burnishing.
  - Wrist motion activations that pivot on the fulcrum finger move the instrument handle from side to side.
  - Side-to-side handle movement is often indicative of blade closure during stroke.
3. *Maintain the adaptation:* Handle is rolled between fingers to keep the cutting edge adapted correctly.

C. Motion Control

Without independent finger movement, the hand, wrist, and arm act as a continuum to activate the instrument.

D. Direction of Strokes

- Select overlapping vertical, oblique (diagonal), or horizontal strokes to accommodate the anatomical features of the tooth surfaces (Figure 38-18, page 593).
- Strokes are applied systematically, not haphazardly.
- Avoid horizontal strokes at the bottom of a pocket to avoid damage to the clinical attachment.

E. Length of Stroke: Within Instrumentation Zone

- Short, smooth, decisive strokes permit accommodation of the cutting edges to changes in the topography of the tooth surface.
- Confine the strokes within a pocket to prevent the need for repeated removal and reinsertion of the curet; prevent trauma to the gingival margin.

VIII. CHANNELS OF STROKES: COVERAGE

A. Make Strokes in Channels (Figure 39-7)

- At the completion of each stroke, move the instrument laterally a very short distance to assure overlap.
- Maintain the same finger rest.

B. Overlap Strokes in Channels

- Ensure complete coverage of every square millimeter of subgingival surface for thorough removal of deposits.

C. Repeat Strokes

- Continue until surface has been completely debrided.

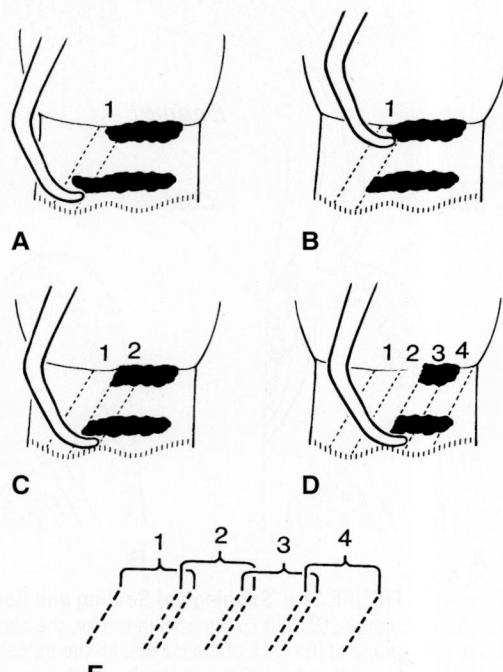

FIGURE 39-7 Channel Scaling. (A) Curet adapted in position for channel 1 stroke from the base of the pocket under the calculus deposit. **(B)** Completion of stroke for channel 1. **(C)** Using an exploratory stroke, the curet is lowered into the pocket and is positioned for calculus removal in channel 2. **(D)** Curet positioned for channel 3. Several strokes in each channel may be needed to ensure complete calculus removal. **(E)** Strokes of each channel overlap strokes of the previous channel. (*Source:* Parr RW, Green E, Madsen L, and Miller S. Subgingival scaling and root planing. Berkeley (CA): Praxis Publishing Co.; 1976.)

IX. PLANE THE ROOT SURFACE

A. Finishing Techniques

- *Purpose:* smoothing the tooth surfaces to lessen immediate recolonization of bacteria.
- *Procedure:* instrumentation is basically the same as for scaling.
- *Application:* only where deemed necessary after exploration with a fine periodontal explorer capable of accessing the farthest reaches of pocket depths.

B. Touch and Pressure

- Specific differences in technique are related to touch and pressure.
  - A lighter grasp will increase tactile sensitivity.
  - Light lateral pressure is applied for maximum sensitivity to minute irregularities of the surface.
  - A lighter stroke can be used for final smoothing of the root surface; increased pressure is not needed.
- Sharp instruments are essential for tactile transmission.

C. Strokes

- Use smooth strokes that overlap systematically.

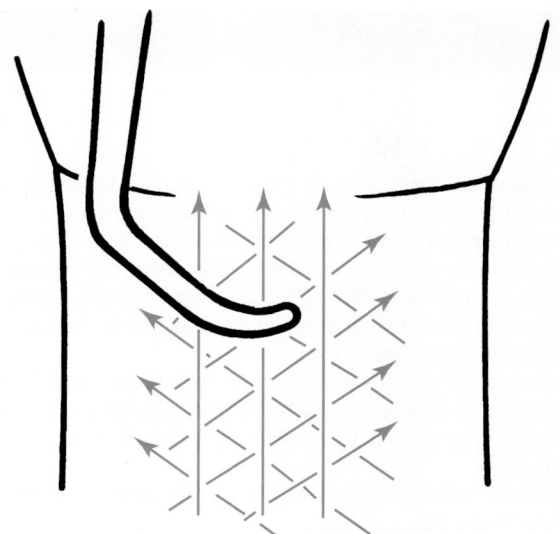

FIGURE 39-8 **Root Surface Strokes.** The use of strokes in vertical and oblique directions with light lateral pressure can help to eliminate grooves left after scaling. A smooth surface results. (*Source:* Parr RW, Green E, Madsen L, and Miller S. Subgingival scaling and root planing. Berkeley (CA): Praxis Publishing Co.; 1976. 42 p.)

- As the surface becomes smoother, longer strokes with reduced pressure help to remove small lines, scratches, or grooves without gouging the surface.
1. *Stroke direction*
   - Multidirectional stroke patterns create the ideal finished surface.
   - Vertical and then oblique strokes may be used **(Figure 39-8)**.
   - Keep horizontal strokes away from the attachment epithelium.
2. *Adaptation*
   - Careful adaptation of the curet to the unique anatomic features of the roots is needed.
   - Convex surfaces, constricted cervical areas, concavities and grooves of the proximal surfaces, and the variations in furcations all require precise adaptation.
   - Minibladed Gracey curets are designed specifically to access and adapt to concavities and convexities where standard-length blades either can span across or protrude beyond (Figure 37-5C).
   - As a surface area becomes smooth, a gradual change in the sound of the instrument stroke may occur. At completion, the instrument may be as quiet as when used on polished enamel.

X. EVALUATION

- Use a subgingival periodontal explorer to examine for completion of calculus removal and smoothness of the treated surfaces.
- Apply explorer in both vertical and diagonal strokes to detect irregularities **(Figure 39-8)**.

- Refine spots of roughness with a sharp curet.
- Adapt curet with light lateral pressure for maximum sensitivity to minute irregularities of the surface. Avoid grooving the treated surface.
- Postcare patient instructions are described in this chapter on page 632.

 # ULTRASONIC AND SONIC SCALING

Ultrasonic and manual nonsurgical instrumentation can produce equivalent results in calculus and dental biofilm removal when the instruments are applied correctly and sensitive posttreatment evaluation is made.[20,21] A blended approach that utilizes both methods of instrumentation is preferred.

- Long-term goals of therapy are accomplished through a blended approach that utilizes both methods of instrumentation.
- The patient benefits from therapy incorporating the strengths of each approach.
- Manual instrumentation was the only method available for the safe removal of supragingival and subgingival calculus until the ultrasonic scaling device was introduced in the 1950s.
- The power-driven scaling device converted high-frequency electrical energy into mechanical energy in the form of rapid vibrations.
- Technologic advances in ultrasonics improved and allowed for rapid calculus removal that resulted in much less hand fatigue for the clinician.
- Later, sonic scalers were developed that worked on the same principle but utilized an air turbine as an energy source.
- Terminology related to power-driven instrumentation is defined in **Box 39-3**.

MODE OF ACTION

Although the main action of the ultrasonic and sonic scalers is mechanical, cavitation and irrigation also play important roles in debridement.

I. MECHANICAL VIBRATION

- Power-driven scaling devices convert electrical energy (ultrasonic) or air pressure (sonic) into high-frequency sound waves.
- Sound waves produce rapid vibrations in the specially designed scaling tips.
- Calculus is incrementally shattered from the tooth surface when the vibrations are applied to the deposit.

II. CAVITATION

- Water is required to dissipate the heat produced at the vibrating tip.

BOX 39-3	Key Words

Ultrasonic and Sonic Instrumentation

Acoustic turbulence: agitation in the fluids surrounding a rapidly vibrating ultrasonic tip; has potential to disrupt the bacterial matrix.

Cavitation: action created by the formation and collapse of bubbles in the water by high-frequency sound waves surrounding an ultrasonic tip.

Ferromagnetic: type of rod with unusually high magnetic permeability used in magnetostrictive ultrasonic unit inserts.

Kilohertz (kHz): a unit of energy equal to 1000 cycles per second.

Lavage: the therapeutic washing of the pocket and root surface to remove endotoxins and loose debris.

Magnetic field: space occupied by magnetic lines of force.

Magnetostrictive: ultrasonic scaling device that generates a magnetic field and produces tip vibrations by the expansion and contraction of a metal stack or rod.

Piezoelectric: ultrasonic scaling device activated by dimensional changes in crystals housed in the handpiece.

Sonic scaler: type of mechanical power-driven scaler that functions from energy delivered by a vibrating working tip in the frequency of 2500 to 7000 cycles per second; driven by compressed air, the handpiece connects directly to a conventional rotary handpiece tubing.

Stack: magnetostrictive inserts made of flat metal strips stacked, or sandwiched, together; metal in stack acts like an antenna to pick up magnetic field and cause vibration.

Transducer: a device that converts energy or power from one form to another.

Ultrasonic scaler: power-driven scaling instrument that operates in a frequency range between 25,000 to 50,000 cycles per second to convert a high-frequency electrical current into mechanical vibrations

---

- Cavitation occurs when the water meets the vibrating tip. Minute bubbles are created that collapse and release energy.[22]
- *Effect of cavitation:* Although the cavitation has little influence on hard deposit removal, it is capable of destroying surface bacteria[23] and can remove endotoxin from the root surface.[24]

III. IRRIGATION

- The water spray penetrates to the base of the pocket[25] to provide a continuous flushing of debris, microorganisms, and endotoxin.
- Oscillation of the ultrasonic tip causes hydrodynamic waves to surround the tip. This acoustic turbulence is believed to have a disruptive effect on surface bacteria.[26,27]
- Ultrasonic debridement following manual instrumentation provides cleansing and rinsing of scaled and root planed surfaces, which can promote healing of soft tissues.

IV. VARIABLE ELEMENTS

Power-driven scaling devices feature varying elements but are mainly distinguished by their frequency output and the direction and pattern of tip motion, as shown in **Figure 39-9**.

- *Amplitude:* distance of tip movement measured in micrometers.
  - Distance of tip movement determines power output of the instrument, which is an adjustable component on all ultrasonic devices.

- *Frequency:* speed of movement.
  - Number of cycles per second (cps) the tip moves.
  - Adjustable component available only on manually tuned ultrasonic devices.
  - Majority of available devices have tuning preset, or "automatic."

ULTRASONIC SCALING DEVICES

I. TWO TYPES

- Magnetostrictive ultrasonic scalers.
- Piezoelectric ultrasonic scalers.

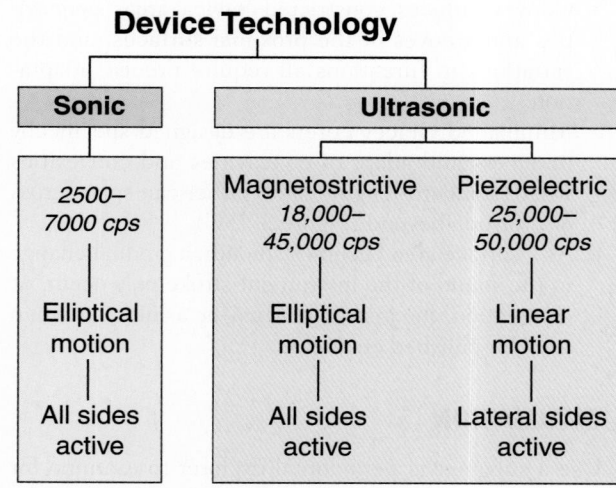

FIGURE 39-9 **Power-Driven Scaling Devices Technology.** For sonic and both magnetostrictive and piezoelectric ultrasonic scalers, the speed [cycles per minute (cps)], the motion (linear or ellipical), and the active part of the tip (lateral sides only or all sides) identified.

II. EQUIPMENT

Ultrasonic scaling devices share certain attributes and are differentiated by others.

A. Unit Parts

- Electric generator
- Handpiece assembly
- Set of interchangeable scaling tip inserts
- Foot control to activate the handpiece

B. Tip Activation

- Vibrations in the tip occur when electric current is applied to the handpiece.

C. Water Source

- Necessary for delivery of water to the handpiece.
- Water is carried through or around the instrument tip.
- Cools tip. Rapid tip movement creates friction and/or temperature increase in the tooth.
- Flushes subgingival debris.

III. MAGNETOSTRICTIVE ULTRASONIC SCALERS

A. Composition

- *Conventional magnetostrictive units:* Utilize a longitudinal stack of metal strips in the handpiece.
- *Ferromagnetic units:* Utilize a fragile ferric rod that generates less heat than the conventional metal stack.

B. Activation

- Vibrations in the tip occur when electric current is applied to the handpiece.
- A magnetic field is created; with expansion and contraction of metal strips in the handpiece.

C. Tip Motion

- Conventional tip moves in an elliptical pattern; all surfaces of the tip are active.
- Ferromagnetic tip rotates 360° in three different planes; equal effectiveness on all sides of the tip.

D. Tip Shape

Cross-section of tip is round.

E. Frequency

- Conventional units range from 18,000 to 45,000 cycles per second (cps).
  - Older units are designed to operate at 25,000 cps and are called 25-kilohertz (kHz) machines.
  - Newer units are designed to operate at 30,000 cps and are called 30-kHz machines.
- Ferromagnetic units operate at 42,000 cps.

IV. PIEZOELECTRIC ULTRASONIC SCALERS

- *Composition:* Scaler devices feature a ceramic rod in the handpiece.
- *Activation:* by dimensional changes in quartz or metal alloy crystal transducers housed in the handpiece.
- *Tip motion:* moves in a linear pattern, forward and backward.
  - Only the lateral surfaces of the tip are active.
  - Handpiece position will adjust at each line angle to maintain adaptation of the lateral surface of the tip to the tooth; accomplished by pivoting the wrist to approximate a 90° turn of the instrument to move from facial or lingual surfaces to proximal surfaces and back again.
- *Technique:* placement and movement of the tip is specific.
  - Position the lateral surface of the tip in contact with the tooth.
  - Use only the terminal 2–3 mm of the tip's lateral surface.
  - Keep terminal lateral surface adapted at all times around curvatures and line angles using wrist pivot.
- *Tip shape:* cross section of tip varies from trapezoidal with angular edges to round to bladed.
- *Frequency*
  - Varies according to manufacturer
  - Ranges from 25,000 to 50,000 cps

SONIC SCALING DEVICES

I. EQUIPMENT: UNIT PARTS

- Handpiece.
- Interchangeable scaling tips.
- Handpiece attaches directly to the dental unit and is activated with the conventional handpiece foot control.

II. TIP ACTIVATION

A. Tip Motion

- Driven by compressed air from the dental unit rather than electrical energy.
- Moves in an elliptical pattern.
- All surfaces of the tip are active.

B. Amplitude

- Less powerful than ultrasonic scalers.

C. Frequency

- Producing vibrations at the tip; range between 2,500 and 7,000 cps.

- Because of fewer vibrations produced, calculus removal is more difficult.

D. Water Source

- Water is required to cool the friction between the instrument tip and the tooth surface.
- Heat is not generated by the scaling tip.

PURPOSES AND USES FOR POWER-DRIVEN SCALERS

I. INDICATIONS FOR USE

- Removal of supragingival calculus and tenacious stains.
- *Subgingival periodontal debridement, including*:
  A. removal of calculus, attached biofilm, and endotoxins from the root surface;
  B. removal of unattached biofilm from the sulcular space.[28]
- *Initial debridement*
  A. For a patient with necrotizing ulcerative gingivitis or other conditions that can be relieved by removal of deposits.
  B. Loose debris and microorganisms are first removed by rinsing, brushing, and flossing during patient instruction to prevent or reduce contaminated aerosol production.
- Debridement of furcation areas following manual instrumentation.[29,30]
- Debridement of deposits before oral surgery.
- Removal of orthodontic cement; debonding.
- Removal of overhanging margins of restorations.

II. CONTRAINDICATIONS

A. Systemic Health Conditions

- *Communicable disease:* Patient with a communicable disease that can be transmitted by aerosols, such as tuberculosis.
- *Susceptibility to infection*
  - Compromised patient with marked susceptibility to infection.
  - Examples: immunosuppression from disease or chemotherapy, uncontrolled diabetes, debilitation, or kidney or other organ transplant.
- *Respiratory risk:* patient with a respiratory risk. Septic material and microorganisms from biofilm and periodontal pockets can be aspirated into the lungs.[31]
  - History of chronic pulmonary disease, including asthma, emphysema, or cystic fibrosis.
  - History of cardiovascular disease with secondary pulmonary disease or breathing problem.
- *Swallowing difficulty*
  - Patient with a swallowing problem or prone to gagging.

- Examples: amyotrophic lateral sclerosis, muscular dystrophy, paralysis, multiple sclerosis.
- *Cardiac pacemaker*
  - Some newer devices have protective coverings. Consultation with the patient's cardiologist is necessary.

B. Oral Conditions

- *Avoid demineralized areas*
  - Ultrasonic vibrations can remove the delicate remineralizing cover of a demineralized area.
- *Exposed dentinal surfaces*
  - Tooth structure can be removed in excess and create sensitivity.
  - The smear layer can be removed and dentinal tubules uncovered, which can increase sensitivity or aggravate existing sensitivity.
- *Children*
  - Young, growing, developing tissues are sensitive to ultrasonic vibrations.
  - Primary and newly erupted permanent teeth have large pulp chambers. Vibrations and heat from the ultrasonic scaler may damage pulp tissue.

III. PRECAUTIONS

A. Damage to the Integrity of Restorations

- *Porcelain:* fracturing; loss of marginal integrity.[32,33]
- *Amalgam:* surface defects; loss of marginal integrity.[34,35]
- *Composites:* surface alterations.[36]

B. Titanium Implant Abutments

Ultrasonic instrumentation will damage titanium surfaces unless the tip insert is covered with a specially designed plastic sheath.[37,38]

IV. RISK CONSIDERATIONS

A. Clinician

- *Cumulative trauma*
  - It has been estimated that dental hygienists apply over 32 tons of scaling forces per year using over 25,000 scaling strokes for calculus removal.[39,40]
  - Many dental hygienists suffer from symptoms related to cumulative trauma.
  - Powered scaling actually reduces the force needed to remove deposits, and it can reduce the risk of carpal tunnel syndrome and other musculoskeletal disorders.
- *Magnetic fields*
  - Ultrasonic scalers produce weak, time-varying magnetic fields similar to those produced by common household appliances.
  - There is no scientific evidence that cumulative exposure to weak, time-varying magnetic fields has caused any biological harm to any dental personnel.[41]

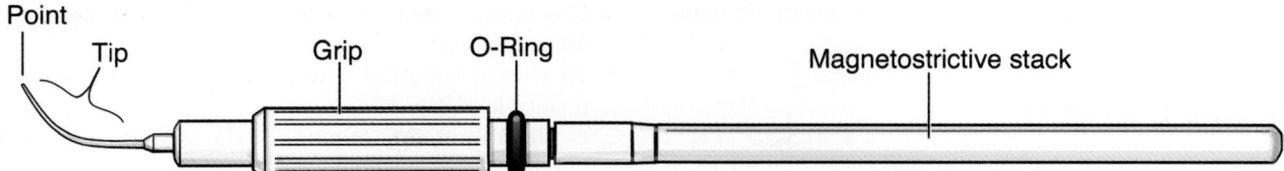

FIGURE 39-10 **Ultrasonic Handpiece Insert.** With parts labeled.

B. Patient

■ *Heat production*
  ▪ Potential damage to the pulp tissue needs to be kept in mind during instrumentation.[42]
  ▪ Constant motion of the instrument, correct angulation, and ample water for cooling are essential to safe operation.
■ *Hearing shifts*
  ▪ Extended exposure to noises above a certain level, such as the noise of a high-speed handpiece or an ultrasonic scaler, may be damaging.
  ▪ Temporary hearing shifts have been demonstrated for a group of patients.[43]

INSTRUMENT TIP DESIGN

I. PARTS

The parts are illustrated in **Figure 39-10**. The design of the instrument tip will vary according to the intended use. **Figure 39-11** shows examples of various tip designs.

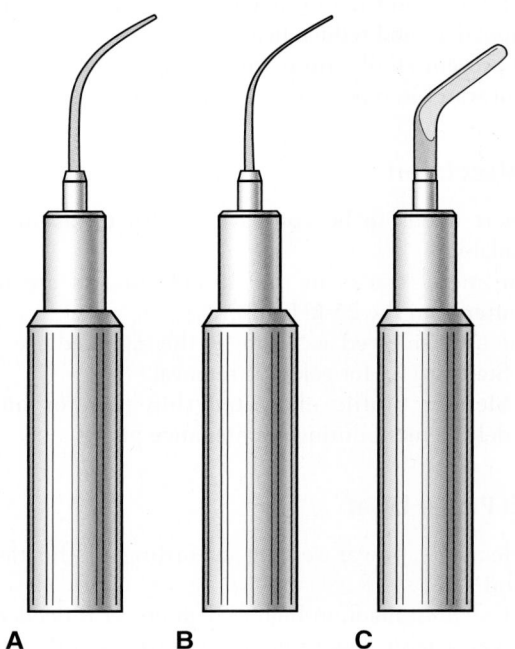

FIGURE 39-11 **Ultrasonic Tip Designs. (A)** Straight tip with internal flow water delivery. **(B)** Thinner tip. **(C)** Beavertail for supragingival surfaces needing removal of heavy calculus or cement.

II. SIZE AND TYPE

A. Conventional or Standard Tip

■ Traditional ultrasonic and sonic tips, bulkier than most curet tips. Also called *universal* tips.
■ Generally used for moderate to heavy deposit removal from supragingival or relatively shallow subgingival surfaces.
■ Standard tips for both magnetostrictive and piezoelectric devices may be used on any power setting.

B. Periodontal or Narrow-Profile Tip

■ Thinner and longer tips provide better access to subgingival surfaces.
■ Allow superior coverage of deep pockets and furcations.
■ Most magnetostrictive thin tips must be used on low to medium power only.
■ Piezoelectric thin tips may be used on high power, which will not burnish calculus.
■ Tip design innovations continue to emerge in answer to the demands of advanced nonsurgical therapy.
■ Bladed and beveled tips are capable of removing calculus rapidly.
■ Diamond-coated tips used on low power are effective for fine scaling and root planing.

C. Plastic or Carbon Composite Tip[44]

■ A close-fitting plastic sheath fits over the metal working end to protect vulnerable restorative surfaces such as titanium abutments of implants, or esthetic materials surfaces.
■ Dentin and titanium surfaces can be safely instrumented with the plastic tip. A light, gentle activation is all that is needed to remove soft and mineralizing deposits.

III. SHAPE

■ *Universal:* Tip slightly curved in one direction; to be used throughout the dentition.
■ *Contra-angled:* Instrument tips have curvatures to left and right designed to adapt to posterior surfaces of the teeth.
■ *Beavertail:* Designed to be used on supragingival surfaces for the removal of heavy calculus, stain, and orthodontic cement.

■ *Thin periodontal:* Straight or contra-angled tip designed for subgingival instrumentation.

IV. WATER DELIVERY

■ *External tube:* An external tube delivers the water to the tip of the instrument.
■ *Internal tube:* Water is delivered from the unit to cool the tip through the internal structure of the insert.

CLINICAL PREPARATION

I. DENTAL HYGIENE CARE PLAN

A. Review Patient's Medical History and Treatment Records

B. Oral Examination

Obtain current periodontal probings. Review the care plan, radiographs, and chart to determine the following:

■ Location of deposits
■ Depth of pockets and soft tissue attachment topography
■ Presence of exposed furcations

C. Instrumentation Plan

■ Plan a systematic sequence.
■ Complete one quadrant before starting another, instrumenting each tooth to completion.

II. INFECTION CONTROL MEASURES

A. Personal Protective Equipment

■ The clinician and assistant wear protective eyewear, high-efficiency bacterial face mask, gloves, and protective outerwear.
■ Use of a face shield as well as a regular mask is needed for added protection against aerosols.
■ Use of a surgical cap to prevent contamination of hair is recommended.
■ Masks need to be changed often—a maximum of 20 minutes, or at the first sign of moisture.

B. Flush Water Lines[45]

■ Biofilm forms on the internal surfaces of dental tubing, as found in the dental unit and ultrasonic unit.
■ Opportunistic pathogens can colonize and replicate on the internal surface.
■ Risk of exposure to dental personnel through the aerosol emerging in the vicinity of the treatment area to beyond 20 feet.

■ Risk of exposure to the patient through aspiration and/or bacteremia.
■ To reduce bacterial contamination, water lines are flushed as follows:
  ■ Flush for 2 to 3 minutes at the beginning of each day.
  ■ Flush for 20 to 30 seconds between patients.
  ■ Flush before sterile insert is placed in the handpiece.

C. High-Volume Evacuation

■ Deposition of tooth-associated microorganisms into the pulmonary system during ultrasonic scaling can result in pulmonary infection.[31]
■ Use of high-volume evacuation will reduce aspiration of contaminated aerosols by both the patient and the clinician.
■ An assistant is required when a high-volume evacuator is used.
■ A special high-volume evacuator attachment provides suction around the handpiece tip and reduces aerosol contamination in the treatment room.[46,47]

III. ULTRASONIC UNIT PREPARATION

A. Establish Power and Water Connections

B. Flush Lines

C. Fill Ultrasonic Handpiece With Water

■ Hold upright as handpiece is filled and insert is placed.
■ Fill with water before placing the insert to eliminate trapped air and reduce heat.
■ To prevent sterile insert from being flushed with stagnant water in pipes.

D. Select Insert

■ Insert needs to be compatible with ultrasonic unit available.
■ The metal stacks in the 30-kHz inserts are much shorter than the 25-kHz inserts.
■ The tip is selected according to the intended use.
  ■ Standard tip for calculus removal.
  ■ Slender profile elongated thin tips for biofilm debridement during maintenance phase.

E. Set Power Level

■ Select the power setting according to the task at hand.
  ■ *Calculus:* medium-high to high power is needed.
  ■ *Soft deposit:* low to medium power is sufficient for removal of attached and unattached biofilm.
■ Consistent use of the unit on the lowest power setting for all case types will burnish the calculus present.

F. Adjust Water

- Water provides cooling and irrigation.
- Proper water setting will create a fine mist at the tip of the instrument.
- Increase water if heat is produced.

G. Use of an Antimicrobial Solution

- Some ultrasonic units have reservoirs so an antimicrobial solution can be used as the coolant since the lavage of ultrasonics can penetrate to the base of the pocket.[25]
- Antimicrobial solutions will reduce the number of pathogens present in the contaminated aerosol.[48,49]

IV. SONIC UNIT PREPARATION

- Flush water lines in slow-speed-handpiece line for 2 minutes.
- Attach sonic handpiece to slow-speed-handpiece line.
- Select and screw sonic tip into handpiece.

V. PATIENT PREPARATION

A. Review Health History

- Check to ensure that any patient requiring preprocedural antibiotic has taken the prescribed medication. Bacteremia is produced in a high percentage of patients treated by powered instrumentation, as well as manual instrumentation.[50]
- Identify any contraindications to ultrasonic instrumentation.

B. Explain Procedure

- Describe and demonstrate sound and spray, vibration, and the purpose for use.
- Request hearing-impaired patient to turn off a hearing aid; ultrasonic use creates interference and feedback in hearing aids.

C. Provide Protection for Patient

- Safety glasses to prevent eye infections or injury.
- Fluid-resistant drape over patient to keep moisture from skin and clothing.

D. Preprocedural Rinse

- Ultrasonic and sonic instrumentation generates aerosols that are heavily contaminated by microorganisms.[51]
- Prior to treatment, patients are directed to rinse with an antimicrobial mouthrinse for 30 seconds to decrease incidence of bacteremia.[52]
- The use of chlorhexidine is preferred for the preprocedural rinse because of its substantivity.

E. Patient Position

Place the patient in a supine position for maximum visibility.

F. Patient Breathing

- Explain to the patient, and request breathing/air exchange through the nose only.
- Reduces potential for aspiration of oral pathogens into lung tissue.
- Allows water to pool for evacuation with saliva ejector.
- Less fogging of mouth mirror.
- More comfort for patient.

G. Pain Control

Prepare to use topical or local anesthetic as necessary.

H. Water Control

- Prepare to use evacuation with saliva ejector or high-volume evacuator with assistant as indicated by the severity and degree of sepsis and communicability of infection from the patient.
- An evacuation system requires proper disinfection before use.
- Shape and position saliva ejector so that the patient can hold it in place to collect water that is pooling in the mouth.

INSTRUMENTATION

As with manual instrumentation, power instrumentation depends on skill and technique. Because tactile sensitivity is reduced or absent when power instrumentation is used, knowledge and awareness of tooth morphology assists the clinician in debriding periodontal pockets efficiently and safely.

Ultrasonic instrumentation is technique dependent. Care in adapting the terminal 3-mm portion of the working end to the tooth surface and methodical activation using sufficient power to disrupt the mineralized deposit are necessary.

I. PRINCIPLES FOR TECHNIQUE

A. Power Setting

- *Low power*
  - While more comfortable for the patient, low power is not capable of removing calculus completely.
  - Deposit can become burnished on the root surface and leave a polished exterior surface that is difficult to detect and remove.

- ■ Remnants of burnished calculus can harbor pathogenic contaminants.
- ■ Pathogenic contaminants remain despite cavitation and lavage provided through the ultrasonic tip.
- ■ *High to medium power*
  - ■ Calculus can be removed using higher power settings, provided the proper technique is employed.
  - ■ Use of anesthesia permits maximum thoroughness while keeping the patient comfortable.

B. Transfer of Energy

- ■ The full length of the tip is vibrating, but only the terminal few millimeters will transfer maximum energy capable of disrupting calculus.

C. Adaptation

- ■ Position side of tip against tooth, with the few millimeters nearest the end of the tip closely adapted on the surface at all times **(Figure 39-12)**.
- ■ May be difficult to accomplish, since the end segment of the tip is generally straight in contrast to anatomical curvatures of the tooth anatomy.

D. Activation

- ■ Adequate time is needed for energy to transfer from the active tip to the deposit to break up the mineralized component effectively.
- ■ Speed of movement is critical to this transfer.
- ■ The tip is moved constantly at a slow to moderate pace.

II. ULTRASONIC SCALING

A. Grasp

- ■ Use a modified pen grasp.
- ■ A light grasp will increase tactile sensitivity.
- ■ The weight of the cord tends to pull on the handpiece and place additional strain on the wrist. Manage cord drag by the following:
  - ■ Loop the cord and hold it between the ring finger and little finger.
  - ■ Drape the cord over the shoulder.

B. Fulcrum/Rest

- ■ A hard tissue fulcrum is not required because force and pressure against the tooth surface are not indicated.
- ■ A gentle finger rest is used to stabilize and guide the instrument tip in anterior segments.
- ■ Extraoral and soft tissue rests allow for proper access and adaptation to deeper posterior segments.

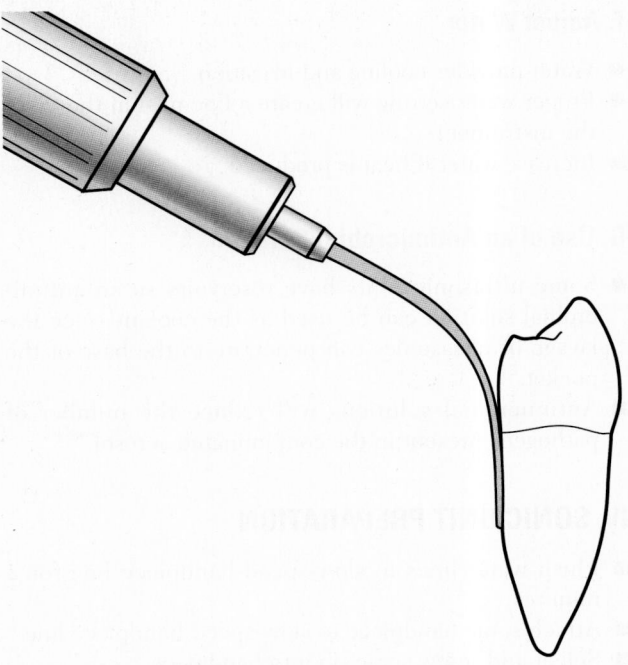

FIGURE 39-12 Adaptation of Ultrasonic Tip. The side of the point of a tip is placed parallel to the tooth surface to prevent damage to the tooth structure. Damage occurs when the point is held perpendicular to the surface.

C. Adaptation

- ■ Keep the side of the instrument tip closely adapted to the tooth surface **(Figure 39-12)**.
- ■ Do not hold the tip perpendicular to the tooth surface at any time because damage to the tooth surface can result.
- ■ *Narrow periodontal pockets*
  - ■ Narrow subgingival pockets interfere with proper adaptation and impede visibility.
  - ■ When instrumenting narrow pockets use an insert with appropriate length and limited width.
  - ■ Direct the tip apically and confirm access to the attachment prior to activating the tip.

D. Stroke

- ■ Keep the instrument tip moving at a moderate to slow pace with a feather-light touch at all times to prevent the following:
  - ■ Scratches or gouging on the tooth surface.
  - ■ Excessive heat build-up.
  - ■ A shock-like effect to the patient.
- ■ Use featherlike pressure to prevent tooth damage. Excessive lateral pressure can result in the following:
  - ■ Damage to the tooth surface.
  - ■ Dampening and deactivation of the tip vibrations.
  - ■ Burnishing of calculus.

- *Overlap strokes*
  - For comprehensive coverage of all surfaces.
  - Strokes may be horizontal, vertical, oblique, or a combination.
- Procedure when the tip binds in an embrasure.
  - Deactivate the power; remove the instrument tip from the embrasure.
  - Reposition the instrument and reactivate the power.

II. WATER CONTROL

A. Foot Pedal

- Release the foot pedal at regular intervals to aid in water control.
- Stop periodically to evaluate tooth surfaces.

B. Mirror Use

- Water is continuously sprayed onto the mirror surface, making indirect vision difficult.
- Wipe the wet surface of the mirror with a gloved finger to coalesce the drops into a clear wet surface. When water is allowed to pool on the surface in this manner, a clearer image of the working area can be seen through the water.

IV. MANUAL SCALING

- Complete the procedure with manual instruments directly following ultrasonic instrumentation.
- Check subgingival areas with a subgingival explorer.
- Remove remaining subgingival irregularities and smooth the surface with curets.

V. EVALUATION

A. Use a Periodontal Subgingival Explorer

- To evaluate the effectiveness of instrumentation periodically during treatment.
- There may be areas of root contour where it is not possible to adapt the ultrasonic insert tip, thus leaving portions of the root surface untreated.
- Portions of the root that cannot be accessed by the ultrasonic tip must be instrumented using curets that will adapt to the root surface; mini-bladed Gracey curets are well suited for this purpose.

B. The Ultrasonic Tip Without Power Can Be Used as a Probe Only

- To confirm access to the soft tissue attachment.
- DO NOT use the insert tip to evaluate the tooth surface.
- There is insufficient tactile sensitivity to accomplish a careful assessment of the root surface smoothness with the insert.

VI. TROUBLESHOOTING

There may be a number of reasons for the ultrasonic instrument to produce unacceptable instrumentation. The causative factor is analyzed to remedy the problem.

A. Tip Wear

- As an ultrasonic tip is used over a period of time, the length of the tip is reduced. With each millimeter of tip length lost, there is a corresponding loss of power.
- Tips need to be checked periodically for wear and replaced when length has reached a point beyond which the tip is incapable of producing sufficient vibration.
- *To monitor tip wear:*
  - use a tip wear indicator template provided by the manufacturer,
  - reserve one of each tip in use as a prototype to compare length reduction,
  - check for loss in length; a 2–3 mm loss in length renders the tip ineffective for calculus removal.

B. Improper Adaptation

- Failure to adapt the terminal few millimeters of the tip to the tooth surface.
- Root morphology has many curvatures featuring convex and concave surfaces.
- Straight instruments do not adapt well to curved surfaces.
- Curets, specifically mini-bladed Gracey curets, are designed to conform to root contours.
- Supplement ultrasonic instrumentation with manual instrumentation to access the highly curved portions of the root.

C. Stroke Too Rapid

- Moving the tip too quickly across the tooth surface.
- Keep tip moving slowly and methodically.
- Brisk tip movement is ineffective for deposit removal.

D. Inadequate Coverage

- Failure to keep strokes confined to close, overlapping channels.
- Moving the tip in a random, scribbling pattern can treat effectively only those limited portions of the root surface that were contacted by the moving tip.
- Move the tip in overlapping segments or channels that cover each square millimeter of root surface.

E. Tip Pressure

- Exerting pressure with the tip against the tooth surface.

- The tip is held with only a light but secure contact and close adaptation against the tooth surface.
- Lateral pressure will render the vibrations ineffective due to a dampening effect.

OVERHANGING RESTORATIONS

I. OVERHANGING MARGINS

Overhangs may occur on any tooth surface, supragingivally or subgingivally. Proximal surfaces overhangs result primarily from

- improper placement of the matrix band and/or wedge,
- incorrect manipulation of the dental material,
- finishing errors.

II. IDENTIFICATION

A. Clinical

An overhang is identified by the:

- relation to the gingival margin (supragingival or subgingival),
- location on specific tooth surface: enamel, cementum, or dentin,
- size or extent,
- information from the patient relative to floss breakage and food impaction.

B. Radiographic

- Limited to proximal surfaces viewed in the radiograph.
- Visibility changed by angulation of the x-ray.
- Supplement radiographic examination with a clinical examination using an explorer.
- Use magnification to detect dental caries adjacent to an overhang.

III. EFFECTS OF OVERHANGING RESTORATIONS

A. Relationship to Periodontal Disease and Dental Caries

An overhang or marginal irregularity is a significant iatrogenic contributing factor because it can do the following:

- Provide a niche where microorganisms that cause periodontal infections and dental caries can proliferate.
- Catch and tear dental floss.
- Render the area inaccessible to a toothbrush and other dental biofilm-removing aids; hinder the patient from disease control procedures.
- Increase the severity of existing inflammation.[53–55]
- Increase the chance of adjacent bone loss.[53,56]
- Retain debris and microorganisms contributing to halitosis and a general lack of oral sanitation.

B. Benefits of Overhang Removal

- Efficient use of dental floss and other interdental cleaning devices.
- Improvement in periodontal health when combined with scaling, root planing, and dental biofilm control.[54,57]

IV. INDICATIONS TO MAINTAIN OR REPLACE THE RESTORATION

All overhanging restorations are corrected or removed and replaced for the health of the periodontium. Whether an overhang can be recontoured or needs to be replaced with a new restoration requires a professional decision.

A. Indications for Continued Maintenance of the Restoration

- The tooth anatomy can be maintained or improved to conform to normal contour.
- The overhang is small or moderate in size.
- The proximal contact is intact.
- No adjacent secondary dental caries or fractures of the margin are present.
- The overhang is accessible for necessary instrumentation to finish and polish without damaging the adjacent tooth structure or traumatizing the gingival tissues.

B. Indications for Removal and Replacement of the Restoration

- The overhang is extensive and would require excessive appointment time.
- Secondary marginal or recurrent dental caries is present.
- The contact area requires restoration.
- Fractures, chips, cracks, or broken margins are apparent.
- When replacement is delayed, a gross overhang is reshaped and smoothed to enable the patient to remove dental biofilm more completely.

V. OVERHANG REMOVAL

A. Procedural Overview

- Remove excess amalgam.
- Finish all cavosurface margins to ensure they are continuous and smooth.
- Smooth all surfaces of the restoration.

B. Manual Instruments

General suggestions for use:

- Select on basis of accessibility of the filling, amount of reduction required, and surface finish indicated.

■ Instruments: chisel, file, scalers, curets, unwaxed extra-fine filament floss.
■ *Technique*
1. Maintain sharp instruments.
2. Remove excess amalgam in small increments to prevent fracture.
3. Work deliberately to prevent damage to gingival tissue and surrounding tooth surfaces, especially cementum.
4. Use finite control on all strokes.
5. Use the tooth surface as a guide to contour the restoration.
6. Move a bladed instrument parallel to, or slightly toward, the margin of the prepared tooth.
7. Keep instruments in contact with the tooth surface to reduce risk of ditching.

C. Procedure

■ *Chisel*
1. Hold the instrument with a modified pen or a palm grasp.
2. Position the blade across the tooth structure and amalgam; activate chisel horizontally across the junction.
3. Use short, well-controlled, overlapping shaving strokes; remove amalgam in small increments to prevent fracture risk.
4. For proximal adaptation, move chisel away from gingiva to prevent pushing bits of amalgam into the tissue; evacuate continuously.
■ *File*
1. Use a *restorative file* for overhang removal; reserve periodontal files for root planing only.
2. Position file perpendicular to the long axis of the tooth on the proximal surface and activate horizontal strokes.
3. Use coarser file for bulk of amalgam; refine margin smoothness with finer file.
4. Extend strokes across amalgam and tooth to prevent leaving a defect.
5. Use short, controlled strokes with light to moderate pressure.
6. File use is always followed by finishing with a curet.
■ *Scaler*
1. Use only a strong scaler; tip can break when extra force is applied.
2. Using a metal cutting edge on metal dulls the instrument.
■ *Curet*
1. *Universal curet:* an aid for smoothing proximal surface.
2. Use vertical strokes with moderate pressure as final finishing.
3. Cross oblique strokes over the junction of the material and the tooth.

■ *Floss*
1. Use unwaxed extra-fine filament floss to ensure the overhang has been removed.
2. Insert floss through the contact area.
3. Curve floss around the tooth surface and gently move it coronally over the margin; the floss no longer catches on a properly finished surface.

D. Power-Driven Instruments

Ultrasonic instrumentation can be used to remove overhanging margins in concert with manual instruments.
1. *Beavertail design:* horizontal strokes on proximal surface.
2. *Standard tip:* vertical strokes on proximal surface.
3. Use medium to high power for bulk of removal; then switch to manual instruments to finish.

COMPLETION OF INITIAL THERAPY

■ After each treatment using nonsurgical instrumentation, an immediate evaluation is made and special instructions are given to the patient for the initial tissue healing period.
■ A follow-up telephone call to the patient during the evening after the appointment can be a welcome gesture that conveys professional responsibility and concern.
■ A short-term follow-up appointment is scheduled in a minimum of 2 weeks when initial healing will be in progress.
■ After health has been attained, it must be maintained. Planning for a long-term maintenance program is described in Chapter 47 on page 733.

I. IMMEDIATE EVALUATION

A. Teeth

■ Observation and exploration reveal the immediate effects of instrumentation on the teeth.
■ An objective has been to produce smooth tooth surfaces, free from deposits.
■ The effect of specific instrumentation is to facilitate the patient's self-care by removing local factors, particularly calculus and overhanging fillings, that encourage dental biofilm retention.

B. Gingiva

■ The gingival changes are not apparent immediately after instrumentation.
■ Tissue regeneration and initial healing begin in a few days, and by 2 weeks, the area can be gently probed. Maturation of connective tissue and keratinization of epithelium take much longer.

■ The objective of treatment is to *create an environment in which the gingival tissue can heal and be maintained in health by the patient.*

II. EXAMINATION

When scaling is accomplished over a series of appointments, each previously scaled quadrant or area is examined and rescaled as needed. Visual and tactile methods are applied carefully to each tooth surface.

A. Visual

■ Compressed air is used with a mouth mirror and adequate lighting to examine the supragingival areas and just below the gingival margins.
■ Transillumination methods are applied.

B. Tactile

■ An evaluation by exploring immediately after completion of instrumentation is made to ascertain that the tooth surfaces are smooth and that all detectable calculus has been removed.

III. INSTRUCTION AFTER SCALING AND ROOT PLANING

Personalized instructions are provided for each patient at the end of each dental hygiene and periodontal appointment. Instruction pertaining to periodontal dressings and sutures is outlined in Table 42-2 (page 671). Many of the same principles can be applied for postcare instruction when a dressing has not been applied.

IV. PRINTED TAKE-HOME INSTRUCTIONS

Personalized printed instructions help to give the patient a handy reference. Verbal instructions alone can easily be forgotten or misinterpreted by even the most conscientious patient.

An added personal note or underlining of significant parts of the printed materials can let a patient sense the caring attitude of the professional team.

A. Information to Include

■ Possible discomfort to expect
■ Rinsing
■ Toothbrushing
■ Eating
■ Where to call in case of problem or question

B. Rinsing

A warm solution is soothing to the tissues and improves the circulation, thereby helping healing.

■ *Solutions suggested for use*
   1. *Hypertonic salt solution:* Level 1/2 teaspoonful of table salt in 1/2 cup (4 ounces) of warm water; provides 3 or 4 mouthfuls for holding and swishing thoroughly.
   2. *Sodium bicarbonate solution:* Level 1/2 teaspoonful of baking soda in 1 cup (8 ounces) of warm water.
   3. *Directions for salt or bicarbonate solutions:* Every 2 hours; after eating; after toothbrushing; before retiring.
■ *Chlorhexidine 0.12%:* Chlorhexidine rinsing is advised following instrumentation for necrotizing ulcerative gingivitis, necrotizing ulcerative periodontitis, and advanced periodontitis,
   1. *Directions:* twice daily, after breakfast and before going to bed, without eating after rinsing to take advantage of the substantivity property of chlorhexidine.
   2. Rinsing is not a substitute for personal biofilm removal with toothbrush and interdental aids.

C. Toothbrushing

The use of a soft brush may be recommended for a few days after scaling and root planing. The patient needs to understand the significance of daily biofilm disruption/removal.

D. Eating

Dietary and nutritional factors are discussed.

■ Patients who are anesthetized are instructed to avoid chewing solid food until the anesthetic has worn off to avoid trauma to the tongue, cheek, and lips.
■ If the tissues are tender during healing, use bland foods lacking in strong, spicy seasonings, as well as continuing use of nutritional foods to promote healing.
■ Foods for a liquid or a soft diet are suggested in Chapter 54 on page 832 to 833.

EFFECTS OF NONSURGICAL INSTRUMENTATION

■ The essential components of successful nonsurgical instrumentation are thorough subgingival debridement by the clinician and effective dental biofilm control by the patient.
■ The focus of treatment and the aims and expected outcomes were described earlier in this chapter on pages 609 to 610.

- Tissue response is the most significant measure of success in periodontal debridement.
- Tissue response is manifested by clinical features commonly referred to as the endpoints of therapy.

I. CLINICAL ENDPOINTS

- *Bleeding on probing:* eliminated.
- *Probing depths:* reduced.
- *Attachment levels:* same or improved.
- *Inflammation:* resolved.
- *Gingival appearance:* size reduced, color normal.
- *Subgingival microflora:* lowered in numbers, delay in repopulation.
- *Dental biofilm control record:* improvement in scores approaching 100% biofilm-free.
- *Tooth surface:* smooth; no biofilm-retentive irregularities.
- *Quality of life factors:* oral comfort with freedom from pain.

II. HEALING

A. Factors Affecting Healing

- Severity of the infection and clinical features at the start of treatment.
- Noncompliance of the patient
  - To dental biofilm control.
  - To follow the complete treatment plan.
- *Tobacco use:* smoking.[58]
- Systemic influences
  - Diabetes.
  - *Lowered defense:* immunocompromised as, for example, in HIV/AIDS, cancer chemotherapy.
- Root surface irregularities from incomplete debridement: retained calculus, endotoxins, and microorganisms.

B. Healing Process

- *Resolution of inflammation:* Edema recedes, necrotic cells are cleared away, and tissue regenerates.
- *Clinical attachment:* A long epithelial attachment can be expected.

III. EFFECT ON MICROORGANISMS

A. Changes in Pocket Flora[59,60]

- The subgingival bacterial flora is changed after debridement, as shown in **Table 39-1**.
- Before instrumentation for treatment of periodontitis, the subgingival microorganisms are primarily anaerobic, gram-negative, motile forms.
- After scaling and root planing, the total number of subgingival organisms decreases substantially.

A shift to aerobic, gram-positive, nonmotile forms occurs.

B. Effect of Conversion of Microorganisms

- The disease-producing gram-negative pocket microorganisms are changed to a health-producing gram-positive flora.
- The gingiva reflects the changes. Gingival bleeding on probing is lessened, and the color, size, shape, and other characteristics assume a normal appearance.

C. Repopulation

- Without personal daily biofilm control, the microorganisms can return to pretreatment levels within an average of 42 days.[61]
- With biofilm control, the repopulation of the pocket takes longer, even in susceptible patients.
- In many patients, nonsurgical periodontal therapy results in a gingival condition that can be maintained free from reinfection.

D. Endotoxins

- Endotoxins are lipopolysaccharides (LPSs) released from gram-negative bacterial cell walls.
- They occur in the bacteria covering the cementum and superficially in the cementum itself. Endotoxins have been shown to be toxic to human cells.[62] Endotoxins do not penetrate deeply into cemental surfaces.[1,2]
- Retained endotoxins are held by calculus not removed during instrumentation as well as by new microorganisms recolonizing on the surfaces.

FOLLOW-UP EVALUATION

- The real evaluation, the true test of successful treatment, cannot be made until at least 2 weeks after initial therapy (scaling and root planing) has been completed.
- At that time, the response of the gingival tissue to therapy is apparent.

I. ASSESSMENT PROCEDURE

A. Periodontal Probing

- Complete probing is performed and documented.
- Bleeding points are noted as probings are made and documented in the periodontal record.

- Patient biofilm control efforts are evaluated.
  - Obtain biofilm score after the soft tissue visual examination has been completed.
  - Provide feedback for the patient's efforts and the degree of improvement noted as well as areas needing further attention.

B. Tactile Evaluation

- Areas demonstrating bleeding points are carefully assessed with a periodontal explorer for residual calculus deposits.
- Pockets of 5 mm or deeper need an explorer with a long terminal shank as shown in Figure 15-13, page 235).
- Residual calculus can be expected on any subgingival surface that demonstrates bleeding on gentle probing.
- Special checks for difficult-to-access areas.
  - Concavities and depressions of the root anatomy.
  - Subgingival margins of crowns, fixed partial denture, or overhanging restoration.
  - Furcation invasions.

II. REINSTRUMENTATION

A. Remove Remaining Calculus

- Use only optimally sharpened instruments.

B. Anticipate Effects

- Smooth root surfaces that are free of calculus create a biologically compatible root surface that can support healing in the overlying tissues.

III. RESPONSE TO TREATMENT

- Once treatment has been completed and the follow up evaluation is made, a decision is made as to the relative success of the therapy.
- The patient has either reached the point of being able to be managed for the present under the care of the dental hygienist, or may require more extensive treatment.
- In case of advanced disease that has not responded adequately to nonsurgical therapy, a referral to a periodontist may be necessary as described in Chapter 47 on page 736.

IV. MAINTENANCE INTERVAL DETERMINED

- Assessment findings indicate the relative success of therapy delivered.

- On the basis of the findings, a determination is made as to recommended intervals for subsequent maintenance appointments.
- Factors taken into account include the following:
  1. Soft tissue response to instrumentation and degree of healing.
  2. Changes and/or stabilization in probing depth.
  3. *Patient factors:* use of tobacco; systemic influences such as diabetes.
  4. Currently demonstrated biofilm control efforts; level of skill.
  5. Motivation and responsibility assumed for daily personal oral self-care.
  6. Psychosocial factors; stress.

INSTRUMENT MAINTENANCE

I. MANUAL SCALERS AND CURETS

A. Examine for Wear While Sharpening

- Reserve thinned or shortened curets to use for conscientious, motivated maintenance patients with shallow sulci and minimal calculus.
- Heavier bladed, newer curets are indicated for application of strong lateral pressure necessary for initial therapy, root preparation, and moderate to heavy accumulations of calculus.
- Handle all instruments with care. Avoid damage, breakage, and dulling of sharp cutting edges; instrument cassettes protect instruments from wear and tear during the sterilization process.

II. ULTRASONIC TIPS

- Avoid dry heat sterilization; use steam or chemical vapor autoclave.
- Insert tips wear with use and a schedule for monitoring them is needed.
- Worn out tips are incapable of removing deposit; calculus is only burnished.
- Worn out tips can cause damage to tooth surfaces.
- Check at intervals (appropriate to extent of use) and replace.

III. BROKEN INSTRUMENTS

The procedure to follow when an instrument blade tip breaks in a patient's mouth during treatment will be in accord with the dentist's own policy.[63] *The principal objective in the location of a broken instrument tip is to know positively that the tip has been removed* (**Figure 39-13**). A general procedure is suggested in **Box 39-4**.

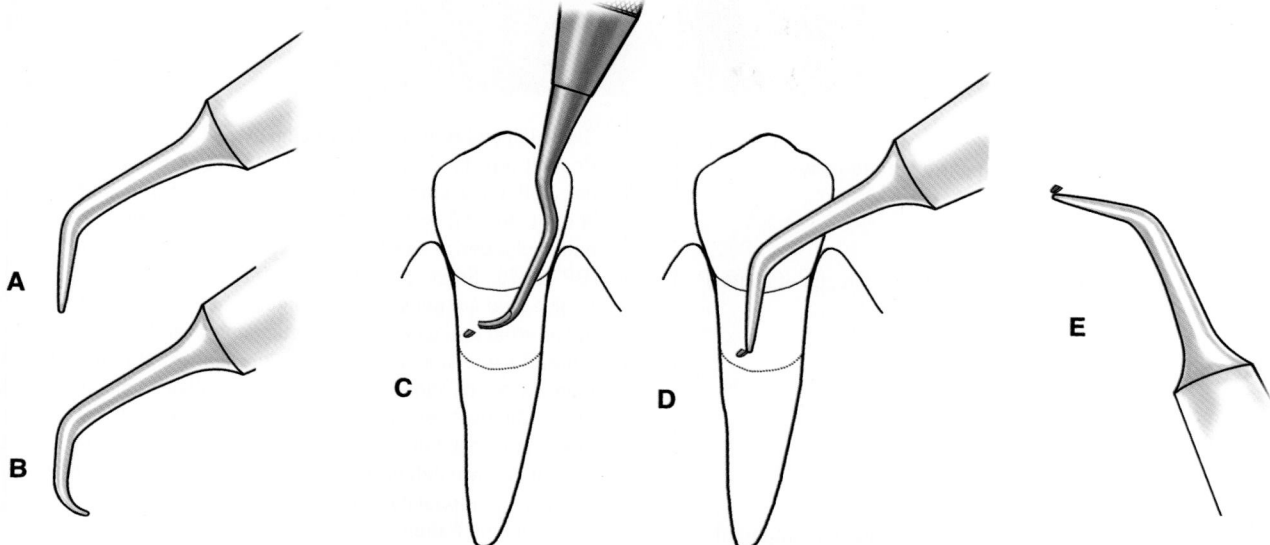

FIGURE 39-13 **Broken Instrument Tip Retrieval. (A)** and **(B)** Two shapes of the "Periotriever" Magnetic instruments: (A) for straight entrance to pocket and (B) shaped to enter furcations. **(C)** Curet in pocket with broken tip. **(D)** Magnetized Retriever in pocket searching for broken tip. **(E)** Curet tip removed from pocket attached to the Retriever. (Source: Schwartz M. The prevention and management of the broken curet. *Compend Cont Educ Dent.* 1998 Apr;19(4):418–20, 422, 424–5.)

DOCUMENTATION

Documentation for the second in a series of appointments for a quadrant of scaling and root debridement with local anesthesia.

■ Complete health history and assessment examination findings.

■ Record new blood pressure
■ Oral preliminary examination for (1) healing and progress of the treatment of the previously treated quadrant, with comments from the patient and (2) specific reexamination of quadrant to be treated that day.
■ Note patient's biofilm successes: provide instructions for care of newly treated area.
■ A sample progress note may be reviewed in **Box 39-5**.

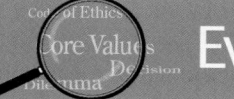 # Everyday Ethics

Lorna and Caroline practice as hygienists in the same office approximately 2 ½ days per week. Lorna graduated from dental hygiene school about 15 years ago, while Caroline was licensed just 3 years ago. They generally had their own patients that were scheduled with the same hygienist. One day Mrs. Border, a patient routinely scheduled with Lorna, showed up in Caroline's appointment book because she wanted to fit in her regular maintenance appointment before going to live with her daughter for several months. The receptionist scheduled her with the first available hygienist.

Caroline reviewed the patient's medical history and recorded the blood pressure. During the gingival examination, as Caroline began to probe, she found rough areas that she first assumed were part of the tooth surfaces. Upon further instrumentation, the areas turned out to be deep calculus. Caroline worked diligently but needed to re-appoint Mrs. Border

for a second visit. The patient was outraged and complained that Caroline "should have used the sprayer-machine like Lorna usually does."

Questions for Consideration:
1. Is this an ethical dilemma or an issue for Caroline? How or why? While respecting both the patient's autonomy and Lorna's role as a professional, Caroline realizes the deep calculus could not all have formed since the previous appointment.
2. How can Caroline proceed to address this problem? She assumes Mrs. Border will make her next appointment with Caroline and possibly complain to the dentist.
3. Using the questions in Table V-1 (in Section V, Introduction, page 362), outline 3 or 4 possible avenues for Caroline to consider in resolving this difficult situation.

BOX 39-4	Care of a Broken Instrument

Preparatory Planning
- Discuss with dentist during early practice days.
- Determine practice policy.

Objective
Know positively that the broken segment (i.e., tip of scaler) has been completely removed

Immediate Action
- Cease procedure, retain retraction.
- Do not move patient's head.
- Isolate with gauze sponge.
- Do not use air/water syringe.
- Adjust saliva ejector to opposite side.
- Do not alarm the patient by describing what happened.

Examination of Area
- Do not dry with air.
- Use careful, gentle retraction to examine the immediate area including the floor of the mouth and Mucobuccal fold
- Blot the gingival tissue dry with a cotton roll to examine around the tooth
- Use transilluminating light or mouth light
- Examine gingival sulcus
  1. Use a curet applied gently with a spoon-like stroke
  2. Take great care not to push the tip into the base of the pocket (in case the broken segment is there)

Treatment
- Apply a magnetized retrieving instrument (Figure 39-13).
- Consult with dentist for assistance in accord with previously discussed policy.
- Prepare a radiograph of the area.
- When not found during any of above procedures:
  A. Arrange for a periodontal surgical procedure

Source: Schwartz M. The prevention and management of the broken curet. *Compend Cont Educ Dent.* 1998 Apr;19:418.

BOX 39-5	Example Progress Note

Gloria (26 yrs) returned after being away for 2 years in the Peace Corps in Africa. Said she had tried hard to care for her teeth daily, but safe water was never assured, and she ran out of floss without a place to shop for more. No basic changes in health history; vitals all within normal (BP 121/70). Smokes ½ pack a day (at most); has planned to give it up but not yet until she gets back to work. External/internal oral exam clear. Teeth: generalized brownish cigarette stain and areas of calculus: slight supragingival mand. anterior, slight to moderate subgingival in molar areas. Gingiva: see probe charting with mostly 2–3 mm and 4 mm mesial of several molars with bleeding where the subgingival calculus was found. Treatment plan for check on personal care procedures; scaling and root debridement. Patient asked about advice on bleaching which was discussed, especially to wait until she quit smoking. She will decide after the appointments for dental hygiene therapy. Appointment made in 2 weeks.

Signed: _____, RDH Date: _____.

Factors To Teach The Patient

- The significance of dental biofilm to periodontal infection.
- The nature, occurrence, and etiology of calculus; its role as a biofilm reservoir.
- The importance of and necessity for complete removal of calculus to the health of the oral tissues in the prevention of periodontal infections.
- Basic reasons for need and the advantages of multiple appointments to complete the scaling and root planing.
- The rationale for follow up evaluation following the completion of scaling and root planing.
- Relationship of personal oral self-care measures to accumulation/maturation of dental biofilm.
- The importance of the patient's role in maintenance of therapeutic gains.
- The limits of what can be accomplished nonsurgically and the rationale for referral to a specialist.
- The rationale for combining manual instrumentation with ultrasonic instrumentation.
- The harmful effects of overhanging margins: producing a niche for biofilm that cannot be cleansed, contributing to gingival disease and caries, and the necessity of overhang removal.

References

1. Nakib NM, Bissada NF, Simmelink JW, Goldstine SN. Endotoxin penetration into root cementum of periodontally healthy and diseased human teeth. *J Periodontol.* 1982 Jun;53(6):368–78.
2. Moore J, Wilson M, Kieser JB. The distribution of bacterial lipopolysaccharide (endotoxin) in relation to periodontally involved root surfaces. *J Clin Periodontol.* 1986 Sep;13(8):748–51.
3. Smart GJ, Wilson M, Davies EH, Kieser JB. The assessment of ultrasonic root surface debridement by determination of residual endotoxin levels. *J Clin Periodontol.* 1990 Mar;17(3):174–8.
4. Chiew SY, Wilson M, Davies EH, Kieser JB. Assessment of ultrasonic debridement of calculus-associated periodontally-involved root surfaces by the limulus amoebocyte lysate assay: An in vitro study. *J Clin Periodontol.* 1991 Apr;18(4):240–4.
5. Nyman S, Westfelt E, Sarhed G, Karring T. Role of "diseased" root cementum in healing following treatment of periodontal disease: A clinical study. *J Clin Periodontol.* 1988 Aug;15(7):464–8.
6. Corbet EF, Vaughan AJ, Kieser JB. The periodontally involved root surface. *J Clin Periodontol.* 1993 Jul;20(6):402–10.
7. Quirynen M, Bollen CM. The influence of surface roughness and surface-free energy on supra- and subgingival plaque formation in man: A review of the literature. *J Clin Periodontol.* 1995 Jan;22(1):1–14.

8. Leknes KN. The influence of anatomic and iatrogenic root surface characteristics on bacterial colonization and periodontal destruction: A review. *J Periodontol.* 1997 Jun;68(6):507–16.

9. Vandekerckhove BN, Bollen CM, Dekeyser C, Darius P, Quirynen M. Full- versus partial-mouth disinfection in the treatment of periodontal infections. Long-term clinical observations of a pilot study. *J Periodontol.* 1996 Dec;67(12):1251–9.

10. Mongardini C, van Steenberghe D, Dekeyser C, Quirynen M. One stage full- versus partial-mouth disinfection in the treatment of chronic adult or generalized early-onset periodontitis. I. Long-term clinical observations. *J Periodontol.* 1999 Jun;70(6):632–45.

11. Quirynen M, Mongardini C, DeSoete M, Pauwels M, Coucke W, van Eldere J, van Steenberghe D. The role of chlorhexidine in the one-stage full-mouth disinfection treatment of patients with advanced adult periodontitis. Long-term clinical and microbiological observations. *J Clin Periodontol.* 2000 Aug;27(8):578–89.

12. Greenstein G. Full-mouth therapy versus individual quadrant root planing: A critical commentary. *J Periodontol.* 2002 Jul;73(7):797–812.

13. Perry DA, Taggart EJ. Occurrence rate of acute periodontal abscess following scaling procedures. *J Dent Res.* 1997;76(Spec 2569):335.

14. Bender IB, Naidorf IJ, Garvey GJ. Bacterial endocarditis: a consideration for physician and dentist. *J Am Dent Assoc.* 1984 Sep;109(3):415–20.

15. Pallasch TJ, Slots J. Antibiotic prophylaxis and the medically compromised patient. *Periodontol. 2000.* 1996;10:107.

16. Ramfjord SP, Caffesse RG, Morrison EC, Hill RW, Kerry GJ, Appleberry EA, Nissle RR, Stults DL. Four modalities of periodontal treatment compared over five years. *J Periodontal Res.* 1987 May;22(3):222–3.

17. Badersten A, Nilvéus R, Egelberg J. Effect of nonsurgical periodontal therapy. I. Moderately advanced periodontitis. *J Clin Periodontol.* 1981 Fab;8(1):57–72.

18. Lindhe J, Nyman S, Karring T. Scaling and root planing in shallow pockets. *J Clin Periodontol.* 1982 Sep;9(5):415–8.

19. Glickman I. *Clinical periodontology.* 4th ed. Philadelphia: Saunders; 1972. 625 p.

20. Oosterwaal PJ, Matee MI, Mikx FH, van't Hof MA, Renggli HH. The effect of subgingival debridement with hand and ultrasonic instruments on the subgingival microflora. *J Clin Periodontol.* 1987 Oct;14(9):528–33.

21. Badersten A, Nilvéus R, Egelberg J. Effect of nonsurgical periodontal therapy. II. Severely advanced periodontitis. *J Clin Periodontol.* 1984 Jan;11(1):63–76.

22. Walmsley AD, Laird WR, Williams AR. A model system to demonstrate the role of cavitational activity in ultrasonic scaling. *J Dent Res.* 1984 Sep;63(9):1162–5.

23. Baehni P, Thilo B, Chapuis B, Pernet D. Effects of ultrasonic and sonic scalers on dental plaque microflora in vitro and in vivo. *J Clin Periodontol.* 1992 Aug;19(7):455–9.

24. Walmsley AD, Walsh TF, Laird WR, Williams AR. Effects of cavitational activity on the root surface of teeth during ultrasonic scaling. *J Clin Periodontol.* 1990 May;17(5):306–12.

25. Nosal G, Scheidt MJ, O'Neal R, Van Dyke TE. The penetration of lavage solution into the periodontal pocket during ultrasonic instrumentation. *J Periodontol.* 1991 Sep;62(9):554–7.

26. McInnes C, Engel D, Martin RW. Fimbria damage and removal of adherent bacteria after exposure to acoustic energy. *Oral Microbiol Immunol.* 1993 Oct;8(5): 277–82.

27. McInnes C, Engel D, Moncla BJ, Martin RW. Reduction in adherence of Actinomyces viscosus after exposure to low-frequency acoustic energy. *Oral Microbiol Immunol.* 1992 Jun;7(3):171–6.

28. Copulos TA, Low SB, Walker CB, Trebilcock YY, Hefti AF. Comparative analysis between a modified ultrasonic tip and hand instruments on clinical parameters of periodontal disease. *J Periodontol.* 1993 Aug;64(8):694–700.

29. Takacs VJ, Lie T, Perala DG, Adams DF. Efficacy of 5 machining instruments in scaling of molar furcations. *J Periodontol.* 1993 Mar;64(3):228–36.

30. Leon LE, Vogel RI. A comparison of the effectiveness of hand scaling and ultrasonic debridement in furcations as evaluated by differential dark-field microscopy. *J Periodontol.* 1987 Feb;58(2):86–94.

31. Suzuki JB, Delisle AL. Pulmonary actinomycosis of periodontal origin. *J Periodontol.* 1984 Oct;55(10):581–4.

32. Lee SY, Lai YL, Morgano SM. Effects of ultrasonic scaling and periodontal curettage on surface roughness of porcelain. *J Prosthet Dent.* 1995 Mar;73(3):227–32.

33. Vermilyea SG, Prasanna MK, Agar JR. Effect of ultrasonic cleaning and air polishing on porcelain labial margin restorations. *J Prosthet Dent.* 1994 May;71(5):447–52.

34. Rajstein J, Tal M. The effects of ultrasonic scaling on the surface of Class V amalgam restorations—a scanning electron microscopy study. *J Oral Rehabil.* 1984 May;11(3):299–305.

35. Sivers JE, Johnson GK. Comparison of effects of ultrasonic and sonic instrumentation on amalgam restorations. *Gen Dent.* 1989 Mar–Apr;37(2):130–2.

36. Bjornson EJ, Collins DE, Engler WO. Surface alteration of composite resins after curette, ultrasonic, and sonic instrumentation: an in vitro study. *Quintessence Int.* 1990 May;21(5):381–9.

37. Gantes BG, Nilvéus R. The effects of different hygiene instruments on titanium surfaces: SEM observations. *Int J Periodontics Restorative Dent.* 1991;11(3):225–39.

38. Rapley JW, Swan RH, Hallmon WW, Mills MP. The surface characteristics produced by various oral hygiene instruments and materials on titanium implant abutments. *Int J Oral Maxillofac Implants.* 1990 Spring;5(1):47–52.

39. White DJ, Cox ER, Arends J, Nieborg JH, Leydsman H, Wieringa DW, Dijkman AG, Ruben JR. Instruments and methods for the quantitative measurement of factors affecting hygienist/dentist efforts during scaling and root planing of the teeth. *J Clin Dent.* 1996;7(Spec 2):32–40.

40. Liskiewicz ST, Kerschbaum WE. Cumulative trauma disorders: an ergonomic approach for prevention. *J Dent Hyg.* 1997 Summer;71(4):162–7.

41. Bohay RN, Bencak J, Kavaliers M, MacLean D. A survey of magnetic fields in the dental operatory. *J Can Dent Assoc.* 1994 Sep; 60(9):835–40.

42. Abrams H, Barkmeier WW, Cooley RL. Temperature changes in the pulp chamber produced by ultrasonic instrumentation. *Gen Dent.* 1979 Sep–Oct;27(5):62–4.

43. Möller P, Grevstad AO, Kristoffersen T. Ultrasonic scaling of maxillary teeth causing tinnitus and temporary hearing shifts. *J Clin Periodontol.* 1976 May;3(2):123–7.

44. Gantes BG, Nilvéus R, Lie T, Leknes KN. The effect of hygiene instruments on dentin surfaces: scanning electron microscopic observations. *J Periodontol.* 1992 Mar;63(3):151–7.

45. Barbeau J, Tanguay R, Faucher E, Avezard C, Trudel L, Cote L, Prevost AP. Multiparametric analysis of waterline contamination in dental units. *Appl Environ Microbiol.* 1996 Nov;62(11):3954–9.

46. Harrel SK, Barnes JB, Rivera-Hidalgo F. Reduction of aerosols produced by ultrasonic scalers. *J Periodontol.* 1996 Jan;67(1): 28–32.

47. King TB, Muzzin KB, Berry CW, Anders LM. The effectiveness of an aerosol reduction device for ultrasonic scalers. *J Periodontol.* 1997 Jan;68(1):45–9.

48. Reynolds MA, Lavigne CK, Minah GE, Suzuki JB. Clinical effects of simultaneous ultrasonic scaling and subgingival irrigation with chlorhexidine. Mediating influence of periodontal probing depth. *J Clin Periodontol.* 1992 Sep;19(8):595–600.

49. Taggart JA, Palmer RM, Wilson RF. A clinical and microbiological comparison of the effects of water and 0.02% chlorhexidine as coolants during ultrasonic scaling and root planing. *J Clin Periodontol.* 1990 Jan;17(1):32–7.

50. Bandt CL, Korn NA, Schaffer EM. Bacteremias from ultrasonic and hand instrumentation. *J Periodontol.* 1964 May–Jun;35:214.

51. Legnani P, Checchi L, Pelliccioni GA, D'Achille C. Atmospheric contamination during dental procedures. *Quintessence Int.* 1994 Jun; 25(6):435–9.

52. Fine DH, Mendieta C, Barnett ML, Furgang D, Meyers R, Olshan A, Vincent J. Efficacy of preprocedural rinsing with an antiseptic in reducing viable bacteria in dental aerosols. *J Periodontol.* 1992 Oct;63(10):821–4.

53. Gilmore N, Sheiham A. Overhanging dental restorations and periodontal disease. *J Periodontol.* 1971 Jan;42(1):8–12.

54. Highfield JE, Powell RN. Effects of removal of posterior overhanging metallic margins of restorations upon the periodontal tissues. *J Clin Periodontol.* 1978 Aug;5(3):169–81.

55. Pack AR, Coxhead LJ, McDonald BW. The prevalence of overhanging margins in posterior amalgam restorations and periodontal consequences. *J Clin Periodontol.* 1990 Mar;17(3):145–52.

56. Jeffcoat MK, Howell TH. Alveolar bone destruction due to overhanging amalgam in periodontal disease. *J Periodontol.* 1980 Oct; 51(10):599–602.

57. Rodriguez-Ferrer HJ, Strahan JD, Newman HN. Effect on gingival health of removing overhanging margins of interproximal subgingival amalgam restorations. *J Clin Periodontol.* 1980 Dec;7(6):457–62.

58. Preber H, Bergström J. The effect of non-surgical treatment on periodontal pockets in smokers and non-smokers. *J Clin Periodontol.* 1986 Apr;13(4):319–23.

59. Listgarten MA, Helldén L. Relative distribution of bacteria at clinically healthy and periodontally diseased sites in humans. *J Clin Periodontol.* 1978 May;5(2):115–32.

60. Slots J, Mashimo P, Levine MJ, Genco RJ. Periodontal therapy in humans. I. Microbiological and clinical effects of a single course of periodontal scaling and root planing, and of adjunctive tetracycline therapy. *J Periodontol.* 1979 Oct;50(10):495–509.

61. Mousqués T, Listgarten MA, Phillips RW. Effects of scaling and root planing on the composition of the human subgingival microbial flora. *J Periodontal Res.* 1980 Mar;15(2):144–51.

62. Aleo JJ, De Renzis FA, Farber PA, Varboncoeur AP. The presence and biologic activity of cementum-bound endotoxin. *J Periodontol.* 1974 Sep;45(9):672–5.

63. Schwartz M. The prevention and management of the broken curet. *Compend Contin Educ Dent.* 1998 Apr;19(4):418–20, 422, 424–5.

CHAPTER 40

Nonsurgical Periodontal Therapy: Supplemental Care Procedures

STACY A. MATSUDA, RDH, BS, MS
ESTHER WILKINS, BS, RDH, DMD

Chapter Outline

NONSURGICAL PERIODONTAL THERAPY

Two essential components of successful therapy are complete subgingival scaling with root debridement by the dental hygienist and effective daily dental biofilm control by the patient. The objective is to eliminate or at least suppress the pathologic microorganisms in the subgingival area to promote healing and hence control the infection.

■ Other components of nonsurgical therapy include activities to supplement care of the major treatment.
■ Supplemental care procedures are selected in accord with the special needs of each patient.

■ The need, the procedures, and the expected outcomes are carefully explained to the patient.
■ The patient learns to accept responsibility and to understand that periodontal disease can be managed, not cured.
■ The success of all periodontal therapy depends on the patient's adherence to periodic professional maintenance appointments and daily personal biofilm control.
■ In this chapter, rationale is described for instrumentation to treat advanced periodontal disease, professional irrigation, and local delivery of antimicrobials.
■ Box 40-1 defines key words and related terminology.

BOX 40-1	Key Words

Nonsurgical Periodontal Therapy

Antibiotic: a form of antimicrobial agent produced by or obtained from microorganisms that can kill other microorganisms or inhibit their growth; may be specific for certain organisms or may cover a broad spectrum.

Antimicrobial therapy: use of specific chemical or pharmaceutical agents for the control or destruction of microorganisms, either systemically or at specific sites.

Attachment: with reference to the *clinical attachment level,* which is the position of the periodontal attached tissue at the base of a sulcus or pocket as measured from a fixed point.

> **New attachment:** the union of connective tissue or epithelium with a root surface that has been deprived of its original attachment apparatus; the new attachment may be epithelial adhesion and/or connective tissue adaptation or attachment, and it may include new cementum.

> **Reattachment:** the reunion of epithelial and connective tissues with root surfaces and bone occurs after an incision or injury.

Bioabsorbable: available for absorption by the body.

Biodegradable: susceptible of degradation by biological processes, as by bacterial or other enzymatic action.

Cannula: tubular instrument placed in a cavity to introduce or withdraw fluid.

Chemotherapy: treatment by means of chemical or pharmaceutical agents.

Controlled release: local delivery of a chemotherapeutic agent to a site-specific area; may be a patch to be worn on the skin or a polymeric fiber, such as that used to deliver an agent to a periodontal pocket.

Endoscopy: a minimally invasive diagnostic procedure used in medicine to examine inaccessible tissues by inserting a fiber-optic tube into the body.

Infection: invasion and multiplication of microorganisms in body tissues.

> **Endogenous infection:** caused by microorganisms that are part of the normal microbiota of the skin, nose, mouth, and intestinal and urogenital tracts.

> **Exogenous infection:** caused by organisms acquired from outside the oral cavity or the host.

> **Opportunistic infection:** occurs in a systemically or locally impaired host; opportunistic pathogens may not be highly virulent, but they can cause disease when the host defense is altered.

Open scaling and root planing: instrumentation performed after the area has been exposed by tissue removal or the tissue is separated and laid back as a flap; visibility and accessibility allow more thorough treatment.

PARQ (Procedures, Alternatives, Risks/benefits, and Questions): used to explain therapies planned that address the patient's problem(s), to answer all questions and obtain their consent.

Refractory: not responding to usual treatment.

I. PATIENT NEEDS

A. Patient With Uncomplicated Gingivitis

- Complete scaling.
- Patient compliance in personal daily biofilm removal.
- Effect: can bring about a reversal of inflammation, and health can be maintained.

B. Patient With Early Periodontitis

- Control of infection may be attained through nonsurgical periodontal therapy.
- Maintaining the healthy state requires continuing routine appointments for professional scaling and supervision of the patient's biofilm removal methods.

C. Patients With Moderate to Advanced Periodontal Conditions, or Patients With Poor Response to Routine Therapy

- Supplemental therapeutic measures may be needed.
- Specialized instruments may be required for deep pockets, furcations, and complex anatomical features of involved diseased root surfaces.

D. Patients That Require Surgical or Other Advanced Periodontal Therapy

- Certain periodontal conditions of patients of all degrees of disease severity will require surgical or other advanced therapeutic procedures.
- For these patients, complete periodontal scaling and root planing (root preparation) prepare the tissues for the added treatment.
- Examples:
  1. *Mucogingival defects:* periodontal plastic surgery.
  2. *Exposed root surfaces:* connective tissue grafting; free gingival grafting.
  3. *Crown lengthening:* functional, restorative, or esthetic.
  4. *Regenerative procedures:* bone grafting.

II. SUPPLEMENTAL CARE PROCEDURES

- Pharmacologic agents as an adjunct to mechanical therapy.
- Supplemental patient care described in other chapters of this book includes:
  - Smoking cessation assistance.
  - Desensitization of teeth.

- At-home rinsing, irrigation, other selective use of antimicrobials, and fluorides (dentifrice, water fluoridation).
- Care for dental implants and prostheses.
- Dental caries prevention: fluoride applications and other preventive measures, especially for root caries prevention for the patient with periodontal recession.
- Correction of biofilm-retaining irregularities; overhang removal when not included in the routine tooth preparation procedures.
- Dietary analysis for all special needs.
- Personal counseling for patients with systemic conditions for which periodontal infection is a risk factor (pregnancy, cardiovascular disease, diabetes).

ADVANCED INSTRUMENTATION

Definitive root debridement strategies that address advanced stages of disease include:

- Specialized debridement instruments.
- Selection and sequence of instruments.
- Definitive debridement of furcations.
- Endoscopic root preparation.

I. SPECIALIZED DEBRIDEMENT INSTRUMENTS

- Clinical attachment loss of 4–6 mm and greater exposes contours of the root that complicate nonsurgical instrumentation.
- Longitudinal grooves, proximal depressions, and concavities and convexities of root morphology make comprehensive debridement covering every square millimeter of tooth surface difficult to accomplish.
- Examples of instruments for problem areas:
  - Mini-bladed area-specific curets.
  - Periodontal files.
  - Diamond-coated files.
  - Precision-thin ultrasonic tips/inserts.

II. SELECTION AND SEQUENCE OF INSTRUMENTS

A. The order in which instruments are selected and used can have an effect on the efficiency and quality of final product, similar to the woodworking process. Heavy coarse grit sanders are always used prior to finer grain tools in order to achieve a uniformly smooth surface.

B. Instrument selection sequence is recommended as follows, in this specific order:
  1. Standard ultrasonic tips/inserts used on moderate to high power.
  2. Sickle scalers and/or periodontal files.
  3. Universal curets.
  4. Gracey curets.
  5. Mini-bladed area-specific and/or Gracey curets.

  6. Micro-mini-bladed Gracey curets.
  7. Diamond files—*used with light pressure only.*
  8. Precision-thin ultrasonic tips/inserts for final finishing.

III. DEFINITIVE DEBRIDEMENT OF FURCATIONS

The complex morphology of a furcation necessitates meticulous care during root preparation. Skillful use of specialized instruments designed for use in furcations can enhance treatment outcomes.

Essential components of furcation debridement include:

A. Optimum blade sharpness and contour.
B. Instrumentation sequence observed.
C. Instrumentation fundamentals observed:
  1. Close adaptation of blade and/or tip/insert to the root surfaces.
  2. Confined, precision movement of blade and/or tip/insert.
D. Use of specialized instruments:
  1. Mini-bladed hoes and furcation curets: *specialized semi-lunar blades—use with light pressure.*
  2. Mini-bladed Gracey numbers 5–6, 11–12, 13–14.
  3. Micro-mini-bladed Gracey numbers 1–2, 11–12, 13–14.
  4. Diamond files: *use with light pressure only.*
E. Precision-thin ultrasonic tips/inserts: *use at low power for final finishing.*
F. Definitive assessment following instrumentation:
  1. Use specific periodontal explorer with lightest pressure to assess root texture for uniform smoothness.
  2. Examples:
    - TU-17 explorer shown in Figure 15-13 (page 229).
    - Extended 3A explorer shown in Figure 15-12 (page 229).

IV. ENDOSCOPIC ROOT PREPARATION

The dental endoscope is a device developed to visualize below the gingival margin for use during diagnosis and instrumentation for treatment of periodontally diseased root surfaces.

A. Objectives

- Visualization of the root surface during instrumentation.
- Explore, instrument, and evaluate the root surface using indirect visual observation on the device monitor.
- Increase the effectiveness and thoroughness of root debridement.[1,2]
- Augment subjective data collection with objective confirmation.

B. Description

- **Subgingival probe:** adapted to provide fiber-optic imaging with magnification of 24×–48×.

- **Sheath** to provide a sterile barrier between the patient and the endoscope.
- **Peristaltic pump** to provide irrigation to the working field.
- **Lamp** to provide illumination to the working field.
- **Video camera** to capture images of the working field for display.
- **Video monitor** for live viewing of the working field.
- **Specialized probes, curets,** and **retracting instruments** to maximize tissue visualization.

C. Indications for Use

- During maintenance to detect and remove remaining deep burnished calculus deposits, which are the cause of continued bleeding on probing.
- Advanced root therapy for patients unable or unwilling to have recommended surgical procedures.

D. Advantages

1. *Quality of end product*—Enhance the quality of instrumentation by providing an objective means of evaluating root surface.
2. *Tactile sensitivity*—Over a period of time, instill a greater tactile sense in the clinician, improving subjective evaluation skill.
3. *Patient education*—Create a new means of engaging, motivating, and educating the patient in the treatment.
4. Provide opportunity for noninvasive, definitive root therapy:
   - When access is limited during routine instrumentation.
   - For sites unresponsive to traditional nonsurgical therapy.
   - In anterior regions where preservation of soft tissue is necessary for optimum esthetics.
   - When surgical therapy may be contraindicated for the patient.
5. Provide confirmation of clinical findings that might otherwise go undiagnosed or require surgical intervention.
   - Root fractures.
   - Restorative post perforations.
   - Open margins.
   - Subgingival caries.
   - Residual cement.
   - Anatomical anomalies.

E. Disadvantage

- *Learning curve:* Using the endoscope to visualize root accretions is of significant benefit, but a level of proficiency with advanced instrumentation must still be developed to remove all deposits completely.

ANTIMICROBIAL TREATMENT

I. OBJECTIVES OF ANTIMICROBIAL THERAPY

- By arresting the infection using antimicrobial drugs, further loss of periodontal attachment and other periodontal tissue destruction caused by microorganisms can be prevented.
- Treatment using antimicrobials aims to suppress and eliminate pathogenic microorganisms to allow the recolonization of the microbiota that are compatible with health.

II. TYPES OF DELIVERY OF ANTIMICROBIALS

A. Systemic Administration

Systemic administration of antibiotics is well known and highly successful in the world of medical care. Antibiotics have saved the lives of many people with generalized infectious diseases.

B. Local Delivery

The knowledge that periodontal diseases are site-specific infections has led to the development of methods for placing antimicrobials directly at the site of the infection—the pocket (see **Table 40-1** for examples). Irrigation and controlled-release methods will be described.

SYSTEMIC DELIVERY OF ANTIBIOTICS

I. ACTION OF SYSTEMICALLY ADMINISTERED ANTIBIOTIC

- In contrast to locally applied agents placed directly into a pocket, antibiotics administered systemically reach the pathogenic organisms in the pocket through the circulation.
- The antibiotic is absorbed into the circulation from the intestine. From the bloodstream, the drug is passed into the body tissues.
- The antibiotic enters the periodontal tissues and passes into the pocket by way of the gingival sulcus fluid.
- The systemically administered drug is in a diluted form by the time it reaches the pathogenic microorganisms, where the destruction is taking place.

II. SELECTION OF ANTIBIOTIC

- Ideally, the specific microorganism that is causing a certain periodontal disease needs to be determined, and the antibiotic that is selected needs to be specific for that organism.[3]
- Microbiological testing is available and can be used to guide clinical decisions.

TABLE 40-1	LOCAL DELIVERY ANTIBIOTICS		
	ARESTIN	**ATRIDOX**	**PERIOCHIP**
Active Ingredient	Minocycline HCl (1 mg)	Doxycycline hyclate (10%)	Chlorhexidine Gluconate (2.5 mg)
Method of Delivery	Unit-dose cartridge inserts into cartridge handle.	Doxycycline hyclate (10%); single use syringe suspended in 450 mg of ATRIGEL [poly(DL-Lactide): NMP].	Gelatin chip is inserted into dried tissue using standard cotton forceps.
Mechanism of Action	Exerts antimicrobial activity by inhibiting protein synthesis in the bacterial cell wall that causes leakage and destroys the cell.	Subgingival controlled release; upon contact with crevicular fluid, the liquid product solidifies and then permits controlled release for a period of 7 days.	Bactericidal: chlorhexidine reacts with microbial cell surface, destroying cell membrane integrity, penetrating the cell to precipitate cytoplasm, after which the cell dies.
Indications	As an adjunctive therapy to scaling and root planing for reduction of pocket depth and bleeding on probing in patients with adult periodontitis.	For use in the treatment of chronic adult periodontitis for reduction in probing depth, reduction in bleeding on probing, and a gain in clinical attachment.	As an adjunct to scaling and root planing for reduction of pocket depth in patients with adult periodontitis.
Contraindications	Sensitivity to minocycline and/or tetracycline; children; pregnant or nursing women.	Sensitivity to doxycycline or any of the tetracycline class.	Sensitivity to chlorhexidine.

- An example of specific treatment in current practice is the use of tetracyclines in combination with mechanical debridement to treat *Aggregatibacter actinomycetemcomitans* in aggressive periodontitis.[4]
- Periodontal diseases are caused by mixed infections of microorganisms. The pathogens tend to work in clusters, that is, in combination with other organisms.
- Selective identification of specific organisms that match with specific antibiotics has been accomplished to a limited degree.

III. LIMITATIONS

- The precautions and adverse effects, as well as the acquisition of antibiotic resistance by the organisms, preclude the widespread use of systemic antibiotics for periodontal problems.
- Limitations include the following:
  - Side effects of certain antibiotics.
  - Potential for the development of resistant strains.
  - Local concentration diluted by the time the drug reaches the pathogens; drug is "wasted" in that it covers a large area not needing the treatment.
  - Superimposed infection can develop, such as candidiasis.
  - Low compliance of the patient in following the prescription for the required number of days.

IV. USE OF SYSTEMIC THERAPY

- Most periodontal infection does not require systemic therapy except when there is systemic involvement shown by generalized symptoms such as lymphadenopathy and fever.
- Examples of acute inflammatory conditions characterized by pain or discomfort and infection that may call for systemic therapy include the following:
  - Necrotizing ulcerative gingivitis.
  - Necrotizing ulcerative periodontitis.
  - Periodontal abscess formation.
  - Pericoronal abscess formation (pericoronitis).
  - Combined periodontal/endodontic lesions (abscesses).

Treatment using systemic antibiotics is a selective procedure.[5]

PROFESSIONAL SUBGINGIVAL IRRIGATION

- Professional subgingival irrigation used in conjunction with periodontal instrumentation is an adjunctive treatment targeting pathogens remaining in the subgingival environment.
- Therapy is based on the premise that delivery of antimicrobial agents may enhance the effects of treatment by scaling and root planing.

■ Irrigation into a pocket can reduce the numbers of microorganisms left behind following instrumentation.
■ Studies have shown that repopulation of the subgingival microflora can occur within weeks after treatment.[6]
■ Overall reduction of subgingival flora depends on the ability of the clinician to remove subgingival biofilm and calculus definitively. Total removal is difficult in deep pockets and areas of complex root morphology.
■ Irrigation with an antimicrobial agent provides a supplemental therapeutic step that may result in additional clinical benefits.[7]
■ Used in conjunction with definitive scaling and root planing in moderate to advanced case types, irrigation has been shown to facilitate posttreatment healing.

I. DELIVERY METHOD

A presterilized disposable cannula, with a side port, multiple side ports, or end release **(Figure 40-1A)**, is used with one of the following:

■ Disposable hand syringe.
■ Specially designed jet irrigator.
■ Air-driven irrigation handpiece.

II. PROCEDURE

■ Prepare the cannula by bending it slightly as it is uncovered **(Figure 40-1B)**.
■ Insert the cannula subgingivally **(Figure 40-1C)**.
■ Allow the irrigant to fill the pocket.
■ Apply circumferentially, releasing solution at three points on the facial surface and three on the lingual surface.
■ Irrigate all teeth, quadrants, or specific selected sites as dictated by the patient's need.

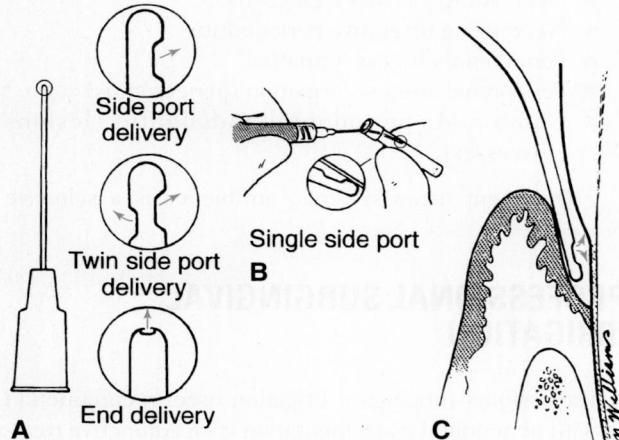

FIGURE 40-1 **Professional Irrigation. (A)** Types of cannula tips with side-port or end-delivery openings. **(B)** Prepare the cannula for use by bending the sterile tip within the encasement to make the insertion easier. **(C)** With knowledge of each probing depth, insert the cannula gently to near the bottom of a pocket. No force should be used.

III. RECOMMENDATIONS FOR USE

A. Preprocedural Delivery

An antimicrobial agent can aid in reducing the numbers of microorganisms to prevent aerosol contamination during instrumentation.

B. Initial Therapy: Postprocedure Irrigation

Periodontal microorganisms are killed with full-strength povidone–iodine or equal parts povidone–iodine and water retained in subgingival sites for at least 5 minutes.[8,9] Moderate to advanced case types being scaled and root planed by sextant or quadrant can be treated with an antimicrobial wash of 10% povidone–iodine to facilitate more rapid healing and minimize postoperative discomfort.

■ Only a minimal amount of solution is needed.
■ Use an endo syringe to draw up a small amount of povidone–iodine.
■ Advance the tip at least 3 mm below the gingival margin and apply just a trickle of solution into the subgingival area of teeth (by sextant) once they are scaled to completion.[10]
■ Let solution remain in place undisturbed for 5 minutes, during which time the solution is reapplied. At the end of 5 minutes, the solution can be rinsed with suction.

C. Maintenance Phase: Postprocedure Irrigation

■ Patient with site(s) not responding to traditional periodontal care.
■ Patient with gingivitis superimposed on periodontitis.
■ Patient with areas inaccessible to mechanical instrumentation because of root contour, furcations, or depth of pocket when open scaling and root planing are not alternatives.

IV. ANTIMICROBIAL AGENTS

■ A variety of antimicrobial agents, saline solution, and water have been researched for professional irrigation with varying results.
■ Products used include chlorhexidine gluconate, povidone–iodine and water, essential oil mouth rinses, and stannous fluoride.[7,10–13]
■ Studies demonstrate professional subgingival irrigation using 10% povidone–iodine to have a positive effect in cases of severe chronic periodontitis and postprocedure healing of initial therapy.

V. SPECIAL CONSIDERATIONS

A. Antibiotic Premedication

■ Subgingival irrigation can produce a bacteremia. Professional irrigation requires premedication in patients susceptible to the effects of bacteremia.

■ When irrigation is selected as a specific form of treatment for a patient susceptible to bacterial endocarditis, the periodontal tissues are brought to health first. The usual procedure for all dental appointments is followed.

B. Irrigation Pressure

■ Professional irrigation systems usually control the amount of pressure.
■ Caution is exercised when irrigating with a disposable syringe because pressure may exceed the safety level for the oral tissues.

LOCAL DELIVERY OF ANTIMICROBIALS

The concept of a controlled local delivery for treatment of periodontal pathogens in a pocket infection was developed over many years by Goodson and coworkers[14] with the introduction of a subgingival tetracycline fiber. Improvements in probing depth, clinical attachment level, bleeding on probing,[15–17] and reduction of sites with periodontal pathogenic microorganisms[18] laid important groundwork for continuing research and development in local delivery agents.

■ Local delivery means that the medication used to treat the periodontal infection is concentrated at the site of the infection.
■ The infecting pathogenic microorganisms are located in the depths of the pockets and the surrounding tissue.
■ Although irrigation does deliver the medication to the pocket, its therapeutic benefit is temporary and limited because of the constant turnover and cleansing taking place in the pocket.
■ Controlled delivery refers to providing the medication over an extended period of time by being held in the pocket and released slowly.
■ Slow-release methods are used in a variety of ways. The nicotine patch, used to assist a person trying to break a smoking addiction, is an example.

I. REQUIREMENTS

A local delivery method can place high concentrations of the antimicrobial in an infected pocket. To be successful, the medication must[19]:

■ Be of a concentration that will act on the microorganisms causing the infection.
■ Reach all areas of the pocket to the very bottom and into furcations.
■ Stay in contact long enough in the effective concentration for the antimicrobial action to take place.
   A. *Comparison with systemic:* When systemic treatment is used, much less of the antimicrobial

medication reaches the actual site of the infection where the pathogens are concentrated because the agent becomes diluted as it passes through the system.

II. USES FOR SLOW-RELEASE LOCAL DELIVERY[20]

■ Local delivery devices have the potential to enhance therapy at sites unresponsive to conventional treatment.
■ Antimicrobials used in individual sites may be considered by the clinician according to their discretion and professional judgment.

A. At Initial Therapy

■ Periodontal diseases result from local infection with a pathogenic microflora.
■ The periodontal pocket is generally teeming with microorganisms and may also contain subgingival calculus, which further acts to harbor bacteria.
■ Scaling and root planing are highly effective procedures for controlling periodontal infections, reducing inflammation, and reducing probing depths.
■ The adjunctive use of local antimicrobials may enhance the effect of the mechanical instrumentation, particularly in areas of compromised access such as furcations and deep concavities. Research has shown that the adjunctive use of a controlled-release antimicrobial increases the effect of scaling and root planing.[21]

B. Adjunctive Treatment: At Reevaluation

■ For the minority of sites that do not respond to basic therapy and may be designated as refractory, chronic, or aggressive periodontitis, a local delivery method can be selected.
■ At the completion of initial periodontal therapy, a reevaluation is made at the first maintenance appointment.
   ▪ Areas that do not respond to additional scaling and root planing cannot be considered as treated to completion.
   ▪ Bleeding upon provocation is indicative of ulceration in pocket epithelial lining—a local infection calling for further definitive treatment.
■ Unless and until residual calculus is removed, the local infection will not resolve.
■ Local drug delivery treatment may be used as a temporary measure to limit further destruction until definitive therapy eliminating the source of infection can be rendered.

C. Recurrent Disease

1. Over time during the maintenance phase of therapy, pockets can recolonize.

2. Recurrence of periodontal infection usually occurs in localized pockets, particularly deep concavities and areas of complex root morphology where comprehensive debridement is most challenging.
   - Partially scaled, residual calculus that is burnished cannot be detected clinically and leads the clinician to assume that adequate instrumentation has been accomplished.
   - Burnished calculus becomes recolonized with pathogenic microbes soon after debridement, permitting the infection to sustain following an initial, partial improvement.
3. Infection recurrence was historically attributed to the patient's lack of diligence in their home oral self-care measures to remove dental biofilm on a daily basis. However, endoscopic imaging has provided visual confirmation that chronic, recurring periodontal infection is associated with burnished calculus left on the root.
4. Bleeding upon provocation may be barely discernible, presenting as pinpoint emergence well after insertion of the probe.
5. The slightest bleeding signifies residual burnished calculus from insufficient instrumentation, a condition beyond the patient's control and unrelated to effectiveness or diligence at home with oral self-care.

D. Peri-implantitis

The ailing or failing implant may respond to a localized slow-release antimicrobial.[22–24]

E. Periodontal Abscess

- After incision and drainage has been established, a locally delivered, sustained-release antimicrobial may aid the healing process.

F. Preparation for Periodontal Surgery

- Preconditioning the tissue and lessening the severity of the infection can contribute to less bleeding during surgery and smoother, more rapid healing.

III. TYPES OF LOCAL DELIVERY AGENTS

- Available for treatment of periodontal infections are bioabsorbable polymers, minocycline and doxycycline, and a chlorhexidine chip.
- Subgingival drug therapy can be applied as a supplement or adjunctive procedure after meticulous scaling and root debridement has been completed and the results evaluated.
- For all products, the manufacturer's advice and directions are followed.

MINOCYCLINE HYDROCHLORIDE

Bioresorbable minocycline hydrochloride is delivered in powdered microsphere form to be placed in periodontal pockets to aid in pocket depth reduction.[25] The treatment is used in conjunction with scaling and root planing.

I. DESCRIPTION

- Unit dose cartridge contains 1 mg minocycline in a gel carrier.
- Sustained release 14 days.
- Refrigeration not needed.
- Does not block the flow of subgingival fluid.
- Contraindications:
  - Patients sensitive to tetracycline.
  - Women who are pregnant.

II. ADMINISTRATION

A. Site Selection

- Use as an adjunct to scaling and root planing.
- Probing depth of at least 5 mm.

B. Cartridge Loading

- Insert unit cartridge into dispenser handle.
- Exert slight pressure.
- Twist cartridge until it snaps securely into place.

C. Tip Preparation

1. Cartridge tip can be manipulated to reposition the angle for difficult-to-reach areas.
2. Leave cap covering the cartridge in place prior to manipulating the angle to prevent agent from being inadvertently expelled.
3. Tip opening can be narrowed for ease of subgingival insertion if needed.
   - Remove cap.
   - Using the end of a mirror handle, gently compress the last millimeter of the tip.

D. Delivery of Agent

1. Place cartridge tip into the site selected for treatment.
2. Keep tip parallel to the long axis of the tooth as it enters the periodontal pocket **(Figure 40-2)**.
3. Do not force the tip down to the base of the pocket.
4. Gently press thumb ring of handle to express the agent while withdrawing cartridge tip away from the base of the pocket.
5. With delivery complete, retract thumb ring and remove cartridge with free hand.
   - Discard contaminated cartridge.
   - Sterilize handle prior to reuse.

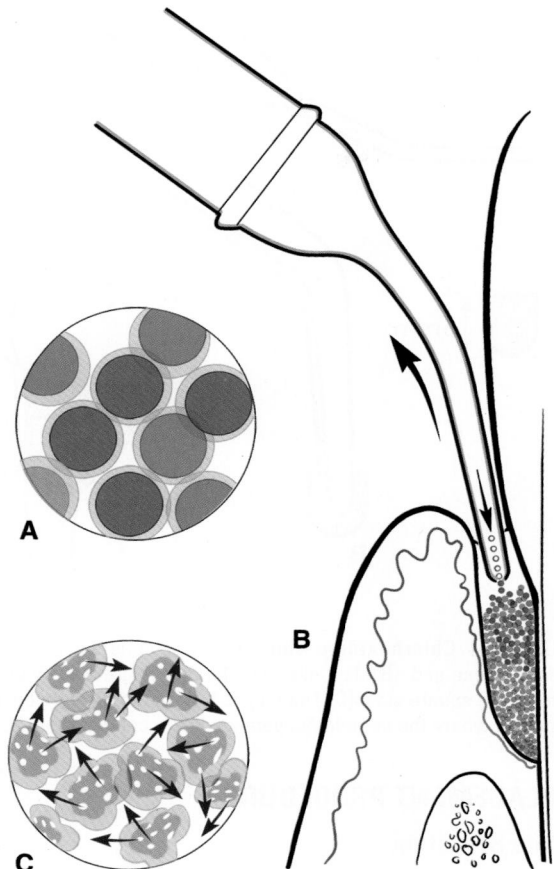

FIGURE 40.2 **Minocycline HCl. (A)** Minocycline microspheres intact within cannula, prior to application. **(B)** Deposition: cannula is withdrawn from periodontal pocket as plunger is depressed. **(C)** Once deposited, microspheres dissipate, releasing activated minocycline HCl into the subgingival space.

6. The bioadhesive microspheres activate and adhere on contact with moisture.
7. Caution patient to avoid disruption of activated material within pocket.

III. POSTTREATMENT INSTRUCTIONS

Instruct patient on proper care of treated areas. Give written guidelines to prevent misunderstanding.
1. Avoid touching treated area(s).
2. Wait at least 12 hours to use a toothbrush after treatment.
3. Do not use interdental cleaners or floss between teeth that have been treated for at least 10 days.
4. Avoid eating hard, crunchy, or sticky foods that could disturb retention of the product.
5. Schedule a follow-up appointment for continuing maintenance care.

IV. MAINTENANCE APPOINTMENTS

1. Probe carefully to evaluate treated area(s).
2. Reinforce home oral self-care measures and adherence to continuing care.

3. Repeat treatment as needed until definitive therapy removes source of infection.

DOXYCYCLINE POLYMER

Biodegradable doxycycline polymer in liquid form is delivered by cannula into a pocket and solidifies on contact with the dampness of the sulcus fluid. Beneficial effects include reduction of probing depths, gain of attachment, and destruction of periodontal pathogenic microorganisms.[26,27] However, gingival fluid flow is blocked at the site of application. Product literature mentions a 6% incidence rate of abscess formation.

I. DESCRIPTION

A. Equipment

1. *Syringe.* Containing liquid 10% doxycycline hyclate.
2. *Cannula.* Blunt ended, 23-gauge, narrow diameter.

B. Preparation of Agent

1. *Mixing.* Two syringes are coupled and the substances are passed back and forth until mixed **(Figure 40-3A)**. The manufacturer's instructions are followed with care.
2. *Adapt cannula.* Attach 23-gauge cannula to syringe. As the cap is removed, the cannula is held part way and

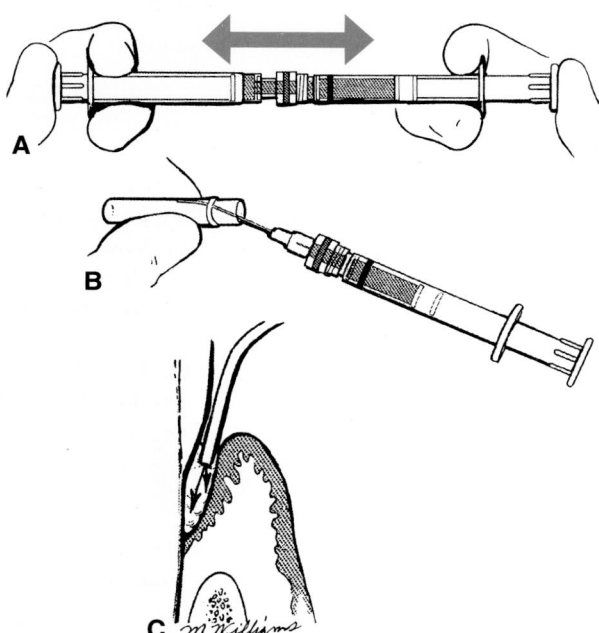

FIGURE 40-3 **Doxycycline Polymer Gel. (A)** Syringes are coupled and the contents passed back and forth until mixed. **(B)** The cannula is attached to the syringe with the agent; as the cap is removed, the cannula is pressed against the side to bend it to an angle appropriate for accessing the pocket to be treated. **(C)** The cannula is inserted to the base of the pocket, and the agent is released to fill the pocket.

bent against the wall of the cover to provide an angle appropriate for insertion into the periodontal pocket **(Figure 40-3B)**.

II. DELIVERY

A. Insert Cannula to Base of Pocket

Express the agent as the cannula is withdrawn to just over the gingival margin **(Figure 40-3C)**.

B. Packing

Use a blunt instrument to pack the agent down. Add more if necessary to fill the pocket. Wet the instrument to prevent sticking to the agent.

C. Hardening of Agent

On contact with the moisture of the pocket, the agent will harden.

D. Periodontal Dressing

Placing a dressing over the area aids retention.

E. Patient Instruction

- Prevent accidental removal.
- Routine brushing and other self-care on all other areas.

F. Appointment for Removal of Dressing

- Evaluate tissue; evaluate biofilm removal.
- Plan routine maintenance.

CHLORHEXIDINE CHIP

- The chlorhexidine chip is intended for use as an adjunctive therapy with scaling and root debridement.[28]
- Chlorhexidine as an agent for local delivery has the advantage over the antibiotics in that there is no potential for the development of bacterial resistance.
- As with doxycycline polymer, gingival fluid flow is blocked at the site of application. Product literature mentions a 6% incidence rate of abscess formation.

I. DESCRIPTION

1. *Size:* 4 by 5 mm and 0.35-mm thick **(Figure 40-4A)**.
2. *Shape:* rectangular, rounded at one end (resembling a baby's fingernail).
3. *Contents:* matrix of hydrolyzed gelatin with 2.5 mg chlorhexidine gluconate incorporated; color is orange-brown.
4. Controlled delivery; biodegradable; maintains a high level of chlorhexidine for 7 to 10 days. The gingival sulcus fluid concentration is greater than 125 µg/mL for 8 days.

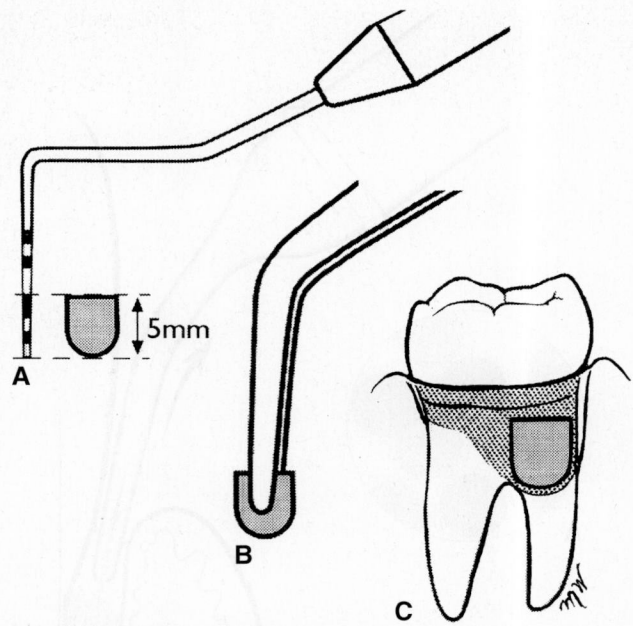

FIGURE 40-4 Chlorhexidine Chip. (A) The chip is 5 mm × 4 mm rounded at one end. **(B)** For insertion, the chip is grasped by cotton pliers on the square side. **(C)** The chip is inserted to the very base of the pocket where the periodontal pathogens are concentrated.

II. PLACEMENT PROCEDURE

A. Site Selection

1. *Pocket Depth.* The chip is contained within the pocket, so since the chip is 5-mm long, pockets of more than 5 mm are indicated for treatment.
2. *Chips Placed.* More than one pocket can be treated in the same appointment on the same side, preferably in the same quadrant for the comfort and convenience of the patient's postcare.

B. Chip Care and Preparation

1. Store product at controlled room temperature 15° to 25°C (59° to 77°F).
2. Packaged in cartons of 10 chips and 20 chips. Each chip is packaged individually in a separate compartment of an aluminum blister pack.

C. Steps in Placement

1. Isolation.
   - Position cotton rolls and saliva ejector.
   - Dry the area with a sponge to prevent wetting chip during placement. Chip may start to soften and become more difficult to place if it gets wet before placement in the pocket.
2. Insertion.
   - Hold chip with cotton pliers; position chip with round side away from the cotton pliers **(Figure 40-4B)**.
   - Insert the chip to the bottom of the pocket; position at the deepest part **(Figure 40-4C)**.

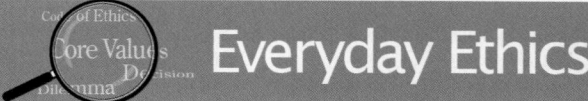

Everyday Ethics

At the first 3-month maintenance appointment for Mrs. Orban, who had had a series of six sextant appointments for deep scaling and root planing with anesthesia, the tissue still showed many areas of inflammation, with probing depths of more than 4 mm and bleeding on gentle probing. She had received repeated personal instructions on daily oral care at each of the appointments, and yet she never achieved a favorable score on her biofilm disclosing tests.

Gretchen, the dental hygienist, showed her new charting of probing and oral tissue review to Dr. Finley, and they both examined the original radiographs. Gretchen had made two vertical bitewings for the molar areas at this current appointment.

Gretchen told Dr. Finley that she thought the best procedure would be to refer Mrs. Orban to the periodontist. "I think she will take her periodontal infection more seriously. She never acts as though she believes what I tell her," Gretchen said. "She still talks as though she is here just to have her teeth 'cleaned,' as she calls it." Dr. Finley agreed to recommend the periodontist, and he personally explained the choice of treatment to the patient. Mrs. Orban definitely told them she was not going to a periodontist under any circumstance and asked for further treatment only from Dr. Finley.

Questions for Consideration

1. What ethical issues may be involved when a patient asks a general practitioner to take over treatment that needs referral to a periodontal specialist? Is this an ethical issue or dilemma? Explain the rationale.
2. How do the ethical core values (in Section II Introduction, Table II-1, page 38) have application in this scenario?
3. Use the steps for making a decision (page 10) to outline two or more plans for action that Gretchen and Dr. Finley can use in this difficult situation.

D. Action

1. Chip biodegrades in 7 to 10 days.
2. Approximately 40% of the chlorhexidine may be released within the first 24 hours, and the rest over the following 7 to 10 days.

E. Patient Instructions

1. Avoid disturbing the area. Do not use dental floss at the site of the insertion for 10 days.
2. Brush all other teeth and clean interdentally as usual.
3. Although some mild to moderate sensitivity may be expected during the first week after placement, contact the clinic or office promptly if pain, swelling, or other problem occurs.

F. Maintenance Appointments

1. Appoint patient for a periodontal maintenance appointment in 3 months.
2. Evaluate probing depth and clinical attachment levels.
3. Ascertain that patient is maintaining a high level of dental biofilm control.

DOCUMENTATION

Patients being treated for advanced and/or unresponsive periodontal disease have a minimum of the following documented in the permanent record:

■ Complete patient health history update, blood pressure, and patient's chief concern or complaint.
■ Findings of extraoral/intraoral examination and periodontal examination; status as compared to last appointment.

BOX 40-2	Example Progress Note

Sue L. came for 3-week follow-up after deep scaling and root planing by quadrant to check healing and determine need for further treatment. After preliminary brief health history review and blood pressure determination, tissue healing was evaluated and pocket examinations made. Periodontal probing was charted along with bleeding points. Exploring found a few areas of deep roughness accompanied by localized bleeding; Hirschfeld files were used to remove the localized calculus remaining as indicated by localized minor bleeding points, on D #14 and terminal distal #18, followed by mini curets. Decision to place minocycline HCl in deep furcation with 5–6 mm pocketing; obtained patient consent after PARQ. One cartridge Minocycline placed mid-facial and DL #14. Instructed patient in aftercare; patient to return in 4 weeks for tissue check and reprobe, and then in 3 months for continuing periodontal maintenance.

Signed: _____, RDH Date: _____.

■ Treatment planned/explained to patient and patient consent; treatment rendered.

■ Dispensation: instructions to patient and next treatment planned/time interval.

■ A sample progress note is included in **Box 40-2**.

Factors To Teach The Patient

■ What a periodontal pocket is and why it needs to be treated.

■ The success of all periodontal therapy depends on the daily personal dental biofilm control by the patient.

■ The necessity of removing all traces of subgingival deposits for reestablishing periodontal health.

■ The limitations of scaling and root planing (SRP) with regard to what can be accomplished nonsurgically.

■ The rationale for and importance of postcare evaluation following SRP.

■ The significance of residual bleeding upon probing post-treatment.

■ The rationale for chemotherapeutic agents used to control disease.

■ How to use the home irrigator; relation between home irrigation and professional irrigation in the dental office.

References

1. Geisinger ML, Mealey BL, Schoolfield J, Mellonig JT. The effectiveness of subgingival scaling and root planing: an evaluation of therapy with and without the use of the periodontal endoscope. *J Periodontol.* 2007 Jan;78(1):22–8.

2. Michaud RM, Schoolfield J, Mellonig JT, Mealey BL. The efficacy of subgingival calculus removal with endoscopy-aided scaling and root planing: a study on multirooted teeth. *J Periodontol.* 2007 Dec;78(12):2238–45.

3. Van Winkelhoff AJ, Rams TE, Slots J. Systemic antibiotic therapy in periodontics. *Periodontol 2000.* 1996 Feb;10:45–78.

4. Slots J, Rosling BG. Suppression of the periodontopathic microflora in localized juvenile periodontitis by systemic tetracycline. *J Clin Periodontol.* 1983 Sep;10(5):465–86.

5. Slots J, Jorgensen MG. Effective, safe, practical and affordable periodontal antimicrobial therapy: where are we going, and are we there yet? *Periodontol 2000.* 2002;28:298–312.

6. Mousqués T, Listgarten MA, Phillips RW. Effect of scaling and root planing on the composition of the human subgingival microbial flora. *J Periodont Res.* 1980 Mar;15(2):144–51.

7. Southard SR, Drisko CL, Killoy WJ, Cobb CM, Tira DE. The effect of 2% chlorhexidine digluconate irrigation on clinical parameters and the level of *Bacteroides gingivalis* in periodontal pockets. *J Periodontol.* 1989 Jun;60(6):302–9.

8. Slots J. Selection of antimicrobial agents in periodontal therapy. *J Periodont Res.* 2002 Oct;37(5):389–98.

9. Rams TE, Slots J. Local delivery of antimicrobial agents in the periodontal pocket. *Periodontol 2000.* 1996 Feb;10:139–59.

10. Wunderlich RC, Singelton M, O'Brien WJ, Caffesse RG. Subgingival penetration of an applied solution. *Int J Periodontics Restorative Dent.* 1984;4(5):64–71.

11. Schmid E, Kornman KS, Tinanoff N. Changes of subgingival total colony forming units and black pigmented bacteroides after a single irrigation of periodontal pockets with 1.64% SnF2. *J Periodontol.* 1985 Jun;56(6):330–3.

12. Mazza JE, Newman MG, Sims TN. Clinical and antimicrobial effect of stannous fluoride on periodontitis. *J Clin Periodontol.* 1981 Jun;8(3):203–12.

13. Schlagenhauf U, Stellwag P, Fiedler A. Subgingival irrigation in the maintenance phase of periodontal therapy. *J Clin Periodontol.* 1990 Oct;17(9):650–3.

14. Goodson JM, Haffajee A, Socransky SS. Periodontal therapy by local delivery of tetracycline. *J Clin Periodontol.* 1979 Apr;6(2):83–92.

15. Newman MG, Kornman KS, Doherty FM. A 6-month multi-center evaluation of adjunctive tetracycline fiber therapy used in conjunction with scaling and root planing in maintenance patients: clinical results. *J Periodontol.* 1994 Jul;65(7):685–91.

16. Kerry G. Tetracycline-loaded fibers as adjunctive treatment in periodontal disease. *J Am Dent Assoc.* 1994 Sep;125(9):1199–203.

17. Vandekerckhove BN, Quirynen M, van Steenberghe D. The use of tetracycline-containing controlled-release fibers in the treatment of refractory periodontitis. *J Periodontol.* 1997 Apr;68(4):353–61.

18. Lowenguth RA, Chin I, Caton JG, et al. Evaluation of periodontal treatments using controlled-release tetracycline fibers: microbiological response. *J Periodontol.* 1995 Aug;66(8):700–7.

19. Goodson JM. Controlled drug delivery: a new means of treatment of dental diseases. *Compend Contin Educ Dent.* 1985 Jan;6(1):27–32, 35–6.

20. Killoy WJ, Polson AM. Controlled local delivery of antimicrobials in the treatment of periodontitis. *Dent Clin North Am.* 1998 Apr;42(2):263–83.

21. Greenstein G, Polson A. The role of local drug delivery in the management of periodontal diseases: a comprehensive review. *J Periodontol.* 1998 May;69(5):507–20.

22. Salvi GE, Persson GR, Heitz-Mayfield LJ, Frei M, Lang NP. Adjunctive local antibiotic therapy in the treatment of periimplantitis II: clinical and radiographic outcomes. *Clin Oral Implants Res.* 2007 Jun;18(3):281–5.

23. Persson GR, Salvi GE, Heitz-Mayfield LJ, Lang NP. Antimicrobial therapy using a local drug delivery system (Arestin) in the treatment of peri-implantitis. I: Microbiological outcomes. *Clin Oral Implants Res.* 2006 Aug;17(4):386–93.

24. Renvert S, Lessem J, Dahlén G, Renvert H, Lindahl C. Mechanical and repeated antimicrobial therapy using a local drug delivery system in the treatment of peri-implantitis: a randomized clinical trial. *J Periodontol.* 2008 May;79(5):836–44.

25. Williams RC, Paquette DW, Offenbacher S, et al. Treatment of periodontitis by local administration of minocycline microspheres: a controlled trial. *J Periodontol.* 2001 Nov;72(11):1535–44.

26. Polson AM, Garrett S, Stoller NH, et al. Multi-center comparative evaluation of subgingivally delivered sanguinarine and doxycycline in the treatment of periodontitis. II. Clinical results. *J Periodontol.* 1997 Feb;68(2):119–26.

27. Garrett S, Adams D, Bandt C, et al. Two multi-center clinical trials of subgingival doxycycline in the treatment of periodontitis. *J Dent Res.* 1997;76(Spec):153.

28. Stabholz A, Sela MN, Friedman M, Golomb G, Soskolne A. Clinical and microbiological effects of sustained release chlorhexidine in periodontal pockets. *J Clin Periodontol.* 1986 Sep;13(8):783–8.

CHAPTER 41

Acute Periodontal Conditions

DONNA J. STACH, RDH, MED
ESTHER M. WILKINS, BS, RDH, DMD

Chapter Outline

INTRODUCTION

Acute periodontal diseases are clinical conditions of rapid onset that involve the periodontium or associated structures.

■ They are characterized by pain or discomfort and infection.

■ They may or may not be related to existing gingivitis or periodontitis and may be either localized or generalized, with possible systemic manifestations.[1]

■ The dental hygienist frequently participates in clinical treatment procedures for acute gingival and periodontal lesions.

■ Key words for acute conditions are defined in Box 41-1.

TYPES OF NECROTIZING PERIODONTAL DISEASES

■ Necrotizing ulcerative gingivitis (NUG) and necrotizing ulcerative periodontitis (NUP) are acute,

BOX 41-1	Key Words

Acute Periodontal Conditions

Abscess: localized collection of pus in a circumscribed or walled-off area formed by the disintegration of tissues.

Acute: runs a relatively short course; produces pain and local inflammation.

Chronic: slow development with little evidence of inflammation; usually an intermittent pus discharge; may follow an acute abscess.

Gingival: localized in the gingiva or interdental papilla but not involving bone.

Periapical: circumscribed collection of pus around the apex of a tooth root; results from pulpal necrosis; also called **endodontic**.

Periodontal: localized in the periodontal tissues; also called **lateral** or **parietal.**

Fetor oris: foul, offensive odor from the mouth; halitosis.

Fistula: a pathologic sinus or abnormal passage that leads from an abscess to the surface of the gingiva or mucosa.

Gum boil: a lay term for a circumscribed swelling in the tissue over the alveolar process, usually at the level of the root apices; may break and drain periodically, thus preventing pain.

Herpetic gingivostomatitis or primary herpetic gingivostomatitis: A viral infection (herpes simplex) of the oral mucosa.

Linear gingival erythema: gingivitis in the HIV-positive patient; characterized by a well-demarcated band of intense erythema at the gingival margin, not associated with dental biofilm, and which does not respond to conventional biofilm removal procedures.

Malaise: feeling of general indisposition, uneasiness, discomfort; may be early indication of illness.

Necrosis: death of tissue; morphologic changes indicative of cell death caused by enzymatic degradation.

Necrotizing periodontal diseases (NPD): A collective term that includes both necrotizing ulcerative gingivitis (NUG) and necrotizing ulcerative periodontitis (NUP) since they may be different stages of the same disease.

Pericoronitis: gingival inflammation around the crown of an incompletely erupted tooth; most frequently occurs about a mandibular third molar.

Pseudomembrane: false membrane; false layer of tissue that covers a surface.

Purulent: accompanied by or containing pus.

Sinus tract: a channel that connects with an abscess or suppurating area.

Ulceration: formation or development of an ulcer with loss of epithelial surface and sloughing of necrotic inflammatory tissue.

Vesiculation: formation or presence of vesicles, small fluid filled blister-like elevations on the skin or mucosa.

---

inflammatory, destructive diseases that are usually related to diminished systemic resistance to bacterial infection of the periodontal tissues.

- They are subcategories of necrotizing periodontal diseases (NPD) and may be different stages of the same infection.[2]
- Other names that have been used include necrotizing gingivitis (NG), acute necrotizing ulcerative gingivitis (ANUG), trench mouth, Vincent's infection, Vincent's disease, and ulceromembranous gingivitis.
- Although NUG may occur at any age, it is usually seen among young people between ages 15 and 30 years.
- It is rare in children under 10 years of age in the United States, but it is not uncommon in young children from low socioeconomic groups studied in sub-Saharan Africa and in some developing countries.[3,4]
- Predisposing factors include: malnutrition, emotional stress, cigarette smoking, poor oral hygiene and lowered resistance to infection including HIV infection.

I. NECROTIZING ULCERATIVE GINGIVITIS (NUG)

A. Basic Characteristics

- Gingival inflammation limited to the free gingiva with ulceration of one or more interdental papilla tips.
- Clinical signs include redness, pain and bleeding.

B. HIV-Positive Patient

Linear gingival erythema with ulceration of tips of interdental papillae.[5]

II. NECROTIZING ULCERATIVE PERIODONTITIS

A. Basic Characteristics

- Destructive infection of periodontal tissues with ulceration of interdental papillae, cratering of interdental bone and soft tissue, and clinical attachment loss.
- Condition can become chronic or recur episodically.

B. HIV-Positive Patient

- An increased incidence of NUG/NUP has been diagnosed in HIV-positive patients.
- A more severe, rapidly progressive breakdown of the periodontium occurs with ulceration of interdental papillae, cratering of interdental bone, clinical attachment loss, and presence of exposed bone with sequestration in the most severe involvement.
- Because of the rapid breakdown, necrosis, and tissue recession with severe attachment loss, the condition usually is not associated with deep pockets.[5]

III. NECROTIZING STOMATITIS

Necrosis may extend beyond the tooth-supporting tissues and cause bone destruction and sequestration. Severe disease may resemble noma or cancrum oris.

IV. CANCRUM ORIS (NOMA)

Orofacial gangrenous necrosis destroys the hard and soft tissues of the oral and para-oral structures and is believed to be an extension of untreated NUP. It is predisposed by malnutrition and debilitating systemic illness.[3,4]

CLINICAL RECOGNITION

I. INITIAL SIGNS AND SYMPTOMS

The patient with NUG or NUP reports

- Sudden onset.
- Pain and soreness caused by slight pressure, such as during chewing and toothbrushing; may be intensified by hot or highly seasoned foods. Gentle probing may produce an exaggerated pain response.
- Bleeding that occurs spontaneously or on slight pressure.
- Poor appetite.
- Metallic or other unpleasant taste.
- Fetid odor.

II. CHARACTERISTIC CLINICAL FINDINGS

A. Interdental Necrosis

- Ulceration of the papillae produces craterlike defects in the col area.
- In early disease, only the tips of papillae are involved, followed by progressive destruction of entire papillae and extension to the marginal gingiva facially and lingually **(Figure 41-1)**.

B. Pseudomembrane

- A pseudomembrane forms over the necrotic area. It is a gray, loose, necrotic slough that, when wiped off, exposes a red and shiny hemorrhagic gingiva.
- The pseudomembrane consists primarily of fibrin, necrotic tissue, leukocytes, and masses of microorganisms.
- It is not always present

C. Extent

The membranous ulceration may be seen locally, that is, between two or three teeth, or it may be generalized throughout both maxillary and mandibular arches.

D. Other Clinical Findings

- Debris and biofilm that collect profusely because the patient avoids brushing the sensitive teeth and gingiva.

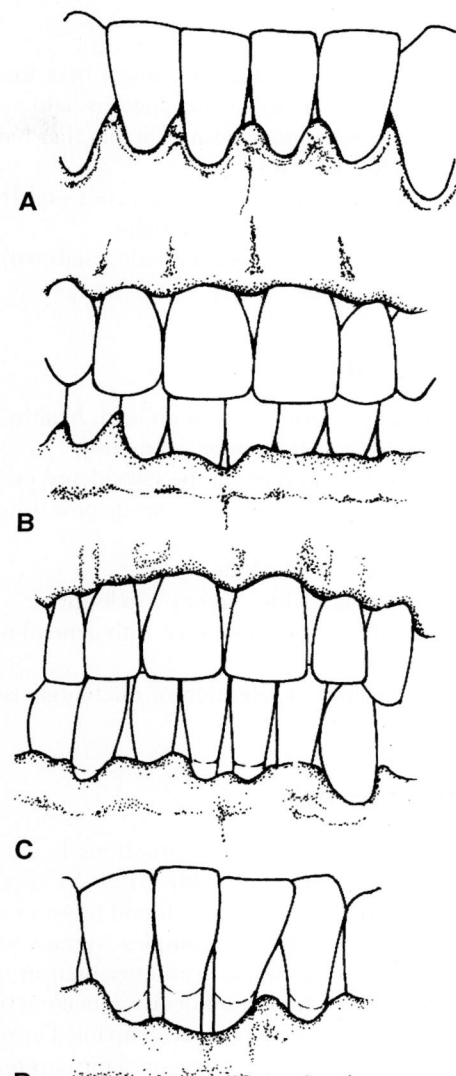

FIGURE 41-1 Necrotizing Ulcerative Gingivitis/Periodontitis. (A) Early lesion with blunted papillae and interdental necrosis. **(B)** Increased destruction with loss of interdental tissue; rolled margins of the gingiva. **(C)** More advanced destruction with recession and interdental cratering. **(D)** Very advanced lesions, with loss of attached gingiva, recession, and tooth mobility.

- Fetor oris (bad breath) that is often severe. It is caused by necrotic tissue, stagnant saliva, and breakdown products of blood and debris.
- Increased salivation.

E. Signs of Systemic Involvement

Examination is made to detect the presence of the following:

- Malaise.
- Lymphadenopathy of submandibular and cervical nodes.
- Possible elevation of body temperature.

RISK FACTORS

- NUG is an infectious disease caused by a fusospirochetal complex of microbes that develops and increases in association with predisposing factors that have lowered the body's defenses.
- Major risk factors are stress, neglected oral hygiene, inadequate diet, and tobacco smoking.
- NUG is not contagious between individuals with a normal immune system.

I. LOCAL FACTORS

- NUG is rarely, if ever, seen in a clean, healthy, cared-for, and professionally supervised mouth.
- Many of the factors that can be considered predisposing are the same as those that predispose to chronic marginal gingivitis.
- Predisposing factors include
  A. Preexisting gingivitis and/or periodontitis.
  B. Inadequate personal oral care with general neglect.
  C. Tobacco use.
  D. Factors related to retention of microorganisms and deposits.

II. STRESS FACTORS

- Acute anxiety related to life situations is a common characteristic of patients with NPD. In susceptible people, the condition has been found to occur or recur during periods of stress. Examples include students during examination periods, military men in combat, and people during important decision-making times.
- Emotional stress is frequently accompanied by poor oral care, improper diet, excessive smoking, overexertion, interrupted sleep, and other deviations in health habits.

III. SYSTEMIC: DISEASE-RESISTANCE FACTORS

- Dietary and nutritional inadequacies; vitamin deficiencies.
- Recent illnesses or immunocompromised; frequent upper respiratory infections, infectious mononucleosis, pernicious anemia, hepatitis, leukemia, and HIV infection.
- Side effects of chemotherapy and radiation.
- Fatigue; insufficient sleep.

ETIOLOGY

- NUG and NUP are acute inflammatory conditions with a characteristic microflora.
- The bacteria in a healthy individual do not result in disease.
- A reduced host response or immunosuppressed condition is an important factor in the disease pathogenesis.

I. MICROBIOLOGY[6]

- Of the many types of organisms found in NUG lesions, fusiform bacilli and medium-sized spirochetes predominate.
- The constant flora has been shown to include *Treponema* and *Selenomonas* species, *Prevotella intermedia, Porphyromonas gingivalis,* and *Fusobacterium* species.

II. COURSE OF DEVELOPMENT

A. Clinical Characteristics of the Lesion

- NPD is superimposed on gingivitis or periodontitis.
- Ulceration and necrosis begin in the interdental papilla.
- Both epithelial tissue and connective tissue are involved.
- The disease process progresses to involve the entire papilla and, eventually, the marginal gingiva on the facial and lingual surfaces.
- The pseudomembrane covering the lesion is a necrotic slough of the surface epithelium. It contains leukocytes, bacteria, epithelial cells, and fibrin. When the pseudomembrane is lifted, the red inflamed connective tissue can be seen.
- Connective tissue shows the signs of acute inflammation. It is hyperemic and filled with leukocytes, and its capillaries are engorged resulting in bright red marginal gingiva, which bleeds on slight manipulation and is painful.
- Malodor is common.
- Localized lymphadenopathy, fever, and malaise may be present.

B. Microscopic Examination

Four zones in the lesion have been described from observations made by electron microscopy.[7] All layers contain spirochetes.

- *Bacterial zone.* The most superficial zone consists primarily of a mass of varied bacteria, including a few spirochetes.
- *Neutrophil-rich zone.* Under the bacterial zone is a layer of leukocytes, predominantly neutrophils. Microorganisms, including many spirochetes, are found among the leukocytes.
- *Necrotic zone.* This zone contains disintegrating tissue cells, many spirochetes, and other bacteria.
- *Spirochetal infiltration zone.* In this nonnecrotized layer where tissue components are still preserved, spirochetes have invaded, but other microorganisms have not.

DENTAL HYGIENE CARE

- Patient instruction and motivation for self-care are needed along with skillful subgingival instrumentation.
- After the initial symptoms have subsided, complete therapy is needed.
- The tissue destruction usually has left the gingiva deformed, with interdental flattening or cratering.

■ Surgical treatment may be needed to restore a physiologic form that can be maintained by the patient in the plan to prevent recurrence of the disease.

I. PREPARATION FOR DENTAL HYGIENE DIAGNOSIS

Initially, certain data must be collected for making the diagnosis and care plan. Basic information needed is suggested by the steps described here.

A. History

1. *Record the chief complaint.* The history of the current disease is described by date of onset, duration, symptoms as reported, and what self-treatment the patient has already performed.
2. *Record whether this is a recurrence.* If so, note details of previous episodes and the treatment given.
3. *Obtain information needed for preliminary treatment*
   A. Conditions needing medical consultation.
   B. Need for premedication for pre-existing condition.
   C. Allergies.
4. *Use knowledge of predisposing factors for NPD to gather pertinent information*
   ■ Tobacco habits.
   ■ Recent illnesses or types of therapy may explain a lowered resistance.
   ■ Record of immediately previous 24-hour food intake. When the mouth has been sore and eating has been painful, a diet recording may not be typical of the patient's usual intake. Later, a 5-day or week-long food record will be requested as part of the continuing prevention program.
   ■ Variations of normal sleeping hours and routine; stress.

B. Examination

1. *Record the patient's temperature*
2. *Extraoral examination*
   ■ Palpate submandibular and cervical nodes.
   ■ Observe face and skin to determine whether flushed, damp.
   ■ Observe signs of malaise.
3. *Oral examination*
   ■ Without instrumentation, a preliminary examination can be made and the overall appearance of the gingival tissue recorded.
   ■ The dentist may prefer to see the gingiva as it appears initially, before instrumentation or rinsing, to make the diagnosis and prepare the treatment plan.

II. CARE PLAN

The dental hygiene care plan is formulated within the total treatment plan. Only a partial treatment plan is made until after the acute phase of the disease has passed.

A. Systemic Treatment

■ Directions concerning diet, rest, and other systemic influences.
■ Multivitamin supplements are sometimes prescribed.
■ After the diagnosis is made, the dentist determines whether systemic antibiotic therapy is indicated. Except for a patient who requires antibiotic coverage to prevent infective endocarditis or for joint replacement, antibiotics are prescribed conservatively.

B. Relief of Acute Symptoms Is the First Therapeutic Goal

■ Personal care instructions for rinsing, brushing, and limiting use of tobacco.
■ Supragingival debridement of all teeth and gingiva.
■ Subgingival scaling started. This is one of the rare times that full-mouth gross or nondefinitive scaling is indicated; usually with an ultrasonic instrument.
■ Chlorhexidine 0.12% rinse twice daily.

C. Basic Therapy

1. *Preventive program*
   ■ Instruction for prevention of recurrence of NPD; eliminate tobacco use.
   ■ Dietary analysis and counseling.
   ■ Self-care fluoride, professional application when indicated for caries.
2. *Complete scaling and debridement*
3. *Reduction or elimination of predisposing factors to NPD*
   ■ Removal of overhanging margins and other biofilm retention factors.
   ■ Restoration of teeth and contact areas.
4. Evaluation for periodontal surgery. Need for restoration of tissue contour and elimination of craters.
5. Restoration of occlusion. Prosthetic replacements and all other dental needs.

CARE FOR THE ACUTE STAGE

A series of appointments for a typical patient with NPD is outlined here. The number of appointments and the exact procedure at each appointment depend on the severity of the disease and the response of the gingiva as treatment progresses. Initially tissue may be very painful to touch.

■ Four or five closely spaced appointments may be needed during the acute stage, depending on the probing depths, the extent of calculus deposits and pain response of patient during instrumentation.
■ The basic objective is to debride the teeth thoroughly to encourage soft tissue healing.
■ A series of full mouth or gross debridements may be used during the acute phase.

■ When the acute stage has subsided, a regular appointment plan is established for a comprehensive periodontal evaluation and treatment and continued supervision.

I. ACUTE PHASE: FIRST APPOINTMENT

A. Patient Instruction

■ Explain local causes and control measures.
■ Demonstrate biofilm with a disclosing agent.
■ Show biofilm removal procedures, using a soft brush moistened with warm water.

B. General Debridement

■ Clean away loose debris: apply hydrogen peroxide (3% solution mixed with equal parts of water) with cotton pellets at proximal areas; request patient to rinse.
■ Avoid use of compressed air or water spray to prevent reaction from sensitivity and dispersion of contaminated aerosols.
■ Use topical anesthetic, local anesthesia or nitrous oxide-oxygen sedation as needed to manage pain.
■ Use manual or ultrasonic instruments for scaling; use high speed evacuation to manage aerosols. Ultrasonic instrumentation may be preferred as it applies less pressure to the gingiva and the flushing of the pockets may help healing.

C. Subgingival Instrumentation

The gingiva responds sooner with definitive scaling.

■ Perform instrumentation with ultrasonic or sharp instruments carefully but thoroughly.
■ Have assistant evacuate continuously to prevent contaminated aerosols and to protect the patient from inhaling microorganisms.
■ Irrigate and evacuate frequently to clear all debris and calculus removed during instrumentation.

D. Patient Instruction

■ *Instructions for home use.* Instructions for home procedures are carefully explained. Written directions are needed.
■ *Instructions for continuing care.* Inform the patient that treatment will not be complete when the pain is eliminated. Explain the underlying gingival or periodontal infection and how NPD recurs if the periodontal condition is not treated.
■ *Rinsing directions*
   A. Vigorous rinsing with warm water or weak saline solution is necessary every hour during the period of acute symptoms.
   B. Using 3% hydrogen peroxide with equal parts of water is preferred by some clinicians. If used, it should be

recommended for only a few days and then discontinued.
   C. Rinsing with chlorhexidine (0.12%) twice daily continues: use 0.5 ounce after brushing after breakfast, and after brushing and flossing before retiring; swish between the teeth for 1 minute.
■ *Toothbrushing*
   A. Use a soft nylon brush gently, but thoroughly.
   B. Clean the teeth as much as possible especially before going to bed.
   C. When a softbrush is not given to the patient at the clinic or office, write down the names of specific brushes for the patient to purchase.

E. Introduce Tobacco Cessation

■ *Inform patient.* Describe the effect of smoked or smokeless tobacco on the oral cavity, with special emphasis on facts about the gingival tissues.
■ *Avoiding tobacco products.* The heavy smoker who is not ready for cessation can be requested to limit the use while treatment for NPD is under way.

F. Diet

■ Recommend frequent, small, nutritious meals that incorporate daily requirements from the *MyPlate* guidelines (in Chapter 34, page 499).
■ A liquid or soft bland diet is advised for the first day, particularly for the patient with systemic symptoms or pronounced sensitivity when chewing. A diet of soft solids can be used on the second day.
■ The choice of foods needs to include increased amounts of meat and milk groups and of fruits and juices.
■ Avoid highly seasoned foods and alcoholic beverages.

II. ACUTE PHASE: SECOND APPOINTMENT (IDEALLY THE NEXT DAY)

A. Patient Examination

■ *Changes.* A remarkable improvement usually can be seen within 24 hours, with pain and discomfort lessened, the pseudomembrane gone, and tissue enlargement reduced.
■ *Toothbrushing.* Apply disclosing agent and show patient missed areas. Emphasize thorough coverage of the entire dentition, using sulcular brushing.

B. Scaling and Root Debridement

■ Deplaque the full mouth.
■ Continue procedures from the previous appointment after checking areas previously treated. Use local anesthesia or other pain management as needed.
■ The objective is to be as thorough as possible because biofilm retained over residual calculus and altered cementum can keep the tissues from healing completely.

C. Instruction: Second Day

■ *Rinsing.* When healing is progressing favorably, change rinsing schedule to every 2 hours.

■ *Proximal surfaces.* The use of floss or a small interdental brush is advised and should be emphasized at this or the third appointment, depending on the readiness of the patient and the tissue. Other proximal cleaning devices may be useful. When the interdental embrasures are open as a result of papillary necrosis **(Figure 41-1C** and **41-1D)**, an interdental brush or other device is indicated. The importance of complete biofilm removal is explained.

■ *Diet.* A liquid diet usually is not indicated after the first day, and the patient can use the soft solids diet or a regular diet adapted with bland foods that will not irritate the healing tissues.

■ *Instructions.* Provide specific written instructions.

III. SUCCESSIVE APPOINTMENTS

After the acute stage, regular appointments for basic treatment are planned. The gingiva is evaluated, and repeated scaling and debridement is performed as needed to complete that part of the treatment.

A. Complete Assessment

The complete plan for dental care is prepared, and the patient is instructed for continued treatment.

B. Recurrence of NUG/NUP

■ When the gingival and bony craters that remain after the initial healing phase are not treated, they are vulnerable to continuing disease and episodic recurrence of NPD. Biofilm and debris can collect readily in the misshapen proximal areas, and these areas are difficult to clean with routine biofilm control techniques. Gingival craters invite further tissue breakdown, leading to periodontal pocket formation.

■ Surgical treatment is explained to the patient. When bony craters exist, treatment may involve flap surgery with osseous reshaping.

PRIMARY HERPETIC GINGIVOSTOMATITIS (PHG)

A viral infection of the oral mucosa caused by *Herpes simplex*. It may be mistaken for necrotizing periodontal disease (NPD). Characteristics for differential diagnosis are shown in **Table 41-1**. Additional information on herpesvirus diseases can be found in Chapter 4 (page 50).

ETIOLOGY

I. MICROBIOLOGY

■ Causative agent is *Herpes simplex* virus (HSV); usually HSV1 but HSV2 possible and clinically the same.

TABLE 41-1	COMPARISON BETWEEN NECROTIZING PERIODONTAL DISEASE (NPD) AND PRIMARY HERPETIC GINGIVOSTOMATITIS (PHG)	
	NPD	**PHG**
Cause	Bacteria and lower immunity	*Herpes simplex* virus
Who	Young adult	Child
Where	Interdental papilla. Rarely beyond periodontium	Entire oral mucosa including gingiva
Signs & Symptoms	Ulcerations, necrotic tissue, and gray pseudomembrane Fetor oris Sometimes fever	Multiple vesicles followed by small round fibrin-covered ulcerations Fetor oris Fever
How Long	1–2 days if treated	1–2 weeks
Contagious	No	Yes
Treatment Focus	Behavior modification to support immune system Biofilm control Complete debridement	No specific treatment Counseling for nutrition, fluid intake, biofilm control Avoid contact (contagious)
Immunity to Recurrence	No	Partial
Long-Term Effect	Permanent damage to periodontal tissue	No permanent tissue change

- HSV1 is spread by infected saliva or active perioral lesions. Saliva can contain and transmit the virus when infected individuals are asymptomatic.
- Two patterns of clinically evident infections:
  A. Primary infection
  1. When an individual without antibodies is initially exposed,
  2. Typically at a young age,
  3. May be symptomatic but most often is asymptomatic,
  4. Virus enters a latent state usually in the trigeminal ganglion.
  B. Secondary or recurrent infection
  1. Occurs when latent virus is reactivated.
  2. Most frequent location is at the vermilion border and adjacent skin of the lips where it is known as herpes labialis, cold sore or fever blister.
- HSV has a short period of viability in the external environment.

II. PATHOGENESIS

- PHG is a primary infection of HSV in an individual without antibodies
- Occurs most often in children from 6 months to 6 years but usually between ages 1–3.
- Can occur at any age.
- Usual incubation period is 3–9 days.
- PHG is self-limiting and resolves in 7–14 days with or without treatment.
- Primary infection is usually asymptomatic (subclincal) or may manifest as pharyngitis that mimics a common cold or may be mistaken as a difficult teeth episode.
- Transmission is by physical contact with contaminated saliva or an active lesion often by kissing, shared utensils or contaminated hands.

CLINICAL RECOGNITION

I. INITIAL SIGNS AND SYMPTOMS

- Onset is abrupt.
- Initial symptoms may include any combination of the following: anterior cervical lymphadenopathy, fever (103–105°F), sore throat, malaise, irritability, headache, drooling, nausea, refusal of food (anorexia), sore mouth.

II. ORAL PRESENTATION

- Oral lesions may be simultaneous with lymphadenopathy and fever or may follow after 1–2 days.
- A generalized sore mouth develops.
- Gingiva is painful, erythematous, enlarged and may have spontaneous bleeding from the gingival sulcus.
- Any oral mucosal site can be involved both keratinized and nonkeratinized mucosa.

- Affected mucosa develops numerous pinhead-sized vesicles, which are often missed because they collapse or rupture quickly to form small superficial red ulcers.
- Initial ulcers enlarge slightly or may coalesce to from a larger, shallow irregular ulceration.
- Central area of the ulcer is covered by yellow fibrin and is surrounded by a red ring of inflammation.
- Number of lesions is highly variable.
- Affected gingival often has punched-out erosions at the midfacial of the free gingival margin.
- Lips and perioral skin are often involved.

III. RESOLUTION

- Fever typically subsides after 2 days.
- Oral lesions begin to heal 3 days after appearance.
- Mild cases resolve in 5–7 days with more severe cases lasting 2 weeks.
- Lesions heal completely and without scaring.

IV. DIAGNOSIS

- Is usually based on clinical presentation.

MANAGEMENT AND TREATMENT CONSIDERATIONS

- Primary goal is pain relief and maintenance of nutrition and hydration.
- Antiviral medication may be considered[8]; antiviral medication is most effective during the earliest phase of viral infection and is rarely identified soon enough in PHG.
- Medical consult or referral may be indicated especially if secondary infection or dehydration is suspected.
- Reassure that condition is self-limiting; usually of 1–2 weeks duration.
- Advise that *Herpes simplex* virus is contagious during the acute stages of the disease especially when vesicles or ulcerated lesions are present.
- Treatment recommendation: Avoid dental treatment including debridement of the teeth because of the infective nature of the virus both to the clinician and to other areas of the patient's mucosa. Oral/dental debris and biofilm accumulation does not contribute to the continuation of the condition as they do in necrotizing periodontal diseases.
- Patient counseling includes instruction in adequate nutrition and fluid intake. Dehydration is the most common cause of hospitalization of small children with PHG.
- Normal oral hygiene is discontinued during the few days of the acute painful stage; gentle oral hygiene can begin again during healing.

PALLIATIVE TREATMENT

1. Soft diet of bland warm or cold foods.
2. Cold foods such as ice cream or sherbet may be soothing.
3. Avoid acidic or carbonated drinks.
4. Warm saline and bicarbonate rinses (½ teaspoon table salt, ½ teaspoon baking soda, 8 ounces warm water) swished, held in the mouth for a few minutes then expectorated. Can be used after meals and at bedtime in place of toothbrushing during the most painful phase.
5. Topical anesthetic rinses or application to help relieve pain.
   - Diphenhydramine elixir and an antacid such as Kaopectate or Maalox mixed in equal parts.
   - Viscous lidocaine, Diphenhydramine elixir and an antacid such as Kaopectate or Maalox mixed in equal parts.
   - Can be mixed at a compounding pharmacy.
   - Instruct patient to swish a teaspoonful for 30–60 seconds and expectorate.
   - Especially helpful before meals.
   - Caution about swallowing difficulties due to numb mouth.

PERIODONTAL ABSCESS

- An abscess is a localized purulent inflammatory lesion.
- Gingival and periodontal abscesses occur within the periodontal tissues. An abscess is called *gingival* when it is located in the marginal area or interdental papilla and *periodontal* when it is in the deeper periodontal tissues. They may be acute or chronic.
- They may also be known as *lateral abscesses* because they occur along the lateral surfaces of teeth.

I. DEVELOPMENT OF A PERIODONTAL ABSCESS

- Pus collects in the tissue as a result of bacterial infection.
- The infection may be a complication of an existing periodontal disease, or it may be an immediate result of microorganisms from biofilm forced into the tissue by some form of trauma.
- The body's reaction is to send large numbers of defense cells to the area, particularly polymorphonuclear leukocytes (PMNs), which are major constituents of the purulent exudate (pus) that collects.
- Pus is a thick fluid product of inflammation. It contains many living and dead PMNs mixed with debris from cells and tissues that have been destroyed by the enzymes released by the PMNs. Unless there is a means for drainage, the pus collects and forms an abscess.
- A sinus or fistula may form. Drainage may occur through the sinus and release the pressure within the abscess, thereby relieving the pain the patient may experience.

II. ETIOLOGIC FACTORS

A. Periodontal Pockets

- Deep pockets of chronic inflammatory periodontal infection provide an environment for abscess formation. Intrabony pockets, pockets that extend into bifurcation or trifurcation areas, and complex pockets that develop in winding or irregular shapes are particularly susceptible to becoming closed and, therefore, susceptible to abscess formation.

B. Instrumentation

- Instrumentation applied within the pocket and the effects of the instrumentation may be the precipitating factors that initiate abscess formation.
- Incomplete scaling in the depth of a pocket may allow the tissue at the opening of the pocket to heal, tighten, and prevent drainage from the infectious material deep in the pocket.
- Biofilm and calculus remaining in the sealed off part of the pocket attract the collection of more bacteria and PMNs, and an abscess develops.

C. Trauma

- Foreign objects may enter by way of the sulcus or pocket and become embedded along with microorganisms. The infection leads to abscess formation.[9]
- Implanted or impacted material such as a popcorn husk, small fish bone or shellfish fragment, seeds, seed coverings, or other material from food; or oral hygiene devices such as a toothbrush bristle or filament or a sliver from a toothpick.

D. Patient Susceptibility to Infection

- The possibility for abscess formation within the gingival tissue is increased from any of the etiologic factors that have been mentioned when the patient's resistance to infection is lowered.
- Patients with uncontrolled diabetes or who are receiving immunosuppressive medication are examples of those at greater risk.

III. CLINICAL SIGNS AND SYMPTOMS

Even though clinical manifestations may vary, the classic signs and symptoms are listed here.

A. Gingival Appearance

- The area of the abscess is enlarged, with a red, shiny, smooth surface.
- The abscess may appear domelike or pointed, and on slight digital pressure, pus may appear.

B. The Tooth

- *Sensitivity.* The tooth may be slightly mobile and sensitive to percussion. When extruded, it may be sensitive to touching the tooth in the opposing jaw.
- *Pulp vitality test.* Pulp testing usually reveals a vital tooth, responding within the normal range.
- *Radiographs.* A radiolucency may be noted along the lateral wall beside the tooth, but such a finding is variable. No bone loss shows in early lesions. The amount of bone destruction and the location of the abscess influence the possible radiographic findings.

C. General Physical Condition

- Occasionally, a patient shows evidence of systemic involvement, such as a slight elevation in body temperature, malaise, and lymphadenopathy.

D. Chronic Abscess

- In the chronic state, a sinus tract usually opens on the gingival surface and drains periodically.
- Before drainage, the patient may have a dull pain from the pressure of the fluid within the abscess area.
- Acute symptoms may be expected from time to time unless definitive periodontal therapy is completed.

IV. COMPARISON OF PERIAPICAL (ENDODONTIC) AND PERIODONTAL ABSCESSES

The dentist often needs to make a differential diagnosis between a periodontal abscess and a periapical abscess of pulpal origin. Certain signs and symptoms are similar for both. A few of the potentially distinguishing findings are noted here.

A. Pulpal Abscess

- Nonvital response to pulp test; sensitivity to percussion.
- May have no periodontal pocket.
- Swelling related to apex of tooth with or without fistulous tract.
- Pain often severe; may be difficult to locate specifically.

B. Radiographic Examination

- Early stages of either a periapical or a periodontal abscess are not evident in a radiograph.
- A widening of the periodontal ligament space may appear.

C. Combined Periodontal/Periapical (Endodontic) Lesion

- Combined periodontal and endodontic lesions (abscesses) occur. Communication between a deep periodontal pocket and an apical lesion is not unusual.

- Communication may exist between a periodontal pocket and the pulp by way of a lateral or accessory canal through the dentin, often in the area of a furcation.
- Etiology: the lesion may originate primarily from pulpal inflammation expressing itself through the periodontal tissues or bacteria from a deep periodontal pocket may invade the pulp. It may be a sequel of a fractured tooth.

V. CARE PLAN

Two phases of treatment are used for the patient with a periodontal abscess. The first is for immediate relief of acute symptoms, and the second is the definitive diagnosis and treatment followed by preventive maintenance. The entire plan is explained to the patient at the outset.

A. Objectives of Emergency Treatment

- Relieve pain.
- Establish drainage.
- Determine need for systemic antibiotic therapy, local antibiotic delivery not recommended.
- Manage patient comfort.

B. Review Medical History

Determine necessary preappointment precautions, such as the need for antibiotic premedication.

C. Examination for Systemic Involvement

Antibiotic medication may be prescribed by the dentist when systemic involvement is definite.

- Determine and record the patient's body temperature.
- Examine submandibular and neck nodes for lymphadenopathy.

D. Provide Anesthesia

- When the abscess is confined to the gingival area, and the drainage may be expected to cause little if any discomfort, a topical anesthetic may suffice.
- Usually, block anesthesia is indicated.

E. Methods for Drainage

1. *Via pocket or sulcus opening*
   - Local anesthetic injection for pain management.
   - Isolate the area, swab with a topical antiseptic, and use a probe to gain admission into the sulcus or pocket.

- Gently probe circumferentially until an opening into the abscess is found.
- Drainage usually begins promptly.
2. *Curet area*
  - Use a curet to open the area, and locate and remove a foreign body irritant when it is known to be present from the history obtained from the patient.
  - Scaling and debridement are performed as needed.

F. Posttreatment Instructions and Follow-Up

- Rinsing with warm saline solution every 2 hours is advised; OTC analgesics as needed.
- The patient returns for observation in 24 to 48 hours. Relief from pain and discomfort can be expected and appointments for definitive treatment planned.
- Biofilm control instruction is initiated or continued, and scaling and debridement are completed.

G. Anticipated Results

- Acute symptoms are resolved.
- Pain relief occurs within a short time following the initiation of drainage because the pressure is released from within the abscessed area.
- Extruded tooth returns to its normal position.
- Swelling is reduced.
- Temporary comfort is obtained for the patient; the lesion is reduced to a standard chronic lesion that requires additional treatment.

- If drainage is not complete, an acute lesion may develop into a lesion with a chronic sinus or pocket drainage.

VI. DEFINITIVE THERAPY

- Whatever pocket elimination procedures are indicated need to be completed within a reasonable time to prevent further complications.
- Careful and regular dental biofilm control with scaling and debridement are essential on a maintenance basis.

DOCUMENTATION

Documentation is the permanent record for each appointment when a patient presents with complaint of pain. It includes a minimum of the following factors:

- Description of signs, symptoms, location, and duration of condition.
- Diagnosis or differential diagnosis.
- Treatment plan.
- Description of treatment.
- Description of patient education and postoperative instructions.
- Future plan.
- An example progress note documenting an appointment for a patient with necrotizing ulcerative gingivitis (NUG) is located in **Box 41-2**.

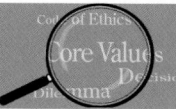# Everyday Ethics

Mr. Rufus, who has been a patient in the office for many years, shows up this afternoon without an appointment because he is suddenly having mouth pain and a "horrible metallic taste." When he speaks to her, Sue, the dental hygienist, is overtaken by a strong mouth odor. Dr. Janus is on vacation this week, but according to the laws of her state, Sue practices under **general supervision** and may provide dental hygiene care for a patient of record even when the dentist is not in the office. Sue seats Mr. Rufus in the dental chair to assess the situation.

Sue determines that there have been no changes in Mr. Rufus' health history, but he describes the heart-breaking details of his divorce proceedings. He confides in Sue that he has hardly eaten or brushed his teeth for weeks.

Sue begins an extraoral and intraoral examination, but Mr. Rufus says it is too painful for her to retract his cheeks and lips. During the brief examination, she noticed punched out papillae and pseudomembrane formation over much of his gingiva. She immediately suspects necrotizing ulcerative gingivitis (NUG), or perhaps necrotizing ulcerative periodontitis (NUP).

Questions for Consideration
1. Which of the core values (Table II-1, page 38) apply to this scenario? Discuss their meaning in this kind of situation. How are "informed consent" or "implied consent" involved when you review what Sue did to help Mr. Rufus?
2. Is it ethical for Sue to develop a DENTAL HYGIENE DIAGNOSIS that is related to her clinical observations? Is it legal for Sue to provide acute phase (first appointment) care for Mr. Rufus today, even though Dr. Janus is not in the office? Why or why not?
3. Mrs. Rufus, who comes in for her appointment later in the month, does not share any information about the divorce. However, she asks Sue why Mr. Rufus was billed for several appointments this time just to "clean his teeth." What ethical principles guide how Sue responds to any questions Mrs. Rufus might ask?

BOX 41-2	**Example Progress Notes: Patient With NUG**

23-year-old male has a nonsignificant medical history and no medications. Smokes 1 pack/day. Chief complaint-painful bleeding gums of 4 days duration. Reports high stress levels recently.

Tissue appearance: marginal gingiva is bright red, glossy, slightly enlarged throughout, easy bleeding with slight contact. The papilla between 3–4, 4–5, and 28–29 have yellowish gray coating. Patient has pronounced oral malodor. Tissue is so painful to touch that full mouth probing was deferred to a future appointment. Bone levels look normal on radiographs.

Dental hygiene diagnosis is necrotizing ulcerative gingivitis (NUG).

Treatment plan: Today—gentle full mouth debridement of supragingival biofilm and calculus and patient education. Second appt. tomorrow to begin debridment with local anesthesia. Definitive period evaluation after pain subsides. Patient gave consent.

Treatment: Pre-tx rinse with CHX; debridement with hydrogen peroxide:water mix (50:50) applied generously to the gingival with a cotton swab; supragingival ultrasonic instrumentation of all teeth. Patient was somewhat uncomfortable but said to continue and generally tolerated procedure well. High-speed evacuation was used to manage aerosol.

Etiology of NUG was explained to pat.; probable contributing factors in his case are stress, heavy cigarette smoking, lack of sleep and poor nutrition plus a long-standing gingivitis, poor biofilm control and lack of professional care. Patient committed to the following behavior modifications: Get at least 6 hrs of sleep a night, eat 3 meals a day and add one fruit and vegetable a day, take a multivitamin daily. He did not think he could reduce stress at this time. We discussed smoking cessation, he is not interested now but willing to talk about it again in future.

Gave him a very soft TB. Did demo and return of gentle Bass brushing technique with instructions to do 2×/day.

Next visit: tomorrow to assess healing, evaluate biofilm control and behavior modification. Modify as needed and add flossing. Full mouth biofilm removal and begin definitive debridement with local anesthesia on right side.

Signed: _____, RDH Date: _____

Factors To Teach The Patient

- Premature discontinuation of treatment for NUG because acute signs have subsided can lead to recurrence of the infection.
- The role of diet, rest, and dental biofilm control in the prevention of NUG.
- The avoidance of an oral irrigating device in the presence of acute inflammatory conditions. Microorganisms may be forced into the tissues beneath a pocket, and bacteremia can be produced.

References

1. American Academy of Periodontology. Parameter on acute periodontal diseases. *J Periodontol*. 2000 May;7(5 Suppl):863–6.
2. Lang N, Soskolne WA, Greenstein G, Cochran D, Corbet E, Meng HX, Newman M, Novak MJ, Tenenbaum H. Consensus report: necrotizing periodontal diseases. *Ann Periodontol*. 1999 Dec;4(1):78.
3. Enwonwu CO, Falkler WA Jr, Phillips RS. Noma (cancrum oris). *Lancet*, 2006 Jul;368(9530):147–56.
4. Taiwo JO. Oral hygiene status and necrotizing ulcerative gingivitis in Nigerian children. *J Periodontol*. 1993 Nov;64(11):1071–4.
5. Greenspan JS. Periodontal complications of HIV infection. *Compend Cont Educ Dent Suppl*. 1994 Nov;(18):S694–8.
6. Loesche WJ, Syed SA, Laughon BE, Stoll J. The bacteriology of acute necrotizing ulcerative gingivitis. *J Periodontol*. 1982 Apr;53(4):223–30.
7. Listgarten MA. Electron microscopic observations on the bacterial flora of acute necrotizing ulcerative gingivitis. *J Periodontol*. 1965 Jul–Aug;36:328–39.
8. Nasser M, Fedorowicz Z, Khoshnevisan MH, Shahiri Tabarestani M. Acyclovir for treating primary herpetic gingivostomatitis. *Cochrane Database Syst Rev*. 2008 Oct;(4):CD006700.
9. Gillette WB, Van House RL. Ill effects of improper oral hygiene procedure. *J Am Dent Assoc*. 1980 Sep;101(3):476–80.

CHAPTER 42

Sutures and Dressings

MARILYN CORTELL, RDH, MS
ESTHER M. WILKINS, BS, RDH, DMD

Chapter Outline

Many periodontal surgical procedures require sutures and dressings. The dental hygienist will often participate in the patient's initial preparation and postcare; therefore, knowledge of the surgical and posttreatment procedures will support continuity of treatment. Key words related to sutures and dressings are defined in **Box 42-1**.

SUTURES

A suture is a strand of material used to ligate blood vessels and approximate tissue. Sutures are necessary in many oral surgical procedures when a surgical wound must be closed, a flap positioned, or tissue grafted.

Through the centuries, a wide range of suture materials has been used, including silk, cotton, linen, and animal tendons and intestines. Today's suture materials are designed for specific procedures, thus decreasing potential for postsurgical infections while providing patient comfort and convenience.

I. FUNCTIONS OF SUTURES

- Close periodontal wounds and secure grafts in position
- Assist in maintaining hemostasis

BOX 42-1	Key Words

Sutures and Dressings

Border mold: the shaping of the peripheries of a dressing by manual manipulation of the tissue adjacent to the borders (e.g., lips, cheeks) to duplicate the contour and size of the vestibule.

Chemical cure: mode of self-cure or setting of a dressing in which the ingredients unite in a chemical process that starts as soon as the blending is complete; the setting time is influenced by warm temperature and the addition of an accelerator.

Coapt: to approximate, as the edges of a wound; bring edge to edge with no overlap.

Eugenol: constituent of clove oil; used in early periodontal dressings with zinc oxide for its alleged antiseptic and anodyne properties; more recently found to be toxic, to elicit allergic reactions, and to hinder, more than promote, healing.

Hemostasis: the termination of bleeding by mechanical or chemical means or by the complex coagulation process of the body that consists of vasoconstriction, platelet aggregation, and thrombin and fibrin synthesis.

Hydrolysis: a process in which water slowly penetrates the suture filaments, causing breakdown of the suture's polymer chain. Hydrolyzation yields a lesser degree of tissue reaction.

Ligation: application of a wire or thread (suture) to hold or constrict tissue.

Septic: presence of potentially pathogenic microorganisms; opposite of **Asepsis:** absence of infectious material.

Suture: a stitch or series of stitches made to secure apposition of the edges of a surgical or traumatic wound.

Suture apposition: a suture that holds the margins of an incision close together.

Swage: the fusion of a suture material to the needle, which allows for a smooth eyeless attachment. The suture will then pass through the tissue as smoothly as possible.

Tensile strength: amount of strength the suture material will retain throughout the healing period. As the wound gains strength, the suture loses strength.

Visible light–cure: light activation using a photocure system; shorter curing time than self-cure (chemical cure); does not start setting until the light is activated, thereby allowing longer working time for adapting the dressing material.

- Reduce posttreatment discomfort
- Promote primary intention healing
- Prevent underlying bone exposure
- Protect healing surgical wound from foreign debris and trauma

II. CHARACTERISTICS OF SUTURE MATERIALS

- Sterile
- Handle comfortably and easily
- Pass through tissue with minimal trauma
- Cause little or no tissue reaction throughout healing
- Possess a high tensile strength

III. CLASSIFICATION OF SUTURE MATERIALS

A. By Number of Strands

- *Monofilament suture:* single strand of material
- *Multifilament suture:* several strands twisted or braided together

B. By Material Used

- *Natural:* capable of causing adverse tissue reaction
- *Synthetic:* developed to reduce tissue reactions and unpredictable rates of absorption commonly found in natural sutures

C. By Absorption Properties

1. *Absorbable sutures:* approximate tissue until wound heals sufficiently to endure normal stress
   - Natural absorbable sutures: digested by body enzymes
     Examples: surgical gut, chromic gut
   - Synthetic absorbable sutures: broken down by hydrolysis, a process in which water slowly penetrates the suture filaments, causing a breakdown of the suture's polymer chain. Hydrolyzation yields a lesser degree of tissue reaction.
     Examples: polyglactin (Vicryl™), poliglecaprone (Monocryl™), polydioxanone (PDS™ II)
2. *Nonabsorbable sutures:* not digested by body enzymes or hydrolyzation; must be removed within specific time period
   - Natural nonabsorbable
     Example: silk
   - Synthetic nonabsorbable
     Examples: nylon (Ethilon™), polyester (Ethibond™), polypropylene (Prolene™) polytetrafluoroethylene (ePTFE) (Gore-Tex™)

D. By Diameter of Suture Material

- Diameters range from 1–0 to 11–0.
- More zeros, smaller the diameter.
- Fewer zeros, larger the diameter.
- Example: 3–0 is larger than 5–0.

TABLE 42-1	SELECTION OF SUTURE MATERIAL
SUTURE TYPES	**SPECIFIC DENTAL PROCEDURES**
Silk, non resorbable, braided	Periodontal flaps and closure
Nylon, monofilament	Periodontal flaps and closure
Polyester, braided	Periodontal flaps and closure
Gut, resorbable	Extraction socket, bone grafting
Resorbable preferred: Nonresorbable used when pain and swelling may be anticipated	Implant flap closure

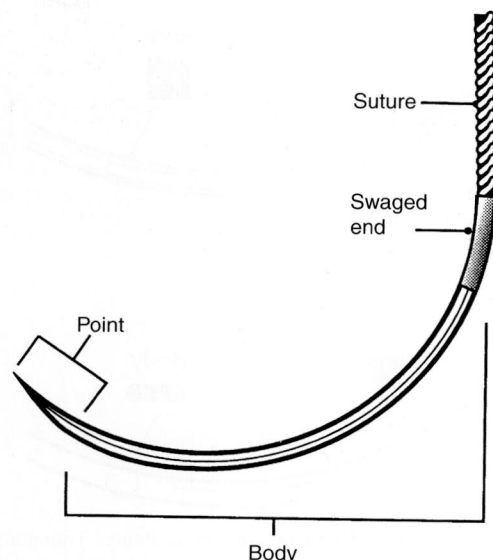

FIGURE 42-1 **Suture Needle Components.**

IV. SELECTION OF SUTURE MATERIAL

Choosing the appropriate suture material for a specific procedure is critical both for patient comfort and tissue health. Suture selection is based on

- preference of surgeon
- delicacy of tissue
- cosmetic implications
  Examples of suture types surgeons may use for specific procedures are found in **Table 42-1**

NEEDLES

Many types of suturing needles are available. Their use and selection are primarily based on specific procedures, location for use, and clinician's preference.

I. NEEDLE COMPONENTS

A. Swaged End (Eyeless)

Swaged allows suture material and needle to act as one unit **(Figure 42-1)**.

B. Body

- *Shape/curvature:*
  - straight
  - half-curved
  - curved 1/4, 3/8, 1/2, 5/8 **(Figure 42-2)**
- *Diameter:* gauge or size; finer for delicate surgeries. The body is the strongest part of the needle that is grasped with the needleholder during the surgical procedure. The swaged end is the weakest part of the body.

C. Point

- The point of the needle extends from the extreme tip of the needle to the widest part of the body.
- Each needle point is designed and manufactured to penetrate tissue with the highest degree of sharpness.

II. NEEDLE CHARACTERISTICS

A. Material

Most needles are made of stainless steel formulated and sterilized for surgical use.

B. Attachment

- Majority of needles are permanently attached to suture material.
- Eliminates need for threading and unnecessary handling.

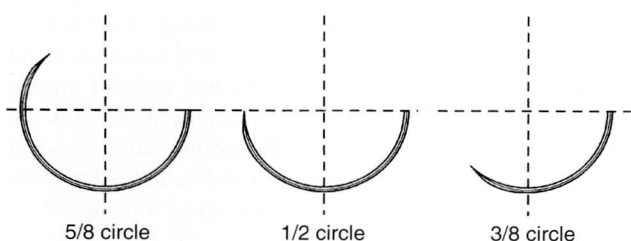

5/8 circle   1/2 circle   3/8 circle

FIGURE 42-2 **Suture Needles.** A curved needle is manipulated with a needleholder. The 3/8 curve is most effective for closure of skin and mucous membranes and is a needle of choice in many dental and periodontal surgeries.

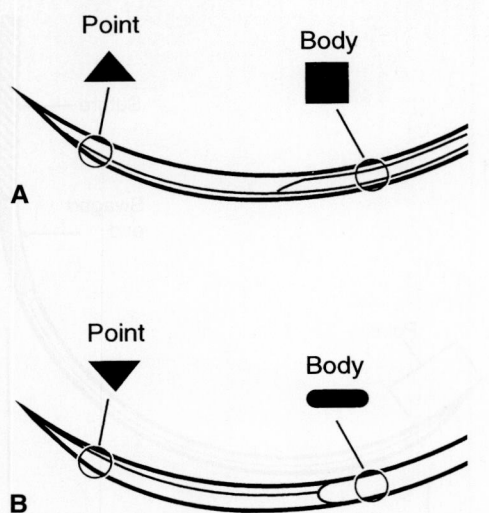

FIGURE 42-3 **Suture Needles.** Shapes of Points. Triangle shows cross section of needle point. **(A)** Conventional cutting with third cutting edge on the inside of the needle curvature. **(B)** Reverse cutting with third cutting edge on the outer curvature of the needle, used for difficult-to-penetrate tissue, such as skin.

C. Cutting Edge (Figure 42-3)

■ *Reverse cut:* It has two opposing cutting edges, with a third located on outer convex curve of needle.
■ *Conventional cut:* It consists of two opposing cutting edges and a third within the concave curvature of the needle.

D. Requirements

■ Needle point is designed to meet the needs of specific surgical procedures.
■ Surgical needles are intended to carry suture material through tissues with minimal trauma.
■ Needle points are sharp enough to penetrate tissues with minimal resistance.
　■ Rigid enough to resist bending, yet are flexible.
　■ Sterile and corrosion resistant.

KNOTS

The book *Surgical Knots and Suturing Techniques*[1] describes a variety of surgical knots. Only a few are used in dentistry. The type of knot used will depend on the specific procedure, the location of the incision, and the amount of stress the wound will endure. Surgeons and square knots are most frequently used in dentistry, with the square knot being the easiest and most reliable.

I. KNOT CHARACTERISTICS

■ A knot is tied as small as possible.
■ Completed knot needs to be firm to reduce slipping.

■ Excessive tension is avoided to prevent breakage or trauma to the tissue.

II. KNOT MANAGEMENT

■ Tie knots on facial aspect for easier access for removal.
■ Leave 2- to 3-mm suture "tail" to assist in locating at the time of removal.

III. SUTURING PROCEDURES

Many different patterns of suturing are used. Assisting and observing during the surgical procedure can be an educational experience for the dental hygienist.

　General types of sutures frequently used in the oral cavity are described here briefly.

A. Blanket

Each stitch is brought over a loop of the preceding one, thus forming a series of loops on one side of the incision and a series of stitches over the incision **(Figure 42-4A)**. It is also called a continuous lock. This stitch is used, for example, to approximate the gingival margins after alveolectomy.

B. Interrupted

Figure 42-4B shows a series of interrupted sutures.

C. Continuous Uninterrupted

A series of stitches tied at one or both ends. Examples of sutures that may be applied in a series are the sling or suspension and the blanket.

D. Circumferential

A term applied to a suture that encircles a tooth for suspension and retention of a flap.

E. Interdental

Where the flaps are on both the lingual and facial sides, interdental ligation joins the two by passing the suture through each interdental area **(Figure 42-4C)**. Coverage for the interdental area can be accomplished by coapting the edges of the papillae.

F. Sling or Suspension

■ When a flap is only on one side, facial or lingual, the sutures are passed through the interdental papilla, around the tooth, and into the adjacent papilla **(Figure 42-4D)**.
■ The suture is adjusted so that the flap can be positioned for correct healing.

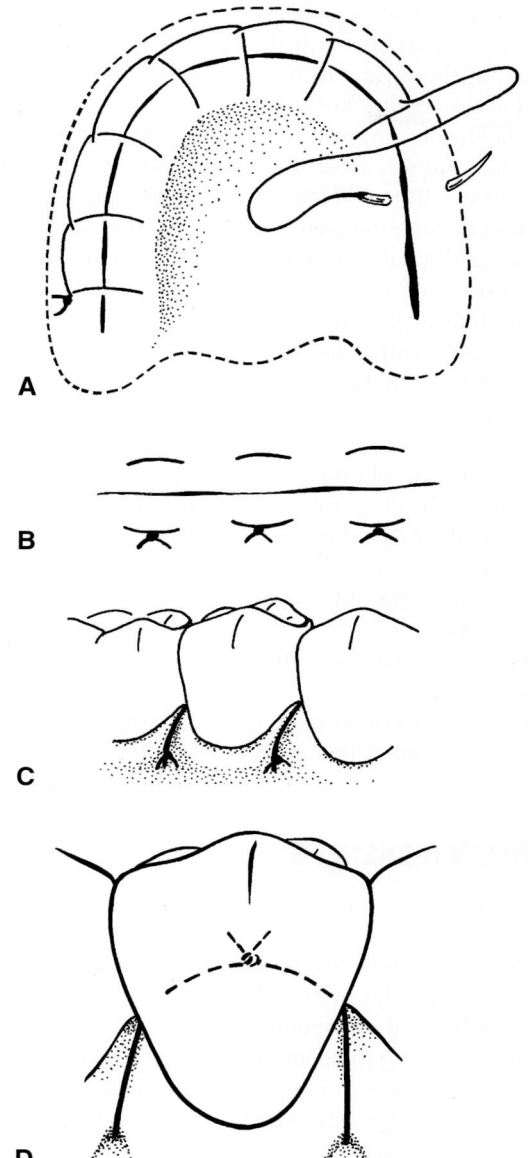

FIGURE 42-4 **Types of Sutures. (A)** Blanket stitch. **(B)** Interrupted, individual sutures. **(C)** Interdental individual sutures. **(D)** Sling or suspension suture tied on the lingual (*dotted line*).

PROCEDURE FOR SUTURE REMOVAL

Sutures are scheduled for removal 7 days after the surgery or no longer than 14 days to prevent tissue infection and promote healing. Chlorexidine rinsing is continued.

I. REVIEW PREVIOUS DOCUMENTATION

- Medical history
- Surgical procedures
- Patient reactions to healing
- Current surgery: number and type of sutures placed

II. SUPPLIES FOR SUTURE REMOVAL

- Mouth mirror
- Cotton pliers
- Curved sharp scissors with pointed tip (suture scissors)
- Gauze sponges
- Topical antiseptic
- Topical anesthetic: type that can be applied safely on an abraded or incompletely healed area to be used
- Cotton pellets
- Saliva ejector tip

III. PREPARATION OF PATIENT

A. Patient History Check

Suture removal can cause bacteremia.[2,3] High-risk patients may need antibiotic premedication for suture removal. Consultation with patient's physician is indicated.

B. Patient Examination

- Observe healing tissue around the suture(s).
- Record any deviations in color, size, shape of the tissue, adaptation of a flap, or coaptation of an incision healing by first intention.

C. Preparation of the Sutured Area

- Sutures placed without a dressing may have a crust over them at the time of removal. Apply a water-based gel with a cotton swab or pellet, and in a short time, the crust will soften and can be wiped away. If the suture is removed with the crust, it can cause unnecessary patient discomfort.
- Debride and rinse the area to remove debris particles, using a cotton-tipped applicator or a cotton pellet dipped in 3% peroxide. Follow with another rinse, or wipe gently with a gauze sponge.
- Place and adjust saliva ejector.
- Retract and pat area with gauze sponge to remove surface moisture.
- Swab area with topical antiseptic. Maintain retraction to prevent dilution.
- Apply topical anesthetic.

D. Retraction

- Three hands are really needed for efficient clinical procedure: one for retraction, one for cotton pliers to hold and remove the suture, and one for cutting the suture.
- When an assistant is not available, a cotton roll placed in the vestibule may provide enough retraction along with the finger rest and little finger of the nondominant hand holding the cotton pliers.

IV. STEPS FOR REMOVAL

The suture removal procedure described here and illustrated in **Figure 42-5** is for a single interrupted suture. The same principles apply for the ends and each segment of a continuous suture, wherever septic suture material can pass through the soft tissue.

1. Grasp the suture knot with the cotton plier held in the nondominant hand. Gently draw the suture up about 2 mm and hold with slight tension (**Figure 42-5A**). A finger rest is needed for control.

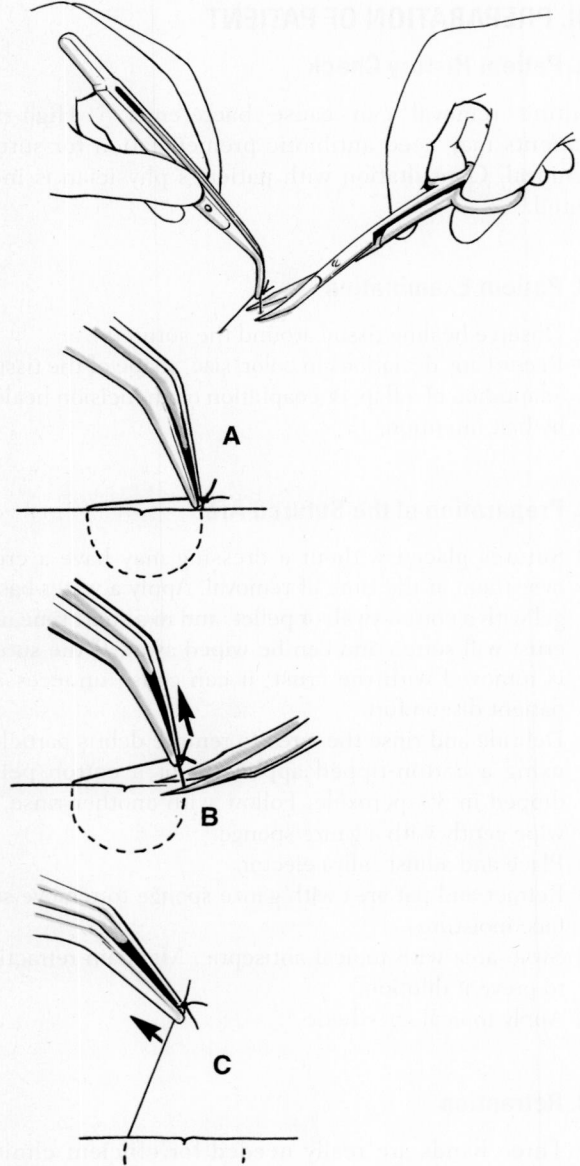

FIGURE 42-5 **Suture Removal. (A)** Suture grasped by pliers near the entrance into tissue. **(B))** Suture pulled gently up while scissor is inserted close to the tissue. Suture is cut in the part previously buried in the tissue. **(C)** Suture is held up for vertical removal. **(D)** Suture is pulled gently to bring it out on the side opposite from where it was cut. The object is to prevent the external part of the suture from passing through the tissue and introducing infectious material.

2. Insert tip of sharp scissors under the suture, slightly depress the tissue with the back of the scissor blade, and cut the suture in the part that was previously buried in the tissue (**Figure 42-5B**).
3. Hold knot end up with the cotton plier and pull gently to allow suture to exit through the side opposite where it was cut (**Figure 42-5C**). This prevents any part of the exposed contaminated segment of the suture from passing through the tissue and introducing infectious material.
4. Withdraw gently and steadily (**Figure 42-5D**).
5. Place each suture on a sponge for final counting, and proceed to remove the next suture.
6. Count the total number of sutures removed. The number of sutures removed should correspond to the number of sutures placed.
   - During healing, sutures can become loosened, misplaced, or occasionally covered by tissue.
   - The effect of a remaining suture can lead to infection and possible abscess around the suture left behind.
7. Apply gauze sponge with slight pressure on bleeding spots.
8. Request patient to close on the sponge while dressing is readied (when a dressing replacement is indicated).

V. SAFETY MEASURES

1. Count sutures; compare number placed with number removed.
2. Observe all tissue and record observations, noting any adverse reactions or bleeding.
3. Record patient's comments.
4. Sutures are not to be left longer than 7 to 14 days.
5. Use caution when removing a periodontal dressing to prevent tearing a suture that may have become embedded in the dressing.
6. Provide proper postappointment instructions both verbally and in writing.

PERIODONTAL DRESSINGS

A dressing may be placed over the surgical wound following periodontal surgery. Dressings are not used to cure the wound but to protect the tissue. Some clinicians use dressings for all surgical procedures, some occasionally, and some others rarely.

I. PURPOSES AND USES

- Provide protection for a surgical wound against external irritation or trauma.
- Help prevent posttreatment bleeding by securing initial clot formation.
- Support mobile teeth during healing.

- Assist in shaping or molding newly formed tissue, in securing a flap, or in immobilizing a graft.

II. CHARACTERISTICS OF ACCEPTABLE DRESSING MATERIAL

An acceptable dressing material has the following characteristics:

- Preparation, placement, and removal will take place with minimal discomfort to the patient.
- Material adheres to itself, teeth, and adjacent tissues, and maintains retention within interdental areas.
- Provides stability and flexibility to withstand distortion and displacement without fracturing.
- Is nontoxic and nonirritating to oral tissues.
- Possesses a smooth surface that will resist accumulation of dental biofilm.
- Will not traumatize tissue or stain teeth and restorative materials.
- Possesses an aesthetically acceptable appearance.

TYPES OF DRESSINGS

Traditionally, dressings were classified into two groups: those that contained eugenol and those that did not. With the development of new products, "noneugenol-containing" dressings have been reclassified into chemical-cure and visible light–cure materials. They are available as ready-mix, paste–paste, or paste–gel preparations.

I. ZINC OXIDE WITH EUGENOL DRESSING

A. Basic Ingredients

- *Powder:* zinc oxide, powdered rosin, and tannic acid. In the past, formulas used asbestos fiber as a binder. Because airborne asbestos is a recognized pulmonary health hazard, dental team members responsible for mixing periodontal dressings frequently may become overexposed. Asbestos fiber is no longer an acceptable ingredient of dressings.
- *Liquid:* eugenol, with oil (such as peanut or cottonseed) and thymol.

B. Examples

Well-known dressings are Ward's WondrPak and Kirkland Periodontal Pack.

C. Advantages

- *Consistency:* firm and heavy—provides support for tissues and flaps
- *Slow setting:* extended working time
- *Preparation and storage:* can be prepared in quantity and stored (frozen) in work-size pieces

D. Disadvantages

- *Taste:* sharp, unpleasant taste
- *Tissue reaction:* irritating; hypersensitivity reactions can occur. An allergic reaction to eugenol or rosin has been reported.
- *Consistency:* The dressing is hard, brittle, and breaks easily. Rough surface encourages dental biofilm retention.

II. CHEMICAL-CURED DRESSING

The ingredients of commercial products are trade secrets, but general information about available dressings can be found. Two examples of chemical-cured dressings are PerioCare™ and Coe-Pak™.

A. Basic Ingredients

- *PerioCare*™: Paste–gel mix
  - Paste: zinc oxide, magnesium oxide, calcium hydroxide, and vegetable oils
  - Gel: resins, fatty acids, ethyl cellulose, lanolin, calcium hydroxide
- *Coe-Pak*™: Paste–paste mix.
  - Base: rosin, cellulose, natural gums and waxes, fatty acid, chlorothymol, zinc acetate, and alcohol
  - Accelerator: zinc oxide, vegetable oil, chlorothymol, magnesium oxide, silica, synthetic resin, and coumarin
  - Coe-Pak™ is available in a hard and fast set.

B. Advantages

- *Consistency:* pliable, easy to place with light pressure
- *Smooth surface:* comfortable to patient; resists biofilm and debris deposits
- *Taste:* acceptable
- *Removal:* easy, often comes off in one piece

III. VISIBLE LIGHT–CURED DRESSING

Visible light–cured (VIC) dressing (*Barricaid*™) is available in a syringe for direct application or from a mixing pad for indirect application. The same light-curing unit used for composite restorations and sealants is also used for this curing process.

A. Basic Ingredients

Gel ingredients include polyester urethane dimethacrylate resin, silanated silica, visible light–cured photoinitiator and accelerator, stabilizer, and colorant.

B. Advantages

- *Color:* more like gingiva than most other dressings
- *Setting:* does not begin until activated by the light-curing unit (Exposure before placement is limited

as daylight in a room may begin the activation process.)

■ *Removal:* easy, often comes off in one piece

IV. COLLAGEN DRESSINGS

■ Absorbable collagen dressings used to promote wound healing.

■ Special use in periodontal surgery for a collagen patch dressing: for protection of graft sites of the palate during healing.

■ One form prepared in a bullet shape to use for deep biopsy sites.

■ Available in individual unit sterile packages.

■ Collagen dressing may be placed on clean moist or bleeding wounds.

CLINICAL APPLICATION

I. DRESSING PLACEMENT

A. General Procedure

For all types of dressing, follow the manufacturer's instructions. Each product has unique properties that require special handling.

B. Retention

1. Mold the dressing by pressing at each interproximal site. Do not extend over the height of contour of each tooth.
2. Border mold to prevent displacement by the tongue, cheeks, lips, or frena.
3. Check the occlusion and remove areas of contact.

II. CHARACTERISTICS OF A WELL-PLACED DRESSING (FIGURE 42-6)

Dressings placed in keeping with biologic principles contribute to healing and are tolerated more comfortably by the patient. A satisfactory dressing has the following characteristics:

■ Is secure and rigid. A movable dressing is an irritant and can promote bleeding.

■ Has as little bulk as possible, yet is bulky enough to give strength.

■ Locks mechanically interdentally and cannot be displaced by action of tongue, cheek, or lips.

■ Covers the entire surgical wound without unnecessary overextension.

■ Fills interdental area and adequately covers the treated area to discourage retention of debris and dental biofilm.

■ Possesses a smooth surface to prevent irritation to cheeks and lips while resisting debris and biofilm retention.

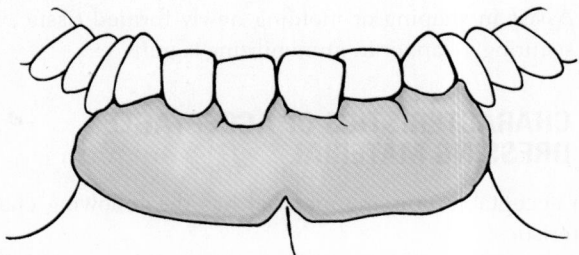

FIGURE 42-6 Periodontal Dressing. A dressing must cover the surgical wound without unnecessary overextension and fill interdental areas to lock the dressing between the teeth. It is molded in the vestibule and around frena to allow movement of the lips, cheeks, and tongue with no displacement of the dressing.

III. PATIENT DISMISSAL AND INSTRUCTIONS

■ Patient is not dismissed until bleeding or oozing from under a dressing has ceased.

■ Written instructions are necessary to reinforce those that are provided verbally. **Table 42-2** lists items to discuss with the patient before discharge.

DRESSING REMOVAL AND REPLACEMENT

During healing, epithelium covers a wound in 5 to 6 days, and complete restoration of epithelium and connective tissue can be expected by 21 days. The dressing may be left in place from 7 to 10 days, as determined by the surgeon.

Keep the following factors relative to dressings in mind:

■ If the dressing becomes dislodged before the removal appointment, the healing tissue needs to be evaluated.

■ When the dressing remains intact for 4 or 5 days, replacement may not be necessary.

■ When replacement is indicated, the dressing is replaced in its entirety rather than patched.

■ Instruct the patient to proceed with daily frequent biofilm removal and rinsing using an antimicrobial agent.

■ Schedule patient's follow-up appointment.

I. PATIENT EXAMINATION

■ Question patient about and record posttreatment effects or discomfort. Record length of time the dressing remained in place.

■ Examine the mucosa around the dressing and record its appearance.

II. PROCEDURE FOR REMOVAL

1. Insert a smooth instrument under the border of the dressing and gently apply lateral pressure.
2. Watch for sutures that can get lodged in the dressing. They may need to be cut.
3. Remove fragments of dressing gently with cotton pliers to avoid scratching the thin epithelial covering of the healing tissue.

TABLE 42-2	INSTRUCTIONS FOR POSTTREATMENT CARE	
FACTOR	**INSTRUCTIONS TO PATIENT**	**PURPOSE OF INSTRUCTION**
Information for the Patient About the Dressing	■ Dressing will protect the surgical wound. ■ Do not disturb the dressing. ■ Allow it to remain until the next appointment.	■ An informed patient is more likely to be more compliant.
Care During the First Few Hours	■ Dressing will not set for a few hours. ■ Do not eat anything that requires chewing. ■ Use only cool liquids. ■ Stay quiet and rest.	■ Dressing will become hard. ■ Do not touch it or disturb it.
Anesthesia	■ Be careful not to bite lip or cheek. ■ Avoid foods that require chewing until anesthesia has worn off.	■ Prevent trauma to lips and cheeks. ■ Rest and be quiet.
Discomfort After Anesthesia Wears Off	■ Fill the prescription and follow directions. ■ Do not take more than directed. ■ Avoid aspirin. ■ Call the dental office if pain persists.	■ Pain control ■ Aspirin can interfere with blood-clotting mechanism. ■ The patient will be more prepared to manage any postoperative discomfort when appropriately informed.
Ice Pack or Cold Compress	■ Apply every 30 min for 15 min; or 15 minutes on, then 15 min off. ■ Use as directed only.	■ Prevent swelling from edema
Bleeding	■ Slight bleeding within the first few hours is not unusual. ■ Do not suck on the area or use straws. ■ Blood clot is left alone.	■ When bleeding seems persistent or excessive, please call the dental office immediately.
Dressing Care and Retention	■ Avoid disturbing the dressing with the tongue or trying to clean under it. ■ Small particles may chip off, which is no problem unless sharp edges irritate the tongue or the dressing becomes loose. ■ Call the dentist if the entire dressing or a large portion falls off before the fifth day. ■ Rinse with a saline solution; rinse with chlorhexidine 0.12% morning and evening after brushing teeth.	■ Dressing is needed for wound protection. ■ Epithelium covers wound by fifth or sixth day in normal healing.
Use of Tobacco and Tobacco Products	■ Do not smoke; avoid all tobacco products. ■ A heavy smoker must make every effort to decrease quantity of tobacco used.	■ Heat and smoke irritate the gingiva and delay healing.
Rinsing	■ Do not rinse on the day of the treatment ■ Second day: Use saline solution made with 1/2 teaspoon (measured) in 1/2 cup of warm water every 2 to 3 h. ■ Begin chlorhexidine 0.12% b.i.d.	■ Might disturb blood clot. ■ Saline cleanses and aids healing.
Toothbrushing and Flossing	■ Continue to maintain optimal personal oral care in untreated areas. ■ Lightly brush occlusal surface over dressing material. ■ Use soft brush with water, and carefully clean film from dressing. ■ Clean the tongue.	■ Dental biofilm control essential to reduce the number of oral microorganisms ■ Odor and taste control ■ Oral sanitation

(continued)

TABLE 42-2	INSTRUCTIONS FOR POSTTREATMENT CARE (*Continued*)	
FACTOR	**INSTRUCTIONS TO PATIENT**	**PURPOSE OF INSTRUCTION**
Diet	■ Use highly nutritious foods for healing. ■ Follow the MyPlate guide (Figure 34-1, page 499) ■ Use soft-textured diet. ■ Avoid highly seasoned, spicy, hot, sticky, crunchy, and coarse foods.	■ Healing tissue requires a healthy diet and specific comfort foods. ■ Use soft foods to protect the dressing from breakage or displacement.
Mastication	■ Avoid foods that require excessive chewing. ■ Chew only on the untreated side. ■ Use ground meat or cut meat into small, bite-sized pieces.	■ To protect the dressing while it protects the surgical site.

4. Observe tissue and record its appearance. Note any deviations from normal healing that is expected within the number of days.
5. Use a scaler for removal of fragments adhering to tooth surfaces; use a curet for particles near the gingival margin. All calculus and roughness is eliminated to prevent new dental biofilm retention.
6. Syringe with a gentle stream of *warm* water. Warm diluted mouthrinse may soothe the traumatized area.

III. PROCEDURAL SUGGESTIONS FOR DRESSING REPLACEMENT

1. Use a topical anesthetic to prevent patient discomfort.
2. Use a soft dressing with minimal pressure during application.

IV. DENTAL BIOFILM CONTROL FOLLOW-UP

Biofilm control follow-up is essential after final dressing removal.

1. Use a soft brush on the treated area, paying careful attention to biofilm removal at the gingival margin. Use usual methods for all other areas of the mouth.
2. Increase intensity of care on the treated area each day, with a return to uncompromised oral hygiene procedures by 3 or 4 days.
3. Rinse with chlorhexidine 0.12% during the healing period twice daily and gently force liquid between the teeth.
4. Recommend a dentifrice with sodium fluoride for root caries prevention to be used regularly and indefinitely.
5. If the patient experiences postsurgical sensitivity, recommend a dentifrice containing a desensitizing agent. Other suggestions for coping with sensitivity may be found in Chapter 43, pages 683 to 685.

V. FOLLOW-UP

The return for observation of the surgical areas can be scheduled in 1 to 2 weeks, depending on the patient's progress and treatment planning.

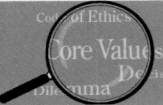 Everyday Ethics

Miss Lin arrived for a suture removal appointment with Marilyn, the dental hygienist, and immediately explains the discomfort she is feeling. When asked why she didn't come in sooner to have the area observed, she said it was so close to the removal appointment she might as well wait. Marilyn notes from the record that no dressing was placed. The area appeared inflamed, with a slight cyanotic appearance circumscribing the suture area. The patient prerinsed with a 0.12% chlorhexidine, and Marilyn began removing the sutures. Moderate bleeding and discomfort were present.

Upon removal, Marilyn noted that only three sutures could be found, but four had been placed. When she conferred with Dr. Wynn, the dentist, Marilyn was told to dismiss the patient and "prepare a prescription for an antibiotic to prevent an infection. Eventually the suture will be absorbed by body tissues."

Questions for Consideration

1. Given the sequence of events, what issues of ethical principles may be applied?
2. Does it seem clear that the patient understood the postoperative instructions? What suggestions do you have to improve communication?
3. Was the treatment provided within an acceptable standard of care for this patient? Which of the core values have application here? (See Section II Introduction, Table II-1, page 38).
4. Prepare examples of progress notes that you suggest Marilyn could write in the permanent record for Miss Lin's appointment. Which example would you prefer and why?

BOX 42-2 | **Sample Progress Note**

Patient presents with dressing fully intact between teeth 11 and 15. Topical anesthetic used. Tissue bled slightly during removal. Removed 4 sutures; checked with 4 sutures placed (see progress note of previous appointment). Patient responded well. Dr. examined and patient discharged with postremoval instructions.

Signed: _____, RDH Date: _____.

DOCUMENTATION

Detailed documentation is required at each patient visit. The appointment is dated and signed by the attending clinician.

1. At the time of surgical treatment include in the patient's permanent record at least the following:
   - Vital signs
   - Anesthesia: type, location, number and size of carpules, and patient response to anesthesia
   - Sutures: type, location, number placed
   - Dressing: specific type and area placed
   - Instructions to patient at dismissal
   - Signature by attending surgeon and surgical assistant

2. Dressing and suture removal
   - Tissue examination: tissue response
   - Patient comments of posttreatment effects, discomfort
   - Number of sutures removed: compare with number placed
   - Patient instruction for continued care
   - Signature by attending dental hygienist

3. A sample progress note may be reviewed in **Box 42-2**.

Factors To Teach The Patient

- Explanations for the items in **Table 42-2**.
- Care of the mouth during the period after treatment while wearing a periodontal dressing.
- Reasons for not using aspirin for pain relief.
- Inform and explain why tobacco use is detrimental and delays healing. Encourage cessation of use of all forms of tobacco.
- Discuss the importance of regular maintenance after treatment is formally over.

References

1. Giddings FD. *Book of surgical knots and suturing techniqes.* 3rd ed. Fort Collins (CO): Giddings Studio Publishing; 2009.
2. King RC, Crawford JJ, Small EW. Bacteremia following intraoral suture removal. *Oral Surg Oral Med Oral Pathol.* 1988 Jan;65(1): 23–7.
3. Giglio JA, Rowland RW, Dalton HP, Laskin DM. Suture removal-induced Bacteremia: a possible endocarditis risk. *J Am Dent Assoc.* 1992 Aug;123(1):65–70.

Dentin Hypersensitivity

TERRI S. I. TILLISS, RDH, MS, MA, PHD
JANIS G. KEATING, RDH, MA

Chapter Outline

HYPERSENSITIVITY DEFINED
I. Stimuli that Elicit Pain Reaction
II. Characteristics of Pain from Hypersensitivity

ETIOLOGY OF DENTIN HYPERSENSITIVITY
I. Anatomy of Tooth Structures
II. Mechanisms of Dentin Exposure
III. Hydrodynamic Theory
IV. Neural Activity

NATURAL DESENSITIZATION
I. Sclerosis of Dentin
II. Secondary Dentin
III. Smear Layer
IV. Calculus

PATIENTS AND THEIR PAIN
I. Patient Profile
II. The Pain Experience

DIFFERENTIAL DIAGNOSIS
I. Differentiation of Dentin Hypersensitivity Pain
II. Data Collection by Interview
III. Diagnostic Techniques and Tests

HYPERSENSITIVITY MANAGEMENT
I. Assessment Components
II. Educational Considerations
III. Treatment Hierarchy
IV. Reassessment

ORAL HYGIENE CARE AND TREATMENT INTERVENTIONS
I. Mechanisms of Desensitization
II. Behavioral Changes
III. Desensitizing Agents and Theorized Mode of Action
IV. Self-Applied Measures
V. Dental Professional Measures
VI. Additional Considerations

DOCUMENTATION

EVERYDAY ETHICS

FACTORS TO TEACH THE PATIENT

REFERENCES

The dental hygienist is often the first oral health professional to become aware of the presence of hypersensitive teeth when a patient presents for care. Individuals who suffer from hypersensitivity may be clearly uncomfortable during dental hygiene treatment, since exposure to stimuli such as a cold water spray and contact with metal instruments can elicit the pain of hypersensitive teeth.

- Episodes of hypersensitivity outside the dental setting are often reported.
- Activities of daily living such as eating or drinking cold foods or beverages may cause pain.
- Patients will ask the dental hygienist to explain the cause and treatment for the discomfort of dentin hypersensitivity.

- Hypersensitivity is often difficult to diagnose because the presenting symptoms can be confused with other types of dental pain with a different etiology.
- Management of hypersensitivity can be a challenge because there are numerous treatment approaches with varying degrees of efficacy.
- Knowledge of the predisposing factors that lead to gingival recession and to loss of enamel or cementum and dentin is necessary if patients are to prevent conditions that cause dentin hypersensitivity or exacerbate it.
- Box 43-1 provides definitions for terms relating to hypersensitivity.

BOX 43-1	Key Words

Dentin Hypersensitivity

Abfraction: wedge- or V-shaped cervical lesion created by the stresses of lateral or eccentric tooth movements during occlusal function, bruxing, or parafunctional activity resulting in enamel microfractures.

ADA: American Dental Association.

Burnishing: repeated rubbing of a tooth surface with a tooth pick or wooden stick.

Dentin hypersensitivity: transient pain arising from exposed dentin, typically in response to a variety of stimuli that cannot be explained as arising from any other form of dental defect or pathology and that subsides quickly when stimulus is removed.

FDA: Food and Drug Administration.

Hydrodynamic theory: currently accepted mechanism for pain impulse transmission to the pulp as a result of fluid movement within the dentin tubule, which stimulates the nerve endings at the dentinopulpal interface.

Intertubular dentin: dentin that is located between dentinal tubules.

Intratubular or peritubular dentin: increased deposition of minerals into tubules that become more mineralized with increasing age, resulting in thicker, sclerotic dentin.

Iontophoresis: a means of applying medications with the assistance of a small electric current to impregnate with ions of soluble salts; used in dentistry to transfer fluoride ions into the tooth.

Neural depolarization mechanism: reduction of the resting potential of the nerve membrane so that a nerve impulse is fired. At rest, the inner surface of the nerve fiber is negatively charged and impermeable to sodium ions. A stimulus temporarily alters the membrane, making it permeable so that potassium leaks out and sodium rushes into the nerve fiber. This mechanism is known as the sodium-potassium pump. The reversal of electrical charge, or **depolarization**, creates the nerve impulse. The process then reverses, and the membrane potential is restored, or **repolarized**.

Osmosis: the passage of fluids and solutions of lesser concentration through a selective membrane to one of greater solute concentration.

OTC: over the counter.

Patent: open, unobstructed.

Secondary dentin: dentin that is secreted slowly over time after root formation to "wall off" the pulp from fluid flow within dentinal tubules following a stimulus; results in narrower pulp chamber and root canals.

Smear layer: has been referred to as "grinding debris" from instrumentation or other devices that are applied to the tooth; consists of microcrystalline particles of cementum, dentin, tissue, and cellular debris; serves to plug tubule orifices.

Tertiary/reparative dentin: a type of dentin formed along the pulpal wall or root canal as a protective mechanism in response to trauma or irritation, such as caries or a traumatic cavity preparation.

HYPERSENSITIVITY DEFINED

There are specific characteristics associated with dentin hypersensitivity. One definitive characteristic is that the pain of hypersensitivity is elicited by a stimulus and alleviated on its removal. Numerous types of stimuli can lead to the pain response in individuals with exposed dentin surfaces.

I. STIMULI THAT ELICIT PAIN REACTION

- *Tactile* : contact with toothbrush and other oral hygiene devices, eating utensils, periodontal and dental instruments, and friction from prosthetic devices such as denture clasps.
- *Thermal*: temperature change caused by hot and cold foods and beverages, and cold air as it contacts the teeth. Cold is the most common stimulus for pain.
- *Evaporative*: dehydration of oral fluids as from high-volume evacuation or applying air to dry teeth during intraoral procedures.
- *Osmotic*: alteration of osmotic pressure in dentinal tubules due to isotonic solutions of sugar and salt.

- *Chemical*: acids in foods and beverages such as citrus fruits, condiments, spices, wine, and carbonated beverages; acids produced by acidogenic bacteria following carbohydrate exposure; acids from gastric regurgitation.

II. CHARACTERISTICS OF PAIN FROM HYPERSENSITIVITY

- Sharp, short, or transient pain of rapid onset.
- Cessation from pain on removal of stimulus.
- Presents as a chronic condition with acute episodes.
- Pain in response to a nonnoxious stimulus, one that would not normally cause pain or discomfort.
- Discomfort that cannot be ascribed to any other dental defect or pathology.[1]

ETIOLOGY OF DENTIN HYPERSENSITIVITY

A review of tooth anatomy facilitates an understanding of the mechanism of hypersensitivity.

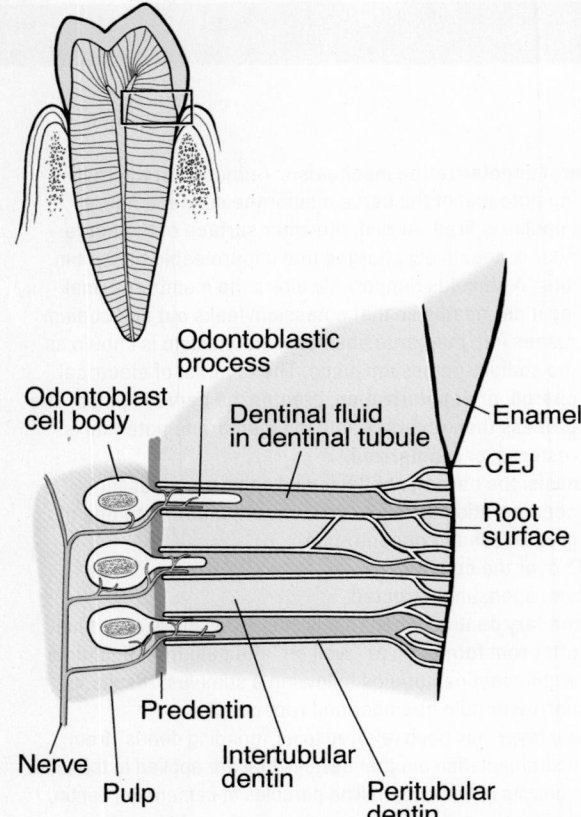

FIGURE 43-1 Relationship of Dentin Tubules and Pulpal Nerve Endings. Nerve endings from the pulp wrap themselves around the odontoblasts that extend only a short distance into the tubule. Fluid-filled dentin tubules transmit fluid disturbances through the mechanism known as hydraulic conductance.

I. ANATOMY OF TOOTH STRUCTURES

A. Dentin

■ The portion of the tooth covered by enamel on the crown and cementum on the root.
■ Composed of fluid-filled dentinal tubules that narrow and branch as they extend from the pulp to the dentinoenamel junction (**Figure 43-1**).
■ The only portions of the dentinal tubules that are innervated with nerve fiber endings from the pulp chamber are those closest to the pulp.
■ Tubules in sensitive areas are wider and more numerous.[2]

B. Pulp

■ Highly innervated with nerve cell fiber endings that extend just beyond the dentinopulpal interface of the dentinal tubules.[3]
■ Body portions of odontoblasts (dentin-producing cells) located adjacent to the pulp extend their processes from the dentinopulpal junction a short way into each dentinal tubule.

C. Nerves

■ Nerve fiber endings extend just beyond the dentinopulpal junction[4] and wind around the odontoblastic processes as shown in **Figure 43-1**.
■ Nerves react via the same neural depolarization mechanism (sodium potassium pump), which characterizes the response of any nerve to a stimulus.

II. MECHANISMS OF DENTIN EXPOSURE

■ The sequential events of gingival recession, loss of cementum or enamel, and subsequent dentin exposure can result in hypersensitivity, as seen in **Figure 43-2**.
■ Loss of enamel or cementum can expose dentin gradually or suddenly as in tooth fracture.
■ As a result of the lower mineral content of cementum and dentin compared with enamel, demineralization occurs more rapidly and at a lower critical pH.
■ Acute hypersensitivity may occur with sudden dentin exposure since gradual exposure allows for the development of natural desensitization mechanisms such as smear layer or sclerosis. After many years, secondary or reparative dentin may have formed, which also protects the pulp.

A. Factors Contributing to Gingival Recession and Subsequent Root Exposure

The occurrence of gingival recession has a multifactorial etiology.

■ Effects of improper oral hygiene self-care.
■ Use of a medium or hard filament toothbrush.
■ Frequent or aggressive use of the toothbrush and/or other oral hygiene devices.
■ An anatomically narrow zone of attached gingiva is more susceptible to abrasion that can lead to recession and subsequent cemental exposure.

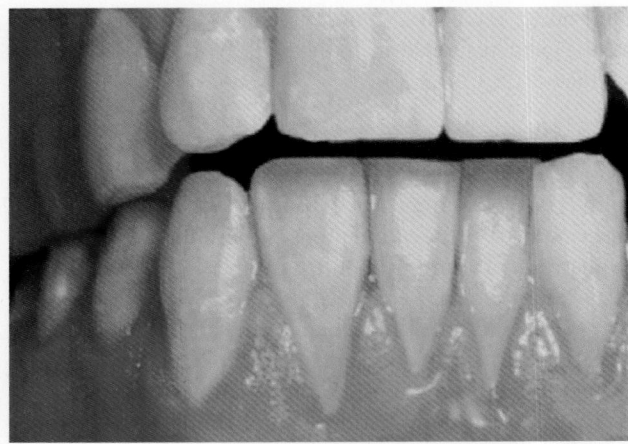

FIGURE 43-2 Gingival Recession of Mandibular Incisors. Note severe recession on the left central incisor and moderate recession on the right central and lateral incisors. If the thin cemental layer of the exposed root surface is lost, dentin hypersensitivity can develop.

- Facial orientation of one or more teeth may increase susceptibility to recession.
- A tight and short labial or buccal frenum attachment that pulls on gingival tissues during oral movement.
- Scaling and root debridement procedures that resolve tissue inflammation with the objective of tissue shrinkage.
- Subgingival instrumentation involving excessive scaling and debridement in shallow sulci.[5]
- Tissue destructive patterns of periodontal diseases, including periodontitis and necrotizing ulcerative gingivitis (NUG); junctional epithelium migrates apically in response to inflammatory factors leading to connective tissue breakdown and loss of periodontal attachment.
- Periodontal pocket reduction surgical procedures to reduce pocket depth can alter the architecture of gingival tissues.
- Periodontal surgery procedures such as crown lengthening, repositioning of gingival tissues, or tooth extractions that can affect gingival coverage of adjacent teeth.
- Orthodontic tooth movement may result in loss of periodontal attachment.
- Restorative procedures, such as crown preparation, that abrade marginal gingival tissues.
- Metal jewelry used in an oral piercing of the lip or tongue that repeatedly traumatizes the adjacent facial or lingual gingival tissue and may lead to gingival recession and bone loss around the involved teeth.

B. Factors Contributing to Loss of Enamel and Cementum

Loss of tooth structure rarely develops from a single cause but rather from a combination of contributing factors.

- Cementum at the cervical area is thin and easily abrades when exposed.
- Enamel and cementum do not meet at the cemento–enamel junction (CEJ) in about 10% of teeth, leaving an area of exposed dentin, as shown in Figure 16-2 (page 250).

C. Attrition and Abrasion

- Erosion from dietary acids, such as citrus fruits/juices, wine, and carbonated drinks.[6]
- Dietary acid intake results in an immediate drop in oral pH; after normal salivary neutralization, a physiologic pH of 7 re-establishes within minutes; differs from acid production that requires a longer recovery.
- Frequency of acid consumption is a critical factor; holding or "swilling" of acidic agents, holding low pH foods such as fruits against teeth, or continual snacking increases risk of developing erosion.
- Hypersensitivity has been suggested as a direct clinical outcome of erosion.[7]
- Brushing with a dentifrice immediately after consumption of acidic foods and beverages further abrades the already demineralizing tooth surface.[7]

- Gastric acids from conditions such as gastric reflux, morning sickness, or self-induced vomiting (bulimia) repeatedly expose teeth to a highly acidic environment.

D. Abfraction

- A wedge-shaped cervical lesion that is not well understood. The etiology of abfraction has been both supported and questioned.[8,9] Clinical evidence is lacking.[10,11]
- A cervical lesion caused by occlusal stresses or tooth flexure from bruxing.
- Microscopic portions of the enamel rods chip away from the cervical area of the tooth resulting in loss of tooth structure **(Figure 43-3)**.
- Lesion appears as a wedge- or V-shaped cervical notch.
- Is a co-factor with abrasion.

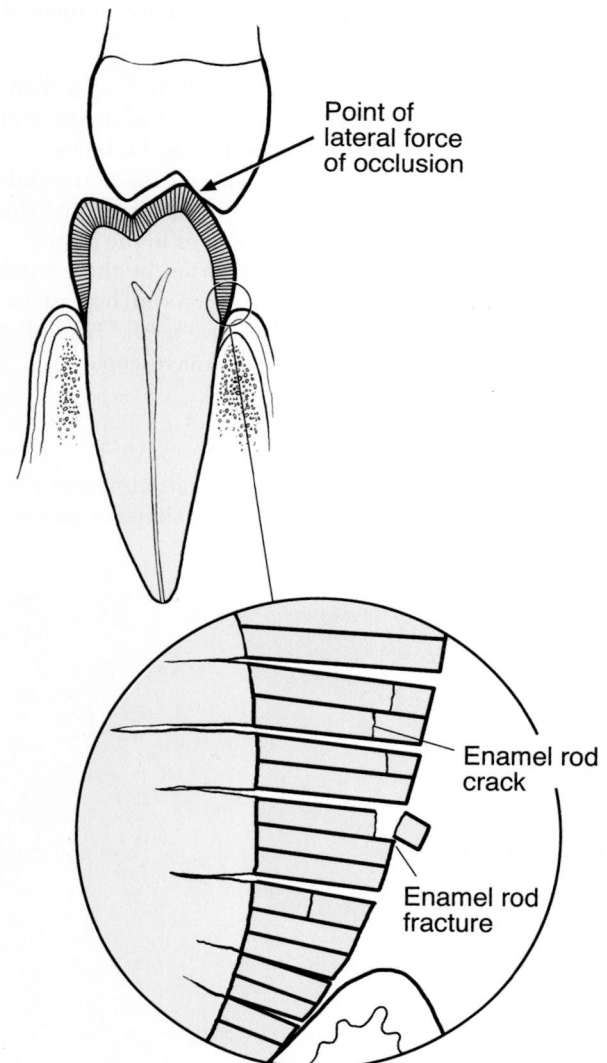

FIGURE 43-3 Process of Abfraction. Lateral occlusal forces stress the enamel rods at the cervical area, resulting in enamel rod fracture over time. In an advanced stage, a wedge- or V-shaped cervical lesion is visible. Although minute cracks in the enamel rods may not be clinically evident, the tooth can exhibit hypersensitivity.

E. Other Factors

- Crown preparation procedures that remove enamel or cementum can expose dentin at the cervical area.
- Instrumentation during scaling or root debridement procedures.
- Frequent or improper stain-removal techniques, where abrasive particles abrade and wear away the cementum and dentin.
- Root surface caries.
- Interproximal removal of enamel using a sandpaper disk or strip to create additional space for orthodontic movement of crowded teeth, also known as "enamel stripping."

III. HYDRODYNAMIC THEORY

Hydrodynamic theory is the currently accepted explanation for transmission of stimuli from the outer surface of the dentin to the pulp.

- Developed by Brannstrom in the 1960s,[12] who theorized that a stimulus at the outer aspect of dentin will cause fluid movement within the dentinal tubules.
- Fluid movement creates a pressure on the nerve endings within the dentinal tubule, which transmits the pain impulse by stimulating the nerves in the pulp.
- Credibility for this theory is supported by the greater number of widened dentin tubules seen with hypersensitive teeth compared with nonsensitive teeth.[2] **Figure 43-4** depicts open dentinal tubules at the microscopic level.

IV. NEURAL ACTIVITY

- Pain is registered by the depolarization/neural discharge mechanism that characterizes all nerve activity.

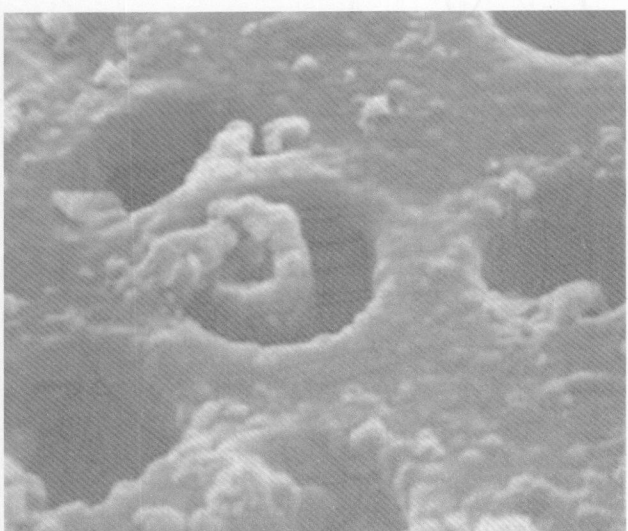

FIGURE 43-4 **Open Dentin Tubules.** Open dentin tubules as seen in dentin hypersensitivity surround a partially occluded tubule (center) viewed with scanning electron microscopy.

- The sodium-potassium pump is responsible for depolarizing the nerve as potassium leaves the nerve cell and sodium enters it.

NATURAL DESENSITIZATION

Hypersensitivity can decrease over time, even without treatment interventions, because nature provides several mechanisms that gradually reduce hypersensitivity. It can be a challenge to determine the true benefits of treatment regimens, since desensitization also occurs naturally. There are several mechanisms by which desensitization can occur naturally over time.

I. SCLEROSIS OF DENTIN

- Occurs by mineral deposition within tubules as a result of traumatic stimuli, such as attrition or dental caries.
- Creates a thicker, highly mineralized layer of peritubular dentin (deposited within the periphery of the tubules).
- Results in a smaller-diameter tubule that is less able to transmit stimuli through the dentinal fluid to the nerve fibers at the dentinopulpal interface.

II. SECONDARY DENTIN

- Deposited gradually on the floor and roof of the pulp chamber after teeth are fully developed. It is secreted more slowly than primary dentin that formed before tooth eruption; both types of dentin are created by odontoblasts.
- Creates a "walling off" effect between the dentinal tubules and the pulp to insulate the pulp from dentin fluid disturbances caused by a stimulus such as dental caries.
- As aging occurs, secondary dentin accumulates, resulting in a smaller pulp chamber with fewer nerve endings and less sensitivity.

III. SMEAR LAYER

- Consists of organic and inorganic debris that cover the dentinal surface and the tubules.[13]
- Accumulates following scaling and root instrumentation, use of toothpaste (abrasive particles), cutting with a bur, attrition, or abrasion (burnishing with a toothbrush or toothpick, or other device).
- Occludes the dentinal tubule orifices, forming a "smear plug" or a natural "bandage" that blocks stimuli.
- The nature of the smear layer changes constantly since it is subject to effects such as mechanical disruption from ultrasonic debridement, or dissolution from acid exposure.
- Smear layer may have a positive or negative effect. It is protective since loss of smear layer increases the risk

for hypersensitivity, but may interfere with reattach-ment of periodontal tissues.

IV. CALCULUS

- Provides a protective coating to shield exposed dentin from stimuli.
- Post debridement sensitivity can occur after removal of heavy calculus deposits; dentinal tubules may become exposed as calculus is removed.

PATIENTS AND THEIR PAIN

Individuals react differently to pain based on factors such as age, gender, situation and context, previous experiences, pain expectations, and other psychological and physiological parameters.

I. PATIENT PROFILE

The prevalence of hypersensitivity varies due to differences in the stimulus, and whether data are gathered by patient report or standardized clinical examination. Patient accounts may not represent true hypersensitivity since the pain can be confused with other conditions.

A. Prevalence of Hypersensitivity

- Hypersensitivity is experienced by 8–30% of the adult population.[14] Greatest incidence is reported at 20–40 years of age.[15]
- Higher prevalence has been reported in periodontally involved populations.[14]
- Incidence and severity declines with advancing age, due to the effects of sclerosis and secondary dentin.[16]
- Gingival recession and subsequent loss of enamel/cementum is more prevalent as one ages.[17,18] This same correlation with aging does not occur for dentin hypersensitivity.
- Hypersensitivity, when measured objectively, occurs equally between men and women[19] although women report more hypersensitivity than men.[20]

B. Teeth Affected

- Located most often at the cervical one-third of the facial surfaces of premolars and mandibular anterior teeth.[15,19]
- Can occur on any tooth exhibiting predisposing factors.

II. THE PAIN EXPERIENCE

A. Pain Perception

- Stimuli that affect the fluid flow within the dentinal tubules can activate the terminal nerve endings near to or surrounding the dentinal tubules; activation of these nerve fibers elicits the pain response.

- The degree of pain is not always in direct proportion to the amount of recession, the percentage of tooth structure loss, or to the quality or quantity of stimulus.
- Pain, a subjective phenomenon, is experienced differently by individuals. Many diverse variables such as stress, fatigue, and health beliefs can impact pain perception.

B. Impact of Pain

- Hypersensitivity can manifest as acute or chronic pain; acute pain may lead to anxiety, whereas chronic pain may be associated with depression.
- Stress may exacerbate the pain response.
- Persistent discomfort from dentin hypersensitivity may affect one's quality of life.

DIFFERENTIAL DIAGNOSIS

Etiology of pain can be systemic, pulpal, periapical, restorative, degenerative, or neoplastic. A differential diagnosis can rule out other causes of pain before treating for hypersensitivity. Skilled interviewing combined with diagnostic techniques and tests contributes to the differential diagnosis. Signs, symptoms, and specific clinical assessments utilized to differentiate a variety of conditions characterized as tooth pain are detailed in **Table 43-1**.

I. DIFFERENTIATION OF DENTIN HYPERSENSITIVITY PAIN

- Hypersensitivity pain elicited by a non-noxious stimulus, such as cold water, can mimic pain elicited by a noxious agent, such as cavitated dental caries.
- When the stimulus is removed the pain of hypersensitivity subsides.
- It is difficult to distinguish between the pain of hypersensitivity and other causes of dental pain when both are in the mild to moderate range. Many types of dental pain can be intensified by thermal, sweet, and sour stimuli.
- Chewing pain (occlusal pressure) can be indicative of pulpal pathology.
- Pulpal pain is severe, intermittent, and throbbing. The pain results from deep dental caries, pulpal inflammation, vertical tooth fracture, or infection, and may occur without provocation and persist after stimulus is removed.

II. DATA COLLECTION BY INTERVIEW

- Utilize direct, open-ended questions.
  A. Establish the location, degree of pain, onset/duration, source of stimulus, intensity, and relieving factors related to the painful response; patients may have difficulty characterizing the pain.
  B. Ask trigger questions as suggested in **Box 43-2** to elicit detailed information to characterize the pain and assist in the dental hygiene diagnosis.

TABLE 43-1	DIFFERENTIAL DIAGNOSIS OF TOOTH PAIN

CONDITION	SIGNS AND SYMPTOMS	CLINICAL ASSESSMENT
Dentinal hypersensitivity	Thermal, mechanical, evaporative, osmotic, chemical sensitivity Sharp, sudden, transient pain	Clinical examination: gingival recession and loss of tooth structure
Caries extending into dentin	Thermal sensitivity Pain on pressure Pain with sweets	Clinical examination, Radiographic examination
Pulpal caries	Thermal sensitivity Severe, intermittent or throbbing pain Pain on chewing	Clinical examination Radiographic examination
Fractured restoration	Thermal sensitivity Pain on pressure	Clinical examination
Fractured tooth	Thermal sensitivity Pain on pressure	Occlusal examination Transillumination
Recently placed restoration	Thermal sensitivity Pain on pressure	Dental history Clinical examination Occlusal examination
Occlusal trauma	Chemical sensitivity Thermal sensitivity Pain on pressure Mobility	Occlusal examination
Pulpitis	Severe, intermittent throbbing pain	Thermal and electric pulp tests Percussion
Sinus infection	"Nondescript" tooth pain Nasal congestion (drainage) Sinus pressure Headache	Clinical examination, including extraoral sinus palpation Radiographic examination
Galvanic pain	Sudden, sharp stabbing pain on tooth to tooth contact	Examination for contact between restoration of dissimilar nonprecious metals
Periodontal ligament inflammation	Pain on chewing	Percussion Clinical examination, including palpation for apical tenderness
Abfraction	"Cratered" areas of enamel or dentin at CEJ in the shape of a wedge- or V-shaped notch	Clinical examination Occlusal examination

- Establish rapport, combined with effective listening and counseling skills to develop treatment/management strategies.
- Record a thorough dental history, including pain chronology, nature, location, aggravating and alleviating factors, and history of dental treatment/restorations.

III. DIAGNOSTIC TECHNIQUES AND TESTS

When patients have difficulty in describing and localizing their pain, the following diagnostic techniques and tests can aid in differentiating among the numerous causes of tooth pain.

- Visual assessment of tooth integrity and surrounding tissues.
- Palpation of extra- and intraoral soft tissues.
- Evaluation of nasal congestion, drainage, or sinus expressed as tooth pain.
- Occlusal examination: Use marking paper to detect a premature contact or hyper-function following placement of a new restoration.
- Radiographic assessment to determine signs of pulpal pathology, vertical tooth fracture or other irregularities of the teeth or surrounding structures.
- Percussion: Use instrument handle to tap lightly on each tooth. A pain response may indicate pulpitis.

BOX 43-2	Trigger Questions for Data Collection

- Which tooth or teeth surfaces is/are sensitive?
- On a scale from 1 to 10, what is your pain intensity, with 10 being the most painful?
- How long does the pain last?
- What is the word that best describes the pain: sharp, dull, shooting, throbbing, persistent, constant, pressure, burning, intermittent?
- Does it hurt when you bite down (pressure)?
- On a scale from 1 to 10, how much does the pain impact your daily life?
- Is the pain stimulated by certain foods? Sweet? Sour? Acidic?
- Does sensitivity result from hot or cold food or beverages?
- Does discomfort stop immediately on removal of the painful stimuli, such as cold food or beverage, or does it linger?
- How effectively are you managing the stress in your life? Does stress impact your life? If so, how are you managing the stress?

- Mobility testing to detect trauma or periodontal pathology.
- Pain from biting pressure: Use a bite stick to assess pain from biting pressure indicative of tooth fracture.
- Transilluminate with a high-intensity focused light to enhance visualization of a cracked tooth; dye may also indicate a fracture line.
- Pulpal pathology can be assessed with thermal and electric pulp tests.

HYPERSENSITIVITY MANAGEMENT

When the differential diagnosis indicates dentinal hypersensitivity, the dental hygiene care plan includes further assessment and patient education combined with treatment interventions.

I. ASSESSMENT COMPONENTS

- Determine extent and severity of pain.
  A. Solicit a self-report of symptoms, including the eliciting stimuli.
  B. Quantify and record the baseline pain intensity using objective measures such as the Visual Analog Scale (VAS) and/or the Verbal Rating Scale (VRS), as described in Box 43-3.
- Help patient to explore improper oral hygiene self-care procedures that may contribute to loss of gingiva or tooth structure.
- Instruct patient in utilizing a diet analysis to assess the frequency of acidic food and beverage intake; correlate intake with timing of toothbrushing.
- Explore parafunctional habits, such as bruxing, that may contribute to abfraction.
- Have patient self-assess stress levels and explore stress-reduction efforts.

II. EDUCATIONAL CONSIDERATIONS

- Provide education regarding etiology and contributing factors. Explain the natural mechanisms for resolution of hypersensitivity over time.
- Discuss realistic self-care measures that the patient is likely to maintain. Involve the patient in technique demonstrations.

BOX 43-3	Subjective Pain Assessment Form

Name: _____
Date: _____
Teeth: _____

VAS—Visual Analog Scale
Please place an "X" on the line at a position between the two extremes to represent the level of pain that you experience.

No Discomfort |———————————————| Severe Discomfort

VRS—Verbal Rating Scale
Please describe the pain you experience on a scale from 0 to 3:

0 = No discomfort/pain, but aware of stimulus

1 = Slight discomfort/pain

2 = Significant discomfort/pain

3 = Significant discomfort/pain that lasted more than 10 seconds

- Minimal application time
- Easy application procedure
- Does not endanger the soft tissues
- Inexpensive
- Requires few dental appointments
- Does not cause pulpal irritation or pain
- Rapid and lasting effect
- Causes no staining
- Consistently effective
- Acceptable taste

- Utilize effective communication and motivational interviewing skills to increase compliance and to decrease patient anxiety. (See Chapter 3, Motivational Interviewing, page 29).

III. TREATMENT HIERARCHY

- There are two basic treatment goals:
  - Pain relief.
  - Modification or elimination of contributing factors.
- Address mild to moderate pain with conservative approaches or agents; more severe pain requires an aggressive approach.
- Sequence treatment approaches from the most conservative and least invasive measures to more aggressive modalities.
- Prognosis of pain resolution is difficult to predict due to variable success with different treatment options among individuals.
  - Historically, a vast array of treatment approaches have been utilized with varying degrees of success; no one best method has been identified.
  - A trial-and-error approach may be necessary until a particular treatment option is found to be most effective.
  - Classical characteristics of an ideal desensitizing agent are still relevant today. They are listed in **Box 43-4** and can be useful evaluation criteria when selecting a desensitizing agent.
- Treatment options that include both self-care measures and professional interventions have synergistic effects with the same objective of reducing hypersensitivity.

IV. REASSESSMENT

- Evaluate treatment interventions.
  - Allow sufficient time to elapse (2–4 weeks) to evaluate effectiveness of treatment recommendations; assess and reinforce behavioral changes.
  - Repeat the VAS and/or the VRS to compare changes in pain perceptions from baseline.

- Persistent pain may require systematic use and comparison of pain relief from various desensitizing interventions and agents.

ORAL HYGIENE CARE AND TREATMENT INTERVENTIONS

I. MECHANISMS OF DESENSITIZATION

Desensitization agents and self-care measures disrupt the pain transmission as described by the hydrodynamic theory in one of two ways:[21]

- Prevent nerve depolarization that interrupts the neural transmission to the pulp. This physiologic process forms the basis for potassium-based products.[22]
- Prevent a stimulus from moving the tubule fluid by occlusion of dentin tubule orifices or reduction in diameter of the tubule lumen.

II. BEHAVIORAL CHANGES

Encourage habits that allow tubules to remain occluded or that occlude patent tubules.

- Help patient to commit to appropriate oral hygiene and dietary habits before or in conjunction with self-applied or professionally applied desensitizing agents. Use a motivational interviewing approach when possible.
- Educate the patient that it may take 2–4 weeks to decrease sensitivity, with some products.

A. Dietary Modifications

- Have patient analyze acidic food and beverage habits that incite pain due to dissolution of the smear layer that had covered open dentinal tubules.[23] Examples include citrus fruits and juices, acidic soda/cola beverages, sharp flavors and spices, pickled foods, wines, and ciders.
- Help patient identify patterns when brushing is sequenced immediately after consuming acidic foods and beverages to eliminate the combined effects of erosion and abrasion, which can accelerate tooth structure loss.[24]
- Explore use of proprietary mouthrinses with patient since many have acidic formulations that can contribute to erosion.
- Provide professional treatment referrals for patients with eating disorders or systemic conditions that repeatedly create an acidic oral environment such as bulimia or acid reflux.
- The acidic environment created by bulimia and acid reflux can be neutralized by rinsing with water (particularly fluoridated water) or an alkaline rinse such as bicarbonate of soda in water.

■ Counsel patient to eliminate extremes of hot and cold foods and beverages to avoid discomfort.

B. Dental Biofilm Control

■ In the presence of dental biofilm, the dentinal tubule orifices increase to three times the original size; with reestablishment of biofilm control measures, there is a 20% decrease in size.[25]
■ The presence/amount of dental biofilm on exposed root surfaces does not directly correlate with the degree of dentin sensitivity,[16] suggesting that biofilm composition maybe a factor.

C. Toothbrush Type and Technique

■ Use of a soft or ultra-soft toothbrush and focused brushing on one or two teeth at a time.
■ Help patient analyze toothbrushing technique to avoid long horizontal strokes over several teeth to prevent further recession and loss of tooth structure.
■ Identify sequencing for brushing various areas of the mouth and adjust by beginning in least sensitive areas and ending with more sensitive areas because the toothbrush filaments are stiffer and brushing is more aggressive in the initial phases of brushing.
■ Explore option of brushing with the non-dominant hand, if dexterity permits; nondominant hand exerts less pressure than the dominant hand.
■ Help patient investigate current toothbrush grip. Adjust to a modified pen grasp rather than a traditional palm grasp to reduce the amount of pressure applied.
■ Explore receptivity to use of a power toothbrush because it removes dental biofilm effectively with less than half the pressure of a manual toothbrush; an individual using a manual toothbrush typically exerts 200–400 grams of pressure, while a power toothbrush user usually exert 70–150 grams of pressure.[26] Some power toothbrushes have a self-limiting mechanism to reduce filament action if too much pressure is applied.
■ Promote dental biofilm control measures that are meticulous, yet gentle, and do not contribute to abrasion of hard or soft tissues are recommended and demonstrated.

D. Burnishing

A wooden toothpick is repeatedly rubbed over the root surface with moderate pressure.

■ The toothpick may be dipped into fluoride dentifrice or other desensitization agents, although it is the burnishing process that forms a smear layer over dentin, occluding the dentinal tubule orifices.[27]

Figure 43-5 shows placement of a toothpick.

■ May stimulate the production of secondary or reparative dentin, although this is a very slow process.

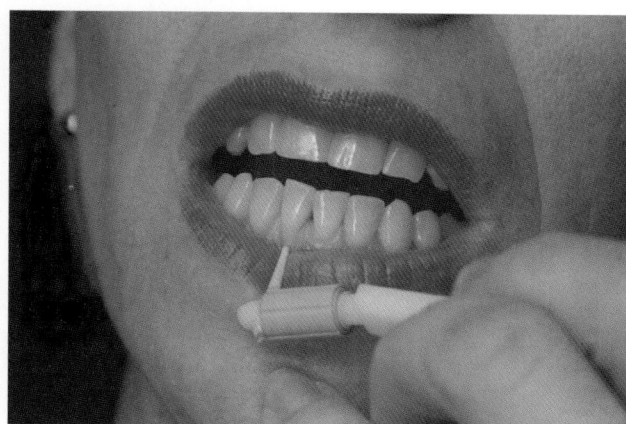

FIGURE 43-5 Burnishing Sensitive Root Surface. A small amount of a fluoride agent or fluoride dentifrice can be burnished into the sensitive area with a toothpick or wooden point. Moderate pressure with a "rubbing" or circular stroke is applied. A toothpick holder facilitates effective use of a toothpick to burnish an exposed root surface.

E. Eliminate Parafunctional Habits

■ Help patient assess bruxing and clenching behaviors and whether additional treatment is indicated.
■ Determine need for occlusal adjustments to eliminate abfractive forces.
■ Coach patient to monitor occurrence of subconscious parafunctional behaviors and levels of stress. Identify indications for stress reduction protocols.

III. DESENSITIZING AGENTS AND THEORIZED MODE OF ACTION

A. Potassium Salts

■ Formulations containing potassium chloride, potassium nitrate, potassium citrate, or potassium oxalate reduce depolarization of the nerve cell membrane and transmission of the nerve impulse.[22]
■ Potassium nitrate dentifrices containing fluoride are widely used[22] and readily available over the counter.

B. Fluorides

■ Precipitate calcium fluoride (CaF_2) crystals within the dentinal tubule to decrease the lumen diameter.[24]
■ Create a barrier by precipitating CaF_2 at the exposed dentin surface,[28] to block open dental tubules.

C. Oxalates

■ Block open dental tubules.[29]
■ Oxalate salts such as potassium oxalate and ferric oxalate precipitate calcium oxalate crystals to decrease the lumen diameter.[29]

D. Gluteraldehyde

■ Coagulates proteins and amino acids within the dentinal tubule to decrease the dentinal tubule lumen diameter.[29]

■ Can be combined with HEMA, a hydrophilic resin, which seals tubules.[29]

■ Creates calcium crystals within the dentinal tubule to decrease the lumen diameter.[30]

E. Calcium Phosphate Technology

■ Advocated for use as a caries control agent to reduce demineralization and increase remineralization by releasing calcium and phosphate ions into saliva for deposition of new tooth mineral (hydroxyapatite)[31] Most likely to be effective for those with poor salivary flow and consequent deficient calcium phosphate levels.[32]

■ These agents that support remineralization could lessen dentinal hypersensitivity by occluding dentinal tubule openings. Most studies in support of calcium phosphate technology are animal model, *in vitro*, or *in situ* designed studies. One *in vivo* study found that there was a reduction in bleaching-induced sensitivity at days 5 and 14 when ACP was added to a bleaching gel.[33] Randomized controlled trials that adhere to clinical research standards are still indicated for calcium phosphate technologies.[34]

■ Amorphous calcium phosphate (ACP)
  ■ Theorized to plug dentinal tubules with calcium and phosphate; promotes an ACP reservoir within the saliva.
  ■ Enhances fluoride delivery in calcium and phosphate-deficient saliva[32]
  ■ Reported to remineralize acid erosion and abrasion, improve enamel luster and surface smoothness, reduce hypersensitivity[32]

■ Calcium sodium phosphosilicate (CSP) (NovaMin®)
  ■ Contains sodium and silica in addition to calcium and phosphorous.
  ■ Delivered in solid bioactive glass particles that react in the presence of saliva and water to release calcium and phosphate ions to create a calcium phosphate layer that crystallizes to hydroxyapatite.
  ■ Reacts with saliva; sodium buffers the acid, and calcium and phosphate saturate saliva to fill demineralized areas with new hydroxyapatite
  ■ Claims include remineralizing enamel and dentin, positive impact on acid erosion and abrasion, a bacteriocidal effect, and reduction in hypersensitivity
  ■ A clinical trial comparing a CSP and a potassium nitrate toothpaste, using a visual analogue scale (VAS) found the CSP paste to be significantly better at reducing dentin hypersensitivity.[35]

■ Casein phosphopeptide-amorphous calcium phosphate (CPP-ACP or Recaldent™)
  ■ CPP is a milk-derived protein that stabilizes ACP and allows it to be released during acidic challenges.
  ■ Benefits are described as remineralization of acid erosion and caries inhibition by promoting fluoride uptake in plaque biofilm.

F. Arginine and Calcium Carbonate Technology

■ This desensitization approach occludes the dentinal tubules utilizing arginine, a naturally occurring amino acid, bicarbonate (pH buffer), and calcium carbonate.

■ Marketed as a prophylaxis paste to be applied before instrumentation, using a slow speed handpiece with a rubber cup and moderate pressure.

■ Randomized controlled trials that adhere to clinical research standards are still necessary.

IV. SELF-APPLIED MEASURES

A. Dentifrices

■ 5% potassium nitrate and fluorides separately or in combination are the active desensitizing agents in OTC sensitivity-reducing dentifrices. Studies have suggested that some of the desensitizing effects of dentifrices may be due to the blocking action of the abrasive particles.[22]

■ Tartar control dentifrices may contribute to increased tooth sensitivity for some individuals, although the mechanism is unclear.

■ Prescription strength dentifrices are available containing highly concentrated fluoride (5,000 ppm fluoride) combined with an abrasive to facilitate extrinsic stain control. This formulation is also available with the addition of potassium nitrate.

B. Gels

■ 5,000 ppm fluoride gels (available by prescription) are brushed on for generalized hypersensitivity or can be burnished into localized areas of sensitivity.

■ Contain no abrasive agents for biofilm and stain control.

■ Can be self-applied with custom or commercially available fluoride or bleaching trays.

V. DENTAL PROFESSIONAL MEASURES

A. Tray Delivered Fluoride Agents

■ Sodium or stannous fluoride is applied utilizing a tray delivery system.

■ Select trays of adequate height and fill with sufficient fluoride agent to cover the cervical areas of the tooth.

B. Fluoride Varnishes

■ 5% sodium fluoride varnish maintains prolonged contact with the tooth surface by serving as a reservoir to release fluoride ions in response to pH changes in saliva and biofilm.[36]

■ Does not require a dry tooth surface, which is advantageous since drying the tooth can be a painful procedure for a patient with dentin hypersensitivity.

- A microbrush is used to apply the varnish to the exposed dentin surface.
- Oral hygiene self-care is avoided for several hours to allow the fluoride to stay in contact with the tooth surface for as long as possible, preferably overnight.

C. 5% Gluteraldehyde

- Formulation can be applied to the affected tooth surface with the use of a microbrush.
- Cotton roll isolation is used to prevent excess flow into soft tissues since contact with soft tissues may cause gingival irritation.

D. Oxalates

- Oxalate preparations are applied (burnished) to a dried tooth surface.
- They may provide immediate and short-, rather than long-term relief.

E. Unfilled or Partially Filled Resins

- Used to cover patent dentinal tubules.
- Resins are applied following an acid etch step that may remove the smear layer, with the potential for discomfort. Local anesthetic may be necessary for this procedure.
- The tooth surface must be dehydrated before resin application, which can create discomfort necessitating the use of local anesthesia.

F. Dentin-Bonding Agents

- Obturation of the tubule opening; does not require use of acid etch or dehydration; a single application may protect against further erosion for 3–6 months
- Methylmethacrylate polymer is a common dentin sealer.

G. Composite/Glass Ionomer

- Glass ionomer can be placed in the presence of moisture so drying the tooth is not necessary.
- Preparation of the tooth surface is required for retention of the restoration.

H. Soft Tissue Grafts

- Surgical placement of soft tissue grafts can cover a sensitive dentinal surface.
- Results are somewhat unpredictable.

I. Iontophoresis

- A low-voltage electric current utilizing electricity to impregnate ions into the tooth; used most often in conjunction with fluoride products.

- Iontophoresis has been shown to enhance desensitization beyond the effect of the agent alone.[37]

J. Lasers

- Four types of lasers have been used to treat hypersensitivity. A review of 31 published papers using the four types of lasers demonstrated from 5 to 100% effectiveness.[38]
- Lasers can close previously open dentinal tubules and alter the tubules' contents through coagulation protein precipitation or the creation of insoluble calcium complexes.[39]
- Long-term, *in vivo* studies are needed to establish safety and efficacy of laser use for dentin hypersensitivity. The FDA has not approved these devices for this therapeutic modality.

VI. ADDITIONAL CONSIDERATIONS

A. Periodontal Debridement Considerations

1. *Preprocedure*
   - Explain potential for sensitivity resulting from calculus removal and/or instrumentation of teeth with areas of exposed cementum or dentin.
   - Patients are likely to respond more favorably to treatment when they know what might occur.
   - During scaling and root planing procedures:
   - When multiple teeth in the same treatment area are hypersensitive, local anesthetics and/or nitrous oxide analgesia can be utilized.
   - Desensitizing agents that are marketed for immediate relief from severe hypersensitivity can be used.
2. *Postprocedure*
   - Professional applied desensitization agents can be used.
   - Patient is instructed in daily oral health behavior changes and use of self-applied desensitizing agents.

B. New Developments

- The search for the ideal desensitizing agent is ongoing.
- Keeping abreast of evidence-based scientific research is necessary as new products are developed; *in vivo* research protocols are needed to support clinical application.

C. Tooth Whitening–Induced Sensitivity

Tooth whitening agents, such as carbamide peroxide, may contribute to increased dentinal hypersensitivity (Table 45-3, page 715).

- Thought to be due to the by-products of 10% carbamide peroxide (3% hydrogen peroxide and 7% urea) readily passing through the enamel and dentin into the pulp, which occurs in a matter of minutes. A reversible pulpitis is caused from the dentin fluid flow and pulpal contact of the material, which changes the osmolarity, without apparent harm to the pulp.[40]

- Hypersensitivity may dissipate over time, lasting from a few days to several months.
- Exposed dentin and preexisting dentin hypersensitivity increase risk for hypersensitivity secondary to whitening.
- Sensitivity can last from a few days to several months.
- Some whitening products contain fluoride or potassium nitrate to minimize or prevent sensitivity.
- Recommendations to prevent or reduce tooth whitening–induced sensitivity:
  - Use of a potassium nitrate, fluoride, or other desensitization product before, or concurrently with whitening. Home-use whitening products are usually less concentrated than professionally applied in-office treatment options, with less risk of development of hypersensitivity.
  - Allow for a "recovery period" between whitening sessions during which desensitizing agents can be used. Decrease frequency of use by whitening every second or third day.

DOCUMENTATION

The permanent record for a patient with a history of tooth sensitivity needs to include at least the following information:

- Medical and dental history, vital signs, extra- and intraoral examinations, consultations, and individual

BOX 43-5	Example Progress Note

Patient complains of pain when eating/drinking cold foods/beverages. There is facial gingival recession of 1–2 mm throughout the mandible, although discomfort seems to be focused bilaterally at the facial of the mandibular premolar areas. Advised patient to rinse with fluoridated water thoroughly immediately after her morning glass of grapefruit juice and to avoid brushing immediately after ingesting citrus fruits or beverages anytime. Recommended purchase and use of an OTC potassium nitrate-containing dentifrice. Explained that relief from the dentifrice can take between 2–4 weeks. Applied fluoride varnish to exposed root surfaces. Advised to re-contact the office if pain persists or worsens.

Signed: _____, RDH Date: _____.

progress notes for each appointment and maintenance appointments.
- For dentin hypersensitivity: identification of teeth involved, differential diagnosis, and all treatments, along with patient instruction for ideal oral self-care, diet and other recommendations for prevention.
- Outcomes and post-treatment directions.
- An example of a progress note for the patient with hypersensitive dentin may be reviewed in **Box 43-5**.

Everyday Ethics

Marcy, the dental hygienist, practices with Dr. Goldman, who only schedules time to examine a patient at alternate dental hygiene visits unless requested for special needs. Mrs. Stuart arrives for her dental hygiene appointment but is not scheduled to see Dr. Goldman until her next visit. She is complaining of discomfort "on the lower back teeth" when she chews and when she eats or drinks something cold. The pain may last up to an hour.

When she completes the scaling and debridement, Marcy determines that Dr. Goldman is running behind schedule. She knows it will be difficult to get him to come to her treatment room to examine her patient in a timely manner and that will make her late for her next patient, who is due any minute. Marcy gives Mrs. Stuart a sample of desensitizing toothpaste and suggests they will see how it is at the next appointment. Marcy then advised Mrs. Stuart to "Call if it gives you more trouble." The patient is not classified as having a periodontal condition, and for dental caries she is considered low to medium risk. Her next visit will be in 4 months.

Questions for Consideration

1. How do each of the core values (Table II-1 page 38) have application in this event? Does the question of informed consent enter this discussion? Explain why or why not.
2. What ethical issues can arise if Marcy and Dr. Goldman do not take time during this appointment to assess Mrs. Stuart's situation completely and establish a differential diagnosis?
3. Answer the questions provided in the "questioning" column of Table V-1 (page 362) to determine at least two ethical alternative actions Marcy could have taken.

Factors To Teach The Patient

- Etiology of gingival recession.
- Activities and habits that may contribute to dentin hypersensitivity.
- Mechanisms of dentin tubule exposure, which can allow various stimuli to trigger pain response.
- Natural desensitization mechanisms that may improve sensitivity over time.
- Appropriate oral hygiene self-care techniques, such as using a soft toothbrush and avoiding a vigorous brushing technique that may contribute to gingival recession and subsequent abrasion of root surfaces.
- Connection between an acidic diet and dentin sensitivity; need to eliminate specific foods and beverages that can cause sensitivity.
- Toothbrushing is not recommended immediately after consumption of acidic foods or beverages.
- The challenges of managing hypersensitivity, hierarchy of treatment measures, and variability in resolution of pain.

References

1. Addy M. Etiology and clinical implications of dentine hypersensitivity. *Dent Clin North Am.* 1990 Jul;34(3):503–14.
2. Absi EG, Addy M, Adams D. Dentine hypersensitivity. The development and evaluation of a replica technique to study sensitive and non-sensitive cervical dentine. *J Clin Periodontol.* 1989 Mar;16(3):190–5.
3. Frank RM. Attachment sites between the odontoblast process and the intradentinal nerve fibre. *Arch Oral Biol.* 1968 Jul;13(7):833–4.
4. Thomas HF, Carella P. Correlation of scanning and transmission electron microscopy of human dentinal tubules. *Arch Oral Biol.* 1984;29(8):641–6.
5. Dufour LA, Bissell HS. Periodontal attachment loss induced by mechanical subgingival instrumentation in shallow sulci. *J Dent Hyg.* 2002 Summer;76(3):207–12.
6. Prati C, Montebugnoli L, Supp P, Valdre G, Mongiorgi R. Permeability and morphology of dentin after erosion induced by acidic drinks. *J Periodontol.* 2002;74(4):428–36.
7. Absi EG, Addy M, Adams D. Dentine hypersensitivity. The effect of toothbrushing and dietary compounds on dentine in vitro. *J Oral Rehabil.* 1992 March;19(2):101–110.
8. Staninec M, Nalla RK, Hilton JF, Ritchie RO, Watanabe LG, Nonomura G, Marshall GW, Marshall SJ. Dentin erosion simulation by cantilever beam fatigue and pH change. *J Dent Res.* 2005 Apr;84(4):371–5.
9. Litonjua LA, Andreana S, Bush OJ, Tobias TS, Cohen RE. Wedged cervical lesions produced by toothbrushing. *Am J Dent.* 2004 Aug;17(4):237–40.
10. Estafan A, Furnari PC, Goldstein G, Hittelman E. In vivo correlation of noncarious cervical lesions and occlusal wear. *J Prosthet Dent.* 2005 Mar;93(3):221–6.
11. Bartlett DW, Shah P. A critical review of non-carious cervical (wear) lesions and the role of abfraction, erosion, and abrasion. *J Dent Res.* 2006 Apr;85(4):306–12.
12. Brannstrom M, Linden LA, Astrom A. The hydrodynamics of the dental tubule and of pulp fluid. A discussion of its significance in relation to dentinal sensitivit. *Caries Res.* 1967;1(4):310–7.
13. Eldarrat AH, High AS, Kale GM. In vitro analysis of "smear layer" on human dentine using ac-impedance spectroscopy. *J Dent.* 2004 Sep;32(7):547–54.
14. Taani Q, Awartani F. Clinical evaluation of cervical dentin sensitivity (CDS) in patients attending general dental clinics and periodontal specialty clinics (PSC). *J Clin Periodontol.* 2002 Feb;29(2):118–22.
15. Gillam DG, Aris A, Bulman JS, Newman HN, Ley F. Dentine hypersensitivity in subjects recruited for clinical trials: clinical evaluation, prevalence and intra-oral distribution. *J Oral Rehabil.* 2002 Mar;29(3):226–31.
16. Addy M, Pearce N. Aetological, predisposing and environmental factors in dentine hypersensitivity. *Arch Oral Biol.* 1994;39 Suppl:33S–38S.
17. Beck JD, Hunt RJ, Hand JS, Field HM. Prevalence of root and coronal caries in a non-institutionalized older population. *J Am Dent Assoc.* 1985 Dec;111(6):964–7.
18. Bissada NF. Symptomology and clinical features of hypersensitive teeth. *Arch Oral Biol.* 1994;39(Suppl):31S–32S.
19. Fischer C, Fischer RG, Wennberg A. Prevalence and distribution of cervical dentine hypersensitivity in a population in Rio De Janeiro, Brazil. *J Dent.* 1992 Oct;20(5):272–6.
20. Zakrzewska JM. Women as dental patients: are there any gender differences? *Int Dent J.* 1996 Dec;46(6):548–57.
21. Addy M. Dentine hypersensitivity: new perspectives on an old problem. *Int Dent J.* 2002;52(Suppl 1):367.
22. Orchardson R, Gillam DG. The efficacy of potassium salts as agents for treating dentin hypersensitivity. *J Orofac Pain.* 2000 Winter;14(1):9–19.
23. Correa FO, Sampaio JE, Rossa C, Orrico SR. Influence of natural fruit juices in removing the smear layer from root surfaces—an in-vitro study. *J Can Dent Assoc.* 2004 Nov;70(10):697–702.
24. Orchardson R, Gilla DC. Managing dentin hypersensitivity. *J Am Dent Assoc.* 2006 July;137(7):990–8.
25. Kawasaki A, Ishikawa K, Sug T, Shimizu H, Suzuki K, Matsuo T, Ebisu S. Effects of plaque control on the patency and occlusion of dentine tubules in situ. *J Oral Rehabil.* 2001 May;28(5):439–49.
26. Van Der Weijden GA, Timmerman MF, Reijerse E, Snoek CM, Van Der Velden U. Toothbrushing force in relation to plaque removal. *J Clin Periodontol.* 1996 Aug;23(8):724–9.
27. Pashley DH, Leibach JG, Horner JA. The effects of burnishing NaF/kaolin/glycerin paste on dentin permeability. *J Periodontol.* 1987 Jan;58(1):19–23.
28. Ritter AV, de L Dias W, Miguez P, Caplan DJ, Swift EJ Jr. Treating cervical dentin hypersensitivity with fluoride varnish: a randomized clinical study. *J Am Dent Assoc.* 2006 Jul;137(7):1013–20.
29. Haywood VB. Dentine hypersensitivity: bleaching and restorative considerations for successful management. *Int Dent J.* 2002;52(Suppl 1):376.
30. Pashley DH, Kalathoor S, Burnham D. The effects of calcium hydroxide on dentin permeability. *J Dent Res.* 1986 Mar;65(3):417–20.
31. Featherstone JD. The continuum of dental caries—evidence for a dynamic disease process. *J Dent Res.* 2004;83(Spec No C):C39–42.
32. Chow L, Wefel JS. The dynamics of de-and remineralization. *Dimensions Dent Hyg.* 2009;7(2):42–6.
33. Giniger M, MacDonald J, Ziemba S, Felix H. The clinical performance of professionally dispensed bleaching gel with added amorphous calcium phosphate. *J Am Dent Assoc.* 2005 Mar;136(3):383–92.
34. Yengopal V, Mickenautsch S. Caries-preventive effect of casein phosphopeptide-amorphous calcium phosphate (CPP-ACP): a meta-analysis. *Acta Odontol Scand.* 2009 Aug;21:1–12.
35. Pradeep AR, Sharma A. Comparison of clinical efficacy of a dentifrice containing calcium sodium phosphosilicate to a dentifrice containing potassium nitrate and to a placebo on dentinal hypersensitivity: a randomized clinical trial. *J Periodontol.* 2010 Aug;81(8):1167–73.

36. Shen C, Autio-Gold J. Assessing fluoride concentration uniformity and fluoride release from 3 varnishes. *J Am Dent Assoc.* 2002 Feb;133(2):176–82.

37. Singal P, Gupta R, Pandit N. 2% Sodium fluoride iontophoresis compared to a commonly available desensitizing agent. *J Periosontaol.* 2005 Mar;76(3):351–7.

38. Kimura Y, Wilder-Smith R, Yonaga K, Matsumoto K. Treatment of dentine hypersensitivity by lasers: a review. *J Clin Periodontol.* 2000 Oct;27(10):715–21.

39. Pashley DH. Potential for dentin hypersensitivity: in-office products. In: Addy M, Embery G, Edgar WM, Orchardson R, eds. *Clinical advances in restorative dentistry.* London: Informa Healthcare; 2000. pp. 351–365.

40. Schulte JR, Morrissette DB, Gasior EJ, Czajewski MV. The effects of bleaching application time on the dental pulp. *J Am Dent Assoc.* 1994 Oct;125(10):1330–5.

CHAPTER 44

Extrinsic Stain Removal

CAREN M. BARNES, RDH, BS, MS

Chapter Outline

INTRODUCTION

After treatment by scaling, root planing, and other dental hygiene care, the teeth are assessed for the presence of remaining dental stains and dental biofilm. The use of cleaning and polishing agents for stain and dental biofilm removal is a "selective procedure." Polishing is "selective" in that the teeth that need to be polished and the clean-ing or polishing agent used must be *selected* based on the patient's individual needs.

■ Preliminary examination of each tooth will reveal that the surfaces to be treated may be tooth structure (enamel, or with recession cementum or dentin) or when restored, a variety of dental materials (metal or esthetic, tooth-color restorations).

■ Preservation of the surfaces of both the teeth and the restorations is of primary importance during all cleaning and polishing procedures.

■ Stain removal will require the use of prophylaxis polishing agents that contain various abrasive grits. The smallest, least abrasive grit is used for the stain present.

■ Patients with no stain present will not require polishing with abrasive polishing pastes.

■ Some patients will not consider their teeth "cleaned" unless they have been polished. This situation is ideal for using a cleaning agent that will not abrade the dental hard tissues, but will remove dental biofilm and the patient's teeth will have the same clean feeling as they would if an abrasive prophylaxis paste were used.

■ The use of the coarsest prophylaxis paste available on all patients is contraindicated. To think that the use of the coarsest paste available will remove the heaviest to the lightest stain present is the wrong approach to polishing.

■ *One size grit prophylaxis paste is not appropriate for every patient and is unethical and clinically the wrong choice. To use such a practice is to ignore a patient's individual needs, worsen hypersensitivity, and cause significant damage to esthetic restorations.*

■ The longevity, esthetic appearance, and smooth surfaces of dental restorations depend on appropriate care by the dental hygienist and the daily personal care by the patient.

■ It is a responsibility of the dental hygienist to be current in knowledge of the procedures to prevent damage to the restorations during professional healthcare appointments.

■ The dental hygienist is responsible for educating the patient about proper personal daily care that will con-tribute to the maintenance of the restorations, such as recommending the least abrasive dentifrices.[1,2]

■ Terms related to extrinsic stain removal are defined in **Box 44-1**.

PURPOSES FOR STAIN REMOVAL

Stains on the teeth are not etiologic factors for any disease or destructive process.

■ The removal of stains is for esthetic, not for health, reasons.

■ Stain removal procedures have been an integral part of the oral prophylaxis since the inception of tooth cleaning procedures and patients have come to expect to have their teeth polished as a part of the oral prophylaxis.

■ The American Dental Hygienists' Association and the Academy of Periodontology include tooth polishing in their definitions of the term "oral prophylaxis."[3,4]

■ Key words related to stain removal, polishing, instruments, coronal polishing, air-powder polishing, cleaning agent, prophylaxis polishing agent, tribiology, two-body abrasion and three-body abrasion are defined in **Box 44-1**.

SCIENCE OF POLISHING

■ Within the science of abrasion, the mechanisms of polishing that require the use of abrasive particles are part of tribiology, the science of interacting surfaces in relative motion.

BOX 44-1	Key Words

Extrinsic Stain Removal

Abrasion: wearing away of surface material by friction.

Abrasive: a material composed of particles of sufficient hardness and sharpness to cut or scratch a softer material when drawn across its surface; available in various particle sizes.

Air-powder polisher: air-powered device using air and water pressure to deliver a controlled stream of specially processed sodium bicarbonate slurry through the handpiece nozzle; also called air abrasive, air polishing, air-powered abrasive, or airbrasive.

Binder: substance used to hold abrasive particles together; examples are ceramic bonding used for mounted abrasive points, electroplating for binding diamond chips for rotary instruments, and rubber or shellac for soft discs.

Coronal polishing: polishing of the anatomic crowns of the teeth to remove dental biofilm and extrinsic stains; does not involve calculus removal.

Glycerin: clear, colorless, syrupy fluid used as a vehicle and sweetening agent for drugs and as a solvent and vehicle for abrasive agents.

Grit: with reference to abrasive agents, grit is the particle size.

Polishing: the production, especially by friction, of a smooth, glossy, mirror-like surface that reflects light; a very fine agent is used for polishing after a coarser agent is used for cleaning.

p.s.i: pounds per square inch.

r.p.m.: revolutions per minute.

Slurry: thin, semi-fluid suspension of a solid in a liquid.

Three-body abrasion: which loose abrasive particles (the abrasive particles in prophylaxis polishing paste) move in the interface space between the surface being polished and the polishing application device.

Two-body abrasion: Two-body abrasive polishing involves abrasive particles attached to a medium (polishing application device) that move directly against the surface being polished.

Tribiology: Tribiology incorporates the study and application of the principles of friction, lubrication, and wear as they apply to polishing.

■ Tribiology incorporates the study and application of the principles of friction, lubrication, and wear.[4,5] Polishing is intended to produce intentional, selective and controlled wear. Within the science of tribiology, polishing is considered to be two-body abrasive polishing or three-body abrasive polishing.

■ Two-body abrasive polishing involves the abrasive particles attached to a medium, such as a rubber cup impregnated with abrasive particles that would not require a prophylaxis polishing paste.

■ Three-body abrasive polishing is the type most commonly used by dental hygienists, in which loose abrasive particles (the abrasive particles in prophylaxis polishing paste) move in the interface space between the surface being polished and the polishing application device (rubber cup or brush).[6–8]

EFFECTS OF CLEANING AND POLISHING

Attention is given to the positive and negative effects of polishing so that evidence-based scientific decisions can be made for the treatment of each patient. *Professional judgment based on a patient's needs and requests determines when a service is to be included in a dental hygiene care plan and if services are warranted, they will be selected carefully.*

I. PRECAUTIONS

■ As with all gingival manipulation with instruments, including a toothbrush,[9,10] bacteremia can be created during the use of power-driven stain removal instruments. Rotation of the rubber cup can force microorganisms into the tissues.

■ An inflammatory response can be expected, and bacteria may gain access to the bloodstream to create a bacteremia.

■ The response is a normal expectation and not of concern in healthy patients.

■ It is a concern for a patient who requires prophylactic antibiotic coverage before dental treatment; another reason why the medical history is such an essential part of patient assessment and is recorded before all treatments.

■ The medical history is reviewed and updated at each succeeding appointment.

■ For patients at risk, particularly those with damaged or abnormal heart valves, prosthetic valves, and other conditions listed in Chapter 9 on page 131, antibiotic prophylaxis may be required as specified by the patient's cardiologist.

II. ENVIRONMENTAL FACTORS

A. Aerosol Production

■ Aerosols are created during the use of all rotary instruments, including a prophylaxis handpiece with a rub-

ber cup to hold polishing paste, and the air and water sprays used during rinsing.[11]

■ The biologic contaminants of aerosols stay suspended for long periods and provide a means for disease transmission to dental personnel, as well as to succeeding patients.

■ Use of power-driven instruments is limited when a patient is known to have a communicable disease, a serious or chronic respiratory disease, or is immunocompromised.

■ Standard personal protective procedures are used.

B. Spatter

■ Protective eyewear is needed for all dental team members and for the patient.

■ Serious eye damage has occurred because of spatter from a polishing paste or from instruments.[12]

III. EFFECT ON TEETH

A. Removal of Tooth Structure

■ Polishing with coarse abrasive prophylaxis pastes may remove a few μm of the outer enamel. There is no research that has definitively determined a range of the amount of the outer enamel that potentially can be removed, which is further justification for using the least abrasive prophylaxis paste necessary to meet the patient's needs for polishing procedures.

■ The fluoride-rich outer surface of the enamel is necessary for protection against dental caries[13] and care is taken for it to be preserved. The use of a cleaning agent in place of an abrasive prophylaxis polishing agent will prevent the removal of the outermost layer of enamel.

B. Areas of Demineralization

■ *Demineralization areas:* Polishing demineralized white spots of enamel is contraindicated. More surface enamel is lost from abrasive polishing over demineralized white spots than over intact enamel.[14]

■ *Remineralization:* Demineralized areas of enamel can remineralize as these areas are exposed to fluoride from saliva, water, dentifrices, and professional fluoride applications. Since remineralization cannot be detected visually, it is necessary to remember that polishing procedures can interrupt enamel surface remineralization.

C. Areas of Thin Enamel, Cementum, or Dentin

■ Areas of thin enamel are contraindicated for polishing. Amelogenesis imperfecta is an example of thin enamel resulting from imperfect tooth development in Chapter 21 (pages 309 to 310).

■ *Exposure of dentinal tubules:* cementum and dentin are softer and more porous than enamel, so greater amounts of their surfaces can be removed during polishing than from enamel. When cementum is exposed

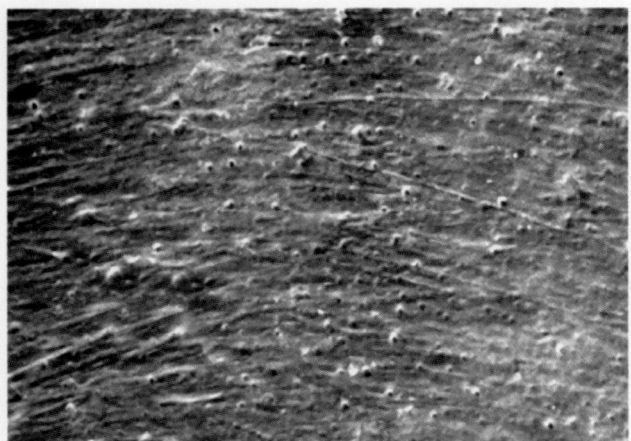

FIGURE 44-1 Scanning electron photomicrograph of a composite restoration polished with coarse prophylaxis paste.

because of gingival recession, polishing of the exposed surfaces is avoided.

■ Smear layer can be removed and dentinal tubules exposed.[15]

■ When surface structure is removed, unnecessary tooth sensitivity can result.[16]

D. Care of Restorations and Implants

■ Use of coarse abrasives may create deep, irregular scratches in restorative materials that will make them retain stain and biofilm more readily. **Figure 44-1** shows a scanning electron photomicrograph of a much damaged surface of a composite restoration polished with a rubber cup and coarse prophylaxis paste. The deep scratches created by the abrasive particles can be seen readily.

■ Microorganisms collect and colonize on a rough surface much more rapidly than on a smooth surface.[17]

■ It is imperative that prophylaxis polishing agents are not used on restorative materials. Polishing pastes not intended for use on restorative materials can destroy the surface integrity of the dental material.[18] The only safe material that will not damage the surface characterization of a restoration is a cleaning agent or a polishing agent that is recommended by the manufacturer of the restorative materials.[18,19]

E. Heat Production

■ Steady pressure with a rapidly revolving rubber cup or bristle brush and a minimum of wet abrasive agent can create sufficient heat to cause pain and discomfort for the patient.

■ Damage to the pulp by the heat has not been documented. The pulps of children are large and may be more susceptible to heat.

■ The rules for the use of cleaning or polishing agents are:

■ Use light pressure, slow speed of the rubber cup.

■ Use a moist agent.

■ Cleaning or polishing agents are never to be used as dry powders applied directly on teeth.

IV. EFFECT ON GINGIVA

■ Trauma to the gingival tissue can result, especially when the prophylaxis angle is run at a high speed with heavy pressure and the rubber cup is applied for an extended period adjacent to gingival tissues.

■ Stain removal after gingival and periodontal treatments, including scaling and root planing, is not recommended on the same day. The diseased lining of the pocket usually has been removed during scaling and inadvertent curettage, leaving the pocket wall wide open ready to receive abrasive particles and microorganisms that can become embedded out of reach of the most careful irrigation and rinsing.

INDICATIONS FOR STAIN REMOVAL

I. TO REMOVE EXTRINSIC STAINS NOT OTHERWISE REMOVED DURING TOOTHBRUSHING AND SCALING

A. Patient Instruction

■ Discuss source of stain and how it can be prevented.

■ Encourage patient to make necessary habit changes, especially to seek counseling for smoking cessation if that is the cause of the patient's stain. Tobacco cessation is described in Chapter 33 on page 489.

■ Practice toothbrushing to remove stains incorporated in dental biofilm.

■ Example of patient's own stain removal: The patient can be taught that chlorhexidine stain can be prevented and/or lessened with dental biofilm removal during personal oral care procedures. The less dental biofilm the patient has, the less chlorhexidine may stain the teeth.

B. Scaling and Root Planing

■ In addition to the use of cleaning or polishing agents during polishing procedures, stains can also be removed during scaling and root planing instrumentation.

■ Example: Black line stain has been identified as a type of calculus. It is described in Chapter 21, on page 307.[20]

II. TO PREPARE THE TEETH FOR CARIES-PREVENTIVE PROCEDURES

A. Placement of Pit and Fissure Sealant

■ Follow manufacturer's directions. Sealants vary in their requirements.

■ Avoid commercial oral prophylaxis pastes that contain glycerin, oils, flavoring substances, or other agents.

Glycerin and oils can prevent an optimum acid-etch and interfere with the adherence of the sealant to the tooth surface, causing the sealant to fail.

■ Air-powder polishing is one method of choice for preparing tooth surfaces for sealants (in Chapter 36, page 546).[21,22]

■ An alternative is the use of a plain, fine pumice mixed with water when precleaning is determined to be necessary (page 704). After the use of pumice, the patient needs to rinse thoroughly to remove the particles.

B. Professional Application of Fluoride Varnishes, Solutions, or Gels

■ Complete tooth polishing is not necessary before fluoride application.[23]

■ Biofilm and debris removal can be accomplished adequately by the patient using a toothbrush and dental floss, after complete calculus removal.

■ The pellicle on the tooth surface does not act as a barrier to fluoride, and fluoride uptake in the enamel from a fluoride application is similar whether the teeth are brushed by the patient or polished with an oral prophylaxis cleaning or polishing agent.[23]

III. TO CONTRIBUTE TO PATIENT MOTIVATION

Removal of biofilm is a *daily* procedure carried out *by the patient*. When accomplished thoroughly at least twice daily and for some patients three times daily, infection can be controlled, the sanitation of the mouth maintained, and staining can be prevented.

A. Development of Biofilm

■ It is known that pellicle returns to cover the teeth within minutes after complete polishing.

■ Biofilm begins to collect on the pellicle within 1 or 2 hours, increasing in thickness until, by 12–24 hours, biofilm is thick enough to show clearly when a disclosing agent is applied.

■ Undisturbed, biofilm may begin to calcify within a few days in a calculus-susceptible patient.

B. Motivation

Smooth polished tooth surfaces may contribute in part to the following effects:

■ Help the instructed patient to obtain more satisfactory results from self-care procedures. A smooth surface can be easier to achieve once the patient understands what a biofilm and debris-free mouth feels likes after having the teeth professionally polished with a cleaning or polishing agent.

■ Show the patient the appearance and feeling of a clean mouth for motivational purposes. The change in behavior, or the true learning, can be obtained through patient participation in the use of a disclosing agent and personal visualization of the biofilm followed by removal of the biofilm with floss and toothbrush.

CLINICAL APPLICATION OF SELECTIVE STAIN REMOVAL

The decision to polish teeth is based on the individual patient's needs.

I. SUMMARY OF CONTRAINDICATIONS FOR POLISHING

The following list suggests some of the specific instances in which polishing either can be performed with a cleaning agent or is contraindicated.

A. No Unsightly Stain

■ Polishing is a procedure that is based on the patient's individual needs. If no stain is present, polishing with an abrasive polishing agent is not justified; however, this is an ideal situation for using a cleaning agent.

■ When polishing is indicated, the choice of the appropriate cleaning or polishing agent is also *selective*, based on the individual needs of the patient. Some stains can be removed with cleaning agents that will not abrade enamel.

■ If cleaning agents will not remove the stain that is present, the obvious choice is the least abrasive polishing agent that will remove the stain.

■ Appearance is important to patients, but maintaining the integrity of the tooth surface for disease prevention is more important.

■ When the need for polishing is indicated and a cleaning agent is not the appropriate agent to use, it is imperative that the proper procedure be used for the application of abrasive prophylaxis polishing pastes; the least abrasive paste that can be used is selected.

■ When the abrasive paste is a medium, coarse, or extra coarse paste, those pastes need to be followed by the use of the next least abrasive paste in succession until the final paste used is fine paste.

B. Characteristics of Patients at Risk for Dental Caries

Patients at risk for dental caries need extra fluoride to protect their tooth surfaces and fluoride-rich enamel surfaces need to be preserved. Examples include:

■ Rampant caries, nursing caries, root caries, all ages
■ Noncavitated dental caries in early stages of demineralization
■ Xerostomia, from any reason

C. Patients With Respiratory Problems

Polishing procedures typically require the rinsing of the patient's mouth several times throughout the procedure.

■ Care is taken to minimize the spray from the air-water syringe as much as possible as the aerosols are contraindicated for such conditions as asthma, emphysema, cystic fibrosis, lung cancer, patients requiring oxygen, or when breathing is a problem.
■ This caution also applies to the use of air-powder polishers and spatter from prophylaxis polishing pastes.

D. Tooth Sensitivity

■ Abrasive agents can uncover ends of dentinal tubules in areas of thin cementum or dentin.
■ The polishing of dentin and cementum is contraindicated and needs to be avoided to every extent possible.

E. Restorations

■ Restorations and titanium implants may be scratched by abrasive prophylaxis polishing pastes.
■ A cleaning agent will not scratch restorative materials or titanium implants.[19]
■ When the clinician charts the patient's existing restorations and reviews current radiographs, attention is paid to chart the location of restorations, especially esthetic restorations that are tooth colored.
■ Tooth-colored restorations need to be polished with a cleaning agent, a polishing paste specifically formulated for use on esthetic restorations, or the paste recommended by the manufacturer of the restorative material.[18]

F. Conditions That Require Postponement for Later Evaluation

■ When instruction for personal biofilm removal (daily care) has not yet been given or when the patient has not demonstrated adequate biofilm control.
■ Soft spongy tissue that bleeds on brushing or gentle instrumentation.
■ Immediately following deep subgingival scaling and root planing because abrasive particles can become embedded in the pocket wall and interfere with healing.
■ Communicable disease potentially disseminated by aerosol.

II. SUGGESTIONS FOR CLINIC PROCEDURE

A. Give Instruction First

■ Daily dental biofilm removal to assist in dental stain control.
■ Explain to the patient that drinking coffee, tea, and color-added soft drinks is responsible for most dental stains.

■ Patients need information about the types of dentifrices that are safe for stain control and those that are contraindicated due to excessive abrasiveness or chemical harshness.
■ Tobacco cessation introduction when stain is primarily from tobacco use (in Chapter 33, page 489).

B. Remove Stain by Scaling

■ Whenever possible, stains can be removed during scaling, root planing, and debridement.
■ Assist in planning a preventive plan for stain control.

C. Stain Removal Techniques

■ Cleaning agent or low-abrasion oral prophylaxis paste.
■ Use the lightest pressure necessary for stain removal.
■ Low-speed handpiece.
■ Minimal heat production.
■ Soft rubber cup
■ Rubber cup at 90° to tooth surface with intermittent light applications.

CLEANING AND POLISHING AGENTS

There are two distinct types of agents used for "polishing" teeth; one is a cleaning agent, the other is a polishing agent.[1]

I. POLISHING AGENTS

■ Traditionally, abrasive agents have been applied with polishing instruments to remove extrinsic dental stains and leave the enamel surface smooth and shiny.
■ Polishing agents act by producing scratches in the surface of the tooth or restoration created by the friction between the abrasive particle and the softer tooth or restorative surface.
■ The cleaning and polishing process progresses from coarse abrasion to fine abrasion until the scratches are smaller than the wavelength of visible light, which is 0.05 μm.[1]
■ When scratches this size are created, the surface appears smooth and shiny—the smaller the scratches, the shinier the surface.
■ Unless the abrasive agent has been specially formulated for esthetic restorative surfaces, the use of prophylaxis polishing pastes is contraindicated for application to any esthetic restorative surfaces.[24,25]

II. CLEANING AGENTS

■ Unlike polishing agents, cleaning agents are round, flat, nonabrasive particles, and do not scratch surface material but produce a higher luster than polishing agents.
■ The most readily available cleaning agent (ProCare®, Young Dental Mfg. Earth City, MO) is made of a combination

of feldspar, alkali (sodium and potassium) and aluminum silicates. This feldspar, sodium-aluminum silicate cleaning agent is formulated into a powder and can be mixed with water or sodium fluoride to make a paste for cleaning.[26,27]

■ Because of the extremely low level of abrasion, cleaning agents can be used on any tooth surface, restorative surface, or implant surface without fear of creating deep scratches.

■ One prophylaxis polishing paste is not appropriate for all tooth and restorative surfaces; only specially formulated agents for polishing restorative surfaces are used when polishing restorations, especially esthetic restorations.

■ Cleaning agents will not harm restorative surfaces and any other polishing agent selected for restorative surfaces is selected based on the formulation and appropriateness for the restorative material.[28]

■ Dental hygienists must be mindful that many esthetic restorations are virtually undetectable due to color and surface match; therefore, it is imperative that the patient's dental chart and radiographs be examined to locate the esthetic restorations before applying polishing agents.

III. FACTORS AFFECTING ABRASIVE ACTION WITH POLISHING AGENTS

During polishing, sharp edges of abrasive particles are moved along the surface of a material, abrading it by producing microscopic scratches or grooves. The rate of abrasion, or speed with which structural material is removed from the surface being polished, is governed by hardness and shape of the abrasive particles, as well as by the manner in which they are applied.

A. Characteristics of Abrasive Particles

1. *Shape:* Irregularly shaped particles with sharp edges produce deeper grooves and thus abrade faster than do rounded particles with dull edges.
2. *Hardness:* Particles must be harder than the surface to be abraded; harder particles abrade faster.
   ■ When comparing the hardness of tooth structures, it is interesting that many of the abrasives used in prophylaxis polishing pastes are 10 times harder than the tooth structure to which they are applied.[28]
   ■ **Table 44-1** provides a comparison of the Mohs Hardness Value of dental tissues compared to agents commonly used in prophylaxis polishing pastes and substances used in cleaning agents. It is notable that enamel has a hardness value of half of some of the abrasive agents used in prophylaxis polishing pastes.
3. *Body strength:* Particles that fracture into smaller sharp-edged particles during use are more abrasive than those that wear down during use and become dull.
4. *Particle size (grit)*
   ■ The larger the particles, the more abrasive they are and the less polishing ability they have.

TABLE 44-1	MOHS HARDNESS VALUE OF DENTAL TISSUES COMPARED TO COMMONLY USED POLISHING ABRASIVE PARTICLES
DENTAL TISSUES	**MOHS HARDNESS VALUE**
Enamel	5
Dentin	3.0–4.0
Cementum	2.5–3.0
ABRASIVE AGENTS IN POLISHING PASTES	**MOHS HARDNESS VALUE**
Zirconium silicate	7.5–8.0
Pumice	6.0–7.0
Silicone carbine	9.5
Boron	9.3
Aluminum oxide	9
Garnet	8.0–9.0
Emery	7.0–9.0
Zirconium oxide	7
Perlite	5.5
Calcium carbonate	3
Aluminum silicates	2
Sodium	0.5
Potassium	0.4

*The Mohs hardness value of enamel, cementum and dentin compared to the Mohs hardness value of abrasive materials commonly used in prophylaxis polishing pastes. The Mohs hardness value is indicative of a material's resistance to scratching. Diamonds have a maximum Mohs value of 10; talc has a minimum of Mohs hardness of 1.

■ Finer abrasive particles achieve a glossier finish.

■ Abrasive and polishing agents are graded from coarse to fine based on the size of the holes in a standard sieve through which the particles will pass.

■ The finer abrasives are called powders or flours and are graded in order of increasing fineness as F, FF, FFF, and so on.

■ Particles embedded in papers are graded 0, 00, 000, and so on.

B. Principles for Application of Abrasives

1. *Quantity applied:* The more particles applied per unit time, the faster the rate of abrasion.
   ■ Particles are suspended in water or other vehicles for frictional heat reduction.

- Dry powders or flours represent the greatest quantity that can be applied per unit of time.
- Frictional heat produced is proportional to the rate of abrasion; therefore, the use of *dry agents* is *contraindicated* for polishing natural teeth because of the potential danger of thermal injury to the dental pulp.

2. *Speed of application:* The greater the speed of application, the faster the rate of abrasion.
   - With increased speed of application, pressure must be reduced.
   - *Rapid abrasion* is *contraindicated* because it increases frictional heat.

3. *Pressure of application:* The heavier the pressure applied, the faster the rate of abrasion.
   - *Heavy pressure* is *contraindicated* because it increases frictional heat.

4. *Summary:* When cleaning and polishing are indicated after patient evaluation, the following are observed:
   - Use wet agents.
   - Apply a rubber polishing cup, using low speed.
   - Use a light, intermittent touch.

IV. ABRASIVE AGENTS

The abrasives listed here are examples of commonly used agents. Some are available in several grades, and the specific use varies with the grade. For example, while a superfine grade might be used for polishing enamel surfaces and metallic restorations, a coarser grade would be used for laboratory purposes only.

Abrasives for use daily in a dentifrice necessarily are of a finer grade than those used for professional polishing accomplished a few times each year.

A. Silex (Silicon Dioxide)

- *XXX Silex:* Fairly abrasive.
- *Superfine Silex:* Can be used for heavy stain removal from enamel.

B. Pumice

Powdered pumice is of volcanic origin and consists chiefly of complex silicates of aluminum, potassium, and sodium. Pumice is the primary ingredient in commercially prepared prophylaxis pastes. The specifications for particle size are listed in the *National Formulary*[29] as follows:

- *Pumice flour or superfine pumice:* Least abrasive, and may be used to remove heavy stains from enamel.
- *Fine pumice:* Mildly abrasive.
- *Coarse pumice:* Not for use on natural teeth.

C. Calcium Carbonate (Whiting, Calcite, Chalk)

- Various grades are used for different polishing techniques.

D. Tin Oxide (Putty Powder, Stannic Oxide)

- Polishing agent for teeth and metallic restorations.

E. Emery (Corundum)

Not used directly on the enamel.

- *Aluminum oxide (alumina):* The pure form of emery. Used for composite restorations and margins of porcelain restorations.
- *Levigated alumina:* Consists of extremely fine particles of aluminum oxide, which may be used for polishing metals but are destructive to tooth surfaces.

F. Rouge (Jeweler's Rouge)

- Iron oxide is a fine red powder sometimes impregnated on paper discs.
- It is useful for polishing gold and precious metal alloys in the laboratory.

G. Diamond Particles

- Constituent of diamond polishing paste for porcelain surfaces.

V. CLEANING INGREDIENTS

- Particles for cleaning agents differ from abrasive agents in shape and hardness.
- Particles used for cleaning agents include feldspar, alkali and aluminum silicate.

A. Clinical Applications

Numerous commercial preparations for dental prophylactic cleaning and polishing preparations are available. Clinicians need more than one type available to meet the requirements of individual restorative materials.

B. Packaging

- Commercial preparations are in the forms of pastes or powders.
- Some are available in measured amounts contained in small plastic or other individual packets that contribute to the cleanliness and sterility of the procedure.
- Selection of a preparation is based on qualities of abrasiveness, consistency for convenient use, or flavor for patient pleasure.

C. Enhanced Prophylaxis Polishing Pastes

Additives are included in prophylaxis polishing pastes to provide a specific function, such as enhancing the mineral surface of enamel, diminishing dentin hypersensitivity, or tooth whitening.

1. *Fluoride prophylaxis pastes*
   - Application of fluoride by use of fluoride-containing prophylaxis polishing pastes **cannot** be considered a substitute for or the equivalent of a conventional topical fluoride treatment.
   - There is no scientific evidence that the amount of fluoride in prophylaxis paste is sufficient to have a preventive effect for dental caries. The fluoride ions in the prophylaxis paste mix with the saliva; fluoride is not burnished into enamel with prophylaxis paste.
   - *Enamel surface:* The greatest benefit of fluoride as a prophylaxis polishing paste additive occurs when the fluoride ions in the prophylaxis paste are released into the saliva.
   - The fluoride ions that become mixed in the saliva may become incorporated into the hydroxyapatite structure of the tooth, thus aiding in the remineralizing of the tooth and improving enamel hardness.
   - *Clinical application:* Use only an amount sufficient to accomplish stain removal to prevent a child patient from swallowing unnecessary fluoride. The paste may contain 4,000 to 20,000 p.p.m. fluoride ion.[30]
2. *Amorphous calcium phosphate and other forms of calcium and phosphate*
   - Amorphous calcium phosphate and other formulations of calcium and phosphate, as an additive to prophylaxis polishing pastes, have been shown to hydrolyze the tooth mineral to form apatite.
   - When these additives are included in oral prophylaxis paste, the benefit is not solely from burnishing them into the tooth surface.
   - When prophylaxis polishing pastes containing calcium and phosphate become mixed with saliva, the mineral ions may become incorporated into the hydroxyapatite structure of the tooth, thus aiding in remineralizing the tooth and improving enamel hardness.
   - Polishing agents containing amorphous calcium phosphate have the potential to enhance tooth smoothness and the luster of the enamel surface.[31,32]
3. *Fluoride, calcium, and phosphate*
   - Fluoride, calcium, and phosphate prophylaxis pastes have an edge over those pastes that contain calcium and phosphate only, in that there are three minerals that can be incorporated into the teeth. Just as with the pastes that contain amorphous calcium and phosphate, the mineral ions, including the fluoride ions, may become incorporated into the hydroxyapatite structure of the tooth, thus aiding in remineralization to improve enamel hardness.
4. *Tooth whitening*
   - In addition to removing extrinsic stains, there are commercially available prophylaxis polishing pastes that contain 35% hydrogen peroxide to provide a whitening benefit.
   - A hydrogen peroxide gel is applied to the tooth and then "polished" into the tooth surface with a rubber cup and prophylaxis polishing paste.[33]
   - Prophylaxis polishing pastes with the hydrogen peroxide additive are not intended to be a primary delivery system for professional tooth whitening but can be used as an aid to maintain whitening results.
5. *Dentin hypersensitivity*
   - Topical desensitizing products work either by occluding dentinal tubules thereby blocking fluid flow or by interfering with nerve transmission.
   - Topical products that occlude dentinal tubules do so by physically occluding the tubules.
   - The desensitizing products that block nerve transmission utilize the active ingredient 5% potassium nitrate (KNO_3). Potassium nitrate blocks nerve transmission by penetrating the dentinal tubules and depolarize the nerve endings, which prevents repolarization and the sensation of pain.[34-36]
   - Dentifrices for patients that have dentinal hypersensitivity have long been available and some prophylaxis polishing pastes have been formulated for this purpose.
   - Prophylaxis polishing pastes that contain arginine, calcium, and bicarbonate/carbonate or Novamin® (active bioglass) have the purpose of minimizing dentin hypersensitivity. Mixing these ingredients produces arginine bicarbonate and calcium carbonate. When applied with a rubber cup these adjunctive ingredients can aid in sealing the dentinal tubules.[37]

 PROCEDURES FOR STAIN REMOVAL (CORONAL POLISHING)

I. PATIENT PREPARATION FOR STAIN REMOVAL

A. Instruction and Clinical Procedures

- Review medical history to determine premedication requirements.
- Determine the time that the patient had taken the prescription. When the initial part of the appointment (scaling and related procedures) has been lengthy, the benefit from the premedication may have passed.
- Review intraoral charting and radiographs. The intraoral chart and radiographs need review before any polishing procedures to locate all restorations. Some tooth-colored restorations are so artfully created and color-matched that they are almost impossible to detect without vision enhancement.
- After review, a plan for polishing can be made that includes the appropriate polishing agents for the restorations that are present.
- Practice biofilm control.
- Complete scaling, root planing, and overhang removal.

- Inform the patient that polishing is a cosmetic procedure, not a therapeutic one.
- After scaling and other periodontal treatment, an evaluation is made to determine the need for stain removal of teeth, polishing restorations, and dental prostheses.
- Check all restorations to ensure that the correct polishing agent has been selected.
- Explain the difference between cleaning and polishing agents.

B. Explain the Procedure

- Describe the noise, vibration, and grit of the polishing paste.
- Explain the frequent use of rinsing and evacuation with the saliva ejector.

C. Provide Protection for Patient

- Safety glasses worn for scaling are kept in place to prevent eye injury or infection.
- Fluid-resistant drape over patient to keep moisture from skin and clothing.

D. Patient Position

- The patient is positioned for maximum visibility.

E. Patient Breathing

- Explain to the patient and request breathing exchange through the nose only.
- Reduce potential for aspiration of oral pathogens into the lungs
- Allow water to pool for evacuation with saliva ejector.
- Less fogging of mouth mirror.
- Enhanced patient comfort.

II. ENVIRONMENTAL PREPARATION

Environmental factors are described in Chapters 4, 5, and 6.

A. Procedures to Lessen the Extent of Contaminated Aerosols

- Clear the water that will be used for rinsing. Flush water through the tubing for 2 minutes at the beginning of each work period and for 30 seconds after each appointment.
- Request that the patient rinse with an antimicrobial mouthrinse to reduce the numbers of oral microorganisms before starting instrumentation.
- Use high-velocity evacuation.

B. Protective Barriers

- Protective eyewear and coverall are necessary for the patient.
- The clinician wears the standard barrier protection, namely, eyewear, mask, gloves, and clinic gown to cover clothing.

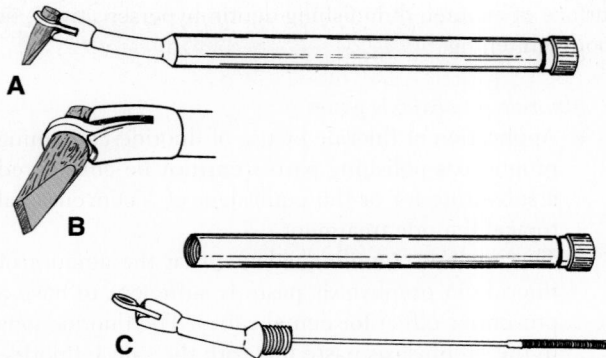

FIGURE 44-2 Porte Polisher. (A) Assembled instrument shows position of wood point ready for instrumentation. **(B)** Working end shows wedge-shaped wood point inserted. **(C)** Disassembled, ready for autoclave.

THE PORTE POLISHER

1. *Design*
   - The porte polisher is a prophylactic manual instrument designed especially for extrinsic stain removal or application of treatment agents such as for hypersensitive areas.
   - It is constructed to hold a wood point at a contra-angle. The wood points may be cone or wedge shaped and made of various kinds of wood, preferably orangewood. **Figure 44-2** illustrates a typical porte polisher.
2. *Grasp:* The instrument is held in a modified pen grasp, Figure 38-13 (page 587), or palm grasp, as shown in Figure 38-14 (page 588).
3. *Application:* The wood point is applied to the tooth surface using firm, carefully directed, massaging, circular or linear strokes to accommodate the anatomy of each tooth.
   - A firm finger rest and a moderate amount of pressure of the wood point provide protection for the gingival margin and efficiency in technique.
4. *Features*
   - The porte polisher is useful for instrumentation of difficult-to-access surfaces of the teeth, especially malpositioned teeth.
   - No heat generation, no noise compared with powered handpieces, and minimal production of aerosols.
   - The porte polisher is readily portable and therefore is useful in any location, for example, for a bedridden patient.

THE POWER-DRIVEN INSTRUMENTS

I. HANDPIECE

- A handpiece is used to hold rotary instruments.
- The three basic designs are straight, contra-angle, and right angle.

- Instruments have been classified according to their rotational speeds, designated by revolutions per minute (r.p.m.) as high speed and low (or slow) speed.
- Handpiece must be maintained and sterilized according to manufacturer's directions

A. Ultra or High Speed

- *Speed:* 100,000 to 800,000 r.p.m.; air-driven.
- *Uses:* For cavity preparation and other restorative preparations.
- *Fiberoptic light:* Better visibility is provided when a fiberoptic light is built into the head of the handpiece. The beam of light is projected onto the field of operation when the handpiece is activated.
- Ultra and high speed handpieces operate at very high speeds and therefore are **not** used for cleaning or polishing teeth with a prophylaxis angle and rubber cup.

B. Low Speed

- *Speed:* Typical range is up to 5,000 r.p.m. for low-speed handpieces manufactured for dental hygienists. Other low speed handpieces may have a higher range of r.p.ms.; air-driven.
- Lowest speeds are used for polishing and finishing procedures.

- Low speed handpieces are used for cleaning or polishing the teeth with a prophylaxis angle and rubber cup.

II. TYPES OF PROPHYLAXIS ANGLES

- Types of prophylaxis angles are described in **Table 44-2**.
- Contra- or right-angle attachments to the handpiece for which polishing devices (rubber cup, bristle brush) are available.
- Contra-angle prophylaxis angles may have a longer shank and a wider angle between the rubber cup and shank to allow for greater reach when polishing posterior teeth and surfaces.
- Disposable with rubber cup impregnated with polishing agent abrasive particles embedded in the rubber cup.[1]
- Stainless steel with hard chrome, carbon, steel or brass bearings.
- **Figure 44-3** shows examples of disposable for one-time use[38] contra-angle and right-angle prophylaxis angles and a stainless steel prophylaxis angle.
- Stainless steel prophylaxis angles that are sealed will not allow saliva and debris into the head of the angle nor will they allow grease and debris to leak out of the head of the angle.[39,40]
- Unless they are disposable, only instruments that can be sterilized are selected. Stainless steel or any other type of metal autoclavable prophylaxis angle must

TABLE 44-2	TYPES OF PROPHYLAXIS POLISHING ANGLES

COMPARISON OF DISPOSABLE PROPHYLAXIS ANGLES AND STAINLESS STEEL PROPHYLAXIS ANGLES*

TYPE OF ANGLE	DISPOSABLE PROPHYLAXIS ANGLE	DISPOSABLE ANGLE WITH ABRASIVE IMPREGNATED RUBBER CUP	STAINLESS STEEL PROPHYLAXIS ANGLE
Maintenance and Care	One-time use, discard	One-time use, discard	Requires maintenance, Sterilization
Attachments	Supplied with rubber cup from the manufacturer	Supplied with rubber cup from the manufacturer that is impregnated with one type of abrasive	Accepts variety of attachments: cups, brushes and cone shaped rubber points
Screw-in or Snap-on Rubber Cups	Usually screw-in type cup		Will accept screw-in or snap-on cups and brushes
Advantages	Requires no maintenance or sterilization	Requires no additional prophylaxis paste	Can be used hundreds of times if maintained properly
Disadvantages	Not package with other attachments; Creates refuse that is not biodegradable	Must have water and/or saliva as lubricant; Creates refuse that is not biodegradable	Does require time to clean and maintain

*A comparison of the features of a disposable prophylaxis angle to a disposable prophylaxis angle with abrasive-impregnated rubber cup and a sterilizable stainless steel prophylaxis angle.

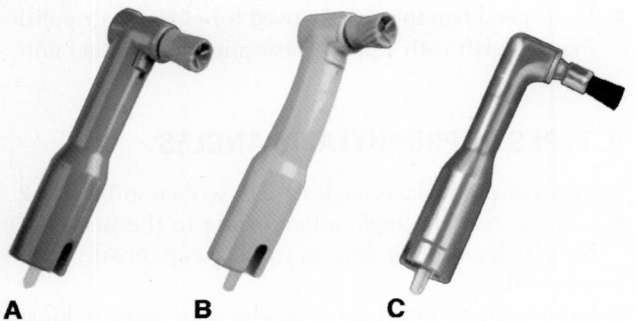

A **B** **C**

FIGURE 44-3 **Prophylaxis Angles. (A)** Disposable right-angled prophylaxis angle with rubber cup attached. **(B)** Disposable contra-angled prophylaxis angle with an attached rubber cup impregnated with a polishing agent (abrasive particles). **(C)** Sterilizable stainless steel prophylaxis angle holding a cleaning or polishing brush on a mandrel.

be sterilized after every use and the manufacturer's instructions followed for the proper maintenance and care as well as the correct sterilization procedures.

III. PROPHYLAXIS ANGLE ATTACHMENTS

A. Rubber Polishing Cups

- *Types.* **Figure 44-4** shows several types of rubber polishing cups from which to choose. The internal designs and sizes have the same purpose, which is to aid in holding the prophylaxis polishing paste in the rubber cup while polishing. The ideal rubber cup design retains the prophylaxis polishing paste in the cup and will release the paste at a steady rate.
  - *Slip-on (snap-on):* with ribbed cup to aid in holding polishing agent.
  - *Threaded (screw type):* with plain ribbed cup or flange (webbed) type.
  - Mandrel mounted.

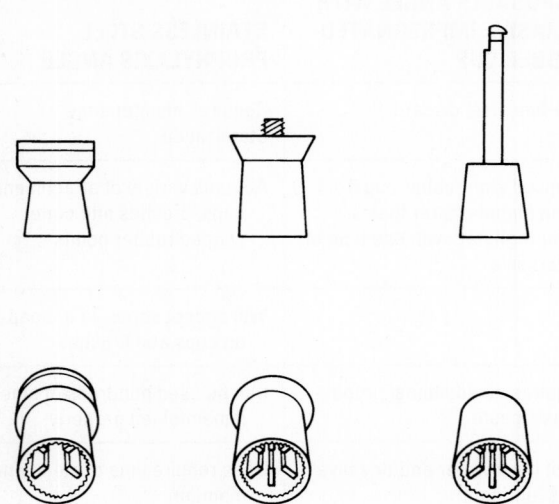

A **B** **C**

FIGURE 44-4 **Rubber Cup Attachments. (A)** Slip-on or snap-on for button-ended prophylaxis angle. **(B)** Threaded for direct insertion in right angle. **(C)** Mandrel stem for latch-type prophylaxis angle.

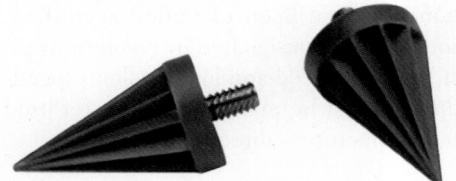

FIGURE 44-5 **Flexible Rubber Point has screw connection for a prophylaxis angle.** Made with ribs or grooves to carry cleaning or polishing agent to difficult-to-reach areas.

- *Materials*
  A. *Natural rubber:* more resilient; adapts readily to fit the contours of the teeth.
  B. *Synthetic:* stiffer than natural rubber.

B. Bristle Brushes

- *Types*
  A. *For prophylaxis angle:* slip-on or screw type.
  B. *For handpiece:* Mandrel mounted.
- *Materials:* synthetic.

C. Rubber Polishing Points

- **Figure 44-5** shows an example of a rubber point that screws into a prophylaxis angle.
- *Material:*
  Natural rubber: Flexible so that tip adapts to proximal surfaces, embrasures, and around orthodontic bands and brackets.
- *Use:* Because the ribs for holding the prophylaxis polishing paste onto the rubber polishing point are on the external surface, the polishing paste will have to be reapplied frequently.

IV. USES FOR ATTACHMENTS

A. Handpiece With Straight Mandrel

- Dixon bristle brush (type C, soft) for polishing removable dentures.
- Rubber cup on mandrel for polishing facial surfaces of anterior teeth.

B. Prophylaxis Angle With Rubber Cup, Brush, or Rubber Point

- *Rubber cup:* for removal of stains from the tooth surfaces and polishing restorations.
- *Brush:* for removing stains from deep pits and fissures and enamel surfaces away from the gingival margin. A brush is contraindicated for use on exposed cementum or dentin.
- *Rubber polishing point;* for removing stains and biofilm from proximal surfaces, embrasures, and around orthodontic bands and brackets.

USE OF THE PROPHYLAXIS ANGLE

I. EFFECTS ON TISSUES: CLINICAL CONSIDERATIONS

- Can cause discomfort for the patient if care and consideration for the oral tissues are not exercised to prevent unnecessary trauma.
- Tactile sensitivity of the clinician while using a thick, bulky handpiece is diminished and unnecessary pressure may be applied inadvertently.
- The greater the speed of application of a polishing agent, the faster the rate of abrasion. Therefore, the handpiece is applied at a low r.p.m.
- Trauma to the gingival tissue can result from too high a speed, extended application of the rubber cup, or use of an abrasive polishing agent.
- Tissue damage and the need for antibiotic premedication for risk patients are described in Chapter 9 on page 131.

II. PROPHYLAXIS ANGLE PROCEDURE

- Apply the polishing agent only where it is needed, that is, where there is unsightly stain. Contraindications are listed on page 693.
- As with all oral procedures, a systematic order is followed.

A. Instrument Grasp

Modified pen grasp (Figure 38-13, page 587).

B. Finger Rest

- Establish a fulcrum firmly on tooth structure or use an exterior rest.
- Use a wide rest area when practical to aid in the balance of the large instrument. For example, place cushion of rest finger across occlusal surfaces of premolars while polishing the molars.
- Avoid use of mobile teeth as finger rests.

C. Speed of Handpiece

- Use lowest available speed to minimize frictional heat
- Adjust r.p.m. as necessary.

D. Use of Rheostat

- Apply steady pressure with foot to produce an even, low speed.

E. Rubber Cup: Stroke and Procedure

- Observe where stain removal is needed to prevent unnecessary rubber cup application.
- Fill rubber cup with polishing agent, and distribute agent over tooth surfaces to be polished before activating the power.
- Establish finger rest and bring rubber cup almost in contact with tooth surface before activating power source.
- Using slowest r.p.m., apply revolving cup at a 90° angle lightly to tooth surfaces for 1 or 2 seconds. Use a light pressure so that the edges of the rubber cup flare slightly. The rubber cup needs to flare slightly underneath the gingival margin and onto the proximal surfaces.
- Move cup to adjacent area on tooth surface; use a patting or brushing motion.
- Replenish supply of polishing agent frequently.
- Turn handpiece to adapt rubber cup to fit each surface of the tooth, including proximal surfaces and gingival surfaces of fixed partial dentures.
- Start with the distal surface of the most posterior tooth of a quadrant and move forward toward the anterior; polish only the teeth that require stain removal. For each tooth, work from the gingival third toward the incisal third of the tooth.
- When two polishing agents of different abrasiveness are to be applied, use a separate rubber cup for each.
- Rubber cups cannot be sterilized and are used only for one patient and then discarded. The same is true for rubber polishing points and polishing brushes that fit onto prophylaxis angles; they are disposable and meant for one-time use only.

F. Rubber Polishing Points (Figure 44-5)

- Rubber polishing points can be used around orthodontic bands and brackets, on fixed bridges and in wide interproximal spaces or embrasures.
- Rubber points are loaded with the cleaning or polishing agent in the grooves around the sides. The rubber points will need to be replenished frequently with paste after use on every 1 to 2 teeth.

G. Bristle Brush

- Bristle brushes are used selectively and limited to occlusal surfaces.
- Lacerations of the gingiva and grooves and scratches in the tooth surface, particularly the roots and aesthetic restorations can result when the brush is not used with caution.
- Soak stiff brush in hot water to soften bristles.
- Distribute mild abrasive polishing agent over occlusal surfaces of teeth to be polished.
- Place fingers of nondominant hand in a position that both retracts and protects cheek and tongue from the revolving brush.
- Establish a firm finger rest and bring brush almost in contact with the tooth before activating power source.
- Use slowest r.p.m. as the revolving brush is applied lightly to the occlusal surfaces only. Avoid contact of the bristles with the soft tissues.

- Use a short stroke in a brushing motion; follow the inclined planes of the cusps.
- Move from tooth to tooth to prevent generation of excessive frictional heat. Avoid overuse of the brush. Replenish supply of polishing agent frequently.

H. Irrigation

- Irrigate teeth and interdental areas thoroughly several times with water from the syringe to remove abrasive particles. Avoid heavy water pressure to prevent forcing particles into the tissue.
- The rotary movement of the rubber cup or bristle brush tends to force the abrasive into the gingival sulci, thereby creating a potential source of irritation to the soft tissues.

POLISHING PROXIMAL SURFACES

- Care must be exercised in the use of floss, tape, and finishing strips.
- Understanding the anatomy of the interdental papillae and their relationship to the contact areas and proximal surfaces of the teeth is prerequisite to the prevention of tissue damage.
- As much polishing as possible of accessible proximal surfaces is accomplished during the use of the rubber cup in the prophylaxis angle.
- This can be followed by the use of dental tape with polishing agent when indicated.
- Finishing strips are used only in selected instances, when all other techniques fail to remove a stain.

I. DENTAL TAPE AND FLOSS

A. Features

- Floss and tape are described in Chapter 28 on page 411.
- The wax covering affords some protection for the tissues, facilitates the movement of the floss or tape, prevents excessive absorption of moisture, and helps prevent shredding.
- Dental tape is flat and has relatively sharp edges, whereas floss is round. Either floss or tape may injure the tissue when used incorrectly or carelessly.
- The use of dental floss or tape for dental biofilm control on proximal tooth surfaces is an essential part of self-care by the patient.

B. Uses During Cleaning and Polishing

- Techniques for tape and floss application are described in Chapter 28 on pages 412 to 413 and illustrated in Figures 28-3, 28-4, and 28-5.
- The same principles apply whether the patient or the clinician is using the floss.
- Finger rests are used to prevent snapping through contact areas.

- *Stain removal with dental tape*: Polishing agent is applied to the tooth, and the tape is moved gently back and forth and up and down curved over the area where stain was observed.
- *Cleaning gingival surface of a fixed partial denture*: A floss threader is used to position the floss or tape over the gingival surface. Floss threaders are described and illustrated in Chapter 31 pages 450 and 451. The agent is applied under the pontic, and the floss or tape is moved back and forth with contact on the bridge surface.
- *Flossing*: Particles of abrasive agent can be removed by rinsing and by using a clean length of floss applied in the usual manner.
- *Rinsing and irrigation*: Irrigate with water-spray syringe to clean out all abrasive agent.

II. FINISHING STRIPS

A. Description

- Finishing strips are also known as linen abrasive strips.
- They are thin, flexible, and tape-shaped.
- Available in four widths: extra narrow, narrow, medium, and wide.
- Made of linen or plastic, with one smooth side and the other side that serves as a carrier for abrasive agents bonded to that side.
- "Gapped" strips are available with an abrasive-free portion to permit sliding the strip through a contact area without abrading the enamel.
- Available in extra fine, fine, medium, and coarse grit. *Only extra narrow or narrow strips with fine grit are suggested for stain removal, and then only with discretion.*

B. Use

- *For stain removal on proximal surfaces of anterior teeth; When other techniques are unsuccessful.*
- *Precautions for use*
  - Edge of strip is sharp and may cut gingival tissue or lip.
  - Use of a finishing strip is limited to enamel surfaces.

C. Technique for Finishing Strip

- *Grasp and finger rest*
  - A strip no longer than 6 inches is most conveniently applied.
  - Grasp and finger rest must be well controlled.
  - Protection of the lip by retraction with the thumb and index finger holding the strip is a helpful safety measure.
- *Positioning*
  - Direct the abrasive side of the strip toward the proximal surface to be treated as the strip is worked slowly and gently between the teeth with a slight sawing motion.
  - Bring strip just through the contact area. If the strip breaks, immediately use floss to remove particles of abrasive.

- When a space is clearly visible through an embrasure and the interdental papilla is missing, a narrow finishing strip may be threaded through. Prepare strip by cutting the end on a diagonal to facilitate threading.
- *Stain removal*
  - Press abrasive side of strip against tooth. Draw back and forth in a 1/8-inch arc two or three times, rocking on the established fulcrum.
  - Remove strip. Do not attempt to turn the strip while it is in the interdental area.
- *Dental floss:* Follow each application of a finishing strip with dental floss to remove abrasive particles.

AIR-POWDER POLISHING

- Principles of selective stain removal are applied to the use of the air-powder polishing system. After biofilm control instruction, instrumentation, and periodontal debridement are completed, follow with an evaluation of a need for stain removal.

I. PRINCIPLES OF APPLICATION

- Air-powder systems manufactured by several companies are efficient and effective methods for mechanical removal of stain and biofilm.[41,42]
- Air-powder systems use air, water, and specially formulated powders to deliver a controlled spray that propels the particles to the tooth surface. Only powders approved by each air-powder polishing manufacturer are used in each brand of air-powder polishing unit. The use of an unapproved powder in an air-powder polishing unit could void the warranty on the unit.[43]
- The equipment is operated using inlet air pressure between 40 and 100 psi and inlet water pressure between 20 and 60 psi. Internal airpolishing unit air and water pressures will vary according to manufacturer and are not to be adjusted from their original settings.
- The orifice of the handpiece nozzle is kept in a constant circular motion, with the nozzle tip 4 to 5 mm away from the enamel surface.
- The spray is angled away from the gingival margin.
- The periphery of the spray may be near the gingival margin, but the center is directed at an angle less than 90° away from the margin.
- Complete directions for care of equipment and preparation for use of the device are provided by the individual manufacturer.

II. SPECIALLY FORMULATED POWDERS FOR USE IN AIR-POWDER POLISHING

A. *Sodium bicarbonate*[43]
  - Sodium bicarbonate is the original powder used in air-powder polishing.
  - It is specially formulated with scant amounts of calcium phosphate and silica to keep it free flowing.
  - The Mohs hardness number for sodium bicarbonate is 2.5 and the particles average 74 μm in size.
  - Warning: over-the counter sodium bicarbonate cannot be used in air polishing equipment as it will clog the unit.
  - The *only* type of sodium bicarbonate that can be used in air-powder polishing units is the type specially formulated for air-powder polishing.
  - Sodium bicarbonate air-powder is available with flavorings. However, the patient will taste the salt and smell the flavor.
B. Aluminum Trihydroxide
  - Aluminum trihydroxide was the first air-powder developed as an alternative to sodium bicarbonate for patients who are sodium bicarbonate intolerant.[44]
  - Aluminum trihydroxide has a Mohs hardness value of 4 and the particles range in size from 80 to 325 μm.
C. *Glycine*
  - Glycine is an amino acid. For use in powders, glycine crystals are grown using a solvent of water and
  - sodium salt.
  - Glycine particles for use in airpolishing have a Mohs hardness number of 2 are 20 μm in size.
D. *Calcium carbonate*
  - Calcium carbonate is a naturally occurring substance that can be found in rocks.
  - It is a main ingredient in antacids, and is also used as filler for pharmaceutical drugs.
  - Calcium carbonate has a Mohs number of 3.[43]
E. *Calcium sodium phosphosilicate (Novamin)*
  - Calcium sodium phosphosilicate (Novamin) is a bioactive glass and has a Mohs hardness number of 6, making it the hardest air polishing particle used in air powder polishing powders.[43] The particles vary from 25 to 120 μm in size.

III. USES AND ADVANTAGES OF AIR-POWDER POLISHING

- Requires less time, is ergonomically favorable to the clinician, and generates no heat.[42–43,45]
- Sodium bicarbonate is less abrasive than traditional prophylaxis pastes, which makes the air-powder polisher ideal for stain and biofilm removal. However, some air-polishing powders are much more abrasive than sodium bicarbonate and should only be used on surfaces that they will not damage.[43]
- Removal of heavy, tenacious tobacco stain and chlorhexidine-induced staining.[41–43,45]
- Stain and biofilm removal from orthodontically banded and bracketed teeth[46,47] and dental implants.[48,49]
- Before sealant placement or other bonding procedures.[21,22]
- Root detoxification for periodontally diseased roots by the periodontist during open periodontal surgery.[50,51]

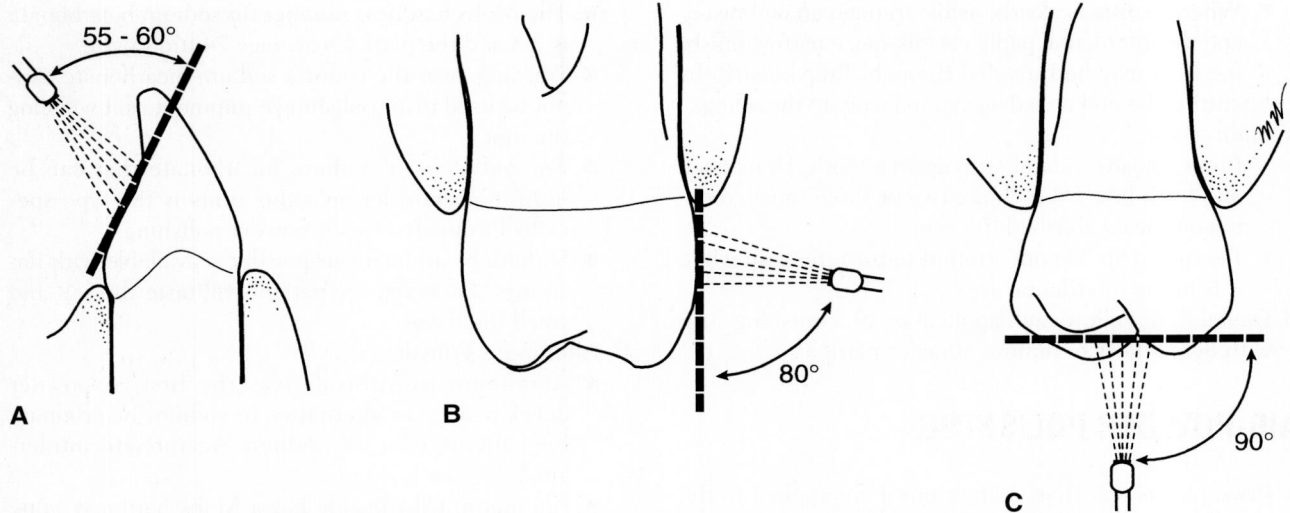

FIGURE 44-6 **Air-Powder Polishing.** Direct the aerosolized spray for **(A)** the anterior teeth at a 60° angle. **(B)** the posterior teeth facial and lingual or palatal at an 80° angle. **(C)** the occlusal surfaces at a 90° angle to the occlusal plane.

IV. TECHNIQUE

Proper angulation of the air-powder polishing handpiece is essential to reduce the amount of inherent aerosols created[52–54] and to remove stain and biofilm without iatrogenic soft tissue trauma.

A. For Anterior Teeth

■ Place the handpiece nozzle at a 60° angle to the facial and lingual surfaces of anterior teeth **(Figure 44-6A)**.

B. For Posterior Teeth

■ Place the handpiece nozzle at an 80° angle to the facial and lingual surfaces **(Figure 44-6B)**.

C. For Occlusal Surfaces

■ Place the handpiece nozzle at a 90° angle to the occlusal plane **(Figure 44-6C)**.

D. Incorrect Angulation

■ Incorrect angulation of the handpiece is probably the single most common cause of excess aerosol production.
■ The handpiece nozzle is never directed into the gingival sulcus or into a periodontal pocket with little bony support remaining, as this could result in facial emphysema (also known as a subcutaneous emphysema.)
■ Facial emphysemas occur due to the abnormal introduction of air into subcutaneous tissues or interstitial spaces.[43]
■ Facial emphysemas can be prevented by avoiding the use of compressed air or compressed air and water

around extraction sites,[55] small areas open to subcutaneous tissues, such as small incisions or lacerations or surgical wounds. Therefore the use of high speed handpieces during third molar extractions,[56] air/water syringes near extraction or surgical sites or lacerations,[57–59] and airpolishing[60,61] spray is avoided in these areas.

■ Facial emphysemas exhibit symptoms such as facial swelling, a "crackling" sensation of the face and neck area when touched, tenderness and pain. If detected early, patients with facial emphysemas usually require observation, antibiotics, and analgesia.[43] **Box 44-2** Contains a list of the sequelae that can develop as a result of compressed air forced into soft tissues of the head and neck. **Box 44-3** contains a list of sequelae that can develop as a result of a facial emphysema.

■ The closer the nozzle is held to the enamel, the more spray will deflect back into the direction of the clinician.

BOX 44-2	Sequelae That Can Develop as a Result of Compressed Air Forced Into Soft Tissues of the Head and Neck

Bilateral pneumothorax
Cerebral air embolism
Cervicofacial emphysema
Facial emphysema
Mediastinal emphysema
Pneumediastinum
Pneumothorax
Retropharyngeal emphysema

BOX 44-3	Sequelae That Can Develop as a Result of Facial Emphysema

Bilateral pneumothorax
Cerebral air embolism
Embolism
Pneumediastinum
Pneumothorax
Thrombosis

- When a clinician directs the handpiece at a 90° angle toward a facial, buccal, and some lingual surfaces, the result is an immediate reflux of the aerosolized spray back onto the clinician.
- Changing the angle of incidence to the proper angulations of 60° and 80° will result in a change in the angle of the reflection, thus reducing the amount of reflux of aerosolized spray.

V. RECOMMENDATIONS AND PRECAUTIONS

A. Aerosol Production

A copious spray containing oral debris and microorganisms is produced. As with all contaminated aerosols, a health hazard can exist. Suggestions for minimizing contamination and the effects of the aerosols include the following:

- Patient uses a preprocedural antibacterial mouthrinse.[62]
- High-volume evacuation is needed, using a wide tip held near the tooth where the spray is released from the nozzle or using a high-volume scavenger attachment for a high-volume evacuation suction tip or saliva ejector.[52–54]

B. Protective Patient and Clinician Procedures

- Use protective eyewear, protective gown, and hair cover.
- Lubricate patient's lips to prevent drying effect of the sodium bicarbonate using a nonpetroleum lip lubricant.
- Do not direct the spray on the gingiva, directly into the gingival sulcus or other soft tissues, which can create patient discomfort, undue tissue trauma, or more seriously, a facial emphysema.
- Avoid directing the spray into periodontal pockets with bone loss or into extraction sites as a facial emphysema can be induced.

VI. RISK PATIENTS: AIR-POWDER POLISHING CONTRAINDICATED

The information from the patient's medical history is used and appropriate applications made. Antibiotic premedication is indicated for all the same patients who are at risk for any dental hygiene procedure (Chapter 9, page 131).

A. Contraindications[43]

- Physician-directed sodium-restricted diet (for sodium bicarbonate powder only).
- Respiratory disease or other condition that limits swallowing or breathing, such as chronic obstructive pulmonary disease.
- Patients with end-stage renal disease, Addison's Disease or Cushing's Disease.
- Communicable infection that can contaminate the aerosols produced.
- Immunocompromised patients.
- Patients taking potassium, anti-diuretics, or steroid-therapy.

B. Other Contraindications

- *Root surfaces:* Avoid routine polishing of cementum and dentin. They can be removed readily during air-powder polishing.[63]
- *Soft, spongy gingiva:* The air-powder can irritate the free gingival tissue, especially if not used with the recommended technique. When heavy stain calls for the use of an air-powder polisher, instruct the patient in daily bacterial biofilm removal. Following scaling and periodontal debridement, postpone the stain removal until soft tissue has healed.
- *Restorative materials:* The use of air-powder polishing on composite resins, cements, and other nonmetallic materials can cause removal or pitting.[18,19,26,63] **Table 44-3** provides a guide as to which restorative materials can be safely treated with air-powder polishing agents,

TABLE 44-3	RECOMMENDATIONS FOR USE OF AIR POLISHING ON RESTORATIVE MATERIALS	
	POLISHING POWDER CONTAINING	
RESTORATIVE MATERIAL	**SODIUM BICARBONATE**	**ALUMINUM TRIHYDROXIDE**
Amalgam	Yes	No
Gold	Yes*	No
Porcelain	Yes*	No
Hybrid composite	No	No
Microfilled composite	No	No
Glass ionomer	No	No
Compomer	No	No
Luting agents	No	No

*Only if margin is avoided.

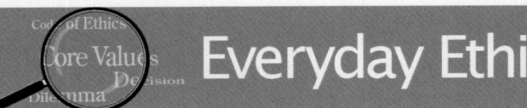

Everyday Ethics

Mr. Jackson, the 62-year-old chief executive officer of a major oil company, presents for his routine 3-months' maintenance with Carol, his dental hygienist of several years. Mr. Jackson is meticulous about his appearance and is always handsomely dressed. He is well known internationally and frequently seen in the news media being interviewed and having pictures taken for news articles.

   Mr. Jackson had a complete cosmetic restoration of his teeth a year ago. Previously his teeth had been stained by the numerous cups of tea he drank every day. He has had porcelain veneers placed on his maxillary anterior teeth, and all restorations are now tooth colored. The color match of the restorations to his teeth is perfect. Unfortunately, Mr. Jackson has not cut back on drinking tea and during her assessment, Carol notes that generalized stain is starting to discolor most of the new restorations. Before the cosmetic restorations were placed, Carol used a coarse prophy paste to eliminate the tea stains and now Mr. Jackson asks her to

"just use that gritty stuff again." He states that he absolutely does not want his teeth to appear stained.

Questions for Consideration
1. What role does each of the Dental Hygiene Core Values play as Carol contemplates a course of action to take in this situation?
2. What alternative actions are available that would respect Mr. Jackson's rights as well as allow Carol to provide treatment that meets standards of care?
3. What financial or legal considerations will Carol need to consider as she determines her course of action?

---

the sodium bicarbonate powder, and the aluminum trihydroxide powder.[38] Significant damage to margins of dental castings has been shown.[50]

DOCUMENTATION

Documentation for a patient receiving tooth stain removal as part of the Dental Hygiene Care Plan for a maintenance appointment would include a minimum of the following:

BOX 44-4	Example Progress Note

Tom came in for regular maintenance appt, grinning to shown his new implant crown and other esthetic restorations (not distinguishable from the color of the teeth). After update on medical history, medications, no changes. Blood pressure (115/75); extra-intraoral exams (all ok); perio exam with complete probing (see chart: a few 3–4 mm, 2 bleeding points (at 4 mm) with rough (calculus); calculus mand ant.; minimal biofilm with yellowish staining. Gave Tom new toothbrush with tongue cleaner on back, and demonstrated the tongue cleaner. Went over places he had been missing on his teeth and gingiva. Calculus removal. Checked his dental records for the material used for the various restorations and selected a mild polishing agent, no abrasive. Next regular appointment 4 months made at front desk.

Signed: _____, RDH Date: _____.

- Review patient medical history with questions to determine health problems, recent medical examinations and treatments, and changes in medications.
- *Current clinical examination findings:* intraoral, extraoral, periodontal, and dental.
- *With dental charting:* identification of dental materials used in restorations that can influence choice of polishing agents. Identification would require use of radiographs and the intraoral dental charting.
- Dental hygiene examination for state of patient's personal daily self-care, calculus and biofilm deposits, sources for dental stains, products used for oral care, and dietary factors influencing the dentition and all oral tissues: Questions answered about best choices for various products
- A sample progress note may be reviewed in **Box 44-4.**

Factors To Teach The Patient

- How dental biofilm and stains form on the natural teeth and their replacements.
- The meaning of selective polishing and why it is not necessary to polish all teeth at every appointment when daily care is effective.
- Stains and biofilm removed by polishing can return promptly if biofilm is not removed faithfully on a schedule of two or three times each day.
- Polishing agents used during professional coronal polishing are too abrasive for daily home use.

References

1. Barnes CM. The science of polishing. *Dimensions Dent Hyg*. 2009 Nov;7(11):18–20, 22.

2. Liljeborg A, Tellefsen G, Johannsen G. The use of a profilometer for both quantitative and qualitative measurements of toothpaste abrasitivity. *Int J Dent Hyg*. 2010 Aug;8(3):237–43.

3. American Academy of Periodontology. Glossary of periodontal terms. 3rd ed. Chicago: American Academy of Periodontology; 1992. 40 p.

4. American Dental Hygienists' Association. Position paper on the oral prophylaxis. Chicago: ADHA; 1998. Available from: www.adha.org/profissues/prophylaxis.htm

5. Jeffries SR. Abrasive finishing and polishing in restorative dentistry: a state-of-the-art review. *Dent Clin North Am*. 2007 Apr;51(2):379–97.

6. Hutchings IM. Abrasion process in wear and manufacturing. Proceedings of the Institution of Mechanical Engineers. *Part J: J Eng Tribol*. 2002;216(2):55–62.

7. Rémond G, Nockolds C, Phillips M, Roques-Carmes C. Implications of polishing techniques in quantitative x-ray microanalysis. *J Res Natl Inst Stand Technol*. 2002 Nov–Dec;107(6):639–62.

8. Williams JA. Wear and wear particles: some fundamentals. *Tribiology Int*. 2005;38(10):863–70.

9. Fine DH, Furgang D, McKiernan M, Tereski-Bischio D, Ricci-Nittel D, Zhang P, Araujo MW. An investigation of the effect of an essential oil mouthrinse on induced bacteraemia: a pilot study. *J Clin Periodontol*. 2010 Sep;37(9):840–7.

10. Lucas V, Roberts GJ. Odontogenic bacteremia following tooth cleaning procedures in children. *Pediatr Dent*. 2000 Mar–Apr;22(2):96–100.

11. Cristina ML, Spagnolo AM, Sartini M, Dallera M, Ottria G, Perdelli F, Orlando P. Investigation of organizational and hygiene features in dentistry: a pilot study. *J Prev Med Hyg*. 2009 Sep;50(3):175–80.

12. Farrier SL, Farrier JN, Gilmour AS. Eye safety in operative dentistry. A study in dental practice. *Br Dent J*. 2006 Feb;200(4):218–23.

13. Featherstone JD. Prevention and reversal of dental caries: role of low level fluoride. Community Dent Oral Epidemiol. 1999 Feb;27(1):31–40.

14. Honório HM, Rios D, Abdo RC, Machado MA. Effect of different prophylaxis methods on sound and demineralized enamel. *J Appl Oral Sci*. 2006 Apr;14(2):117–23.

15. Kubinek R, Zapletalova Z, Vujtek M, Novotný R, Kolarova H, Chmelickova H. Examination of dentin surface using AFM and SEM. In: Méndez-Vilas A, Díaz J, eds. *Modern research and educational topics in microscopy*. Vol. 2. Zurbarán, Spain: Formatex; 2007. pp. 593–8.

16. Miglani S, Aggarwal V, Ahuja B. Dentin hypersensitivity: recent trends in management. *J Conserv Dent*. 2010 Oct–Dec;13(4):218–24.

17. Anusavice KJ. Phillips' science of dental materials. 11th ed. St Louis: Saunders; 2003. Chapter 13, Finishing and polishing materials, p. 352.

18. Barnes CM. Polishing esthetic restorative materials. *Dimensions Dent Hyg*. 2010 Jan;8(1):24, 26–8.

19. Barnes CM. Care and maintenance of esthetic restorations. *J Prac Hyg*. 2004 Jul–Aug;14:19–22.

20. Essex GA Predilection for Polishing. *Dimensions Dent Hyg*. 2005 Mar;3(3):36, 8.

21. Scott L, Greer D. The effect of an air polishing device on sealant bond strength. *J Prosthet Dent*. 1987 Sep;58(3):384–7.

22. Ahovuo-Saloranta A, Hiiri A, Nordblad A, Mäkelä M, Worthington HV. Pit and fissure sealants for preventing dental decay in the permanent teeth of children and adolescents. *Cochrane Database Syst Rev*. 2008 Oct 8;(4):CD001830. Review.

23. Azarpazhooh A, Main PA. Efficacy of dental prophylaxis (rubber cup) for the prevention of caries and gingivitis: a systematic review of literature. *Br Dent J*. 2009 Oct 10;207(7): E14.

24. Barnes CM, Covey DA, Walker MP, Johnson WW. Essential selective polishing: the maintenance of aesthetic restorations. *J Prac Hyg*. 2003 Sep–Oct;12(5):18–24.

25. Barnes CM. Care and maintenance of esthetic restorations. *J Prac Hyg*. 2004 Jul–Aug;14:19–22.

26. Putt MS, Kleber CJ, Davis JA, Schimmele RG, Muhler JC. Physical characteristics of a new cleaning and polishing agent for use in a prophylaxis paste. *J Dent Res*. 1975 May–Jun;54(3):527–34.

27. Putt MS, Kleber CJ, Muhler JC. Enamel polish and abrasion by prophylaxis pastes. *J Dent Hyg*. 1982 Sep;56(9):38, 40–3.

28. Barnes CM. Adapting polishing procedures to maintain aesthetic restorations. *J Prac Hyg*. 2005 Apr;15:22.

29. United States Pharmacopeia. The national formulary. Rockville (MD): United States Pharmacopeia Convention: 1995. 1342 p.

30. Burrell KH, Chan JT. Fluorides. In: *American Dental Association, Council on Scientific Affairs. ADA guide to dental therapeutics*. 3rd ed. Chicago: ADA; 2003. 238 p.

31. Tung MS, Eichmiller FC. Amorphous calcium phosphates for tooth mineralization. *Compend Contin Educ Dent*. 2004 Sep;25(9 Suppl 1):9–13.

32. Tung M, Malerman R, Huang S, McHale WA. Reactivity of prophylaxis paste containing calcium phosphate and fluoride salts. *J Dent Res*. 2005;84(Special Issue A),Abstract #2156, IADR Abstracts, 2005.

33. Daniels A. Professionally applied enhanced polishing agents. *J Prac Hyg*. 2006 Apr;15:26.

34. Wolff MS, Kleinberg I. Duration of reduction of dentinal hypersensitivity after prophylaxis with a calcium/arginine bicarbonate carbonate paste. *J Dent Res*. 2003;82(Special Issue)Abstract 180.

35. Canadian Advisory Board on Dentin Hypersensitivity. Consensus-based recommendations for the diagnosis and management of dentin hypersensitivity. *J Can Dent Assoc*. 2003 Apr;69(4):221–6.

36. Addy M. Dentine hypersensitivity: new perspectives on an old problem. *Int Dent J* 2002;52(5 Suppl 1)367–75.

37. Mattana D. Reducing dentin Hypersensitivity. *J Prac Hyg*. 2006 Apr;15:24.

38. Barnes CM, Fleming LS. An in vitro evaluation of commercially available disposable prophylaxis angles. *J Dent Hyg*. 1991;65(9):438–41.

39. Barnes CM, Anderson NA, Li Y, Caufield PW. Effectiveness of steam sterilization in killing spores of Bacillus stearothermophilus in prophylaxis angles. *Gen Dent*. 1994 Sep–Oct;42(5):456–8.

40. Barnes CM, Anderson NA, Michalek SM, Russell CM. Effectiveness of sealed dental prophylaxis angles inoculated with Bacillus stearothermophilus in preventing leakage. *J Clin Dent*. 1994;5(2):35–7.

41. Gutmann ME. Air polishing: a comprehensive review of the literature. *J Dent Hyg*. 1998 Summer;72(3):47–56.

42. Weaks LM, Lescher NB, Barnes CM, Holroyd SV. Clinical evaluation of the Prophy-Jet as an instrument for routine removal of tooth stain and plaque. *J Periodontol*. 1984 Aug;55(8):486–8.

43. Barnes CM. An in-depth look at air polishing. *Dimensions Dent Hyg*. 2010 Mar;8(3):32, 34–6, 40.

44. Barnes CM, Covey DA, Walker MP, Ross JA. An in vitro evaluation of the effects of aluminum trihydroxide delivered via the Prophy Jet on dental restorative materials. *J Prosthet Dent*. 2004 Sep;13(3):166–72.

45. Orton GS. Clinical use of an air-powder abrasive system. *Dent Hyg*. 1987 Nov;61(11):513–18.

46. Barnes CM, Russell CM, Gerbo LR, Wells BR, Barnes DW. Effects of an air-powder polishing system on orthodontically bracketed and banded teeth. *Am J Orthod Dentofac Orthop*. 1990 Jan;97(1):74–81.

47. Shultz PH, Brockmann-Bell SL, Eick JD, Gross KB, Chappell RP, Spencer P. Effects of air-powder polishing on the bond strength of orthodontic bracket adhesive systems. *J Dent Hyg*. 1993 Feb;67(2):74–80.

48. Barnes CM, Fleming LS, Mueninghoff LA. An SEM evaluation of the in-vitro effects of an air-abrasive system on various implant surfaces. *Int J Oral Maxillofac Implants*. 1991 Winter;6(4):463–9.

49. Barnes CM, Toothaker RW, Ross J. Polishing dental implants and dental implant restorations. *J Prac Hyg*. 2005;14(8):6–8.

50. Berkstein S, Reiff RL, McKinney JF, Killoy WJ. Supragingival root surface removal during maintenance procedures utilizing an air-powder abrasive system or hand scaling. An in vitro study. *J Periodontol*. 1987 May;58(5):327–30.

51. Agger MS, Hörsted-Bindslev P, Hovgaard O. Abrasiveness of an air-powder polishing system on root surfaces in vitro. *Quintessence Int*. 2001 May;32(5):407–11.

52. Barnes CM. The management of aerosols with airpolishing delivery systems. *J Dent Hyg.* 1991 Jul–Aug;65(6):280–2.

53. Harrel SK, Barnes JB, Rivera-Hidalgo F. Aerosol reduction during air polishing. *Quintessence Int.* 1999 Sep;30(9):623–8.

54. Worrall SF, Knibbs PJ, Glenwright HD. Methods of reducing bacterial contamination of the atmosphere arising from use of an airpolisher. *Br Dent J.* 1987 Aug;163(4):118–19.

55. Tan WK. Sudden facial swelling: subcutaneous facial emphysema secondary to use of air/water syringe during dental extraction. *Singapore Dent J.* 2000 Dec;23(1 Suppl):42–4.

56. Davies DE. Pneumomediastinum after dental surgery. Anaesth Intensive Care. 2001 Dec;29(6):638–41.

57. Josephson GD, Wambach BA, Noordzji JP. Subcutaneous cervicofacial and mediastinal emphysema after dental instrumentation. *Otolaryngol Head Neck Surg.* 2001 Feb;124(2):170–1.

58. Yang SC, Chiu TH, Lin TJ, Chan HM. Subcutaneous emphysema and pneumomediastinum secondary to dental extraction: a case report and literature review. *The Kaohsiung J Med Sci.* 2006;22(12):641–5.

59. Heyman SN, Babayof I. Emphysematous complications in dentistry, 1960–1993: an illustrative case and review of the literature. *Quintessence Int.* 1995;26(8):535–43.

60. Arai I, Aoki T, Yamazaki H, Ota Y, Kaneko A. Pneumomediastinum and subcutaneous emphysema after dental extraction detected incidentally by regular medical checkup: a case report. Oral Surg Oral Med Oral Pathol Oral Radiol Endod. 2009;107(4): e33–8.

61. Finlayson RS, Stevens FD. Subcutaneous facial emphysema secondary to use of the Cavi-Jet. *J Periodontol.* 1988 May;59(5):315–17.

62. Fine DH, Mendieta C, Barnett ML, Furgang D, Meyers R, Olshan A, Vincent J. Efficacy of preprocedural rinsing with an antiseptic in reducing viable bacteria in dental aerosols. *J Periodontol.* 1992 Oct;63(10):821–4.

63. Atkinson DR, Cobb CM, Killoy WJ. The Effect of an air-powder abrasive system on in vitro root surfaces. *J Periodontol.* 1984 Jan;55(1): 13–18.

CHAPTER 45

Tooth Bleaching

PAMELA S. KENNARD, BSN, RDH, MA

Chapter Outline

INTRODUCTION

There are many different causes and colors for tooth stains and discolorations. As described in Chapter 21, stains may be intrinsic, within the tooth structure itself, extrinsic, directly on the tooth surface, or in the dental pellicle or biofilm attached superficially on the surface.

In conjunction with learning about tooth bleaching, a review of Chapter 21 is recommended.

Patients of all ages have concerns about the appearance of their teeth. They ask questions about discolorations and how they can be removed. Tooth bleaching may improve a patient's appearance and contribute to a patient's self-confidence in daily life.

Motivation to improve overall oral health can be a significant benefit.

I. BLEACHING VERSUS WHITENING

The terms bleaching and whitening have been used interchangeably, but two separate descriptions can define them more accurately.[1]

- Tooth whitening refers to use of abrasive agents contained in a dentifrice to remove extrinsic stain.
- Bleaching involves free radicals and the breakdown of pigment, which occurs in the tooth bleaching procedures.
- Key words and abbreviations are defined in **Box 45-1**.

II. VITAL TOOTH BLEACHING VERSUS NONVITAL TOOTH BLEACHING

- External tooth bleaching is used for both vital and nonvital teeth.
- Vital teeth can be stained intrinsically and extrinsically.
  - Agents for bleaching are applied to the external surfaces of the teeth.
  - Color change can extend into the dentin to produce a whitened tooth.
- Nonvital teeth become intrinsically stained by blood breakdown products, or agents from root canal therapy.[1]

- Nonvital tooth bleaching is a procedure performed by a dentist after root canal therapy using rubber dam or other type of isolation. The bleaching agents are introduced into the pulp chamber.
- The color of a single tooth is lightened to help it blend with the adjacent teeth.

III. HISTORY

A. Nonvital Tooth Bleaching

- Bleaching of discolored, nonvital teeth was first described as early as 1864.[2,3]
- In 1961 the "walking bleach" method was introduced. The "walking bleach" method sealed a mixture of sodium perborate and water into the pulp chamber and retained it there between the patient's visits.[4]
- By 1963 the "walking bleach" was modified using water and 30–35% hydrogen peroxide instead of the sodium perborate and water. Result: improved lighter color of nonvital teeth.[2]

B. Vital Tooth Bleaching

- In the 1960s, tooth lightening was observed after orthodontic patients used an antiseptic which contained carbamide peroxide to promote tissue healing due to gingivitis.[2,5]

BOX 45-1	**Key Words**

Tooth Bleaching

Abfraction: the pathologic loss of hard tooth substance caused by biomechanical loading forces. The loss is thought to be due to flexure and chemical fatigue degradation of enamel and/or dentin at a location distant from actual point of loading. (See Figure 43-3 for additional explanation).

Bleaching: a cosmetic dental procedure that uses a free radicals and breakdown of pigments to whiten teeth.

Block-out resins: light-cured resin materials that can be used as a rubber dam substitute during bleaching procedure or on study models to create space to hold bleaching material on custom trays.

Color: a phenomenon of light or visual perception that enables the differentiation of otherwise identical objects. Usually determined visually by measurement of hue, saturation, and luminous reflectance of light.

Esthetic: pertaining to the study of beauty and the sense of beautiful; objectifies beauty and attractiveness, elicits pleasure.

Extrinsic: external, extraneous, as originating from or on the outside.

Iatrogenic: resulting from the activity of a clinician; disorders induced in a patient by the clinician.

Intrinsic: from within, incorporation of a colorant within a material.

Laser bleaching and ultraviolet light system: dental office procedure that uses light in combination with hydrogen peroxide to activate bleaching materials and reduce the time necessary to produce a lighter color of teeth; use of rubber dam or protective light-cured resin on soft tissue required for use as well as eye protection.

Microabrasion: a proven method for treating tooth discolorations by microreduction of superficial enamel through various methods of mechanical and/or chemical actions.

NGVB: Acronym for night guard vital bleaching, which requires development of a custom tray that allows for administration and containment of tooth bleaching material such as carbamide peroxide or hydrogen peroxide.

Potassium nitrate: active ingredient in many anti-sensitivity dentifrices.

Psoralen: a compound that absorbs ultraviolet radiation, and is used to treat skin problems such as psoriasis, eczema, or alopecia.

Synergism: when the combined effect of the interaction of elements produces a greater total effect than the sum of the individual elements.

Translucency: having the appearance between complete opacity and complete transparency; partially opaque.

Whitening: use of abrasive agents in the dentifrice that results in whitening of teeth. Has also been used to describe the process of bleaching.

- In the 1980s lighter tooth color was noted after advising patients to use carbamide peroxide in customized trays for antiseptic purposes following periodontal surgery.[5]
- In 1989 the use of carbamide peroxide for the primary purpose of tooth bleaching was introduced.[6] Use of a custom tray was advocated to maintain the bleaching gel on the tooth surface for an extended time. The procedure was known as nightguard vital bleaching (NGVB).
- According to the American Dental Association Council on Scientific Affairs,[7] no significant, long-term oral or systemic health risks have been associated with professional at-home tooth bleaching materials containing 10% carbamide peroxide or 3.5% hydrogen peroxide when professionally supervised.

MECHANISM OF BLEACHING VITAL TEETH

The bleaching process is being studied and still is not fully understood. The color of the teeth will be influenced by thickness of enamel and underlying color of dentin.

I. TOOTH STRUCTURE

- Enamel is composed of rods that form a crystalline lattice structure, the enamel matrix.
- Dentin, largest portion of the tooth, underlies enamel; dentin color is either yellow or gray, which shows through the enamel.
- Bleaching products penetrate enamel and dentin, and can reach the pulp within 5–15 minutes.[7,8]
- Pulpal necrosis was noted when material was combined with excessive heat or trauma. No pulpal damage to teeth occurs without heat or trauma exposure.[9]

II. HYDROGEN BREAKDOWN/STAIN BREAKDOWN

- Unstable hydrogen peroxide breaks down into highly unstable free radicals. The breakdown products of carbamide peroxide and hydrogen peroxide are shown in the flowchart in **Figure 45-1**.
- Free radicals break larger pigmented organic molecules in the enamel matrix into smaller, less pigmented constituents.
- Oxidation, from the oxygen released from bleaching products into dentin and enamel, results in a color change affecting the optical qualities of the tooth color.[10]
- Higher product concentration and contact time results in more rapid bleaching.

III. TOOTH COLOR CHANGE WITH BLEACHING

- Color of both dentin and enamel are changed, but primarily the dentin color is changed.[10]

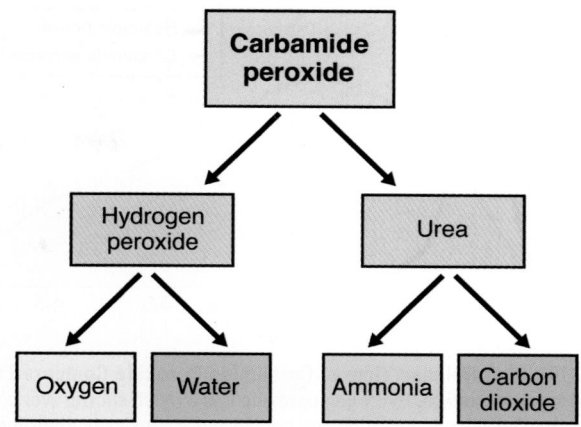

FIGURE 45-1 **Hydrogen Peroxide and Carbamide Peroxide Product Breakdown.** Flowchart to show breakdown of bleaching products. Hydrogen peroxide breaks down into oxygen and water; carbamide peroxide breaks down into hydrogen peroxide and urea which further break down as shown.

- Each tooth reaches its maximum color change. Additional bleaching product or contact time will not necessarily result in a lighter color[10]
- Teeth become dehydrated immediately, during, and after product administration. A lighter shade can result temporarily.
- Color will stabilize approximately two weeks after bleaching[10,11]

MATERIALS USED FOR VITAL TOOTH BLEACHING

- Both hydrogen peroxide and carbamide peroxide are used to lighten extrinsic color of vital teeth.
- Hydrogen peroxide is approximately three times stronger than carbamide peroxide.[5]
- Hydrogen peroxide has a short working time; carbamide peroxide has an extended working time.[8] **Figure 45-2** compares the release or duration time of carbamide peroxide with that of hydrogen peroxide.
- The chemicals are used alone or in combination with each other.
- Bleaching materials need an appropriate viscosity to flow over the tooth surface but not so excessive as to spread onto gingival and other oral tissues.

I. HYDROGEN PEROXIDE

- Oxygen ions break the bonds of the stain molecules into smaller, more soluble molecules.
- Active agent in most bleaching systems is hydrogen peroxide in a 15–35% concentration.
- Hydrogen peroxide is used directly or produced through a chemical reaction when carbamide peroxide breaks down.[11]
- Hydrogen peroxide has a lower pH than carbamide peroxide, which may result in demineralization when used for longer treatment times than recommended.

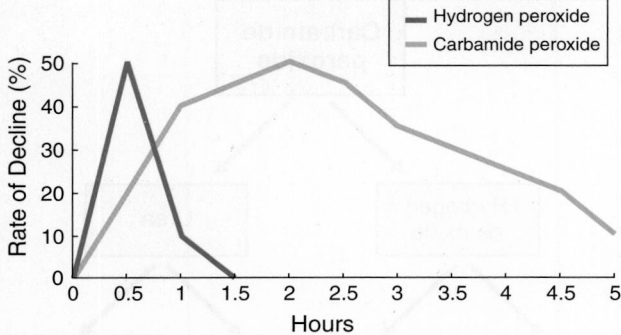

FIGURE 45-2 Release Time of Carbamide Peroxide Compared to Hydrogen Peroxide. Hydrogen peroxide has a much shorter working time than carbamide peroxide and causes more sensitivity. Hydrogen peroxide releases all of the peroxide within 1.5 hours. Carbamide peroxide releases the peroxide over a much longer time. Hydrogen peroxide is approximately three times stronger than carbamide peroxide. (Figures courtesy of Dr. Van Haywood. Reprinted from: Haywood VB. Treating sensitivity during tooth whitening. *Compend Contin Educ Dent*. 2005 Sep;28(9 Suppl 3):11–20. © 2005, AEGIS Publications, LLC. Used with permission).

Hydrogen peroxide takes less time per day, but more days to change tooth color effectively.[7]
■ Higher concentrations of hydrogen peroxide result in greater sensitivity, and greater color relapses after termination of bleaching[12]
■ Longer wait is required before composite bonding resin is placed.
■ High acidic nature of hydrogen peroxide results in dentin changes that never recover.[12]

II. CARBAMIDE PEROXIDE

■ Carbamide peroxide breaks down into hydrogen peroxide and urea. As shown in the flowchart **(Figure 45-1)** urea may further break down into ammonia with high pH to facilitate bleaching.
■ Carbamide peroxide is slow release: 50% of peroxide released in 2–4 hours and remainder of peroxide in 2–6 hours resulting in less sensitivity.[8] In **Figure 45-2** the release time of carbamide peroxide compared with hydrogen peroxide is shown.
■ At neutral pH, 10% carbamide peroxide solution is both safe and effective as a bleaching agent.[13]
■ Carbamide peroxide takes fewer days but more contact time.[1]

III. ADDITIONAL INGREDIENTS IN VITAL TOOTH BLEACHING SYSTEMS

A. Desensitizers

■ Materials to reduce the sensitivity side effect of bleaching are added to bleaching systems.
■ Materials can be incorporated into the bleaching gel, applied to teeth before bleaching, or given for use in trays before, during, and after treatment.

■ Material used:
  A. Potassium nitrate creates a calming effect on pulp by affecting the transmission of nerve impulses.[8]
  B. Sodium fluoride.
  C. Calcium phosphate and amorphous calcium phosphate aid in remineralization.[8]

B. Other Ingredients

■ Carbopol: A water-soluble resin used as a thickening agent, which prolongs the release of hydrogen peroxide from carbamide peroxide and promotes quicker results.
■ Glycerin: a gel to thicken and control the flow of bleaching agent to prevent overextending onto gingival tissues.
■ Sodium hydroxide: a chemical base
■ Flavoring

IV. INTERACTIONS WITH BLEACHING AGENTS[1]

■ Coffee, tea may compromise treatment. Advise patient to avoid.
■ Use of tobacco may compromise treatment; may have additive carcinogenic effect when combined with hydrogen peroxide. Advise patient to avoid.
■ Heavy use of alcohol-containing products may have additive carcinogenic effect when combined with hydrogen peroxide. Advise patient to avoid.

SAFETY

I. TOOTH STRUCTURE

■ Both hydrogen peroxide 3.5% and carbamide peroxide 10% are considered safe to lighten the color of teeth when professionally monitored.[7]
■ Up to two thirds of patients will experience transitory mild to moderate tooth sensitivity.[7]
■ Hydrogen peroxide at concentrations such as 30% or higher will remove the enamel matrix and create microscopic voids that scatter light. That can result in an increase in whiteness until remineralization occurs and color partly relapses.[1]
■ Carbamide peroxide 10% will cause fewer changes in the enamel matrix.[1]

II. SOFT TISSUE

■ Hydrogen peroxide is caustic and may cause burning and bleaching of the gingiva and any exposed tissue.[2]
■ 10% hydrogen peroxide concentration or higher has greater incidence of gingival irritation.[7]
■ Ill-fitting or overfilled tray may cause product spillage onto soft tissues resulting in tissue burning.
■ Studies have not demonstrated a risk to oral cancer.[2]

III. RESTORATIVE MATERIALS

- Restorative material color such as porcelain or composite materials will not be changed by bleaching.
- After bleaching, restorative procedures need to be delayed for 2 weeks to allow for color stabilization[12]
- Bonding needs to be delayed for 2 weeks due to significantly reduced bonding strength associated with recently bleached tooth surface.[12]
- Bleaching chemicals that contain hydrogen peroxide may have a negative effect on restorations and restorative materials due to lower pH, although impact does not require the renewal of the restoration.[10]
- May increase mercury release from amalgam restorations giving off a green hue.[10]
- May increase solubility of some dental cements.[14]

IV. SYSTEMIC

- Peroxides have mutagenic potential and may boost effects of known carcinogens such as alcohol; avoidance of use of known carcinogens is recommended while using bleaching products.[1]
- The use of tooth-bleaching products containing hydrogen peroxide or carbamide peroxide has not been proven to increase the risk of oral cancer in the general population, including those persons who are alcohol abusers and/or heavy cigarette smokers.[7]
- Accidental ingestion of small amounts can cause sore throat, nausea, vomiting, abdominal distention, and ulcerations of the oral mucosa, esophagus, and stomach.[2]
- Drugs that may be associated with photosensitivity and hyperpigmentation when light-activated whitening agents are used are described in **Box 45-2**.

V. CONTRAINDICATIONS ASSOCIATED WITH BLEACHING

A. Personal Factors

- Teeth that are at an acceptable shade, which is subjective.
- Patients with unrealistic personal expectations.

BOX 45-2 | **Drugs Associated With Potential Photosensitivity and Hyperpigmentation**

- Acne medications
- Anticancer drugs
- Antidepressants
- Antiparasitics
- Antipsychotics
- Diuretics
- Hypoglycemic
- Nonsteroidal anti-inflammatory drugs

BOX 45-3 | **Issues Associated With Light Activated Bleaching**

All contraindications noted are for bleaching with a light. Contraindicated for patients who are:

- Light sensitive
- Taking a photosensitive medication
- Receiving photochemotherapeutic drugs or treatments such as psoralen and ultraviolet radiation

Exposure to ultraviolet radiation produced by some lights is avoided by those with increased risk or have a history of skin cancer, including melanoma.

- Patients who are unable to be compliant with treatment will not achieve optimal results.
- Patients with tooth conditions that do not respond favorably to vital tooth bleaching.

B. Special Needs Patients

Children and Adolescents

- Caution with patient selection and safety concerns with children and adolescents.
- The American Academy of Pediatric Dentistry[15] discourages full-arch cosmetic bleaching for patients with a mixed dentition, but encourages judicious use of vital and nonvital bleaching due to the negative self-image that may arise from a discolored tooth or teeth.
- Current ADA recommendations for children and adolescent use includes
  - delaying treatment until after permanent teeth have erupted.
  - use of a custom-fabricated tray to limit amount of bleaching gel.
  - close supervision.[7]

C. Contraindicated

- Pregnant and lactating women are contraindicated for use of bleaching products.
- Patients taking photosensitive medications (Box 45-2)
- Laser light/power bleaching would be contraindicated for some patients as described in **Box 45-3**.

EFFICACY

- Both hydrogen peroxide and carbamide peroxide will lighten tooth color effectively. As noted in **Table 45-1**, selected tooth conditions will not respond to tooth bleaching; some tooth conditions will respond slowly.
- The initial color of the teeth and the type of stain present will affect the final color change.
- Specific indications for bleaching and the methods of treatments are listed in **Table 45-2**.

TABLE 45-1	DECISION-MAKING FOR TOOTH BLEACHING	
TOOTH CONDITION	**RESPONSE TO TOOTH WHITENING**	**SPECIAL CONSIDERATIONS**
Yellow Color	Normally excellent.	Resistant yellow may be tetracycline stain.
Enamel White Spots	Do not bleach well or may get lighter during whitening.	Eventually background color lightens resulting in less noticeable white spots. Goes through splotchy stage before background color whitens. Microabrasion may lessen white spots if less than one third through enamel.
Brown Fluorosis Stains	Respond 80% of the time.	Microabrasion techniques done after whitening and color stabilization may improve final result.
Nicotine Stains	Require longer treatment.	May take 2–3 mo of nightly application.
Tetracycline Stains	Multi-colored band may not respond well. Gray most difficult. Dark grays only get lighter. Dark cervical has poorest prognosis.	Requires 2–12 mo of daily whitening.
Minocycline Stains	Will respond; will take longer than yellow stain.	Type of tetracycline stain. Gives gray hue.
Root Exposure	Does not respond to whitening.	Better treated with periodontal coverage.
Dentinogenesis Imperfecta and Amelogenesis Imperfecta	No significant improvement with bleaching.	Inherited condition resulting in defective dentin and enamel, respectively.
Microcracks	Become whiter than rest of tooth.	Bright light or magnification required during assessment to view; may appear streaky during whitening process.
Anterior Lingual Amalgams	Become more visible after bleaching.	Replacement with very light composite restoration before bleaching.
Dental Caries	Not to be bleached.	Decay removal; temporary restoration followed by bleaching and final restoration after color stabilization; carbamide peroxide will increase sensitivity and is bacteriocidal.
Dark Canines	Require longer bleaching.	Isolated canine treatment until color match.
Attrition	Incisal edges do not respond.	Composite restorations added to incisal edges after bleaching.
Aging	Excellent.	More youthful appearance; root surfaces exposure likely.
Translucent Teeth	Bleaching will increase translucency at incisal.	Translucent areas will appear darker after whitening due to contrast.

I. FACTORS THAT INFLUENCE OUTCOME[1,10]

- Initial tooth color: the darker the initial color, the more difficult to lighten.
- Patient age: Attrition, incisal, and occlusal wear through enamel exposes the darker underlying dentin.
- Concentration of bleaching agent.
- Ability of agent to reach the stain molecules.
- Duration of contact of the active bleaching agent: longer duration, the greater the degree of bleaching.
- Number of applications that the agent is applied to obtain desired results: darker teeth tend to require more treatment applications.
- Temperature of agent: heat will result in faster oxygen release, but speed of color change may not be altered.

TABLE 45-2	INDICATIONS FOR TOOTH BLEACHING AND METHODS OF TREATMENT
INDICATION	**METHOD TO TREAT**
Discolored, Endodontically Treated Tooth	Internal bleaching; in-office or walking.
Single or Multiple Discolored Teeth	External bleaching: in-office 1–3 visits or custom trays worn 2–6 wk.
Surface Staining	Brushing with whitening dentifrice.
Isolated Brown or White Discoloration, Shallow Depth in Enamel	Microabrasion followed by neutral sodium fluoride applications.
White Discoloration on Yellowish Teeth	Microabrasion followed by custom tray whitening.

■ Nicotine stains: require 1–3 months of nightly treatment due to the tenacity of the stain.

II. TETRACYCLINE, MINOCYCLINE, FLUOROSIS STAINING

A. Tetracycline and Minocycline Staining

■ Tetracycline particles incorporate into dentin during calcification of unerupted teeth through chelation with calcium resulting in discolored dentin that is resistant to bleaching.[16]

■ Minocycline, a derivative of tetracycline, can discolor erupted teeth.[14]

■ Tetracycline and minocycline staining severity varies. A comparison of before and after bleaching of brown tetracycline staining is shown in **Figure 45-3**.

A. *First category staining*: Light-yellow to light-gray responds to bleaching.

B. *Second category staining*: darker, more extensive yellow-gray responds to extended bleaching time.

C. *Third category staining*: intense dark gray-blue banding stains. Severe third category staining may require porcelain veneers for satisfactory esthetic result.

D. Some tetracycline stains will require 1–12 months to achieve a satisfactory result

B. Fluorosis

■ Fluorosis results from ingesting excessive fluoride during tooth development resulting in white or brown spots on teeth.

■ Bleaching does not change white spots, but lightens the background color making the contrast less noticeable.

■ White spots go through a splotchy stage during bleaching but will return to baseline.[12]

■ Amorphous calcium phosphate (CCP-ACP) may be effective in lessening the white spots if lesion is less than one-third through enamel.[13]

■ Brown discoloration responsive to bleach 80% of the time.[13]

III. LONGEVITY OF RESULTS

■ Darkening or relapse of the tooth shade is expected after bleaching.

■ Relapse of shade occurs almost immediately as newly bleached, dehydrated teeth rehydrate.

■ As months and years pass, teeth may discolor and darken again, especially if stain-inducing activities continue.

■ To maintain shade, periodic bleaching procedures are performed or repeated.

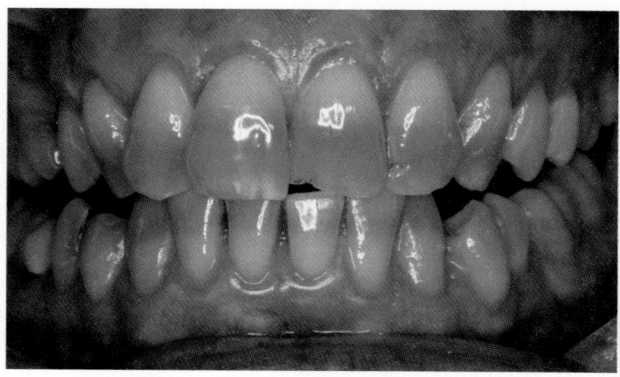
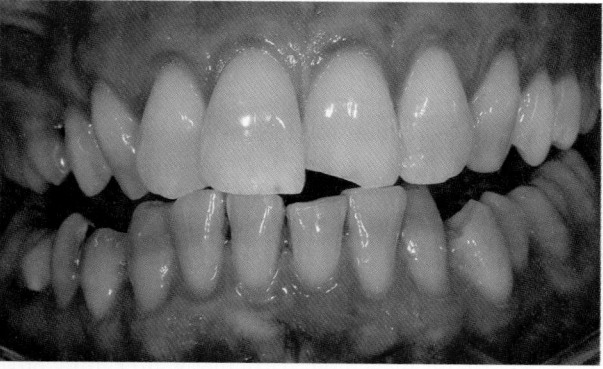

A   B

FIGURE 45-3 **Before and after Bleaching of Brown Tetracycline-Stained Teeth. (A)** Patient before treating. **(B)** Patient treated with 10% carbamide peroxide for 2 months. Some tetracycline-stained teeth will require up to 12 months to achieve improved results. Those with severe gray stain or banded staining may require porcelain veneers to achieve an acceptable cosmetic result. (Images courtesy of Dr. Van Haywood. Reprinted from: Haywood VB. The "bottom line" on bleaching 2008. *Inside Dentistry.* 2008 Feb;4(2):2–5. © 2008, AEGIS Publications, LLC. Used with permission.)

IV. ADDITIONAL BENEFITS OF BLEACHING

■ Hydrogen peroxide used in bleaching has temporary additional effects that includes an antimicrobial action that may lead to a reduction in biofilm and improved gingival health.[17]

■ Improved motivation to have higher standards of personal daily oral hygiene while participating in bleaching procedures.

■ Carbamide peroxide may assist with caries control due to raising pH levels to 8 during application.[18]

■ Carbamide peroxide has been shown to be bacteriocidal to cariogenic bacteria which benefits elderly xerostomic patients, and orthodontic patients.

REVERSIBLE SIDE EFFECTS OF BLEACHING

I. SENSITIVITY

A. The most common side effect of bleaching is tooth tingling and sensitivity.

B. Aching sensation can occur because of insult of peroxide on nerves: a reversible pulpitis.[8]

　■ Primarily occurs in the first 2 weeks of treatment and may last days to months after cessation of bleaching.

　■ Resolves completely as teeth become accustomed to bleaching

　■ Not correlated with increased wear time[8]

　■ Lower concentrations have been used for up to 12 months and do not exhibit greater sensitivity[8]

　■ Patients with prior history of tooth sensitivity may be more at risk to develop sensitivity during bleaching.

II. VULNERABLE TOOTH SURFACES

■ Exposed root surfaces and dentin appear to increase risk of developing sensitivity and need to be protected from bleaching material.

■ Teeth with unrestored abfraction lesions tend to have more sensitivity.

■ Addition of desensitizing materials decreases sensitivity.

■ Treatments to reduce tooth sensitivity are listed in **Table 45-3**.

IRREVERSIBLE TOOTH DAMAGE[1]

I. ROOT RESORPTION

■ Can occur after bleaching, particularly after intracoronal, nonvital tooth bleaching, when heat is applied during the technique.

■ Internal and external resorption may become apparent several years after bleaching.

■ Occurs usually in cervical third of the tooth.

■ Cause may be related to a history of trauma.

TABLE 45-3	DESENSITIZATION PROCEDURES FOR BLEACHING
PRETREATMENT	■ Brush on or use with tray a desensitizing toothpaste containing potassium nitrate, without sodium lauryl sulfate, which removes smear layer from dentin, beginning 2 wk before whitening. ■ Use toothpaste with prescription strength sodium fluoride. ■ Use toothpaste that includes calcium carbonate.
DURING	■ Continue to use desensitizing toothpaste, which includes sodium fluoride or potassium nitrate, daily between treatments. ■ Increase time intervals between treatments. ■ Reduce exposure time of bleaching materials ■ Limit the amount in tray to prevent tissue contact.
POSTBLEACHING	■ Sensitivity diminishes with time. ■ Continue daily use of desensitizing dentifrice. ■ Have professional fluoride varnish application. ■ Avoid foods and beverages with temperature extremes or that contain acidic elements.

■ May lead to tooth loss.

■ Bleaching agents are not placed on exposed cementum to avoid complications.

II. TOOTH FRACTURE

■ May be related to removal of tooth structure or reduction of the microhardness of dentin and enamel.

■ May lead to tooth loss.

III. DEMINERALIZATION

■ Patient with over-the-counter product may not seek or follow professional advice and attempt to get the teeth whiter by using the product more than recommended.

■ Demineralization with slight surface pitting can result.

■ Remineralization may be possible if started early enough.

■ Remineralization procedures are described in Chapter 26 on page 383.

MODES OF VITAL TOOTH BLEACHING

■ A comparison of the advantages and disadvantages of professionally applied and professionally dispensed/professionally monitored systems and the over-the-counter systems are listed in **Table 45-4**.

TABLE 45-4	COMPARISONS OF MODES OF TOOTH BLEACHING SYSTEMS	
METHODS	**ADVANTAGES**	**DISADVANTAGES**
Professionally Applied Utilizing Laser/ Ultraviolet Light System Procedure	■ Comprehensive ■ Treatment may be combined with trays and professional grade home bleaching materials ■ Product selection ■ Patient education ■ Follow-up, evaluation of effectiveness ■ Sensitivity treatment ■ Compliance guaranteed ■ Quickest result	■ Higher cost
Professionally Dispensed Includes Professional Grade Product and Trays	■ Comprehensive ■ Dental exam ■ Appropriate patient ■ Selection ■ Product selection ■ Patient education ■ Follow-up, evaluation of effectiveness ■ Sensitivity treatment ■ Choice of comfortable time and place for application ■ Quicker result	■ Cost ■ Longer time to whiten than professionally applied
Over-the-Counter	■ Lowest cost ■ Immediate start ■ Easier access to purchase	■ No comprehensive exam ■ Slowest whitening ■ Non-customized delivery ■ Results and tissue response not monitored ■ Over-the-counter products have short exposure times which limits effects ■ Unsupervised ■ Compliance issues

■ The different methods of tooth bleaching can achieve similar, effective results although the mode of delivery, length of treatment, and ease of treatment vary.

I. PROFESSIONALLY APPLIED

■ Professionally applied bleaching is performed with high concentrations of 30–40% hydrogen peroxide or 35–44% carbamide peroxide.
■ Some systems use activation or enhancement with a light or heat source.
   ▪ Teeth are not anesthetized in order to monitor heat-provoked sensitivity.
   ▪ Heat applied or produced by the use of light may cause an adverse effect such as necrosis of the pulp of the tooth.
   ▪ The additional issues associated with the use of a light-activated whitening are listed in **Box 45-3**.
■ Treatment may take one to six applications for preferred results.
■ Time for each application varies between the different products; ranges from 30- to 60-minute treatment.
■ Bleaching gels are administered in a professional treatment room. They are not for at-home use.

■ Rubber dam or an equivalent technique, such as a liquid light-cured resin dam, is applied to isolate the caustic agents from contact with soft tissues.
■ Care must be taken to assure the liquid light-cured resin dam is in the interproximal spaces to protect gingival tissue.
■ Improvements in paint-on rubber dams, cheek, lip retractors, and lower concentrations of peroxide have made in-office bleaching safer for patient and dentist.
■ Laser-safe/ultraviolet light protection of eyes for all in treatment room is required.
■ Gingival sensitivity or irritation may occur.
■ Laser/Power bleaching treatment plan may also involve use of trays for home use.

II. PROFESSIONALLY DISPENSED/ PROFESSIONALLY MONITORED

■ Also called nightguard vital bleaching (NGVB), external bleaching, at-home bleaching.
■ Tray preparation:
   ▪ An impression of the teeth is taken to prepare the cast for fabrication of the tray.
   ▪ Thin, vacuum-formed custom trays are made for each dental arch to be bleached.

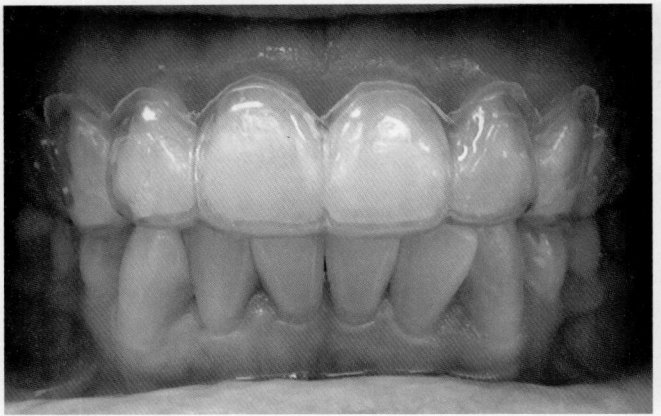 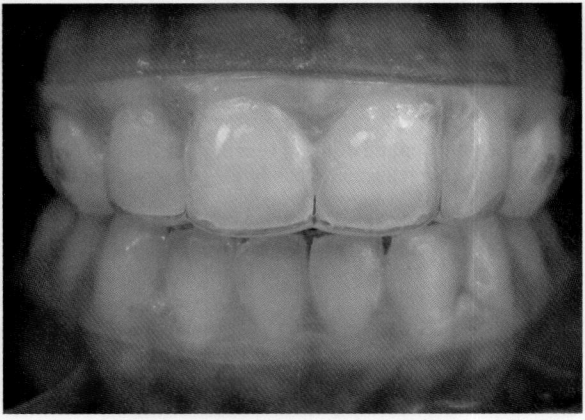

A   B

FIGURE 45-4 **Scalloped and Unscalloped NGVB Tray Designs.** Either scalloped or unscalloped trays may be used. **(A)** Scalloped trays aim to protect the gingiva and exposed root surfaces. **(B)** Unscalloped trays are more comfortable and take less preparation time. Patients need to be warned to avoid overfilling trays.

- Trays are fitted to the patient and adjusted to ensure bleaching material will not come into contact with soft tissues.
- As shown in **Figure 45-4**, trays are either scalloped at gingival margin or unscalloped and trimmed at mucogingival line. Appendix A of Reference 10 shows the preparation of the trays.
- Nonscalloped trays seal better, use less material, and are more comfortable.
- Patient instruction:
  - Patient is given instructions and bleaching materials for use in the trays at home.
  - Once or twice daily application for 1–2 weeks is usually recommended if lack of sensitivity and other side effects permit.
  - Patient retains the trays after completion of bleaching to reuse for touch-ups as needed.
  - Professionally dispensed bleaching products are commonly recommended after professionally applied bleaching procedures to maintain and promote results.

III. OVER-THE-COUNTER PRODUCTS

- Also called "at-home" or "self-directed" products.
- When asked about use of the self-directed product, a dental hygienist can stress the need for professional examination and supervision; the products can cause harm if misused, may irritate tissues or cause systemic illness if ingested.
- May be recommended to help maintain results of professionally applied and professionally dispensed methods of bleaching.

A. Methods of Bleaching

1. Preparation
- Patient informs dental professional of proposed use to discuss risks and possible interaction with any proposed dental treatment.

- Patient is advised to have thorough oral evaluation before use of the products, as well as appropriate dental and periodontal treatment including calculus, stain, and biofilm removal.
- Delivered through various packaging, viscosities, and flavors.

2. Strips
- Hydrogen peroxide is delivered on polyethylene film strips.
- Strips are placed on the teeth up to two times per day for 30 minutes for about 2 weeks.

3. Prefabricated Trays
- Thin membrane tray loaded with bleaching agent is adapted to maxillary or mandibular arch.
- Usually worn 30–60 minutes daily for 5–10 days.

4. Paint-on
- Carbamide peroxide is incorporated into a thick gel that is painted on the teeth selected to be bleached.
- An advantage to this method is that individual teeth may be bleached.

5. Dentifrice
- Used to help keep teeth cleaner, therefore look whiter.
- Some have more abrasive materials to remove extrinsic stains.
- Due to short exposure time, the bleaching agent in the dentifrice has little effect on staining.
- Some contain hydrogen peroxide; others contain agents that may deter further attachment of stains to the teeth.

6. Mouthrinse
- Content of alcohol is avoided in selection of mouthrinse.

NONVITAL TOOTH BLEACHING

- Also called "walking bleach" procedure, internal bleaching.
- Bleaching of a single, endodontically treated tooth that is discolored can be accomplished by nonvital tooth bleaching procedures.
- Alternative to more invasive correction, such as a post and core with crown, of single, discolored, endodontically treated tooth.
- Performed by a dentist.
- Requirements for procedure:
  - Healthy periodontium.
  - Successfully obturated root canal filling.
  - Root canal filling is sealed off with a restorative material before treatment to prevent bleaching agent from reaching periapical tissue.
- Hydrogen peroxide and/or sodium perborate is placed in the pulp chamber, sealed, and left for 3–7 days, as outlined in **Box 45-4**.

BOX 45-4	**Procedure for Nonvital Tooth Bleaching**

Periodontally healthy, endodontically treated tooth:

1. Photograph of the tooth to be bleached with shade guide.
2. Perform prophylaxis to remove extrinsic stain and calculus.
3. Probe circumferentially to determine the outline of the CEJ.
4. Rubber dam isolation is applied to prevent contamination of root canal therapy.
5. Prepare access cavity. Remove all endodontic obturation material, sealer, cement, and necessary restorative material without removing more dentin than necessary.
6. Remove 2–3 mm of obturation material from the root canal to level below the crest of the gingival margin.
7. Irrigate access cavity with copious amount of water and dry well without desiccating.
8. Root canal therapy is sealed off, commonly with glass ionomer cement or other filling material.
9. Medicament is placed in pulp chamber.
10. Pulp chamber is sealed with a temporary restoration.
11. Patient returns in 3–7 days for evaluation.

Above procedure is repeated several times until desired result is obtained.

   To finalize procedure:

1. Rubber dam isolation.
2. Temporary restoration on medicament is removed.
3. Pulp chamber is irrigated thoroughly with water.
4. Coronal restoration is placed; generally a composite material.
5. Photograph tooth with corresponding shade guide for records.

- Hydrogen peroxide and sodium perborate may be synergistic and very effective in bleaching the tooth.
- The process is repeated until a satisfactory result is obtained.
- Once satisfactory result is obtained the pulp chamber is sealed with glass ionomer cement.
- Appoint patient 2 weeks later to place permanent, bonded, composite-resin restoration in access cavity to allow dissipation of residual oxygen that would interfere with efficacy of bonding agent.
- If unsuccessful after repeated attempts, techniques for vital tooth bleaching can be tried or an alternative restorative procedure, such as a post and core, with crown.
- Results usually last longer than external tooth bleaching.
- There is no universal standard for what is considered acceptable esthetics.
- Personal background, culture, and a society's and patient's image of esthetics are factors.
- The dentist initially may not identify a patient's esthetic issues in the same way that the patient identifies them.
- Care is taken to communicate and agree about the course of treatment and the expected result of treatment before the start of bleaching.

DENTAL HYGIENE PROCESS OF CARE

I. PATIENT ASSESSMENT

A. Review of medical history; identify any contraindications for bleaching.
B. Complete dental assessment including the following:
  - Complete extraoral and intraoral examination including oral cancer screening.
  - Updated radiographs. Cavitated dental caries is contraindicated for bleaching.
  - A lesion is prepared and restored with a temporary restoration to be replaced with permanent matching restoration upon completion of bleaching.
  - Updated radiographs to identify abscesses or nonvital teeth which would require endodontic therapy before bleaching.
  - Periodontal examination including areas of recession. Cementum needs to be protected from bleaching material to avoid potential internal and/or external resorption.
  - Obtain photographic record of tooth shade without lipstick or strong clothing colors that may interfere with accurate assessment. Use canine for base color. Color will be gray or yellow. Confirm with patient. **Figure 45-5** illustrates using a shade guide.
C. Identify those factors that would lead to a guarded prognosis for bleaching including:
  - History or presence of sensitive teeth.
  - Extremely dark gingival third of tooth visible during a smile.

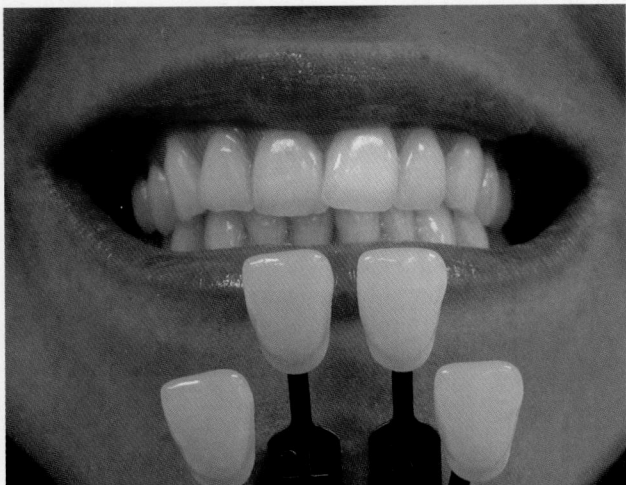

FIGURE 45-5 **Digital Photographic Record of Tooth Shade.** Patient's shade taken, recorded, and photographed in natural light or color-corrected lighting after extrinsic stain removal before bleaching. Several manufacturers provide color ranges with as many as 29 shades. Electronic digital shade guides provide objective records. Patient's shade and photograph are recorded at each visit while in bleaching treatment. (Photo courtesy of author).

- Extensive white spots that are very visible.
- Temporomandibular joint dysfunction or bruxism that would make wearing NVB uncomfortable and potential for aggravating condition.
- Very translucent teeth that would become less esthetic due to increased translucency.

D. Identify contraindications for at-home whitening including the following:
- Unrealistic expectations.
- Unwillingness or unable to comply with at-home treatment routines.
- Excessive existing restorations not requiring replacement.
- Inability to tolerate the taste of the product.
- Pregnancy or lactation.

II. DENTAL HYGIENE DIAGNOSIS

Identify patient with dissatisfaction in appearance of tooth color that would likely respond positively to tooth bleaching and has no contraindications.

III. DENTAL HYGIENE CARE PLAN

A. *Dental hygiene therapy* with complete removal of all supra- and subgingival calculus and stain along with personal care instruction.
B. *Patient education*
   1. Procedure, product chosen based on patient need.
   2. Tooth sensitivity treatment and sensitivity prevention.
   3. Emphasis on the following:
      - Effective daily biofilm removal before bleaching material use to prevent additional extrinsic stain accumulation.
      - Use of nonabrasive whitening dentifrice.
      - Removal of excess bleaching material after use.
      - Avoidance of over-filling tray to protect soft tissue and exposed cementum.
      - Avoidance of foods that stain teeth, coffee, alcohol, and use of tobacco to maximize results.
      - Avoidance of swallowing bleaching material due to irritation of materials to mucosa.
C. Choose appropriate bleaching method
   1. Discussion of procedure, risks, and realistic results
   2. Plan with patient for anticipated needs after bleaching, such as replacement of existing tooth-colored restorations that will not match after bleaching.
   3. Obtain informed consent listing procedure and risks with patient's signature (in Chapter 24, page 358).

IV. IMPLEMENTATION

- Review instructions for use and patient education items previously listed.

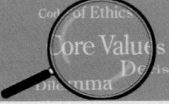

Everyday Ethics

Julia is a 12-year-old dental hygiene patient who is quite verbal about the appearance of her "dark front tooth." As part of the oral care instructions, Theresa, the dental hygienist, begins to discuss possible options of nonvital bleaching to lighten the tooth. Julia becomes visibly excited and wants to whiten the tooth right away. Following Dr. Leonard's examination, Theresa brings Julia's mother in to discuss the possibility of whitening. The mother quickly tells Julia "You don't want to do that, it's probably too expensive."

Questions for Consideration
1. Is it ethical to discuss treatment options with a child patient before informing the parent or guardian who will make the decision for treatment? Explain.
2. Consider the Steps in Resolving an issue or dilemma (in Chapter 1, page 10). What are the rights of each of the individuals involved in this situation? Are there any conflicts of interest that Theresa must identify as she works through the steps in resolving this issue?
3. What financial, legal, or cultural factors need consideration if Theresa is to identify an alternative approach that will lead to a positive outcome? Describe her possible approaches.

- *Dental hygiene therapy:* removal of all calculus deposits, and extrinsic stains.
- Pretreatment desensitization when indicated. Recommended procedures for pretreatment, during treatment and postbleaching are listed in **Table 45-3**.
- Premedication with anti-inflammatory pain medication when indicated for sensitivity.
- Preparation of trays; impression and construction
  - Wet teeth before taking impression to ensure teeth are not dehydrated.
  - Monitoring appointments as needed to assess patient compliance, results, sensitivity.

V. EVALUATION, PLANNING FOR MAINTENANCE

- At routine appointments, compare tooth color with tooth color guide. Take follow-up photos as appropriate for records.
- Color from bleaching relapses with time.
- Plan for repeat of bleaching process at appropriate intervals.

DOCUMENTATION

Documentation in the patient's permanent record when planning tooth bleaching includes a minimum of the following:

- Current oral conditions
- Consent to treat related to tooth whitening
- Services provided including necessary records for tooth shade
- Impressions and preparation of the trays
- Demonstration of tray filling, positioning, timing, and cleaning
- Instructions given to patient
- Planned follow-up care and appointments
- Patient problems or complaints expressed
- An example of a progress note is shown in **Box 45-5**.

 **Factors To Teach The Patient**

- Why a complete oral cancer screening and dental examination, including radiographs and periodontal evaluation, is performed before any form of whitening is initiated.
- During bleaching, teeth and gingival tissues may become sensitive for a period of time.
- If sensitivity is experienced, use a desensitizing product, discontinue bleaching, or delay next treatment.
- Regardless of method, color relapse occurs in a relatively short period of time.
- Excessive use of bleaching products may be harmful. Follow manufacturer's directions.
- Existing tooth-colored restorations will not change color, therefore may not match and may need to be replaced after bleaching.

BOX 45-5	Example Progress Note

Patient presents for 6-month maintenance visit. All extrinsic stains removed. Patient expressed dissatisfaction with tooth color. Patient presents with no contraindications for tooth whitening process. Radiographs and dental exam reveal absence of cavitated caries. Patient educated on procedure, cost, benefits and limitations of whitening process. Patient agreed to proceed with treatment. Consent to treat signed (and filed with this permanent progress note); copy of consent to treat given to patient. Written instructions provided to patient. Color shade C1. Appears to have yellow stain only. Record photographs obtained. Impressions for NGVB tray obtained. Patient has history of tooth sensitivity. Patient instructed to brush with potassium nitrate product for 2 weeks before beginning whitening process, begin whitening with carbamide peroxide 10% every other day. Patient scheduled for follow-up appointment 2 weeks after whitening process initiated.

Signed: _____, RDH Date: _____.

References

1. Byrne BE, McIntyre F. *ADA/PDR guide to dental therapeutics.* 5th ed. Chicago: American Dental Association; 2009. Chapter 12, Bleaching Agents; p. 351.
2. Dahl JE, Pallesen U. Tooth bleaching—a critical review of the biological aspects. *Crit Rev Oral Biol Med.* 2003 Jul;14(4): 292–304.
3. Truman J. Bleaching of non-vital discolored anterior teeth. *Dent Times.* 1864;1:69.
4. Spasser HF. A simple bleaching technique using sodium perborate. *NY State Dent J.* 1961 Aug-Sep;27:332.
5. Mokhlis GR, Matis BA, Cochran MA, Eckert GJ. A clinical evaluation of carbamide peroxide and hydrogen peroxide whitening agents during daytime use. *J Am Dent Assoc.* 2000 Sep; 131(9):1269–77.
6. Haywood VB, Heymann HO. Nightguard vital bleaching. *Quintessence Int.* 1989 Mar;20(3):173–6.
7. ADA Council on Scientific Affairs. *Tooth whitening/bleaching treatment considerations for dentists and their patients.* Chicago: American Dental Association; 2009 Sep. 12 p.
8. Haywood VB. Treating sensitivity during tooth whitening. *Compend Contin Educ Dent.* 2005 Sep;26(9 Suppl 3):11–20.
9. Cooper JS, Bokmeyer TJ, Bowles WH. Penetration of the pulp chamber by carbamide peroxide bleaching agents. *J Endod.* 1992 Jul; 18(7):315–7.
10. Haywood VB. Tooth whitening indications and outcomes of nightguard vital bleaching. Chicago: Quintessence; 2007. Chapter 1, Diagnosis and treatment planning for bleaching; p. 1–26.

11. Sweeney MR. Tooth whitening. In: Gladwin M, Bagby M, editors. *Clinical aspects of dental materials*. Philadelphia: Lippincott, Williams & Wilkins; 2009. p. 212–22.

12. Haywood VB. The "bottom line" on bleaching 2008. *Inside Dent*. 2008 Feb;4(2):2–5.

13. Shannon H, Spencer P, Gross K, Tira D. Characterization of enamel exposed to 10% carbamide peroxide bleaching agents. *Quintessence Int*. 1993 Jan;24(1):39–44.

14. Bowles WH, Bokmeyer TJ. Staining of adult teeth by minocycline by septic proteins. *J Esthet Dent*. 1997;9(1):30–4.

15. American Academy of Pediatric Dentistry Council on Clinical Affairs. Policy on dental bleaching for child and adolescent patients. *Pediatric Dent*. 2005–2006;27(7 Suppl):46–8.

16. Mello HS. The mechanism of tetracycline staining in primary and permanent teeth. *J Dent Child*. 1967 Nov;34(6):478–87.

17. Marshall K, Berry TG, Woolum J. Tooth whitening: current status. *Compend Contin Educ Dent*. 2010 Sep;31(7):486–92, 494–5.

18. Haywood VB. Bleaching and caries control in elderly patients. *Aesthetic Dent Today*. 2007 Oct;1(4):42–4.

Evaluation

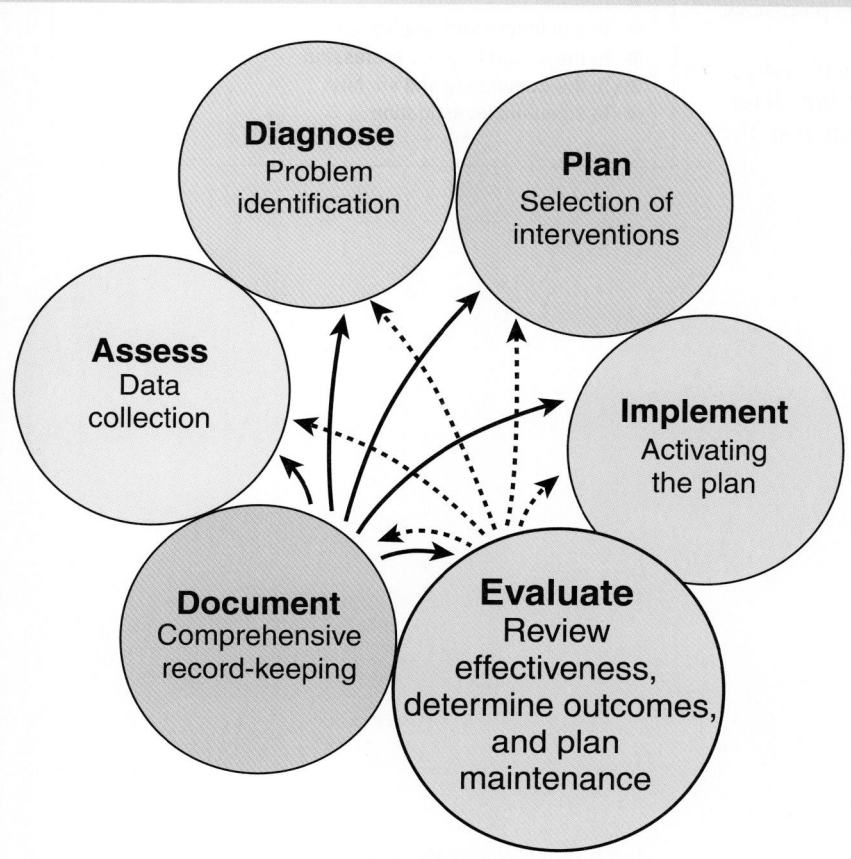

FIGURE VII-1 **The Dental Hygiene Process of Care**

INTRODUCTION

Evaluation of treatment outcomes relies on the careful re-collection with assessment data and comparison of the information with baseline data to determine further treatment needs and appropriate periodontal maintenance interval. Collection and analysis of assessment data at each maintenance appointment allows comparison with both previous and future observations in order to determine changes in the patient's oral health status over time.

THE DENTAL HYGIENE PROCESS OF CARE

The Dental Hygiene Process of Care continues with the next step of evaluation. Evaluation is an essential component of every step in the cycle, as illustrated by the arrows in **Figure VII-1**. The dental hygienist who evaluates each step in the process during each patient appointment will assure that attention is paid to any changing circumstance that affects patient care or treatment outcomes.

As the cycle of the process of patient care, continues:

■ The evaluation step proceeds again to the collection of assessment data that determines whether the oral health goals identified in the patient's care plan have been met.
■ A new care plan, based on evaluation data will address further treatment or preventive needs and/or determine the proper maintenance interval to support the patient's oral health status.

■ During the maintenance appointment, the process will be used to determine if the patient's needs have changed and to plan and implement interventions that meet those needs.

ETHICAL APPLICATIONS

It is beneficial to evaluate an ethical situation involving treatment outcomes or self-evaluation of professional skills and abilities based on the *Standards of Professional Responsibility* outlined in the ADHA Code of Ethics and listed in **Box VII-1** below. The ethical dental hygienist will assess how a particular decision could potentially affect each of the facets that comprise the professional role of a dental hygienist and will evaluate a choice of action that acknowledges each area of professional responsibility.

BOX VII-1	Standards of Professional Responsibility

Professional dental hygienists acknowledge the following responsibilities:

■ To ourselves as individuals and professionals
■ To family and friends
■ To patients
■ To employers and employees
■ To the dental hygiene profession
■ To the community and society
■ To scientific investigation

CHAPTER 46

Principles of Evaluation

CHARLOTTE J. WYCHE, RDH, MS

Chapter Outline

PRINCIPLES OF EVALUATION

Evaluation of treatment and oral health education outcomes is sometimes considered the final step in providing evidence-based dental and dental hygiene care.[1,2] However, as illustrated in the dental hygiene process of care **Figure VII-1**, page 723, ongoing evaluation at each step provides feedback that determines success or indicates need to modify procedures throughout the process.

Key terms related to evaluation are defined in **Box 46-1**. For the most part, principles of evaluation and definitions for related terminology have been developed for educational[3,4] and community-based program[5] evaluation, but the basic principles can be adapted for assessment of clinical and patient education outcomes as well.

I. PURPOSE OF EVALUATION

Evaluation is a systematic determination of worth, value, or significance.[6] Evaluation of dental hygiene care includes assessment of outcomes for both treatment and preventive interventions. Ideally, evaluation measures are enacted at each step in the dental hygiene process of care as shown in **Figure VII-1**.

- *Formative evaluation,* information collected during any dental hygiene appointment, provides ongoing feedback that will allow the dental hygienist to monitor patient needs (e.g., need for pain control) and adapt to changes in the patient's general health or oral health status during care.
- *Immediate evaluation,* for example use of an explorer to check for residual calculus or evaluating to make

BOX 46-1 | **Key Words**

Evaluation

Data: information collected during the evaluation procedure that is analyzed to determine oral health outcomes related to dental hygiene interventions.

Evaluation design: a description of the purpose, plans, and strategies that will be needed to gather, process, and interpret the data used to determine treatment outcomes.

Evaluation methods: data collection procedures and strategies that are selected to determine whether or not expected outcomes related to patient specific oral health goals identified in the dental hygiene care plan have been met. (See Figure 24-1, page 354.)

Expert witness: a person licensed to perform treatment in a specific health profession or with specialized knowledge, beyond that of the average person, in an area of treatment; a source for determining legal professional standard of care in a court case.

Feedback: communication that occurs among all individuals participating in the patient's care, including the dentist, the dental hygienist, the patient and the patient's physician or caregiver, if necessary. Giving and receiving feedback creates trust and ensures that those involved in all aspects of patient care stay informed at every step.

Formative evaluation: ongoing evaluation to monitor each step in the dental hygiene process of care; ongoing feedback that determines any needed changes in the dental hygiene care plan prior to the completion of a treatment sequence.

Indicators: benchmarks used to measure or test changes. In evaluating dental hygiene interventions, indicators can be quantitative (such as measurement of probing depth or plaque scores) or qualitative (such as patient expressions of satisfaction or ability to perform self-care routines).

Objectives: measurable goals; the expected outcomes of clinical treatment, patient education, counseling, or oral hygiene instruction/home care interventions identified in the patient care plan.

Outcomes assessment: a measure of the effectiveness of dental hygiene clinical and educational interventions in meeting oral health goals identified in the patient care plan.

Standard of care: criteria or protocols that define the minimal quality of care required to defend against a legal dispute against the practice of one's profession; usually established by federal laws, state and local statutes and codes and/or testimony from an "expert witness," and is supported by guidelines or recommendations documents published by professional associations.

Summative evaluation: formal, standardized evaluation procedures conducted at the end of a treatment series; includes determination of periodontal maintenance interval and/or identification of further treatment needs.

---

sure there has been no undue tissue trauma at the end of a scaling and root planing procedure, will help make sure patient care goals have been met at each appointment.

- *Ongoing evaluation* of tissue changes and patient self-care abilities during a multiappointment treatment sequence can provide information regarding the need for modifications in the original patient care plan.

- *Summative evaluation* at the end of a sequence of planned dental hygiene interventions determines whether the oral health goals stated in the patient's care plan have been met.

- Assessing the outcome of both clinical and preventive interventions at the completion of a treatment cycle identifies need for further treatment and adapted self-care protocols.

- The evaluation process also helps to determine the appropriate maintenance interval to maintain an achieved increase in oral health status.

II. EVALUATION DESIGN

- A plan for evaluation of patient care outcomes includes informal monitoring, feedback, and modifications in

patient care provided during each patient appointment.

- Methods for evaluating the success of dental hygiene treatment have traditionally included re-collection of the new clinical data, such as probing depths and areas of bleeding that are used to compare with the patient's health status at the beginning of treatment.

- The evaluation process includes measures that assess the extent to which disease prevention and health promotion interventions have been effective.

- A comparison of pre- and posttreatment values indicates areas of success or areas of need for further intervention.

III. EVALUATION PROCESS

- When writing the dental hygiene care plan, indicators (evaluation measures) that will evaluate each oral health goal and objective set in the plan can be determined.

- Following treatment, new complete assessment data is documented.

- An evidence-based decision-making approach[1] is used to determine any necessary modifications to the

ongoing treatment sequence or to plan maintenance care.
- Document in the patient's record all assessment findings and any planned modifications for treatment or oral health education.

EVALUATION BASED ON GOALS AND OUTCOMES

The dental hygiene care plan establishes individualized immediate and long-range patient goals for each dental hygiene intervention. The treatment, education, and self-care instruction goals listed in the patient's care plan provide the basis for evaluating whether expected outcomes have been achieved at each level.

Outcomes that can be evaluated following the completion of dental hygiene treatment and patient education in each area of a three part plan for care are listed in **Box 46-2**. Selected outcomes can be used to develop goals for patient care when writing the dental hygiene care plan.

BOX 46-2	Expected Outcomes Following Dental Hygiene Interventions

Gingival/Periodontal Health Outcomes
- Reduced dental biofilm
- Smooth tooth surfaces with calculus removed
- Reduced probing depths
- No bleeding on probing
- Resolution of erythematous tissue
- Reduced swelling and edema
- No further loss in attachment level
- Decrease or no change in mobility

Dental Caries Risk Outcomes
- No new cavitated lesions
- Demineralized/noncavitated areas resolved
- Reduced intake of cariogenic foods/beverages
- Dental sealants placed
- Increased fluoride use

Prevention Outcomes
- Elimination of iatrogenic factors (calculus, restoration overhangs)
- Increased percentage of biofilm-free areas
- Patient demonstration of recommended oral care procedures
- Compliance with daily care recommendations
- Compliance with recommended maintenance care interval
- Tobacco-free status achieved
- Modification/stabilization of systemic risk factors

EVALUATION OF CLINICAL (TREATMENT) OUTCOMES

- Final evaluation of dental hygiene treatment outcomes is made after initial therapy (scaling and root planing) has been completed, when the response of the gingival tissue to therapy is apparent.
- When a treatment sequence consists of multiple appointments, evaluation of the previously treated areas at each subsequent appointment allows immediate intervention in an area that shows poor response to the previous treatment.
- The clinical examination instruments and procedures used for initial assessment as well as evaluation assessment are more completely described in Chapter 15 on page 224.
- Methods for evaluating treatment outcomes are as follows.

I. VISUAL INSPECTION

- Obtain biofilm score after the soft tissue visual inspection has been completed so that use of disclosing solution does not interfere with soft tissue examination, as described in Chapter 14 on page 215.
- Gingival examination looks for changes in tissue color, size, shape (contour) and consistency and compares them to examination findings documented prior to treatment.
- Visual examination can also determine whether a goal related to caries risk, such as restorative treatment or sealants has been completed.

II. PERIODONTAL PROBING

- A complete probing is performed and documented using a form that allows comparison with pretreatment assessment data.
- Bleeding points are noted as probings are made and documented in the periodontal record.

III. TACTILE EVALUATION

- All tooth surfaces, particularly in areas demonstrating bleeding points, are assessed with a periodontal explorer for residual calculus deposits and other iatrogenic factors.
- Use of an explorer with a long terminal shank (as shown in Figure 15-13, page 235) is needed for areas with pockets of 5 mm or deeper.
- Residual calculus can be expected on any subgingival surface that demonstrates bleeding on gentle probing.
- Smooth root surfaces that are free of calculus create a biologically compatible root surface that can support healing in the overlying tissues.
- Special checks for difficult-to-access areas include:
    - concavities and depressions of the root anatomy,
    - subgingival margins of crowns, fixed partial denture, or overhanging restoration,
    - furcation invasions.

EVALUATION OF HEALTH BEHAVIOR OUTCOMES

- The evaluation of health behavior outcomes determines:
  - The patient's response to the clinician's counseling and education interventions.
  - Development of oral self-care skills.
- The dental hygiene care plan establishes self-care and health behavior goals that are determined in collaboration with the patient.
- If the evaluation process indicates that goals have not been met, the data collected during evaluation can provide a baseline from which the dental hygienist can again collaborate with the patient to develop new or next step goals.
- Methods for evaluating self-care and health behavior outcomes are as follows.

I. VISUAL INSPECTION

- Patient biofilm control is evaluated using the same dental indices used to determine original biofilm levels.
- Self-care skills are evaluated by observing a demonstration of each skill by the patient.

II. INTERVIEW EVALUATION

- Patient interviewing techniques can be used to determine whether each goal established by the patient for health behavior change and daily self-care has been met.
- Patient interview and discussion can be used to evaluate the success of factors associated with patient comfort during treatment, patient understanding of recommendations and self-care instructions, or effectiveness of the clinician's communication approaches.

COMPARISON OF ASSESSMENT FINDINGS

Analysis and comparison of pretreatment and evaluation data determines the relative success of the therapy. Analysis of evaluation findings and comparison with findings from initial assessment can help determine whether the patient:

- Is able to be managed for the present under the care of the dental hygienist, requiring determination of a continuing care interval and development of a new dental hygiene care plan.
- Has not responded adequately to nonsurgical therapy and referral for specialized periodontal care may be necessary (Chapter 40, page 640).
- On the basis of the findings, a determination is made as to recommended intervals for subsequent maintenance appointments.

BOX 46-3	Factors Considered When Determining Need for Retreatment, Referral, or Maintenance Interval

- Soft tissue response to instrumentation and degree of healing
- Changes and/or stabilization in probing depth and attachment loss
- Patient health behaviors, such as use of tobacco
- Systemic influences on oral health status, such as diabetes
- Level of skill and effectiveness in biofilm control
- Motivation and responsibility assumed for daily personal oral self-care
- Psychosocial factors that can affect oral status, such as stress

- Additional factors taken into account when determining next steps for patient care are listed in **Box 46-3**.

STANDARD OF CARE

- In addition to evaluating individual patient outcomes at all points in the dental hygiene process of care, the dental hygienist is responsible for evaluating personal adherence to a professional standard of practice.
- Standards of care in dentistry evolved from early court cases that established a ruling of negligence when healthcare providers failed to possess a minimum standard of special knowledge and ability, as well as adhere to reasonable and recognized standards while providing patient care.[7]
- Three sources for determining standard of care in a legal dispute are listed in **Box 46-4**.
- Failure to provide a minimally acceptable level of patient care is considered to be professional negligence.

BOX 46-4	Three Sources for Determining Standard of Care in a Legal Dispute

- Opinion of expert witnesses
- Journals, guidelines, or other published documents from recognized professional associations or other authoritative sources
- Federal, state, or local statutes and/or regulations

Source: Curley AW. The legal standard of care. *J Am Coll Dent.* 2005 Winter;72(4):20–22.

TABLE 46-1	STANDARDS FOR CLINICAL DENTAL HYGIENE PRACTICE	
STANDARD	**DESCRIPTION**	**CRITERIA FOR EVALUATING ADHERENCE TO STANDARD**
Standard 1 ASSESSMENT	Ongoing collection and interpretation of patient data	■ Collect personal, dental and health history. ■ Provide comprehensive clinical examination. ■ Assess risks to general and oral health.
Standard 2 DENTAL HYGIENE DIAGNOSIS	Analysis and critical decision making	■ Analyze and interpret all data. ■ Determine patient needs. ■ Incorporate dental hygiene diagnosis into overall dental treatment plan.
Standard 3 PLANNING	Making clinical decisions within the context of ethical and legal principles	■ Identify, prioritize, and sequence interventions. ■ Coordinate resources and collaborate with other health care providers. ■ Present plan and explain rationale, risks benefits, expected outcomes, alternatives, and prognosis to patient. ■ Obtain informed consent or refusal.
Standard 4 IMPLEMENTATION	Delivery of dental hygiene interventions.	■ Review, implement, and modify care plan and plan for continuing care. ■ Communicate with patient.
Standard 5 EVALUATION	Reviewing and documenting outcomes throughout the process of care	■ Use measurable criteria. ■ Communicate with patient. ■ Collaborate with other health care providers.
Standard 6 DOCUMENTATION	Complete and accurate recording of information	■ Document all components of care objectively, legibly, concisely, and accurately. ■ Recognize ethical and legal aspects of recordkeeping. ■ Respect and protect patient information.

Source: American Dental Hygienists' Association. Standards for clinical dental hygiene practice. Chicago: ADHA; 2008. pp. 6–9. [cited 2011 Feb 22]. Available from: www.adha.org/downloads/adha_standards08.pdf

■ Standards for delivery of dental hygiene care are defined by the ADHA Standards for Clinical Dental Hygiene Practice, based on the Dental Hygiene Process of Care and summarized in **Table 46-1**.

■ *The American Academy of Periodontology Parameters of Care* (Chapter 23, page 345) and the *Center for Disease Control Guidelines for Infection Control in Dental Health-Care Settings* (Appendix IV, page 1096) as well as a variety of other documents published by both dental and dental hygiene professional associations are additional sources used for establishing a professional standard of care in dentistry and dental hygiene.

■ Adherence to a professional dental hygiene standard of care is enhanced through continuous evidence-based inquiry and pursuit of life-long learning.

■ The professional dental hygienist recognizes that standards of care change over time as new knowledge is introduced and becomes commonly accepted by the profession and the public. Dental hygienists need to update and have knowledge of current practice standards.

SELF-ASSESSMENT AND REFLECTIVE PRACTICE[8–13]

Ongoing self-assessment of skills and current knowledge is an essential component of evaluating clinical practice. Although self-assessment and reflection in health care practice have been studied mainly in educational settings, there is evidence to suggest that development of these skills can help assure quality and positive outcomes in the delivery of patient care.

I. PURPOSE

■ Self-assessment of personal clinical and communication skills and knowledge can guide the dental hygiene practitioner toward an evidence-based approach to finding new information that supports best-practice interventions for patient care.

■ Reflecting on clinical experiences contributes to development of critical thinking skills that can help the practitioner determine and implement new and more successful approaches for patient care.

■ Self-assessment can assist the dental hygienist to determine a need to enhance specific clinical skills and abilities, or develop a plan for continuing education that supports personal professional goals.

II. SKILLS AND METHODS

■ Key skills for reflective practice include:
  ■ perceptive self-awareness,
  ■ judgment and self-assessment,
  ■ critical analysis and synthesis,
  ■ access to and application of new knowledge,
  ■ feedback and evaluation (continued reflection).
■ Methods for informal assessment of professional practice include individual reflection (thinking about one's own practice habits) or discussing clinical issues with colleagues.

■ Reflective practice can also take on a more formal aspect, as in maintaining a written "critical incident" journal.

III. A "CRITICAL INCIDENT" APPROACH

A formal approach used to evaluate dental hygiene practice takes the form of answering questions about a specific situation, often called a critical incident, that prompts the practitioner to look for answers.

■ Three steps, sometimes referred to as the "What? So What? Now What" approach, can be used to structure written reflective journal entries or can also be used to guide a less formal means of thoughtful personal self-assessment.
■ The approach to reflective self-assessment includes a basic progression of reflective actions with questions

TABLE 46-2	COMPONENTS OF A "CRITICAL INCIDENT" APPROACH TO REFLECTION AND SELF-ASSESSMENT		
STEP	**SUMMARY/DEFINITION**	**SOME EXAMPLE QUESTIONS FOR GUIDING REFLECTION**	**CLINICAL PRACTICE EXAMPLE**
DESCRIPTION "What?"	Brief description of what happened and what effect the situation had on those involved in the incident.	What about the situation triggered a need to evaluate what happened? Who was involved? How did those involved feel about or react to the incident What about this situation is interesting to explore further?	Patient presents for evaluation following scaling and root planing. Residual calculus, resulting in areas of bleeding and need for patient to return for re-treatment of those areas. Patient is not happy about need for re-treatment. Dental hygienist is concerned about skill in calculus removal.
ANALYSIS "So What?"	Reflective phase which involves analysis and critical thinking to identify: ■ Potential causes and factors that influenced outcome of the situation ■ Gaps related to standards of good practice ■ Changes that need to be made in current practice ■ New knowledge required	Why did this happen? What gaps in knowledge or skill influenced the outcome? Does the knowledge base need to be updated? Were patient and/or clinician's goals met during this situation? How were values or ethical standards related to or applied during this situation?	The dental hygienist analyzes the situation using some of the questions in the previous column, and realizes that this is not the first time the personal patient care goal for complete calculus removal at each appointment has not been met. Recently, while participating in an advanced instrumentation continuing education course, it became clear that the problem is not deficient scaling and root planing skills. Instrument sharpening skills have not been updated (or applied) recently.
APPLICATION "Now What?"	Summary of insights or learning from the situation and a plan for addressing need for new knowledge or alternative action.	What was learned? What next steps can be taken to produce a different outcome in a future situation?	The dental hygienist learned that instrumentation skill alone might not be all that is necessary to meet the goal of complete calculus removal. Next steps: find an instrument-sharpening "how-to" booklet to begin practicing sharpening and attend a continuing education workshop related to instrument sharpening at the first opportunity.

for each step that can help guide thinking about the situation from a variety of perspectives.

- The steps and a brief clinical practice example are provided in **Table 46-2**. The same steps and similar questions can be used to guide self-assessment reflection about situations involving communication skills, patient education approach, or adherence to ethical and legal standards of practice.

DOCUMENTATION

I. PATIENT CARE OUTCOMES

- Evaluation of such factors as patient comfort, communication efforts, and treatment safety and efficacy is ongoing and occurs at each patient appointment. Documentation in the patient record provides guidance for future patient interactions.
- Documentation of outcomes evaluation following clinical dental hygiene treatment is similar to the documentation of clinical data during initial assessment. Evaluation data following treatment are recorded in an identical format to the pretreatment assessment data, which facilitates comparison and analysis of outcomes.
- **Box 46-5** has an example progress note that documents evaluation of a patient care situation.

BOX 46-5	**Example Progress Note for Ongoing Evaluation of Patient Comfort During Treatment**

Patient presents for 3rd in a series of appointments scheduled for scaling and root planing. Pt complaint: following both of the previous appointments, his back has significantly bothered him because of laying back so far in the dental chair for such a long time period. Analyzed the problem through discussion and decided together that placing a small cushion (or his jacket) beneath his knees as well as briefly bringing the chair to an upright position every 15 minutes could help to alleviate his discomfort.

Completed 2nd quadrant scaling and provided flossing instruction as indicated in the patient's care plan for this appointment while using the new "comfort protocol." He indicated that he felt much better during this treatment session. Re-evaluate at the next appointment, scheduled in 2 weeks.

Signed: _____, RDH Date: _____.

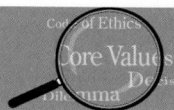

Everyday Ethics

Mrs. Midoun called in this morning and scheduled during a cancelled appointment time in the afternoon. She states that she is in a hurry and just wants her teeth "shined up" as her daughter is graduating this weekend. Salima one of three dental hygienists in the practice, has not provided care previously for Mrs. Midoun. She quickly scans the patient record, noticing that Mrs. Midoun had received scaling and root planing treatments in all four quadrants that was completed three months ago. Although she had signed a consent form for treatments that outlined the entire sequence of appointments, including evaluation, Mrs. Midoun had cancelled that appointment at the last minute and never rescheduled it.

Salima explains that, before providing any further dental hygiene care, it would be necessary to complete the posttreatment evaluation. Mrs. Midoun objects strenuously to "wasting time" with evaluation of her previous treatment. She states that her oral health is much better now and she notices very little bleeding. Mrs. Midoun states emphatically that, unless Salima cleans her teeth today, she will "just leave now and find another office" where they will clean her teeth. Dr. Kim is out of the office and Salima hesitates, not knowing quite how to handle the situation without consulting him.

Questions for Consideration
1. Is this an ethical issue or a dilemma? Explain.
2. What are Mrs. Midoun's rights in this situation? What core values need to be considered during Salima's decision making process?
3. What alternative decisions can Salima make about interventions she will provide at Mrs. Midoun's appointment today that will meet the standards of care for dental hygiene practice?

I. SELF-ASSESSMENT AND REFLECTION

Self-assessment and reflective evaluation of personal professionalism and learning can be documented in several ways. Two suggestions are as follows:

- Regular written entries in a professional practice reflection journal that describe and critically analyze a variety of clinical, ethical, and professional situations the dental hygienist has found meaningful. Over time, this ongoing record will reflect how the practitioner's professional skills, actions, and knowledge have been enhanced through the process of reflective practice.
- A clinical practice portfolio can be developed that documents a variety of factors related to professional development and self-evaluation of dental hygiene practice. A portfolio may contain artifacts such as:
  - Case presentations describing care provided for patients with special needs.

Factors To Teach The Patient

- The need for evaluation to establish the basis for "next step" treatment and maintenance decisions.
- Types of evaluation measures and indicators that measure outcomes for each goal.
- How outcomes from dental hygiene interventions are used to determine further treatment needs and maintenance interval.

- A personal practice philosophy that indicates ethical parameters that impact how the dental hygienist provides care.
- Goals for future continuing education and courses taken or planned for reaching those goals.

References

1. Forrest JL, Miller SA. Evidence-based decision making—a new term for a new concept. *Dimensions Dent Hyg.* 2005 Sep;3:12.
2. Niederman R, Richards D. Evidence-based dentistry: concepts and implementation. *J Am Col Dent.* 2005 Winter;72(4):37.
3. Hamm RW. Educational evaluation: theory and a working model. *Education.* 1988 Spring;108:404.
4. Chambers DW, Glassman P. A primer on competency-based evaluation. *J Dent Educ.* 1997 Aug;61:651.
5. Baker QE, Davis DA, Gallerani R, Sanchez V, Viadro C. An Evaluation Framework for Community Health Programs. Durham (NC): The Center for the Advancement of Community-Based Public Health; 2000, pp. 63–65. Available from: www.cbph.org.
6. Centers for Disease Control and Prevention. Framework for Program Evaluation in Public Health. *MMWR.* 1999 Sep;48:24.
7. Graskemper JP. The standard of care in dentistry: where did it come from: How has it evolved? *J Am Dent Assoc.* 2004 Oct;135(10):1449–55.
8. Arkins S, Murphy K. Reflection: a review of the literature. *J Adv Nurs.* 1993 Aug;18(8):1188–92.
9. Cirocco M. How reflective practice improves nurses' critical thinking ability. *Gastroenterol Nurs.* 2007 Nov–Dec;30(6):405–13.
10. Gwozdek AE, Klausner CP, Kerschbaum WE. Online directed journaling in dental hygiene education. *J Dent Hyg.* 2009 Winter;83(1):12–17.
11. Wetmore AO, Boyd LD, Bowen DM, Pattillo RE. Reflective blogs in clinical education to promote critical thinking in dental hygiene students. *J Dent Educ.* 2010 Dec;74(12):1337–50.
12. Asselin ME. Reflective narrative: a tool for learning through practice. *J Nurses Staff Dev.* 2011 Jan–Feb;27(1):2–6.
13. Jackson SC, Murff EJ. Effectively teaching self-assessment: preparing the dental hygiene student to provide quality care. *J Dent Educ.* 2011 Feb;75(2):169–79.

CHAPTER 47

Maintenance

ESTHER M. WILKINS, BS, RDH, DMD
ANNA MATSUISHI PATTISON, RDH, MS

Chapter Outline

INTRODUCTION

The overall purposes of treatment are to arrest disease and provide oral health, function, and comfort for the patient. After a series of active treatments, when evaluation shows that the soft tissue is in optimum health and the dentition has been restored in function, the patient enters a new phase of treatment for continuing supervision and care.

- Maintenance in dental hygiene means continuing care.
- The patient needs to understand that oral diseases do recur, but *control* is possible through combined personal and professional effort.
- Lifelong preservation of the teeth and their supporting structures is a realistic goal.
- Initially the success of the program depends on the understanding by the patient of the maintenance procedure.
- One way to help the patient become aware is by including the concept of the maintenance phase in the initial care plan.
- Terms associated with preventive maintenance are defined in **Box 47-1**.

I. PURPOSES OF THE MAINTENANCE PROGRAM

- Continue the healthy state attained during active therapy.
- Prevent recurrence of previous infections
- Prevent new disease from starting.
- Monitor educational and behavioral changes.
- Monitor clinical signs of health and disease including periodontal infections, and oral mucosal lesions, and the stages of dental caries from demineralization, noncavitated and cavitated lesions.
- Provide specialized instruction for new implants, prostheses, orthodontic appliances, and various restorations.
- Offer motivational encouragement for self-care and self-evaluation **(Box 47-2)**.

II. APPOINTMENT INTERVALS

A. Frequency Planning

- No fixed schedule by which all patients can be maintained in oral health is possible because the frequency depends on the needs of each patient.

BOX 47-1	Key Words

Maintenance

Compliance: action in accordance with request; extent to which a person's health behaviors coincide with dental/medical health advice. Also called **adherence**.

Consultation: the joint deliberation, usually for diagnostic purposes, between two or more practitioners or between a patient and a practitioner.

Disease activity: ongoing dynamic process that results in loss of clinical attachment and alveolar supporting bone; an area is quiescent when a diseased site becomes inactive or stable without treatment.

End points: criteria for completion of a particular procedure; therapeutic end points generally have been reached when the clinical signs of the treated pathologic condition have been eliminated or reduced.

PMT: periodontal maintenance therapy; also called preventive maintenance, supportive periodontal treatment.

Recall: system of appointments for the long-term maintenance phase of patient care; the system is carried out by computer, telephone, and/or mail.

Refractory: resistant, not responding to routine therapy.

Remission: diminution or abatement of the symptoms of a disease; the period during which the diminution occurs.

Response diagnosis: the diagnosis made at a reevaluation spaced for a period of time after treatment (or a series of treatments); diagnosis that shows the response to prior treatment.

Risk factor: a characteristic, habit, or predisposing condition that makes an individual susceptible to, or in danger of acquiring, a certain disease or disability.

SPT: supportive periodontal therapy; procedures performed at selected intervals as an extension of periodontal therapy to assist the patient in maintaining oral health; includes complete assessment, review of and/or additional instruction in dental biofilm control, and such clinical procedures as scaling and root planing; also called preventive maintenance, periodontal maintenance therapy.

■ Appointment intervals may vary from 2 to 6 months. The time interval is reevaluated periodically and changed in accord with changing needs.

B. Factors to Consider in Determining Maintenance Frequency

■ Risk for periodontal disease activity.
■ Risk for dental carious lesions.
■ Risk for oral cancer: tobacco and alcohol users.
■ Predisposing diseases, conditions, and behaviors for periodontal diseases including diabetes, HIV/AIDS, host genetic factors, smoking, and stress.
■ Compliance: keeping appointments, personal daily biofilm control.

BOX 47-2	Purposes and Outcomes of Dental Hygiene Periodontal Therapy

■ Resolve inflammation
■ Eliminate bleeding on probing
■ Restore lost tissues to normal contour and texture
■ Create environment for healing
■ Arrest disease progression
■ Preserve esthetics
■ Provide patient comfort
■ Encourage patient self-care
■ Create environment that deters recurrence of infection
■ Motivate patient to cooperate in continuing care

■ Previous treatment: patient who has had previous disease, either dental caries or periodontal infection, is at a greater risk for recurrence.
■ Local factors: rate of calculus formation.
■ Restorative complications: implants, prosthetic replacements.

C. Special Appointment Requirements

Intervals of 2 or 3 months are required for many patients. A few are mentioned here.

■ *Periodontitis.* Patients who have completed initial nonsurgical or surgical periodontal therapy. The first maintenance appointment is dated from the completion of the initial scaling and root planing (or nonsurgical therapy).
■ *Cognitive or physical disability.* Managing the toothbrush and other oral care devices may be difficult; when the disability involves the mouth area, opening the mouth may be a problem.
■ *Diabetes.* Diabetes or other disease can predispose patients to lowered resistance to infection; tissues must not be allowed to develop advanced disease.
■ *Cardiovascular disease or other condition.* Brushing is a difficult procedure to carry out and only short appointments at the dental office can be tolerated because of the fatigue factor.
■ *Patient undergoing extensive dental care.* The gingival or periodontal treatment may be completed or nearly completed by the time appointments for restorative phases of treatment are under way. The first maintenance appointment needs to be dated from the completion

of the initial gingival and periodontal treatment. When extensive restorative, prosthetic, or other treatment is in progress, frequent tissue maintenance during long-term therapy is essential.

■ *Rampant dental caries.* Appointment for continuation of a caries control effort includes topical fluoride applications, dietary supervision, and personal care factors for biofilm control.

■ *Orthodontic therapy.* Appliances make cleaning and biofilm control difficult; frequent topical fluoride applications may be indicated; response of gingival tissue to irritants can be marked.

D. Periodontal Maintenance Therapy (PMT)[1]

Any of the types of patients who have been mentioned and many of the patients with special needs described in Section VIII of this book may have a potentially recurrent periodontal infection or may have had periodontal corrective surgical therapy. Four categories of PMT have been defined:

■ *Preventive PMT:* To prevent the initiation of disease in individuals without periodontal infection.

■ *Trial PMT:* To provide an interim study period for borderline patients with conditions that must be observed and further evaluated before a decision can be made as to whether corrective surgery may be necessary or whether maintenance is possible without further advanced disease therapy.

■ *Compromise PMT:* To slow the progress of disease in patients for whom corrective surgery and other advanced treatment are indicated but cannot be implemented for reasons of health, economics, or other personal factors.

■ *Posttreatment PMT:* To prevent the recurrence of disease and maintain the state of periodontal health attained during periodontal therapy. Such therapy may have been nonsurgical or surgical.

MAINTENANCE APPOINTMENT PROCEDURES

The dental hygiene process of care is described in Chapter 1 and is illustrated in Figure VII-1. As with preparation of the initial dental hygiene care plan in Chapter 24 (page 351), the steps in the process of care apply for the *maintenance dental hygiene care plan.*

I. ASSESSMENT

■ Preparation of data follows the same plan as that for a new patient.

■ At every maintenance appointment, whether at 3, 6, or any other number of months, a patient of any age needs a complete reassessment, progress diagnosis, and maintenance care plan.

A. Review of Patient History

■ Supplementary questions are asked to determine the present state of health with emphasis on changes since the previous appointment.

■ Recent illnesses, current medications, and other pertinent new data.

B. Vital Signs

■ Blood pressure determination (Chapter 10, page 139).

C. Extraoral and Intraoral Examination

A thorough extraoral and intraoral examination for oral disease is made and recorded in Chapter 11 (pages 145 to 151 and Table 11-1).

D. Radiographs

■ Radiographs are not taken routinely.

■ The frequency of radiographic surveys is in accord with the dentist's determination of an individual patient's need (Table 12-4, page 175).

E. Periodontal Examination

■ Observe and record: gingival color, size, shape, recession; mucogingival changes.

■ Complete probing: bleeding on probing, attachment levels, compare with previous probings and check for all changes since treatment was completed.

■ Occlusion, fremitus, mobility.

■ Calculus: distribution, amount.

F. Examination of the Teeth

■ Integrity of restorations and sealants.

■ Dental caries: demineralization, early dental caries, and cavitated lesions.

■ Sensitivity: location

G. Evaluation of Oral Cleanliness and Adequacy of Self-Care Measures

■ Relate biofilm on teeth as observed after applying a disclosing agent to areas of gingival redness, enlargement, and other signs of inflammation.

H. Examination of Specific Areas

■ Areas of special problems include endodontically treated teeth, postsurgical areas, implants, occlusal factors, and prosthetic appliances.

II. MAINTENANCE CARE PLAN

A care plan is outlined on the basis of new dental hygiene diagnosis and evaluation of the patient's oral condition. A patient in any of the maintenance categories will require a basic care plan such as suggested later. Supplemental procedures may be needed.

A. Oral Hygiene Instruction/Motivation

- During continuing care, the patient is considered a co-therapist.
- Compliance in faithful personal daily care is a major feature in the total program if etiologic factors are to be kept under control.

B. Periodontal Scaling and Debridement

- Periodontal pocket examination with bleeding on probing indicates need for deep scaling and root planing.
- Plan for type of anesthetic: local anesthesia or subgingival gel.
- Plan for number of appointments.
- Local delivery of antimicrobials for isolated persistent deep pockets (Chapter 40, page 644).
- For repeated areas of bleeding on probing: endoscopic examination is indicated.

C. Dental Caries Control

- Prevention with attention to root caries; fluoride applications and diet modifications.
- Implement or monitor previously introduced remineralization protocol (Chapter 26, page 383).

D. Supplemental Care Procedures

- Smoking cessation assistance (Chapter 33, page 489).
- Desensitization of sensitive areas.
- Special care for implants and fixed prostheses.
- Referral for retreatment evaluation.

III. CRITERIA FOR REFERRAL TO A PERIODONTIST

A. Referral From General Practice

General practice dentists frequently may include periodontal surgical therapy in their practices while others refer all the severe or complicated periodontal cases to the specialist periodontist. Three points during patient care when the dental hygienist in a general practice may confer with the dentist to determine the need for referral to a periodontist are suggested as follows:

- *Initially* when a patient new to the practice is first examined and severe advanced periodontitis is evident, or the patient has an uncommon periodontal disease such as an aggressive periodontitis (formerly called "juvenile periodontitis"), necrotizing ulcerative gingivitis or periodontitis, or a drug-induced gingival enlargement (such as phenytoin for seizures).
- *Later during the reevaluation* after periodontal quadrant scaling for a nonresponsive or refractory type of moderate or advanced periodontal condition (or any of the conditions mentioned earlier).
- *During maintenance.* If there is continued or recurrent bleeding or suppuration on probing, increasing pocket depth, increasing mobility or migration of teeth, or recurrent periodontal abscesses.

B. Criteria for Referral During Maintenance

During the maintenance therapy, any of the types of patients mentioned above may still need referral. Other cases may include:

- Pocket depth that prohibits access for complete debridement during dental hygiene periodontal therapy.
- Furcation involvements and other deep or complex anatomical areas that cannot be instrumented successfully by nonsurgical methods.
- Mucogingival problems; lack of attached gingiva near healthy receded gingival margin.
- Periodontal disease that is refractory, or not responsive to thorough, usual treatment.

RECURRENCE OF PERIODONTAL DISEASE

- Recurrence of signs and symptoms of periodontal infection indicates recolonization of periodontal pathogens.
- Recolonization of a pocket can occur within an average of 42 days.[2] Without daily personal dental biofilm control and regular professional supervision and maintenance procedures, infection can recur. How soon after the completion of treatment it may reappear will vary with each patient depending on a number of contributing factors.

I. CONTRIBUTING FACTORS

A. Insufficient Personal Care

- Inadequate biofilm control.
- Needs more frequent reminders.

B. Lack of Compliance With Maintenance Appointments

- *Patient decision*: Misunderstanding of importance; personal reasons.
- *Professional laxity*: Insufficient patient counseling; inadequate recall system.

C. Incomplete Professional Treatment

■ *Scaling and debridement*: Incomplete, especially in areas of difficult access such as furcations and deep proximal pockets.
■ *Biofilm retention*: Neglect to remove or replace over-hanging restorations and other areas that trap biofilm and foster bacterial growth.

D. Tobacco Use[3]

■ Encourage tobacco use cessation.
■ Tobacco influences disease progression.

E. Systemic Diseases

■ Diabetes mellitus,[4] HIV/AIDS, and certain other systemic diseases influence healing and may control factors related to bone loss and severity of infections.

F. Genetic Factors[5,6]

■ Risk assessment may include testing for genetic factors.

II. REINFECTION

■ Transmission of periodontal microorganisms has been shown.[7,8]
■ Colonization in the recipient depends on the number, frequency of exposure, and virulence of the organisms.

ADMINISTRATION METHODS

■ Methods for administration of a maintenance plan vary.
■ For any plan, individual file information includes name, address, telephone numbers, and instructions concerning appointment frequency and available or preferred day and time.
■ The data may be kept on 3 × 5 or 4 × 6-inch file cards or in a computer.

I. PREBOOK METHOD

■ Make each patient's appointment before the patient leaves the current appointment.
■ An appointment card is given to the patient, who is asked to enter it on the calendar ahead of time.
■ An envelope is prepared for mailing a duplicate card 10 days to 1 week before the scheduled appointment. The card requests the patient to call to confirm.
■ For unconfirmed appointments, a call to the patient the day before is made.

II. MONTHLY REMINDERS

■ By this system, individual data are filed alphabetically by the last name of the patient under the month when the patient is due.

■ Each month the cards are pulled and reminders are mailed or telephoned well in advance.

III. COMPUTER ASSISTED

■ Computers can be helpful in maintaining appointment systems. Either the prebook or the monthly reminders can be used in combination with a computer.
■ Data stored on a computer can be readily accessible.
■ Computers are capable of printing address labels so that postal cards can be mailed monthly or envelopes containing the prebook appointment card can be sent at the appropriate time.

DOCUMENTATION

For the permanent patient's record at least the following needs to be recorded for a patient who is scheduled for routine continuing care:

■ Medical, dental, medications, histories updated with each continuing care appointment.
■ Complaints and questions patients may express of significance to the treatment given and the personal self-care expected by the patient.
■ Findings during routine examinations including vital signs, extraoral and intraoral, periodontal, dental, temporomandibular joint, occlusion, and all special examinations following individual treatments for other reasons.
■ A sample progress note may be reviewed in **Box 47-3**

BOX 47-3	Example Progress Note

Ms. Kitt was right on time and apologized for not being able to clean after lunch; she asked for a toothbrush and went to the ladies' room. That was such a remarkable behavior change since she started with us 4 years ago that it needed to be recorded in her permanent record! Medical, dental and medication reviews, no changes. BP 135/60, Extra- and intraoral nothing remarkable. Made vertical bitewings for molar areas as planned for once a year. Periodontal examination with probing revealed mesial 19 still with BOP in 4 mm pocket. Treated under local for another root scaling in that quadrant after reviewing her personal flossing and interdental brush technique. Dr. Jay recommended CHX rinse before going to bed and dipping her interdental brush in CHX in conjunction with the rinsing, especially for #19.
  Next appt 3 mos.

Signed: _____, RDH Date: _____.

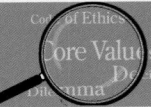

Everyday Ethics

There were two full-time dental hygienists in the practice. Jeanette had been there more than 15 years, and Wilma less than a year. Wilma had previously practiced with a periodontist in another city for 6 years, and she joined this practice shortly after she moved here. Each hygienist had instruments of their own preference and cared for them relative to sharpening and preparation for the autoclave. Patients usually had appointments with the same dental hygienist. Jeanette scheduled a maintenance for 45 minutes, whereas Wilma never felt she had time enough even with an hour.

Occasionally, certain long-standing patients who had been with Jeanette for many years would be scheduled with Wilma when Jeanette could not be in the office.

As Wilma saw more of Jeanette's regular patients, she began to see a pattern of subgingival calculus that could not have formed since the previous 3 or 4 months' maintenance appointment. She had decided to ask the secretary to have Jeanette's patients wait for her return for their appointments.

Ms. Doubleday had already been scheduled and came for her appointment the next day. After the usual history review, periodontal charting, and treatment started, Wilma had to tell the patient that she needed two appointments and wanted to complete her scaling with local anesthesia. The patient was confused after having only short appointments faithfully and wanted to know whether to reschedule with Jeanette to finish since Jeanette would be back from her vacation soon.

Questions for Consideration

1. Is this an ethical issue or a dilemma? Explain. How do the core values (Table II-1, page 38) apply in this scenario?
2. Using the step procedure for solving an issue or a dilemma (page 10), suggest various possible actions for Wilma.
3. Prepare possible answers Wilma could use for her reply to Ms. Doubleday's immediate question.

Factors To Teach The Patient

■ Purposes of follow-up and maintenance appointments.
■ Relationship of personal oral care habits to the maintenance of cleanliness provided through professional scaling and debridement.
■ Importance of keeping all maintenance appointments.

References

1. Schallhorn RG, Snider LE. Periodontal maintenance therapy. *J Am Dent Assoc.* 1981 Aug;103:227.
2. Mousqués T, Listgarten MA, Phillips RW. Effects of scaling and root planing on the composition of the human subgingival microbial flora. *J Periodontal Res.* 1980 Mar;15:144.
3. MacFarlane GD, Herzberg MC, Wolff LF, Hardie NA. Refractory periodontitis associated with abnormal polymorphonuclear leukocyte phagocytosis and cigarette smoking. *J Periodontol.* 1992 Nov;63: 908–913.
4. Grossi SG, Skrepcinski FB, DeCaro T, Zambon JJ, Cummins D, Genco RJ. Response to periodontal therapy in diabetics and smokers. *J Periodontol.* 1996 Oct;67(10 Suppl):1094–1102.
5. Hart TC, Komman KS. Genetic factors in the pathogenesis of periodontitis. *Periodontol 2000.* 1997;14:202.
6. Kornman KS, diGiovine FS. Genetic variations in cytokine expression: a risk factor for severity of adult periodontitis. *Ann Periodontol.* 1998 Jul;3(1):327–328.
7. Von Troil-Lindén B, Torkko H, Alaluusua S, Wolf J, Jousimies-Somer H, Asikainen S. Periodontal findings in spouses: a clinical, radiographic and microbiological study. *J Clin Periodontol.* 1995 Feb;22(2):93–99.
8. Zambon JJ. Periodontal diseases: microbial factors. *Ann Periodontol.* 1996 Nov;1(1):829–925.

Patients With Special Needs

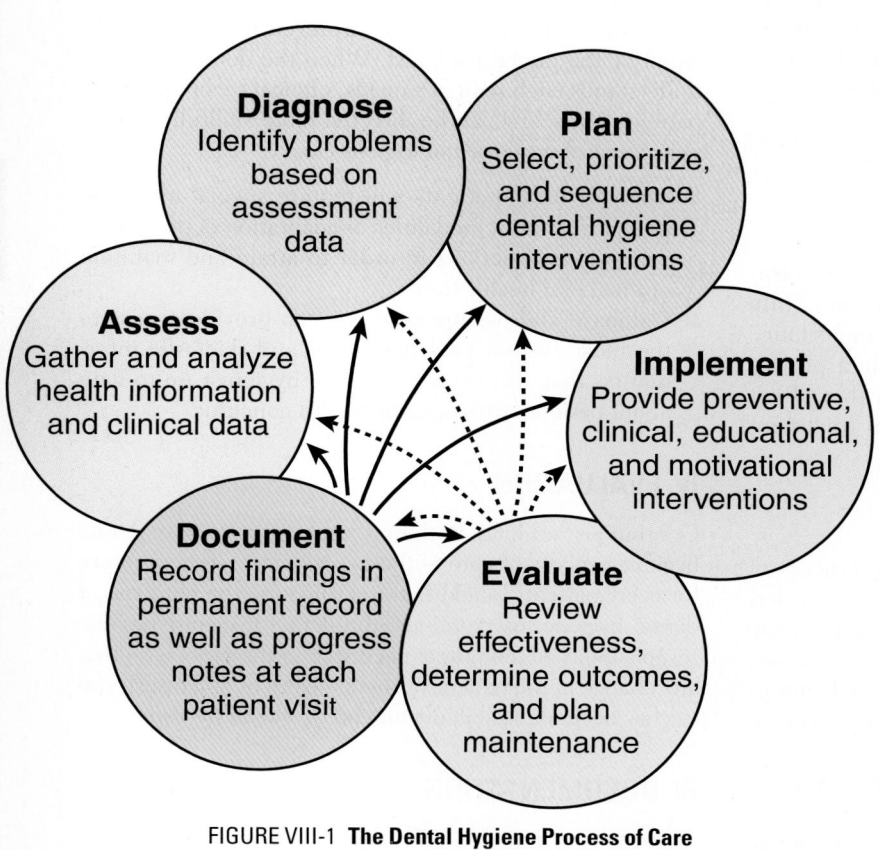

FIGURE VIII-1 **The Dental Hygiene Process of Care**

INTRODUCTION

The dental hygienist's obligation is to see that no patient needs special rehabilitative dental or periodontal services because of any condition that could have been prevented by dental hygiene care.

For every patient, dental hygiene interventions are selected and patient management strategies are considered according to individualized needs. Certain patients have significant concerns related to their age group and/or unusual health factors that may complicate the plan for dental hygiene care. Such patients may require more skillful application of dental hygiene knowledge and ability in order to accomplish a comparably favorable outcome.

- Optimum oral health is frequently a contributing factor in maintaining or restoring optimum systemic health and enhancing quality of life.
- Oral health may have assumed less importance because other health problems have demanded so much attention. For some, neglect has intensified the need for oral care.
- Patients with chronic disabling conditions or advanced stages of disease may not be able to perform self-care regimens independently or access dental care in traditional practice settings.

Patients who will be considered in the following chapters include patients with specific oral and general systemic conditions. Variations with respect to age and degree of physical and/or mental disability are also considered.

THE DENTAL HYGIENE PROCESS OF CARE

The chapters in Section VIII attempt to integrate learning from other areas of medical and social sciences into the Dental Hygiene Process of Care. The importance of each step in the process is enhanced when providing care for a patient with health concerns that affect patient management or increase risk for poor treatment outcomes (**Figure VIII-1**).

I. ASSESSMENT

The assessment phase of the dental hygiene process of care becomes particularly important when considering patients with health concerns. The interrelationship between oral conditions and systemic diseases is revealed through a patient's personal, dental, and medical histories and identified by clinical changes noted during extraoral and intraoral examinations.

Identifying and understanding the individualized needs of each patient requires attention to general health status, physical and cognitive capabilities, emotional, vocational, economic, and social issues as well as oral problems.

- Basic psychological needs can influence the outcome of treatment, as does the patient and/or caregiver attitude toward dental and dental hygiene care.
- Oral manifestations may be evident in association with certain acute and chronic systemic diseases.
- Certain oral findings can suggest the possibility of an undiagnosed systemic disease.

II. DENTAL HYGIENE DIAGNOSIS AND CARE PLANNING

Analyzing assessment data to diagnose patient problems and plan for dental hygiene interventions can be complicated if the patient has a complex, multifaceted medical history. New research that links periodontal infections with systemic conditions provides the basis for emphasis on periodontal health and a preventive approach.

- Risk factors for periodontal infections also may be risk factors for systemic conditions.
- Periodontal infection is a risk factor for many systemic conditions.
- Certain systemic conditions are risk factors for periodontal conditions.

III. IMPLEMENTATION

Every individual described in the chapters of this section can benefit from treatment and preventive services provided by the dental hygienist. When the dental hygienist understands each patient's needs, clinical techniques and patient counseling can be directed more skillfully to provide *comprehensive dental hygiene care*.

- Many of these patients will require special modification of treatment modalities or adaptation of preventive care and instructions in order to attain and maintain optimal oral health status.
- Database and on-line searches can provide access to the most current evidence-based and scientific information that will keep the dental hygienist up-to-date about patients with specific health concerns.

IV. EVALUATION

Continuous evaluation during each step of the dental hygiene process of care is the key to successful outcomes for every patient. In addition to evaluating the outcome of dental hygiene interventions, the dental hygienist has the responsibility to monitor at each step in the process so that any change in the patient's general health or oral health status has been identified, documented, and addressed.

IV. DOCUMENTATION

Thorough, complete, and accurate documentation of all assessment data, dental hygiene interventions, and patient management strategies during each patient visit

TABLE VIII-1	ETHICAL CONCERNS FOR TREATMENT OPTIONS	
QUALITY OF LIFE	**DEFINITION**	**APPLICATION EXAMPLES**
Competency	The patient's ability to make choices about dental and dental hygiene care.	Educates the patient based on intellectual capacity so autonomous consent can be given.
Surrogate	Described as a "substitute" or proxy with regard to healthcare decisions.	Acknowledges a "Durable Power of Attorney" for a patient, where applicable.
Advanced Directives	Individuals may write their choices for limiting health care in the event that they are unable to make choices in the future.	Examples include a "Living Will," "Do Not Resuscitate" (DNR) order, and "Patient Values" history.

is essential to assure evaluation of the quality and effectiveness of patient care for individuals with significant health concerns. Comprehensive patient records can also provide a means of communication between professional team members relative to successful patient management strategies.

ETHICAL APPLICATIONS

The complex medical and dental conditions of certain patients may translate into a need to identify unique treatment approaches. Dental hygiene professionals consider not only the quality of care provided to patients but also their quality of life in general. Increasingly, medically compromised patients are ambulatory and appear in a dental practice or clinic for maintenance and preventive procedures. A dental hygienist may also provide care in alternative settings such as a long-term care facility or the patient's home.

The ethical dental hygienist:

- Selects dental hygiene interventions that are consistent with the patient's physical, mental, and personal capabilities.
- Ensures that all appropriate persons are included in all chairside discussions, if someone other than the patient is responsible for making treatment decisions.
- Understands what the patient and/or caregiver values in terms of dental care.
- Instructs patients and/or caregivers about oral hygiene problems and needs related to their systemic disorders and medications.
- Documents all information in the patient's permanent record.
- Reviews progress notes for any updates or changes in the patient's status.

Table VIII-1 provides an overview of some ethical concerns to be considered when presenting treatment options to patients with special needs.

The Pregnant Patient

ESTHER M. WILKINS, BS, RDH, DMD
NANCY SISTY LePEAU, RDH, MS, MA

Chapter Outline

During pregnancy, attention is focused on good health practices for the mother. She is concerned for the health of her baby and for herself. This alertness to total health, of which oral health is a significant part, provides an unusual opportunity to help the patient learn principles that may be applied to the future care of the child.

■ The term *prenatal care* refers to the supervised preparation for childbirth that helps the mother enjoy optimum health during and after pregnancy and provides the maximum chance for the baby to be born healthy.

■ Such a program involves the combined efforts of the obstetrician and/or midwife, the nurse practitioner, the dentist, the dental hygienist, the dietitian, and the expectant parents.

■ Key words for study with this chapter are defined in Box 48-1.

SOURCES FOR PATIENTS

■ Obstetricians, family practitioners, and nurses in private and public health settings need to recommend dental and periodontal examinations early in pregnancy.

■ Referrals may bring many women to the private dental practice or clinic who would not have had a regular plan for obtaining professional service.

■ Many of these women have not known the advantages of personal habits of daily care and diet related to the health of the oral tissues. Numerous misconceptions are counteracted when providing up-to-date information about the relationship of pregnancy and oral health.

■ Women who do not receive routine oral health care may appear for emergency dental services and may be receptive to a program of care and instruction to prevent further emergencies.

BOX 48-1	Key Words

Pregnancy

Amniocentesis: a testing procedure on fluid aspirated from the amniotic sac to detect chromosomal abnormalities and metabolic disorders.

Amniotic sac: the innermost of the membranes enveloping the embryo *in utero;* **amniotic fluid** fills the sac in which the embryo is free to move and is protected against mechanical injury.

Anticipatory guidance: the term applied to teaching ahead of time so that untoward, unfavorable conditions can be prevented.

Cesarean section: delivery of a fetus by incision through the abdominal wall and uterus.

Embryo: developing organism from conception to approximately the end of the second month.

Epulis: nonspecific term referring to a growth on the gingiva.

Estradiol: the most potent natural estrogen in humans; the circulating blood level of estradiol rises during the follicular phase of the reproductive cycle and drops when ovulation occurs (see Figure 51-2, page 792).

Fetus: developing organism from the second month after conception to birth.

Gestation: the period of pregnancy.

Granuloma: nonspecific term applied to a nodular inflammatory lesion containing macrophages and surrounded by lymphocytes.

"Pyogenic" granuloma: a misnomer because it does not contain pus, but contains blood vessels and inflammatory cells.

In utero: within the womb; not yet born.

Infant: child younger than 1 year of age.

Intrapartum: occurring during childbirth.

Midwife: a person who attends a woman during delivery.

Nurse–midwife: a registered nurse specializing in midwifery; requires additional education and special licensure in certain states and countries.

Obstetrics: the branch of medicine that has to do with the care of the pregnant woman during pregnancy and parturition.

Obstetrician: physician who practices obstetrics.

Parturition: childbirth; labor; giving birth.

Placental abruption: sudden or unexpected breaking off of the connection between uterine and fetal mucous membranes.

Postpartum: pertaining to the period following childbirth or delivery.

Premature birth: birth that occurs before the expected delivery date; denotes an infant born prior to 37 weeks of gestation.

Puerpera: woman who has just given birth to a child.

Pyogenic: producing pus.

Teratogen: nongenetic factors that cause malformations and disease syndromes in utero.

Teratogenic agent: any drug, virus, or irradiation exposure that can cause malformation of the fetus.

Trimester: a period of 3 months; one-third of a pregnancy.

- The dental hygienist in public health, especially maternal and child health clinics participates in community educational programs with public health nurses. In these programs some less informed women may learn of the need for professional dental and dental hygiene care and education during pregnancy.
- Key words with their definitions that relate to the health of a pregnant woman are given in **Box 48-1.**

FETAL DEVELOPMENT

- Pregnancy is arbitrarily divided into three periods of 3 months each called the first, second, and third trimesters.
- Normal pregnancy, or period of gestation, is approximately 40 weeks. Premature birth refers to a birth before 37 weeks' gestation.
- Physiologic changes in the mother are related to nearly every bodily system.
- Early development of the embryo is greatly influenced by heredity and the general health of the mother.

I. FIRST TRIMESTER

- During the first trimester, the embryo is highly susceptible to injuries and malformations.
- Teratogenic effects can be produced by many sources, including maternal poor nutrition, infections, and drug intake.
- All organ systems are formed (organogenesis) during the first trimester. By 12 weeks, the fetus moves and swallows.

A. Oral Cavity Development Includes the Teeth, Lips, and Palate

- Tooth buds develop between the fifth and sixth weeks. Initial mineralization occurs from the fourth to the fifth month (Table 49-8, page 762).
- Lips form during the fourth to the seventh week and the palate forms between the eighth and the twelfth week.
- Cleft lip is apparent by the eighth week; cleft palate, by the twelfth week (page 777).

II. SECOND AND THIRD TRIMESTERS

- The organs are completed, and growth and maturation continue.
- Fetal weight changes from 1 ounce at 3 months to an average of 7.5 pounds at birth.

III. FACTORS THAT CAN HARM THE FETUS

A. Infections

- Protection from infectious diseases is necessary because damage to and infection of the fetus can result.
- Women of childbearing age need to take advantage of all available vaccines prior to conception.
- Defects, deformities, and life-threatening infections in the fetus can result from infection acquired during pregnancy or during delivery and after birth.
- Rubella (German measles), rubeola, varicella, herpes viruses, hepatitis B (in Chapter 4, pages 45 to 50), human immunodeficiency virus (HIV) infection (in Chapter 4, pages 54 to 55), syphilis (congenital syphilis), and gonorrhea all can have serious effects on the fetus.
- Severe periodontitis can be a significant risk factor for preterm delivery with low birth weight. A pregnant mother with advanced periodontal infection may have a 7.5 to 7.9-fold increased risk for a preterm low-birth-weight infant.[1,2] All sources of chronic infection can be potential risk factors.

B. Medications and Other Drug Use

- Ideally, no medications or other drugs are good to be used during pregnancy. Nearly all drugs can pass across the placenta to enter the circulation of the developing fetus.
- Many drugs have teratogenic effects.
- **Table 48-1** lists selected drugs with examples of their possible effects on the fetus.
- *Effect of Tetracycline*
  A. Tetracycline is well known for intrinsic staining of tooth structure.
  B. The effect occurs during mineralization of the primary teeth beginning at about 4 months of gestation and of the permanent teeth near and after birth (page 762).
  C. When an antibiotic is required during pregnancy, a choice other than tetracycline can be made.
- *Therapy for HIV Infection*
  A. Prevention of perinatal HIV transmission and health for the fetus and neonate are considered with the plan for optimal healthcare for the mother with HIV/AIDS infection.
  B. Some antiretroviral medications are not withheld because of pregnancy.[3] Consideration by the mother can be given to withholding the antiretroviral treat-

ment during the first 14 weeks of pregnancy. That is the period of maximal organogenesis and risk for teratogenicity.

C. Drugs of Abuse

- Adverse effects of controlled substances, alcohol, and tobacco products are included in **Table 48-1**. There are many serious effects from their use.
- Information on the effects of alcohol use during pregnancy and Fetal Alcohol Syndrome is included in Chapter 64 on pages 972 and 973.
- The effects of tobacco use on pregnancy and assistance for smoking cessation are found in Chapter 33, page 489.

D. Herbal Dietary Supplements

- Herbal dietary supplements are not regulated by the Federal Drug Administration. The public is free to purchase them over the counter to self-medicate.
- Questions about use of herbal supplements, their amount, and duration need to be included when taking a routine medical history. Information about possible problems when taking the supplements can be presented to the patient.
- Common uses are for colds, burns, headaches, allergies, rashes, depression, insomnia, and premenstrual syndrome.
- Several remedies have implications for dental/dental hygiene treatment, such as:
  A. Echinacea used for upper respiratory infections (colds) activates cell-mediated immunity: may cause allergic reactions, decreased effectiveness of immunosuppressants, and immunosuppression with long-term use.
  B. Valerian used for insomnia and stress has a sedative effect and may increase the sedative effect of anesthetics and, with long-term use, may increase anesthetic requirements.[4]

ORAL FINDINGS DURING PREGNANCY

I. GINGIVAL INFLAMMATORY CHANGES

- Primarily an exaggerated response of the tissues to dental biofilm.
- When the periodontal tissues are in good health and the patient uses adequate personal oral care measures for biofilm control, major adverse gingival changes are not expected.
- Reaction to the physiologic changes of pregnancy, as well as to the influence of the increased circulating levels of female sex hormones.
- Trauma, poor oral hygiene, and local irritation from calculus or prostheses may be contributory factors.

TABLE 48-1	DRUGS CONTRAINDICATED DURING PREGNANCY AND BREAST-FEEDING	
CLASSIFICATION	**DRUGS PRESCRIBED FOR TREATMENT***	**POSSIBLE ADVERSE EFFECTS ON FETUS AND INFANT**
Anticoagulant	Warfarin (Coumadin) (D) Dicumarol (D)	Hemorrhagic fetal death Birth malformations
Anticonvulsant	Barbiturates (phenobarbital) (D) Phenytoin sodium (D) Trimethadione (D) Valproate sodium (D)	Congenital malformations Developmental delays Fetal phenobarbital syndrome Fetal hydantoin syndrome Fetal trimethadione syndrome Fetal valproate syndrome
Antimicrobial	Streptomycin (B) Tetracycline (D)	Toxic action on ear: 8th cranial nerve damage Bone growth inhibition; intrinsic dental stain
Antineoplastic	Cyclophosphamide (Cytoxan) (D) Mercaptopurine (D) Methotrexate (D)	Multiple anomalies; fetal death
Hormone	Clomiphene (Clomid) (X) Estrogenic substances (X) diethylstilbestrol (X) Prednisone (C) Progesterone (X)	Increased anomalies; neural tube defects Cancer of the vagina and cervix; genital tract anomalies; congenital heart defects
Psychotrophic	Antianxiety: Chlordiazepoxide (Librium) (D) Diazepam (Valium) (D) Meprobamate (Miltown) (D) Antimanic Lithium carbonate (D)	Low heart rate, muscle tone, respiration; poor sucking reflex Taken near term may cause neonatal withdrawal syndrome or cardiorespiratory instability Lethargy, cyanosis, teratogenic (dose related)
Drugs of Abuse	Alcohol	Fetal alcohol syndrome (Chapter 64, page 972) Spontaneous abortion; low birth rate Mental retardation
	Cocaine prenatal exposure inhale free-base vapors (postpartum)	Decreased birth weight; prematurity Fetal growth retardation; microcephaly Teratogenic effects Increased rate of seizures
	Narcotics heroin methadone methamphetamine	Decreased birth weight Withdrawal symptoms Convulsions; sudden infant death Intrauterine-growth retardation; enters breast milk
	Tobacco cigarette smoking involuntary smoking Environmental	Low birth weight, prematurity, miscarriage, still birth, infant mortality Sudden infant death syndrome Children: increased respiratory infections and symptoms Deficiencies in physical growth, intellectual development Higher incidence in mortality rate of infant and child

*United States Food and Drug Administration (FDA) categorizes drugs and their relation to pregnancy as: **A.** No risk demonstrated to fetus in any trimester. **B.** No adverse effects in animals; no human studies available. **C.** Only given after risks to fetus are considered; animal studies have shown no adverse reactions, no human studies available. **D.** Definite fetal risks; may be given in spite of risks if needed in life-threatening conditions. **X.** Absolute fetal abnormalities; not to be used at any time in pregnancy.

■ Gingival reaction in pregnancy may be seen by the second month.
■ When left untreated, the gingival inflammation continues as the hormones rise to a maximum level by the eighth month.

■ Symptoms abate after the birth of the child, but a completely healthy condition does not necessarily result. A patient with a gingival disturbance during pregnancy continues to have the disturbance, even if to a somewhat lessened degree, after the birth.

II. GINGIVITIS

A. Clinical Appearance

- Shows characteristics of inflamed tissues, including enlargement, redness, smooth and shiny surface
- Bleeding on probing

B. Predisposing Factors

- Local irritation and infection because of poor oral hygiene leaving dental biofilm on the teeth and gingiva
- Hormonal changes during pregnancy that may alter the tissue reaction[5,6]
- Increased proportions of *Prevotella intermedia* have been found in gingivitis and elevated serum levels of the hormones of pregnancy (estrogen and progesterone).[7]

III. GINGIVAL ENLARGEMENT

A. Oral "Pyogenic" Granuloma

- Benign, inflammatory lesion; also called an epulis gravidarum, a pregnancy granuloma, or a pregnancy tumor.[8–10]
- The use of the word tumor is misleading; the lesion is not a tumor but a hyperplasia and also occurs in men and nonpregnant women.
- When the lesion is removed during pregnancy, there is some tendency for recurrence.

B. Clinical Appearance

- The lesion appears as an isolated, discrete, soft, round enlargement near the gingival margin usually associated with an interdental area, as shown in **Figure 48-1**.
- It forms in a mushroom-like shape with a smooth, glistening surface.
- The pressure of the lip or cheek tends to flatten it.
- The color depends on the vascularity and may be purplish-red, magenta, or deep blue, sometimes dotted with red.

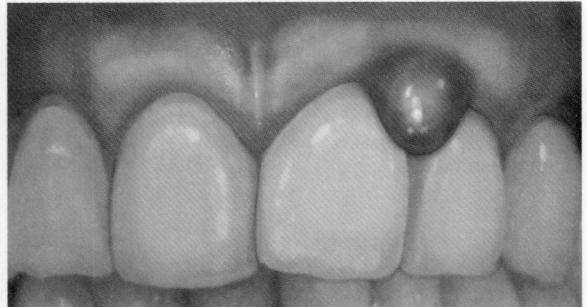

FIGURE 48-1 Artist's painting to show characteristics of a "Pyogenic" Granuloma or "Pregnancy Tumor." Isolated, discrete, round, soft enlargement near the gingival margin; smooth, glistening surface, purplish-red in color.

C. Symptoms

- Bleeds readily with slight trauma.
- Painless unless it becomes large enough to interfere with occlusion and mastication.

D. Significance

- Interference during mastication: can contribute to inadequate nutritive intake for mother and baby because of discomfort when chewing.
- Provides a site for bacterial growth; potential development of periodontal attachment loss and eventual bone destruction.
- Results in bleeding and pain: may interfere with routine dental biofilm removal using toothbrush and interdental aids.
- Creates undesirable esthetic effects.

IV. ENAMEL EROSION

A. Development

- Morning sickness with vomiting over an extended period can lead to demineralization and acid erosion primarily on the maxillary palatal surfaces.

B. Recommendations for the Patient

- Eat small amounts of nutritious yet non-cariogenic foods throughout the day.
- Use a sodium bicarbonate rinse after vomiting to neutralize acid.
- Chew gum containing xylitol after eating.
- Use gentle toothbrushing and low abrasive fluoride toothpaste to prevent damage to demineralized tooth surfaces.

ASPECTS OF PATIENT CARE

I. ASSESSMENT

A. Early Appointment

- Dental hygiene appointments are scheduled as early in pregnancy as possible.
- Anticipatory guidance is mandatory relative to the effects of drugs, tobacco use, and periodontal infection on the development and subsequent health of the infant.
- The first few months may be challenging for the mother-to-be because pregnancy provides an emotional experience with many adjustments.
- The second trimester is considered the safest for general dental treatment.
- Dental hygiene care needs to start much earlier to keep the gingival tissues in optimum health and prevent oral infections.

B. Medical History: Other Health Problems Need Identification During Examination

■ Gestational Diabetes: First recognition during pregnancy; needs insulin adjustment and careful supervision.[11] More information is included with Chapter 68 page 1044.

■ Cardiovascular diseases can involve serious complications. Women with hypertension have greater risk for fetuses with intrauterine growth retardation, placental abruption, and a 15 to 20% increase for superimposed preeclampsia later in gestation.

■ **Adolescent health:** When the expectant mother is an adolescent, her own special needs differ from those of a mature woman. Aspects of adolescent development are described in Chapter 51, page 787.

C. Consultations

■ Contact with the patient's physician and/or obstetrician is necessary for integrating general and oral care. All routine dental treatment is acceptable unless the patient's obstetrician advises otherwise.

■ When a patient seeks dental and dental hygiene care and is not under the care of a physician, she is urged and assisted to obtain medical supervision for her health and the health of her baby.

II. RADIOGRAPHY

A. Universal Safety Factors

■ Radiographs are not made for any patient unless necessary.

■ With contemporary safety factors of modern radiography, the patient can be assured that essential radiographs can be made without question during pregnancy.

■ When they are required during pregnancy, the patient is covered with a lead apron, a thyroid collar, and a second apron for the back to prevent secondary radiation from reaching the abdomen.

■ All current methods for radiation safety and protection are applied, including optimum filtration, collimation, use of the fastest film, and extended target film distance.

B. Exposures

■ Determine the minimum number of film exposures that will produce the required diagnostic information; the same procedure for all patients.

■ The use of a paralleling technique does not require angulation directed toward the patient's abdomen.

■ Careful and skillful film placement, angulation, processing, and all phases of technique prevent the need

for remaking radiographs that are not acceptable for diagnosis.

III. OVERALL TREATMENT CONSIDERATIONS

A. Dental Hygiene Care Goal

■ The dental hygienist who is well informed about dental care can motivate the patient and alleviate fears related to certain services.

■ Patients often consult with the dental hygienist for reassurance and interpretation of the dentist's recommendations and procedures.

■ Gingival disease need not be expected when the patient is motivated to practice conscientious self-care procedures for oral cleanliness and daily dental biofilm control. This calls for a specific appointment plan for scaling and disease control instruction.

■ A concentrated plan for dental caries control is indicated. A multiple fluoride program and limitation of cariogenic foods are basic to the preventive efforts.

B. Dental Care

■ *Elective Treatment:* Postpone until second trimester or early third trimester.

■ *Restorative.* Complete restorative needs with permanent restorative materials. One important contraindication for the use of temporary restorations is that after the baby is born, the mother may be too busy to attend to appointments because of added family responsibilities or return to career employment.

C. Appointment Planning

■ Frequency
  ▪ Monthly appointments or appointments three times during the 9-month period may be required.
  ▪ Appointment frequency depends on the patient's needs as well as ability and motivation to maintain a healthy oral environment.

■ Individual Appointments
  ▪ Patients are more comfortable with short appointments.
  ▪ A series of appointments is indicated when calculus deposits are heavy.

■ Postpartum Maintenance Appointments
  For the patient who has not been on a regular maintenance plan prior to pregnancy, emphasis is placed on motivating the patient to continue regular appointments for dental hygiene and dental care after the baby is born.

D. Clinical Care

■ Common physical changes can be identified that affect appointment procedures.

TABLE 48-2	APPOINTMENT ADAPTATIONS FOR THE PRENATAL PATIENT
CHARACTERISTIC	**DENTAL HYGIENE IMPLICATION**
Fatigues easily, may even fall asleep	Short appointments; several in series, as needed Work with an assistant to accomplish more at each appointment
General awkwardness because of new shape and weight gain	Attend to details, such as gently lowering and straightening chair for patient Make sure rinsing facilities are convenient; or preferably, an assistant attends to evacuation
Frequent urination	Allow sufficient appointment time for interruptions Suggest at beginning of appointment that patients mention the need for interruption
Discomfort of remaining in one position too long	Position the patient on her left side and not in supine or Trendelenburg position **(Figure 48-2)**
Backache	Interrupt in middle of appointment to allow patient to change position Assistance with evacuation during intraoral instrumentation can shorten appointment time
Faintness and dizziness	Be prepared for emergency (Table 69-4, page 1077)
Adverse reaction to strong smells and flavors	Recommend less strong-flavored dentifrice
Exaggerated reactions to odors and flavors of medicaments and other office materials	Determine particularly obnoxious odors for an individual patient and remove them; check office ventilation
Unpleasant taste in mouth	Advise: nonalcoholic mouth rinse; use a neutral sodium fluoride rinse Demonstrate tongue cleaning in Chapter 27 (page 402)
Nausea and vomiting (first trimester)	Do not brush right after vomiting. Rinse generously with water after vomiting to remove acid from the teeth.
Gagging	Recommend a small toothbrush Turn head down over sink while brushing; helps to relax throat and allow saliva to flow out Take care in instrument and radiographic film placement
Physician's recommendation for alleviation of nausea symptoms: frequent eating of small amounts of foods	Encourage use of non-cariogenic foods
Unusual food cravings	If cravings are for sweets, clearly define relationship of frequent nibbling of cariogenic foods to dental caries Provide list of nutritious non-cariogenic snacks.

■ Nearly every woman is bothered by one or more minor complaints at some time during her pregnancy.

■ Attention to details provides the patient with comfort and motivates her to continue oral care.

■ **Table 48-2** lists common physical changes of pregnancy and suggests appointment considerations.

E. Patient Positioning[12]

1. *Effect of Supine Position.*
   ■ The weight of the developing fetus in the uterus bears down directly on the major vessels, the aorta, and the inferior vena cava.
   ■ The vessels are pressed between the spinal column and the uterus.
   ■ During the third trimester, symptoms of circulatory insufficiency can appear when venous return is decreased.

2. *Supine Hypotensive Syndrome: Emergency*[13]
   ■ Patient is lying in supine position
   ■ Abrupt fall in blood pressure
   ■ Bradycardia, sweating, nausea, weakness, air hunger
   ■ Symptoms caused by impaired venous return resulting from pressure of the uterus with developing baby on the inferior vena cava.
   ■ Leads to decrease in blood pressure, reduced cardiac output, and loss of consciousness

3. *Emergency Treatment*
   ■ *Roll the patient over to her left side to relieve pressure of uterus on vena cava*
   ■ *Blood pressure will return to normal promptly*

4. Alternate Positions **(Figure 48-2)**.
   ■ Elevate the right hip to displace the uterus to the left. Use a pillow or rolled-up blanket **(Figure 48-2A)**.
   ■ Patient lies on left side **(Figure 48-2B)**

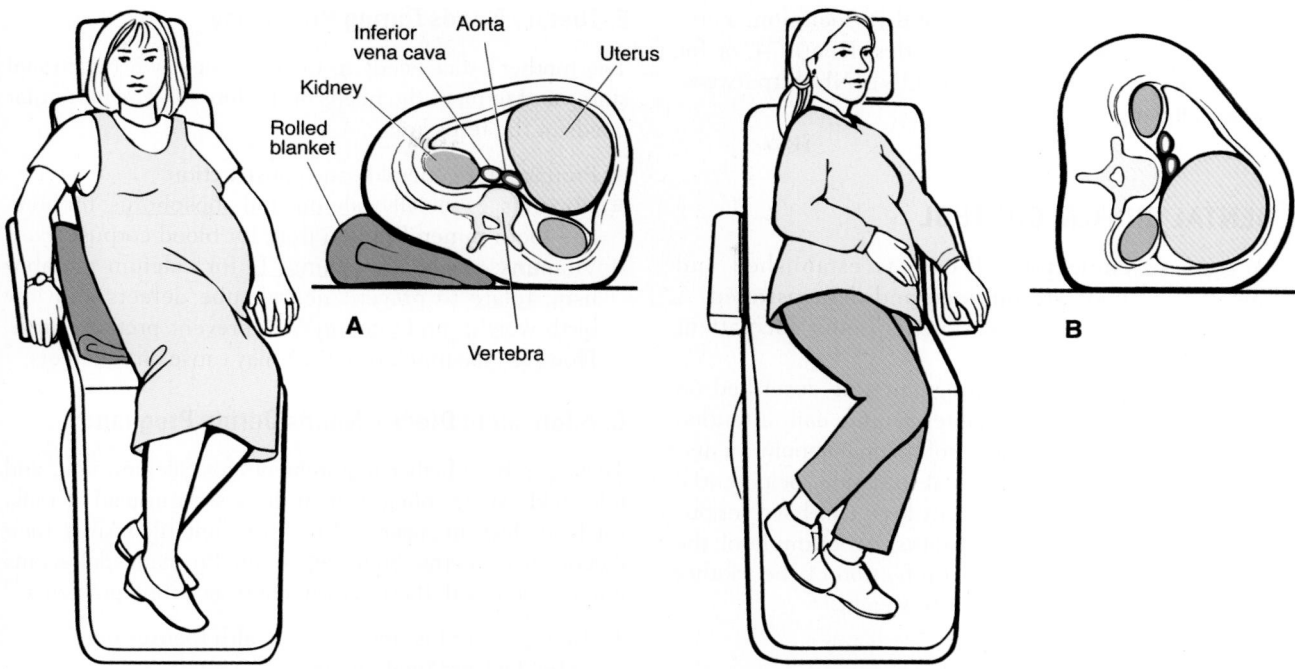

FIGURE 48-2 **Positions During Pregnancy.** The supine position allows the weight of the developing fetus to bear down directly on the major vessels. **(A)** Patient lies on left side with a pillow or blanket roll to elevate right hip. **(B)** Patient turned farther to left. Note position of uterus in cross sections of the abdomen.

IV. DENTAL HYGIENE CARE

A. Preventive Care

- Preventive care needs priority attention, beginning with information and motivation.
- Areas of food impaction are corrected, and all overhanging restorations are reshaped or replaced.
- All nonsurgical procedures are carefully and thoroughly completed.
- Complicated elective surgical periodontal treatment is deferred.

B. Preventive Measures

- When a patient has gingival enlargement and inflammation, instruction in biofilm control and other preventive measures including diet and eating patterns is needed.
- At the follow-up appointments, evaluation with disclosing agent is made and instruction is continued.

C. Instrumentation

- **Careful instrumentation for complete calculus removal is indicated.**
- The use of ultrasonic scalers is not contraindicated for reasons related to pregnancy. Refer to Chapter 39, page 623 for other potential contraindications.
- If stain removal is needed, the use of an abrasive cleaning paste is postponed until the tissue has responded to the biofilm control measures.

D. Anesthesia

- After consultation with the patient's physician, nitrous oxide/oxygen may be used in moderation.
- Nitrous oxide–oxygen sedation is widely used in childbirth and other appointments required during pregnancy.
- If used in the second or third trimester, precaution is required, including the length minimized to 30 minutes with oxygen percentage at 50%.

PATIENT INSTRUCTION

- The emphasis on general health during pregnancy provides the ideal setting for instructions relative to many aspects of oral health for the mother, her expected child, and other family members.
- New developments in disease prevention and control need to be explained.
- Helping the mother learn what to expect before the infant arrives is essential and may be found in Table 49-1, anticipatory guidance: birth to 24 months (page 756).
- Reading material that supplements personal discussions can contribute to patient understanding and cooperation. Printed materials concerning the prevention of periodontal infections and dental caries and the development and care of children's teeth are available from the American Dental Association. An ADA product catalog for the current year may be obtained by

writing to the American Dental Association, catalog sales, P.O. Box 776, St. Charles, IL 60174, or for ordering THE ADA CATALOG ONLINE: http://www.adacatalog.org/.)

I. DENTAL BIOFILM CONTROL

■ A rigid schedule for self-care is established and specific methods are outlined and demonstrated. A series of instructional sessions is better for patient learning.

■ Gingival changes during pregnancy, as described on pages 744 to 746 in this chapter, require daily attention by the patient and periodic professional appointments.

■ Severity of existing periodontal infection, or potential for the initiation of attachment loss, can have serious effects on both mother and fetus. An example of the possible effect of periodontal infection of the mother on the fetus is preterm low birth weight.[1,2]

II. SMOKING CESSATION

■ Use of tobacco, alcohol, and substances of abuse during pregnancy can have severe influences on the developing fetus as well as on the child after birth.

■ Pregnancy is an ideal time to motivate a patient to quit smoking and avoid the use of other harmful substances. The mother focuses on making changes because she wants to do her very best for a healthy child.

■ Explain increased risks for reduced birth weight, spontaneous abortions, perinatal deaths, and sudden infant death syndrome.

■ Explain the effects of second-hand and third-hand smoke on the fetus and child after birth.

■ Present the steps in a cessation program, as described in Chapter 33, page 489.

III. DIET

■ Instruction is provided in prevention of dental caries and maintenance of the health of the supporting structures of the teeth.

■ The use of a varied diet containing the essential protective food groups, with a minimum of cariogenic foods, is necessary. The MyPlate Food Guide is shown in Chapter 34 on page 499.

A. Purposes of Adequate Diet During Pregnancy

■ To maintain daily strength and feeling of well-being.

■ To provide the essential building materials for the developing fetus.

■ To protect and promote the health of the oral tissues of the mother.

■ To minimize postpartum problems.

B. Dietary Needs During Pregnancy

The mother's diet needs to maintain her own nutritional status and to meet the needs of the fetus.[14] The particular needs of the fetus are:

■ Proteins, for general tissue construction.

■ Minerals, especially calcium and phosphorus, for bone and tooth mineralization; iron, for blood corpuscles.

■ Vitamins, especially vitamin D for calcium metabolism, folate to prevent neural tube defects and low birth weight, and vitamin A to prevent preterm birth. However, too much vitamin A may cause birth defects.[15]

C. Adolescent Dietary Needs During Pregnancy

Teenagers have higher requirements for calcium, iron, and folic acid. Many young women drink soda instead of milk, eat foods high in sugar and fat, or voluntarily restrict their diet due to concerns about weight gain. Pregnant adolescents often present with these same dietary needs and problems.[14]

1. Taking a diet history for oral health focuses on:
   ■ Intake from food groups
   ■ Number and types of snacks per day
   ■ Frequency of cariogenic foods
   ■ Intake of sweetened beverages, particularly soda with sugar
   ■ Use of sugar-containing chewing gum
2. Dietary recommendations for oral and general health include:
   ■ A healthy diet from the fruit, vegetable, grain, meat and meat alternatives, and dairy food groups
   ■ 1300 mg of calcium per day or four servings of calcium-rich foods
   ■ Iron and folic acid supplements and iron- and folate-rich foods
   ■ Healthy snacks
   ■ Substitution of water for soda drinks with caffeine and sugar
   ■ Use of sugarless chewing gum with xylitol after eating

IV. DENTAL CARIES CONTROL

A. Incidence During Pregnancy

■ Some patients believe that they have more dental caries during and because of pregnancy.

■ Research has shown that this is not true and that any relationship is indirect.

■ Factors that result in dental caries formation are the same during pregnancy as at other times (Figure 34-4 and page 506).

B. Factors That May Contribute to Apparent Increase in Dental Caries Rate

■ *Previous Neglect.* A patient may not have kept a regular dental appointment plan. The existing dental caries during pregnancy may represent years of accumulation.

- *Diet During Pregnancy.* Possible increase in intake of cariogenic foods:
  - Unusual cravings may be for sweet foods.
  - Frequency of eating: patient may be eating every few hours for prevention of nausea, and those foods may be cariogenic.
- *Neglect of Personal Oral Care Procedures.* Patient may lack interest in daily dental biofilm removal or be lax about rinsing (with water) immediately following intake of a cariogenic food.
- The smell of toothpaste or the act of brushing may precipitate nausea and reduction in oral care.

C. Calcium and the Mother's Teeth

- The misconception concerning the withdrawal of calcium from the mother's teeth and its relationship to dental caries is widespread.
- It is necessary to review the known facts because the patient's beliefs may need clarification. In discussing the problem with the patient, a summary of the process of dental caries initiation can be helpful.
- Minerals contained in the erupted tooth enamel and dentin are not available, and no removal of minerals can occur by way of the pulp.
- Minerals are removed from the external surface of the enamel and exposed root surface in the process of demineralization. Demineralization is due to incomplete daily dental biofilm removal and overexposure to fermentable carbohydrates, rather than the effects of pregnancy.
- Minerals contained within the alveolar bone are available, as they are from other bones of the body. When the mother's diet does not contain sufficient calcium and phosphorus, her own reserve may be utilized. The metabolism of calcium is complex.
- Most calcium and phosphorus of bones and teeth is added to the fetus during the third trimester. The incidence of dental caries in the mother is not different during that period, although the carious lesions may be larger if the teeth have been neglected throughout the pregnancy.

D. Relationship of Fluoride

No direct evidence shows that prenatal fluoride intake by the mother influences the rate of dental caries in the child.[16–18]

V. FLUORIDE PROGRAM

- *Professional Topical Application*
  A. All patients can benefit from a topical application of fluoride solution, gel, or varnish after scaling and root planing.
  B. Applications can be indicated, especially for patients with a tendency toward demineralization and those

with numerous restorations. Risk factors determination is described on page 380 and Table 26-1, page 381.
- *Self-applications*
  A. A fluoride dentifrice is recommended for all patients to be used at least two times daily, after breakfast and before going to bed.
  B. Other fluoride recommendations are individualized according to patient need.
  C. A daily nonalcoholic fluoride mouth rinse, gel tray, or other mode of application is essential for some patients; review how to rinse thoroughly (Box 29-4, page 431).
  D. A comprehensive fluoride effort can be particularly helpful for the pregnant adolescent.

SPECIAL PROBLEMS FOR REFERRAL

I. DEPRESSION DURING PREGNANCY

Childbearing years place women at greatest risk for depression.[19] Oral healthcare professionals can learn to identify signs and symptoms of depression in pregnant patients. Treatment for depression and dental hygiene care for individuals with depression are described on page 956 in Chapter 63.

A. Signs of Depression

- Depressed mood; loss of interest or pleasure in ordinary activities
- Fatigue and disturbed sleep
- Loss of appetite
- Difficulty making decisions
- Feelings of worthlessness and suicidal thoughts[20]

B. Impact on Health of the Fetus

- Higher tendencies for preeclampsia
- Longer labor
- Low birth rate
- Preterm delivery

C. What to Do

1. Explain that depression is a biologically based illness caused by a chemical imbalance in the brain.
2. Indicate that depression is treatable, and when treated, can improve the quality of life.
3. Refer the patient to the physician of record or a community mental health resource center.

II. DOMESTIC VIOLENCE

A. Identification

Identification, assessment, and intervention with victims of domestic violence can be a significant part of a dental visit (Chapter 61, page 936).

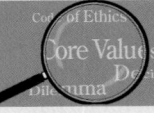

Everyday Ethics

Anna, the dental hygienist, welcomed her patient Julie, a 20-year-old single woman. She is in the first trimester of pregnancy and was referred by a nurse from the Maternal and Child Health Clinic. Anna notices the way Julie holds a hand over her mouth when she talks. Julie's history appears negative except for smoking about a half pack of cigarettes daily. Examination reveals multiple carious lesions, heavy calculus, and 4- to 5-mm proximal probing depths in several molar areas. After making the radiographic survey and presenting initial patient instruction, there was time for one quadrant of scaling. Follow-up appointments were scheduled for dental hygiene and with the dentist. Julie does not show up for any of the appointments.

Questions for Consideration

1. Which of the dental hygiene core values (Table II-1, Section II Introduction, page 38) apply to this situation? Explain.
2. What is the role of the dental hygienist, if any, to make further contact with this patient, and why? How will she go about it?
3. Describe two or three courses of action and the possible outcomes of the situation through a dental hygiene care plan.

B. Most Common Sites of Injury

- Head
- Face
- Neck

C. Obstetrical and Other Manifestations

- Obstetrical: miscarriages and spontaneous or multiple abortions
- Possible substance abuse
- Depression
- Suicide attempts[21]

D. What to Do

1. Address the issue with the patient
2. Refer to the Domestic Violence Intervention Program in the community if a case of domestic violence is suspected[22]

DOCUMENTATION

Documentation for the pregnant patient includes a minimum of the following:

- Note a carefully prepared medical history, medications taken, use of tobacco, alcohol, or illicit drugs, history of gestational diabetes, miscarriage, hypertension, and morning sickness.
- Note consults and answers when requested, including general physician and obstetrician.
- Note oral examination findings with areas of concern that need treatment and follow-up.
- Note changes from previous examinations with respect to personal oral care by the patient and record for the record types of instruction provided.
- A sample progress note may be found in **Box 48-2**.

BOX 48-2	**Example Progress Note**

Goldie is in her second trimester now. We had advised 3-week exams with oral hygiene, but she already skipped 2 of them. Today: Blood Pressure 130/80 mm Hg. Gingiva soft and spongy with new calculus. Says her two older children (both under age 5 years) require a lot of attention and she gets very tired.

We had discussed appointments for the two older children previously and she brought that up today saying she couldn't bring them on the same day ("they might tear the place apart").

Went over her toothbrushing again and I advised a power brush to help her get her gingiva back in health. Demonstrated on dentoform for proximal surfaces. She promised to come in 4 weeks next. Said her husband was complaining at all the bills for extra visits "so I had better try treating my gums myself as you have told me."

Signed: _____, RDH Date: _____

Factors To Teach The Patient

- The relationship of oral health of the mother to the general health of the fetus and newborn.
- The serious effects of tobacco and other drugs on the health of the fetus, the infant, and the child.
- Reasons for dental hygiene appointments early during pregnancy, at regular intervals throughout pregnancy, and after birth of the baby.
- Reasons for scheduling dental care appointments during pregnancy in the second trimester or early in the third trimester.
- The rationale for maintaining good personal oral hygiene care to control dental biofilm throughout the pregnancy and after the baby's birth.
- Self-examination of the oral cavity to evaluate the effectiveness of daily dental biofilm removal and the health of the soft tissues.
- Reasons for limiting fermentable carbohydrate intake and maintaining a healthy diet from the fruit, vegetable, grain, meat, and meat alternatives, and dairy food groups.

References

1. Offenbacher S, Katz V, Fertik G, Collins J, Boyd D, Maynor G, McKaig R, Beck J. Periodontal infection as a possible risk factor for preterm low birth weight. *J Periodontol.* 1996 Oct;67(10 Suppl):1103–13.

2. Gibbs RS, Romero R, Hillier SL, Eschenbach DA, Sweet RL. A review of premature birth and subclinical infections. *Am J Obstet Gynecol.* 1992 May;166(5):1515–28.

3. Watts DH. Management of human immunodeficiency virus infection in pregnancy. *N Engl J Med.* 2002 Jun;346(24):1879–91.

4. Ang-Lee MK, Moss J, Yuan CS. Herbal medicines and perioperative care. *JAMA.* 2001 Jul;286(2):208–16.

5. Loe H. Periodontal changes in pregnancy. *J Periodontol.* 1965 May–Jun;36:209–17.

6. Otomo-Corgel J. Chapter 43, Periodontal therapy in the female patient. In: Newman MG, Takei HH, Klokkevold PR, Carranza FA, eds. *Carranza's clinical periodontology.* 10th ed. Philadelphia: Saunders; 2006. p. 636–49.

7. Kornman KS, Loesche WJ. The subgingival microbial flora during pregnancy. *J Periodont Res.* 1980 Mar;15(2):111–22.

8. Fehrenbach MJ, Lemborn UE, Phelan JA. Inflammation and repair. In Ibsen OA, Phelan JA. *Oral pathology for the dental hygienist.* 3rd ed. Philadelphia: Saunders; 2000. p. 75.

9. Pindborg JJ. *Atlas of diseases of the oral mucosa.* 5th ed. Philadelphia: Saunders; 1992. p. 286–8.

10. Carranza FA, Hogan EL. Gingival enlargement. In: Newman MG, Takei HH, Klokkevold PR, Carranza FA, eds. *Carranza's clinical periodontology.* 10th ed. Philadelphia: Saunders; 2006. p. 373–90.

11. Moore PA, Orchard T, Guggenheimer J, Weyant RJ. Diabetes and oral health promotion: a survey of disease preventive behaviors. *J Am Dent Assoc.* 2000 Sep;131(9):1333–41.

12. Tarsitano BF, Rollings RE. The pregnant dental patient: evaluation and management. *Gen Dent.* 1993 May–Jun;41(3):226–34.

13. Little JW, Falace DA, Miller CS, Rhodus NL. *Dental management of the medically compromised patient.* 7th ed. St. Louis: Mosby; 2008. p. 268–78.

14. Harper LF, Faine MP. Nutrition in pregnancy, infancy, and childhood. In: Palmer CA, ed. *Diet and nutrition in oral health.* 2nd ed. New Jersey: Prentice Hall; 2007. p. 344–65.

15. Oakley GP, Erickson JD. Vitamin A and birth defects. Continuing caution is needed. *N Engl J Med.* 1995 Nov;333(21):1414–5.

16. Driscoll WS. A review of clinical research on the use of prenatal fluoride administration for prevention of dental caries. *ASDC J Dent Child.* 1981 Mar–Apr;48(2):109–17.

17. Thylstrup A. Is there a biological rationale for prenatal fluoride administration? *ASDC J Dent Child.* 1981 Mar-Apr;48(2):103–8.

18. Bawden JW, editor. Changing patterns of fluoride intake. Workshop. Chapel Hill, April 23–25, 1991. *J Dent Res.* 1992 May;71(5):1214–27.

19. Monacs R, Cohen LS. Depression during pregnancy: diagnosis and treatment options. *J Clin Psychiatry.* 2002;63(7 Suppl)24.

20. American Psychiatric Association. *Diagnostic and statistical manual of mental disorders (DSM-IV-TR).* 4th ed. Washington: APA; 2000. p. 422–3.

21. McFarlane J, Parker B, Soeken K, Bullock L. Assessing for abuse during pregnancy. Severity and frequency of injuries and associated entry into prenatal care. *JAMA.* 1992 Jun;267(23):3176–8.

22. Love C, Gerbert B, Caspers N, Bronstone A, Perry D, Bird W. Dentists' attitudes and behaviors regarding domestic violence. The need for an effective response. *J Am Dent Assoc.* 2001 Jan;132(1):85–93.

Pediatric Oral Health Care: Infancy Through Age 5

TERESA BUTLER DUNCAN, RDH, BS
NANCY SISTY LEPEAU, RDH, MS, MA

Chapter Outline

Oral health for infants and young children up to 5 years depends primarily on parental interventions.

- Parents are counseled and given the information needed to assess their child's oral health status.
- They are taught how to intervene and to anticipate the child's oral health needs at various ages and stages of growth and development.
- Healthcare professionals provide education through anticipatory guidance before a child's birth and at regular intervals thereafter. **Box 49-1** defines key words associated with this chapter.

ACCESS TO PARENTS, INFANTS, AND YOUNG CHILDREN

I. LOCATIONS FOR CONTACT WITH PARENTS

- Hospitals: prenatal and birthing classes.
- Public and private community health centers.
- Daycare and preschool centers.
- Pediatrician and family practice offices.
- Home health providers for education and anticipatory guidance in high-risk families.

BOX 49-1	Key Words

Pediatric Oral Health Care: Infants Through Age 5

Anticipatory guidance: provide information to parents and caregivers on what to expect in a child's current and next developmental stage so that the child's needs can be anticipated and properly managed.

Dental home: establish a dentist of record in the community early in childhood for continuous and comprehensive preventive interventions, dental hygiene, and dental care.

Grazing: eating or drinking at will throughout the day or evening.

Infant: child younger than 1 year of age.

Neonate: newborn.

Neonatal: refers to the period immediately following birth and continuing through the first month of life.

Nonnutritive sucking: sucking fingers, thumb, pacifiers, or other objects for comfort.

Premature birth: birth that occurs before the expected delivery date; denotes an infant born before 37 weeks of gestation.

Sippy cup: a special cup with a lid that may have a straw or a drinking projection to teach a young child to drink.

Toddler: child from age 1 year to approximately 3 years of age.

Wean: to discontinue breast- or bottle-feeding; to nourish the infant with other food.

II. GOALS OF EARLY ACCESS

- Assist parents in establishing a dental home for the child.
- Educate parents on prevention of oral diseases, early problem identification, and oral hygiene.

III. ROLE OF HEALTHCARE PROFESSIONALS

- Many children have visited a child healthcare professional many times before age 3.
- Healthcare professionals, including community health workers and health educators, need to be trained to examine the mouths of infants and children for early childhood dental caries, dental biofilm, gingivitis, oral pathologies, and evidence of orofacial trauma and/or possible abuse.
- Guide parents to be aware of and to attend to their infant and children's oral health needs.[1,2]
- Identify problems and refer infants and young children to a dental hygienist and dentist.

IV. FIRST DENTAL AND DENTAL HYGIENE CONTACT

- Infants need to be seen by a dentist and dental hygienist by 6 months or after the eruption of the first primary tooth and by no later than age 1 year.[3]
- Emphasis is placed on early intervention before serious oral health problems can develop.[4]
- Educate parents and emphasize prevention.

V. REGULAR DENTAL HOME VISITS

A. Frequency

Visits to the dental hygienist and the dentist are scheduled according to the child's specific needs. The usual appointment plan for children with little or no oral disease is every 6 months.

B. Scheduling

The best time to schedule visits is early in the morning or after naps when the child is not tired and is more apt to listen and cooperate.

C. Purposes

Appointments are planned for assessment, prevention, and introduction to dental hygiene.

- Develop rapport with the child and the family.
- Initiate positive preventive measures, such as fluoride usage, appropriate feeding practices, and daily dental biofilm removal.
- Discover, intercept, and recommend changes in any parental practices that may be detrimental to the child's oral health.

VI. ANTICIPATORY GUIDANCE

- Anticipatory guidance in oral health counseling helps parents learn what to expect of a child during the current and next developmental stage.[5]
- Essential information tailored to the child's individual needs is provided to parents verbally and in writing.
- Teach parents what constitutes good oral health care and how to anticipate the child's future requirements.
- Present proper expectations of what children are able to do at each age level to allow for more positive interactions between parent and child.
- Developmental milestones, nutrition and feeding, oral hygiene measures, dental caries prevention, health and safety precautions, and treatment measures are outlined in **Table 49-1** (Birth to 24 Months) and in **Table 49-2** (Age 2 Through 5 Years).[6]
- Additional recommendations are presented in *Oral Health Considerations for Infants* (page 767) and *Oral Health Considerations for Toddlers and Preschoolers* (page 770).

TABLE 49-1	ANTICIPATORY GUIDANCE: BIRTH TO 24 MONTHS		
AREA OF CONCERN	**BIRTH TO 6 MONTHS**	**6–12 MONTHS**	**12–24 MONTHS**
Developmental Milestone	■ Eruption of first tooth ■ Pattern of eruption	■ Pattern of eruption ■ Expected new teeth	■ Check tooth contacts ■ Close contacts: teach parents to floss
Nutrition and Feeding	■ Relation of improper bottle/breast feeding to initiation of dental caries ■ No propping of bottles in bed ■ Avoid use of bottle as pacifier ■ Breast feeding passage of alcohol and drugs to infant ■ Discuss weaning	■ Begin weaning ■ Discontinue bottle feeding by age 1 year ■ Use small regular cup ■ Avoid at-will access to bottle or sippy cup ■ Discuss sugar use, sugar retention, and caries initiation ■ Discuss consumption of sugar-sweetened beverages ■ Snacking safety (aspiration) ■ Avoid use of food for behavior modification	■ Review prior content covered ■ Nutrition, snacking based on child's diet ■ Reduce snacking frequency ■ Review snacking safety ■ Avoid food as reward for behavior modification ■ Avoid dependence on sippy cup
Oral Hygiene and Caries Prevention	■ Oral health of parents; *Streptococcus mutans* transmission ■ Clean ridges after each feeding (soft, wet cloth or gauze) ■ Use of brush (water only) ■ Position of infant for brushing	■ Use of brush ■ Review position of infant for brushing ■ Parents look for signs of disease ■ Importance of maintaining primary dentition	■ Disclose for dental biofilm ■ Review brushing ■ Parents are the role models ■ Parents look for signs of disease
Fluoride Information	■ Explain the relation of fluoride to teeth ■ Anticipate need to supplement ■ Check water supply for fluoride content at home and daycare	■ When water supply is deficient, prescribe supplement (see **Table 49-5**) ■ Discuss compliance ■ Review manner of storage: cool, dry, out of reach ■ Possible fluoride varnish application	■ Update fluoride status ■ Store fluoride products out of reach of children ■ Use of small, thin smear of fluoride dentifrice on brush ■ Need for fluoride varnish application
Trauma Prevention	■ Car seat safety	■ Discuss highest accident rate is 1–2 years ■ Car seat safety ■ Trauma proofing ■ Confirm emergency access to dental provider	■ Car seat safety ■ Discuss oral electrical burns and child-proofing home ■ Care of avulsed tooth
Habits/Function Behaviors	■ Discuss teething ■ Discuss nonnutritive sucking	■ Discuss oral/head and neck signs of child abuse	■ Effects of continued thumb, finger, or pacifier sucking
Environmental (Passive) Smoke	■ Detrimental at all ages; smoking parents must start tobacco cessation program	■ Provide smoke-free environment	■ Children need smoke-free environment
Dental/Dental Hygienist Visit	■ Provide rationale for timing of baby's first dental visit ■ Explain what happens at first dental visit ■ Encourage parents to make appointments for their own dental care to eliminate *Streptococcus mutans* and maintain oral health	■ Schedule first dental visit within 6 months of eruption of first tooth ■ Provide information about how to make the first dental/dental hygiene visit a happy experience ■ Review need for parents to complete their own dental care	■ Home preparation for dental visit ■ Frequency depends on parent compliance with home preventive measures ■ Parents emphasize helping-caring nature of dentist/dental hygienist ■ Toothbrush dental biofilm removal ■ Discuss findings and recommendations with parents

Source: Nowak AJ, Casamassimo PS. Using anticipatory guidance to provide early dental intervention. *J Am Dent Assoc.* 1995 Aug;126(8):1156–63.

TABLE 49-2	ANTICIPATORY GUIDANCE: AGE 2 THROUGH 5 YEARS	
AREA OF CONCERN	**2–3 YEARS**	**4–6 YEARS**
Developmental Milestone	■ Primary dentition complete ■ Evaluate occlusion for possible crowding, overbite, overjet ■ Bruxing and occlusal wear ■ Discuss sealants for primary molars	■ Discuss exfoliation of primary teeth ■ Eruption patterns and expected new permanent teeth ■ Discuss sealants for first permanent molars
Nutrition and Feeding	■ Suggest snacks from fruit, vegetable, dairy and meat groups ■ Limit juice intake to 4 ounces	■ Snacking: suggest healthy snacks ■ Limit juice and soda
Oral Hygiene and Caries Prevention	■ Parents continue to assist ■ Ask about problems ■ Lift upper lip when brushing ■ Brush morning and night ■ Review signs of disease	■ Parents continue to assist ■ Review signs of disease
Fluoride Information	■ Parents control toothpaste ■ Evaluate changes in diet and water ■ Make appropriate fluoride recommendations ■ Possible fluoride varnish applications	■ Parents continue toothpaste control ■ Check fluoride status ■ Varnish applications
Trauma Prevention	■ Provide trauma management plan at daycare or preschool ■ Discuss head and neck, oral signs of child abuse ■ Review safety measures	■ Trauma management plan at school ■ Discuss bike safety ■ Discuss child abuse ■ Review safety measures
Habits/function Behaviors	■ Nonnutritive sucking may still be present ■ Discuss elimination of thumb/finger sucking	■ Eliminate thumb/finger sucking
Environmental (Passive) Smoke	■ Smoke free environment required	■ Smoke free environment required
Dental/Dental Hygiene Visit	■ Need regular care every 6 months unless need for greater frequency identified ■ Emphasize helping/caring nature of dentist/dental hygienist ■ Use disclosing solution to identify dental biofilm ■ Toothbrush or rubber cup dental biofilm removal ■ Radiographic evaluation if indicated ■ Discuss findings and recommendations with parents	■ Need regular care ■ Radiographic evaluation if indicated ■ Emphasize helping/caring nature of providers ■ Use disclosing solution to identify dental biofilm ■ Assess for calculus requiring scaling ■ Rubber cup polishing ■ Discuss findings and recommendations with parents

Source: Nowak AJ, Casamassimo PS. Using anticipatory guidance to provide early dental intervention. *J Am Dent Assoc.* 1995 Aug;126(8):1156–63.

VII. BARRIERS TO DENTAL CARE

■ Lack of knowledge about prevention.
■ Language.
■ Cost.
■ Fear.
■ No dental home.
■ Dentist does not see children under age 3 years.
■ Dentist's hours do not fit into parents'/caregivers' schedules.

■ Dentist does not accept dental insurance.
■ Transportation.

ASSESSMENT

I. INTERVIEW

Parents can be seated in a quiet, private place so that they are able to concentrate and feel comfortable while supplying the information requested. After rapport is established with the parents, an explanation is given as to why the information is needed and the following factors are addressed:

A. Family Configuration

- Number of people in the household and their relationship to the child.
- Family members who work outside the home and the time spent with the child at home.
- Other caregivers, the time periods, and location.
- Socioeconomic status and educational level of parents or guardians.

B. Prenatal and Perinatal History

- Physician of record and frequency of visits.
- History of chronic/infectious diseases.
- Prenatal care provided for mother.
- Problems in pregnancy or delivery, including prematurity or low term birth weight.
- Drugs, alcohol consumed during pregnancy.
- Use of tobacco during pregnancy.

C. Medical History of the Child

- Family history of chronic/infectious disease.
- Genetic, developmental, metabolic diseases.
- Hospitalizations/surgeries and reasons.
- Allergies or reactions to medications.
- Frequency of ear infections.
- History of high fevers.
- Current medications.

D. Dental History of the Parents and Children

- Dentist of record for the family and the frequency of visits for the parents and children.
- Dental caries and periodontal disease experience of parents and children.
- Tooth eruption patterns of parents and children.

- Parents' personal oral hygiene habits.
- Teething problems exhibited by child.
- Deep pits and fissures in primary molars and no spacing.

E. Feeding Patterns Infant (Birth to 1 Year)

- Breast/bottle fed.
- Formula used and fluoride content of water used for preparation.
- Frequency and method of feeding.
- Problems with feeding.
- Problems with sleeping.
- Pacifier, thumb, or finger sucking.
- Other liquids besides formula or milk in bottle/sippy cup.
- Age other children in family were weaned.

F. Feeding Patterns Toddler (1–3 Years) and Preschool Child (3–5 Years)

- Number of snacks per day and time period.
- Types of snacks provided.
- Amount of juice or other sweet drinks consumed per day.
- Use and content of bottle/sippy cup.
- Availability of snacks without supervision.
- Problems with eating, including likes and dislikes.
- Special diet prescribed or initiated by parent.

G. Fluoride Exposure

- History of exposure to fluoride.
- Fluoride level of current water supply, including childcare environments (check public health department records).
- Well water (have water tested for fluoride level).
- Use of nonfluoridated bottled water or water systems using reverse osmosis.
- Type of toothpaste, amount, and frequency of use.
- Parental control of fluoride toothpaste.
- Use of fluoride supplementation (**Table 49-3**).

TABLE 49-3	FLUORIDE SUPPLEMENTS DOSAGE SCHEDULE (MGF/DAY)*		
	WATER FLUORIDE CONCENTRATION (PPM)		
AGE OF CHILD (YEARS)	**LESS THAN 0.3**	**BETWEEN 0.3 AND 0.6**	**GREATER THAN 0.6**
Birth–6 mo	0	0	0
6 mo–3 yr	0.25 mg	0[†]	0[†]
3–6 yr	0.50 mg	0.25 mg	0
6–16 yr	1.0 mg	0.5 mg	0

*2.2 mg sodium fluoride provides 1 mg fluoride ions.
[†]Infants receiving their total diet from breast-feeding need a 0.25 mg supplement.
Source: Recommendations from the American Dental Association, Chicago, IL.

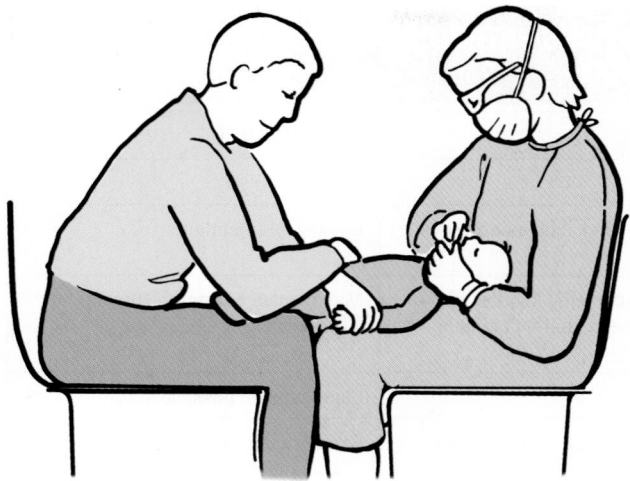

FIGURE 49-1 **Infant Dental/Dental Hygiene Visit.** The clinician makes the oral examination, discusses oral findings, and demonstrates proper oral care for the parent. The position of the infant then is reversed so that the parent is provided the opportunity to position the child and demonstrate proper oral care.

II. INFANT ORAL EXAMINATION

A. Oral Examination: Positioning for Access

- Seat parent and clinician knee to knee.
- Place child's head on the lap of the examiner, as seen in **Figure 49-1**.

B. Examination Sequence

- Examine the child's head and neck, legs, and arms for evidence of abuse. Signs of abuse are described in Chapter 61 on page 932.
- Ask the parent to control the child's extremities while the oral soft tissues are assessed **(Tables 49-4 and 49-5)**.[7]
- If teeth are present, lift the upper lip to observe in the condition of the anterior teeth.
- Examine all teeth for evidence of biofilm, discoloration.
- Look for malformations **(Figure 49-2)** and dental caries **(Figure 49-3)**.
- Show parents the findings and inform them of the significance.
- Make referrals to the dentist if evidence of pathology is noted **(Tables 49-4** and **49-5** and Table 17-2, page 264).

III. TODDLER/CHILD ORAL EXAMINATION

A. Preparing the Child for the Dental Visit

- Make the dental office or clinic visit as pleasant as possible for the child.
- Children are told that the dental hygienist and dentist help them take good care of their teeth.
- Parents are instructed to avoid using negative words, such as "hurt, pain, do not be scared."
- When the child is not present, parents are asked if the child has any fears or has had any prior negative experiences.

TABLE 49-4	ORAL SOFT AND HARD TISSUE CONDITIONS/PATHOLOGY IN INFANTS (1 TO 6 MONTHS)		
CONDITIONS	**FINDINGS**		**SIGNIFICANCE**
Soft Tissue			
Pseudomembranous candidiasis (thrush)	Mucosa or tongue; white, curd-like plaques; wipe-off leaving red and raw area		Discomfort; antifungal medication
Congenital epulis	Maxillary anterior ridge; pink, smooth, pedunculated mass; present at birth		Benign; spontaneous involution or surgical excision
Bohn's nodule	Buccal and lingual aspects of dental ridge; mucous gland remnant; smooth, translucent nodules		No treatment Shed spontaneously
Epstein's pearls	Palate near raphe; smooth, translucent nodules		No treatment
Dental lamina cysts	Crest of maxillary and mandibular ridges; dental lamina origin; smooth, translucent		No treatment
Bifid uvula	Cleft in uvula		Evaluate for possible submucous palatal cleft
Ankyloglossia	Short lingual frenum; may limit tongue mobility		Surgical reduction if interferes with nursing
Teeth			
Natal teeth	85% mandibular primary incisors; present at birth; commonly occur in pairs		Familial tendency; remove if mobile or have sharp edges causing injury
Neonatal teeth	Erupt within 30 days after birth		Same as above

Source: McDonald RE, Avery DR, Dean JA. *Dentistry for the child and adolescent.* 8th ed. St. Louis: Mosby; 2004. pp. 137–138, 154–155, 183–185, 423.

TABLE 49-5	ORAL SOFT AND HARD TISSUE CONDITIONS/PATHOLOGY IN CHILDREN APPROXIMATELY 6 MONTHS TO 5 YEARS	
CONDITIONS	**FINDINGS**	**SIGNIFICANCE**
Soft Tissue		
Eruption cysts	Translucent, smooth; may appear blue to blue-black if bleeding in cystic space	Usually no treatment
Mucocele	Lower lip, floor of mouth, buccal mucosa most common in order of occurrence; fluid-filled vesicle or blister; trauma, tearing of minor salivary duct	May resolve or require surgical excision
Traumatic ulcer	Reaction to puncture wound	Clean wound; possible suture
Alveolar abscess	Smooth, red or yellowish nodule; tender; primary teeth-more diffuse infections; may be acute or chronic	Radiographic evaluation, drainage and antibiotic may be required
Primary herpetic gingivostomatitis	High fever, 102–104°F; regional lymphadenopathy; diffuse, swollen erythematous gingiva; vesicles form painful ulcers	Resolves in 7–10 days
Geographic tongue	Red, smooth areas devoid of filliform papillae on dorsum of tongue; margins well-developed, slightly raised; pattern changes	No treatment; brush tongue to reduce bacteria
Verruca vulgaris	Multiple white sessile lesions; finger-like projections, rough surface; human papilloma virus in origin	May resolve spontaneously or require excision
Teeth		
Enamel hypoplasia	Disturbance of enamel matrix during tooth development; irregular to round pits of varying size on enamel, usually in a row; multiple causes	Esthetics
Fluorosis	Infrequent in primary dentition; usually seen in cervical region of second primary molars	Daily biofilm removal
White-spot lesions	Opaque enamel, usually cervical and proximal areas of teeth at contacts; earliest clinical sign of the carious process; indicates that the surface and underlying enamel are demineralized	Need fluoride for remineralization; daily biofilm removal
Fused teeth	Usually limited to anterior teeth; union of two independently forming primary tooth buds; familial tendency	Possible caries at point of fusion; may be absence of one of corresponding permanent teeth
Gemination	More common in primary teeth; invagination of single tooth germ; bifid crown on single root; crown appears wide	None

Source: McDonald RE, Avery DR, Dean JA. *Dentistry for the child and adolescent.* 8th ed. St. Louis: Mosby; 2004. pp. 105–108, 115–120, 139–140, 150–151, 155, 182, 418–422.

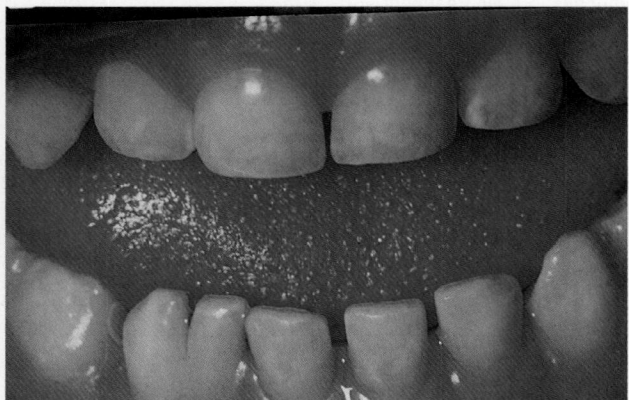

FIGURE 49-2 **Developmental Disturbance of Primary Teeth.** Gemination of mandibular right lateral incisor caused by invagination of a single tooth germ and resulting in a notched and grooved crown. Note the presence of six mandibular anterior teeth.

B. Positioning

Older children are able to sit in a dental chair. The size of the chair usually can be modified by removing the headrest and a portion of the backrest.

C. Parental Involvement

- Plan the assessment and treatment.
  - Determine the expected developmental milestones of the child according to the chronological age, as outlined in **Tables 49-6** and **49-7**.[8,9]
  - Ask parents to identify actual developmental milestones so that proper management can be initiated during the appointment.
  - Ask parents to provide a general statement regarding the child's temperament and ability to cooperate.

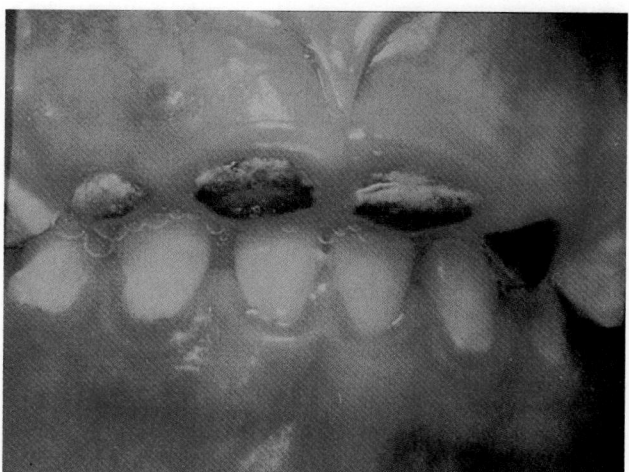

FIGURE 49-3 **Severe Early Childhood Caries (ECC).** Nearly complete loss of tooth structure of maxillary incisors. Note the abscess on the gingival tissues between the maxillary right central and lateral incisor, and the moderate cervical plaque on the mandibular incisors.

- Evaluate if the parent needs to accompany the child.
  1. At the first visit, a parent often accompanies the child to the treatment room.
  2. Advise the parent to let the dental hygienist/dentist explain about the dental or dental hygiene procedure.
  3. Instruct the parent to offer nonverbal reassurance for the child.
  4. Ask the parent if there are any questions regarding the treatment.
  5. When appropriate, explain that the child is ready to go to the treatment room unaccompanied.

D. Gingival Evaluation

- *Healthy gingiva* in the primary dentition has the following characteristics:
  - Color is pink or slightly red.
  - Tissue appearance is thick, rounded or rolled, and shiny.

- Tissue adaptation is not tight to the teeth and less fibrous than in the permanent dentition.
- Interdental papillae on spaced anterior teeth are flat or saddle-shaped.
- A col is present between facial and lingual papillae on posterior teeth in contact.
- *Unhealthy gingiva* exhibits swelling, redness, and bleeding on brushing or debriding.

E. Dental Caries Evaluation

1. Anterior Teeth
- Retract the lips to expose all of the teeth from the facial aspect.
- Look for white-spot lesions, or demineralization, along the cervical areas and on proximal tooth surfaces. Run the side of the tip of the explorer lightly over the area to assess for an intact surface, and, if present, initiate caries control for remineralization.
- Observe discolored areas or dental caries interproximally using direct vision or transillumination.
- Look for the presence of demineralization or cavitation on smooth surfaces.

2. Posterior Teeth
- Observe the pits and fissures of the primary molars to determine if they are shallow or deep and need sealants.
- Look for dark discolorations in the pits and fissures and on proximal surfaces.
- Look for open dental carious lesions on occlusal and smooth surfaces.

F. Occlusion

1. Evaluation
- Lack of spacing between primary teeth.
- Malposed, crowded, or congenitally missing teeth.
- Tooth eruption delays as compared with normal averages in **Table 49-8**.

TABLE 49-6	MILESTONES IN CHILD DEVELOPMENT: BIRTH TO AGE 18 MONTHS		
AREAS	**BIRTH TO 6 MONTHS**	**6–12 MONTHS**	**12–18 MONTHS**
Language	■ 0–2 months: quiets to sound ■ Reflects displeasure at noises ■ Coos and babbles	■ Says dada or mama ■ Understands name ■ Pays attention to verbalization	■ Repeats a few words ■ Says two or more words ■ Uses expressions, "uh,oh" ■ Points to few body parts ■ Follows one-step directions
Motor	■ 2 months: head control ■ 6 months: transfer hand to hand ■ Grasps with forearm (ulnar grasp)	■ 7–9 months: sits ■ 9–10 months: plays pat-a-cake ■ Waves bye, bye	■ Pincer grasp ■ Gives toys on request ■ 15–18 months: good use of cup and spoon
Social/Emotional	■ 2 months: gazes at human face ■ Alert to voices	■ Inhibited by word "no" ■ Separation anxiety ■ Stranger awareness	■ Separation anxiety and stranger awareness continue

Source: Goldson E, Reynolds A. Chapter 2: Child development and behavior. In: Hay WW, Levin MJ, Sondheimer JM, Deterding RR. *Current pediatric diagnosis and treatment.* 19th ed. New York: McGraw Hill; 2008. pp. 66–83.

TABLE 49-7	MILESTONES IN CHILD DEVELOPMENT: 18 MONTHS TO 5 YEARS			
AREAS	**18 MONTHS TO 2 YEARS**	**2–3 YEARS**	**3–4 YEARS**	**5 YEARS**
Language	■ Has up to 50 words and 2-word sentences ■ Talks to self ■ Hums or sings simple songs ■ Says names of familiar objects ■ Listens to short rhymes	■ Up to 500 words ■ Converses using simple 2- to 3-word phrases and sentences ■ Responds to simple directions	■ 75–80% of speech understandable ■ Knows location words ■ Likes familiar stories repeated over and over ■ Knows what, who, why questions	■ Five-word sentences ■ Conversations more mature ■ Links past and present events
Motor	■ Feeds self ■ Uses straw ■ Walks well ■ Helps wash hands ■ Seats self in chair	■ Dresses with supervision ■ Holds crayon in fist	■ Feeds self well ■ Takes off jacket ■ Holds crayon with fingers	■ Fine motor coordination maturing ■ Buttons clothing ■ May be able to tie shoelaces
Social/ Emotional	■ Likes to imitate ■ Independent ■ Difficulty waiting ■ Shy with strangers ■ Likes adult attention ■ May exhibit anger and temper tantrums	■ Likes to see and touch ■ Attached to parent ■ Rarely shares ■ Self-help skills of interest	■ Likes to please ■ Responds to commands	■ Distinguishes fantasy from reality ■ Likes pretend play ■ Longer attention span ■ Tolerates parent separation

Source: Goldson E, Reynolds A. Chapter 2: Child development and behavior. In: Hay WW, Levin MJ, Sondheimer JM, Deterding RR. *Current pediatric diagnosis and treatment.* 19th ed. New York: McGraw Hill; 2008. pp. 66–83.

TABLE 49-8	TOOTH DEVELOPMENT AND ERUPTION: PRIMARY TEETH				
	TOOTH	**HARD TISSUE FORMATION BEGINS (WEEKS *IN UTERO*)**	**ENAMEL COMPLETED (MONTHS AFTER BIRTH)**	**ERUPTION (MONTHS)**	**ROOT COMPLETED (YEAR)**
Maxillary	Central incisor	14	1½	10 (8–12)	1½
	Lateral incisor	16	2½	11 (9–13)	2
	Canine	17	9	19 (16–22)	3¼
	First molar	15½	6	16 (13–19 boys) (14–18 girls)	2½
	Second Molar	19	11	29 (25–33)	3
Mandibular	Central incisor	14	2½	8 (6–10)	1½
	Lateral incisor	16	3	13 (10–16)	1½
	Canine	17	9	20 (17–23)	3¼
	First molar	15½	5½	16 (14–18)	2¼
	Second Molar	18	10	27 (23–31 boys) (24–30 girls)	3

Source: Reprinted with permission from Lunt Lunt RC, Law DB. A review of the chronology of deciduous teeth. *J Am Dent Assoc.* 1974;89:372.

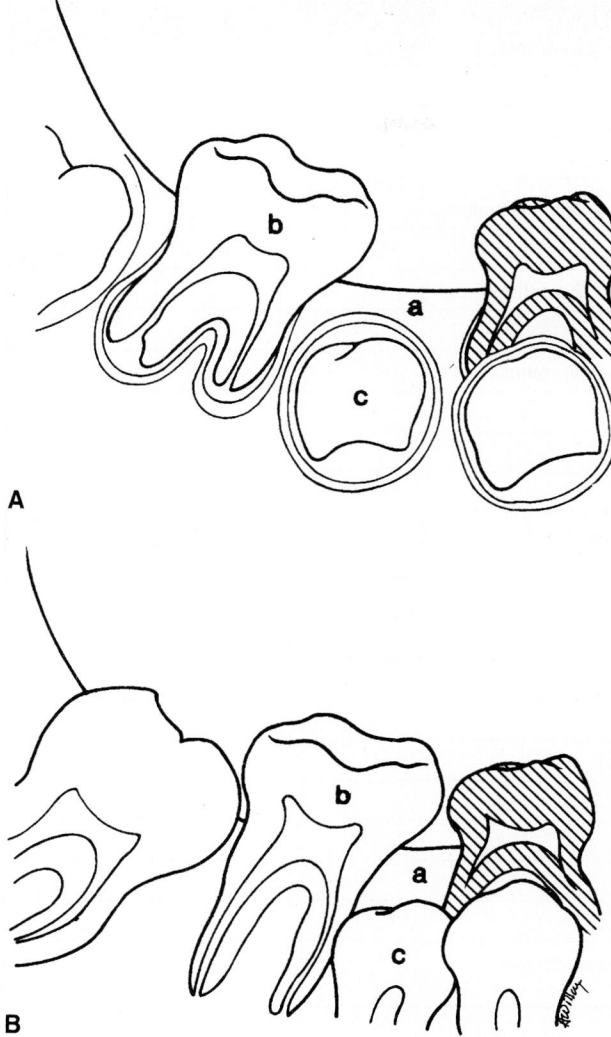

A

B

FIGURE 49-4 **Premature Loss of Second Primary Molar. (A)** Developing first permanent molar (*b*) inclines and drifts mesially into the space (*a*) from which the second primary molar was removed. Developing second premolar (*c*) is crowded. **(B)** Space from which molar was removed (*a*) is nearly closed by the mesial drift and eruption of the first permanent molar (*b*). Developing second premolar (*c*) is closed in and prevented from eruption. Note that the second permanent molar has impacted against the first molar.

- Discrepancies between the size of the teeth and the size of the mouth.
- Early loss of primary molars: this condition, if untreated, usually disrupts the eruption and alignment of permanent molars and premolars, as depicted in **Figure 49-4**.

2. Indications for Referral
- Severely crowded, malposed, or congenitally missing teeth.
- Overbite, overjet, or crossbites.
- Early loss of primary molars requires placement of a space maintainer to preserve arch length and allow for proper eruption of permanent teeth.

IV. RADIOGRAPHIC EVALUATION OF PRIMARY DENTITION

A. Indications for Radiographic Exposures

- Primary molars are close together and interfere with visualization and exploration.
- Trauma.
- Suspected pathology.
- Problems with growth and development.

B. Use of Leaded Apron and Thyroid Collar

Protection is required because children are more susceptible than are adults to low-level radiation.

C. Film Size

Film size is determined by the size of the mouth. Normally, one pediatric-sized film is used on each side to assess the primary molars.

D. Cooperation

Cooperation of the child is required and will depend on age and past experiences.[10]

V. ORAL RISK ASSESSMENT

Risk factors[5,11,12] for early childhood oral disease are identified from the interview with the parents or guardians and oral examination.

- Review caries risk indicator/factors and complete CAMBRA risk assessment for ages 0–5 years as shown in **Table 49-9**.[13]
- Assign caries risk status of low, medium, or high.
- Evaluate risk factors for gingivitis: visible biofilm, mouth breathing, crowded teeth.

TREATMENT PLANNING AND CONSENT

The dental hygiene diagnosis is used to develop the dental hygiene care plans (Chapter 24, page 351). Before treatment, the care plan is discussed with the dentist in order to integrate the dental hygiene plan into the comprehensive dental treatment plan.

- Inform parent/guardian of findings from the assessment and present the care plan both orally and in writing.
- Have parents/guardians sign an informed consent before treatment (Chapter 24, page 358).

DENTAL HYGIENE CARE

I. ORAL PROPHYLAXIS

A. Purpose of the Oral Prophylaxis

- Provide a positive and enjoyable introductory experience.

TABLE 49-9	CAMBRA ASSESSMENT TOOL FOR DENTAL PROVIDERS (0–5)

Caries Risk Assessment Form for Age 0–5.

Patient Name_____ ID#_____ Age____ Date_____

Initial/base line exam date_____ Caries recall date_____

Respond to each question in sections 1, 2, 3, and 4 with a checkmark in the Yes or No column.

1. Caries Risk Indicators—Parent Interview**	YES	NO	Notes
a. Mother or primary caregiver has had active dental decay in the past 12 months.			
b. Child has recent dental restorations (see 5b below)			
c. Parent or caregiver has low SES (socioeconomic status) and/or low health literacy			
d. Child has developmental problems			
e. No dental home/episodic dental care			
2. Caries Risk Factors (Biological)—Parent Interview**			
a. Child has frequent (> 3 × dly) between-meal snacks of sugars/cooked starch/sugared beverages			
b. Child has saliva-reducing factors present incl.			
1. Medications (e.g., some for asthma or hyperactivity)			
2. Medical (Cancer Treatment) or Genetic Factors			
c. Child continually uses bottle-contains fluids other than water			
d. Child sleeps w/bottle or nurses on demand.			
3. Protective Factors (Nonbiological)—Parent Interview			
a. Mother/caregiver decay-free last 3 years.			
b. Child has a dental home and regular dental care.			
4. Protective Factors (Biological)—Parent Interview			
a. Child lives in a fluoridated area or takes fluoride supplements by slowly dissolving or as chewable tablets.			
b. Child's teeth are cleaned w/fluoridated toothpaste daily			
c. Mother/caregiver chews/sucks xylitol gum/lozenges 2–4 × daily			
5. Caries Risk Indicators/Factors—Clinical Examination of Child**			
a. Obvious white spots, decalcifications or obvious decay present on the child's teeth			
b. Restorations placed in the last two years in/on child's teeth			
c. Plaque is obvious on the child's teeth and/or gums bleed easily			
d. Child has dental or orthodontic appliances present, fixed or removable: e.g., braces, space maintainers, obturators			
e. Risk factor: Visually inadequate saliva flow—dry mouth			
**If yes to any one of 1a, 1b, or 5b or any two in categories 1, 2, 5, consider performing bacterial culture on mother or caregiver and child. Use this as a base line to follow results of antibacterial intervention.	Parent/Caregiver Date:		Child Date:
a. Mutans streptococci (Indicate bacterial level: high, medium, low)			
b. Lactobacillus species (Indicate bacterial level: high, medium, low)			

Child's overall caries risk status: (CIRCLE)	Extreme	Low	Moderate	High

Recommendations given Yes___ No____ Date Given_____ Date follow up:_____

SELF-MANAGEMENT GOALS:_____

_____

Practitioner Signature_____ Date:_____

Reprinted with permission from Ramos-Gomez FJ, Crall J, Gansky SA, Slayton RL, Featherstone JD. Caries risk assessment appropriate for the age 1 visit (infants and toddlers). *J Calif Dent Assoc.* 2007;35(10):687–702.

- Remove biofilm, stain, and calculus for gingival health and to facilitate visual examination of the teeth.
- Educate parents and children regarding proper, daily biofilm control procedures and other preventive measures.
- Teach parents how to examine their child's mouth for biofilm, gingivitis, dental caries, or injury.

B. Type of Oral Prophylaxis

The type of oral prophylaxis provided for the child depends on the age and oral findings.

- Many children under 3 years require only a wet toothbrush for dental biofilm removal.
- Remove calculus, stain, and heavy dental biofilm not removed during toothbrush instruction.
- Disclosing agent is essential for assessment and education.

II. CAMBRA: CARIES MANAGEMENT BY RISK ASSESSMENT

Caries management by risk assessment (CAMBRA) is a system designed to manage and prevent dental caries.

A. Principles

- Modification of the oral flora to favor oral health by use of topical antibacterial agents
- Patient education
- Promotion of remineralization of non-cavitated lesions by use of topical fluorides
- Minimal restorative intervention of cavitated lesions and defective restorations[14]

B. Steps

- Complete CAMBRA risk assessment.
- Implement treatment guidelines shown in **Table 49-10**.[13]

C. Role of the Dental Hygienist

- Risk assessment
- Radiograph exposure
- Salivary testing
- Varnish application
- Sealant application
- Patient/parent education[15]

III. FLUORIDE VARNISH APPLICATION

A. Indications

- Fluoride varnish reduces the risk of inadvertent ingestion in children under age 6 years. Professional strength topical gels and foams are not recommended for this age group.[16]

- Fluoride varnish is used on infant and young children's teeth at risk for early childhood caries.[17,18]
- Fluoride varnish application is recommended for children at moderate and high risk for dental caries beginning at age 1 year.[16,19] Fluoride varnish has been shown to reduce the incidence of early childhood caries.[20]

B. Positioning

- The knee-to-knee position is helpful for fluoride varnish application in young children **(Figure 49-1)**.
- Older children are seated in the dental chair in a reclined position.

C. Application

- Tooth preparation usually requires brushing only unless there is calculus that requires removal.
- Requires a light source, gauze squares or cotton rolls for drying, and applicators such as cotton swabs or a disposable brush.
- Unit dose packages for children are recommended. Stir the varnish to completely mix the fluoride.[21]
- Wipe teeth dry with the gauze or cotton roll and apply the varnish to cover the teeth.
- Instruct parents to have the child avoid hard foods and brushing the teeth until the next day or at least 4–6 hours after application.
- Recommend application at least two times per year and more frequently for children at highest risk for dental caries.

IV. CHILD MANAGEMENT

A. Establish Rapport

The purpose of the visit is to teach appropriate behaviors and to prevent management problems. Cooperation is usually gained by smiling and talking to establish rapport.

B. Show, Tell, and Do

- Each piece of equipment and step of the procedure is shown and explained to the child before it is used (show, tell, and do).[22]
- Use fun names for the equipment such as the "elevator chair," "tooth feeler," "tooth mirror," "slurpy straw," and "waterfall."
- Keep explanations brief and do the procedures as quickly as possible.
- Four- and five-year-olds enjoy holding a hand mirror to watch what you are doing, which often distracts them from possible anxiety and fear of the unknown.

C. Crying

- Stop the procedure if the child cries.
- Comfort the child by telling him or her it is all right to cry.

TABLE 49-10 | **CAMBRA TREATMENT GUIDELINES (0–5 YEARS)**

Caries Management by Risk Assessment (CAMBRA) Clinical Guidelines for Patients

RISK LEVEL	SALIVA TEST	ANTIBACTERIALS	FLUORIDE	FREQUENCY OF RADIOGRAPHS	FREQUENCY OF PERIODIC ORAL EXAMS (POE)	XYLITOL AND/OR BAKING SODA§	SEALANTS‡	EXISTING LESIONS
Low risk	Optional (Base-line)	Not required or if saliva test was performed; treat main caregiver accordingly	Not required	After age 2: Bitewing radiographs every 18–24 mos.	Every 6–12 mos. To re-evaluate caries risk AND ANTICIPATORY GUIDANCE†		Optional	
Moderate risk	Recommend	Not required or if saliva test was performed; treat main caregiver accordingly	OTC fluoride-containing toothpaste twice daily (a pea-sized amount) Sodium fluoride treatment gels/rinses	After age 2 bitewing radiographs every 12–18 mos.	Every 6 mos. to re-evaluate caries risk AND ANTICIPATORY GUIDANCE	Xylitol gum or lozenges. Two sticks of gum or two mints 4 × dly for the caregiver. Xylitol food, spray or drinks for the child.	Sealants for deep pits and fissures after two yrs. age. High fluoride conventional glass ionomer is recommended.	Lesions that do not penetrate the DEJ and are not cavitated should be treated w/fluoride toothpaste and fluoride varnish
High risk*	Required	Chlorhexidine 0.12% 10 ml. rinse for main caregiver of the infant or child for one week each mo. Bacterial test at every caries recall. Health provider might brush infant's teeth with CHX	Fluoride varnish at initial visit and caries recall exams. OTC fluoride-containing toothpaste and calcium phosphate paste combo twice daily Sodium fluoride treatment gel/rinses.	After age 2; Two size #2 occlusal films and 2 bitewing radiographs every 6–12 mos. or until no cavitated lesions are evident	Every 3 mos. To re-evaluate caries risk and apply fluoride varnish AND ANTICIPATORY GUIDANCE	Xylitol gum or lozenges. Two sticks of gum or two mints 4 × daily for the caregiver. Xylitol food, spray or drinks for the child.	Sealants for deep pits and fissures after two years of age. High fluoride conventional glass ionomer is recommended.	Lesions that do not penetrate the DEJ and are not cavitated should be treated w/fluoride toothpaste and fluoride varnish. ART might be recommended.
Extreme risk*	Required	Chlorhexidine 0.12% 10 ml. rinse for one minute daily at bedtime for 2 wks. each mo. Bacterial test at every caries recall. Health provider might brush infant's teeth with CHX	Fluoride varnish at initial visit and caries recall and after prophylaxis or recall exams. OTC fluoride-containing toothpaste and calcium phosphate paste combo twice dly. Sodium fluoride treatment gel/rinses.	After age 2; Two size #2 occlusal films and 2 bitewing radiographs every 6 mos. or until no cavitated lesions are evident	Every 1–3 months. To re-evaluate caries risk and apply fluoride varnish and anticipatory guidance	Xylitol gum or lozenges. Two sticks of gum or two mints 4 × dly for the caregiver. Xylitol food, spray or drinks for the child.	Sealants for deep pits and fissures after two yrs. age. High fluoride conventional glass ionomer is recommended.	Holding care with glass ionomer materials until caries progression is controlled (ART). Fluoride varnish and anticipatory guidance/ self-management goals.

*Pediatric patients with one (or more) cavitated lesions are high-risk patients.
*Pediatric patients with one (or more) cavitated lesions and hyposalivary or special needs are extreme risk patients.
*Pediatric patients with daily medication such as inhalers or behavioral issues will have diminished salivary function.
†Anticipatory guidance–"Anticipatory discussion becomes an integral part of each visit for care." AAPD
‡ICDAS protocol presented by Jenson et al. This issue may be helpful on sealant decision.
§Xylitol is not good for pets (esp. dogs)
For all risk levels. Pediatric patients through their caregiver must maintain good oral hygiene and a diet low in frequency of fermentable carbohydrates.
Patients with appliances (RPDs orthodontics) require excellent oral hygiene together w/intensive fluoride therapy. Fluoride gel to be placed in removable appliances. Caries risk assessment appropriate for the age 1 visit (infants and toddlers).
Source: Reprinted with permission from Ramos-Gomez FJ, Crall J, Gansky SA, Slayton RL, Featherstone JD. Caries risk assessment appropriate for the age 1 visit (infants and toddlers).
J Calif Dent Assoc. 2007;35(10):687–702.

- The clinician's use of voice is extremely important: use a pleasant and modulated tone.
- Avoid raising the voice. This frightens the child and indicates that the provider has lost control.
- Continuous crying after the aversive stimulus is removed means the child is fearful.
- If crying ceases, ask if the child is ready to begin again and then reinitiate the show, tell, and do routine.

D. Positive Reinforcement

- Use positive verbal reinforcement during the appointment, such as "Super," "You are doing great," "What a great helper," "Great job," "I knew you could do it," "Well done."
- Provide brief breaks in the procedure for compliance and cooperation.

E. Lack of Cooperation

Reschedule the appointment if the child is unable to cooperate.

V. REFERRAL

- Appropriate referrals are made when problems are identified that require intervention by other health providers.
- Conditions that require referral include evidence of systemic illness, pathology, child abuse or neglect, failure to provide safety measures, substance abuse in the family, and evidence of poor parenting skills.[5]

ORAL HEALTH CONSIDERATIONS FOR INFANTS

I. NONNUTRITIVE SUCKING

A. Normal Sucking

- Infants engage in nonnutritive sucking patterns during the first year of life and beyond.
- They may suck on their thumb, fingers, or pacifiers for comfort.
- Inform parents that such sucking is normal and acceptable behavior.[23]

B. Pacifier Selection and Use

- The use of pacifiers has been shown to decrease the incidence of sudden infant death syndrome (SIDS). The American Academy of Pediatrics Task Force on SIDS recommends the use of a pacifier throughout the first year of life. For breastfed infants, delay introduction until 1 month old.[24]
- Solid construction so that it cannot be pulled apart. **Figure 49-5** shows two types of pacifiers, one has an orthodontic nipple and the other a nonorthodontic.

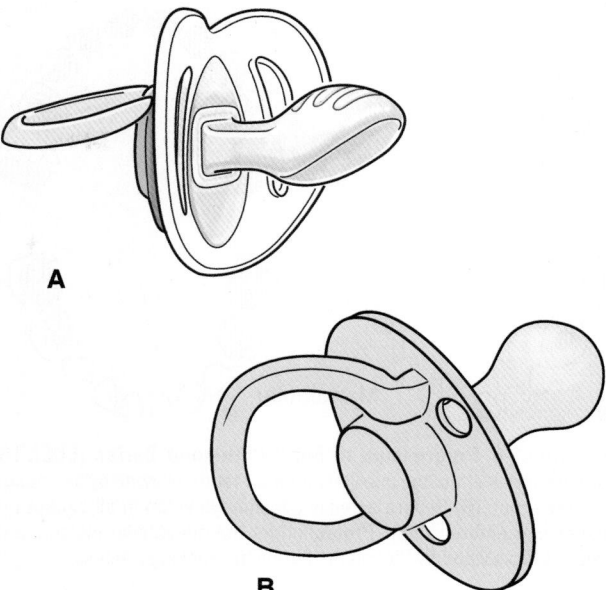

FIGURE 49-5 Criteria for Selecting Pacifiers. Two styles of pacifier nipples: **(A)** orthodontic and **(B)** conventional. True orthodontic pacifiers expand to support the palate and maintain natural tongue posture. It is important to select the appropriate bulb size for each stage of development (0–3, 3–6, 6–18 months). Criteria for selection of a safe pacifier: size of shield is wider than child's mouth (at least 1¼ inches) in diameter; shield has air vents; plastic portion is of sturdy construction to prevent separation and possible choking; nipple is checked frequently for cracking and stickiness, at which time pacifier is replaced.

The orthodontic nipple is designed to be more like a mother's breast nipple during nursing.
- Nontoxic material.
- Ventilated shield larger than the child's mouth to prevent swallowing.
- Not tied to the crib, child's clothing, or around the neck or hand which could lead to strangulation.
- Not cleaned in the parent's/caregiver's mouth since caries-producing bacteria could be transferred to the infant who has teeth.[25]
- Clean in warm, soapy water or sterilize. Replace regularly.

II. BOTTLE/BREAST-FEEDING

A. Bottle

- Put only formula or milk in the bottle.
- Hold the child during feeding.
- Avoid placing the child in bed with a bottle.
- Do not put juice or other sweet liquids in the bottle. Give juice in a sippy cup.
- Do not use the bottle as a pacifier.

B. Breast

- Do not allow prolonged, at-will breast-feeding after teeth erupt.
- If the infant sleeps with the mother, do not allow suckling at will after the eruption of teeth.

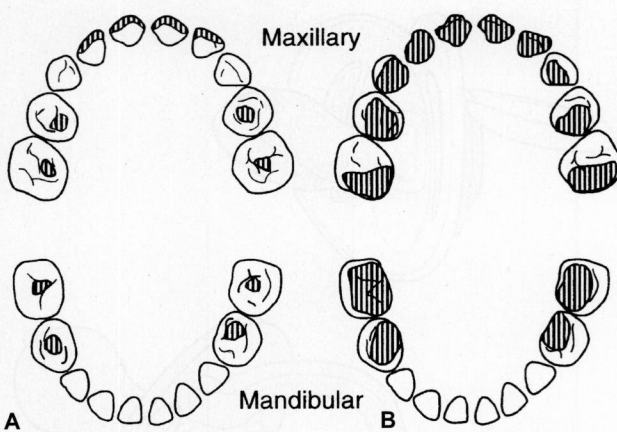

FIGURE 49-6 **Progression of Early Childhood Caries (ECC). (A)** Earliest caries affect the maxillary anterior teeth followed by the molars as they erupt. **(B)** Severe extensive lesions develop in all except the mandibular anterior teeth. Protection for the mandibular incisors and canines is provided by the tongue during the sucking process.

■ When the infant falls asleep after sucking, milk collects around teeth and causes demineralization. Dental carious lesions are most often seen first in the maxillary anteriors as seen in **Figure 49-6.**

III. TEETHING

A. Eruption Patterns

■ Tell parents/caregivers when to expect teeth to erupt.
■ Provide a table of primary tooth eruption patterns, as shown in **Table 49-8.**
■ Explain that eruption patterns vary widely and are familial in nature.

B. Teething Behaviors

■ Excessive chewing and drooling.
■ Irritability.
■ Change in appetite.
■ Interrupted sleep patterns.
■ Crying.
■ Fever or diarrhea usually are not symptoms and require consultation with a physician to assess the presence of a systemic illness.[2]

C. Palliative Measures

■ Chewing on objects
  ■ Cold wash cloth.
  ■ Hard, solid teething ring.
  ■ Rub gums with clean finger.
■ Numbing solutions
  ■ Over-the-counter numbing solutions are not recommended.
  ■ Products contain a strong anesthetic that is difficult to control.
  ■ May numb the entire oral cavity and, if swallowed, suppress the gag reflex.[2]

IV. EARLY CHILDHOOD CARIES (ECC)

■ Dental disease exhibited in primary teeth of infants and very young children is termed early childhood caries.
■ Baby bottle tooth decay is one form and is usually seen in children who routinely have been given a bottle when going to sleep or who have experienced prolonged at-will breast-feeding.
■ Other names for this condition are nursing caries, baby bottle caries, and rampant caries.[26]
■ Children experiencing caries as infants or toddlers are at higher risk for developing caries in primary and permanent teeth in the future.[27,28]

A. American Academy of Pediatric Dentistry Definitions[3]

1. ECC
■ One or more decayed, missing (due to caries), or filled tooth surfaces in any primary tooth.
■ Child 71 months of age or younger.

2. Severe ECC
■ Smooth surface caries in children younger than age 3.
■ Cavitated, missing, or filled smooth surfaces in primary maxillary anterior teeth in children ages 3–5. dmfs score of ≥4 (age 3), ≥5 (age 4), or ≥6 (age 5) also indicates Severe ECC.

B. Prevalence
■ Dental caries in children 2–5 years old is increasing. 28% of 2–5 year olds have dental caries.[29]
■ High numbers of teeth are affected in preschool children with caries experience.[30]

C. Microbiology
■ Colonization of mutans streptococci (MS) has been shown to occur before tooth eruption and as early as birth.[31,32]
■ High levels of MS in saliva and dental biofilm are a strong risk indicator for ECC.[33]
■ Transfer of MS from parent, caregiver, sibling, or other child by saliva sharing behaviors to the infant or young child.[25,31]
■ *Lactobacilli* in large numbers in the dental biofilm.
■ Avoid saliva sharing behaviors such as kissing on the mouth, tasting food before feeding, cleaning dropped pacifier by mouth, and sharing of cups, toys or utensils.[19]

D. Risk Factors

The areas of concern related to risk factors are listed in **Tables 49-1 and 49-2.** Teaching the parents about the cause and effects of early childhood caries is a significant part of anticipatory guidance **(Tables 49-1** and **49-2).**

E. Predisposing Factors

- Placing bottle/sippy cup in bed.
- Bottle contains sweetened milk or other fluid sweetened with sucrose.
- Prolonged at-will breast- or bottle-feeding as a sleep or behavioral control.
- Ineffective or no daily biofilm removal from the teeth.

F. Effects

- Maxillary anterior teeth and primary molars are the first to be affected, as noted in **Figures 49-3** and **49-6**.
- As the baby falls asleep, pools of sweet liquid can collect around the teeth.
- While the sucking is active, the liquid passes beyond the teeth.
- The nipple covers the mandibular anterior teeth; hence, they are rarely affected.

G. Recognition

- Demineralization or white-spot lesions may be noted along the cervical third of the maxillary anterior teeth and proximal surfaces when the upper lip is lifted, as described on page 378.
- At a later stage, cavitation occurs and the lesions appear brown or dark brown. Eventually, the crowns may be destroyed to the gum line, abscesses may develop, and the child may suffer severe pain and discomfort. An advanced stage of dental caries is shown in **Figure 49-3**.
- Teach parents to lift lip and look in the infant's mouth for white or brown spots on the teeth.[19]

V. DAILY DENTAL BIOFILM REMOVAL

A. Demonstrate Biofilm Removal

- Wiping/brushing is demonstrated by the clinician while the parent/caregiver observes.
- Move the child's head to the lap of the parent and ask the parent to demonstrate the procedures. Make appropriate suggestions for changes.

A. Gaining Access and Cooperation

- Infants may cry, fuss, and squirm during oral health care.
- Parents use a knee-to-knee position to control the child's head, arms, and feet as depicted in **Figure 49-1**. Other positions are shown in Figure 56-13 on page 870.
- One parent can cradle the infant's head with one arm and wipe or brush with the opposite hand.
- Visibility and access can be improved if the child is placed on a bed or changing table.
- Singing, talking, and smiling during this oral cleaning help the child associate the process with a pleasant experience.

B. Wiping Before Tooth Eruption

- Oral health needs before tooth eruption include daily, gentle wiping of gum ridges, inside of cheeks, lips, and tongue with a clean, wet cloth or gauze.
- Infants become accustomed to the oral care routine through this daily activity.
- Parents often elect to do the wiping at bath time.

C. Toothbrushing

- When the first tooth erupts, teeth are brushed twice daily with an age-appropriate sized toothbrush and a small "smear" of fluoridated toothpaste or plain water.[3,19]
- For children at moderate or high caries risk, brush teeth with a small "smear" of fluoridated toothpaste until approximately 2 years of age. For children at low caries risk, water may be used.[19]
- Lift lip to brush anterior teeth.
- Recommend a good quality toothbrush with soft and end-rounded filaments.
- Emphasize brushing teeth in the morning and before bed.
- Replace the brush when filaments are frayed or bent, usually every 2–3 months.

VI. ANTIBACTERIAL AGENTS

- Antimicrobial mouthrinses are not recommended for young children due to the potential for ingestion.
- Main caregiver of the child may rinse once daily rinsing with 0.12% chlorhexidine for 1–2 weeks per month to decrease cariogenic bacteria.[13]

VII. FLUORIDE SUPPLEMENTATION

- Discuss fluoride requirements at 6 months according to the guidelines specified in **Table 49-3**.
- Review all dietary sources of fluoride to estimate exposure to systemic fluoride.
- History information regarding fluoride exposure directs decisions regarding fluoride supplementation.
- Have well water tested for fluoride levels.
- Consult with the child's dentist to make this decision.
- When fluoride tablets are recommended, the child should be encouraged to chew, swish, and swallow or suck the tablets. This will optimize topical benefits of the fluoride supplement.[34]

VIII. USE OF XYLITOL

- Xylitol inhibits mutans streptococci, reduces plaque formation and bacterial adherence, and inhibits demineralization.
- Use of xylitol chewing gum by mothers can prevent dental caries in children by preventing the transmission of mutans streptococci.[35,36]
- Xylitol gum or mints should be consumed 3–5 times per day. The effective daily dose of xylitol is 6–10 g.[37]

IX. FEEDING PATTERNS

A. Introducing the Cup

A small, plastic cup is introduced to the child when the child is ready developmentally, usually 8–12 months. The goal is to discontinue use of the bottle by 12 months of age.

B. Diet and Health

- High risk dietary practices seem to be established early, by 12 months of age, and continue through childhood.[38] Therefore, dietary counseling should be conducted during the prenatal and perinatal periods.
- Teach about the relationship between frequent and large amounts of sweetened beverage intake and dental caries and obesity.[39,40]
- Provide healthy snacks from the grain, vegetable, fruit, meat and meat alternatives, and dairy groups between meals.
- Limit intake of fermentable and retentive carbohydrate foods.
- Rinse the child's mouth with water immediately following the dispensing of sweetened medications. Medications such as those used for ear infections and nutritional supplementation often are made with a sugar or a syrupy base to disguise medication flavors.

ORAL HEALTH CONSIDERATIONS FOR TODDLERS AND PRESCHOOLERS

I. ACCIDENT AND INJURY PREVENTION

The greatest incidence of injury to the primary dentition occurs at 2–3 years of age.[41] Toddlers have increased mobility and developing coordination and as a result are subject to injuries. House structures/furniture such as floors, steps, tables, and beds are most commonly associated with dental injuries in children under age 7 years.[42] Parents can be taught to protect the child by close supervision, anticipating problems, and making the environment safe by removing dangers. Written information regarding what to do in the event of a traumatic oral injury makes parents feel more prepared. Table 69-5 (page 1081) provides information on a dislocated jaw, facial fracture, and tooth forcibly displaced or avulsed.

II. SUPERVISED BRUSHING AND FLOSSING

A. Establish a Routine

- Make suggestions as to how to establish and maintain a brushing routine.
- Recommend brushing in the morning after breakfast and before bedtime.
- Specify that the most critical time for dental biofilm removal is before bedtime.

B. Gaining Cooperation

- At these ages, the child is becoming more independent.
- Parents can provide a fun activity by making up and singing a brushing song.
- For 2- to 3-year-olds, teach them to take turns when brushing by using the phrase, "It's your turn to brush," followed by, "It's my turn to brush."
- To gain better cooperation, connect brushing with a fun activity such as first, we brush teeth and then, we read a story.
- Provide disclosing agent and 2- or 3-minute timers to be used for motivation during brushing.

C. Parental Supervision

- Parents keep fluoride toothpaste out of reach of the child and are in charge of placing the proper amount of toothpaste on the toothbrush.
- Until the child develops fine motor coordination, and is able to effectively remove biofilm, the parents/caregivers assist the child in cleaning the teeth by doing the brushing and flossing. The time to cease assistance depends on parental/caregiver assessment and varies markedly from child to child.
- Parents teach the child to brush and follow up with effective and complete biofilm removal.
- Parents floss closely approximated primary teeth to remove biofilm from proximal surfaces.
- Parents are taught how to examine the mouth for signs of gingival inflammation, dental caries, and injury.

III. FLUORIDE

A. Assessments Needed to Recommend Supplements and Topical Applications

- Source and fluoride levels of the child's water supply.
- Type of toothpaste used and frequency of brushing.
- Effectiveness of personal oral health care.
- Dietary patterns and caries experience.
- Confirm fluoride needs with dentist to finalize care plan (Table 49-3).

B. Toothpaste

- Children's toothpastes manufactured in the United States contain the same amount of fluoride as adult toothpastes, whereas manufacturers in several other countries around the world reduce the amount of fluoride in children's toothpastes. Parents/caregivers are informed that they need to prevent problems by controlling the amount of toothpaste used and placing it out of the child's reach.
  - Young children may swallow large amounts of the toothpaste during brushing, which could cause dental fluorosis in developing teeth.[43]

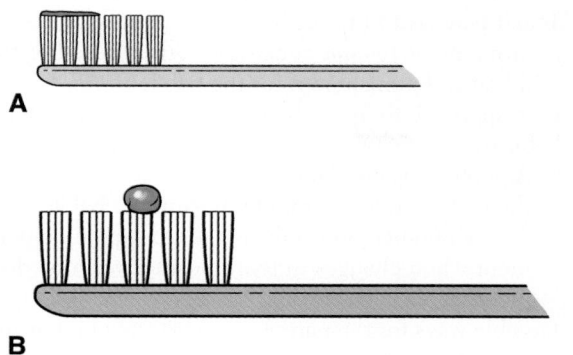

FIGURE 49-7 Dentifrice for a Child under 2 and 2 to 5 Years of Age. For children with moderate or high caries risk under 2 years of age, a parent is instructed to place a small smear of fluoridated toothpaste on a child sized brush **(A)**. For all children ages 2 through 5 years of age, the appropriate size is that of a small pea **(B)**. The paste is spread in a thin layer over the brush surface and then spread over all of the teeth before brushing.

- The use of fluoride toothpaste by young children has been shown to cause mild fluorosis. This relationship is most pronounced at about 24 months of age.[44]
- Children like the taste of toothpaste and may eat a large amount at one time that could result in acute fluoride toxicity.
- Instructions for parents:
  - For children with moderate or high caries risk under 2 years of age, a small "smear" of fluoridated toothpaste is dispensed on an age appropriate sized toothbrush by the parent.[3,45]
  - For children, ages 2 through 5 years, a small, pea-sized amount of toothpaste is used and spread the length of the brush head[3,45] **(Figure 49-7)**.
  - Spread the toothpaste from the brush on all of the teeth before brushing.
  - Teach the child to lean over the sink so that collected saliva and fluoride toothpaste can drip in the sink and be spat out.
  - Continue to control the toothpaste and keep it out of reach.

C. Fluorosis

- The most critical time for fluorosis to develop in primary teeth as a result of excessive fluoride intake is during the middle of the first year of life.[46]
- The primary second molar could show evidence of fluorosis along the cervical margin.[46] Identification of primary fluorosis should alert the dental hygienist to the likelihood of fluorosis of the permanent incisors.[47]
- Esthetically significant permanent teeth are most susceptible to fluorosis during the first 1–3 years of life.[48] The most critical time for dental fluorosis of maxillary

permanent incisors to occur is when the child is 22–26 months of age.[45]

IV. ORAL MALODOR

A. Causes

- Bacteria at the base of the tongue.
- Bacteria between the teeth.
- Postnasal drip.[49]

B. What to Teach Parents

- Explain bacterial causes.
- Emphasize thorough dental biofilm removal through daily brushing of the teeth.
- Teach how to floss the child's teeth.
- Show how to brush gently the dorsum of the tongue in Chapter 27, page 402.

V. DIETARY AND FEEDING PATTERN RECOMMENDATIONS

- Children need a series of small, healthy meals during the day.
- Healthy snacks include foods from the grain, vegetable, fruit, meat and meat alternatives, and dairy groups that do not promote tooth decay.
- Sweetened foods and drinks are limited and provided at mealtimes rather than between meals.

VI. GRAZING ON THE SIPPY CUP

- Do not allow the child to sip milk or sweet liquids at will, which promotes demineralization.
- Have the child sit in a chair and complete a drink when thirsty.
- Put any remaining drink away until the child is thirsty again.
- Juice intake is limited to no more than 4–6 ounces per day for children between the ages of 1 and 6 years.[50]
- Parents or caregivers avoid giving young children carbonated soda drinks that promote demineralization and may contribute to childhood obesity.[38]
- Parents or caregivers avoid using food as a reward for behavior modification.

VII. THUMB AND FINGER SUCKING

- Prolonged thumb and finger sucking habits have been associated with narrow maxillary arch width, anterior open bite, posterior crossbite, increased overjet and decreased overbite.[3]

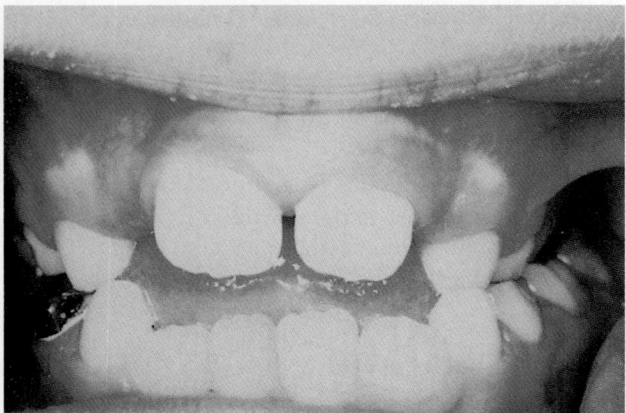

FIGURE 49-8 Effects of Prolonged Thumb Sucking on Teeth.
Anterior openbite with posterior crossbite.

- Encourage parents to help children stop finger or thumb sucking by age 3 years. Intervention is initiated before the time of the eruption of the maxillary anterior permanent teeth to prevent malocclusion as shown in **Figure 49-8**.[3,11]
- The clinician explains to the child what effects thumb sucking has on the teeth.

- Teach parents to praise the child and provide positive reinforcement for not sucking the thumb rather than scolding and punishment for the habit.
- One approach to use to help the child stop the sucking habit is:
  - A photo is taken to document the current position of the teeth and as a reminder to stop the habit.
  - A new photograph is taken at a subsequent appointment when changes in tooth positions can be documented.
- Possible ways for the parents to assist the child in stopping the habit are:
  - Place a reminder on the thumb or finger at the time the child usually sucks.
  - The reminder may be a band-aid, hand puppet, glove, or fingernail polish on the nail of the thumb or finger.
  - Provide the child with a small piece of satin ribbon or a soft, stuffed animal to stroke as a substitute for the thumb or finger sucking.
  - Use a chart for daily recording of compliance with stars or stickers.
  - Agree upon a reward for stopping the habit for 14 continuous days.

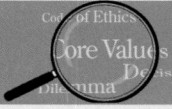

Everyday Ethics

Maria has practiced as a dental hygienist in the office of Dr. Reynolds for three years. Maria recently attended a continuing education course on dental caries risk assessment and prevention. At the course, recommendations from professionally applied topical fluoride: Evidence-based clinical recommendations published by the American Dental Association were reviewed. Maria heard the results of systematic reviews on fluoride varnish, reviewed the ADA's recommendations of fluoride varnish as the only topical fluoride recommended for children under age 6, and learned fluoride varnish can even be used on infants to prevent early childhood caries. Maria is convinced that she needs to be using fluoride varnish on patients of all ages based upon caries risk. Dental hygienists at Dr. Reynolds' office are currently applying 2.0% sodium fluoride foam to patients under age 18. At the weekly staff meeting, Maria presented an overview of fluoride varnish products, key research findings, a cost comparison of varnish versus fluoride tray and foam, and distributed copies of the ADA fluoride recommendations. The following week, Dr. Reynolds told Maria that she had reviewed the fluoride varnish information and decided to continue using the fluoride foam and trays. When Maria asked why, Dr. Reynolds stated, "the increased costs of using fluoride varnish would really add up over a year and increasing patient fees is not an option. Anyway, patients expect to have smooth shiny teeth after a prophylaxis," Dr. Reynolds concluded.

Questions for Consideration
1. Because fluoride varnish is the safest professional fluoride application and recommended by the ADA for children under age 6, how do the ethical principles of beneficence and nonmaleficence apply in this situation?
2. Do clinical recommendations or guidelines from professional associations, such as the ADA, constitute standards of care? Why or why not?
3. Maria has an ethical responsibility to her employer, who has expressed concerns about cost and patient acceptance of this "new" type of fluoride treatment, as well as to her patients. Which questions in the steps for resolving an ethical situation (page 10) might help Maria to balance those responsibilities as she makes a decision about an action to take in continuing this discussion with Dr. Reynolds?

F. Have the child call the clinician to say that the prize has been won.

■ When behavior modification techniques fail, a habit-breaking appliance or solution to coat the thumb may be recommended.

DOCUMENTATION

The following items are documented in the progress notes of children ages 1 through 5.

■ Overall appraisal of physical status and key health history findings.
■ Existing pathology: soft tissue, gingiva, caries, occlusal status.
■ Oral hygiene status and oral risk assessment.
■ Anticipatory guidance given and self/parent care recommendations.
■ Type of appointment: age 1 year initial examination, toothbrush prophylaxis, maintenance, type of topical fluoride applied.
■ Notes on child's behavior and level of cooperation.
■ Treatment planned for next visit.
■ Box 49-2 provides a sample progress note.

 **Factors To Teach The Parents**

■ How the parents' own oral health affects the baby's oral health.
■ How the bacteria that cause dental caries can be transferred to the baby's mouth from parents or other family members.
■ How fluoride makes enamel stronger and more resistant to the bacteria that cause dental caries.
■ Methods to prevent dental caries from developing in a young child's mouth.
■ How feeding methods and snacking patterns can contribute to dental caries.
■ How the parent can examine the infant's/child's mouth and what to look for during the examination.
■ Reasons why the baby's mouth should be examined by an oral health professional at 6 months of age or as soon as the first tooth erupts.
■ Reasons why maintenance of primary teeth is important for oral health, growth, and development.
■ Ways parents can prepare their young children for visits to the dentist and dental hygienist.
■ How parents can prevent accidents and injury in their infants and children.

| **BOX 49-2** | **Example Progress Note** |

Amy Williams, a healthy and active 3-year-old presented for her 1st dental hygiene appointment accompanied by her mother. Amy had been seen by Dr. Hunt for an age 1 examination after she had fallen but showed no effects from the bump and the present examination. Oral examination revealed class I occlusion with normal spacing, gingival enlargement and erythema on lingual surfaces of mandibular molars, light biofilm on lingual of all anterior teeth and heavy biofilm on lingual surfaces of mandibular molars. Amy's mother stated that she has trouble reaching the back teeth when she helps Amy brush. A child sized power toothbrush was recommended and instructions for twice-daily use were given to Amy and Ms Williams. Ms Williams was also instructed to apply only a small pea sized amount of an ADA accepted toothpaste to the brush and to encourage Amy to spit out the toothpaste after brushing. Disclosing agent was applied and areas of biofilm accumulation were shown to patient and parent. Toothbrush prophylaxis was completed followed by an application of 5.0% sodium fluoride varnish and post-op varnish instructions. Though Amy initially appeared anxious, she was cooperative and helpful during treatment. Avoidance of between meal snacking, 3-month fluoride varnish applications, use of disclosing agent to insure complete biofilm removal and use of an ADA accepted fluoride toothpaste were recommended. Next appointment: 3-month maintenance and application of fluoride varnish.

Signed: _____, RDH Date: _____.

References

1. McWhorter AG, Seale NS, King SA. Infant oral health education in US dental school curricula. *Pediatr Dent.* 2001 Sep–Oct;23(5):407.
2. Mueller WA, Abrams RB. Oral medicine and dentistry. In: Hay WW, Hayward AR, Levin MJ, Sondheimer JM. *Current pediatric diagnosis and treatment.* 14th ed. Stamford (CT): Appleton and Lange; 1999. pp. 384–94.
3. American Academy of Pediatric Dentistry. Oral health policies and clinical guidelines. *Pediatr Dent.* 2009;31(6 Reference Manual):44, 96, 97, 119–121, 135.
4. Green M, Palfrey JS, eds. *Bright futures: guidelines for health supervision of infants, children, and adolescents.* 2nd ed. rev. Arlington (VA): National Center for Education in Maternal and Child Health; 2002. Chapter 1, Getting started; pp. 1–15.
5. Casamassimo P, Holt K, eds. *Bright futures in practice: oral health pocket guide.* Washington: National Maternal and Child Oral Health Resource Center; 2004. p. 98.
6. Nowak AJ, Casamassimo PS. Using anticipatory guidance to provide early dental interventions. *J Am Dent Assoc.* 1995 Aug;126(8):1156–63.
7. McDonald RE, Avery DR, Dean JA. *Dentistry for the child and adolescent.* 8th ed. St.Louis: Mosby; 2004. pp. 105–8, 115–20, 137–40, 150–1, 154–5, 182–5, 418–23.
8. Overby KJ. Pediatric health supervision. In: Rudolph AM, Kamei RK, Overby KJ. *Rudolph's fundamentals of pediatrics.* 3rd ed. New York: McGraw-Hill; 2002. pp. 1–69.
9. Goldson E, Reynolds A. Child development and behavior. In: Hay WW, Hayward AR, Levin MJ, Sondheimer JM, Deterding RR. *Current pediatric diagnosis and treatment.* 19th ed. New York: McGraw Hill; 2008. pp. 66–83.
10. Kaakko T, Riedy CA, Nakai Y, Domoto P, Weinstein P, Milgrom P. Taking bitewing radiographs in preschoolers using behavior management techniques. *ASDC J Dent Child.* 1999 Sep–Oct;66(5):320–4.
11. Casamassimo PS, Warren JJ. Examination, diagnosis, and treatment planning of the infant and toddler. In: Pinkham JR, Casamassimo PS, Fields HW, McTigue DJ, Nowak AJ. *Pediatric dentistry: infancy through adolescence.* 4th ed. St. Louis: Elsevier Saunders; 2005. pp. 208–14.

12. Albert DA, Park K, Findley S, Mitchell DA, McManus JM. Dental caries among disadvantaged 3- to 4-year-old children in northern Manhattan. *Pediatr Dent.* 2002;24(3):229–33.

13. Ramos-Gomez FJ, Crall J, Gansky SA, Slayton RL, Featherstone JD. Caries risk assessment appropriate for the age 1 visit (infants and toddlers). *J Calif Dent Assoc.* 2007;35(10):687–702.

14. Young DA, Featherstone JD, Roth JR, Anderson M, Autio-Gold J, Christensen GJ, Fontana M, Kutsch VK, Peters MC, Simonsen RJ, Wolff MS. Caries management by risk assessment: implementation guidelines. *J Calif Dent Assoc.* 2007 Nov;35(11):799–805.

15. Gutkowski S, Gerger D, Creasey J, Nelson A, Young DA. The role of dental hygienists, assistants, and office staff in CAMBRA. *J Calif Dent Assoc.* 2007;35(11):786–9, 792–3.

16. American Dental Association Council on Scientific Affairs. Professionally applied fluoride: evidence-based clinical recommendations. *J Am Dent Assoc.* 2006 Aug;137(8):1151–9.

17. Autio-Gold JT, Courts F. Assessing the effect of fluoride varnish on early enamel carious lesions in the primary dentition. *J Am Dent Assoc.* 2001 Sep;132(9):1247–53.

18. Beltran-Aguilar ED, Goldstein JW, Lockwood SA. Fluoride varnishes. A review of their clinical use, cariostatic mechanism, efficacy and safety. *J Am Dent Assoc.* 2000 May;131(5):589–96.

19. California Dental Association Foundation. Oral health during pregnancy and early childhood: evidence-based guideline for health professionals. *J Calif Dent Assoc.* 2010 Jun;38(6):391–426.

20. Weintraub JA, Ramos-Gomez F, Jue B, Shain S, Hoover CI, Featherstone JD, Gansky SA. Fluoride varnish efficacy in preventing early childhood caries. *J Dent Res.* 2006 Feb;85(2):172–6.

21. Azarpazhooh A, Main PA. Fluoride varnish in the prevention of dental caries in children and adolescents: a systematic review. *J Can Dent Assoc.* 2008;74(1):73–9.

22. Pinkham JR. Patient management. In: Pinkham JR, Casamassimo PS, Fields HW, McTigue DJ, Nowak AJ. *Pediatric dentistry: infancy through adolescence.* 4th ed. St. Louis: Elsevier Saunders; 2005. pp. 394–413.

23. Warren JJ, Levy SM, Nowak AJ, Tang S. Non-nutritive sucking behaviors in preschool children: a longitudinal study. *Pediatr Dent.* 2000 May/Jun;22(3):187–91.

24. American Academy of Pediatrics Task Force on Sudden Infant Death Syndrome. The changing concept of sudden infant death syndrome: diagnostic coding shifts, controversies regarding the sleeping environment, and new variables to consider in reducing risk. *Pediatrics.* 2005 Nov;116(5):1245–55.

25. Kohler B, Andreen I. Influence of caries-preventive measures in mothers on cariogenic bacteria and caries experience in their children. *Arch Oral Biol.* 1994 Oct;39(10):907–11.

26. Tinanoff N, O'Sullivan DM. Early childhood caries: overview and recent findings. *Pediatr Dent.* 1997 Jan;19(1):12–6.

27. Peretz B, Ram D, Azo E, Efrat Y. Preschool caries as an indicator of future caries: a longitudinal study. *Pediatr Dent.* 2003 Feb;25(2):114–8.

28. Foster T, Perinpanayagam H, Pfaffenbach A, Certo M. Recurrence of early childhood caries after comprehensive treatment with general anesthesia and follow-up. *J Dent Child.* 2006 Jan–Apr;73(1):25–30.

29. Dye BA, Tan S, Smith V, Lewis BG, Barker LK, Thornton-Evans G, Eke PI, Beltrán-Aguilar ED, Horowitz AM, Li CH. Trends in oral health status: United States, 1988–1994 and 1999–2004. *Vital Health Stat 11.* 2007 Apr;248:1–92.

30. Tinanoff N, Reisine, S. Update on early childhood caries since the Surgeon General's Report. *Acad Pediatr.* 2009 Jun;9(6):396–403.

31. Wan AK, Seow WK, Purdie DM, Bird PS, Walsh LJ, Tudehope DI. Oral colonization of Streptococcus mutans in six-month-old predentate infants. *J Dent Res.* 2001 Dec;80(12):2060–5.

32. Berkowitz RJ. Mutans streptococci: acquisition and transmission. *Pediatr Dent.* 2006 Mar–Apr;28(2):106–9; discussion 192–8.

33. Parisotto TM, Steiner-Oliveira C, Silva CM, Rodrigues LK, Nobre-dos-Santos M. Early childhood caries and mutans streptococci: a systematic review. *Oral Health Prev Dent.* 2010 Jan; 8(1):59–70.

34. Adair SM. Evidence-based use of fluoride in contemporary pediatric dental practice. *Pediatr Dent.* 2006 Mar–Apr;28(2):133–42; discussion 192–8.

35. Isokangas P, Soderling E, Pienihakkinen K, Alanen P. Occurrence of dental decay in children after maternal consumption of xylitol chewing gum, a follow-up from 0 to 5 years of age. *J Dent Res.* 2000 Nov;79(11):1885–9.

36. Soderling E, Isokangas P, Pienihakkinen K, Tenovuo J, Alanen P. Influence of maternal xylitol consumption on mother-child transmission of mutans streptococci: 6-year follow-up. *Caries Res.* 2001 May–Jun;35(3):173–7.

37. Ly KA, Milgrom P, Rothen M. Xylitol, sweeteners, and dental caries. *Pediatr Dent.* 2006 Mar–Apr;28(2):154–63.

38. Kranz S, Smiciklas-Wright H, Francis LA. Diet quality, added sugar, and dietary fiber intakes in American preschoolers. *Pediatr Dent.* 2006 Mar–Apr;28(2):164–71, discussion 192–8.

39. Harnack L, Stang J, Story M. Soft drink consumption among US children and adolescents: nutritional consequences. *J Am Diet Assoc.* 1999 Apr;99(4):436–41.

40. Strauss RS, Pollack HA. Epidemic increase in childhood overweight,1986–1998. *JAMA.* 2001 Dec;286(22):2845–8.

41. Flores MT. Traumatic injuries in the primary dentition. *Dent Traumatol.* 2002 Dec;18(6):287–98.

42. Stewart GB, Shields BJ, Fields S, Comstock RD, Smith GA. Consumer products and activities associated with dental injuries to children treated in United States emergency departments, 1990–2003. *Dent Traumatol.* 2009 Aug;25(4):399–405.

43. Warren JJ, Levy SM. A review of fluoride dentifrice related to dental fluorosis. *Pediatr Dent.* 1999 Jul–Aug;21(4):265–71.

44. Franzman MR, Levy SM, Warren JJ, Broffitt B. Fluoride dentifrice ingestion and fluorosis of the permanent incisors. *J Am Dent Assoc.* 2006 May;137(5):645–52.

45. ECLKC: Early Childhood Learning & Knowledge Center: A service of the Office of Head Start [Internet]. Washington: Office of Head Start; [cited 2009 Dec 21]. Appendix A: decision support matrix—topical fluoride recommendations; 2007 Oct. 4 p. Available from: http://eclkc.ohs.acf.hhs.gov/hslc/ecdh/Health/Oral%20Health/Oral%20Health%20Program%20Staff/TopicalFluoride.pdf.

46. Levy SM, Hillis SL, Warren JJ, Broffitt BA, Mahbubul Islam AK, Wefel JS, Kanellis MJ. Primary tooth fluorosis and fluoride intake during the first year of life. *Community Dent Oral Epidemiol.* 2002 Aug;30(4):286–95.

47. Levy SM, Warren JJ, Broffitt B, Kanellis MJ. Associations between dental fluorosis of the permanent and primary dentitions. *J Public Health Dent.* 2006 Summer;66(3):180–5.

48. Hong L, Levy SM, Broffitt B, Warren JJ, Kanellis MJ, Wefel JS, Dawson DV. Timing of fluoride intake in relation to development of fluorosis on maxillary central incisors. *Community Dent Oral Epidemiol.* 2006 Aug;34(4):299–309.

49. Amir E, Shimonov R, Rosenberg M. Halitosis in children. *J Pediatr.* 1999 Mar;134(3):338–43.

50. American Academy of Pediatrics, Committee on Nutrition. The use and misuse of fruit juice in pediatrics. *Pediatrics.* 2001 May;107(5):1210.

CHAPTER 50

The Patient With a Cleft Lip and/or Palate

SARA L. BERES, RDH, BA, MS

Chapter Outline

Cleft lip and/or palate are the most common of the many types of congenital craniofacial anomalies.[1] Cleft lip and/or palate may occur as isolated conditions, but frequently occur as part of a syndrome with other birth defects.

■ The prevalence varies between 1 to 2/1000 births, but this ratio varies based on geographic and ethnic distribution.[1]

■ Cleft lip occurs more frequently in males, while cleft palate occurs more frequently in females.[1]

■ The person with a cleft lip and/or palate can be dentally dysfunctional unless extensive habilitative care and supervision from birth is available.

■ An interdisciplinary team of medical and dental specialists is required to provide adequate treatment and family counseling as needed.

■ The dental hygienist can be a member of the team with responsibilities to coordinate dental and periodontal care.

■ Speaking ability and appearance are among the first factors considered when the long-range treatment program is planned because the objective is to help the patient lead a normal life.

■ Dental personnel need to maintain a current list of the health agencies, clinics, and other community resources where the patient and family can obtain assistance for the various phases of treatment and habilitation.

■ Key words relating to cleft lip and/or palate are defined in **Box 50-1**.

BOX 50-1	Key Words

Cleft Lip and/or Palate

Autograft: graft transferred from one part of the patient's body to another part.

Bifid uvula: cleft of the uvula of the soft palate that divides the uvula into two parts (**Figure 50-1**, Class 2).

Cheiloplasty: surgical repair of a lip defect.

Cheilorhinoplasty: plastic surgery of nose and lip.

Cleft lip: a unilateral or bilateral congenital fissure of the upper lip, usually lateral to the midline; can extend into one nostril or both and may involve the alveolar process; caused by defect in the fusion of the maxillary and globular processes.

Cleft palate: a congenital fissure of the palate caused by failure of the palatal shelves to fuse; may extend to connect with unilateral or bilateral cleft lip.

Congenital: present at and existing from the time of birth.

Craniofacial: pertaining to the cranium, the part of the skull that encloses the brain, and the face.

Dentally dysfunctional: abnormal functioning of dental structures.

Graft: tissue that is transplanted and expected to become a part of the host tissue.

Haberman feeder: specialty bottle used for infants with cleft palate.

Heredity: genetic transmission of traits from parents to offspring; the hereditary material, chromosomes, is contained within the ovum and the sperm (23 chromosomes each), which unite when the sperm penetrates the ovum.

Mandibular distraction: method used to increase the length of a micrognathic mandible.

Multifactorial: pertaining to, or arising through the action of, many factors.

Nasoalveolar molding technique (NAM): treatment used for unilateral and bilateral cleft palate to reduce the severity of the cleft in the maxillary gingiva or alveolar ridges and to reduce the deformity of the nose.

Obturator: a prosthesis designed to close a congenital or acquired opening, such as a cleft of the hard palate.

Orthognathic surgery: surgical repositioning of all or parts of the maxilla or mandible.

Orthopedics: branch of surgery dealing with the preservation and restoration of function of the skeletal system, its articulations, and associated structures.

Palatoplasty: plastic reconstruction of the palate.

Premaxilla: anterior part of maxilla that contains the incisor teeth; bilateral cleft lips separate the premaxilla from its normal fusion with the entire maxilla.

Prosthesis: an artificial replacement of an absent part of the human body; a therapeutic device to improve or alter function.

Rehabilitation: the process of restoring a person's ability to live and work as normally as possible after a disabling injury or illness; aims to help the individual to achieve maximum possible physical and psychologic fitness and to regain ability to carry out personal care.

   Habilitation: the same goals and objectives as rehabilitation, but for a person with acquired disability for whom the ability to achieve maximum physical and psychologic fitness is acquired for the first time.

Rhinoplasty: plastic surgery of nose.

Speech aid prosthesis: a prosthetic device with a posterior section to assist with palatopharyngeal closure; also called bulb, speech bulb, or prosthetic speech appliance.

   Pediatric speech aid prosthesis: a temporary or interim prosthesis used to close a defect in the hard and/or soft palate; may replace tissue lost as a result of developmental or surgical alterations; necessary for intelligible speech.

   Adult speech aid prosthesis: a definitive prosthesis to improve speech by obturating (sealing off) a palatal cleft or occasionally assisting an incompetent soft palate.

Syndrome: a combination of symptoms either resulting from a single cause or occurring so commonly together as to constitute a distinct clinical picture.

Tracheostomy: creation of an opening into the trachea through the neck, with insertion of an indwelling tube to facilitate passage of air or evacuation of secretions.

Velopharyngeal insufficiency: anatomic or functional deficiency in the soft palate or the muscle affecting closure of the opening between mouth and nose in speech; results in a nasal speech quality.

Velum: covering structure or veil.

   Velum palatinum: soft palate.

CLASSIFICATION OF CLEFTS

■ Classification is based on disturbances in the embryologic formation of the palate as it develops from the premaxillary region toward the uvula in a definite pattern.

■ Interference with normal development of the palate may occur at one stage level of the embryo and the normal pattern may be reestablished at a later stage.

■ The seven classes are illustrated in **Figure 50-1**. All degrees are found, from an insignificant notch in the mucous membrane of the lip or uvula, which produces no functional disability, to the complete cleft defined by Class 6 of this classification.

ETIOLOGY

I. EMBRYOLOGY[2,3]

■ Cleft lip and palate represent a failure of normal fusion of embryonic processes during development in the first trimester of pregnancy.

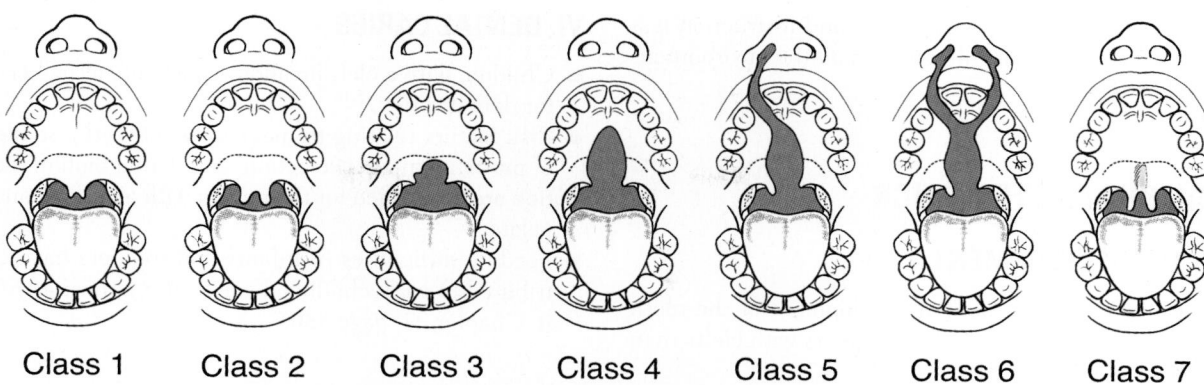

Class 1   Class 2   Class 3   Class 4   Class 5   Class 6   Class 7

FIGURE 50-1 **Classification of Cleft Lip and Cleft Palate.** Class 1. Cleft of the tip of the uvula; Class 2. Cleft of the uvula (bifid uvula); Class 3. Cleft of the soft palate; Class 4. Cleft of the soft and hard palates; Class 5. Cleft of the soft and hard palates that continues through the alveolar ridge on one side of the pre-maxilla; usually associated with cleft lip of the same side; Class 6. Cleft of the soft and hard palates that continues through the alveolar ridge on both sides, leaving a free premaxilla; usually associated with bilateral cleft lip; Class 7. Submucous cleft in which the muscle union is imperfect across the soft palate. The palate is short, the uvula is often bifid, a groove is situated at the midline of the soft palate, and the closure to the pharynx is incompetent.

- Figure 50-2 shows the locations of the globular process and the right and left maxillary processes.
- With normal fusion, no cleft of the lip results.
- Fusion begins in the premaxillary region and continues backward toward the uvula.
- Formation of the lip:
  - Occurs between the fourth and seventh week *in utero.*
  - A cleft lip becomes apparent by the end of the second month *in utero.*
- Development of the palate
  - Takes place during the eighth to twelfth week.
  - A cleft palate is evident by the end of the third month.

II. RISK FACTORS[4]

- Multifactorial genetic and environmental factors can be significant. Rarely, a single factor can be found as the specific cause.
- Early in the first trimester is the significant time for influences due to the environmental factors.
- Environmental factors include:
  - Use of tobacco.[5–7]
  - Alcohol consumption.[8,9]
  - Teratogenic agents: phenytoin, vitamin A (isotretinoin), corticosteroids, drugs of abuse (Table 48-1, page 745).
  - Inadequate diet: vitamins, especially folic acid deficiency.

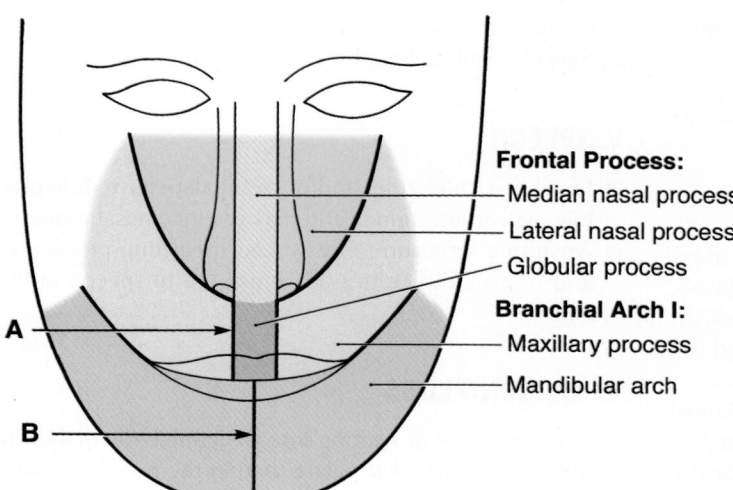

Frontal Process:
— Median nasal process
— Lateral nasal process
— Globular process

Branchial Arch I:
— Maxillary process
— Mandibular arch

FIGURE 50-2 **Developmental Processes of the Face.** The derivations of parts of the face from the frontal process and the branchial arch I. **(A)** Location of cleft lip when fusion of the globular process and a maxillary process fails. **(B)** Cleft of the mandible can occur at the midline. (Redrawn with permission from Melfi, R.C. Permar's oral embryology and microscopic anatomy. 8th ed. Philadelphia: Lea & Febiger; 1988.)

■ Lack of adequate prenatal care and instruction is a risk factor that has influence on all the environmental factors.

ORAL CHARACTERISTICS

I. TOOTH DEVELOPMENT

■ Disturbances in the normal development of the tooth buds occur more frequently in patients with clefts than in the general population.

■ There is a higher incidence of missing and supernumerary teeth, as well as of abnormalities of tooth form.[10]

■ Common missing teeth include maxillary laterals and they usually correspond to the side of the mouth that has the cleft.[11]

II. MALOCCLUSION

■ A high percentage of patients with cleft lip and palate require orthodontic care.

■ Orthodontic treatment may be required after each stage of surgical treatment for cleft palate.

III. OPEN PALATE

■ Before surgical correction, an open palate provides direct communication with the nasal cavity.

■ A cleft lip makes it more difficult for a child to suck on a nipple. Special nipples and bottles have been designed to make feeding easier.

■ A cleft palate may cause formula or breast milk to pass into the nasal cavity. A prosthetic palatal obturator may be constructed to aid during drinking and eating.

IV. MUSCLE COORDINATION

■ A lack of coordinated movements of lips, tongue, cheeks, floor of mouth, and throat may exist.

■ Compensatory habits may be formed by the patient in the attempt to produce normal sounds while speaking.

V. PERIODONTAL TISSUES

■ Dental biofilm accumulation is influenced by the irregularly positioned teeth, inability to keep lips closed, mouth breathing, and the difficulties in accomplishing adequate personal oral care, especially around the cleft areas.

■ Early periodontal disease with loss of bone and clinical attachment at cleft sites is common in adolescents.[12]

■ Periodontal tissue loss in later years is greatest at the cleft sites.[13,14]

VI. DENTAL CARIES

■ Children with a cleft lip and/or palate are at higher risk for dental caries.[15,16]

■ Risk factors relating to malpositioned teeth, problems of mastication, diet selection, and dental biofilm retention are intensified for the person with a cleft lip and/or palate.

■ Feeding difficulties of infants and toddlers have contributed to early childhood caries also known as ECC, in Chapter 22, page 330.

GENERAL PHYSICAL CHARACTERISTICS

I. OTHER CONGENITAL ANOMALIES

■ Incidence of multiple congenital anomalies is high with cleft lip and/or palate.

■ In more than 300 disorders, cleft lip, cleft palate, or both represent one feature of a syndrome.[17,18]

II. FACIAL DEFORMITIES

Facial deformities may include

■ Depression of the nostril on the side with the cleft lip.

■ Deficiency of upper lip, which may be short or retroposed.

■ Overprominent lower lip.

III. INFECTIONS

■ Predisposition to upper respiratory and middle ear infections is common.

IV. AIRWAY AND BREATHING

■ The craniofacial anomalies of the nose and throat area predispose the child with a cleft palate to airway obstruction and breathing problems.[19]

■ Early treatment intervention is necessary for the infant to cope with feeding problems.

■ Speech involves breathing and swallowing.

V. SPEECH[1]

■ Patients with cleft lip and/or cleft palate have difficulty making certain sounds and may produce nasal tones.

■ Anatomic structure, airway and breathing problems, and hearing difficulties all contribute to speech problems.

VI. HEARING LOSS

■ The incidence of hearing loss is significantly higher in individuals with cleft palate than in the noncleft population.

TREATMENT

- Treatment is coordinated by a team of specialists and is based on the patient's progress at each age period.[1]
- Members of the interdisciplinary team are listed in **Box 50-2**.
- The team is responsible for providing integrated case management. Quality and continuity of care are essential.[20]
- The need for attention to gingival health throughout the years of treatment cannot be overemphasized.

I. CLEFT LIP

- Surgical union of the cleft lip is made at 2 to 3 months of age. A general well-known rule for scheduling surgery: when the child is approximately 10 weeks of age, weighs 10 pounds, and has achieved a serum hemoglobin of 10 mg/ml.[1]
- The infant's general health is a determining factor.

A. Purposes for Early Treatment

- Aid in feeding.
- Encourage development of the premaxilla.
- Help partial closure of the palatal cleft.
- Assist families in adjusting to the birth of a child with cleft lip and/or palate.

B. Orthodontics and Dentofacial Orthopedics

- In preparation for cleft closure, orthodontic and orthopedic treatment may be needed to reduce the protrusion and stabilize the premaxilla.[21]

II. CLEFT PALATE

- Primary surgery to close the palate is usually undertaken by age 18 months or earlier when possible.[20]
- The combined efforts of many specialists are required as listed in **Box 50-2**.

A. Goals for Treatment

- Produce anatomic closure.
- Maximize maxillary growth and development.
- Achieve normal function, particularly normal speech.
- Relieve problems of airway and breathing.
- Establish good dental esthetics and functional occlusion.

B. Types of Secondary Surgical Procedures (Box 50-3)

- Secondary surgical care refers to additional surgical procedures after primary closure of the clefts.
- Secondary surgery may involve the lips, nose, palate, and jaws.

BOX 50-2	Interdisciplinary Team for Treatment of Patient With Cleft Lip and/or Palate

DENTAL PROFESSION
Dental hygiene
Oral and maxillofacial surgery
Orthodontics
Pediatric dentistry
Prosthodontics
Implantology
Periodontics

MEDICAL PROFESSION
Anesthesiology
Genetics/dysmorphology
Imaging/radiology
Neurology
Neurosurgery
Ophthalmology
Otolaryngology
Pediatrics
Physical anthropology
Plastic surgery
Psychiatry

ALLIED MEDICAL
Audiology
Diet and Nutrition
Nursing
Genetic counseling
Psychology
Social work
Speech-language pathology
Vocational counseling

- Objectives are to improve function for coherent communication, improve appearance, or both.
- Treatment plans are individualized to fit the needs of the patient.
- Team evaluations on a periodic basis determine the effects of treatment to date and outline the next phase.

BOX 50-3	Types of Secondary Surgical Procedures

- Rhinoplasty and nasal septal surgery for an airway problem.
- Velopharyngeal flap or other pharyngoplasty.
- Closure of palatal fistulae.
- Tonsillectomy and/or adenoidectomy.

C. Use of Bone Grafting[22,23]

■ Bone grafting is used to repair residual alveolar and hard palate clefts.

1. *Alveolar graft*
   ■ Placed before eruption of maxillary teeth at the cleft site.
   ■ Creates a normal architecture through which the teeth can erupt. A need for future prosthetic replacement of missing teeth is reduced.
   ■ Support is provided for teeth adjacent to the cleft areas.

2. *Hard palate graft*
   ■ Provides closure of oronasal fistulae.
   ■ Helps to relieve a compromised airway.

3. *Sources for autogenous bone for graft*
   ■ Rib, iliac crest, skull, mandible, or bone morphogenic proteins.

D. Use of Osseointegrated Implant

After bone grafting, implants can be used to replace individual teeth.

■ Implants also provide support for a complete prosthesis.[24,25]

III. PROSTHODONTICS

A. Types of Appliances[26]

■ *Obturator*: A removable prosthesis may be designed to provide closure of the palatal opening.
■ *Speech Aid Prosthesis*: A removable appliance to complete the palatopharyngeal valving required for speech.

B. Purposes and Functions of a Prosthesis

The prosthesis may be designed to accomplish one or all of the following:

■ Closure of the palate.
■ Replacement of missing teeth.
■ Scaffolding to fill out the upper lip.
■ Masticatory function.
■ Restoration of vertical dimension.
■ Postorthodontic retainer.

IV. ORTHODONTICS

■ Treatment may be initiated as early as 3 years of age, depending on the problems of dentofacial development.
■ Each stage of surgery and other treatment may require orthodontic intervention and follow-up.
■ Final formal orthodontic treatment for realigning the teeth and gaining a functional occlusion may start during the mixed dentition years or later.

■ During the orthodontic treatment period, an intensive program for dental caries prevention and gingival health is supervised.

V. SPEECH THERAPY

■ Training is started with very young children.
■ Emphasis after the surgical or prosthodontic treatment is urgent.

VI. RESTORATIVE DENTISTRY

■ Dental hygienists practicing with a pediatric dentist or general dentist are involved in direct patient care.
■ A major problem can be dental caries, leading to tooth loss. With missing teeth, major difficulties arise related to all phases of treatment.
■ Preservation of the primary teeth has special significance.

DENTAL HYGIENE CARE

■ Preventive measures for preservation of the teeth and their supporting structures are essential to the success of the special care needed for the habilitation of the patient with a cleft lip and/or palate.
■ Each phase of dental hygiene care and instruction, necessary for all patients, takes on even greater significance in light of the magnified problems of the patient with a cleft lip and/or palate.
■ Every attempt is made to avoid the need for removal of teeth, especially around the cleft area. In an area already weakened by lack of bone, the removal of teeth creates further complications.
■ The presence of teeth encourages optimum arch growth.

I. PARENTAL COUNSELING: ANTICIPATORY GUIDANCE

■ Understanding by the patient and the parents of the value of preventive procedures is accomplished through explanation and instruction.
■ When the patient has not had specialized care, the dental team has a responsibility to arrange referral to an available agency, clinic, or private practice specialist.
■ *Anticipatory Guidance*: Items from Tables 49-1 and 49-2, in Chapter 49 (pages 756 and 757), pertain to the parents and infant with a cleft lip and/or palate.
■ Primary concerns are daily dental biofilm removal and prevention of early childhood dental caries.

II. OBJECTIVES FOR APPOINTMENT PLANNING

■ Frequent appointments, scheduled every 3 or 4 months, are usually needed during the maintenance phase of the patient's care.

- *Objectives include* the following:
  - To review dental biofilm control measures.
  - To provide encouragement for the patient to maintain the health of the supporting structures and the cleanliness of the removable prostheses. Care of dental prostheses is discussed on page 453.
  - To remove all calculus and smooth the tooth surfaces as a supplement to the patient's personal daily care procedures.
  - To supervise a dental caries prevention program for both primary and permanent dentitions with fluorides (Box 35-5, page 537) and sealants (Figure 36-2, page 545).

III. APPOINTMENT CONSIDERATIONS

A. Patient Apprehension and Self-Esteem

- A patient who has been seen often in hospital clinics may become "clinic tired" and be very apprehensive about dental and dental hygiene care.
- Lowered self-esteem and difficulties in social interaction have also been noted with a patient with cleft lip and/or palate.[27]

B. Communication

- *Speech:* Speech may be almost indiscernible. With repeated contact, understanding can be developed. Referral for speech assessment, if not already done, is recommended.
- *Hearing:* Depending on the severity of hearing loss, the approach is similar to that for speech difficulties. Suggestions for care of patients with hearing problems are described in Chapter 59 on page 912.

C. Provide Motivation

- Quiet, unresponsive, or bold, rebellious patients can be approached in ways that can help them gain an objective attitude toward oral health.

IV. PATIENT INSTRUCTION

A. Personal Oral Care Procedures

- For a small child, the caretakers may be afraid of damaging the deformed areas or hurting the child if cleaning methods are employed.
- An empathetic approach and plan for continued instruction over a long period is needed.
1. *Personal daily care:* Select toothbrush, brushing method, and auxiliary aids according to the individual needs.
2. *Fluoride:* Instigate daily self-application of fluoride by way of fluoride dentifrice, and diet supplements for a young child in a nonfluoridated community (Table 35-2, page 528).

3. *Rinsing instruction:* Only older children (at least age 6 years, but evaluated for ability to rinse without swallowing) are given mouthrinsing for therapy. Instruction in how to rinse is needed when this procedure is new to the patient (Box 29-4, page 431).
4. *Prosthesis or speech aid:* Halitosis may be a real problem when the prosthesis forms the soft palate and the floor of the nasal cavity. Mucus secreted in the nasal cavity, as well as biofilm, accumulates on the prosthesis. Instruct the patient in the need for frequent removal of prosthesis for cleaning, particularly following eating. The method for cleaning the prosthesis is the same as that for a removable partial denture in Chapter 31, page 453.

B. Diet

- *Need for a varied diet:* Include adequate proportions of all essential food groups (Figure 34-1, MyPlate, page 499).
- *Need for prevention of dental caries:* Limit cariogenic foods, particularly for between-meal snacks.

C. Smoking Cessation

- The patient or family member who smokes or uses any form of smokeless tobacco is informed about the effects of tobacco on all the oral tissues.
- Emphasis on the potential damage to the periodontal tissues can have special significance for the patient with a cleft palate.
- Offer assistance with a smoking cessation program.

V. DENTAL HYGIENE CARE RELATED TO ORAL SURGERY

A. Presurgery (page 825)

- Objectives have particular significance because the patient with a cleft palate is unusually susceptible to infections of the upper respiratory area and middle ear.
- Every precaution is taken to prevent complications.

B. Postsurgery Personal Oral Care

- In certain palate surgical procedures, arm restraints are applied to prevent accidental damage to the repaired region.
- After each feeding (liquid diet for several days, soft diet for the next week), the mouth is rinsed carefully.
- Oral care is needed and accomplished with great care, usually by the parent or caregiver, to avoid damage to the healing suture lines.
- In selected cases, a toothbrush with suction attachment may be useful (page 882).
- Water irrigation using low pressure can also be helpful.

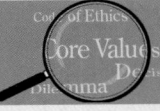

Everyday Ethics

Leona, a dental hygienist, has been delivering dental hygiene care and providing oral health education for Brian's family since they moved to her town right after he was born. Brian, now 8 years old, was born with a bilateral clefting of the lip with partial involvement of the palate. He recently had another surgical procedure completed on his upper lip. Brian's mother Joyce has been very impressed by the extra time that Leona has taken to research and learn about oral clefting. Joyce has depended on the guidance Leona has provided to help the family anticipate and meet Brian's oral health needs before, during, and after each of his multiple surgeries.

Joyce asks Leona to sign up as a hospital volunteer and share her expertise with parents of children who are receiving surgical care for orofacial clefts. Leona hesitates to agree because she really is not sure she has the time to prepare an educational presentation right now. In addition, she is concerned about how much of her limited free time this volunteer position will take.

Questions for Consideration

1. Consider the Basic Beliefs and Fundamental Principles identified in the ADHA Code of Ethics (Appendix I, page 1085). Does Leona have an ethical responsibility to share her professional expertise as a volunteer in her community? Why or why not?
2. Are there elements in the ADHA Code of Ethics that help support Lorna's decision if she decides NOT to volunteer? Explain.
3. What elements in the Canadian (CDHA) or the International (IFDH) Codes of Ethics (Appendices II and III, pages 1089 and 1094) encourage community volunteerism?

DOCUMENTATION

The documentation of care that the patient with cleft lip or palate receives over the individual's lifetime is imperative. Documentation includes the following:

- Description of location, classification, and extent of cleft.
- History and status of surgical interventions.
- Missing teeth and related recommendations for self-care regimens.

- Description of prosthetic appliances and recommendations for daily care regimens.
- A sample progress note is found in **Box 50-4**.

Factors To Teach The Patient

- Parental anticipatory guidance (Tables 49-1 and 49-2).
- Biofilm removal methods for cleft areas.
- Prevention of mouth odors by proper cleaning of tongue and removable appliances.
- Necessity for regular dental hygiene appointments to maintain freedom from infection.
- Resources with addresses for team treatment clinics specializing in craniofacial developmental defects.

BOX 50-4	**Example Progress Note for a Patient With Cleft Lip and/or Palate**

Six year-old patient presents for routine maintenance appointment. Reviewed medical history: patient had a rhinoplasty completed 6 months ago. All vital signs are normal. Extraoral examination: scar on right maxillary lip from cleft lip surgery at age 3 months. Intraoral examination: Unilateral Right Class 5 cleft lip and palate, missing #7 and wears obturator, which was removed during examination, Disclosed to show biofilm, demonstrated modified bass toothbrushing technique and "C" flossing. Showed patient and his mother how to use a proxy brush to clean in-between # 6 and #8 and stressed daily cleaning of obturator. Hand scaled all 4 quads, polish with fine grit prophy paste, floss, and Fluoride Varnish. Gave post-op instructions. Patient tolerated appointment well. Three-month continuing care appointment scheduled.

Signed: _____, RDH Date: _____.

References

1. Robin NH, Baty H, Franklin J, Guyton FC, Mann J, Woolley AL, Waite PD, Grant J, Robin NH, Batty H, Franklin J, Guyton FC, Mann J, Wolley AL, Waite PD, Grant J. The multidisciplinary evaluation and management of cleft lip and palate. *South Med J.* 2006 Oct;99(10):1111–20.
2. Melfi RC, Alley KE. *Permar's oral embryology and microscopic anatomy.* 10th ed. Philadelphia: Lippincott Williams & Wilkins; c2000. Chapter 2, Embryonic development of the face and oral cavity; pp. 25–42.
3. Ten Cate AR. *Oral histology, development, structure, and function.* 7th ed. St. Louis: Mosby, c2008. Chapter 3, Embryology of the head, face, and oral cavity; pp. 32–56.
4. Slavkin HC. Meeting the challenges of craniofacial-oral-dental birth defects. *J Am Dent Assoc.* 1996 May;127(5):681–2.

5. Shaw GM, Wasserman CR, Lammer EJ, O'Malley CD, Murray JC, Basart AM, Tolarova MM. Orofacial clefts, parental cigarette smoking, and transforming growth factor-alpha gene variants. *Am J Hum Genet.* 1996 Mar;58(3):551–61.

6. Little J, Cardy A, Arslan MT, Gilmour M, Mossey PA. United Kingdom-based case-control study. Smoking and orofacial clefts: a United Kingdom-based case-control study. *Cleft Palate Craniofac J.* 2004 Jul;41(4):381–6.

7. Källén K. Maternal smoking and orofacial clefts. *Cleft Palate Craniofac J.* 1997 Jan;34(1):11–16.

8. Werler MM, Lammer EJ, Rosenberg L, Mitchell AA. Maternal alcohol use in relation to selected birth defects. *Am J Epidemiol.* 1991 Oct;134(7):691–8.

9. Lorente C, Cordier S, Goujard J, Aymé S, Bianchi F, Calzolari E, De Walle HE, Knill-Jones R. Tobacco and alcohol use during pregnancy and risk of oral clefts. Occupational Exposure and Congenital Malformation Working Group. *Am J Public Health.* 2000 Mar;90(3):415–19.

10. Menezes R, Vieira AR. Dental anomalies as part of the cleft spectrum. *Cleft Palate Craniofac J.* 2008 Jul;45(4):414–19. Epub 2008 Feb 28.

11. Bartzela TN, Carels CE, Bronkhorst EM, Rønning E, Rizell S, Kuijpers-Jagtman AM. Tooth agenesis patterns in bilateral cleft lip and palate. *Eur J Oral Sci.* 2010 Feb;118(1):47–52.

12. Gaggl A, Schultes G, Kärcher H, Mossböck R. Periodontal disease in patients with cleft palate and patients with unilateral and bilateral clefts of lip, palate, and alveolus. *J Periodontol.* 1999 Feb;70(2):171–8.

13. Brägger U, Schürch E Jr, Salvi G, von Wyttenbach T, Lang NP. Periodontal conditions in adult patients with cleft lip, alveolus, and palate. *Cleft Palate Craniofac J.* 1992 Mar;29(2):179–85.

14. Huynh-Ba G, Brägger U, Zwahlen M, Lang NP, Salvi GE. Periodontal disease progression in subjects with orofacial clefts over a 25-year follow-up period. *J Clin Periodontol.* 2009 Oct;36(10):836–42. Epub 2009 Aug 23.

15. Bokhout B, Hofman FX, van Limbeek J, Kramer GJ, Prahl-Andersen B. Incidence of dental caries in the primary dentition in children with a cleft lip and/or palate. *Caries Res.* 1997;31(1):8–12.

16. Stec-Slonicz M, Szczepańska J, Hirschfelder U. Comparison of caries prevalence in two populations of cleft patients. *Cleft Palate Craniofac J.* 2007 Sep;44(5):532–7.

17. Cohen MM Jr, Bankier A. Syndrome delineation involving orofacial clefting. *Cleft Palate Craniofac J.* 1991 Jan;28(1):119–20.

18. Wyszynski DF, Sárközi A, Czeizel AE. Oral clefts with associated anomalies: methodological issues. *Cleft Palate Craniofac J.* 2006 Jan;43(1):1–6.

19. Perkins JA, Sie KC, Milczuk H, Richardson MA. Airway management in children with craniofacial anomalies. *Cleft Palate Craniofac J.* 1997 Mar;34(2):135–40.

20. American Cleft Palate-Craniofacial Association. *Parameters for evaluation and treatment of patients with cleft lip/palate or other craniofacial anomalies.* Rev. ed. Chapel Hill: American Cleft Palate-Craniofacial Association: 2009. pp. 1–34. [cited 2010 Dec 20]. Available from: http://www.acpa-cpf.org/teamcare/Parameters Rev.2009.pdf

21. Figueroa AA, Polley JW, Cohen M. Orthodontic management of the cleft lip and palate patient. *Clin Plast Surg.* 1993 Oct;20(4):733–53.

22. Kalaaji A, Lilja J, Friede H, Elander A. Bone grafting in the mixed and permanent dentition in cleft lip and palate patients: long-term results and the role of the surgeon's experience. *J Craniomaxillofac Surg.* 1996 Feb;24(1):29–35.

23. Guo, J, Zhang Q, Zou S, Chen J, Ye Q, Deacon SA, Zhao Z. Secondary bone grafting for alveolar cleft in children with cleft lip or cleft lip and palate. *The Cochrane Collaboration.* 2008 Jul; 2(4): 1–8.

24. Jansma J, Raghoebar GM, Batenburg RH, Stellingsma C, van Oort RP. Bone grafting of cleft lip and palate patients for placement of endosseous implants. *Cleft Palate Craniofac J.* 1999 Jan;36(1):67–72.

25. Lund TW, Wade M. Use of osseointegrated implants to support a maxillary denture for a patient with repaired cleft lip and palate. *Cleft Palate Craniofac J.* 1993 Jul;30(4):418–20.

26. Reisberg DJ. Dental and prosthodontic care for patients with cleft or craniofacial conditions. *Cleft Palate Craniofac J.* 2000 Nov;37(6):534–7.

27. Sousa AD, Devare S, Ghanshani J. Psychological issues in cleft lip and cleft palate. *J Indian Assoc Pediatr Surg.* 2009 Apr;14(2):55–8.

The Patient With an Endocrine Disorder or Hormonal Change

PATRICIA A. COHEN, RDH, BS, MS

Chapter Outline

OVERVIEW OF THE ENDOCRINE SYSTEM

The endocrine glands are glands of internal secretion. They secrete highly specialized substances—the hormones—that, with the nervous system, maintain body homeostasis. Some of the influences of the endocrine system on oral health and patient care are described in this chapter. Key words are defined in **Box 51-1**.

I. GLANDS OF THE ENDOCRINE SYSTEM

- The major endocrine glands, shown in **Figure 51-1**, are the pineal, hypothalamus, pituitary, thyroid, parathyroids, thymus, pancreas, adrenals, and gonads.

- The anterior pituitary is called the master gland because it regulates the output of hormones by other glands. In turn, the pituitary itself is regulated by the hormones produced by the other endocrine glands.
- Hormones produced by each of the endocrine glands are listed in **Table 51-1**.

II. HORMONES AND THEIR FUNCTIONS

- Hormones affect a number of major functions and are transported by the blood or lymph.
- Hormones may act directly on body cells or indirectly to control the hormones of other glands.

BOX 51-1	Key Words

Preadolescent to Postmenopausal Patients

Acne vulgaris: a chronic skin disorder with increased production of oil from the sebaceous glands; may be inflammatory or noninflammatory; appears on the face, back, and chest.

Adolescence: the period extending from the time the secondary sex characteristics appear to the end of somatic growth, when the individual is mature.

Amenorrhea: absence of spontaneous menstrual periods in a female.

Circumpubertal: on or around the age of puberty.

Coitus: sexual union; copulation; intercourse.

Dysmenorrhea: difficult and painful menstruation.

Dysphoria: feeling unwell or unhappy, depressed feeling.

Endocrine: pertaining to secretion of a substance directly into blood or lymph rather than into a duct; the opposite on exocrine.

Endometrium: the lining of the uterus.

Endometriosis: a condition of the endometrium that causes pelvic pain.

Epinephrine: a catecholamine hormone that causes the "fight-or-flight" response to physical or emotional stress; increased secretion produces marked dilation of bronchioles and increased blood pressure, blood glucose level, and heart rate.

Gland: organ or structure that secretes or execrates substances.

Gonad: sex gland in which reproductive cells form.

Goiter: enlargement of the thyroid gland, may indicate Grave's disease or Hashimoto's thyroiditis.

Gynecologist: physician who specializes in conditions specific to women, particularly of the genital tract, female endocrinology, and reproductive physiology.

Homeostasis: the tendency of biologic systems to maintain constant internal stability while continually adjusting to external changes.

Hormone: a chemical product of an organ or of certain cells within the organ that has a specific regulatory effect upon cells elsewhere in the body.

Hormone replacement therapy: prescription of a purified or synthetic hormone to correct or prevent undesirable symptoms of menopause.

Libido: sexual urge or desire.

Mastalgia: fullness, soreness, or pain in the breast.

Maturity: state of complete growth.

Menarche: onset of menstruation; may occur from ages 9 to 17 years.

Menopause: the time of life when a woman ceases menstruation; defined as a period of 12 months of amenorrhea in a woman over 45 years of age.

Menses: menstruation.

Myxedema: thickening of the skin, blunting of the senses and intellect, labored speech associated with hypothyroidism.

Norepinephrine: a catecholamine that functions as a neurotransmitter, sending signals from one neuron to another neuron or to a muscle cell.

Oligomenorrhea: menstrual intervals of greater than 45 days.

Premenstrual syndrome: a cluster of behavioral, somatic, affective, and cognitive disorders that appear in the premenstrual (luteal) phase of the menstrual cycle and that resolve rapidly with the onset of menses.

Puberty: period in which the gonads mature and begin to function.

Pubescence: arriving or having arrived at the age of puberty.

Spermatogenesis: the process of male sperm production.

Thyroiditis: inflammation of the thyroid.

Xerostomia: dry mouth.

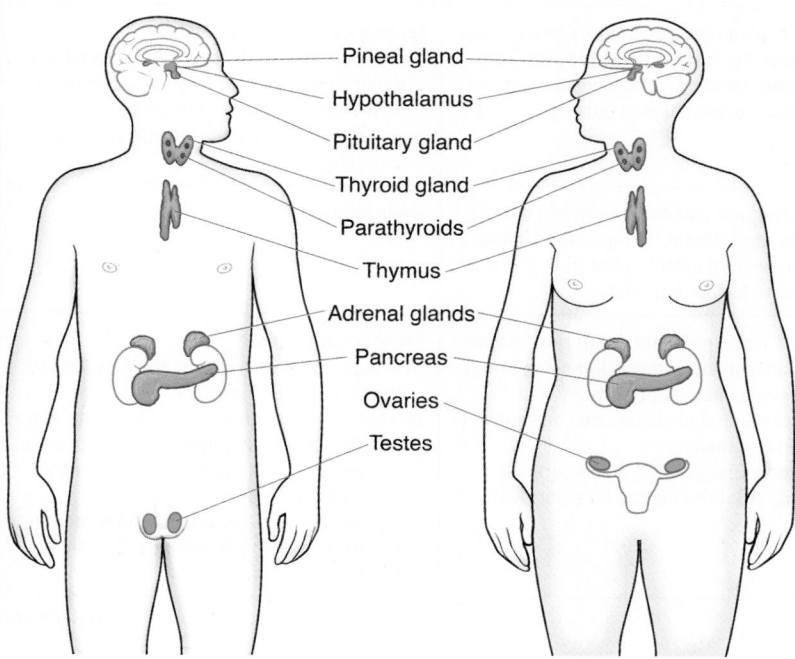

FIGURE 51-1 The Major Endocrine Glands. Illustrated here for both male and female, these glands produce hormones that regulate body systems.

TABLE 51-1	ENDOCRINE GLAND FUNCTIONS AND IMPLICATIONS FOR ORAL HEALTH CARE	
ENDOCRINE GLANDS AND HORMONES	**FUNCTION AND EFFECTS**	**IMPLICATIONS OF IMBALANCE FOR ORAL CARE**
Pineal ■ Melatonin	Controls sleep patterns; may inhibit action of gonadotrophin, which causes development and function of ovaries and testes.	None known.
Hypothalamus ■ Controls hormone production in the pituitary gland.	Communicates with nervous and endocrine systems; stimulates or inhibits pituitary function; creates uterine contractions during labor; aides in water balance, body temperature, appetite, emotions and autonomic functions, including sleep cycle.	See Thyroid below.
Pituitary: divided into two parts: Anterior Pituitary ■ Prolactin (PRL) ■ Growth Hormone (GH) ■ Adrenocorticotropin (ACTH) ■ Thyroid-Stimulating Hormone (TSH) ■ Luteinizing Hormone (LH) ■ Follicle-Stimulating Hormone (LSH) Posterior Pituitary ■ Oxytocin ■ Antidiuretic Hormone (ADH); also called Vasopressin	Called the "master gland" because of great influence on body organs; important for overall well-being. Stimulates milk production, bone growth, stimulates cortisol production by the adrenal gland; stimulates thyroid hormones; regulates testosterone and estrogen; promotes sperm and egg production; affects fertility. Causes milk letdown in nursing mothers; stimulates contractions during childbirth; regulates water balance.	General anesthesia may be contraindicated for some individuals. Mandibular enlargement may cause Class 3 occlusion.
Thyroid ■ Tri-iodothyronine (T3) ■ Thyroxine (T4)	Regulates metabolism, bone status, and blood calcium; increased risk of osteoporosis, hypertension, heart failure, peptic ulcer and diabetes; goiter is enlargement of thyroid gland.	Monitor blood pressure; avoid aspirin; increased risk of periodontitis, oral candidiasis, bleeding gingiva, infection, and poor wound healing with poor thyroid function.
	Hyperthyroid: Grave's Disease is often the underlying cause; accelerated tooth development and potential malocclusion.	Local anesthetics to be avoided; sweating may indicate hypoglycemic reaction.
	Hypothyroid: lethargic and slow to react; coarse dry skin; macroglossia; swollen lips due to myxedema.	Do not use epinephrine if uncontrolled; increased risk of dental caries.
Parathyroid ■ Parathyroid Hormone (PTH)	Controls calcium and phosphorus levels; regulates blood pressure, stress reaction, salt and water balance, bone development and body hair development at puberty.	Monitor blood pressure and heart function (strength and regularity of pulse) at each visit. Chronic illness can cause over secretion of PTH with attendant symptoms such as kidney stones, bone pain, muscle weakness and fatigue.
Thymus ■ Humoral Factor Hormones	Enables lymphocytes to develop into mature T-cells; important in cell-mediated immunity for several months after birth and then serves no further function	None known
Adrenals: made up of two organs: Adrenal Cortex (outer portion): hormones are essential for life. ■ Glucocorticoids (such as Cortisol) ■ mineral Corticoids (such as Aldosterone)	Regulates blood pressure, heart rate, stress reaction, salt and water balance and body hair development at puberty. Danger of adrenal crisis and two diseases related to imbalance: ■ Addison's Disease (too much cortisol) ■ Cushing's Syndrome (too little cortosol)	Monitor vital signs. Oral pigmentation; swollen face may lead to dental inquiry. Increased susceptibility to bacterial infection and delayed wound healing; predisposition for herpes, chicken pox, candidiasis and bacterial infections. Long term immuno-suppression may lead to Kaposi's sarcoma, lymphoma, lip cancer or other complications.

(continued)

TABLE 51-1	ENDOCRINE GLAND FUNCTIONS AND IMPLICATIONS FOR ORAL HEALTH CARE (*Continued*)	
ENDOCRINE GLANDS AND HORMONES	**FUNCTION AND EFFECTS**	**IMPLICATIONS OF IMBALANCE FOR ORAL CARE**
Adrenal Medula (inner portion) hormones not essential for life. ■ Epinephrine (adrenaline) ■ Norepinephrine		In stressful situations (such as dental appointments) may need to increase prescribed steroids.
Pancreas	Regulates blood glucose by way of islets of Langerhans.	Complications related to Type-1 diabetes—see Chapter 68 for more information.
Gonads: Testes ■ Testosterone Ovaries ■ Estrogen ■ Progesterone ■ Inhibin	Produces male and female sexual characteristics; regulates puberty. In the female, regulates the menstrual cycle, pregnancy and menopause	Hormonal changes during the life cycle can increase host response. Loss of ovarian function in the female leads to symptoms of menopause, including hot flashes, thinning of mucosal tissues, mood changes and osteoporosis.

Source: Little JW, Falace D, Miller C, Rhodus NL. Dental management of the medically compromised patient. 7th ed. St. Louis: Mosby Elsevier; 2008. pp. 236–66; Ganda KM. Dentist's guide to medical conditions and complications. Ames, Iowa: Wiley-Blackwell; 2008. p. 257–72; Scully C, Cawson RA. Medical problems in dentistry. 4th ed. Oxford; Boston: Wright; 1998. pp. 265–82.

■ Complex and unified actions of hormones produced by endocrine glands augment and regulate many vital functions, including growth and development, energy production, food metabolism, reproductive processes, and the responses of the body to stress and temperature.

■ Regulation of hormonal secretion is complex, and the mechanisms are not fully understood. Normally, hormones are secreted when needed.

■ The stimulus for hormone secretion is often a chemical signal in the blood; when the hormone is released the signal disappears. As more hormone is required, the signal reappears.

■ This system of "negative feedback" works to provide hormones in optimal amounts and only in response to a need.

■ Both hyposecretion and hypersecretion of a hormone can cause physical and mental disturbances.

III. ENDOCRINE GLAND DISORDERS

■ When diseases affect the glands, the hormones may be underproduced or overproduced, causing physical and biochemical changes that may have profound effects on the body, including the oral cavity.

■ The functions and effects of the endocrine glands and implications for oral health care are listed in **Table 51-1**.

■ Presence or absence of a particular hormone may affect oral structures and may cause the host response to infection, healing, or stress to vary.[1]

■ Many systemic diseases and disorders are risk indicators or risk factors for periodontal disease.

■ Hormonal fluctuations associated with puberty, pregnancy and menopause can affect the periodontium and directly modify the tissue's response to local factors.

ADOLESCENCE AND PUBERTY

I. STAGES OF ADOLESCENCE

The period of life considered adolescence is represented by the years between ages 10 and 21. The adolescent years, which include puberty, are marked by many physical and psychosocial changes.

From a psychosocial aspect, this period can be divided into three overlapping phases:

■ Early adolescence, approximately ages 10 to 13.
■ Middle adolescence, approximately ages 14 to 17.
■ Late adolescence, approximately ages 18 to 21.

II. PUBERTAL CHANGES

Puberty is a dynamic period of development marked by rapid changes in body size, shape, and composition. Some individuals go through changes earlier and faster than others.

Chronologic age is an unreliable indicator because puberty may begin normally in either sex between 9 and 17 years of age, depending on such factors as race, heredity, and nutritional status. Friends of the same age may look quite different from one another because there is a wide range of normal. Females generally begin puberty before males. The secondary sex characteristics begin to appear between 10 and 13 years of age in females, whereas changes in males start at about 13 or 14 years. The major changes are usually complete in 3 to 4 years.

III. PHYSICAL DEVELOPMENT

A. Hormonal Influences

Pituitary hormones control the hormones produced by the ovaries and the testes. The several hormones produced by the ovaries are known collectively as estrogens, and those produced by the testes are called androgens. They are responsible for the development of the sex organs, the accessory sex organs, and the secondary sex characteristics. They have strong physical, mental, and emotional influences throughout the body.

B. Female Development

- Accelerated growth spurt.
- *Development of the sex organs:* fallopian tubes, uterus, vagina, and breasts.
- Appearance of secondary sex characteristics:
  - Growth of pubic and axillary hair.
  - Skeletal development, increased height, enlargement of the pelvis.
  - Fat deposition on the hips.
  - Voice drops one or two tones.
- Beginning of menstruation and ovulation. Menstruation may precede the first ovulation.

C. Male Development

- Increase in size of testes and scrotum and beginning of spermatogenesis.
- *Development of the sex organs:* vas deferens, seminal vesicles, prostate, and penis.
- *Appearance of secondary sex characteristics:*
  - Growth of facial, pubic, and axillary hair.
  - Voice deepens.
- Increased height, increased muscle volume, and mass.

D. Growth Spurt

- Varies in age of occurrence, extent, and duration; usually occurs in females between 11 and 14 years, and in males between 12 and 16 years.
- Overeating with underexercise, along with psychological problems, makes obesity a difficult and serious problem.
- Poor coordination and awkwardness in young adolescents may result from irregular, uneven stages of growth.
- *Teens need three health basics:* fuel, activity, and rest.

IV. PSYCHOSOCIAL DEVELOPMENT

Psychologically and socially, adolescence is the bridge from childhood to adulthood.

A. Changes

During the stages of development, the changes that take place can be grouped under the following topics, as detailed in **Table 51-2**.

- Achievement of independence from parents.
- Assignment of increased importance to body image and acceptance of one's own body image.
- Adoption of peer codes and lifestyles.
- Establishment of sexual, ego, vocational, and moral identities.

B. Relevance in Dental Hygiene Care

- Vital for all health professionals to understand the general patterns of growth and development.
- Insight into changes during adolescence can direct patient teaching.

V. NUTRITIONAL REQUIREMENTS

- Highest of any time in life for males; exceeded only during pregnancy for females.
- Undernutrition is common.
  - *Boys:* due to overactivity and poor food selection.
  - *Girls:* due to voluntary diet restrictions, with poor food selection and fad diets in the attempt to be trim.
  - Teens with a distorted body image may take concern to extremes.
- Eating disorders
  - Anorexia nervosa and/or bulimia, can lead to severe health complications and even death.
  - Successful treatment usually requires an interdisciplinary team approach involving medical care, psychotherapy, and nutrition and family counseling (as described in Chapter 63 on page 961).
- Iron-deficiency anemia
  - Common among teenage girls, particularly after the onset of menstruation.
  - Treated with iron supplements, changes in diet, or both, as described in Chapter 34 on page 1031.

VI. PERSONAL FACTORS

Adolescents are no longer children, yet they have not reached adulthood. They may respond and wish to be treated as adults or as children at different times. They are learning to adapt to body changes, sexual impulses, secondary sex characteristics, and independence. There is no fixed picture. Characteristics listed below are exhibited to one degree or another by many adolescents. Issues can be addressed at the family, school, or individual level.[2]

TABLE 51-2	PSYCHOSOCIAL DEVELOPMENT OF ADOLESCENTS		
TASK	**EARLY ADOLESCENCE APPROX 10–13 YEARS MIDDLE SCHOOL**	**MIDDLE ADOLESCENCE APPROX 14–17 YEARS HIGH SCHOOL**	**LATE ADOLESCENCE APPROX 18–21 YEARS HIGHER EDUCATION OR WORK**
Independence	■ Less interest in parental activities ■ Wide mood swings	■ Peak of parental conflicts	■ Reacceptance of parental values
Body Image	■ Preoccupation with self and pubertal changes ■ Uncertainty about appearance	■ General acceptance of body ■ Concern over making body more attractive	■ Acceptance of pubertal changes
Peers	■ Intense relationships with same-sex friends	■ Peak of peer involvement ■ Conformity with peer values ■ Increased sexual activity and experimentation	■ Peer group less important ■ More time spent in sharing intimate relationships
Identity	■ Increased cognition ■ Increased fantasy world ■ Idealistic vocational goals ■ Increased need for privacy ■ Lack of impulse control	■ Increased scope of feelings ■ Increased intellectual ability ■ Feeling of omnipotence ■ Risk-taking behavior	■ Practical, realistic vocational goals ■ Refinement of moral religious, and sexual values ■ Ability to compromise and to set limits

Adapted with permission from Radzik M, Neinstein LS, ed. Adolescent health care: a practical guide, 5th ed. Baltimore: Lippincott Willams & Wilkins; 2008. Radzik M, Sherer S, Neinstein LS. Psychosocial development in normal adolescents. p. 27.

A. Anxiety

Causes of adolescent anxiety include:

■ Health problems. Younger, less healthy teenagers tend to show greater health concerns.
■ Violence, substance abuse.
■ Sexual issues, peer pressures.
■ Family arguments, divorce.
■ School performance, concern about the future.

B. Increased Self-Interest

■ Have a great deal of concern for themselves and respond best to those who show concern for them.
■ Want attention and tend to reject those who do not listen.
■ Have interest in their own health.

C. Growing Independence

■ Adolescence is a period of rapidly growing independence of thought and action, with conflicts between feelings of dependence and independence.
■ Childhood dependence on parents is gradually given up; the idea of infallibility of parents is lost; teachers and other authority figures are questioned.
■ Personal identity is sought; adolescents are uncertain about their place and role in society.
■ Independence from parents frequently means increased confidence in and respect for other adults outside the family.

■ Teachers, coaches, and health professionals can have a powerful impact at this time.

D. Concern over Physical Characteristics

■ Girls mature earlier than boys; young females are usually taller than their male counterparts. Social problems may result.
■ Increased interest in personal appearance; want to dress and be like their peers.
■ Issues such as delayed growth and delayed sexual development.
■ Obesity may be troublesome. Obesity is a serious health problem and is associated with increased morbidity and mortality.
■ Skin disorders may occur. Acne vulgaris results from overactivity of the sebaceous glands. The impact upon self-esteem can affect social interactions and school performance.

ORAL CONDITIONS

I. DENTAL CARIES

■ Incidence higher during adolescence than other age groups, especially in communities without fluoridation.
■ Related to eating habits: frequency, demands of rapid growth, emotional issues, peer pressures.
■ Cariogenic foods selected: frequent snacks, sweetened carbonated beverages.

II. PERIODONTAL INFECTIONS

Adolescents are at risk for categories of periodontal infections (Tables 16-1 and 16-2, pages 245 and 246). Gingival problems are common in this age group. Careful probing and study of radiographs are indicated for each patient. Emphasis is placed on preventive measures, early assessment, early treatment, and regular maintenance appointments.

A. Biofilm-Induced Gingivitis During Puberty[3]

- Incidence and severity may increase.
- Clinical changes and hormonal changes related to increased dental biofilm.
- Exaggerated response to dental biofilm.

B. Risk Factors for Periodontitis[4]

- Local factors: supragingival and subgingival calculus; dental biofilm accumulations.
- Pathogenic microorganisms, viruses.
- Untreated dental caries and defective restorations.[5]
- Orthodontic appliances.
- Oral hygiene: personal habits of care.
- Infrequent, inadequate dental and dental hygiene care.
- Socioeconomic influences.
- Use of tobacco.
- Systemic diseases such as diabetes and hematological diseases.
- Host immune factors.
- Genetic factors.

C. Destructive Periodontal Diseases

Periodontal diseases in adolescents may be either in the aggressive or chronic classification. Loss of periodontal attachment and supporting bone is evident in 5 to 47% of adolescents around the world.[6]

    The two distinct disease categories are localized aggressive periodontitis (LAP) and generalized aggressive periodontitis (GAP). Both types have a familial tendency and may have a neutrophil dysfunction with a compromised immune response.[7]

- *Localized aggressive periodontitis (LAP)*
  - Characterized by severe bone loss involving the first permanent molars and the incisors, with proximal surface attachment loss on at least two permanent teeth.
  - First diagnosed during the circumpubertal years.
  - Pathogenic microorganism of etiologic importance is the *Actinobacillus actinomycetemcomitans,* a powerful microorganism that can invade tissue.
- *Generalized aggressive periodontitis (GAP)*
  - Characterized by generalized proximal surface attachment loss affecting at least three permanent teeth other than the first molars and incisors.

- Occurs in persons under 30 years of age.
- Microflora found in periodontal pockets of GAP have similarities to the microflora of chronic adult periodontitis.

DENTAL HYGIENE CARE

I. IMPACT OF CARE

- Dental hygiene services provided during adolescence can impact oral health throughout the patient's lifetime.
- The concrete information, education, and guidance from interested and caring health professionals will help form the attitudes and health behavior practices developed by adolescents.
- Influences at this time can have wide-reaching significance throughout life.

II. PATIENT APPROACH

- Communication strategies for motivating adolescent patients are discussed in Chapter 3 on page 29.
- Adolescence is a period of transition and growth spurts. Understanding adolescents, their issues, and their biological changes is critical for promoting health and preventing disease.[8]
- Each situation requires its own approach.
- Health behaviors at this stage of development can have lifelong implications.
- Adolescence is an opportune time to promote health and prevent disease.
- Treat adolescents as adults. Physically, many of them are mature, although their emotional development varies. They are becoming less dependent on the family and paying more attention to the influence of peers.
- Be attentive and show interest in them and their issues. Encourage them to talk, and then listen carefully.
- Avoid lecturing and admonishing. Suggest and advise, but do not become impatient or take offense when they choose to make their own decisions. Adolescents need time to process information about health behavior changes.
- Highlight the positive. Self-concept plays a significant role in mediating changes in dental health behavior. High self-esteem has a strong positive association with oral cleanliness in adolescents.[9,10]
- Question the patient regarding motivations and health behaviors.
- Health, including oral health, may be a serious concern.
- Adolescents need information about their oral health; explanations based on science are generally appreciated.

III. PATIENT HISTORY

- *History questions:* Adolescents may provide their own information for the medical and dental histories. Verification by the parent or guardian for additional details is needed, but not in the same interview with the patient and not without the patient's consent.
- *Responsibility for health:* Adolescents need to take increasing responsibility for their own health. Although the initial dental visit may be at the suggestion of a parent or guardian, every effort is made to focus on the patient.
- *Other health problems:* The patient with diabetes; cardiovascular disease; a mental, physical, or sensory disability; or other systemic involvement requires special adaptations of procedures as described in the various chapters of Section VIII of this book.
- *Medical clearance:* The parent or legal guardian will need to consent to medical clearance for conditions requiring antibiotic coverage, local anesthesia, or other medication for a patient under legal age.
- *Parental approval:* The dental hygiene care plan requires approval by a parent or legal guardian.

IV. ORAL HEALTH ISSUES IN ADOLESCENCE[11]

Dental caries and periodontal infections of the adolescent years have been described. Some examples of other oral problems related to adolescent development and behavior characteristics, including risky health behaviors, are listed here.

- Oral manifestations of sexually transmitted infections (STIs).
- Effects of tobacco use, such as leukoplakia and periodontal damage.
- Effects of cocaine use and other drugs.
- Potential effects of oral contraceptives on periodontal tissues (page 793).
- Oral findings of anorexia nervosa or bulimia (in Chapter 63, pages 961 and 962).
- Traumatic injury to teeth and oral structures may occur. Contact sports and skateboarding are risky behaviors. Automobile and motorcycle accidents can also cause dental injuries.
- Pregnancy and parenting may be issues for the adolescent. The dental hygienist has the opportunity to use anticipatory guidance in educating the patient on important oral health issues (Tables 49-1 and 49-2, pages 756 and 757).
- Piercings in the orofacial region are common. Inform patients who are considering a piercing regarding piercing procedures and related health risks. Patients need education regarding daily hygiene of the piercing site to avoid infection.

V. DENTAL BIOFILM CONTROL

- Educate the patient by explaining the following:
  - A. Causes and prevention of dental caries and periodontal infections.
  - B. Effects of dental biofilm accumulation.
  - C. Purposes of professional calculus removal.
  - D. Daily self-care and its relation to oral tissue health and halitosis prevention.
- The total caries-control program
      For dental caries prevention, adolescents are educated about the beneficial effects of fluoride and the need to restrict the intake of cariogenic foods. The program is outlined and conducted on the basis of these clear-cut preventive measures:
  - A. Instruction in self-care procedures.
  - B. Continuing reassessment over a series of appointments to develop behavioral changes that include daily practices that can be carried over into adult life.

VI. INSTRUMENTATION

- Series of appointments may be required, depending on probing depth and extent of calculus deposits.
- Careful and complete scaling and root planing.
- Removal of all local irregularities, such as inadequate margins of restorations.

VII. FLUORIDE TREATMENT PROGRAM

- A combined fluoride program is indicated for most adolescent patients, particularly for those who have not had the benefit of a fluoridated water supply.
- Fluoride varnish or topical fluoride applications made in conjunction with dental hygiene appointments; self-administered methods include a fluoride dentifrice and a daily fluoride mouthrinse.
- A daily application of a fluoride gel in a custom-made tray may be necessary in selected cases (in Chapter 35, page 532).

VIII. DIET CONTROL

A. Dietary Assessment (Chapter 34, page 507)

A study of the patient's diet and counseling relative to general nutrition and dental caries control can provide important learning experiences for many adolescents. The parent or other person who is responsible for shopping and food preparation is included so that appropriate foods are available. As much responsibility as possible is placed with the adolescent patient.

B. Instruction Suggestions

- *Advise foods from the most recent MyPlate Food Guide in Chapter 34* (page 499): Emphasize foods for growth, energy, clear complexion, wellness, and overall good health.

■ *Emphasize a nutritious breakfast:* Teenagers tend to omit breakfast.
■ *Snack selection:* Advise selecting nutritious foods, with recognition of cariogenic foods. Suggest healthy snacks such as raw fruits and vegetables, nuts, unsweetened milk, use of sugar-free foods when possible, and sugarless chewing gum with xylitol immediately after lunch and dinner.
■ *Suggest reading labels:* Recommend that teens learn how to read nutrition labels and become aware of serving size and nutrition information such as total fat, fiber, and calories.

MENSTRUATION

I. MENSTRUAL CYCLE

The cycle, illustrated in **Figure 51-2** is the period from the beginning of one menstrual flow to the beginning of the next menstrual flow.

A. Cyclic Changes in the Uterus

■ Instigated by hormones
■ Preparation of the endometrium for pregnancy

B. When Conception Does Not Occur

■ Fluid discharged during menstruation.
■ Composed of blood, mucous, endometrial membrane fragments.
■ Length: 3 to 6 days; cycle starts over.

II. CHARACTERISTICS

A. Occurrence

■ Cyclic menstruation occurs from puberty to menopause.
■ Pregnancy and part of breast-feeding disrupt cycle.
■ Cycle complete in about 28 days (range 22 to 35 days).

B. Onset

■ Between ages 9 and 19 years.
■ May occur before the first ovulation.
■ Timing and extent of flow may be irregular for several months or years.

III. IRREGULARITIES

■ Variations are common. Many have no problems.
■ Factors affecting the cycle: changes in climate, changes in work schedule, emotional trauma, acute or chronic illnesses, weight loss, or excessive exercise.
■ Emotional impact: may have a psychological basis.

A. Premenstrual Syndrome

Premenstrual syndrome (PMS) is a distinctive group of physical and emotional changes that may occur 7 to 10 days before menstruation.

■ *Physical symptoms:* fatigue, headache, bloating, mastalgia, skin breakouts, cramps, and food cravings

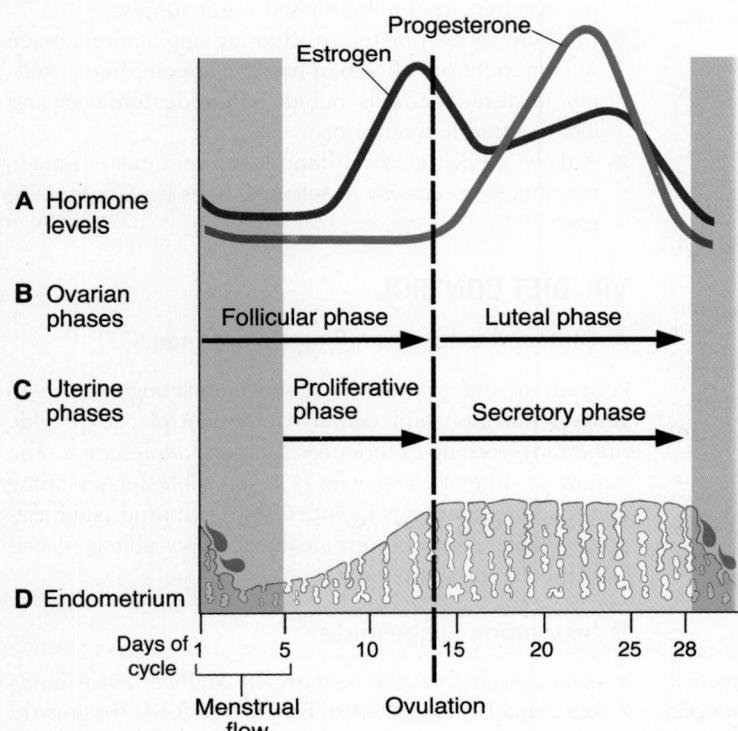

FIGURE 51-2 **Changes During the Menstrual Cycle.** The 28 days of a normal cycle are shown, with ovulation between days 12 and 15 and the menstrual flow between days 1 to 5 and again at day 28. **(A)** Hormonal levels show the estrogen peak shortly before ovulation during the follicular phase of the ovary **(B)** and the proliferative phase of the uterus **(C)**. **(D)** The endometrium builds up at the end of each menstrual flow. This prepares the area for possible implantation of a fertilized ovum.

- *Affective symptoms:* depression, anxiety, irritability, hostility, tearfulness, mood changes, reduced ability to concentrate.
- *Medical management:* medical care for severe symptoms, possibly prescription medication.
- *Self-help methods:* daily exercise, diet modification to eliminate caffeine, salt, alcohol, and simple carbohydrates, stress reduction, and rest; over-the-counter (OTC) medications to manage discomfort.[12]

B. Dysmenorrhea

- *Primary or functional dysmenorrhea:* The organs are normal and there are symptoms of hyperactivity and contractions.
- *Secondary or acquired dysmenorrhea:* Associated with abnormal anatomy of the uterus or as the result of an illness such as endometriosis or pelvic inflammatory disease (PID).
- *Physiologic or psychological factors:* Emotional status, inadequate preparation for the arrival of puberty, poor parental example.

IV. DENTAL HYGIENE CARE

A. Patient History

- Menstruation is normal and healthy; not an illness.
- Terminology for history questions: use "period" or "monthly period."
- Include questions concerning regularity.
- Irregularity may reflect general health problems.

B. Oral Findings[13]

- No specific gingival changes; occasional problems may occur.
- Exaggerated response to local irritants or unusual gingival bleeding may be noted.
- Prevention through dental biofilm control, self-care measures, and removal of calculus at regular maintenance appointments.

HORMONAL CONTRACEPTIVES

Numerous types of hormonal contraceptives are available. Birth control pills, also known as oral contraceptives (OCs) are recognized as a safe and effective method of contraception when they are taken as prescribed. They are used by millions of women throughout the world.

I. TYPES[14]

A. Combination Preparations

- *Estrogen and progestin*
  - Combination of synthetic hormones estrogen and progestin is nearly 100% effective in preventing pregnancy when taken appropriately.

- Oral contraceptives inhibit the release of gonadotropin-releasing hormone, without which the ovum cannot be released from the ovary.
- *Schedule of administration*
  - One pill taken each day for 21 days starting 5 days after the onset of the menstrual flow.
  - For a period of 7 days, a placebo pill is taken.
  - Routine is followed regardless of when menstrual flow starts or stops.

B. Single Preparations: Minipills

- The progestin-only pill has been used when estrogen is contraindicated.
- Pregnancy prevention is slightly less effective with this pill.
- Menstrual cycles tend to be irregular; side effects frequent.

C. Injectable Contraceptive: Depo-Provera™

- Contains synthetic progestin.
- One injection every 12 weeks prevents ovulation.
- Can be helpful for those who have trouble remembering to take a daily pill.

D. Subdermal Implant

- Allows for slow release of hormone.
- Provides effective contraception for 5 years.
- Method of action is similar to injectable.

II. CONTRAINDICATIONS[14]

Contraceptives containing hormones are not usually prescribed for a patient in the presence of the following:

- Circulatory problems, thromboembolic disorders, cerebrovascular disease, coronary heart disease, severe hypertension
- Liver disease
- Cancer of the breast
- Severe migraine headaches
- Pregnancy or lactation

III. SIDE EFFECTS[14]

Side effects may be related to incorrect use of the drug rather than to hormonal effects. Visual problems, mental depression, rashes, and bleeding irregularities occur in some women. The most significant side effects are:

- Cardiovascular (including increased blood pressure)
- Weight gain
- Decreased effectiveness when certain drugs are used, including antibiotics,[15,16] anticonvulsants, and rifampin

IV. EFFECT ON THE GINGIVA

An exaggerated response to dental biofilm and other local irritants has been noted. The gingivitis is similar to that described for pregnancy (in Chapter 48, page 746).

V. APPOINTMENT CONSIDERATIONS

A. Medical History

A record of the use of oral contraceptives is updated with each history review.

B. Inform the Patient

- Potential oral side effects of hormonal contraceptives.
- The need for exceptional personal oral care and regular professional maintenance appointments to prevent complications.

MENOPAUSE

Menopause is the complete and permanent cessation of menstrual flow.

- Menopause generally occurs between the ages of 47 and 55 years.
- The end of fertility due to decreased production of estrogen and progesterone by the ovaries.
- Menopause is usually confirmed when a woman has no menstrual period for 12 consecutive months and there is no other cause for this change.

I. CHARACTERISTICS

Before menopause, menstruation changes in frequency, duration, and amount of flow over a period of about 12 to 24 months. Menopause is accompanied by a number of characteristic physiologic changes. Although many women experience only minor symptoms, a small percent have increased symptoms during menopause.

A. General Symptoms

As ovarian function declines with diminishing estrogen, physiologic changes in body function take place.

1. *Vasomotor reactions*

- Hot flashes, defined as periodic surges of heat involving the whole body; may be accompanied by drenching sweats.
- Hot flash may begin with a headache; proceed to a flushing of the face, with heart palpitations, and dizziness, followed by a chill.
- Episodes may last a few minutes or more than 30 minutes.
- Night sweats and sleeping problems may lead to feeling tired, stressed, or tense.

2. *Vaginal changes*

- Dryness, irritation, and thinning of tissue may occur.
- Frequent vaginal infections may occur.
- Associated with decreased estrogen levels.

3. *Emotional disturbances*

- Alterations in estrogen level may result in mood swings, depression, irritability, and difficulty with concentration or memory.
- Decreased libido and changes in sexual response.
- Some women experience anxiety, tension, and irritability and feel useless.
- Weight gain or increase of body fat around waist.

B. Postmenopausal Effects

- Reproductive organs atrophy.
- Bone problems have been associated with the menopausal patient.
- Skin and mucous membranes decrease in thickness and keratinization, becoming fragile and easily injured.
- Predisposition to conditions including atherosclerosis, diabetes, and hypothyroidism.

II. ORAL FINDINGS

Oral changes can be related to menopause, but they are not a common feature. Control of local factors through preventive dental hygiene appointments for maintenance will supplement daily personal oral care.

A. Gingiva

- Gingival changes associated with menopause usually represent an exaggerated response to dental biofilm.
- Hormonal changes influence oral tissue response.
- Menopausal gingivostomatitis may develop. It may also occur after removal of, or radiation therapy to, the ovaries.

B. Mucous Membranes and Tongue

- Tissue may appear shiny and may vary in color from abnormal paleness to redness.[16] Dryness with burning sensations may be present.
- Burning mouth syndrome may occur.[17]
- Altered salivary composition in some menopausal women may be due to psychological stress.
- Epithelium may become thin and atrophic with decreased keratinization; tolerance for removable prostheses may lessen, especially with xerostomia.
- Taste perception may be altered, described as salty, peppery, or sour.
- Inadequate diet and eating habits may contribute to the adverse changes of the mucosal tissues. The appearance and symptoms frequently resemble those associated with vitamin deficiencies, particularly B vitamins.

C. Alveolar Bone Loss

As a result of systemic osteoporosis, ridge resorption and loss of teeth can occur.[18] Osteoporotic jaws may be unsuitable for conventional prosthetic devices or dental implants.[19]

III. DENTAL HYGIENE CARE

During patient education, a specific relationship of oral conditions to menopause need not be emphasized. Emphasize the need for self-care measures. Because of the importance of local factors, attention is directed to the need for meticulous and daily biofilm control, along with regular and frequent professional care.

A. Appointment Suggestions

The symptoms of physical and emotional changes are kept in mind when planning and conducting the appointment. In treating women entering menopause, consideration is given to the stressful phase of life the patient may be experiencing.

- Rapport begins with the clinician's courtesy, personal attention, and friendly, unhurried manner.
- Give particular attention to details, such as seating the patient promptly, handling materials and instruments efficiently and with calm assurance.
- Consider adjusting the temperature of the room for patient comfort if necessary.

B. Instruction of Patient

- Saliva substitute may be needed to provide relief from xerostomia and aid in the prevention of dental caries.
- Measures for the prevention of periodontal infections can be carefully explained.
- Emphasize reasons for frequent calculus removal as a supplement to meticulous daily self-care.

- Explain the relationship between good general health and oral health.

C. Diet

- Dietary assessment may prove to be a helpful teaching–learning experience by helping the patient identify and correct inadequately balanced food selection (in Chapter 34, page 499).
- Recommend whole grain products, vegetables, and fruits. Choose foods low in fat and cholesterol. Recommend calcium to keep bones strong. Limit alcohol intake to no more than one drink per day for adults.
- Caries prevention through selection of nutritious and noncariogenic foods is especially important for the patient who snacks frequently.

D. Fluoride Therapy

Fluoride recommendations are based on assessment of the patient's caries risk status (Chapter 26, page 383).

DOCUMENTATION

When documenting care for a patient with oral manifestations related to hormonal fluctuations, factors to document include:

- Patient's age and gender.
- Description of the patient's health status related to any endocrine disorder or hormone fluctuations.
- Symptoms and oral manifestations related to hormonal fluctuations.
- Box 51-2 provides an example of a progress note for a patient with an oral manifestation related to reproductive hormone fluctuation.

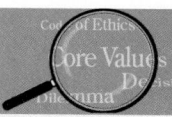

Everyday Ethics

Amy, an 18-year-old female, returns home from her first semester of college and presents with swollen gingiva, weight gain, and stories about considerable amounts of alcoholic beverages being consumed at parties. She also tells Sally, the dental hygienist who has provided care for her since she was a child, that she has just started taking birth control pills and mentions that her mother would be furious if she knew. Sally acknowledges Amy's desire to exercise her independence while away at school but also lectures her extensively on the health consequences of these new behaviors. When she writes her progress notes for the appointment, Sally indicates the term "risky behaviors" in the patient's chart.

Questions for Consideration

1. What ethical issues come into play when Sally considers her responsibility for discussing this situation with Amy's parents, who are financially responsible for her oral health care?
2. Consider what has been entered into the patient's chart—"risky behaviors." What personal values might Sally be bringing into play when she uses this subjective, judgmental statement in writing her progress notes? Has Sally violated Amy's rights by using this documentation style?
3. Using the decision-making steps from Chapter 1 on page 10, prioritize the factors that Sally must address as she determines actions to take in resolving this ethical dilemma.

| BOX 51-2 | **Progress Notes for an Adolescent Patient With Gingivitis** |

Thirteen-year-old female patient reports for routine maintenance appointment. Examination findings include extreme biofilm-induced maxillary anterior gingivitis that appears to be exacerbated by hormonal fluctuations related to patient's irregular menstrual cycle. Patient stated she has stopped flossing because of the bleeding. Motivational interviewing technique discovers that patient values her beautiful smile. Patient agreed to concentrate on careful, complete daily biofilm removal in order to reduce what she called "disgusting and ugly" gingival redness, swelling, and bleeding. Flossing instruction provided. Patient scheduled for 3-month follow-up maintenance appointment.

Signed: _____, RDH Date: _____.

Factors To Teach The Patient

- Self-care procedures that are necessary to maintain good oral health.
- The long-term impact of health behaviors, including lifestyle choices and risk reduction.
- The benefits of fluoride throughout life.
- The importance of nutrition, exercise, and sleep for good health.
- The value of seeking professional help when problems arise.

References

1. Newman MG, Takei HH, Klokkevold PR, Carranza FA. *Carranza's clinical periodontology.* 10th ed. Philadelphia: Saunders; 2006. Chapter 17, Influence of systemic disorders and stress on the periodontium. pp. 284.

2. Resnick MD, Bearman PS, Blum RW, Bauman KE, Harris KM, Jones J, Tabor J, Beuhring T, Sieving RE, Shew M, Ireland M, Bearinger LH, Udry JR. Protecting adolescents from harm: findings from the national longitudinal study on adolescent health. *JAMA.* 1997 Sep;278(19):823–32.

3. Newman MG, Takei HH, Klokkevold PR, Carranza FA. op.cit. p. 285.

4. Albandar JM, Rams TE. Risk factors for periodontitis in children and young persons. *Periodontol 2000.* 2002;29(1):207–22.

5. Albandar JM, Buischi YA, Axelsson P. Caries lesions and dental restorations as predisposing factors in the progression of periodontal diseases in adolescents: a 3-year longitudinal study. *J. Periodontol.* 1995 Apr;66(4):249–54.

6. Hansen BF, Gjermo P, Bellini HT, Ihanamaki K, Saxén L. Prevalence of radiographic alveolar bone loss in young adults: a multinational study. *Int Dent J.* 1995 Feb;45(1):54–61.

7. Armitage GC. Development of a classification system for periodontal diseases and conditions. *Ann Periodontol.* 1999 Dec;4(1):1–6.

8. Susman EJ, Reiter EO, Ford C, Dorn LD. Work group I: developing models of healthy adolescent physical development. *J Adolesc Health.* 2002 Dec;31(6 Suppl):171–4.

9. Regis D, Macgregor ID, Balding JW. Differential prediction of dental health behaviour by self-esteem and health locus of control in young adolescents. *J Clin Periodontol.* 1994 Jan;21(1):7–12.

10. Macgregor ID, Regis D, Balding J. Self-concept and dental health behaviours in adolescents. *J Clin Periodontol.* 1997 May;24(5): 335–9.

11. American Academy of Pediatric Dentistry. 2010–11 Definitions, oral health policies, and clinical guidelines: Guidelines on adolescent oral health care. Revised 2010. Chicago: American Academy of Pediatric Dentistry; revised 2010. pp. 119–26. [cited 2011 Jan 4]. Available from: http://www.aapd.org/media/policies.asp

12. Campbell MA, McGrath PJ. Use of medication by adolescents for the management of menstrual discomfort. *Arch Pediatr Adolesc Med.* 1997 Sep;151(9):905–13.

13. Newman MG, Takei HH, Klokkevold PR, Carranza FA. op.cit., p. 288.

14. Greydanus DE, Patel DR, Rimsza ME. Contraception in the adolescent: an update. *Pediatrics.* 2001 Mar;107(3):562–73.

15. American Dental Association, Council on Scientific Affairs. Antibiotic interference with oral contraceptives. *J Am Dent Assoc.* 2002 Jul;133(7):880.

16. American Dental Association, Health Foundation Research Institute, Department of Toxicology. Antibiotic interference with oral contraceptives. *J Am Dent Assoc.* 1991 Dec;122(12):79.

17. Ciberka RM, Nelson SK, Lefebvre CA. Burning mouth syndrome: a review of etiologies. *J Prosthet Dent.* 1997 Jul;78(1):93–7.

18. Jeffcoat MK, Chesnut CH. Systemic osteoporosis and oral bone loss: evidence shows increased risk factors. *J Am Dent Assoc.* 1993 Nov;124(11):49–56.

19. Friedlander AH. The physiology, medical management and oral implications of menopause. *J Am Dent Assoc.* 2002 Jan;133(1): 73–81.

CHAPTER 52

The Older Adult Patient

ESTHER M. WILKINS, BS, RDH, DMD
JANET H. TOWLE, RN, RDH, BS, MED

Chapter Outline

The number of adults over 65 years of age continues to increase. In 2006, the first of the "baby boom" generation turned 60. They are the first generation to benefit from systemic fluoride in community water supplies and topically in toothpastes. This older population is

- retaining more natural teeth; many with full dentitions.
- placing a high value on maintaining and improving oral health.[1]

Research indicates that the percentage of adults 55 and older seeking dental care is increasing.[2]

- Dental hygienists will be challenged by the complex needs of this aging population.
- As the life span of individuals increases, so does the incidence of chronic diseases.
- Dental hygienists need to be competent in providing safe, preventive, and therapeutic services for the older adult patients in all types of dental practices.

BOX 52-1	Key Words

Elderly Patient

Ageism: discrimination toward/against the aged population.

Aging: the continuous process (biologic, psychologic, social), beginning with conception and ending with death, by which organisms mature and decline.

Alzheimer's disease: a form of irreversible dementia, usually occurring in older adulthood, characterized by gradual deterioration of memory, disorientation, and other features of dementia.

Biologic age: the anatomic or physiologic age of a person as determined by changes in organismic structure and function; takes into account features such as posture, skin texture, strength, speed, and sensory acuity.

Chronologic age: the actual measure of time elapsed since a person's birth.

Dementia: severe mental deterioration involving impairment of mental ability; organic loss of intellectual function.

Dysphagia: difficulty in swallowing.

Emphysema: pathologic accumulation of air in tissues or organs; general use refers to chronic pulmonary emphysema, in which terminal bronchioles become plugged with mucus, the lung and tissue lose elasticity, and breathing difficulties ensue.

Geriatric dentistry: the branch of dentistry that deals with the special knowledge, attitudes, and technical skills required in the provision of oral health care for older adults.

Geriatrics: the branch of medicine that deals with the problems and illnesses of aging and their treatment.

Gerontology: study of the aging process; includes the biologic, psychologic, and sociologic sciences.

Hemostasis: arrest of the escape of blood by either natural (clot formation or vessel spasm) or artificial (compression or ligation) means, or by the interruption of blood flow to a part.

Isolated systolic hypertension: condition in which only the systolic blood pressure is elevated; once thought to be part of the normal aging process; medical intervention is recommended.

Life expectancy: average number of years that a person can be expected to live; expectancy from birth in 1900 averaged 47 years; in 2009, average life expectancy for white females was 80.9 years; black females, 77.4 years; white males, 72.2 years; and black males 70.9 years.*

Lifestyle: relatively permanent organization of activities, including work, leisure, and associated social activities, characterizing an individual.

Osteoid: young bone that has not undergone calcification.

Osteopenia: decreased calcification or density of bone; inadequate osteoid synthesis.

Osteoporosis: low bone mass resulting from an excess of bone resorption over bone formation, with resultant bone fragility and increased risk of fracture.

Polypharmacy: concurrent use of a large number of drugs.

Presbycusis: progressive loss of hearing due to the normal aging process.

Presbyopia: a condition of farsightedness resulting from a loss of elasticity of the lens of the eye due to aging.

Psychologic age: the age of a person as determined by his or her feelings, attitudes, and life perspective.

Senescence: the process of growing old.

Senility: old age; loss of mental, physical, or emotional control; caused by physical and/or mental deterioration.

Sjögren's syndrome: an immunological disorder characterized by insufficient production of the lacrimal gland to produce tears and the salivary glands to produce saliva that results in abnormally dry eyes and mouth.

Tinnitus: ringing, buzzing, tinkling, or hissing sounds in the ear.

---

*Centers for Disease Control and Prevention. Life expectations at birth by race and sex—United States, 2000–2009. *MMWR* 2011 May; 60(18):588.

- An increasing number of dental hygienists will need to specialize in the care of the elderly and be employed in long-term care and resident facilities for the aged.
- Tooth loss increases with age, but not because of age.
- Dental caries and periodontal diseases are the major causes of tooth loss. Periodontal diseases in the older population represent the cumulative effects of long-standing, undiagnosed, untreated, or neglected chronic infection.
- Dental caries as an oral problem for older adults is significant in part because of increases in life longevity, tooth retention, and the adverse oral effects of some medications on saliva production.
- Dental caries may also be related to the belief by many elders in the old paradigm that fluorides are only for children. In fact, water fluoridation and fluoride varnish can provide valuable protection to teeth and exposed root surfaces at all ages.
- Key words relating to older patients are defined in **Box 52-1**.

AGING

I. BIOLOGIC AND CHRONOLOGIC AGE

- When aging is defined from a chronologic viewpoint, the aging population may be recognized as the "older population" (55 years and older), the "elderly" (65 years and older), the "aged" (75 years and older), and the "very old" (85 years and older).[3]

- Biologic age is not synonymous with chronologic age, and, hence, signs of aging appear at different chronologic ages in different individuals. In other words, some people are old at 45 years, whereas others are not old at 75 years.

II. CLASSIFICATION BY FUNCTION

- The degree of general health and physical activity provides a workable classification not based on age.
- Relative to the degree of impairment, older persons may be *functionally independent, frail,* or *functionally dependent.*[4]
- Classification by function is more useful and is defined by Activities of Daily Living (ADL) and Instrumental Activities of Daily Living (IADL) as described in Table 23-3 (page 343).

III. PRIMARY AND SECONDARY AGING[5]

- *Primary aging:* influence of the passage of time on a person, independent of extrinsic influences or disabilities including stress, trauma, or disease.
- *Secondary aging:* growing old in the presence of external influences, with disabilities related to trauma and chronic diseases.

PHYSIOLOGIC AGING

- Primary normal changes with aging are physiologic. They are not to be confused with secondary pathologic influences that accelerate the aging process.
- Each age level brings changes in body metabolism, activity of the cells, endocrine balance, and mental processes. It can be difficult to separate many of these characteristics from pathologic changes.
- In a healthy person, free of chronic diseases and medications with their potential side effects, the tissue changes of aging may be more subtle, appear at a later age, and be influenced by the person's lifestyle.
- Primary physiologic changes that occur as the individual ages are universal, progressive, decremental, intrinsic, and unavoidable.[6] They vary among individuals and among organs and tissues of the same individual.
- During aging, an overall gradual reduction in functional capacities occurs in most organs, with a decrease in cell metabolism and numbers of active cells.
- The following is a summary of selected physiological changes that occur due to the normal aging process.

I. MUSCULOSKELETAL SYSTEM

- Bone volume (mass) decreases gradually after the age of 40.

- Loss of muscle function; diminished muscular strength, and diminished speed of response.
- Curvature of cervical vertebrae due to a decrease in bone density and atrophic changes to cartilage and muscle.
- Joints may stiffen because of loss of elasticity in the ligaments.

II. SKIN

- Thin, wrinkled, and dry, with pigmented spots, loss of tone, and atrophy of the sweat glands.
- Reduced tolerance to temperature extremes and solar exposure is evident.

III. CARDIOVASCULAR SYSTEM[6]

- Decrease in cardiac output; increase in size of left ventricle.
- Blood vessels become less elastic. Lumen of vessels decreases in size with resultant reduction of blood supply to organs, especially the liver and kidneys; increased peripheral resistance.
- Some atherosclerosis is considered normal with aging; diet can be an influence.
- Changes in cardiovasculature do not affect function under normal, unstressful conditions.

IV. RESPIRATORY SYSTEM[6]

- Vital capacity is progressively diminished; decreased pulmonary efficiency and gas exchange.
- Respiratory problems may occur under stressful conditions when demand for oxygen exceeds supply.
- Less effective cough reflex; risk for infections.

V. GASTROINTESTINAL SYSTEM

- Production of hydrochloric acid and other secretions gradually decreases.
- Peristalsis is slowed.
- Decreased absorptive functions can affect nutrition and medications.

VI. CENTRAL NERVOUS SYSTEM

- Intellectual or cognitive function is slowed, not lost.
- Complex tasks may be more difficult.[7]
- Short-term memory declines; long-term memory remains constant.

VII. PERIPHERAL NERVOUS SYSTEM[6]

- Decrease in tactile sensitivity.
- Decreased proprioception (sense of one's position in space); risk for falls.

VIII. SENSES

- *Vision*[6]
  A. Presbyopia.
  B. Decreases in visual acuity (more light needed), peripheral vision, color clarity (problems with blues and greens).
  C. Decreased dilation and constriction of pupils results in difficulty adjusting to changes in light and problems with glare.
- *Hearing*
  A. Presbycusis (hearing loss).
  B. Thicker and dryer cerumen (wax) contributes to hearing loss.
  C. Decrease in ability to hear high frequency tones.
  D. Tinnitus.

IX. ENDOCRINE SYSTEM

- Decrease in thyroid efficiency; decreased basal metabolic rate.
- Altered thermoregulatory system; sensitive to cold; may not respond to infection with increased temperature.

X. IMMUNE SYSTEM[8]

- It is generally accepted that the immune system declines with age. Among individuals the degree of decline varies greatly.
- Nonspecific body defense mechanisms become less effective.
- The activity of B cells and T cells decreases in older age. T cells are most affected.
- With age there may be an increase in autoimmune responses.
- Changes in the immune system result in increased incidence of infections.

PATHOLOGY AND DISEASE

Helping people to learn early in life the health maintenance procedures that prevent the development of chronic illnesses and disabilities is a responsibility of all healthcare personnel.

I. FACTORS THAT INFLUENCE DISEASE

An older person's health status is influenced by many factors. Biologic, environmental, psychosocial, and lifestyle factors influence longevity.

- Genetically, a person may belong to a family that has exhibited resistance to disease factors.
- Individuals may have inherited a specific disease state.
- Healthy dietary habits and regular exercise can prevent or minimize disease.

- The risk factors of smoking, alcohol, and obesity influence disease states.
- Decreased immunologic functioning of aging is a factor in increased susceptibility of both men and women to HIV infection and AIDS.[9]
- Research has shown associations between periodontitis and specific systemic diseases including diabetes mellitus, cardiovascular diseases, and stroke.[10]
- The incidence of disease is higher in individuals from lower educational and socioeconomic backgrounds.

II. RESPONSE TO DISEASE

The diseases that affect the older age group also occur in younger people, but there are differences. Characteristics of the elderly are as follows:

- *Course and severity:* Disease may occur with greater severity and have a longer course, with slower recovery.
- *Pain sensitivity:* may be lessened.
- *Temperature response:* may be altered so that a patient may be very ill without the expected increase in body temperature.
- Healing:
  - Decreased healing capacity.
  - More prone to secondary infection.

III. COMMON CHRONIC CONDITIONS

- Although many seniors function well and live independently in the community, the incidence of chronic diseases increases with advancing age.
- Individuals may have more than one chronic illness.
- The most common chronic conditions are arthritis, hypertension, visual and hearing impairments, cardiovascular diseases, and diabetes.
- Because of the number of chronic conditions, patients may be taking a large number of medications (polypharmacy), which can exacerbate xerostomia and increase the possibility of drug interactions. See Box 25-4 (page 373) for a list of some of the drug groups that promote xerostomia.
- **Box 52-2** lists conditions of particular significance in the elderly.

IV. ALCOHOLISM[11]

1. Due to age-related primary physiological changes older drinkers as compared to younger drinkers:
   - Require less alcohol for adverse effects to occur.
   - Have more severe consequences.
2. Excessive use of alcohol:
   - Exacerbates medical and emotional problems associated with aging.
   - Predisposes a person to adverse drug reactions with medications.
3. Alcohol abuse in seniors is associated with major depressive disorder.

BOX 52-2	Conditions of Significance: Older Adult Patients

Alcoholism
Cardiovascular Conditions
Chronic Obstructive Pulmonary Disease (COPD)
Depression
Diabetes
Hypertension
Isolated Systolic Hypertension[11]
Neurological Disorders
Dementia and Alzheimer's Disease
Parkinson's Disease
Osteoarthritis
Osteoporosis
Sexually Transmitted Diseases
Stroke
Visual Impairments

OSTEOPOROSIS

- Osteoporosis is common in individuals older than age 60, and the incidence increases with age.
- Osteoporosis is a bone disease involving loss of mineral content and bone mass.
- Although most prominent in postmenopausal women, the condition may also occur at other ages and in men.

I. CAUSES

- *Endocrine:* hormonal disturbances; depletion of estrogen after menopause.
- Calcium deficiency or defective absorption of calcium.

II. PREVENTION[12]

Prevention is the first line of defense against osteoporosis.

- Adequate calcium intake during adolescence and early adulthood is critical to forming peak bone mass.
- The minimum requirements for both calcium and vitamin D increase with age.
- Load bearing exercise is necessary to maintain bone mass.

III. RISK FACTORS

A number of risk factors have been identified, some of which usually work together. From the risk factors, a list of methods for long-term prevention can be derived:

- Female gender; positive family history.
- Caucasian or Asian ethnicity (worldwide, Blacks are least affected).
- Low calcium and vitamin D intake (lifelong).
- Early menopause or early surgical removal of ovaries; use of corticosteroids; eating disorders.

- Sedentary lifestyle; lack of exercise.
- Alcohol abuse; tobacco use; high caffeine intake.
- High sodium intake.
- Low body–mass index (BMI).

IV. RELATION TO PERIODONTAL DISEASE[12–15]

- Relationship exists between the reduced bone mineral density of osteoporosis and oral bone loss in skeletal and mandibular bone; oral bone loss pertains to periodontal bone destruction and residual ridge loss in the edentulous person.
- Osteoporosis and periodontal disease have mutual risk factors. Included are smoking, nutritional deficiencies, alcohol use, hormonal status, and others from the aforementioned list of risk factors for osteoporosis.
- Osteoporotic bone is less dense and more readily absorbed; periodontal pathogenic microorganisms can provide the toxic products for increased periodontal breakdown.

V. SYMPTOMS

A. Asymptomatic Period

Osteoporosis develops over many years; a long asymptomatic period of bone change occurs with no clinical symptoms.

B. Clinical Symptoms

- *Backache:* stooping of the posture.
- *Fractures:* hip, compression fractures of spine, ends of long bones.
- *Evidence of bone changes in the mandible:* residual ridge resorption.

VI. TREATMENT

A. Medications[12,16]

A number of medications, with various mechanisms of action, are used to treat osteoporosis. The medications generally, and to different degrees, decrease bone resorption, increase bone formation, or both. Whichever regimen of medications is prescribed, successful treatment and prevention requires simultaneous intake of calcium and vitamin D.

- *Bisphosphonates:* inhibit bone resorption.
- *Selective estrogen receptor modulators (SERMs):* inhibit bone resorption.
- *Calcitonin:* inhibits bone resorption.
- *Parathyroid hormone (PTH):* stimulates bone formation.

B. Activity

- Exercise has a beneficial effect on bone mass.

- Activity and exercise require caution and preventive measures to avoid accidental falls.
- Severe involvement of the spine may require orthopedic support and medication for pain.

C. Behavioral

- Avoidance of smoking and excessive alcoholic intake.

VII. DENTAL HYGIENE MANAGEMENT CONSIDERATIONS

- Do not rush; prevent falls.
- Provide extra time for positioning; provide cushioning.
- Taking bisphosphonates is a contraindication for dental surgery.
- Health promotion opportunities exist for long-term prevention. Encourage:
  - Smoking cessation.
  - Limiting alcohol consumption.
  - Healthy lifestyles involving adequate calcium and Vitamin D intake and routine exercise.

ALZHEIMER'S DISEASE

Dementia is severe impairment of cognitive abilities, notably thinking, memory, and judgment. Alzheimer's disease is a nonreversible type of dementia and the most common of all dementias.

- *Two types:*
  - Early onset: rare, reported in patients in their 30s and 40s.
  - Late onset: most common, people over 65.
- *Etiology unknown:* theories include genetics, environment, nutrition, free radicals, and infectious agents.[17]
- Average duration is 8 to 10 years from onset of symptoms to death.

I. SYMPTOMS

- The common impairments of Alzheimer's disease may be divided into six or seven overlapping stages that may extend up to 20 years.
- In **Box 52-3**, characteristics are divided into the following stages: no impairment, very mild cognitive decline, mild cognitive decline, moderate cognitive decline, moderately severe cognitive decline, severe cognitive decline, and very severe cognitive decline.

II. TREATMENT

- There is no proven treatment to prevent or cure the disease.
- Treatment is designed for supporting the family as well as the patient.
- Requires a prolonged multidisciplinary effort.

- Medications are for patients with mild to moderate symptoms.[17]
  - Cholinesterase inhibitors.
  - The medications slow progression of the disease, temporarily improve cognitive function, and provide some improvement in behavioral symptoms.
- *Medications to address behavioral problems:* antidepressants, antianxiety, and antipsychotics.
- Anticonvulsants for the small percentage who have seizures.

III. MANAGEMENT CONSIDERATIONS

- *Goals of dental hygiene care:*
  - Preserve oral health and function.
  - Provide comfort; prevent disease.
- *Care plan:*
  - Directed at the stage of the disease.
  - Provide comprehensive care in anticipation of future decline in oral health.
- *Undiagnosed patients:* referral to the patient's physician is made when patient's behavior is suspect.

A. Early Stages

- Review of the patient's medical and dental history at each maintenance appointment may reveal lapses in memory and other signs of early disease.
- An early sign may be a slow decline of interest in oral hygiene and personal care.
- Provide routine care with initiation of aggressive preventive regimens.
- Three-month intervals are recommended.
- Topical fluoride applications; fluoride varnish.
- Oral hygiene instruction; involve caregivers early in disease process.

B. Later Stages

- Routine intraoral examination to assess lesions due to cancer, medications, or injury.
- Sedation may be required.
- Possible need for mouth prop and physical restraint.
- Power toothbrushes may improve dental biofilm removal.
- Caregivers assume daily oral care.
- Patient may reside in a long-term care facility. Dental hygienists who specialize in the treatment of this population may oversee care.

SEXUALLY TRANSMITTED DISEASES (STD)

The most common sexually transmitted diseases include chlamydia, syphilis, HIV/AIDS, genital herpes, gonorrhea, and human papilloma virus (HPV). While once thought to be the realm of younger generations, sexually transmitted diseases are on the rise in the elderly populations.

BOX 52-3 | Stages of Alzheimer's Disease

Experts have developed "stages" to describe how a person's abilities change from normal function through advanced Alzheimer's.

It is important to keep in mind that stages are general guides, and symptoms vary greatly. Not everyone will experience the same symptoms or progress at the same rate.

This seven-stage framework is based on a system developed by Barry Reisberg, M.D., clinical director of the New York University School of Medicine's Silberstein Aging and Dementia Research Center.

Stage 1: No impairment (normal function) The person does not experience any memory problems. An interview with a medical professional does not show any evidence of symptoms of dementia.

Stage 2: Very mild cognitive decline (may be normal age-related changes or earliest signs of Alzheimer's disease) The person may feel as if he or she is having memory lapses—forgetting familiar words or the location of everyday objects. But no symptoms of dementia can be detected during a medical examination or by friends, family, or co-workers.

Stage 3: Mild cognitive decline (early-stage Alzheimer's can be diagnosed in some, but not all, individuals with these symptoms) Friends, family, or co-workers begin to notice difficulties. During a detailed medical interview, doctors may be able to detect problems in memory or concentration. Common stage 3 difficulties include:

- Noticeable problems coming up with the right word or name
- Trouble remembering names when introduced to new people
- Having noticeably greater difficulty performing tasks in social or work settings Forgetting material that one has just read
- Losing or misplacing a valuable object
- Increasing trouble with planning or organizing

Stage 4: Moderate cognitive decline (mild or early-stage Alzheimer's disease) At this point, a careful medical interview should be able to detect clear-cut problems in several areas:

- Forgetfulness of recent events
- Impaired ability to perform challenging mental arithmetic—for example, counting backward from 100 by 7s
- Greater difficulty performing complex tasks, such as planning dinner for guests, paying bills, or managing finances
- Forgetfulness about one's own personal history
- Becoming moody or withdrawn, especially in socially or mentally challenging situations

Stage 5: Moderately severe cognitive decline (moderate or mid-stage Alzheimer's disease) Gaps in memory and thinking are noticeable, and individuals begin to need help with day-to-day activities. At this stage, those with Alzheimer's may:

- Be unable to recall their own address or telephone number or the high school or college from which they graduated
- Become confused about where they are or what day it is
- Have trouble with less challenging mental arithmetic; such as counting backward from 40 by subtracting 4s or from 20 by 2s
- Need help choosing proper clothing for the season or the occasion
- Still remember significant details about themselves and their family
- Still require no assistance with eating or using the toilet

Stage 6: Severe cognitive decline (moderately severe or mid-stage Alzheimer's disease) Memory continues to worsen, personality changes may take place, and individuals need extensive help with daily activities. At this stage, individuals may:

- Lose awareness of recent experiences as well as of their surroundings
- Remember their own name but have difficulty with their personal history
- Distinguish familiar and unfamiliar faces but have trouble remembering the name of a spouse or caregiver
- Need help dressing properly and may, without supervision, make mistakes such as putting pajamas over daytime clothes or shoes on the wrong feet
- Experience major changes in sleep patterns—sleeping during the day and becoming restless at night
- Need help handling details of toileting (for example, flushing the toilet, wiping, or disposing of tissue properly)
- Have increasingly frequent trouble controlling their bladder or bowels
- Experience major personality and behavioral changes, including suspiciousness and delusions (such as believing that their caregiver is an impostor) or compulsive, repetitive behavior like hand-wringing or tissue shredding
- Tend to wander or become lost

Stage 7: Very severe cognitive decline (severe or late-stage Alzheimer's disease) In the final stage of this disease, individuals lose the ability to respond to their environment, to carry on a conversation and, eventually, to control movement. They may still say words or phrases.

At this stage, individuals need help with much of their daily personal care, including eating or using the toilet. They may also lose the ability to smile, to sit without support, and to hold their heads up. Reflexes become abnormal. Muscles grow rigid. Swallowing impaired.

(Reprinted with permission from Alzheimer's Association. Stages of Alzheimer's [Internet]. Chicago: Alzheimers'Association; 2011. [updated 2011 Jun 1; cited 2011 July 14.] Available from: http://www.alz.org/alzheimers_disease_stages_of_alzheimers.asp#stage1)

I. INCIDENCE IN OLDER POPULATIONS[18,19,20]

- There has been a 50% rise in the number of men over 40 diagnosed with STDs.
- The most common STD in this demographic is HIV/AIDS with a high percent of all new HIV/AIDS cases in the over 55 years age group.
- *Factors that influence the increase in numbers include:*
  - Increased use of medications to treat erectile dysfunction.
  - Increased divorce rate.
  - People living longer in better health.
  - Sexually active senior women are more prone to acquiring sexually transmitted diseases due to the thinning of the epithelium of the vaginal area and a diminished immune system.
  - Increased number of seniors living in assisted living centers or senior housing communities.
  - Cultural and generational differences may explain why selected seniors are not as knowledgeable about the need for safe-sex practices.
  - Seniors might not practice safe sex since the risk of pregnancy is eliminated.

II. DENTAL HYGIENE MANAGEMENT CONSIDERATIONS

- *Medical referral or consultation*
  - A consultation with the patient's physician may be necessary to determine impact on dental hygiene care.
  - Medications to treat the STD will be determined by the patient's physician.
- *Goals of dental hygiene care:*
  - Open, non-judgmental communication.
  - Increased patient awareness of the transmission of STDs.
  - Importance of discussing this with the physician.
- *Care plan*
  - Include use of safe-sex practices in patient education.

ORAL FINDINGS IN AGING

The oral condition in generally healthy elderly people compares favorably with the oral condition of generally healthy younger people.[21] Healthy tissue features of primary aging need to be separated from the long-term effects of secondary aging because of chronic diseases and their medications.

I. SOFT TISSUES

A. Lips

- *Tissue changes:* Dry, purse-string opening results from dehydration and loss of elasticity within the tissues.

- *Angular cheilitis[22]*
  - Angular cheilitis is not specifically an age-related lesion, but it is seen frequently among elderly persons.
  - Etiologic factors may be candidiasis and vitamin B deficiency.
  - Appears as skin folds with fissuring at the angles of the mouth and can be related to reduced vertical dimension or inadequate support of the lips.
  - Cheilitis in conjunction with dentures is described in Chapter 53 on page 818.

B. Oral Mucosa

- *Atrophic changes:* The tissue may become thinner and less vascular, with a loss of elasticity. Clinically, the smooth shiny appearance is related to thinning of the epithelium.
- *Hyperkeratosis:* White, patchy areas may develop because of irritation from sharp edges of broken teeth, restorations, or dentures, and from use of tobacco.
- *Capillary fragility:* Facial bruises and petechiae of the mucosa are common.

C. Tongue

- *Atrophic glossitis (burning tongue):* The tongue appears smooth, shiny, and bald, with atrophied papillae. The condition is usually related to anemia that results from a deficiency of iron or combinations of deficiencies.
- Elderly people have deficiency anemias more frequently than do those in other age groups because of nutritional factors, but not because of aging specifically.
- *Taste sensations:[23]* Renewal of taste buds is slower in the elderly. The acuity of the perception for salt declines with age. The perception of sweet and sour does not decline with age. Olfactory acuity, which significantly affects taste, declines more than taste.
  - Flavoring agents and spices can be added to foods instead of salt and sugar to enhance taste.
  - Tongue cleaning may increase taste perception for patients with prostheses.
- *Sublingual varicosities*
  - Clinical appearance: Deep, red or bluish nodular dilated vessels on either side of the midline on the ventral surface of the tongue.
  - Significance: Although frequently occurring, these varicosities do not necessarily have a direct relation to systemic conditions.

D. Xerostomia[24]

- Xerostomia is prevalent in the elderly but not a consequence of age.
- Causes of xerostomia include:

- Systemic medications provide the most common influence.
- Autoimmune diseases (Sjögren's syndrome) and other systemic diseases.
- Radiation therapy.

E. Oral Candidiasis[25]

- Oral candidiasis is the most common infection of the oral mucosal tissues.
- Denture stomatitis and angular cheilitis represent the two common forms, as described in Chapter 53, page 818.
- Candidiasis is associated with the use of antibiotics, head and neck radiation therapy, chemotherapy, steroids and other immunosuppressive drugs.
- Medical conditions that alter the immune system, including diabetes and HIV infection permit an overgrowth of the Candida organisms.
- Patients with xerostomia have an increased incidence of candidiasis.

II. TEETH

A. Color

- Darkening or yellowing is the result of changes in the underlying dentin.
- Color changes are from long use of tobacco and beverages such as tea and coffee.
- Dark intrinsic stains from dental restorations may be evident.

B. Dental Pulp[7,26]

- Whether pulpal changes can be considered results of aging is questionable.
- Pulpal changes develop as reactions to wear, dental caries, restorations, bruxism, and other assaults during the elderly person's long life.
- Changes noted here may be observed at younger ages but are seen more frequently in older people.
  - Narrowing of pulp chambers and root canals; increased deposition of secondary and tertiary dentin.
  - Progressive deposition of calcified masses (pulp stones or denticles).
  - Number of blood vessels entering the tooth declines with age.

C. Attrition

- The teeth of elderly people frequently show signs of wear, which may be the long-term effects of diet, occupational factors, or bruxism.
- Attrition may be accompanied by chipping, and teeth may seem more brittle, particularly compared with teeth of young people.

D. Abrasion

- Abrasion at the cervical third of a tooth may be the result of extended use of a hard toothbrush in a horizontal direction with an abrasive dentifrice.
- With current preventive measures, use of soft-textured brushes, and attention to abrasiveness of dentifrices, future generations will be less likely to exhibit such tooth alterations.

E. Root Caries[27]

1. *Prevalence:* Older adults have more root caries than any other age group. Risk factors, not age, are responsible for the number of root surface caries.
2. *Risk factors:*
   - Exposed root surfaces due to:
     - Periodontal infections that cause recession.
     - Horizontal toothbrushing technique.
   - Biofilm retention due to inadequate oral hygiene:
     - Cognitive and physical disabilities that hinder biofilm removal.
     - Inadequate oral care received.
     - Faulty restorations and partial dentures retain cariogenic food substances for biofilm.
   - Xerostomia and medications.
   - High carbohydrate diet; frequency.
   - Combinations of these factors increase the risk.
3. *Effect of fluoride:* Adults with longtime residence in a fluoridated community have substantially fewer root carious lesions than those in a nonfluoridated community. This is especially true for lifelong residents where there has been natural fluoride in the water.[28]
4. Prevention is as important for older adults as it is for all age groups. Emphasis is placed on periodontal health because attachment loss with resultant root exposure needs to be prevented. Caries preventive agents need to be strongly recommended, including the professional application of fluoride varnish.

III. PERIODONTIUM

A. Tissue Changes Related to Aging

1. *Bone*
   - Osteoporosis may be present.[12–15]
   - Depressed vascularity, a reduction in metabolism, and reduced healing ability affect bone.
2. *Cementum*
   - Increased thickness has been demonstrated. In one series of measurements, the average overall thickness of the cementum at 20 years of age was 0.095 mm, whereas cementum from 60-year-old persons measured 0.215 mm.[29]
3. *Gingiva*
   - Most gingival changes can be traced to the effects of infection or to anatomic factors. For example,

gingival recession is common in older individuals. Predisposing factors may be a lack of sufficient attached gingiva or malposition of the teeth.

■ Increased density of blood vessels; blood vessels with active flow decreased.[7]

B. Risk Factors[1]

■ Similar to younger individuals.
■ May be modified by chronic diseases and medications.

C. Clinical Findings

The periodontal tissues reflect the health and disease of the patient over the years.

   Moderate periodontal disease may be more prevalent than advanced disease.[1] One of the following may apply to any patient.

1. *The healthy periodontium:* Healthy tissues that have been maintained over the years may have had a minimum of disease. The radiographs show little if any bone recession, the gingiva are firm, and the appearance is normal. Probing reveals minimal sulcus depth with no bleeding. The teeth are not mobile.
2. *The patient with periodontal infection:* Neglect or omission of preventive measures and therapy over the years may have resulted in a chronic periodontal infection with extension of tissue destruction into the bone, periodontal ligament, and cementum. Loss of attachment, deep periodontal pockets, tooth mobility, and radiographic signs of periodontitis may be present.
3. *The treated patient:* Although the patient was subject to periodontal infection, treatment was completed, and the tissues were maintained in health through personal care and professional supervision. The tissues may show the effects of the treated disease, such as scar tissue. Areas of recession with exposed cementum may also be evident. The teeth are not mobile, especially when occlusal analysis and adjustment has been featured.

DENTAL HYGIENE CARE

As with all patients, the dental hygiene process of care for the elderly is based on patient need. Many elderly people value oral health as a component of overall health and wellness. The following material emphasizes components of the dental hygiene process of care that are of special concern.

■ Care for the older patient needs to be planned in terms of comprehensive, not palliative, treatment.
■ Increasing numbers of the elderly population avail themselves of esthetic dental services.

■ Adaptations need to be made to the process of care when cognitive, sensory, or physical conditions/limitations are present.
■ Long-term maintenance for the prevention of oral disease is the basic objective.

I. BARRIERS TO CARE

A. Lack of Perceived Need

■ Most common reason the elderly do not seek dental care.[2]
■ Older generations believed that a decline in oral health was the result of the aging process.

B. Economic and Access Barriers

■ Fixed income after retirement.
■ Lack of dental insurance; Medicare provides little dental coverage.
■ Transportation problems.
■ Functional disabilities affecting mobility limit access without assistance.

C. Physical/Architectural Barriers

■ Accessibility to the dental office or clinic.
■ Restrictions to access to care for institutional residents.
■ Wheelchair access.
■ Hazards, such as small rugs, which can slide on polished floors; loose corners of rugs, which can be tripped over; and irregularities in floor levels, need to be eliminated.
■ Sitting for extended periods, keeping mouth open, and such might be difficult; provide frequent opportunities to change positions.
■ Consider several short appointments as opposed to extended appointments.
■ Raise the chair to a sitting position slowly due to the possibility of postural hypotension.

II. ASSESSMENT

A. Patient History

Preparation of a careful and detailed medical and dental history takes on particular significance. Suggestions for good communication include the following:

■ Allow sufficient time for reviewing complex histories.
■ Eliminate distracting background music or sounds.
■ Sit facing the patient and speak clearly with a low tone of voice.
■ Speak directly to the patient even when a caregiver is present.
■ Do not call the patient by his/her first name unless the patient suggests doing so.

B. Medications

- Because of the prevalence of chronic diseases, older patients are the largest consumers of both prescription and over-the-counter medications.
- Drug usage and the incidence of adverse drug reactions goes up with age.
- Obtain a complete list. Include herbal and dietary supplements.
- Ask the patient to bring in either the bottles that contain the various medications (over-the-counter as well as prescription items) or a written copy of the labels so that a list may be kept in the patient's record.
- The patient's physician is the best source for an accurate list of prescription medications.
- *References for checking drugs:* Each practice center or clinic needs access to current references, such as the *Physician's Desk Reference (PDR), Merck Manual,* or pharmacology reference Web sites specifically directed to the dental practice.
- Review the list of medications at each maintenance appointment. Changes in health status and medication usage occur.
- Review each medication to determine:
  - Potential adverse side effects. Pay particular attention to effects on the oral cavity such as xerostomia and gingival hyperplasia.
  - Possible drug interactions with products recommended or used during the appointment.
  - Certain medications may require frequent bathroom breaks.

C. Need for Antibiotic Premedication

- Conditions that require prophylactic coverage may be found in the elderly.
- Prosthetic heart valves are susceptible to infective endocarditis.[30]
- Individuals with uncontrolled diabetes or those who receive chemotherapeutic or steroid treatments may have an increased susceptibility to infection.
- A list of conditions for which prophylactic premedication is recommended can be found in Chapter 9 on page 131.

D. Vital Signs

- Blood pressure is determined and recorded at each visit.

E. Intraoral and Extraoral Examination

- The need for careful, periodic examination of the oral mucosa from lips to throat cannot be overstressed at any age, but it is especially crucial for the elderly patient because oral cancer occurs with increasing frequency with advancing years.
- Most oral lesions exist without the patient being aware of them.

- Document lesions with accurate descriptions and comparisons over time.
- When indicated, patient referral for biopsy is planned with the patient.

III. PREVENTIVE CARE PLAN

- Older patients may need frequent appointments to maintain a high level of oral health.
- The content of a care plan resembles that for other age groups with an emphasis on the control of dental biofilm.
- Follow-up to determine complete care, healed gingival tissues, and meticulous daily biofilm removal.
- Give printed oral health instructions to partner or care giver to be posted in bathroom or where the patient will be performing self-care.

DENTAL BIOFILM CONTROL

I. OBJECTIVES

Basic objectives do not differ from those for younger people: Infection needs to be eliminated and controlled. Patients with cognitive, mental, and physical deficits can provide a challenge to the dental hygienist.

II. DENTAL BIOFILM FORMATION

A. Factors Contributing to Accumulation of Biofilm

- Gingival recession with wide embrasures that result from periodontal destruction provides a larger surface area for biofilm retention.
- Exposed cementum with areas of abrasion or dental caries at the cervical third of a tooth can create undercut areas where special adaptation of biofilm removal devices is needed.
- Decreased saliva production reduces or eliminates the cleansing and lubricating effects of saliva.

B. Biofilm Retention and Removal

- Exposed untreated cementum may hold biofilm more readily than does enamel. A smooth root surface is less likely to hold biofilm, and biofilm removal efforts can be more successful.
- Restorations and prostheses provide a more complex dentition for personal care. Biofilm removal requires more time, patience, and motivation.
- Deficient restorations may have overhanging margins that provide areas for biofilm retention.
- Lack of dexterity related to disabling conditions resulting from chronic diseases, such as arthritis and Parkinsonism, makes biofilm removal more difficult. Consider recommending electric toothbrushes and oral irrigators when appropriate.

III. APPROACH TO INSTRUCTION

- Motivation through expression of sincere interest on the part of dental personnel can be an influencing factor in helping the patient to better health.
- Allow sufficient time; do not leave instructions until the end of the appointment.
- When appropriate, include the caregiver in instructions.
- Carefully assess the patient's ability to perform each technique.
- Base instruction on the patient's functional status.
- Work from what the patient already knows.
- Make changes gradually over time.
- Repeated reinforcement and evaluation are critical.

IV. SPECIFIC RECOMMENDATIONS

A. Selection of Dental Biofilm Removal Devices

- Use of a power toothbrush may help patients with impaired hand function.
- Power toothbrushes, recommended for all patients, are often easier for caregivers to manage.
- Adaptations to alter the handle of a manual brush are described in Chapter 56 on page 864.

- Interproximal brushes are recommended for open gingival embrasures. Methods are described in Chapter 27, page 396.

B. Dentifrice Selection

- Fluoride ingredient mandatory for root caries prevention.
- Mild abrasive agent to prevent abrasion of root surfaces.
- Desensitizing ingredient for exposed dentinal tubules.

C. Relief for Xerostomia

- Recommendations are described in Chapter 25 on page 374.
- Provide specific instructions for use of a saliva substitute.

D. Motivation and Instruction

- Instruction and motivation techniques are applied gradually and regularly at frequent intervals for best results.
- Suggestions for adaptations of instruction for elderly patients are listed in **Table 52-1**.

TABLE 52-1	CHARACTERISTICS AFFECTING INSTRUCTION FOR THE ELDERLY PATIENT
CHARACTERISTIC OF THE ELDERLY PATIENT	**SUGGESTIONS FOR PATIENT INSTRUCTION**
Vision impaired	Provide adequate lighting. Provide instructional materials in large print on nonglare paper. Avoid instructional materials in blue and green colors. For the patient who wears prescription eyeglasses, make sure the glasses are worn while instruction is being given. Recommend that eyeglasses be worn at home while performing biofilm control procedures.
Hearing impaired; loss of sensitivity to higher tones	Speak distinctly in normal voice. Look directly at patient while speaking; many are lip readers.
Hearing aid	Reduce background noise; turn off music. Lower or turn off when handpiece is used.
Slowing of voluntary responses Slowing of speed of thought associations Rate of learning slowed, ability to learn not changed Changes in speed of vocalization	Make suggestions gradually, over a series of appointments. Be realistic and practical with expectations; go slowly, anticipate difficulties, give cues and clues. Distinguish between slowness of learning and inability to learn.
Memory difficulties	Provide written instruction; spoken instructions may be forgotten or misunderstood. Provide repeated reinforcement. Give instructions to caregivers.
Apparent frustration with diminished functional abilities	Acknowledge frustration; retain positive attitude; provide repeated reinforcement.
Symptoms of depression	Acknowledge feelings; positive attitude but avoid overly cheerful demeanor; repeated reinforcement.

PERIODONTAL CARE

The incidence and severity of periodontal diseases increase with age as an effect of disease accumulation. The extent of periodontal destruction reflects the length of time the tissues have been exposed to disease-producing factors, primarily biofilm microorganisms.

- Implementation of periodontal care includes complete debridement of calculus and biofilm.
- Follow-up evaluation to assess the need for additional therapy is essential.
- The patient's cognitive, mental, or physical condition may necessitate shorter appointments.
- Quadrant instrumentation with anesthesia may be appropriate.

DENTAL CARIES CONTROL

- Assess diet; diet record covering several days.
- Diet adjustment to eliminate cariogenic foods and make appropriate substitutions.
- Emphasis on prevention of root caries.
- Professionally applied topical fluoride treatments: fluoride varnish.
- *Daily self-applied fluoride therapy:*
  A. Fluoride dentifrice.
  B. Fluoride rinses and gels; custom trays as necessary.
- Chlorhexidine rinses for individuals with high bacterial counts; effective against *Mutans streptococcus* (page 384 in Chapter 26).
- Xylitol chewing gum for patients without chewing and swallowing difficulties.

DIET AND NUTRITION

I. DIETARY HABITS

A. Nutritional Deficiencies

- Dietary and resulting nutritional deficiencies are common in older people.
- Characteristic changes, such as burning tongue, angular cheilitis, and atrophic glossitis, may be related to vitamin B deficiencies.

B. Factors Contributing to Dietary and Nutritional Deficiencies

- Limited budget; living alone or eating alone.
- Not eating regular meals; frequently using nonnutritious snacks.
- Lacking interest in shopping for or preparing food.
- Acuteness of senses (taste, smell) lowered; may seek highly seasoned or sweetened foods.
- Inadequate masticatory efficiency because of tooth loss or dentures that no longer fit properly.
- Adverse food selection may result from social embarrassment over inability to chew.
- Following dietary fads that provide only a limited and unbalanced diet.
- Difficulty in swallowing.
- Alcoholism.

II. DIETARY NEEDS OF THE AGED

The nutritional needs of older persons vary from those of younger persons.

- The number of calories needs to be reduced as a result of decreased energy needs.
- Protein, vitamins, minerals, and water are particularly important for body function, repair, and resistance to disease.
- Increased need for calcium, vitamin D, and folate.
- A necessary objective in geriatric nutrition is to retard the progression of diet-induced chronic diseases. Examples of these are atherosclerosis related to high dietary cholesterol, anemias related to iron and folic acid deficiencies, and osteoporosis resulting from calcium and vitamin D deficiency.
- Fluoride intake over the years is beneficial in the prevention of osteoporosis and fractures of the bones, and water fluoridation is beneficial for direct application to the teeth.

III. INSTRUCTION IN DIET AND ORAL HEALTH

- Dietary analysis by means of a 4- or 5-day record of the patient's diet can provide information to guide recommended changes.
- Patients with cognitive and/or memory deficits may be unable to provide an accurate food diary. If possible, enlist the help of family members or caretakers.
- Minimally, an accurate 24-hour food diary needs to be obtained.
- Recommendations for aging patients are based on establishing a well-balanced diet with limited amounts of cariogenic foods for dental caries prevention.
- Provide patient with dietary educational materials.
- Patient motivation may be enhanced by discussing the relationship of dietary deficiencies to:
  - Lowered resistance to disease
  - Appearance
  - Premature aging

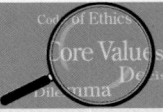 **Everyday Ethics**

Mr. and Mrs. Bracken were among Dr. Roberts' first patients when he began his practice almost 30 years ago. They keep a strict 4-month maintenance plan with the dental hygienist. Rosemary, the new hygienist, is looking forward to meeting and treating the Brackens for the first time as she has heard many wonderful things about this lovely elderly couple.

On completion of the oral examination with Mrs. Bracken, Rosemary recorded significant dental biofilm retention and evidence of xerostomia. She immediately begins to give the patient detailed homecare instructions and asks for a complete listing of medications Mrs. Bracken is taking for her arthritis, angina, and diabetes. Mrs. Bracken left the appointment confused and upset.

Questions for Consideration

1. Which of the ethical core values (Table II-1 in Section II Introduction, page 38) apply in this scenario? Considering that Mrs. Bracken seemed overwhelmed at the end of her appointment, how may Rosemary have erred in her judgment of the patient and the instruction she gave? Suggest alternative approaches.

2. To ensure the autonomy of Mr. and Mrs. Bracken while acknowledging their longevity in the practice, how can the medical status of these patients be clarified?

3. Using the questions in Table V-1 in Section V Introduction (page 362) outline at least 3 alternative care plans that Rosemary could have used for her appointment with Mrs. Bracken.

DOCUMENTATION

The permanent record for an elderly adult needs complete personal health history followed from initial appointment to include a minimum of the following:

- Detailed health history, dental history, medications history and current radiographs with exposure records, extra- and intraoral examination with particular emphasis on oral cancer, vital signs, dental and periodontal clinical examination, record of periodontal probing, occlusion, dental calculus, biofilm scoring, and teeth (restorations, attrition and other hard tissue findings.
- For each professional visit, a summary of current findings and planned treatment as well as outcomes from previous appointment treatments.
- A sample individual progress note may be reviewed in **Box 52-4**.

 **Factors To Teach The Patient**

- To remember to tell the dentist and dental hygienist all changes in personal health, medical care received since the last appointment, and all changes in prescriptions.
- The interrelationship of the systemic and oral health.
- The dentition can last a lifetime. Daily preventive measures and a healthy lifestyle are essential.
- The value of a well-balanced diet with reduced calories and regular exercise to successful aging.
- Importance of drinking fluoridated water when it is available.
- Dental caries is a transmissible disease; therefore, it is urgent to have all cavities restored and dental biofilm cleaned from the teeth every day.

BOX 52-4	Example Progress Note

Mary B returned for first alternating appointment after periodontal therapy. She had had a crown lengthening. The RDH in the periodontal office sent the message that Mary B needed more help with the care for the area of the surgery. Clinical examination showed area to be red and inflamed. Mary B had been rinsing in mild warm salt water. Dora (dental hygienist) had the general dentist look at it, and he advised chlorhexidine rinse. And brush all the other teeth several times a day to get the whole mouth as clean as possible; lots of fruit, Vitamin C and avoid irritating spicy things. Call Friday and let us know how it feels— we can make the appt. to start the crown preparation.

Signed: _____, RDH Date: _____

References

1. Niessen LC, Fedele DJ. Older adults – implications for private dental practitioners. *J Calif Dent Assoc.* 2005 Sep;33(9):695–703.
2. Macek MD, Cohen LA, Reid BC, Manski RJ. Dental visits among older U.S. adults, 1999: the roles of dentition status and costs. *J Am Dent Assoc.* 2004 Aug;135(8):1154–62.
3. World Health Organization. Planning and organization of geriatric services. Report of a WHP Expert Committee. *World Health Organ Tech Rep Ser.* 1974;(548):11.
4. Ettinger RL. The unique oral health needs of an aging population. *Dent Clin North Am.* 1997 Oct;41(4):633–49.
5. Busse EW, Pfeifer E, eds. *Behavior and adaptation in late life.* 2nd ed. Boston: Little, Brown and Company; 1977. Busse EW. Theories of aging. p. 9.
6. Ebersole P, Hess P, Touhy T, Jett K. *Gerontological nursing & healthy aging.* 2nd ed. St. Louis: Mosby; 2005. Chapter 7, Physical changes of aging; p. 84–105.
7. Berg R, Morgenstern NE. Physiologic changes in the elderly. *Dent Clin North Am.* 1997 Oct;41(4):651–68.
8. Saxon SV, Etten MJ. *Physical change and aging. A guide for the helping professions.* 4th ed. New York: Tiresias Press; 2003. Chapter 14, The immune system; p. 294 –5.

9. Woolery WA. Occult HIV infection: diagnosis and treatment of older patients. *Geriatrics.* 1997 Nov; 52(11):51,55–8,61.

10. Persson RE, Persson GR. The elderly at risk for periodontitis and systemic diseases. *Dent Clin North Am.* 2005 Apr;49(2):279–92.

11. Friedlander AH, Norman DC. Geriatric alcoholism: pathophysiology and dental implications. *J Am Dent Assoc.* 2006 Mar;137(3):330–8.

12. Jeffcoat M. The association between osteoporosis and oral bone loss. *J Periodontol.* 2005 Nov;76(11 Suppl):2125–32.

13. Wactawski-Wende J. Periodontal diseases and osteoporosis: association and mechanisms. *Ann Periodontol.* 2001 Dec;6(1):197–208.

14. von Wowern N, Klausen B, Kollerup G. Osteoporosis: a risk factor in periodontal disease. *J Periodontol.* 1994 Dec;65(12):1134–8.

15. Wactawski-Wende J, Grossi SG, Trevisan M, Genco RJ, Tezal M, Dunford RG, Ho AW, Hausmann E, Hreshchyshyn MM. The role of osteopenia in oral bone loss and periodontal disease. *J Periodontol.* 1996 Oct;67(10 Suppl)1076–84.

16. Mulligan R, Sobel S. Osteoporosis: diagnostic testing, interpretation, and correlations with oral health: implications for dentistry. *Dent Clin North Am.* 2005 Apr;49(2):463–84.

17. Little JW. Special patient care. Dental management of patients with Alzheimer's disease. *Gen Dent.* 2005 Jul-Aug;53(4):289–96.

18. Jena AB, Goldman DP, Kamdar AK, Lakdawalla DN, Lu Y. Sexually transmitted diseases among users of erectile dysfunction drugs: analysis of claims data. *Ann Intern Med.* 2010 Jul 6;153(1):1–7.

19. Centers for Disease Control and Prevention. Estimates of New HIV Infections in the United States [Internet]. Atlanta: Centers for Disease Control and Prevention; 2008 Aug 3 [cited 2011 Apr 21]. Available from: http://www.cdc.gov/hiv/topics/surveillance/resources/factsheets/incidence.htm

20. Centers for Disease Control and Prevention. HIV/AIDS Statistics and Surveillance: Basic Statistics [Internet]. Atlanta: Centers for Disease Control and Prevention; 2009 [updated 2011 Feb 28; cited 2011 Apr 21]. Available from: http://www.cdc.gov/hiv/topics/surveillance/basic.htm#hivaidsage

21. Ship JA, Baum BJ. Old age in health and disease. Lessons from the oral cavity. *Oral Surg Oral Med Oral Pathol.* 1993 Jul;76(1):40–4.

22. Langlais RP, Craig CS. *Color atlas of common oral conditions.* 3rd ed. Philadelphia: Lippincott Williams & Wilkins; 2003. Section 5, Intraoral findings by color changes; p. 94.

23. Winkler S, Garg AK, Mekayarajjananonth T, Bakaeen LG, Khan E. Depressed taste and smell in geriatric patients. *J Am Dent Assoc.* 1999 Dec;130(12):1759–65.

24. Atkinson JC, Grisius M, Massey W. Salivary hypofunction and xerostomia: diagnosis and treatment. *Dent Clin North Am.* 2005 Apr;49(2):309–26.

25. Fantasia JE. Diagnosis and treatment of common oral lesions found in the elderly. *Dent Clin North Am.* 1997 Oct;41(4):877–90.

26. Seltzer S, Bender IB. *The dental pulp. Biologic considerations in dental procedures.* 3rd ed. St. Louis: Ishiyaku EuroAmerica; 1990. p. 324–48.

27. Saunders RH, Meyerowitz C. Dental caries in older adults. *Dent Clin North Am.* 2005 Apr;49(2):293–308.

28. Stamm JW, Banting DW, Imrey PB. Adult root caries survey of two similar communities with contrasting natural water fluoride levels. *J Am Dent Assoc.* 1990 Feb;120(2):143–9.

29. Zander HA, Hurzeler B. Continuous cementum apposition. *J Dent Res.* 1958 Nov-Dec;37(6):1035–44.

30. Little JW. Special medical concerns in the dental management of older adults. *Gen Dent.* 2004 Mar-Apr;52(2):152–60.

The Edentulous Patient

ESTHER M. WILKINS, BS, RDH, DMD
KATHRYN RAGALIS DAVIS, RDH, MS, DMD

Chapter Outline

A fully edentulous patient has no teeth. Absence of teeth may be congenital or due to loss from a variety of causes such as a traumatic accident or the progression through years of inadequate oral hygiene practices and periodontal disease. Information about and unique issues associated with the edentulous patient are outlined in this chapter.

- Various combinations are found among denture wearers.
- A partially edentulous patient may have a single arch complete denture opposing an arch with all natural teeth or various fixed or removable partial prostheses.
- An edentulous patient may have dental implants to improve the function and stability of an overdenture dental prosthesis.

- Terminology related to the edentulous patient is defined in **Box 53-1**.

PURPOSES FOR WEARING DENTURES

- Replace missing teeth and adjacent structures
  - Presence of teeth have esthetic role.
  - Restore facial contour including lip support and temporomandibular joint position.
- Provide function
  - Enhance ability to eat a wider variety of foods.
  - Promote proper speech and enunciation.

BOX 53-1	Key Words

Edentulous Patient

Anodontia: a rare condition characterized by congenital absence of all teeth, primary and permanent.

Complete denture prosthodontics: that body of knowledge and skills pertaining to the restoration of the edentulous arch with a removable prosthesis.

Denture: an artificial substitute for missing natural teeth and adjacent tissues.

 Complete denture: a complete removable dental prosthesis that replaces the entire dentition and associated structures of the maxilla or mandible.

 Immediate denture: a complete denture fabricated for placement immediately following the removal of a natural tooth/teeth and/or other surgical preparation of the dental arches.

 Overdenture: a removable denture that covers and is partially supported by one or more remaining natural teeth, roots, and/or dental implants and the soft tissue of the residual alveolar ridge; also called overlay denture.

Denture adhesive: a material used to adhere a denture to the oral mucosa.

Denture characterization: modification of the form and color of the denture base and teeth to produce a more lifelike appearance.

Denture foundation area: the surfaces of the oral structures available to support a denture.

Denture placement: the process of directing a prosthesis to a desired oral location; introduction of a prosthesis into a patient's mouth; other terms used are denture delivery or denture insertion.

Exostosis: bony projection extending beyond the normal contour of a bony surface.

Implant prosthesis: any prosthesis that is supported and retained in part or whole by dental implants.

Prosthesis: an artificial replacement of an absent part of the human body A therapeutic device to improve or alter function.

 Dental prosthesis: artificial replacement of one or more teeth and/or associated dental/alveolar structures.

Resection: excision of a segment of any part; removal of articular ends of one or both bones forming a joint.

TYPES OF REMOVABLE COMPLETE DENTURES[1]

1. *Tissue-supported complete denture:* A removable dental prosthesis that replaces the entire dentition and associated structures of the maxilla or the mandible and rests on the denture foundation area, the mucosal-covered alveolar ridge.

2. *Implant denture:* A complete dental prosthesis that is supported in part or whole by one or more dental implants. The denture itself is not an implantable device.

3. *Overdenture:* A removable prosthesis that rests on one or more remaining natural teeth, tooth roots, and/or dental implants (Figure 31-9, page 461). Also called an overlay prosthesis.

4. *Interim denture prosthesis:* A removable dental prosthesis designed to enhance esthetics, stabilization, and/or function for a limited period, after which it is to be replaced by a definitive prosthesis. Often such prostheses are used to assist in determination of the therapeutic effectiveness of a specific treatment plan or in determining the form and function of the planned definitive prosthesis. Also called a provisional prosthesis.

5. *Immediate denture:* A denture fabricated for placement immediately following the removal of a natural tooth or teeth. An immediate or interim denture tends to loosen after the significant remodeling of bone and soft tissue that follows surgery. Temporarily, the denture may be relined with a soft liner or a tissue conditioning material. The patient may use a denture adhesive until the majority of healing occurs. After approximately 6 months, dentures are remade, relined, or rebased.

6. *Denture for primary teeth*
 ◾ Dentures occasionally must be constructed to replace primary teeth.
 ◾ The teeth may be congenitally missing (anodontia) or may have been extracted due to rampant caries or trauma.
 ◾ Early childhood dental caries can severely break down the teeth soon after eruption.
 ◾ To provide esthetics and function, dentures can be constructed for the accepting child who is able to cooperate.
 ◾ As the permanent teeth begin to erupt, parts of the denture are cut away as in **Figure 53-1**.
 ◾ A supervised caries prevention program is initiated for protection of the permanent dentition.

THE EDENTULOUS MOUTH

I. BONE

A. Residual Ridges

◾ After the teeth are removed, the residual ridges enter into a continuing process of remodeling.

◾ The alveolar bone, which had supported the teeth, undergoes resorption. The rate and amount of bony resorption vary with each individual.

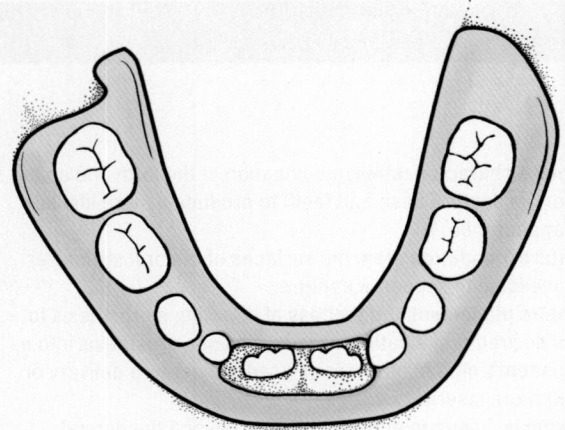

FIGURE 53-1 **Denture for a Young Child.** As permanent teeth erupt, parts of the denture are cut away. Shown is the denture alteration for the erupting permanent mandibular incisors.

- Major bony changes occur during the first year after the teeth are removed, but changes continue throughout life.
- Mandibular bone loss is generally as much as four times greater than maxillary bone loss.[2]
- Bone remodeling and soft tissue healing may make it necessary to have dentures rebased, relined, or remade at intervals.

B. Tori and Exostoses

Benign bony outgrowths may interfere with the fabrication and wearing of dentures. Because of the size, shape, or location, excess bone often needs to be removed surgically before a denture can be constructed.

- *Torus palatinus:* Bony enlargement located over the midline of the palate.
- *Torus mandibularis:* Bony mass generally located on the lingual in the region of the premolars.
- *Exostosis:* A bony protuberance generally located on the buccal aspects of maxilla and/or mandible.

II. MUCOUS MEMBRANE

A. Composition: Mucosa

Oral mucosa is composed of masticatory, lining, and specialized mucosa.

- *Masticatory* mucosa covers the edentulous ridges and the hard palate. The mucous membrane covering the bony ridges is made up of two layers, the lamina propria and the surface-stratified squamous epithelium, which is keratinized in the healthy mouth.
- *Lining* mucosa covers the floor of the mouth, vestibules, and cheeks.
- *Specialized* mucosa covers the dorsal surface of the tongue and contains filiform, fungiform and circumvalate papillae, as shown in Figure 14-2 on page 210.

B. Composition: Submucosa

- Underneath the mucous membrane is the submucosa, which is attached to the underlying bone.
- Composed of connective tissue with vessels, nerves, adipose tissue, and glands.
- The support or cushioning effect for the denture depends on the makeup of the submucosa, which varies in different parts of the mouth.

C. Tension Test

Examine the edentulous mouth by retracting the lips and cheeks using a tension test technique described in Chapter 15 on page 233.

- A line of demarcation similar to the mucogingival junction is apparent, separating the attached tissue over the bony ridge and the loose lining mucosa of the vestibule.
- Frenal attachments can be observed readily.

THE PATIENT WITH NEW DENTURES

I. PATIENT COUNSELING

A. Preparation

- The preparation for denture insertion has to begin well in advance of the day the dentures are delivered.
- Becoming edentulous may be very emotional for a patient and requires effort to learn to adapt and function with the new prosthesis.
- Anticipatory guidance will help the patient gain a clear idea of what to expect and what procedures to follow.
- Successful after-care and denture satisfaction depend to a large extent on conditioning the patient to the adjustments to be made and to the period of practice and learning with the new dentures that can be expected.

B. Adjuncts

Many dental teams prepare their own printed educational materials, whereas others use those available from outside sources.

II. POSTINSERTION CARE

The preliminary counseling is followed through the initial postinsertion appointments to adjust the prosthesis, teach denture hygiene, and arrange for continuing maintenance appointments.

A. Immediate Denture

- The patient is instructed to leave the immediate denture in place for 24 to 48 hours after tooth removal and surgery to aid in the control of bleeding and swelling.

- When the patient returns and the denture is removed, the mouth is rinsed and appropriate instructions are given.
- After initial healing, the denture care and other instructions are similar to those presented in **Table 53-1**.

B. New Dentures Over Healed Ridges

1. *Appointments*
   - Following insertion, appointments are scheduled routinely because adjustments can be expected.
   - The first appointment is made within 24 to 48 hours of the time of insertion.
   - Additional appointments are made in as needed for each individual patient.
2. *Instructions*[3]
   - Many verbal instructions given on the day of insertion may confuse the patient; limit instruction to basic denture care and other procedures of immediate concern.
   - Slow repetition over several periods helps the patient to develop adequate denture management and hygiene habits.
   - Written instruction can be helpful for the patient.
   - Basic information for the new denture wearer is provided in **Table 53-1**.
   - Denture cleaning methods are described with other biofilm control procedures for the care of dental prostheses on pages 456 to 460.

DENTURE-RELATED ORAL CHANGES

The condition of the mucous membranes, salivary glands, and alveolar bone is influenced by dietary and nutritional deficiencies, age, and various chronic diseases. Some of the denture-related changes are listed here.

I. BONE CHANGES

A. Effects of Alveolar Ridge Remodeling

Alveolar ridge remodeling may lead to the following:

- Loss of denture support
- Loss of facial height and lip support
- Increased prominence of the chin
- Temporomandibular joint manifestations
- Occlusal disharmony

B. Compensations by the Patient

- Patients may adapt to the bone changes by making compensating adjustments in the way they wear and manage the dentures.
- Other patients may resort to drugstore remedies, such as pads, adhesives, or self-reline materials, which can be detrimental if used improperly.

- Denture adhesives should never be used to compensate for a poorly designed, poorly constructed, or ill-fitting denture.

C. Treatment by the Dentist

- Dentures need adjusting, repairing, relining, rebasing, or remaking periodically.
- Patients are instructed to seek professional care if any issues relating to denture or oral health arise between scheduled maintenance.

II. ORAL MUCOSAL CHANGES

A. Tissue Reaction

- Tissue under a denture varies considerably among individuals.
- One mouth may have thinning of the mucosa, submucosa, and, particularly, the epithelium with an absence of keratinization, and another may have normal keratinization or hyperkeratinization.

B. Factors That Influence the Mucosa

- Systemic conditions that alter host response.
- Aging, mucosa tends to become thinner.
- Denture and tissue hygiene.
- Wearing the denture constantly.
- Xerostomia.
- Fit and occlusion of the denture itself.

III. EFFECT OF XEROSTOMIA

The causes of xerostomia are described in Chapter 25 on page 373. Diminished salivary flow can influence denture retention and tissue lubrication, as well as reduce the resistance of the oral mucosa to trauma and infection.

- *Lubrication:* The oral mucosa needs saliva for protection against frictional irritation by the denture.
- *Retention:* The film of saliva between the denture and the mucosa contributes to retention and suction of the denture.

IV. SENSORY CHANGES

A. Tactile Sense

- With the dentures in place, sensitivity may be diminished to small objects in the mouth, such as small bones or bits of nutshells.
- Proprioception, which signals how hard to chew and when to stop biting, is lost due to the absence of periodontal ligaments.

B. Taste

- Patients occasionally indicate that food has a different taste since they have been wearing dentures.

TABLE 53-1	PATIENT INSTRUCTION FOR COMPLETE DENTURES
ITEM	**FACTORS TO TEACH**

Food Selection	■ Use foods from the MyPlate Food Guide (page 499, Figure 34-1 Check each day's diet to fulfill needs for a balanced diet appropriate for each individual patient
	■ Select foods to prevent diet deficiency and diet-induced chronic diseases.
	■ New denture wearer:
	  ■ Avoid foods that need incising.
	  ■ Avoid raw vegetables, fibrous meats, and sticky foods until experience has been gained.
	  ■ Cut food into small pieces.
	■ Practiced denture wearer:
	  ■ Select a variety of foods, but do not expect the same efficiency as with the previous denture.

Incision or Biting	■ Use the canine and premolar area. Insert for biting at the angle of the mouth. ■ Push back as the food is incised; do not pull or tear the food in a forward direction.
Chewing	■ Take small portions. ■ Try to chew with some food on each side at the same time to stabilize the denture. ■ Be patient, chew slowly, and practice.
Salivary Flow	■ Anticipate an increased flow of saliva when a new denture is worn.
Speaking	■ Speak slowly and quietly. ■ Practice by reading aloud at home, preferably in front of a mirror. ■ Repeat and practice words that seem the most difficult.
Sneezing, Coughing, Yawning	■ Anticipate loss of denture retention. ■ Cover mouth with hand and handkerchief.
Denture Hygiene	■ Thoroughly clean dentures at least twice each day. ■ Immerse dentures in chemical solution and brush for biofilm removal; rinse thoroughly. ■ Complete denture care is described in Chapter 31 on page 456. ■ Devices to aid a person with a disability are shown in Chapter 56 on page 866–887 and Figure 56-12.
Mucosa	■ Tissues need to rest each day; consult dentist regarding whether it is best to leave the denture out while sleeping or during an alternative time period. ■ Brush and massage the mucosa to clean away biofilm and debris and stimulate circulation.
Storage of Dentures	■ After careful cleaning to remove all bacterial biofilm, store the denture in water (or cleaning solution) in a covered container. ■ Place in a safe place inaccessible to children or house pets. ■ Change water or cleaning solution daily and wash the container.
Over-the-Counter Products	■ Never attempt to alter the denture for relief of discomfort. ■ Do not buy and use self-reline materials, adhesives, or other additives without consulting the dentist. They may be harmful to the dentures and/or the oral tissues. ■ Consult the dentist for advice about all denture problems.
Maintenance	■ Understand the importance of the dentist's examination of the denture fit, occlusion, wear, and the condition of the oral mucosa. ■ First year: expect reline, rebase, or remake of dentures because bone remodeling is greatest during the first year after extraction. ■ Subsequent appointments: an examination each year for most patients, provided the denture hygiene is ideal; other patients in the cancer-susceptible category need an examination every 3 mo.
Seek Care	■ Report any concerns, changes, or problems immediately. ■ Dentures may need adjustments to correct occlusion or traumatic sore spots.

- Taste buds that are located in the tongue papillae are not affected by the dentures.
- Taste buds of the palate are covered by a maxillary denture and therefore are ineffective for taste and temperature perception.
- Dentures may develop thick odoriferous biofilm, which can alter food flavors, if not kept meticulously clean.

DENTURE-INDUCED ORAL LESIONS

When the mouth is examined extraorally and intraorally, the dentures are removed and the mucosa is examined carefully and thoroughly.

- A patient may tell of an area that has been sensitive and thus helpfully call attention to a specific visible lesion.
- A patient may be unaware of chronic mucosal lesions, which are often asymptomatic.
- Because tissue changes can be important indicators of serious disease, such as oral cancer, the intraoral examination must be conducted thoroughly with good illumination.

I. PRINCIPAL CAUSES OF LESIONS UNDER DENTURES

The factors that singly or in combination cause most oral lesions under dentures are:

A. Ill-Fitting Dentures

- Because tissue changes under dentures can occur gradually over a long period, the patient may not be aware of developing disease.
- The patient may not realize or may not have been informed of the importance of having regular professional examinations of the dentures and the oral mucosa.

B. Inadequate Oral Hygiene

- Dentures and the oral mucosa need daily care.
- Neglected dentures can accumulate heavy biofilm and calculus that may irritate the mucosa and cause infection and inflammation.

C. Continuous Wearing of Dentures

- Dentures need to be removed for a part of every day so that the mucosa can have a rest from the pressure of the hard acrylic during occlusion, bruxism, and clenching.
- A rest period allows the tissue to recover in its natural environment, where the tongue and saliva provide a cleansing effect.

II. INFLAMMATORY LESIONS

A. Contributing Factors

The following may occur singly or in combination.

- Denture trauma from the fit, occlusion, or parafunctional habits.
- Inadequate denture hygiene and care of the mucosa.
- Chemotoxic effect from residual cleansing paste or solution not thoroughly rinsed from the denture.
- Allergy to the denture base (rare).
- Continuous denture wearing without relief for the tissues.
- Patient self-treatment with over-the-counter products for relining.
- Tolerance of the tissues to trauma and resistance to infection can be reduced, for example, with nutritional deficiencies, immunosuppression such as chemotherapy, and systemic diseases such as diabetes.

B. Localized Inflammation (Sore Spots)

1. *Appearance:* isolated, red, inflamed area, sometimes ulcerated.
2. *Contributing factors:* trauma from an ill-fitting denture, a rough spot on a denture surface, a tongue bite, or a foreign object caught under the denture.

C. Generalized Inflammation, *Candida albicans* Infection[4]

- Oral candidiasis in the form of *denture stomatitis* is a reoccurring disease common to denture wearers and may be characterized by the following:
  - Generalized redness, inflamed mucosa of the tissues that support the denture
  - Burning sensation
  - Discomfort
  - Unpleasant taste
  - Most denture wearers unaware that condition is present
- Etiology factors include the following:
  - Trauma from ill-fitting, usually maxillary, denture.
  - Continuous denture wearing.
  - Reduced salivary flow.
  - Lack of denture cleanliness.
  - Aging dentures have surface texture favorable to attachment of biofilm.
  - Treatment may include denture adjustments, fabrication of new denture, antifungal medication, and massaging the tissues.
- Patients with the following are more prone to oral candidiasis:
  - Depressed immune system
  - History of head and neck radiation therapy
  - Antibiotic use

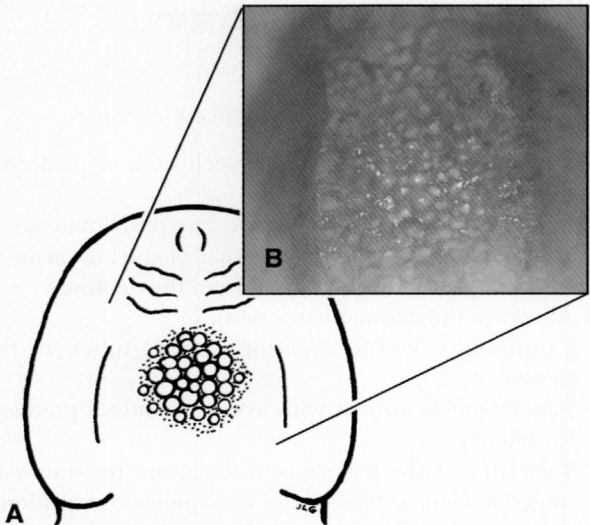

FIGURE 53-2 **Papillary Hyperplasia. (A)** Outline of an edentulous palate shows the characteristic location of papillary hyperplasia within the bony ridges. **(B)** Photograph of inflammatory papillary hyperplasia on hard palate. Courtesy of Michael Kahn, DDS, Chairperson, Oral Pathology, Tufts University, School of Dental Medicine.

III. ULCERATIVE LESIONS

■ Localized ulcerated lesions can be related to an overextended denture border.
■ The ulcer may resemble a cancerous lesion and should be biopsied if it persists longer than expected of a healing traumatic ulcer (7 to 14 days) after the denture is adjusted.

IV. PAPILLARY HYPERPLASIA[5]

A. Appearance

Inflammatory papillary hyperplasia is located on the palate, rarely outside the confines of the bony ridges **(Figure 53-2A)**. The overall lesion appears as a group of closely arranged, pebble-shaped, red, edematous projections **(Figure 53-2B)**.

B. Contributing Factors

The cause is unknown but it is associated with poor denture hygiene, ill-fitting dentures, and possible *C. albicans* infection.

V. DENTURE IRRITATION HYPERPLASIA (EPULIS FISSURATUM)[5]

Long-standing chronic inflammatory tissue appears in single or multiple elongated folds related to the border of an ill-fitting denture.

VI. ANGULAR CHEILITIS[6]

A. Appearance

■ Fissuring at the angles of the mouth, with cracks, ulcerations, and erythema.
■ Moist with saliva or sometimes dry with a crust.

B. Contributing Factors

■ Lack of support of the commissure because of overclosure from loss of vertical dimension of occlusion and by moistness from drooling.
■ Secondarily, a riboflavin deficiency or an infection by *C. albicans* or other organisms may be involved.
■ Prescription antifungal medication may be indicated.

PREVENTION

I. DENTURE HYGIENE

■ Dentures must be cleaned after each meal, as described in Chapter 31 on page 457.
■ Cleansing solutions must be changed daily.

II. ORAL MUCOSA

■ Brush to clean and massage.
■ Perform digital massage.

III. REST FOR THE TISSUES

■ Having the dentures out while sleeping may be the best procedure to provide rest for the oral tissues for many patients. However, the potential for damage to the temporomandibular joint from lack of support needs checking.
■ Daytime for as long a period as possible, such as while bathing.
■ Place dentures in a container with cleaning solution when out of the mouth.
■ Clean and massage the underlying mucosa.

IV. DIET AND NUTRITION

■ Teaching of food selection cannot be overemphasized.
■ Emphasis on foods from the basic food groups as shown in MyPlate, Figure 34-1 on page 499 is necessary.
■ Control of weight and avoidance of foods that are related to specific chronic conditions contribute to long-range oral health.
■ A dietary analysis can provide a foundation for making specific recommendations.
■ Diet problems of the older adult patient are described in Chapter 52 on page 809.
■ Factors that contribute to dietary deficiencies in patients of any age are magnified when dentures are ill fitting or painful and masticatory efficiency is decreased. The patient tends to overlook food value and to select foods that are within the limits of chewing ability or that can be swallowed without chewing.
■ Learning to adapt to an initial denture may affect nutrition. Patient can be instructed to attempt small amounts of a soft diet to relearn to chew.

V. RELIEF FROM XEROSTOMIA

- The use of the various forms of saliva substitutes may be recommended.
- Other suggestions for management of xerostomia are in Chapter 25 on page 374.

VI. DENTAL CARIES CONTROL FOR OVERDENTURE WEARERS

- Meticulous denture hygiene and dental biofilm control for the natural teeth are mandatory.
- Care of the overdenture is described in Chapter 31 on page 461.
- Fluoride dentifrice is used while brushing the teeth. Daily fluoride application is made by placing gel drops inside the overdenture.

MAINTENANCE

The edentulous patient requires regular maintenance appointments for evaluation of the oral tissues and oral cancer screening. Regular maintenance appointments include evaluation of the fit and function of the prostheses, supervision of daily biofilm control for dentures, as well as care of the soft tissues.

I. APPOINTMENT FREQUENCY

A. First Year

After the initial adjustments, the patient can expect the dentures to need reline, rebase, or remake in 6 months to 1 year.

B. Subsequent Maintenance Period

Frequency of maintenance appointments is determined by individual needs and risk factors, as shown in **Table 53-2**. Patients are encouraged to seek care at any time if discomfort or concerns arise with the denture or any tissue area.

II. MAINTENANCE APPOINTMENT

Maintenance procedures are followed with necessary adaptations for the edentulous patient.

A. Procedures

1. Review patient history; make necessary additions to the record.
2. Determine blood pressure.
3. Perform an extraoral and intraoral examination.
4. Examine dentures for cleanliness and evidence of patient care.
5. Ask patient to demonstrate the personal hygiene care procedures used routinely.
6. Supplement with additional demonstration and instruction when the care is less than adequate.
7. Clean the dentures to remove calculus and stain.

B. Procedures for the Dentist

- Review the complete assessment.
- Examine the oral tissues and the fit and occlusion of the dentures.
- Treat as needed.

C. Subsequent Appointment

- Make necessary appointments for continuing current treatment and for maintenance.
- All tissues must be examined at least annually for oral cancer screening and any other changes indicative of oral or systemic disease.

DENTURE MARKING FOR IDENTIFICATION[7]

The need for denture marking is apparent in a variety of situations. A universal system for marking would be ideal. Marking is required by law in some countries and in most states of the United States.

TABLE 53-2	MAINTENANCE RECOMMENDATIONS	
RISK LEVEL	**DESCRIPTION OF PATIENT**	**APPOINTMENT INTERVAL**
Low Risk	■ Healthy individual, healthy life-style and diet, no systemic disease ■ No tobacco or alcohol use ■ Impeccable denture care and hygiene practices	6–12 mo
Moderate Risk	■ All patients in between Low and High Risk	6 mo
High Risk	■ Daily tobacco and alcohol use ■ Previous history of cancer ■ Systemic diseases such as diabetes ■ Medication use such as immunosupressants or those that cause xerostomia ■ Continuously wears denture ■ Any remaining natural teeth and/or implants	3–6 mo

- In forensic dentistry, or for identification of victims of war, such disasters as flood or fire, or transportation catastrophes, the dentition has been used increasingly as a means of identification.
- Dentures provide a method for immediate identification. Prompt identification can be urgent when an individual is found unconscious from illness or injury or is suffering from amnesia as a result of psychiatric or traumatic causes, as well as from Alzheimer's disease.
- The dentures of people in long-term residence or care facilities must be marked. Mislaid dentures can be returned, and mix-ups by the direct care staff can be prevented. An important contribution to an oral health program is to introduce a plan for denture marking.

I. CRITERIA FOR AN ADEQUATE MARKING SYSTEM

Information on the denture must be specific so that rapid identification is possible.

A. Relative to the Denture

- Must have no adverse effects on denture material.
- Must not change the strength, surface texture, or fit of the denture.
- Must be cosmetically acceptable; the label must be placed in an unobtrusive position.

B. Relative to the Procedure

- Readily learned and simple to carry out.
- Inexpensive.
- Durable result. When the information is incorporated during denture processing, indefinite durability can be expected. A surface marker for a denture already in use should be able to withstand denture-cleaning methods for a reasonable period of time.

C. Characteristics of the Material Used

- *Fire and humidity resistant:* When the label is placed inside the posterior section of a denture, the surrounding tongue and maxillofacial parts offer protection except in the most severe conflagration.
- *Radiopaque:* A metal marker can be of use as a means of identification by radiographic examination in the event the radiolucent acrylic denture is accidentally swallowed.

II. INCLUSION METHODS FOR MARKING

A. New Dentures

- A printed enclosure is inserted as a denture is being processed.
- Labels are positioned on the impression surfaces of the maxillary and mandibular dentures **(Figure 53-3)**.
- Cover label, just before the final closure of the flask, with a clear acrylic material.

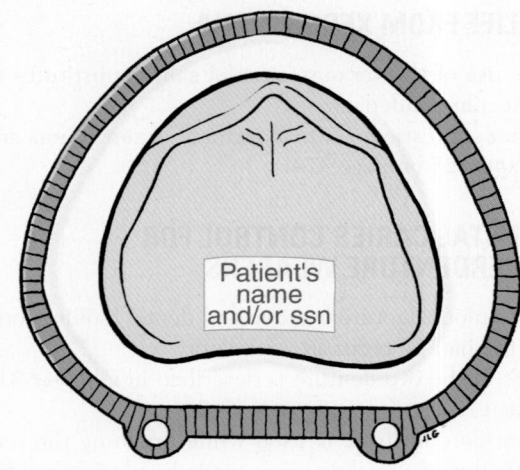

FIGURE 53-3 **Inclusion Marker for New Denture.** The label is inserted on the impression surface as the denture is being processed. In the flasked maxillary denture shown, the marker is positioned near the posterior border.

- A label may be typewritten on onionskin paper or the tissue paper that separates sheets of packaged baseplate wax.[7,8]
- Another system uses a thin metal strip for the insert. Stainless steel matrix bands, orthodontic bands, and thin metal strips (shim stock) have been used.[9]
- *Microchips* can be incorporated for denture marking because of the small size, esthetic acceptability, forensic identification qualities, and information they can contain. They have a higher cost than other methods.[10]
- *Copper vapor laser* has been used to mark dentures with metal frameworks, removable partial dentures, and other metallic restorations.[11]

B. Existing Dentures[12]

1. Clean the dentures thoroughly.
2. Use a No. 6 or 8 round bur and an inverted cone to cut small, shallow, boxlike preparations in the posterior buccal flange of the maxillary denture and the lingual posterior flange of the mandibular denture **(Figure 53-4)**. Do not go through to the impression surface.
3. Print two copies of the patient's name (or other choice of identification) on onionskin paper, and trim the papers to fit the boxlike preparations.
4. Cover the paper with cold-cure clear acrylic and fill to a slight excess; after the acrylic has cured, polish to a smooth finish.

III. SURFACE MARKERS

Surface markers are not as durable, but instruction can be provided for persons not trained in dental laboratory methods. In a skilled nursing facility or other long-term institution that has no resident dentist or dental hygienist, it may be possible to teach a nurse or other staff member to mark dentures of residents as they are admitted. The methods described as follows have been used for this purpose.

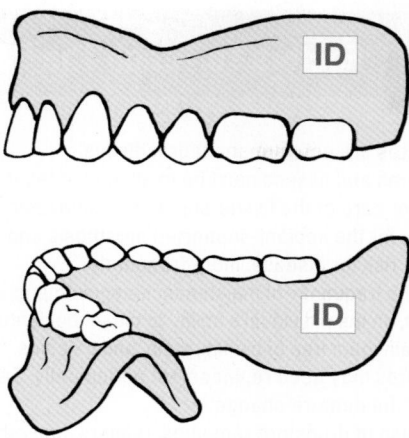

FIGURE 53-4 **Surface Markers for Dentures.** The labels are placed on the external denture surfaces for existing dentures. As shown, the markers are on the maxillary buccal flange and the mandibular lingual flange.

A. Indelible Pen or Ballpoint

■ After cleaning and drying the denture, a small area near the posterior of the outer or polished denture surface is rubbed with an emery board until it is rough (Figure 53-4).

■ Name, initials, or other identification is printed on the roughened area with an indelible pen and dried.

■ Two or three coats of a fingernail acrylic (heavy nail protector) are painted over the area; each layer is dried before applying the next.

■ Surface markings have been found to last at least 6 months.[13]

■ Light-cured materials may also be used.[14,15]

B. Engraving Tool

An engraving tool is used to enter the name on the denture, and the grooves created are darkened with a special pencil before a sealing liquid is applied. Materials are available in a commercial kit.[16]

IV. INFORMATION TO INCLUDE ON A MARKER

■ For residents of a home or institution, using only the person's name and initials should suffice for temporary surface marking.

■ In a community, country, or international situation, the name alone would not provide enough identification, and the social security number, armed services serial number, or the equivalent in other countries can be included.

■ Other identification, such as blood type and vital drug or disease condition, has been suggested.

■ In certain countries, the dentist's registration or hospital number has been used. In Sweden, the patient's date of birth and national registration number have been marked on the dentures.

■ Markings that can provide *immediate* identification are the most significant.

DOCUMENTATION

Every appointment for a patient wearing a denture or having one made or repaired, needs a carefully prepared progress note in the patient's permanent record to include a minimum of the following:

■ Changes in the health history, vital signs, and findings from a careful extra- and intraoral examinations.

■ Patient reports of tissue changes or difficulty with a denture.

■ Observation of the denture, fixed or removable to make necessary changes in the patient's daily care of the denture; new instruction with additional devices or cleaning materials when necessary.

■ A sample progress note may be reviewed in **Box 53-2**.

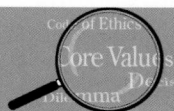 # Everyday Ethics

Mr. Ryan presents for his yearly denture examination and oral cancer screening. He faithfully keeps his appointment every year because the cigarette stains build up on his full upper and lower dentures and he likes the way his dental hygienist, Kaitlin, gets them very clean.

   During this visit, Kaitlin notices a small area on the alveolar ridge under the denture near the area of tooth #29. Mr. Ryan is aware of the lesion and sometimes doesn't wear his lower denture, but he indicates that it doesn't really bother him. Kaitlin informs Mr. Ryan that she will ask the dentist to check the area. Mr. Ryan becomes annoyed at her concern. He clearly states that he just wants to have his denture cleaned and to leave.

Questions for Consideration
1. Since Mr. Ryan has been a heavy smoker for over 40 years, what actions are indicated to document and evaluate the lesion? Which of the core values (Table II-1, in Section II, Introduction, page 38) are evident in this scenario?
2. Is Kaitlin facing an ethical issue or a dilemma? What are Kaitlin's ethical obligations to the patient in communicating the possible serious nature of her findings?
3. Study the questions in Table V-1 in Section V Introduction, page 362 to determine possible avenues Kaitlin may take if Mr. Ryan leaves the office without having the lesion evaluated.

BOX 53-2 | Example Progress Note

Ms Waters came for maintenance; wears complete max. and mand. dentures. Chief complaint: soreness under molar area on left mandibular area. Intraoral examination revealed red area 2 mm by 1 mm on lingual side of ridge near first molar area. Dr. Frye examined and designated sending to pathologist for biopsy. Completed necessary forms with necessary information to give the pathologist. Called and made appointment for Ms Waters. Cleaned the dentures, including scaling calculus on lingual mandibular denture. Discussed agents she uses for cleaning at home, and how often, and advised being sure they are carefully rinsed after using cleaning agents as well as after soaking agents when dentures are out all night. Will call her when biopsy report is available probably within a week.

Signed: _____, RDH Date: _____

Factors To Teach The Patient

- Dentures are not permanent prostheses.
- Dentures and tissues must be examined at least once a year for care of the tissue-supported removable prosthesis; for the implant-supported prosthesis and those at higher risk for disease, more frequently.
- Why the frequency of maintenance appointments depends, in part, on the individual's ability to clean the dentures and maintain them free of biofilm, stain, and calculus.
- Dentures may need replacement periodically. Tissues under the denture change.
- Why use of drugstore remedies, reliners, and other home-applied materials are avoided unless the dentist has provided specific instruction.
- Specific methods of care for dentures.
- Why dentures need to be left out of the mouth overnight in accord with the dentist's directions.
- Where to obtain and how to use a saliva substitute.

References

1. Academy of Prosthodontics Foundation. The glossary of prosthodontic terms. 8th ed. *J Prosthet Dent*. 2005 Jul;94(1):10–92.
2. Tallgren A. The continuing reduction of the residual alveolar ridges in complete denture wearers: a mixed-longitudinal study covering 25 years. *J Prosthet Dent*. 2003 May;89(5):427–35.
3. Clark JW, ed. *Clinical dentistry*. 5th rev ed. Volume 5. Philadelphia: Lippincott; 1984. Chapter 14, Gallagher JB. Insertion and postinsertion care. p. 1–27.
4. Ramage G, Tomsett K, Wickes BL, López-Ribot JL, Redding SW. Denture stomatitis: a role for Candida biofilms. *Oral Surg Oral Med Oral Pathol Oral Radiol Endod*. 2004 Jul;98(1):53–9.
5. Robinson HB, Miller AS. *Color atlas of oral pathology*. 5th ed. Philadelphia: Lippincott; 1990. p. 94–5.
6. Robinson: op.cit., p.141.
7. American Dental Association; Council on Prosthetic Services and Dental Laboratory Relations. *Techniques for denture identification*. Chicago: American Dental Association; 1984. 12 p.
8. Dentsply International, Inc. Method for placing permanent record data in denture base without affecting tissue adaptation. Technical bulletin. York (PA): Dentsply International; [date unknown].
9. Turner CH, Fletcher AM, Ritchie GM. Denture marking and human identification. *Br Dent J*. 1976 Aug 17;141(4):114–7.
10. Rajan M, Julian R. A new method of marking dentures using microchips. *J Forensic Odontostomatol*. 2002 Jun;20(1):1–5.
11. Ling BC, Nambiar P, Low KS, Lee CK. Copper vapour laser ID labelling on metal dentures and restorations. *J Forensic Odontostomatol*. 2003 Jun;21(1):17–22.
12. Bauer TL. Technique for denture identification. *J Indiana Dent Assoc*. 1979 Nov–Dec;58(6):28–9.
13. Deb AK, Heath MR. Marking dentures in geriatric institutions. The relevance and appropriate methods. *Br Dent J*. 1979 May 1;146(9):282–4.
14. Richards EE, Williams JE, Gauthier G. A modified light-cured denture identification technique. *Spec Care Dentist*. 1992 Mar–Apr;12(2):81–3.
15. Lamb DJ. A simple method for permanent identification of dentures. *J Prosthet Dent*. 1992 Jun;67(6):894.
16. Identure, Geri, Inc., P.O. Box 9086, North St. Paul, MN 55109.

CHAPTER 54

The Oral and Maxillofacial Surgery Patient

ESTHER M. WILKINS, BS, RDH, DMD

Oral and maxillofacial surgery is the specialty of dentistry that includes the diagnostic, surgical, and adjunctive treatment of diseases, injuries, and defects involving both the functional and the aesthetic aspects of the hard and soft tissues of the oral and maxillofacial regions.[1] Box 54-1 lists types of treatment included in this specialty.

■ The practice of an oral surgeon may be primarily in a group clinical setting, in a hospital, or in a private practice with outpatient hospital facilities available.
■ With the oral surgeon is a team of specially trained individuals that include surgical assistants, anesthetists, registered nurses, and dental hygienists.
■ Terminology that relates to maxillofacial surgery is defined in Box 54-2.

■ The surgeon is involved with various dental practitioners, including general dentists and specialists.
■ Maxillofacial surgery can be programmed, for example, with prosthodontists, orthodontists, implantologists, and specialists caring for any of the patients suggested by the list in Box 54-1.

Surgery for treatment of diseases and correction of defects of the periodontal tissues is categorized specifically as *periodontal surgery*. Within the scope of periodontal surgery are procedures for pocket elimination, gingivoplasty, treatment of furcation involvements, correction of mucogingival defects, treatment for bony defects about the teeth, and placing implants. Preparation for periodontal surgery is not specifically described in this chapter.

BOX 54-1	Categories of Oral and Maxillofacial Treatments

DENTOALVEOLAR SURGERY
Exodontics
Impacted tooth removal
Alveolar bone surgery: alveoloplasty

INFECTION
Abscesses
Osteomyelitis

TRAUMATIC INJURY
Fractures of jaws, zygoma
Fracture of teeth, alveolar bone

NEOPLASM
Cysts
Tumors

DENTAL IMPLANT PLACEMENT
PREPROSTHETIC RECONSTRUCTION
Maxillofacial prosthetics
Immediate denture

ORTHOGNATHIC SURGERY
Prognathism correction
Facial aesthetics

CLEFT LIP/PALATE

TEMPOROMANDIBULAR DISORDERS (TMD)

SALIVARY GLAND OBSTRUCTION

PATIENT PREPARATION

I. OBJECTIVES

Dental hygiene care and instruction before oral and maxillofacial surgery may contribute to the patient's health and well-being by one or more of the following:

A. Reduce Oral Bacterial Count

- Aid in the preparation of an aseptic field for the surgery.
- Make postsurgical infection less likely or less severe.

B. Reduce Inflammation of the Gingiva and Improve Tissue Tone

- Lessen local bleeding at the time of the surgery.
- Promote postsurgical healing.

C. Remove Calculus Deposits

- Remove a source of dental biofilm retention and thus improve gingival tissue tone.
- Prevent interference with placement of surgical instruments.
- Prevent pieces of calculus from breaking away.
  - Danger of inhalation, particularly when a general anesthetic is used.
  - Possibility of calculus falling into a socket or other surgical area and acting as a foreign body to inhibit healing.

BOX 54-2	Key Words

Oral and Maxillofacial Surgery

Comminution: act of breaking or condition of being broken into small fragments.

Ecchymosis: a hemorrhagic spot, larger than a petechia, in the skin or mucous membrane caused by extravasation of blood; forms a nonelevated, rounded, or irregular purplish patch.

Exodontics: branch of dentistry dealing with the surgical removal of teeth.

Exostosis: benign new growth projecting from the surface of bone.

Intermaxillary fixation: fixation of the maxilla in occlusion with the mandible held in place by means of wires and elastic bands; the healing parts are stabilized following fracture or surgery.

Maxillofacial: pertaining to the jaws and the face.

Maxillofacial prosthetics: the branch of prosthodontics concerned with the restoration of the mouth and

jaws and associated facial structures that have been affected by disease, injury, surgery, or a congenital defect.

Orthognathic surgery: surgery to alter relationships of the dental arches and/or supporting bone; usually coordinated with orthodontic therapy.

Orthognathics: science dealing with the causes and treatment of malposition of the bones of the jaws.

Osteosynthesis: internal fixation of a fracture by mechanical means, such as metal plates, pins, or screws.

Miniplate osteosynthesis: a method of internal fixation of mandibular fractures utilizing miniaturized metal plates and screws formerly made of titanium or stainless steel and currently made primarily of biodegradable or resorbable synthetic materials.

Trismus: motor disturbance of the trigeminal nerve with spasm of masticatory muscles and difficulty in opening the mouth (lockjaw).

D. Instruct in Presurgical Personal Oral Care Procedures

- Reduce inflammation and thus improve tissue tone.
- Help to prepare the patient for postsurgical care.

E. Instruct in the Use of Foods

- Foods that provide the elements essential to tissue building and repair during pre- and postsurgical periods.
- For the patient who will have teeth removed and immediate complete or partial dentures inserted, the importance of a diet containing all essential food groups is emphasized.

F. Interpret the Dentist's Directions

- Explanation is needed for the immediate presurgical preparation with respect to rest and dietary limitations, particularly when a general anesthetic is to be administered.

G. Motivate the Patient Who Will Have Teeth Remaining

- Motivation to prevent further tooth loss through routine dental and dental hygiene professional care and personal oral care procedures.

II. PERSONAL FACTORS

- The extent of the surgery to be performed and previous experiences affect the patient's attitude.
- Many patients who are in the greatest need of presurgical dental hygiene care and instruction may be people who have neglected their mouths for many years. They may have been indifferent to or unaware of the importance of obtaining adequate oral care.
- Visits to a dentist may have been to have a toothache relieved. Their knowledge of preventive measures may be limited.
- A few possible characteristics are suggested here.

A. Apprehensive and Fearful

- Apprehensive and indifferent toward need for personal care of teeth.
- Fearful of all dental procedures, particularly oral surgery and anesthesia.
- Fearful of personal appearance after surgery.

B. Resigned

- Feeling of inevitableness of the situation.
- Lack of appreciation for preserving natural teeth.

C. Discouraged

- Over tooth loss or development of soft tissue lesions.

- Toward time lost from work.
- Toward the financial aspects of dental care.
- Toward inconvenience and discomfort.

DENTAL HYGIENE CARE

I. PRESURGERY TREATMENT PLANNING

A. Initial Oral Preparation

- The pending date for the surgery and the patient's attitude may limit the time to be spent.
- Complete medical and dental history, extraoral and intraoral examination, vital signs, photographs, and radiographs are essential; determine need for prophylactic premedication.
- Develop rapport; explain purposes of presurgical appointments.
- Explain and demonstrate dental biofilm control principles. Demonstrate appropriate technique using new soft toothbrush.
- Perform scaling to prepare for tissue healing; local anesthesia is used as needed.
- Provide postappointment instruction for rinsing with basic saline or with chlorhexidine 0.12% for tissue conditioning.

B. Follow-Up Evaluation

- Complete or continue the scaling.
- More appointments may be needed for patients who will have surgery for oral cancer or who have a cardiovascular or other condition for which all periodontal and dental treatment must be completed before surgery.
- When radiation or chemotherapy will be used following surgery for oral cancer, or when a prosthetic heart valve or total joint replacement will be involved, complete oral care is needed before surgery.
- Scaling and planing is planned for a few weeks after oral surgery. Emphasis must be placed on review and redemonstration of personal daily care.

II. PATIENT INSTRUCTION: DIET SELECTION

- The nutritional state can influence the resistance to infection and wound healing, as well as general recovery powers.
- Nutritional deficiencies can occur because of the inability to ingest adequate nutrients orally.
- Specific recommendations of what to include and not to include in the diet are provided.
- Postsurgical suggestions may differ from presurgical; for example, when difficulty in chewing is a postsurgical problem, a liquid or soft diet may be required.
- When major oral surgery requires hospitalization, tube feeding may be used during the initial healing period.

A. Nutritional and Dietary Needs

Diets outlined are designed to include the essential foods from the MyPlate Guide (Figure 32-1, page 499).

- *Essential for promotion of healing:* Protein and vitamins, particularly vitamin A, vitamin C, and riboflavin.
- *Essential for building gingival tissue resistance:* A varied diet that includes adequate portions of all essential food groups.
- *Essential for dental caries prevention:* Noncariogenic foods. When a patient has not been able to masticate properly, the diet employed frequently may have included many soft and cariogenic foods.

B. Suggestions for Instruction

1. Provide instruction sheets that show specific pre- and postsurgery meal plans. Foods for liquid and soft diets are listed on page 832 in this chapter.
2. Express nutritional needs in terms of quantity or servings of foods so that the patient clearly understands.
3. For the patient who will receive dentures, careful instruction must be provided over a period of time. Information for the patient with new dentures is described in Chapter 53 on page 814 and in Table 53-1 (page 816).
4. When the patient loses the teeth because of dental caries, the diet has likely been highly cariogenic. Emphasis needs to be placed on helping the patient include nutritious foods for the general health of the body and, more specifically, the health of the alveolar processes, which will support the dentures.

III. PRESURGICAL INSTRUCTIONS[2]

At the appointment just before the oral surgery appointment, instructions relative to the surgical procedure are discussed with the patient. The objective is to let the patient know what to expect so that full cooperation is possible. The patient may have concerns about the anesthesia, the surgical procedure, and the outcome.

- Explain the general procedures for anesthesia and surgery.
- Provide printed instructions concerning the following:
  1. *Food and liquid intake:* Specify the number of hours before the time of the surgery when the patient stops further intake of food and fluids.
  2. *Alcohol and medication restrictions:* Certain medications, supplements, and alcohol are not compatible with the anesthetic and drugs to be used during and following the surgical procedure. The patient is instructed to discontinue use.
  3. *Transport to and from the appointment:* When a general anesthetic or light sedation is used, the patient must not drive. Plans for someone to accompany and assist the patient are to be made.
  4. *The night before the appointment:* In addition to food and alcohol restrictions, a good night's rest is advocated.

  5. *Personal items*
     - Clothing: The clothing worn should be loose and comfortable. The sleeves should be easily drawn up over the elbows for taking blood pressure.
     - Care of contact lenses and prostheses. The patient will be asked to remove prostheses, and may be asked to remove contact lenses, so needs to bring containers for their safe keeping.

IV. POSTSURGICAL CARE

A. Immediate Instructions

Printed postsurgical instructions are provided following all oral procedures. The prepared material is reviewed with the patient after surgery. Specific details vary, but basic information for postsurgical instruction sheets includes the following:

1. *Control bleeding:* Keep the sponge in the mouth over the surgical area for 1/2 hour; then discard it. When bleeding persists at home, place a gauze pad or cold wet teabag over the area and bite firmly for 30 minutes.
2. *Rinsing:* Do not rinse for 24 hours after the surgical appointment. Then use warm salt water [1/2 teaspoonful salt in 1/2 cup (4 ounces) of warm water] after toothbrushing and every 2 hours.
3. *Dental biofilm control:* Brush the teeth and floss more than usual. Avoid the surgery site.
4. *Rest:* Get plenty of rest; at least 8 to 10 hours of sleep each night. Avoid strenuous exercise during the first 24 hours, and keep the mouth from excessive movement.
5. *Diet:* Use a liquid or soft diet high in protein. Drink water and fruit juices freely. Avoid foods that require excessive chewing or are acidic.
6. *Pain:* If needed, use a pain-relieving preparation prescribed by the dentist. Adhere to directions.
7. *Icepack:* Following a flap procedure or when swelling is likely to occur, apply icepack (ice cubes in a plastic bag) for 15 minutes followed by 15 minutes off, or apply for 15 minutes after 30 minutes off, as directed by the dentist. Heat is not used for swelling.
8. *Complications:* Include the telephone number to call after office hours, should complications arise; complications may include uncontrollable pain, marked bleeding, temperature rise, difficulty in opening the mouth, or unusual swelling a few days after the surgery.

B. Follow-Up Care

1. The dental hygienist may participate in suture removal, irrigation of sockets, and other postsurgical procedures when the patient returns.
2. Appropriately, instruction concerning biofilm control, rinsing, oral irrigation, and other personal care, as well as diet supervision, can be continued.

PATIENT WITH INTERMAXILLARY FIXATION

- The limited access for personal oral care procedures and the effect of the liquid diet required for most cases define the need for special dental hygiene care for the patient with intermaxillary fixation.
- Attention to rehabilitation of the oral tissues during the period following the removal of appliances takes on particular significance to prevent permanent tissue damage and inadequate oral care habits from being continued indefinitely.
- Descriptions in this section are related to a fractured jaw, but intermaxillary fixation may be required for a variety of corrective surgeries and other conditions, including temporomandibular joint treatment and reconstructive and orthognathic surgeries.
- Regardless of the reason for intermaxillary fixation, instructions for dental hygiene care are similar, and the patient's problems are much the same.

FRACTURED JAW

- The patient with a fractured jaw may be hospitalized.
- A dental hygienist employed in a hospital would be called upon to assume a part of the responsibility for patient care or to give oral hygiene instruction to direct-care personnel.
- After dismissal from the hospital, the patient may require special attention in the private dental office for a long period.
- Treatment of a fractured jaw may be complex, and the patient may suffer considerably, both physically and mentally.
- Basic knowledge of the nature of fractures and their treatment is helpful in understanding the patient's needs.

I. CAUSES OF FRACTURED JAWS

A. Traumatic

Interpersonal violence, sporting injuries, falls, road traffic accidents (including bicycles), and industrial accidents.

B. Predisposing

Pathologic conditions, such as tumors, cysts, osteoporosis, or osteomyelitis, weaken the bone; thus, slight trauma or even tooth removal can cause fracture.

II. EMERGENCY CARE

- Immediate attention must be paid to measures for care of the patient's general condition.
- Monitor breathing, airway, and circulation, and prepare for possible defibrillation (pages 1058 to 1075).
- Hemorrhage, shock, and skull or internal head injuries are next in the sequence of concern.
- Almost any category of emergency care may be required (Tables 69-4 and 69-5, pages 1076 to 1081).
- Although treatment for the fractured jaw must not be postponed for any great length of time, its immediate care takes second place to the vital aspects of patient care.
- Tetanus prophylaxis may be indicated as soon as medical treatment is available.

III. RECOGNITION

A. History

Except for a pathologic fracture, a history of trauma should be available.

B. Clinical Signs

- Pain, especially on movement, and tenderness on slight pressure over the area of the fracture.
- Teeth may be displaced, fractured, or mobile. Because of muscle pull or contraction, segments of the bones may be displaced and the occlusion of the teeth may be irregular.
- Muscle spasm is a common finding, particularly when the fracture is at the angle or ramus of the mandible.
- Crepitation can be heard if the parts of bone are moved.
- Soft tissue in the area of the fracture may show laceration and bleeding, discoloration (ecchymosis), and enlargement.

IV. TYPES OF FRACTURES

A fracture is classified by using a combination of descriptive words for its *location, direction, nature,* and *severity.* Fractures may be single or multiple, bilateral or unilateral, complete or incomplete.

A. Classification by Nature of the Fracture (**Figure 54-1**)

1. *Simple:* has no communication with outside.
2. *Compound:* has communication with outside.
3. *Comminuted:* shattered.
4. *Incomplete:* "Greenstick" fracture has one side of a bone broken and the other side bent. It occurs in incompletely calcified bones (young children, usually). The fibers tend to bend rather than break.

B. Mandibular (Described by Location)

- Alveolar process
- Condyle
- Angle
- Body
- Symphysis

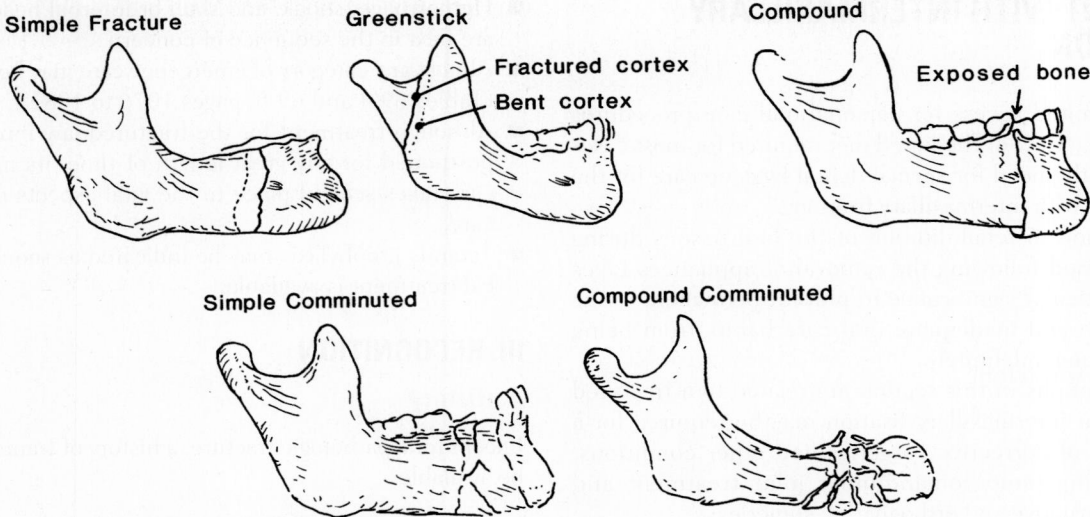

FIGURE 54-1 **Types of Fractures.** (Reprinted with permission from Kruger GO. *Textbook of Oral* and *Maxillofacial Surgery.* 6th ed. St. Louis: Mosby; 1984.)

C. Midfacial

■ *Alveolar process:* The alveolar process fracture does not extend to the midline of the palate.
■ *Le Fort:*[3] The Le Fort classification is used widely to identify the three general levels of maxillary fractures, as shown in **Figure 54-2**.
1. *Le Fort I:* A horizontal fracture line that extends above the roots of the teeth, above the palate, across the maxillary sinus, below the zygomatic process, and across the pterygoid plates.
2. *Le Fort II:* The midface fracture extends over the middle of the nose, down the medial wall of the orbits, across the infraorbital rims, and posteriorly, across the pterygoid plates.
3. *Le Fort III:* The high-level craniofacial fracture extends transversely across the bridge of the nose, across the orbits and the zygomatic arches, and across the pterygoid plates.

V. TREATMENT OF FRACTURES[4,5]

Each fracture differs from the next, and the methods used in treatment vary with the individual case.

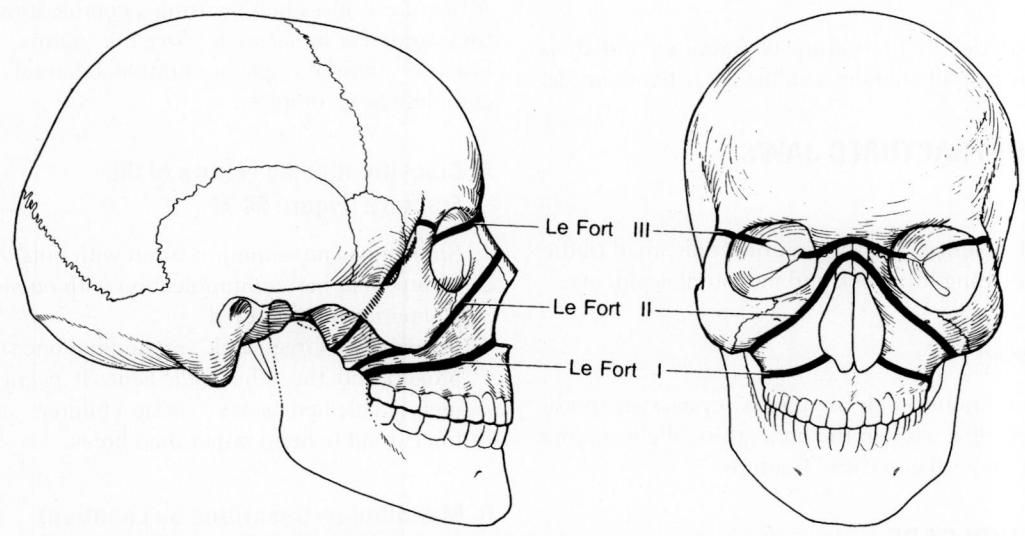

FIGURE 54-2 **Le Fort Classification of Facial Fractures.** *Le Fort I, horizontal fracture above the roots of the teeth, below the zygomatic process, and across the pterygoid plates.* Le Fort II, midface fracture over the middle of the nose and across the intraorbital rims. *Le Fort III, transversely across the bridge of the nose, across the orbits and the zygomatic bone.* (Adapted with permission from Archer WH. *Oral and maxillofacial surgery.* 5th ed. Philadelphia: Saunders; 1975. From Committee on Trauma, American College of Surgeons. Early care of the injured patient. Philadelphia: Saunders; 1972.)

A. Treatment Planning

- Many factors are involved when the oral surgeon selects the methods to be used, particularly the location of the fracture or fractures, the presence or absence of teeth, existing injuries to the teeth, other head injuries, and the general health and condition of the patient.
- All fractures do not require active intervention. Examples are fractures of the condylar and coronoid processes, nondisplaced fractures of an edentulous mandible, and greenstick fractures of children.

B. Basic Treatment

- *Reduction* (open or closed) of the fracture.
- *Fixation* of the fragments.
- *Immobilization* for healing.
- Control of complications of treatment centers around prevention of infections, malunion of the parts, and malocclusion of the dentition.

C. Healing

- Union is affected by the location and character of the fracture.
- Much depends on the patient's general health and resistance, as well as on cooperation.
- Six weeks is considered the average for the uncomplicated mandibular fracture, and 4 to 6 weeks for the maxillary.
- The major cause of complication is infection.

MANDIBULAR FRACTURES

Reduction means the positioning of the parts on either side of the fracture so they are in apposition for healing and restoration of function.

- *Open reduction* refers to the use of a surgical flap procedure to expose the fracture ends and bring them together for healing.
- *Closed reduction* is accomplished by manipulation of the parts without surgery.

I. CLOSED REDUCTION

- The closure of the teeth in normal occlusion for the individual is the usual guide for position of the fracture parts in the dentulous patient.
- To identify the customary relation of the teeth can be difficult, especially in the partially edentulous mouth.

II. INTERMAXILLARY FIXATION (IMF)

After reduction, a method of fixation and then immobilization that has been used for many years is *intermaxillary fixation*. It still is indicated under certain circumstances and in certain parts of the world.

A. Description

- Intermaxillary fixation is accomplished by applying wires and/or elastic bands between the maxillary and mandibular arches **(Figure 54-3)**.
- *Arch bars:* Readymade, contoured arch bars are adapted to fit accurately to each tooth and provide hooks for connecting the arches **(Figure 54-3C)**. A small horizontal elastic may be positioned across the fracture to reduce the lateral displacement **(Figure 54-3D)**.

B. Evaluation: Advantages

- Relative simplicity without surgical requirement: noninvasive.

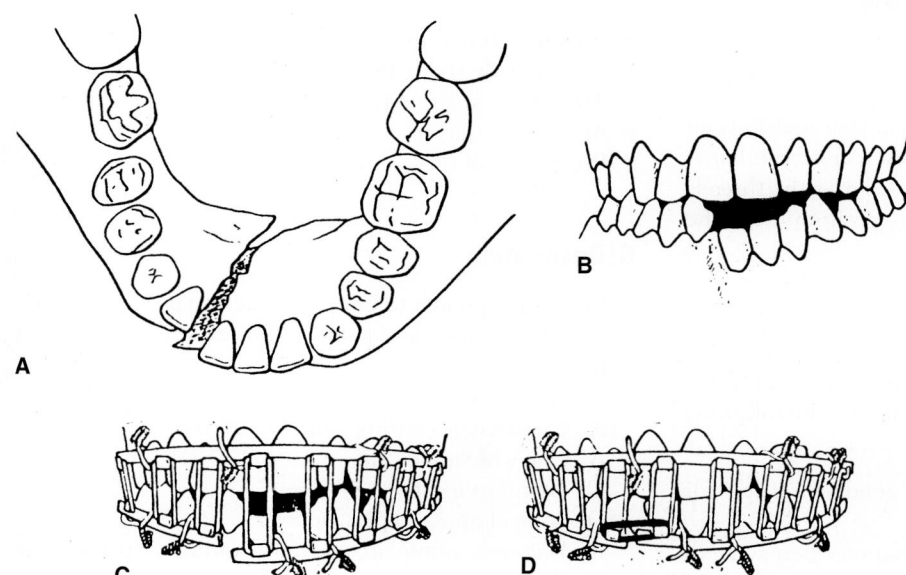

FIGURE 54-3 **Intermaxillary Fixation. (A)** Location of fracture of the mandible. **(B)** Segments of bone on either side of the fracture are displaced by muscle pull or contraction. **(C)** Arch bars with hooks for metal wires or rubber bands positioned to provide a steady pull for fracture reduction. **(D)** Note small horizontal rubber band extending from the hook at the mandibular right central incisor to the mandibular right canine to reduce the lateral displacement. (Adapted with permission from Archer WH. *Oral and maxillofacial surgery.* 5th ed. Philadelphia: Saunders; 1975.)

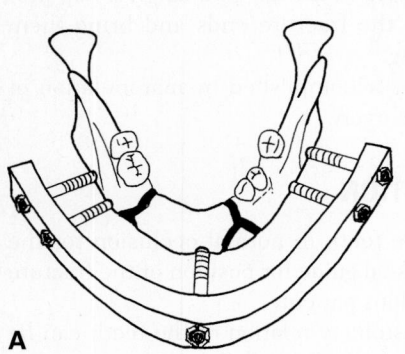

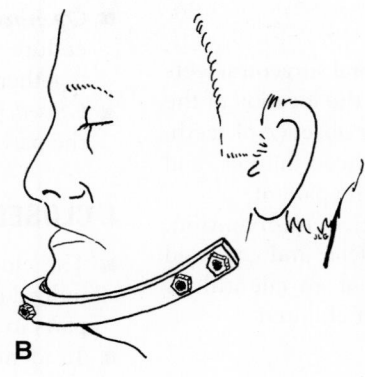

FIGURE 54-4 **External Skeletal Fixation.**
(A) Precision bone screws placed on either side of the fractures shown by heavy black lines. **(B)** Molded acrylic bar positioned over the bone screws and locked into position with nuts.

- Lower cost; shorter hospital stay (depending on other injuries).
- In less developed countries, resources and trained surgeons may be limited.
- Person can return to activity and work sooner; can use outpatient facility for follow-up.

C. Evaluation: Contraindications and Disadvantages

- Patients with chronic airway diseases who cough and expectorate: asthma, chronic obstructive pulmonary diseases.
- Patients who vomit regularly; notably, during pregnancy.
- Patients with a mental illness.
- Dietary problems: patients lose weight with liquid, monotonous diet, often with cariogenic content.
- Oral hygiene and dietary limitations lead to increased dental caries and periodontal infection.

III. EXTERNAL SKELETAL FIXATION (EXTERNAL PIN FIXATION)

A. Description

Two special bone screws are placed via skin incisions on either side of the fracture **(Figure 54-4A)**. An acrylic bar is molded and, while still pliable, is pressed over the threads of the bone screws and locked into position with the screw nuts **(Figure 54-4B)**.

B. Indications

Management of a fracture cannot always be accomplished satisfactorily by intermaxillary wiring alone. The following are indications for external fixation:

- Insufficient number of teeth in good condition for intermaxillary fixation.
- As a supplement to intermaxillary fixation when no teeth are present in the fractured portion of the mandible.

- Loss of bone substance.
  A. When bone substance is lost because of an accident, a gunshot wound, or a pathologic condition, a bone graft may be indicated.[6]
  B. The extraoral fixation is used first to hold the fractured parts in a normal relationship, and then to immobilize the area during healing following the bone graft surgery.
- Certain patients may be unable to have the jaws closed for a long period. Examples of these are:
  - Patient with a vomiting problem, such as during pregnancy.
  - Patient with a mental or physical disability, such as cerebral palsy, epilepsy, or mental retardation.
- Edentulous mandible when the fracture fragments are greatly displaced, when the fracture is at the angle of the mandible, or when the mandible is atrophic or thinned.

IV. OPEN REDUCTION

A. Principles for Treating Skeletal Fractures

- Anatomic reduction
- Functionally stable fixation
- Atraumatic surgical technique
- Active function
- Prevention of infection

B. Description

- Surgical approach to bring the fracture parts together.
- *Anesthesia:* anesthesia selected in accord with patient history.
- Types of systems used for immobilization include:
  A. Transosseous wiring (osteosynthesis)
  B. Plates of various sizes
  C. Titanium mesh
  D. Bone clamps, staples, screws
  E. *Materials:* miniplates, screws, and other parts made of biodegradable or resorbable synthetic materials

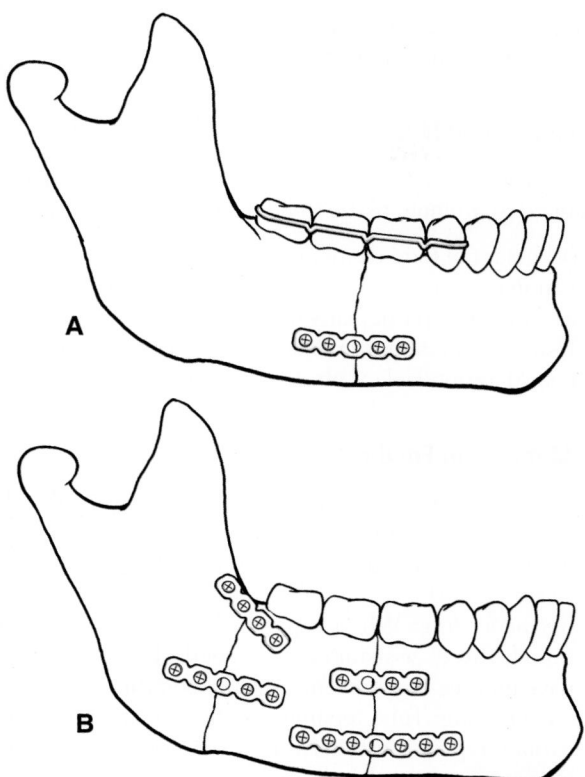

FIGURE 54-5 **Miniplates for Immobilization of Fracture. (A)** Tension band on the teeth to aid in maintaining correct occlusion while miniplate holds fracture ends in apposition. **(B)** Examples of possible positions for miniplates.

C. Clinical Example

- **Figure 54-5** illustrates various positions for miniplates to provide stability for the reduced fracture parts.
- Care is needed so that the screws are not placed over a fracture line or over the roots of teeth and so that they do not infringe on the mandibular canal.

MIDFACIAL FRACTURES

I. PRINCIPLES

- Maxillary fractures are more difficult to manage because of the number of bones, the associated anatomy, and the complications of basal skull fractures.
- Not all midface fractures need fixation following reduction.
- Both function and cosmetics are involved.

II. DESCRIPTION

A. Older Methods

- Internal wire suspension
- External cranial suspension to a stable bone, such as uninvolved zygoma
- Headcaps

B. Current Therapeutic Interventions

- Open reduction with internal fixation
- Use of bone plates of various sizes
- Grafts for reconstruction of midface defects
- Early reconstruction before scarring and soft tissue contracture deform the surrounding area

ALVEOLAR PROCESS FRACTURE

The most common fracture is of the alveolar process, maxillary or mandibular.

I. CLINICAL FINDINGS

- Face: bruising, areas of swelling
- Teeth: fractures, mobility, avulsion, displacement
- Lips and gingiva: bruising, bleeding lacerations from contact with teeth at the time of impact
- Bone fracture: most frequently in anterior

II. TREATMENT

- Replantation of displaced teeth.
- Immobilization with interdental wiring. A temporary fixed splint of acrylic may be placed over the wires. The teeth must be tested periodically for vitality.
- Endodontic therapy may be required later.

DENTAL HYGIENE CARE

I. PROBLEMS

Fixation apparatus, however carefully placed to prevent tissue irritation, interferes with normal function. Identification of possible effects of treatment provides the basis for planning dental hygiene care.

A. Development of Gingivitis or Periodontal Complications

- Thick biofilm formation and food debris accumulation provide sources of irritation to the gingiva.
- Gingivitis can develop in 9 to 19 days.[7]
- Lack of normal stimulation to the circulation of the periodontium and of cleansing effects usually provided by the action of the tongue, lips, and facial muscles contributes to stagnation of saliva and accumulation of debris and bacteria.
- Tender, sensitive gingiva make biofilm control more difficult, even on available surfaces.

B. Initiation of Demineralization

- An appetizing soft or liquid diet is difficult to plan using limited cariogenic foods for dental caries prevention.

C. Loss of Appetite

- Loss of appetite related to monotonous liquid or soft diet may lead to weight loss and lowered physical resistance.
- Secondary infections, including those of the oral tissues, may result.

D. Difficulty in Opening the Mouth

- When the temporomandibular joint has been injured, the patient wearing fixation appliances that involve only the mandible has difficulty in applying a toothbrush to the lingual surfaces of teeth.
- After removal of appliances, all patients have a degree of muscular trismus that limits personal oral care and mastication.

II. INSTRUMENTATION

A. Presurgical

Gross calculus is removed, insofar as possible, before open reduction procedures. Trauma to surrounding soft tissues of lip, tongue, and cheeks limits accessibility.

B. During Treatment

Periodic scaling contributes to oral health. Although access is only from the facial aspect for a patient with intermaxillary wiring, some benefit can be obtained. An assistant provides continual suction during treatment.

C. After Removal of Appliances

A few weeks after removal of appliances, when the patient can open the mouth normally and personal daily oral care has been initiated, complete scaling and planing can be performed.

III. DIET

Many patients with fractured jaws tend to lose weight, which is generally related to an inadequate nutrient and caloric intake. Objectives in planning the diet are:

- To help the patient maintain an adequate nutritional state.
- To promote healing.
- To increase resistance to infection.
- To prevent new carious lesions.

Attention must be given to the patient's willingness and ability to follow the recommendations made. The patient may be in the hospital for a few days to a few weeks, depending on the severity of other injuries. A greater length of time is spent as an outpatient, when the diet is much more difficult to supervise. The patient's understanding of dietary instructions and what is expected may appear more significant than the specific components of the diet recommended.

A. Nutritional Needs

After a surgical fixation procedure, the diet must be planned to promote tissue building and repair.

- All essential food elements.
- Emphasis on protein, vitamins, particularly A and C, and minerals particularly calcium and phosphorus.
- Usual caloric requirements for patient's age, taking into consideration lack of physical exercise and loss of

B. Methods of Feeding

- *Plastic straw:* Liquid is sucked through the teeth or through an edentulous area. Straw can be bent to accommodate a patient who cannot sit up.
- *Spoon feeding:* When a patient's arms are not functional, direct assistance is needed. The mouth may have injuries that prevent sucking food through a straw.
- *Tube feeding:* Tube feeding may be indicated following various types of extensive oral surgery, facial trauma, burns, immobilized fractured jaw, and other conditions that prevent ingesting sufficient calories and nutritional foods by way of the mouth.
  - A nasogastric tube is used. Blenderized food can be prepared, or special tube formulas are available commercially.
  - When commercial preparations are used, contents can be selected to meet the specific nutritional and caloric requirements of an individual patient.

C. Liquid Diet

A *clear liquid* diet to help prevent dehydration may be prescribed initially, but it can be nutritionally inadequate. A *full liquid* diet to provide high protein and other healing elements is of a consistency to be taken by a cup. A *blenderized liquid* diet can be passed through a straw.

- *Indications*
  - All patients with jaws wired together.
  - All patients with no appliance or single-jaw appliance who have difficulty in opening the mouth because of a condition, such as temporomandibular joint involvement or tongue or lip injury, that hinders insertion of food or manipulation of food in the mouth.
- *Examples of foods:* fruit juices, milk, eggnog, meat juices and soups, cooked thin cereals, and canned baby foods. Strained vegetables and meats (baby foods) may be added to meat juices and soups.
- *Use of a blender:* Regular table foods can be mixed in a food blender. With liquid, such as clear soup or milk, added, a fluid consistency can be obtained that will pass through a straw **(Figure 54-6)**.

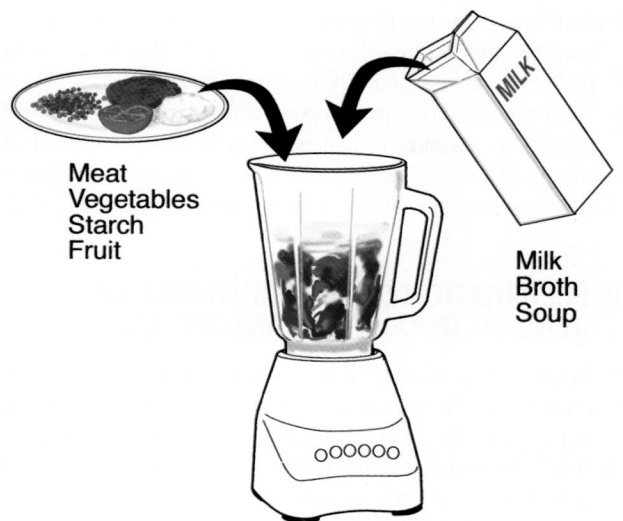

Meat
Vegetables
Starch
Fruit

Milk
Broth
Soup

FIGURE 54-6 **Preparation of a Liquid or Soft Diet.** Regular table foods can be blended with milk or other nutritious liquid.

D. Soft Diet

1. *Indications*
   - Patient with no appliance or with single-jaw appliance without complications in opening the mouth or in movement of the lips and tongue.
   - Patient who has been maintained on liquid diet throughout treatment period. After appliances are removed, the soft diet is recommended for several days to 1 week to provide the stomach with foods that are readily digestible rather than making a drastic change to a regular diet. A soft diet can also aid by protecting tender oral tissues from the rough textures of a regular diet until the tissues have had a chance to respond to softer foods.
2. *Examples of foods*
   - Soft-poached, scrambled, or boiled eggs; cooked cereals; mashed soft-cooked vegetables, including potato; mashed fresh or canned fruits; soft, finely divided meats; custards; plain ice cream.

E. Hints for Diet Planning With the Nonhospitalized Patient

1. Provide instruction sheets that show specific meal plans.
2. Express nutritional needs in quantities or servings of foods.
3. Show methods of varying the diet. A liquid or soft diet is at best monotonous because of the sameness of texture.
4. Encourage limitation of cariogenic foods as an aid to prevention of dental caries.

IV. PERSONAL ORAL CARE PROCEDURES

Every attempt to keep the patient's mouth as clean as possible for comfort and sanitation, and as free of dental biofilm as possible for disease prevention, is made. The extent of possible care depends on the appliances; the condition of the lips, tongue, and other oral tissues; and the cooperation of the patient.

Encouragement must be given to the patient to begin toothbrushing as soon as possible after the surgical procedure, but until the patient is able, a plan for care is outlined for a caregiver.

A. Irrigation

- *Indications:* During the first few days after the surgical procedure, while the mouth may be too tender for brushing, frequent irrigations are required; irrigation also serves as an adjunct to toothbrushing.
- *Method:* In a hospital, irrigations with suction are possible. At home, the patient irrigates with the head lowered over a sink (Box 28-2, page 420).
- *Mouthrinse selection:* The oral surgeon is consulted for specific instructions.
  A. Physiologic saline
  B. Chlorhexidine gluconate
  C. Fluoride rinse

B. Early Mouth Cleansing

While the patient is in the hospital, a soft toothbrush with suction can be used. The toothbrush with suction is described in Chapter 57 on page 882.

C. Personal Care by the Patient

- As soon as possible, the patient is instructed in personal care.
- A toothbrushing method and other aids, such as those used for orthodontic appliances, are recommended and demonstrated, as shown in Chapter 30, page 440.
- Because interdental and proximal tooth-surface care is limited to access only from the facial approach, the choice of devices is limited.[8] Some spaces permit insertion of an interdental brush. With instruction, most patients can use a rubber tip to "pencil" around just under the free gingival margin, as shown in Chapter 28, page 416.
- When the tongue is not injured, the patient can be instructed to use the tongue as an aid in cleaning the lingual surfaces of the teeth and massaging the gingiva.
- The ambulatory patient can use a water irrigator. A low-pressure setting is used, and the spray is directed carefully to prevent tissue injury, as described in Chapter 28, page 420.

D. After Appliances Are Removed

Except for the patient who had practiced good personal oral care before the accident, a step-by-step series of lessons is usually necessary.

A method for daily self-applied fluoride, such as a mouthrinse or brush-on gel, can be introduced along with the use of a fluoride dentifrice. Demineralization and dental caries can result from biofilm retention about the appliances.

DENTAL HYGIENE CARE BEFORE GENERAL SURGERY

■ Completing dental and dental hygiene treatment and bringing the oral cavity to a state of health before surgery have special significance for certain patients who will have surgical procedures other than oral.

■ When emergency surgery is performed, preparation of the mouth is not possible, and postsurgical examination and care may be complicated by various limitations.

■ When surgery is elective, or planned in advance, the patient can be encouraged to have complete dental and periodontal treatment.

■ Types of patients are described briefly here. Other examples are found in the various special patient chapters throughout this section of the book.

I. PATIENTS IN WHOM SURGICAL PROCEDURES AFFECT THEIR RISK STATUS

■ Patients who receive chemotherapeutic agents as partial treatment after surgery for various types of cancer, and others who use immunosuppressant drugs, require special management to prevent complications during dental and dental hygiene appointments.

■ Antibiotic premedication to prevent infective endocarditis and other infections is mandatory for certain patients is described in Chapter 9, page 131.

■ Before surgery for prostheses, transplants, cancer, and other serious conditions, patients can be informed of the need for completing oral care treatments and practicing preventive daily personal care.

II. PREPARATION OF THE MOUTH BEFORE GENERAL INHALATION ANESTHESIA

■ Because the mouth is an entryway to the respiratory chambers, the possibility always exists that bacteria, debris, and fluids may be inhaled from the mouth.

■ Inhalation could occur during the administration of an anesthetic or when the patient coughs.

III. PATIENT WITH A LONG CONVALESCENCE

■ Patients whose surgery requires a long convalescence may be unable to keep a regular maintenance appointment.

■ When the patient has a healthy mouth before the hospitalization and convalescence, the problems of postsurgical oral care are lessened but not eliminated.

■ Instruction for the caregiver may be needed. A home visit by the dental hygienist may be possible.

DOCUMENTATION

The permanent oral care record for most maxillofacial patients needs to include a summary of the hospital care when available, but may start when the patient returns to the general practice.

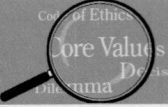 **Everyday Ethics**

Ms. Squires (age 79) was involved in a serious automobile accident that fractured her mandible and required fixation with intermaxillary wiring. Apparently she is here because of pressure from her adult children who have been taking turns tending to her needs. The daughter who accompanied her to this appointment said her bad breath was bothering them even more than her complaining all the time.

This is her first appointment with William, the dental hygienist, since the accident 10 months ago. He documented the moderate amounts of calculus and heavy dental biofilm throughout the mouth. Mrs. Squires demonstrates difficulty opening her mouth and seems fussy and apprehensive when William attempts to go over a toothbrushing procedure and continually asks her to "open wider, please."

Questions for Consideration

1. Which of the dental hygiene core values (Table II-1 in Section II Introduction, page 38) become involved with a patient with such complications? Explain each one.

2. Review the steps for decision making in Chapter 1 (page 10) to help plan and present optimal oral health services to benefit this patient?

3. Describe the role of the dental hygienist in coordinating preventive care with the posttreatment examinations Mrs. Squires has with the oral maxillofacial surgeon?

BOX 54-3	Example Progress Note

Carolyn (age 31) came for her dental hygiene appointment nearly 5 weeks after automobile accident, hospitalization; jaw fracture, and still on crutches for leg fracture. Health history review, vitals, and usual extra- and intraoral clinical examination. Patient complaint: mouth "feels very dirty; can even feel the calculus." Probing revealed several 3–4 mm with bleeding. Patient indicated she is still on mostly softer things, with ground or chopped meat, fish; jaw gets tired from chewing too much and holding mouth open for long. Did maxillary right quadrant scaling and appointed for other quadrants. Suggested jaw exercises using xylitol gum.

Signed: _____, RDH Date: _____

At that time the initial recording needs a minimum of the following:

- Health history, radiographs interpretation, extra- and intraoral findings, vital signs.
- Periodontal review including gingival description, charting of probing depths and overall periodontal review and summary of current needs.
- Risk factors and dental caries review; complete examination for demineralization.
- Care planning for maintenance.
- A sample progress note is available for review in **Box 54-3.**

Factors To Teach The Patient

Accident Prevention
- Always use seat belts in automobiles and other vehicles.
- Use mouthguards and all safety devices during contact sports.
- Wear motorcycle and bicycle helmets.

For the Patient who Will Have General Surgery
- Significance of a clean mouth during general anesthesia.
- Postsurgery oral problems related to specific diseases.

References

1. American Dental Association, Council on Dental Education, Chicago, 1990.
2. Chuong R. Perioperative management of the surgical patient. In: Peterson LJ, editor. *Oral and maxillofacial surgery.* Philadelphia: Lippincott; 1992. p. 63–85.
3. Haskell R. Applied surgical anatomy. In: Rowe NL, Williams JL, editor. *Maxillofacial injuries.* London: Churchill Livingstone; 1985. p. 21–4.
4. Luyk NH. Principles of management of fractures of the mandible. In: Peterson, LJ, editor. *Oral and maxillofacial surgery.* Philadelphia: Lippincott; 1992. p. 407–34.
5. Banks P, Brown A. *Fractures of the facial skeleton.* Oxford: Wright; 2001. Chapter 5, Treatment of fractures of the mandible; p. 81–106.
6. Boyne PJ. *Osseous reconstruction of the maxilla and the mandible.* Chicago: Quintessence; 1997. Bone grafts; p. 64–74.
7. Löe H, Theilade E, Jensen SB. Experimental gingivitis in man. *J Periodontol.* 1965 May-Jun;36:177–87.
8. Phelps-Sandall BA, Oxford SJ. Effectiveness of oral hygiene techniques on plaque and gingivitis in patients placed in intermaxillary fixation. *Oral Surg Oral Med Oral Pathol.* 1983 Nov;56(5):487–90.

The Patient With Cancer

DEBORAH S. MANNE, RDH, RN, MSN, OCN

Chapter Outline

Dental hygiene care of the patient with cancer before, during, and after therapy strives not only to attain but also maintain a patient's oral health at the highest possible level. This contributes to the patient's general health and overall quality of life. Terminology relating to cancer is defined in Box 55-1.

Cancer treatment modalities (radiation therapy, chemotherapy, surgery, and hematopoietic cell transplantation) have the potential to affect the oral cavity significantly. The patient will be under the care of a team of multidisciplinary specialists. Box 55-2 lists the members of the multidisciplinary team.

DESCRIPTION

A. Cancer refers to:
- A group of neoplastic diseases in which there is transformation of normal cells into malignant ones.
- As cancer cells proliferate, the mass of abnormal tissue that is formed enlarges until it takes over the host site. It then sheds cells that spread to distant sites (metastasis).

B. Characteristics of benign and malignant neoplasms are compared in **Table 55-1**.

BOX 55-1	Key Words

Cancer

Alopecia: a loss of hair.

Anaplasia: an irreversible alteration in adult cells toward more primitive (embryonic) cell types; characteristic of tumor cells.

Benign: not malignant (**Table 55-1**).

Biotherapy: use of biological agents to treat cancer.

Carcinogen: an agent that may cause cancer; may be chemical, physical (ionizing radiation), or biologic; biologic carcinogens may be external (for example, viruses) or internal (genetic defects).

Carcinoma: a malignant tumor of epithelial origin.

Chemotherapy: treatment of illness by chemical means, that is, by medication or drugs.

Dysgeusia: distortion of the sense of taste.

Dysplasia: an abnormality of development; in pathology, alteration in size, shape, and organization of adult cells.

Hematologic profile: an analysis of the blood and blood-forming tissues.

Hematopoiesis: formation and development of blood cells.

Hyperbaric oxygen: the patient is placed in a sealed chamber and given pure oxygen through a face mask. At the same time, compressed air is introduced into the chamber to raise the atmospheric pressure to several times normal. This equalizes the pressure inside and outside of the body, thereby flooding the tissues with oxygen. An increase in oxygen to the irradiated tissues can temporarily compensate for the reduction in circulation.

Imaging: the production of diagnostic images, including radiography, ultrasonography, or scintigraphy.

Infiltration: the diffusion or accumulation in a tissue of cells or substances not normal to it or in amounts in excess of normal; in leukemia, for example, white blood cells infiltrate body tissues.

In situ: in its normal place; confined to the site of origin.

Interstitial: pertaining to, or situated in, the interstices (small spaces) of a tissue.

Intrathecal: within a sheath; through the theca of the spinal cord into the subarachnoid space; in leukemia, for example, the location for the delivery of various chemotherapeutic drugs.

Isogenic: having the same genetic constitution; syngeneic.

Leukemia: an acute or chronic progressive malignant neoplasm of the blood-forming organs, marked by diffuse proliferation of immature white blood cells (leukocytes); subsequent reduction in erythrocytes and platelets results.

Lymphadenectomy: excision of one or more lymph nodes.

Malignant: tending to become progressively worse and to result in death; having the properties of anaplasia, invasiveness, and metastasis; said of tumors (**Table 55-1**).

Metastasis: transfer of disease from one organ or part to another not directly connected with it; for example, regional or distant spread of cancer cells from the site primarily involved.

Nadir: the point at which a patient's blood counts reach their lowest level after chemotherapy administration; do not perform any dental care during this time.

Neoplasm: any new and abnormal growth, specifically one in which cell multiplication is controlled and progressive; may be benign or malignant.

Oncology: the sum of knowledge regarding tumors: the study of tumors.

Oral mucositis/stomatitis: inflammation and ulceration of the oral mucous membranes; can increase the risk for pain, oral and systemic infection, and nutritional compromise.

Osteoradionecrosis: blood vessel compromise and necrosis of bone exposed to high-dose radiation therapy, resulting in decreased ability to heal if traumatized and in extreme susceptibility to infection.

Palliative/Palliation: affording relief, but does not cure.

Pancytopenia: abnormal depression of all cellular elements of the blood.

Pleomorphism: occurrence in more than one form; the assumption of various distinct morphologic types by a single organism or cell.

Radiation therapy: the treatment of disease by ionizing radiation; may be external megavoltage or internal by use of interstitial implantation of an isotope (radium).

Radium: a highly radioactive chemical element found in uranium minerals; used in the treatment of malignant tumors in the form of needles or pellets for interstitial implantation.

Relapse: the return of a disease weeks or months after its apparent cessation.

Remission: diminution or abatement of the symptoms of a disease; the period during which such diminution occurs.

Sarcoma: a tumor, often highly malignant, composed of cells derived from connective tissue such as bone and cartilage, muscle, blood vessel, or lymphoid tissue.

Staging: the succinct, standardized description of a tumor with regard to origin and spread. This clinical classification is based on physical assessments, biopsy, imaging, and endoscopy. Each stage (I–IV) consists of three components: T (size of tumor); N (lymph node involvement); and M (presence or absence of distant metastasis).

Stomatoxic: potential for causing oral ulceration/inflammation of the gastrointestinal tract

Trismus: limitations of opening because of spasm and/or fibrosis of the muscles of mastication and/or temporomandibular joint located in the field of radiation.

Xerostomia/salivary gland dysfunction: dryness of the mouth because of thickened, reduced, or absent salivary flow; increases the risk for infection and compromised chewing, speaking, and swallowing. Persistent dry mouth increases the risk for dental caries.

<table>
<tr><td>**BOX 55-2**</td><td>**Multidisciplinary Team for the Care of the Patient With Cancer**</td></tr>
</table>

CANCER SPECIALISTS
Medical oncologist
Radiation oncologist
Surgeon (all subspecialties)
Oncology nurse
Oncology dietician
Oncology social worker

ORAL CARE SPECIALISTS
Dental hygienist
Dentist
Oral surgeon
Periodontist
Endodontist
Oral maxillofacial prosthodontist
Oral pathologist

OTHER HEALTH SPECIALISTS
Speech pathologist
Physical therapist
Occupational therapist
Psychologist/psychiatrist

C. Cancers are classified on the basis of
- the origin of the tissue involved, that is, carcinomas from epithelial tissue, and sarcomas from connective tissue;
- the type of cell from which they arise, namely, an epithelial or connective tissue cell.[1]

D. Staging is
- a succinct, standardized description of a tumor based on origin and spread;
- made up of three components: T (tumor size), N (presence or absence of lymph nodes), and M (presence or absence of distant metastases).

I. INCIDENCE AND SURVIVAL

Cancer is the second leading cause of death in the United States for adults under the age of 85.[2] Survival depends on the following:

- Location and size of the tumor
- Type of cancer
- Presence of distant metastasis
- Tumor sensitivity to treatment
- Physical condition and age of the patient

TABLE 55-1	CHARACTERISTICS OF BENIGN AND MALIGNANT NEOPLASMS	
CHARACTERISTIC	**BENIGN**	**MALIGNANT**
Cell Characteristics	Cells resemble normal cells of the tissue from which the tumor originated	Cells often bear little resemblance to the normal cells of the tissue from which they arose; there is both anaplasia and pleomorphism
Mode of Growth	Tumor grows by expansion and does not infiltrate the surrounding tissues; encapsulated	Tumor grows at the periphery and sends out processes that infiltrate and destroy the surrounding tissues
Rate of Growth	Rate of growth is usually slow	Rate of growth is usually relatively rapid and is dependent on level of differentiation; the more anaplastic the tumor, the more rapid the rate of growth
Metastasis	Does not spread by metastasis	Gains access to the blood and lymph channels and metastasizes to other areas of the body
Recurrence	Does not recur when removed	Tends to recur when removed
General Effects	Is usually a localized phenomenon that does not cause generalized effects unless by location it interferes with vital functions	Often causes generalized effects, such as anemia, weakness, and weight loss
Destruction of Tissue	Does not usually cause tissue damage unless location interferes with blood flow	Often causes extensive tissue damage as the tumor outgrows its blood supply or encroaches on blood flow to the area; may also produce substances that cause cell damage
Ability to Cause Death	Does not usually cause death unless its location interferes with vital functions	Usually causes death unless growth can be controlled

Reprinted with permission from Porth, C., *Pathophysiology: Concepts of Altered Health States,* 2nd ed. Philadelphia, J. B. Lippincott Co., 1986.

II. RISK FACTORS[3]

There are numerous factors that increase a person's risk for developing cancer:

- *Tobacco:* both smoking and spit tobacco are implicated in head and neck cancer, lung cancer, and bladder cancer.
- *Alcohol:* chronic, long-term use especially in combination with tobacco use implicated in head and neck cancer, bladder cancer, and liver cancer.
- *Sunlight:* especially occupations requiring work in the sun such as construction workers, farmers, as well as sunbathers.
- *Environmental/occupational:* exposure to asbestos, radon, coal dust, and chemicals, to name a few.
- *Viruses:* Epstein–Barr virus implicated in Burkett's lymphoma, Hepatitis C implicated in liver cancer, human papillomavirus (HPV) implicated in cervical cancer and cancer of the oral cavity/oropharynx.
- *Socioeconomic:* late diagnosis with poorer prognosis seen in lower socioeconomic populations (inner city, rural, working poor).

III. TYPES OF CANCER[2]

The most common types of cancer are as follows:

Men:

- Prostate
- Lung and bronchus
- Colon and rectum

Women:

- Breast
- Lung and bronchus
- Colon and rectum

IV. HOW CANCER IS TREATED[3,4,5]

Cancer is treated using a variety of different approaches based on the following:

- The location and size of the tumor
- Treatment objectives (cure, control, or palliation)

    The different approaches include

- Surgery
- Chemotherapy
- Radiation therapy
- Hematopoietic cell transplantation
- Hormone therapy
- Vaccine therapy
- Biotherapy
- A combination of two or more of the above

SURGERY

Surgery is the most common form of treatment for solid tumors, both malignant and nonmalignant.

I. INDICATIONS FOR SURGERY[6]

- Tumors that are small in size, localized, and easy to remove.
- Debulk or remove portions of large tumors before treatment (chemotherapy or radiation therapy).
- Provide pain relief or prolong life when no chance of cure is possible (palliation).

CHEMOTHERAPY[7]

Chemotherapy involves the use of drugs that affect the rapidly dividing cancer cell at different points in the cell cycle. The drugs are used as a single agent or in combination. Side effects can be severe and frequently involve the oral cavity.

I. OBJECTIVES

- To destroy cancer cells and keep them from metastasizing.
- To prevent cancer from recurring.
- To provide an improved quality of life.

II. INDICATIONS

- Eliminate a localized tumor too large for surgical removal.
- Treat cancer that has metastasized to other parts of the body.
- Prevent cancer recurrence with maintenance therapy.
- Use before surgery to make a tumor easier to remove completely.
- Extend life when no chance of a cure is possible (palliation).

III. TYPES OF CHEMOTHERAPY[7]

Box 55-3 lists the types of agents used for chemotherapy.

IV. SYSTEMIC SIDE EFFECTS OF CHEMOTHERAPY[8]

Chemotherapy affects both rapidly dividing cancer cells and rapidly dividing normal cells (hair, oral/gastrointestinal

BOX 55-3	Types of Agents Used for Chemotherapy
	Alkylating agents
	Antibiotics
	Antimetabolites
	Plant alkaloids
	Steroids/hormones
	Miscellaneous

mucosa, and bone marrow). This can cause side effects that can range from mild to life threatening. The most common include the following:

- Alopecia (hair loss)
- Myelosuppression (bone marrow suppression causing a reduction in blood counts leading to anemia, leukopenia, and thrombocytopenia)
- Immunosuppression (inhibition of antibody responses resulting from leukopenia)
- Nausea, vomiting, and diarrhea
- Loss of appetite
- Gastrointestinal mucositis

V. ORAL COMPLICATIONS OF CHEMOTHERAPY[4,9]

The following are oral complications resulting from chemotherapy.

- Oral mucositis/stomatitis: an inflammation of the oral mucosa characterized by redness, ulcerations, and pain.
- *Xerostomia:* reduced amount or complete absence of saliva
- *Infections:*
  - Bacterial
  - *Viral:* herpes simplex, varicella zoster, cytomegalovirus
  - *Fungal: Candida albicans*
- *Bleeding:* anywhere in the mouth; spontaneous or induced
- *Neurotoxicity:* mimics toothache; usually bilateral

RADIATION THERAPY[10]

Radiation therapy uses ionizing radiation to treat cancer.

- It impacts the cancer cell's ability to replicate and survive.
- Not all tumors are radiosensitive (ability of the radiation therapy to kill the tumor).
- Head and neck radiation therapy produces acute short-term and chronic long-term effects in the oral cavity.

I. INDICATIONS

- Treat a small localized tumor that is radiosensitive.
- Shrink a large tumor before surgery.
- Assist chemotherapy effect when used concurrently.
- Prevent the spread of cancer or control residual tumor.
- Prevent a recurrence of the cancer.
- Provide symptom/pain relief for bone metastases or palliative therapy.

II. TYPES

- *External beam:* radiation that is applied outside the body. **Figure 55-1** illustrates exposure areas for external radiation.

- *Internal:* The source (such as implants or seeds) of the radiation is placed within the body. Less radiation is delivered to surrounding tissues than when an external source is utilized.

III. DOSES[11]

- Total dose given depends on the type of tumor, treatment goals, and patient's ability to tolerate treatment.
- Total radiation dose is approximately 3,000 to 7,000 centigrays.
- It is divided into equal doses or fractions per day.
- It is given once a day, 5 days a week, for 5 to 12 weeks.

IV. SYSTEMIC EFFECTS[12]

- *Skin reactions:* looks like a bad sunburn
- Fatigue
- Nausea, vomiting, diarrhea, constipation

V. ORAL COMPLICATIONS[4,9]

- Oral mucositis/stomatitis
- Xerostomia
- Radiation caries
- Taste loss
- *Infection:*
  - Bacterial
  - *Viral:* herpes simplex, varicella zoster
  - *Fungal: Candida albicans*
- *Trismus:* inability to open mouth completely
- Osteoradionecrosis

HEMATOPOIETIC CELL TRANSPLANTATION[13,14]

Hematopoietic cell transplantation is used to treat a variety of blood diseases, including leukemia. The purpose is to substitute blood stem cells or bone marrow from a healthy, compatible donor to replace the diseased bone marrow of the patient.

I. TYPES OF TRANSPLANTS[13]

The three basic types of transplants:

- Autolgous—self
- Allogenic—matched donor
- Syngeneic—identical twin

II. STAGES OF THE TRANSPLANTATION PROCESS[13,14]

A. Patient Selection

- *Indications:* patient not responsive to chemotherapy alone; relapse occurs after one or more remissions.

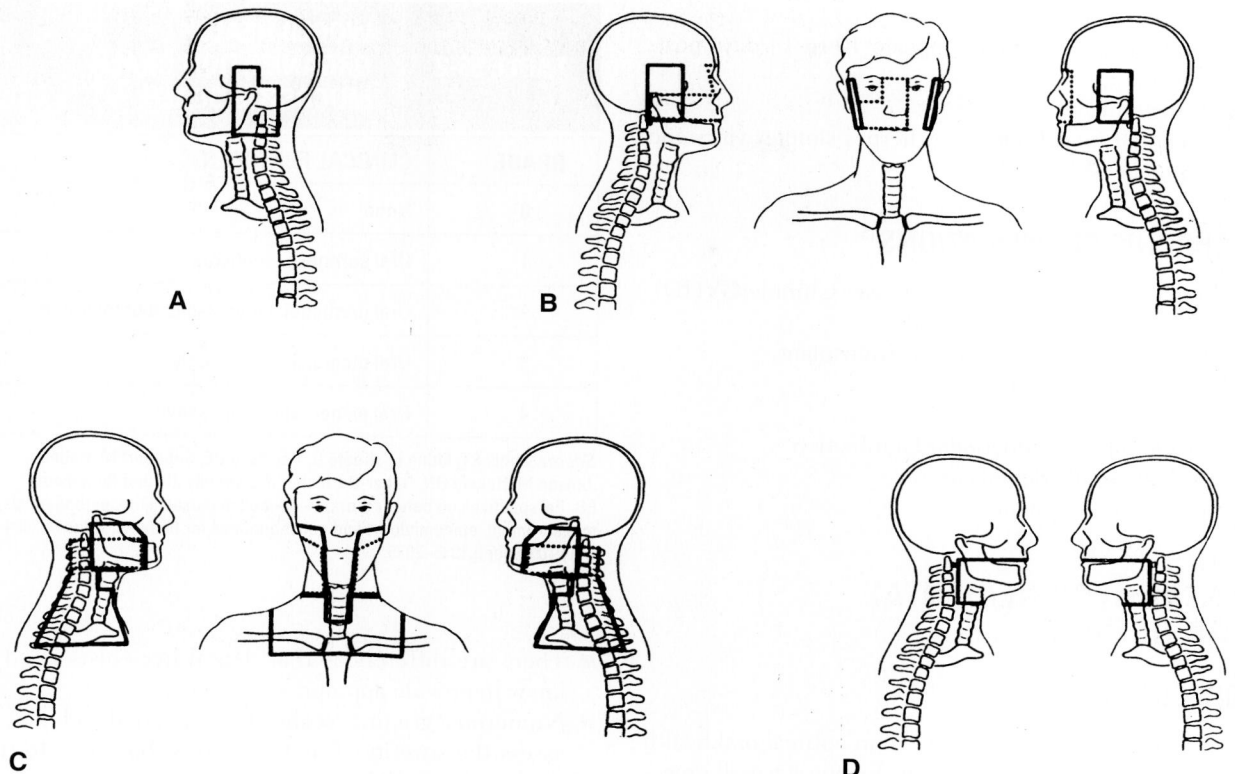

FIGURE 55-1 **Common Fields of Radiation for Head and Neck Tumors.** Dark lines show fields when increased dosages are needed. **(A)** Parotid field. **(B)** Antrum field. **(C)** Oropharynx field. **(D)** Floor of mouth field. (Courtesy of Jansma, J. Oral sequelae resulting from head and neck radiotherapy. Groningen: Drukkerij van Denderen B.V.; 1991.)

■ *Evaluation:* medical and dental assessments completed to ensure patient is free of infection and physically able to undergo the preparative regimen.

B. Donor Regimen

■ Histocompatibility matching
■ Bone marrow aspirated from iliac crest, ribs, or sternum

C. Conditioning of Patient to Receive Bone Marrow Graft

■ Preparative high-dose immunosuppressive regimen: chemotherapy alone or with total body irradiation.
■ *Purposes:*
  ▪ Kill malignant cells
  ▪ Suppress immune system so new marrow will engraft

D. Transplantation

■ Intravenous infusion of donor's marrow

E. Pancytopenic Period

■ All cellular elements of the blood are depressed.
■ Protective isolation for the patient is required; patient is highly susceptible to infection.

■ Function of new marrow (to produce peripheral blood elements) begins after 10 to 20 days.

F. Recovery

■ Immune recovery 3 to 12 months; long-term recovery 1 to 3 years.

III. ACUTE COMPLICATIONS[15]

■ Acute-Graft-Versus-Host Disease (Acute GVHD)
  Description: The donor's T-lymphocytes see the host cell antigens as foreign and react against the host tissue.
  Symptoms:
  ▪ Present during the first 100 days posttransplant.
  ▪ Painful red skin rash starting on the palms of hands and soles of feet and progressing to the upper trunk.
  ▪ Severe, persistent diarrhea.
  ▪ Jaundice, elevated liver enzymes, liver tenderness.
■ *Infection:*
  ▪ Bacterial
  ▪ *Viral:* herpes simplex, varicella zoster, cytomegalovirus
  ▪ *Fungal: Candida albicans*
■ Gastrointestinal, hepatic, cardiac, pulmonary, hematologic, neurologic complications

■ *Oral Complications:*
   ■ *Oral mucositis:* severe; appears 10 to 14 days post-transplant
   ■ Xerostomia
   ■ *Viral and fungal infections:* herpes simplex virus and *Candida albicans*

IV. CHRONIC COMPLICATIONS[15]

■ Chronic-Graft-Versus-Host Disease (Chronic GVHD)
   ■ Affects all organs of the body.
   ■ Can appear up to 2 years posttransplant.
   ■ *Oral Complications:*
      1. Oral mucositis
      2. Oral infection/periodontal infection
      3. Xerostomia/dental caries
      4. Poor oral hygiene

DENTAL HYGIENE/DENTAL PLAN OF CARE[4]

I. OBJECTIVES

It is recommended that patients be in optimal oral health before starting any type of cancer therapy. Overall objectives include the following:

■ Assess the oral cavity for any signs of dental/oral/periodontal infection.
■ Eliminate sources of dental/oral/periodontal infection.
■ Instruct the patient in preventive oral care measures.

II. PERSONAL FACTORS

The very word *cancer* brings fear and anxiety to the patient, and many times is viewed by the patient as *cancer equals death.* This will impact anything taught to the patient. Suggestions include the following:

■ Encourage the patient to bring a friend or family member along to take notes during teaching visits.
■ Provide written instructions appropriate to the reading level of the patient. Make sure they are written in the patient's native tongue.
■ Provide positive reinforcement and be creative in helping the patient maintain optimal oral health.
■ Show acceptance. Acknowledge the appropriateness of the patient's concerns.
■ Practice active listening skills.

III. PATIENT ORAL CARE

The following sections are adapted from the *Oral Complications of Cancer Treatment: What the Oral Health Team Can Do* from the National Institute for Dental and Craniofacial Research (NIH publication no. 02-4372).

■ Similarities exist between the three forms of treatment.

TABLE 55-2	WORLD HEALTH ORGANIZATION ORAL MUCOSITIS SCALE

GRADE	CLINICAL FEATURES
0	None
1	Oral soreness, erythema
2	Oral erythema, ulcers, solid diet tolerated
3	Oral ulcers, liquid diet only
4	Oral alimentation impossible

Source: Sonis ST, Elting LS, Keefe D, Peterson DE, Schubert M, Hauer-Jensen M, Bekele BN, Raber-Durlacher J, Donnelly JP, and Rubenstein EB. Perspectives on cancer therapy-induced mucosal injury: pathogenesis, measurement, epidemiology, and consequences for patients. *Cancer.* 2004 May;100(Suppl):1995–2025.

■ There are differences that dental hygienists need to know to provide appropriate oral care.
■ Numerous grading scales have been developed to assess the severity of oral mucositis, but none for the other oral complications.
■ **Table 55-2** shows an example of one mucositis scale.

A. Pretreatment Therapy

■ It is well-recognized that patients who do intensive personal oral care in preparation for and all during their cancer therapy have a reduced risk for the development of oral complications.
■ Box 55-4 lists the dental hygiene/dental treatment that is to be completed before the start of any cancer therapy.

B. Head and Neck Radiation Therapy[16,17]

■ Patients receiving radiation therapy to the head and neck are at high risk for developing severe oral complications that will affect the patient in the short term and long term.
■ Box 55-5 lists the patient's personal oral care to be followed during treatment.
■ *During radiation therapy:*
   ■ Monitor the patient's personal daily oral care including biofilm removal at least twice daily.
   ■ Monitor the patient's once daily fluoride gel tray usage.
   ■ Monitor the patient for trismus; check for pain or weakness in masticating muscles in the radiation field.
   ■ Instruct the patient to exercise 3 times a day, opening and closing the mouth as far as possible without pain; repeat 20 times.

BOX 55-4	Dental Hygiene/Dental Pretreatment Guidelines for Patients Planning to Undergo Cancer Therapy

DENTAL
- Conduct a pretreatment oral health examination.
- Schedule dental treatment in consultation with the oncologist (medical or radiation).
- Extract teeth with a poor or questionable prognosis at least 2 weeks before the start of cancer therapy.
- Restore or repair indicated teeth before the start of cancer therapy.
- Perform other necessary oral surgery procedures at least 2 weeks before the start of cancer therapy.

DENTAL HYGIENE
- Conduct a pretreatment oral health assessment.
- Schedule dental hygiene treatment in consultation with the oncologist (medical or radiation).
- Perform dental hygiene treatment (periodontal scaling and root planing, polishing, fluoride applications) before the start of cancer treatment.
- Evaluate the patient's oral health knowledge and provide an appropriate oral hygiene regimen based on the cancer therapy being received.
- Prevent tooth demineralization and dental caries:
  A. Instruct the patient in the daily application of fluoride gel at home.
  B. If receiving head-neck radiation therapy, fabricate custom gel-applicator trays for the patient.
  C. Demonstrate application of a 1.1% neutral pH sodium fluoride gel or a 0.4% stannous, unflavored gel for use in the trays.
  D. Use only a neutral pH sodium fluoride gel for porcelain crowns or glass or resin ionomer restorations.
  E. The trays cover all tooth surfaces and are left in the mouth for 5 minutes. Instruct the patient to have nothing to eat or drink for 30 minutes after using the fluoride. Specific technique is located on page 532 in Chapter 35.

BOX 55-5	Patient Oral Care During Treatment

DAILY BIOFILM REMOVAL
- Gently brush teeth, gingiva, and tongue with an extra soft toothbrush and fluoride toothpaste after every meal and at bedtime.
- Floss teeth gently but thoroughly each day.

MOUTHRINSING
- Every 2 to 3 hours while awake, rinse the mouth with a baking soda and water solution, followed by a plain water rinse. (Use 1/4 teaspoon of baking soda in 1 cup of lukewarm water.)
- Avoid mouthrinses containing alcohol because of their drying and irritating effects.

XEROSTOMIA
- Sip water frequently.
- Suck on ice chips or use sugar-free gum or candy.
- Use saliva substitute spray or gel or a prescribed saliva stimulant.
- Avoid lemon glycerin swabs.
- Avoid hot, spicy, salty, or sharp foods.
- Moisten foods with gravy or liquids before eating.

DENTAL CARIES PREVENTION
- Use fluoride toothpaste every day.
- If prescribed, brush teeth with 1.1% neutral NaF gel for 60 seconds after usual tooth cleaning, just before going to bed. Do not eat, drink, or rinse for 30 minutes afterward.
- If using custom-made polyvinyl trays, place gel in trays, apply to teeth, close mouth, and hold in place for 4 minutes. Set timer. Remove trays, expectorate several times, and do not eat or drink for 30 minutes afterward.

ORAL PAIN MANAGEMENT
- Swish, gargle, and spit a capful of prescribed mouthrinse containing topical anesthetic solution 30 minutes before eating.

- *After radiation therapy:*
  - For the first 6 months after cancer treatment, recall the patient for nonsurgical periodontal therapy and review instructions for daily personal oral hygiene every 4 to 8 weeks as needed.
  - Reinforce the importance of daily personal oral hygiene.
  - After mucositis subsides, consult with the radiation oncologist about when to have the dentist make dentures and other appliances.
  - Watch for trismus, demineralization, and caries. Lifelong, daily applications of prescription fluoride (either gel or rinse) are needed for patients with chronic xerostomia.
  - Advise against all oral surgery on irradiated bone, because of the risk of osteoradionecrosis. Tooth extraction, if unavoidable, is conservative, using hyperbaric oxygen therapy first.

C. Chemotherapy[18,19]

The extent of oral complications of chemotherapy depend on

- the degree of oral/periodontal/dental infection present,
- the chemotherapy drugs used and their dosages,
- the concurrent or adjuvant radiation therapy,
- the patient's personal daily oral hygiene.
- *During chemotherapy:*
  - Consult the medical oncologist before any dental or dental hygiene clinical procedures.
  - Ask the medical oncologist to order blood work 24 hours before oral surgery or other invasive procedures

(such as periodontal scaling/root planing). Postpone when the

1. platelet count is less than 50,000/mm^3 or abnormal clotting factors are present,
2. neutrophil count is less than 1,000/mm^3.

- In patients with fever of unknown origin (FUO) as determined by the medical oncologist, check for oral source of viral, bacterial, or fungal infection.
- Encourage thorough oral hygiene measures.
- Before any dental or dental hygiene clinical procedures:
  1. Ensure antibiotic premedication for patients with central venous catheters or peripherally inserted catheters (also known as central lines).
  2. Consult the medical oncologist for preference on using the American Heart Association prophylactic antibiotic regimen or another antibiotic regimen.
  3. Refer to **Box 55-5** for patient oral care during treatment.

- *After Chemotherapy*
  - Place the patient on a dental hygiene/dental maintenance schedule when chemotherapy is completed and all side effects, including immunosuppression, have resolved.

D. Hematopoietic Cell Transplantation[20,21]

Most hematopoietic cell transplant patients develop acute oral complications, especially patients with graft-versus-host disease.

- *After transplantation*
  - Watch for oral infections on the tongue and oral mucosa. Herpes simplex and *Candida albicans* are common oral infections.
  - Continue to monitor the patient's oral health for biofilm control, tooth demineralization, dental caries, and oral infection.
  - Delay elective dental procedures (such as implants) for 1 year.
  - Follow patients for long-term oral complications (mucositis, xerostomia, dental caries). Such problems are strong indicators of chronic graft-versus-host disease.
  - Continue to monitor the patient's oral health for biofilm control, tooth demineralization, dental caries, and oral infection.
  - Follow transplant patients carefully for second malignancies in the oral region.

E. Special Care for Children[22]

Children receiving chemotherapy and/or radiation therapy are at risk for the same oral complications as adults. Other actions to consider in managing pediatric patients include the following:

- Extract loose primary teeth and teeth expected to exfoliate during cancer treatment.

- Remove orthodontic bands and brackets if highly stomatoxic chemotherapy is planned or if the appliances will be in the radiation field.
- Continually monitor craniofacial and dental structures for abnormal growth and development.
- Perform routine daily personal oral care including biofilm removal and fluoride application.
- Try to avoid cariogenic foods and drinks. If these are necessary to improve a child's weight, then have the child rinse with plain fluoridated water after eating or drinking.

DOCUMENTATION

Each patient appointment is carefully documented to include at least the following:

- Cancer diagnosis; type of treatment; treatment start and completion dates.
- Oncologists' names and contact information; note any consults done with the oncologists.
- Oral assessment, clinical care provided, patient teaching on each visit.
- Any oral complications present; grading scaling number of oral mucositis; and what symptom management was prescribed.
- Planned follow-up visit and plan of care with proposed symptom management treatment outcomes.
- **Box 55-6** shows an example of a Progress Note.

BOX 55-6	Example Progress Note

Patient presents for 3-month perio maintenance appointment with oral mucositis grade 4 and severe xerostomia: medical history changes include diagnosis of stage IV floor of mouth (FOM) cancer; lesion found at previous perio maintenance visit and patient went to Otolaryngologist 3 months ago resection surgery performed 10 weeks ago completed 6 weeks of radiation therapy for a total of 62 Gy last week;

Complete oral exam performed; unable to perform perio maintenance due to severe oral mucositis; reviewed oral hygiene; pt is not currently using fluoride; recommendations prescribed: use of extra soft toothbrush and brushing after meals and at bedtime, gentle flossing once daily; use of prescription neutral sodium fluoride once daily as a brush on gel; bland mouthwash of baking soda 1 Tbsp to 8oz glass of warm water three times a day; avoid alcohol containing mouth rinses; plan to see weekly for follow-up until oral mucositis resolves. Next visit begin regiment for managing xerostomia and review current plan and revise as needed.

Signed: _____, RDH Date: _____.

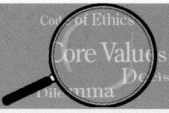

Everyday Ethics

It's the end of the day and all of the patients, staff, and the dentist had left the office. Ashley, the dental hygienist, was reviewing the next day's patient records at the front desk.

The telephone rang and Ashley answered it. It was Gina, the daughter of a longtime patient, Mr. Prisby. Gina, a pediatric registered nurse, lives out of state, but is visiting her 70-year-old father who is undergoing head and neck radiation therapy and chemotherapy treatments for tongue cancer. When she arrived, she was shocked to find her father having difficulty opening his mouth completely and a white coating on the inside of his cheeks. Gina also noticed multiple sores in his mouth. Her father has been unable to eat anything but the softest of foods due to the severe discomfort and dryness. Gina is concerned that her father cannot maintain a healthy weight during treatment. She asks Ashley what the white coating and the sores are in her father's mouth and what can be done for him.

Ashley puts Gina on hold and pulls Mr. Prisby's record. She sees that he had a complete examination and all treatment performed that left him in good dental health 3 months ago, just before he started his cancer treatment. The white coating that Ashley described may be candidiasis and require medication. But she's not sure how to treat the sores Gina sees. Ashley considers whether to refer Gina back to the oncologists treating her father or phoning in the prescription in the dentist's name to save time.

Questions for Consideration

1. What advice can Ashley give to Gina, considering the stipulations of patient confidentiality?
2. Describe the ethical and legal consequences of Ashley phoning in a prescription for Mr. Prisby.
3. What decisions and/or actions are appropriate for Ashley to pursue within the scope of her legal duties at this time?

Factors To Teach The Patient

- How to exercise the jaw muscles 3 times a day to prevent and treat jaw stiffness from head and neck radiation therapy.
- Why to avoid candy, gum, and soda unless they are sugar free.
- Why to avoid spicy or acidic foods, and the use of toothpicks.
- Why to avoid use of tobacco products and alcohol.
- Why the dental hygienist needs to conduct an oral soft tissue screening and complete oral examination at regular frequent intervals.
- How and when to use dental biofilm control methods, gel-tray application, use of saliva substitute, and all other details of personal oral care to reduce oral side effects caused by the disease and/or cancer treatment.
- Ideas for remembering to follow the instructions to keep the mouth healthier and more comfortable during cancer treatment.
- The reasons why a routine schedule of preventive periodontal scaling, fluoride application, and oral hygiene assessment by a dental hygienist contributes to the success of the cancer treatment.

Factors To Teach The Caregiver

- How maintaining optimal oral health throughout treatment will contribute to the successful outcome of cancer therapy.
- The need to report any changes in the oral cavity to the oncologist and/or dentist/dental hygienist.
- Why it is necessary for the patient to receive preventive periodontal scaling, polishing if indicated, fluoride application, and oral hygiene assessment by a dental hygienist on a regular frequent basis.
- Why it is important to support the patient in stopping tobacco and alcohol use.

References

1. Hanahan D, Weinberg RA. The hallmarks of cancer. *Cell.* 2000 Jan; 7;100(1):57–70.
2. Jemal A, Siegel R, Ward E, Hao Y, Thun MJ. Cancer statistics 2009. *CA Cancer J Clin.* 2009 Jul–Aug;59(4):225–49.
3. Lenhard RE, Osteen RT, Gansler T, eds. *Clinical oncology.* Atlanta (GA): American Cancer Society; 2001. Chapter 3, Heath CW, Fontham ETH. Cancer etiology. pp. 37–54.

4. Barker GJ, Barker BF, Gier RE. *Oral management of the cancer patient: a guide for the health care professional.* 6th ed. Kansas City (MO): Biomedical Communications, University of Missouri-Kansas City, School of Dentistry; 2000.

5. Yarbo CH, Frogge MH, Goodman M, Groenwald SL, eds. *Cancer nursing: principles and practice.* 5th ed. Boston: Jones and Bartlett; 2000. Chapter 13, Works CR. Principles of treatment planning and clinical research. pp. 259–71.

6. Yarbo CH, Wujcik D, Gobel BA, eds. *Cancer nursing: principles and practice.* 7th ed. Boston: Jones and Bartlett; 2011. Chapter 11, Gillespie TW. Surgical therapy. pp. 232–48.

7. Yarbo CH, Wujcik D, Gobel BH, eds. *Cancer nursing: principles and practice.* 7th ed. Boston: Jones and Bartlett; 2011. Chapter 15, Tortirice PV. Cytotoxic chemotherapy: principles of therapy. pp. 352–89.

8. Yarbo CH, Wujcik D, Gobel BH, eds. *Cancer nursing: principles and practice.* 7th ed. Boston: Jones and Bartlett; 2011. Chapter 17, Camp-Sorrell D. Chemotherapy toxicities and management. pp. 458–503.

9. Manne DS. Oral mucositis and xerstomia: challenging oral health conditions part I oral mucositis. *Access.* 2006 Jul;20:34–37.

10. Yarbo CH, Wujcik D, Gobel BH, eds. *Cancer nursing: principles and practice.* 7th ed. Boston: Jones and Bartlett; 2011. Chapter 12, Gosselin TK. Principles of radiation therapy. pp. 249–68.

11. Yarbo CH, Wujcik D, Gobel BH, eds. *Cancer nursing: principles and practice.* 7th ed. Boston: Jones and Bartlett; 2011. Chapter 13, Behrend SW. Radiation treatment planning. pp. 269–11.

12. Yarbo CH, Wujcik D, Gobel BH, eds. *Cancer nursing: principles and practice.* 7th ed. Boston: Jones and Bartlett; 2011. Chapter 14, Maher KE. Radiation therapy: toxicities and management. pp. 312–51.

13. Yarbo CH, Frogge MH, Goodman M, eds. *Cancer nursing: principles and practice.* 7th ed. Boston: Jones and Bartlett; 2011. Chapter 18, Ezzone SA. Principles and techniques of blood and marrow transplantation. pp. 504–12.

14. Yarbo CH, Frogge MH, Goodman M, eds. *Cancer nursing: principles and practice.* 6th ed. Boston: Jones and Bartlett; 2005. Chapter 19, Wujcik D, Price K. Techniques of hematopoietic cell transplantation. pp. 479–94.

15. Yarbo CH, Wujcik D, Gobel BH, eds. *Cancer nursing: principles and practice.* 7th ed. Boston: Jones and Bartlett; 2011. Chapter 19, Anderson-Reitz L. Complications of hematopoietic cell transplantation. pp. 513–29.

16. Miller M, Kearney N. Oral care for patients with cancer: a review of the literature. *Cancer Nurs.* 2001 Aug;24(4):241–54.

17. Vissink A, Jansma J, Spïjkervet FKL, Burlage FR, Coppes RP. Oral sequelae of head and neck radiotherapy. *Crit Rev Oral Biol Med.* 2003;14(3):199–212.

18. Köstler WJ, Hejna M, Wenzel C, Zielinski CC. Oral mucositis complicating chemotherapy and/or radiotherapy: options for prevention and treatment. *CA Cancer J Clin.* 2001 Sep–Oct;51(5):290–315.

19. Redding SW. Cancer therapy-related oral mucositis. *J Dent Educ.* 2005 Aug;69(8):919–29.

20. Morimoto Y, Niwa H, Imai Y, Kirita T. Dental management prior to hematopoietic stem cell transplantation. *Spec Care Dent.* 2004 Nov–Dec;24(6):287–92.

21. Westbrook SD, Paunovich ED, Freytes CO. Adult hematopoietic stem cell transplantation. *J Am Dent Assoc.* 2003 Sep;134(9):1224–31.

22. da Fonseca MA. Dental care of the pediatric cancer patient. *Pediatr Dent.* 2004 Jan–Feb;26(1):53–7.

CHAPTER 56

The Patient With a Disability

CHARLOTTE J. WYCHE, RDH, MS
KATHRYN RAGALIS DAVIS, RDH, MS, DMD

Chapter Outline

BOX 56-1	Key Words

Impairment, Disability, Handicap

Americans With Disabilities Act (ADA): the ADA prohibits discrimination on the basis of a disability and requires places of public accommodation and commercial facilities to meet standards of accessibility by removing architectural, transportation, and communication barriers.

AwDA: Americans with Disabilities Act; abbreviation sometimes used to prevent confusion with the ADA (American Dental Association).

Barrier-free: area that is freely accessible to all without discrimination on the basis of a disability; obstacles to passage or communication have been removed.

Behavior modification: an approach to correction of undesirable conduct that focuses on changing observable actions; modification of behavior is accomplished through systematic manipulation of the environmental and behavioral variables related to the specific behavior to be changed.

Behavior therapy: an approach in which the focus is on the patient's observable behavior rather than on conflicts and unconscious processes presumed to underlie the maladaptive behavior; accomplished through systematic manipulation of the environmental and behavioral variables related to specific behavior to be modified.

Deinstitutionalization: returning patients to home and community as quickly as possible after treatment rather than housing them permanently or for long periods in custodial institutions; the elimination of mental health institutions, for example, has been made possible by (1) the use of new medications that control the symptoms of illness and (2) community health centers that serve as support.

Desensitization: the treatment of phobias and related disorders by intentionally exposing the patient, in imagination or real life, to emotionally distressing stimuli; desensitization of a fearful patient to accept dental treatment might consist, for example, of short exposures to the dental chair, instruments, air syringe, and the sound of a handpiece along with building trust in the dental team members.

Developmental disability: a substantial handicap of indefinite duration with onset before the age of 18 years, attributable to mental retardation, autism, cerebral palsy, epilepsy, or other incurable neuropathy.

Disability: (individual dimension) any restriction or lack of ability (resulting from an impairment) to perform an activity in the manner or within the range considered normal for a human being of the same age, sex, and background.

Handicap: (social dimension) a disadvantage for an individual, resulting from an impairment or a disability, that limits or prevents fulfillment of a role that is within the normal range for a human of the same age, sex, and social and cultural factors as the affected individual.

Impairment: (organ or body dimension) any loss or abnormality of psychologic, physiologic, or anatomic structure or function.

Mainstreaming: integration of people with disabilities into their community through programs of rehabilitation; process by which persons with special needs (educational, physical, psychologic) are included within the mainstream of society rather than segregated.

Normalization: making available to all individuals patterns and conditions of everyday life that are as close as possible to the norms and patterns of the mainstream of society.

A patient with a disability may require special attention and adaptations in daily life and during dental and dental hygiene appointments. Some disabilities severely impact the daily activities and function of an individual, which can lead to poor oral hygiene, rampant dental disease, and dental neglect. Box 56-1 supplies key words and definitions pertaining to impairments, disabilities, and handicaps.

- Obtaining access to oral health services can present challenges for both the patient and dental personnel.
- The patient may need to overcome numerous obstacles in daily living before the additional issues of oral self-care and access to dental care are addressed.
- Imagination, ingenuity, flexibility, and persistence are necessary in order to individualize and modify dental hygiene interventions when caring for people with disabilities.
- Patience, calmness, kindness, and empathy are keys to approaching the special needs patient.

DISABILITIES

I. DEFINITIONS AND CLASSIFICATIONS

- The United States Americans With Disabilities Act (ADA) defines an individual with a disability as a person who "has a physical or mental impairment that substantially limits one or more major life activities, has a record of such impairment, or is regarded as having such impairment."[1] The ADA definition usually refers to individuals with an impairment that is permanent or long-term.
- Impairment refers to a loss of structure or function that leads to restriction of ability.
- Handicap refers to a perception that an individual with impairment is disadvantaged in some way.
- The World Health Organization, International Classification of Functioning, Disability, and Health (ICF) is a universal classification of disability and health that provides a standard language and framework for the description of health and health-related states.[2] Table 56-1 lists the ICF categories and descriptions.

TABLE 56-1	INTERNATIONAL CLASSIFICATION OF FUNCTIONING, DISABILITY AND HEALTH (ICF)
PART 1: FUNCTIONING AND DISABILITY	
BODY FUNCTIONS	
Mental Functions	The brain: both global mental functions, such as consciousness, energy and drive, and specific mental functions, such as memory, language, and calculation mental functions.
Sensory Functions	Seeing, hearing, tasting, and touch, as well as the sensation of pain.
Voice and Speech Functions	Producing sounds and speech.
Functions of the Cardiovascular, Hematological, Immunological, and Respiratory Systems	The heart and blood vessels, blood production, immunity, respiration and exercise tolerance.
Functions of the Digestive, Metabolic, and Endocrine Systems	Ingestion, digestion, and elimination, as well as metabolism and the endocrine glands.
Genitourinary and Reproductive Functions	Urination and the reproduction, including sexual and procreative functions.
Neuromusculoskeletal and Movement-Related Functions	Movement and mobility, including functions of joints, bones, reflexes, and muscles.
Functions of the Skin and Related Structures	Skin, skin glands, nails, hair, and related structures.
BODY STRUCTURES	
Structures of the Nervous System	Brain, spinal cord, meninges, and nervous system, including sympathetic and parasympathetic nervous systems.
The Eye, Ear, and Related Structures	Eye socket, eyeball, external ear, middle ear, inner ear, and related structures.
Structures Involved in Voice and Speech	Nose, mouth, pharynx, larynx, and related structures.
Structures of the Cardiovascular, Immunological, and Respiratory Systems	Heart, arteries, veins, and capillaries; central lymphoid tissue (bone marrow, thymus) and peripheral lymphoid tissue (lymph nodes, spleen, mucosa-associated lymphoid tissue); and pharynx, trachea, bronchi, and lungs.
Structures Related to the Digestive, Metabolic, and Endocrine Systems	Salivary glands, esophagus, stomach, intestines, pancreas, liver, gall bladder and ducts, endocrine glands, and related structures.
Structures Related to the Genitourinary and Reproductive Systems	Kidneys, ureter, bladder, pelvic floor, and male and female reproductive structures.
Structures Related to Movement	Head, neck, shoulder, upper and lower extremities, pelvic regions, trunk, musculoskeletal system, and other structures related to movement.
Skin and Related Structures	Skin, skin glands, nails, hair, and related structures.
PART 2: CONTEXTUAL FACTORS	
ACTIVITIES AND PARTICIPATION	
Learning and Applying Knowledge	Learning, applying the knowledge that is learned, thinking, solving problems, and making decisions.
General Tasks and Demands	Carrying out specific single or multiple tasks, organizing routines and handling stress; identifying the underlying features of the execution of tasks under different circumstances.
Communication	General and specific features of communicating by language, signs and symbols, including receiving and producing messages, carrying on conversations, and using communication devices and techniques.

(*continued*)

TABLE 56-1	INTERNATIONAL CLASSIFICATION OF FUNCTIONING, DISABILITY AND HEALTH (ICF) (*Continued*)
PART 2: CONTEXTUAL FACTORS (*Continued*)	
ACTIVITIES AND PARTICIPATION	
Mobility	Moving by changing body position or location or by transferring from one place to another by carrying, moving, or manipulating objects; by walking, running, or climbing; and by using various forms of transportation.
Self-Care	Caring for oneself, washing and drying oneself; caring for one's body and body parts; dressing, eating and drinking; and looking after one's health.
Domestic Life	Carrying out domestic and everyday actions and tasks; acquiring a place to live, food, clothing and other necessities; household cleaning and repairing; caring for personal and other household objects; and assisting others.
Interpersonal Interactions and Relationships	Carrying out the actions and tasks required for basic and complex interactions with people (strangers, friends, relatives, family members and lovers) in a contextually and socially appropriate manner.
Major Life Areas	Carrying out the tasks and actions required to engage in education, work, and employment and to conduct economic transactions.
Community, Social and Civic Life	Actions and tasks required to engage in organized social life outside the family in community, social, and civic areas of life.
ENVIRONMENTAL FACTORS THAT INFLUENCE FUNCTIONING	
Products and Technology	Natural or human-made products or systems of products, equipment, and technology in an individual's immediate environment that are gathered, created, produced, or manufactured.
Natural and Human-Made Changes to Environment	Animate and inanimate elements of the natural or physical environment, and components of that environment that have been modified by people, as well as characteristics of human populations within that environment.
Support and Relationships	People or animals that provide practical physical or emotional support, nurturing, protection, assistance, and relationships to other persons in their home, place of work, school, at play, or in other aspects of their daily activities.
Attitudes	The observable consequences of customs, practices, ideologies, values, norms, factual beliefs, and religious beliefs that influence individual behavior and social life; individual or societal attitudes about a person's value as a human being that may motivate positive, honorific practices or negative and discriminatory practices.
Services, Systems and Policies	Governmental and private programs, infrastructure, regulations, and standards designed to meet the needs of individuals.

II. TYPES OF CONDITIONS

- The causes of disabilities include heredity, systemic disease or disorder, and trauma.
- Some types of impairment can manifest as a stable condition; others may cause progressive disability.
- A temporary disability can result from a physical impairment such as a broken leg or because of a physiologic condition such as the limitations that occur during pregnancy.
- A variety of impairments are found among persons with disabilities, and an individual may have more than one type of disability.
- Many of the diseases and syndromes with symptoms of impairments are described in the various chapters throughout Section VIII of this book.

III. OCCURRENCE

- Approximately one of five persons is affected by a disability; and that number is increasing.[3]
- Progress in medical care has increased initial survival of those born with a disability and increased the survival rate of those experiencing a disabling condition.
- As life expectancy increases, so does the likelihood of acquiring a disability.

IV. BARRIERS TO DENTAL CARE

- People with disabilities experience a diminished oral health status and reduced access to dental services compared to the general population.

TABLE 56-2	EXAMPLES OF BARRIERS TO ACCESS FOR DENTAL CARE		
	PATIENT	**FAMILY, CAREGIVER, GUARDIAN**	**DENTAL PROFESSIONAL**
Attitude Barriers	May not comprehend importance of dental health; may not be aware of needing dental care; may not want to or be able to cooperate.	May not care for own dental health, may be overstressed with other patient health issues that seem more important than dental need.	May not feel adequately trained to or want to or be able to treat safely a physically, cognitively, or medically compromised patient.
Health Literacy Barriers	May not understand the relationship of oral health to systemic health; may have difficulty understanding insurance coverage, locating a provider, making appointments, or completing paperwork.	May not understand the relationship of oral health to systemic health; may have difficulty understanding insurance coverage, locating a provider, making appointments, or completing paperwork.	May not understand that the patient has many barriers to accessing dental care; may not have adequately assessed the patient's health literacy when providing previous care.
Physical Barriers	Fear of not being able to cope with architectural barriers; fear of falling; fear of attracting attention in an embarrassing way.	May not be able to transport patient with wheelchair; may not be able to lift or support patient in car or dental chair.	Office facility or treatment rooms may not provide a barrier-free environment.
Financial Barriers	May have limited income; may not have adequate dental insurance coverage or cannot find a provider who accepts specific insurance.	May not be able to take time from employment to accompany patient to appointments.	Cost of building accessible features or buying specialized equipment; lack of reimbursement for the additional cost of longer appointment times needed for care.

- Progress is being made to ensure adequate access to dental care, but barriers that exist can involve the patient, the family, caregivers, guardians, and dental professionals, as described in **Table 56-2**.
- Having adequate access to dental and dental hygiene services can make a significant contribution to the oral health, well-being, independence, and sense of personal esteem of a patient with a disability.
- Although dental professionals are not always comfortable or confident about providing care for patients with disabilities, training and experience can help.[4]

V. TRENDS IN COMMUNITY-BASED DELIVERY OF SERVICES

A. Overview

- Most individuals with physical and intellectual impairments have community-based living, educational, and work arrangements.
- Barrier-free or assisted-living housing for individuals and staffed community-based residential facilities for group living are available for those who need daily assistance.
- Many home-care and community-based services are available for individuals with disabilities, however access to dental services is still limited by traditional office-based dental care delivery systems.

- New oral health care delivery system models are being proposed to deliver dental services where people live, work, play, go to school, or receive other social services.[5-7]

B. New Models

- Development of delivery system that focuses on screening, triage, prevention, and education, with only complex treatment needs being referred to a private dental office or hospital clinic.
- Integration of oral health into general health and social services systems.
- Integration of licensed "health facilities" in public and private residential facilities and training of staff and other caregivers to play a more major role in oral health.
- Delivery of services in private homes using mobile equipment.
- Expansion of "direct access" regulations[8] that increase the ability of dental hygienists to provide preventive services in alternative settings.
- The development of new mid-level oral health providers trained to provide less complex dental care.
- Use of technology to facilitate consultation between oral health professionals as well as communication between patient and providers.
- Reform of the oral health insurance/Medicaid reimbursement systems to provide enhance payment for extra time needed to provide care for special needs populations.

ORAL MANIFESTATIONS

The two principal oral diseases found in all patients are dental caries and periodontal infections. Some patients have additional oral manifestations. Oral characteristics common with specific a disability or disease are described more completely in the chapters devoted to that particular condition. Examples of types of oral manifestations caused by, or as result of, a patient's disabling condition or the treatment for it are included here.

I. CONGENITAL MALFORMATIONS

An increased incidence of malformations has been observed in patients with developmental disabilities, for example:

- Cleft lip or palate, as described in Chapter 50 on page 775.
- Other craniofacial anomalies, such as malformed jaws, malocclusions, and malposed teeth.
- Tooth defects, such as variations in number and structure, for example, dentinogenesis imperfecta, amelogenesis imperfecta, and enamel hyperplasia.

II. ORAL INJURIES

A. Attrition

Attrition caused by bruxism is common among individuals, for example, with cerebral palsy and intellectual disability.

B. Trauma to Teeth and Soft Tissues

- Trauma to teeth and soft tissues may result from accidents (instability, falling), self-abuse, or seizures.
- Individuals with epilepsy and cerebral palsy are particularly susceptible to accidents. Chipped and fractured teeth and residual scars in the tongue and lips are seen.

III. FACIAL WEAKNESS OR PARALYSIS

- When a patient has muscle weakness or paralysis of one side of the face, bilateral mastication or self-cleaning motion of the tongue may not be possible.
- Biofilm usually collects more heavily, and food debris is retained, on the involved side. Certain patients may have bilateral weakness.
- Drooling or impaired swallowing of saliva is a common feature of some disabling conditions that involve head and neck musculature.[9]

IV. MALOCCLUSION

- Malocclusion is frequently found among persons with developmental disabilities.
- Factors contributing to problems of occlusion include skeletal and muscular deformities, macroglossia, congenitally missing teeth, and such oral habits as tongue thrust and mouth breathing.

V. THERAPY-RELATED ORAL FINDINGS

A. Drug-Induced Gingival Overgrowth

- A patient treated with phenytoin (Dilantin) or other antiepileptic medication may be susceptible to gingival enlargement.
- The amount of gingival enlargement is usually related to the effectiveness of daily biofilm control; effective daily biofilm removal is associated with less enlargement.
- A description of phenytoin-induced gingival overgrowth is included in Chapter 62 on page 945.

B. Chemotherapy

- Oral ulcerations, mucositis, and susceptibility to infection are frequent manifestations following chemotherapy.
- Patients with leukemia have a high incidence of oral manifestations, including lymphadenopathy, gingival changes with bleeding, and petechiae, which are more severe following chemotherapy.

C. Radiation Therapy

- When radiation therapy of the head and neck area involves the salivary glands, xerostomia can result and contribute to an increased incidence of dental caries.
- The symptoms and treatment aspects of radiation therapy are described in Chapter 55 on page 840.

D. Other Medications

- Patients with disabilities may be treated with various medications.
- All side effects of medications, particularly the oral side effects such as xerostomia or increased dental caries risk due to sweetened elixirs, are addressed in planning patient care.

DENTAL AND DENTAL HYGIENE CARE

I. OBJECTIVES

Whether care is being delivered in a traditional private practice, residential or educational facility, or community-based clinical setting the dental team has as its objectives to:

- Motivate the patient and the caregiver to establish and maintain healthy oral tissue with freedom from infection.
- Contribute to the patient's general health through, for example, prevention of tooth loss, which increases the ability to masticate food to prevent malnutrition and increase resistance to infection.
- Prevent the need for extensive dental and periodontal treatment that the patient may not be able to undergo because of lowered physical stamina or the inability to cooperate.

- Prevent the need for dentures or other removable prostheses, which can be hazardous, difficult, or impossible for certain patients to tolerate.
- Aid in personal appearance, the perception of healthy oral status, and social acceptance without halitosis.
- Make dental and dental hygiene treatment pleasant and comfortable.

II. PRETREATMENT PLANNING

Patients with disabilities can be treated in the traditional clinical setting. Only a relatively small number need hospitalization or care in their residence due to difficulties in management, inability to travel, or a systemic condition that requires special medical supervision.

A. Preliminary Contact

- Information may be obtained from the patient, or with legal authority from the guardian, parent, relative, advocate, or other person responsible for the patient.
- The essential information can be obtained in advance by telephone interview, or medical forms can be mailed to the home for completion.
- Advanced information permits the dental team to be prepared to make the appointment a successful and positive experience for the patient and clinician.

B. Legal Guardianship

- When a person is declared incapacitated by a legal process, a guardian is appointed.
- The guardian then provides consent for any treatment, including signatures on consent forms.
- Written proof of legal guardianship is obtained and kept in the patient record.

C. Information to Obtain

- In addition to the usual topics covered by the medical, personal, and dental histories, additional information is requested, using questions listed in **Box 56-2**.
- To avoid unpleasant situations and misunderstanding, ask direct questions about a patient's disability rather than making assumptions.

D. Consultations With Physicians, Other Specialists, and Sources

- Management of a patient with disabilities can be very complex because the patient is medically compromised.
- Consultation with the other professionals involved may be required to help determine a plan for patient treatment and continued care.
- Pertinent information may be obtained from other medical specialists and the social worker.
- Extra time may be required to access information about the conditions and medications before appointment.

BOX 56-2 | **Patient With a Disability: Additional Information to Obtain Before the Appointment**

BASIC INFORMATION
- Has a guardian been legally appointed? Obtain written documentation.
- Is there a caregiver, case worker, or counselor that works with the patient?
- Will someone accompany the patient to appointments?
- Does the patient give consent to discuss care with other individuals?
- Degree of independence, self-care, and way to communication with the patient.

MEDICAL HISTORY
- Specific list of disabilities or disabling conditions
- When diagnosed
- History of treatments, hospitalizations, or institutionalization
- Current medications and other therapy
- Names and addresses of specialists
- Any restrictions, such as dietary or for safety (leg braces, helmet)

DENTAL HISTORY
- Previous dental experiences and patient's attitude
- Difficulties in obtaining appointments, barriers to dental care experienced
- Most recent care: procedures, setting, success
- History of oral infections and oral habits
- Fluoride history, including self- or professionally applied topical methods
- Current home care methods: aids and special devices, frequency, degree of self-care
- Concepts of perceived needs, attitudes, and apparent emphasis on dental care
- Modifications and successful techniques used before and during appointments

SUPPLEMENTAL INFORMATION
Are any of the following affected by disability:
- Muscular coordination, mobility, walking
- Sitting tolerance
- Sitting position
- Ability to cooperate/involuntary movements
- Communication: speech, hearing, vision
- Breathing, including when reclined
- Swallowing, control of saliva
- Bowel or bladder control
- Mental capacities
- Dexterity, ability to brush and floss teeth
- Ability to chew or eat

OPEN-ENDED OTHER INFORMATION
- Does patient require any additional assistance or have any other issues of concern?

E. Interaction With Caregiver

- A patient with a disability may depend on a caregiver for daily life activities.
- Caregivers may or may not be the legal guardian of patient or contact person to plan appointments; if the caregiver is not the legal guardian, the patient is consulted to determine the limits of the caregiver's role.
- Caregivers can be an excellent source of information, help in preparing the patient for the appointment, and suggestions for gaining cooperation from the patient.
- Invite the caregiver to the office before the appointment to see the facility and become familiar with the surroundings and staff.

APPOINTMENT SCHEDULING

I. SPECIAL REQUIREMENTS

- Determine what preparation needs to be taken before appointment to allow time in the schedule, for example, to move furniture, retrieve and set up special equipment, or premedicate the patient.
- Identify special aids the patient must bring to the appointment, such as a transfer board for transfer into the dental chair, hearing aid, dental prostheses, and biofilm control devices currently in use.
- Some individuals with disabilities are accompanied by service dogs, such as guide dogs for the blind and hearing and signal dogs, which are allowed by law into all public buildings and on public transportation. Additional information about guide dogs for the blind is found in Chapter 59 on page 910.

II. TRANSPORTATION

- A patient may rely on the caregiver or another source for transport to an appointment.
- A wheelchair patient may need to reserve a wheelchair transport vehicle and be limited by the time schedule.
- Patient may arrange a ride transportation service that is contacted when the patient has completed the appointment; forms may need to be completed.

III. TIME OF APPOINTMENT

A. Patient

Determine how the patient's daily schedule influences time selection for scheduling appointments. The cooperation of the patient may be decreased if basic routines are disturbed; for example:

- Appointment for the patient with diabetes does not interfere with medication, meal, or between-meal eating schedules.

- The elderly person who rises early may feel better during a morning appointment.
- Patients with arthritis may have greater mobility late in the morning or in the afternoon.
- Child's nap schedule may preclude afternoon appointments.
- Early morning appointment may be difficult for a patient who requires a long time for morning preparation, such as a patient with a spinal cord injury or colostomy.

B. Caregiver

The schedule of the caregiver who accompanies the patient is considered.

C. Dental Facility

- Arrange a time when the patient will not have to wait a long time after arrival.
- Allow sufficient time so that the patient is not rushed; many persons with disabilities cannot hurry.
- Consider incontinence issues and the difficulties and time needed for rest room visits; encourage emptying bladder before entering treatment room.

IV. FOLLOW-UP

The frequency of maintenance appointments for all patients is individualized. Frequent appointments are encouraged for the following reasons:

- To decrease length of single appointment by keeping the oral tissues at an optimum level of health.
- To assist the patient whose disability limits the ability to perform personal oral hygiene adequately.
- To provide motivation through monitoring biofilm and review of procedures for the patient and the caregiver involved.

BARRIER-FREE ENVIRONMENT

- In general, a facility that is barrier-free for a patient in a wheelchair is accessible to all other individuals. The patient in a wheelchair requires more space for turning and positioning.
- Additional features are needed for other specific disabilities, for example, braille floor indicators can be installed beside the numbers on elevators; doorways, steps, and stairways can be outlined with bright colors that contrast with the background for people with limited vision.
- Guidelines and specifications for a barrier-free environment are available. The descriptions that follow represent general features based on governmental regulations for accessibility standards, along with suggested applications for a dental clinic or office.[10]

I. EXTERNAL FEATURES

A. Parking

A reserved area, clearly marked, near the building entrance and 13 feet wide (8-foot car space with 5-foot access aisle) to permit opening car doors for exiting and reboarding.

B. Walkways

- A 3-foot-wide walkway is needed for wheelchair accommodation.
- The surface is solid and nonslip, without irregularities.
- Curb ramps (cuts) from the street and from the parking area are necessary.

C. Entrance

- At least one entrance to the building on ground level accessible by a gently sloping ramp (rise of 1 inch for every 12 inches).
- An easily grasped handrail (height 30–34 inches) is needed on at least one side, and preferably both sides, to accommodate left- and right-handed cane and one-crutch users.

D. Door

The lightweight door with a lever type of handle opens at least 32 inches for a person using a tall crutch and for a wheelchair as shown in **Figure 56-1**.

II. INTERNAL FEATURES

Official regulations specify dimensions for accessibility of all aspects, including passageways, floors, drinking fountains, and restrooms. A few are described here.

A. Passageways

- The passageways are at least 3 feet wide, with handrails along the sides.
- Passageways are free from obstructions, such as hanging signs that a tall blind person could collide.

B. Floors

- Level floors with nonslip surfaces are necessary.
- Thick or small, unattached movable rugs or carpets present obstacles for wheelchairs or walkers and hazards for a patient with crutches, cane, or leg brace.

C. Reception Area

- At least part of the furniture will permit easy access during seating and rising.

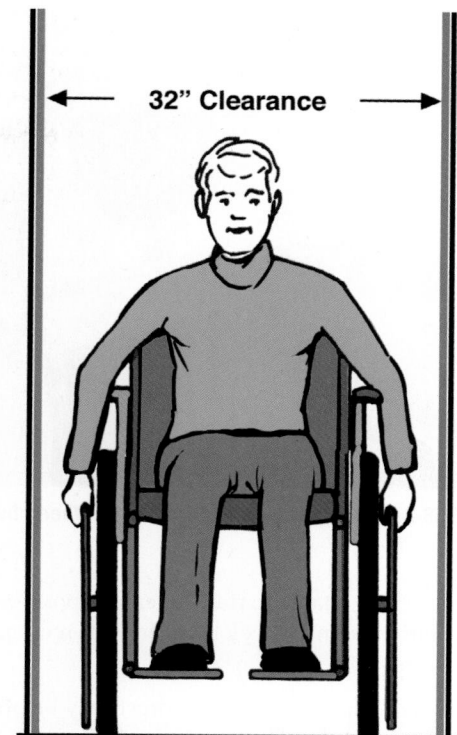

FIGURE 56-1 Wheelchair Accessibility. Wheelchairs designed for adults vary in width from 2 feet 3 inches to 2 feet 8 inches. A clear door width of 32 inches to accommodate these wheelchairs has been accepted as the official regulation.

- Preferred are chairs with 18-inch-high, flat, firm seats, and arms for support when pushing oneself up by the arms.
- Select chairs that do not slide or tip as the person rises.

III. THE TREATMENT ROOM

A. Dimensions

- Space is needed for the dental chair, related dental equipment, and the wheelchair.
- The doorways are at least 32 inches wide.
- The wheelchair is placed beside and parallel to the dental chair for patient transfer. In a small facility, the dental chair can be rotated to allow for turning the wheelchair.
- The dental chair selected is able to be lowered to 19 inches from the floor and accessible from both sides for wheelchair transfer.
- An x-ray machine in the same treatment room can simplify the problems of moving the patient into a separate radiography room.

B. Wheelchair Used During Treatment

When the patient is in a total support wheelchair, transfer to the dental chair may not be advisable. The wheelchair

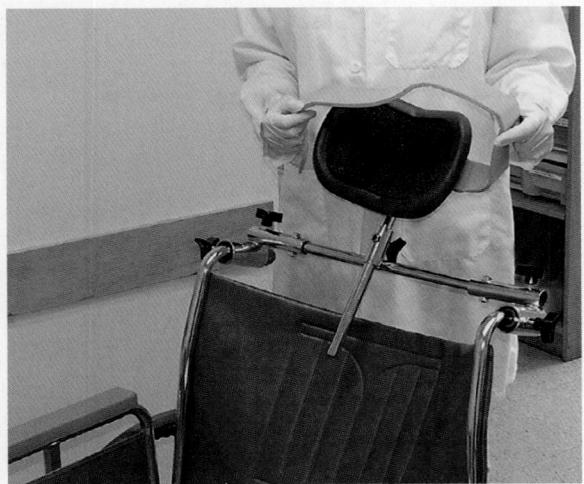

FIGURE 56-2 **Portable Headrest Attached to Wheelchair.**

of a patient who is unable to transfer can be positioned for direct utilization; some wheelchairs are self-reclining and have headrests.

- *Portable headrest:* A portable headrest may be attached to the wheelchair handles, as shown in **Figure 56-2**.
- *Position of dental chair:* The dental chair can be swiveled to permit the wheelchair to be backed up to place the patient's head in a usual treatment position. The dental light can then be directed into the patient's oral cavity and the equipment adjusted for easy access.
- *Wheelchair lift:* An automatic wheelchair lift that tilts the chair back to a usual working position can be obtained for a clinical facility where wheelchair patients are treated frequently.

IV. PATIENT INSTRUCTION

When a teaching area is planned for patient instruction, attention is given to ensure accessibility for a patient in a wheelchair.

A. Dimensions

The tabletop and washbasin built at a height of 32 to 34 inches permit clearance underneath for knees and wheelchair arms, as shown in **Figure 56-3**.

B. Washbasin

- Lever- or blade-type handles on faucets are usable by patients who have difficulty gripping handles or have no hands; prevent burning the patient who cannot sense temperature.
- Hot pipes under the sink are covered or insulated because patients who have no sensation in their legs could be burned.

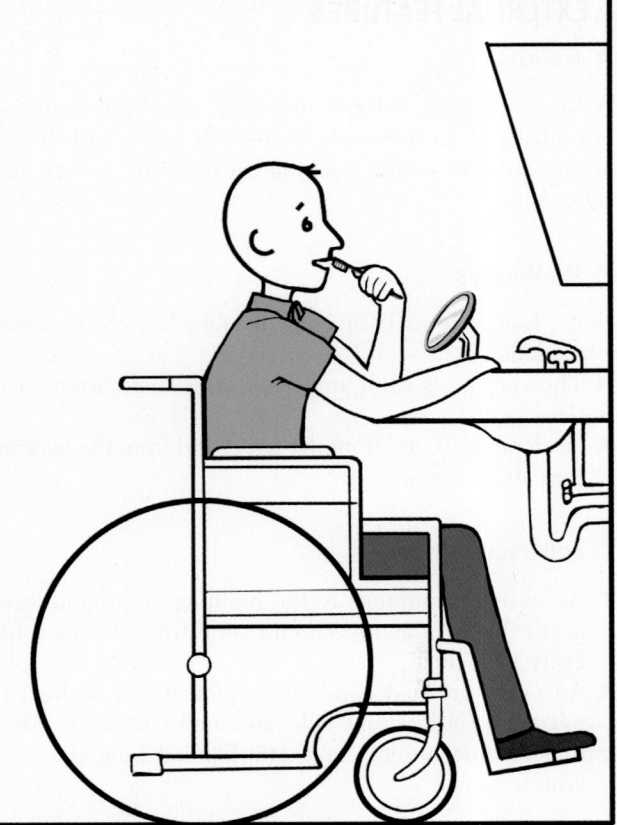

FIGURE 56-3 **Biofilm Control Facility.** The tabletop and washbasin in a patient instruction area or lavatory are built at a height of 32–34 inches to provide clearance underneath for knees of the patient and arms of the wheelchair. Hot pipes under a sink are covered or insulated because patients with no sensation could be burned.

C. Mirror

- Mirrors and dispensers are positioned low; a tilt mirror could provide better viewing of the teeth during instruction for most patients.
- An unattached hand mirror, preferably on a pedestal that tilts, supplements the wall mirror.
- A magnifying mirror can provide an excellent aid for viewing the disclosed biofilm and the devices for biofilm removal.

PATIENT RECEPTION: THE INITIAL APPOINTMENT

The orientation of a patient with a disability paves the way for long-term success of dental and dental hygiene supervision and care.

I. ORIENTATION

- The first appointment includes and, when necessary, may be devoted entirely to a basic orientation to the facilities, the dental chair, and the personnel.

- The examination of the oral cavity is started, and dependent on the degree of patient cooperation, various steps in the assessment may be completed.
- Preventive personal care instructions are initiated, and participation of the caregiver is solicited.
- Several orientation visits may be necessary to acclimate the patient to surroundings and to desensitize.

II. COMMUNICATION

- Basic communication strategies are adapted in order to address the unique needs of the patient with a disability.
- Unless the patient has an extreme cognitive impairment, the patient is always addressed first and the caregiver secondarily.
- The patient's ability to understand what is said is not underestimated; assessment of the patient's cognitive ability is essential and respect is indicated by addressing and making eye contact with the patient.
- Kindness, patience, and empathy will help the clinician build trust; each patient is unique, and members of the dental team can watch, listen, and learn procedures that will develop the patient's cooperation.
- Desensitization techniques and a "show-tell-do" approach, described in Chapter 43 on page 682, can help reduce anxiety, particularly for a patient with cognitive impairment or one who is fearful.
- Parents and other caregivers can explain how best to communicate with the patient.
- The caregiver can help interpret the changing moods of the patient, identify problems, and note changes in behavior that may indicate a dental problem.
- Nonverbal communication using facial expressions, pointing, body language, and demonstration helps certain patients to respond.
- A patient may prefer to write messages on a pad of paper or use sign language, a language board, or other devices the dental personnel can learn to use.

III. PREVENTIVE CARE INTRODUCTION

- Whether or not the assessment and treatment plan are completed at the initial visit, the personal oral daily care program is introduced.
- Find out what the current daily care has been to determine what modifications are needed in daily biofilm removal instruction and diet evaluation.
- The complete instruction and prevention program is described on pages 862 to 868.

WHEELCHAIR TRANSFERS[11]

- Selection of a transfer technique is influenced by the size, weight, and mobility of the patient, along with any special physical conditions and patient preferences.

- The patient may prefer to transfer from the left or the right side of the dental chair, depending on which side of the body is stronger.
- Transfer from the wheelchair can be a frightening experience to the patient owing to fear of falling and injury.
- Always inform the patient of intended actions before starting.

I. PREPARATION FOR WHEELCHAIR TRANSFER

A. Clear the Area

- Before starting a transfer, clear the area: move the clinician's stool, bracket tray, portable unit, and dental light.
- After the transfer, release the wheelchair brake to move it aside.
- In a small treatment room, the wheelchair may be folded and set aside.

B. Special Needs of Patient

- *Chair padding:* Special padding is used in a wheelchair as protection from pressure sores. Depending on the length of the appointment, the patient will decide whether the padding is moved to the dental chair. Pressure sores are described in Chapter 58 on page 889.
- *Bags and catheters:* Patients who do not have control of urine discharge, such as those with paraplegia or quadriplegia, have a bag with tubing for collection. The bag may be attached to the leg of the patient or to the wheelchair. After transfer, the tubing is checked to be sure it is not bent or twisted.
- *Spasms:* Ask the patient about susceptibility to spasms and about procedures to follow for prevention.
- *Advice concerning transfer:* Ask the patient, family member, or caregiver how best the clinician can help during the transfer. The patient is allowed to do as much as possible.

II. MOBILE PATIENT TRANSFER

When a patient can support his or her own weight, the "stand and pivot" technique can be used, as shown in **Figure 56-4**.

A. Position the Wheelchair

Face the wheelchair in the same direction as the dental chair at approximately an angle of 30°; set brakes; remove footrests and wheelchair armrests. The patient will adjust a power-driven chair and set the brakes before turning it off.

B. Prepare Dental Chair

Adjust the dental chair to the same height as or lower than the wheelchair; clear a path for transfer by uplifting the dental chair arm.

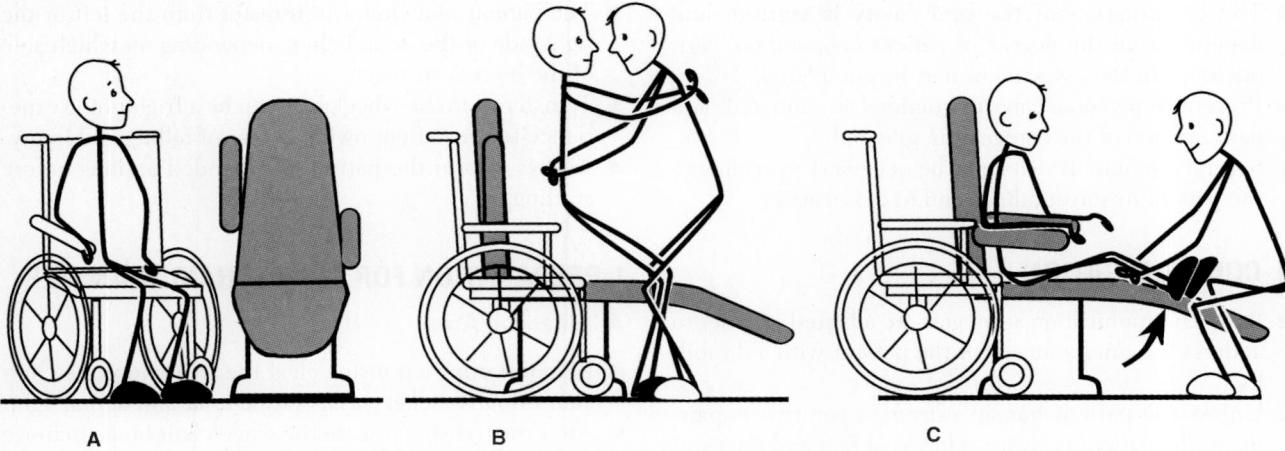

A   **B**   **C**

FIGURE 56-4 **Wheelchair Transfer for a Mobile Patient. (A)** Position the wheelchair at level of or lower than the dental chair; set wheel locks, remove footrests and armrests, and raise the dental chair arm. **(B)** Clinician places feet outside of the patient's feet, grasps the patient around the waist under the arms, locks hands, or grasps belt in back; patient holds clinician around shoulders or neck; patient is lifted up and pivoted to dental chair side. **(C)** Patient is gently lowered to sitting position; dental chair arm is lowered; clinician grasps legs together to lift onto dental chair.

C. Approach to Patient

- Detach patient's safety belt.
- Face the patient and place feet outside the patient's feet for pivoting. Clinician's knees are placed close to or against the patient's knees to prevent buckling.
- Place hands under the patient's arms and grasp the waist belt in back. Patient places arms around clinician's neck or places hands on wheelchair to push up.
- Clinician lifts patient to standing position, as in **Figure 56-4B**.

D. Pivot to Dental Chair

- Pivot together slowly until the patient is backed up to the side of the dental chair, with the backs of the legs touching. The patient is gently lowered to a sitting position. Reposition the arm of the dental chair.
- Grasp the patient's legs together between the ankles and knees, and lift them onto the dental chair, as shown in **Figure 56-4C**.

E. Repeat in Reverse

After the appointment, return the patient to the wheelchair in the reverse order of procedure.

III. IMMOBILE PATIENT TRANSFER

When the patient is unable to support his or her own weight, two aides are required. The parent or other caregiver may serve as the second person.

A. Position the Wheelchair

- Position the wheelchair in the same direction and parallel with the dental chair; set brakes; remove footrests.

- Adjust the dental chair to the same height as or lower than the seat of the wheelchair.
- Move the arm of the dental chair out of the transfer area, and remove the arm of the wheelchair.

B. Aide I

- Aide I is positioned behind the wheelchair.
- Place feet, one on either side of the rear wheel nearest the dental chair; place hands under the patient's arms below the elbows, pressing forearms against the patient's lower thorax area.
- Clasp hands or wrists under the patient's rib cage.

C. Aide II

Aide II may do either of the following, depending on the size and weight of the patient.

- Face patient and grasp hands under the patient's knees.
- Face dental chair; place one arm under the thighs and the other under the calves of the lower legs.

D. Transfer

On a prearranged signal and a steady motion, lift and gently transfer the patient to the dental chair.

E. Repeat in Reverse

After the appointment, the patient is returned to the wheelchair in the reverse order of procedure.

IV. SLIDING BOARD TRANSFER

A patient may bring a sliding board or one may be kept in the office or clinic. A transfer board is shown in **Figure 56-5**.

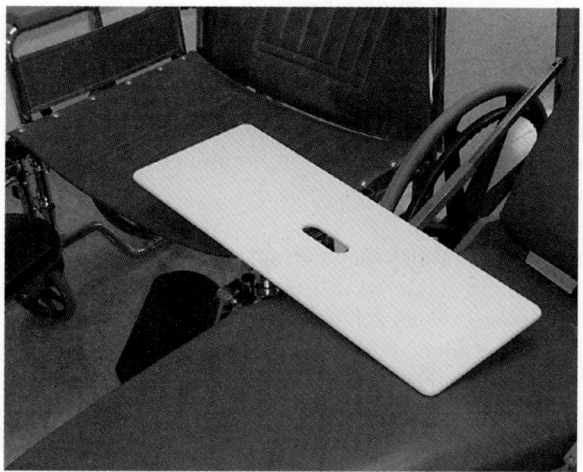

FIGURE 56-5 **Transfer Board.** Transfer board placement between wheelchair and dental chair.

A. Position the Wheelchair

- Position the wheelchair in the same direction as and parallel with the dental chair; set the brakes; remove the footrests.
- Adjust the seat of the dental chair to slightly lower than the wheelchair seat.
- Move the arm of the dental chair out of the transfer area, and remove the arm of the wheelchair.

B. Adjust the Sliding Board

- Patient or clinician places the sliding board well under the hip of the patient.
- The board is extended across the dental chair.

C. Transfer

- Patient shifts weight, balances on hands, and walks the buttocks across the board. The clinician can assist or do the transfer by holding the patient under the axillae. Two persons are needed when the patient is heavy or less mobile.
- Board is removed and replaced after the appointment.

D. Repeat in Reverse

Dental chair is positioned slightly higher than the wheelchair seat for the return transfer.

ASSISTANCE FOR THE AMUBLATORY PATIENT

- A patient may walk with one or more assistive aids such as braces, a cane, crutches, or a walker.
- Certain patients do better without assistance because they have developed their own method of balancing;

many patients gain balance by holding both hands on the partially flexed forearm of a person walking beside them.

I. SEATING THE PATIENT

- Ask patient how much and what kind of assistance is needed.
- Raise chair slightly above the patient's knee level and adjust chair arm out of the way.
- Stand aside or assist while patient moves until back of legs touch chair and then bends knees to lower into dental chair.
- If assistance is needed grasp ankles, lift legs, and turn patient into dental chair.
- Remove assistive aides and store out of the way; service dogs that accompany a patient are allowed to lie quietly nearby during the dental appointment.

II. THE SEATED PATIENT

- After telling the patient, tilt chair back slowly. Balance can be precarious while sitting as well as standing; patient may fall forward.
- If necessary, position supportive padding to maintain patient comfort.

III. RISING FROM THE CHAIR

- After telling patient, slowly raise the chair to upright position, with the seat slightly higher than the patient's knee level to minimize need to bend knees when rising.
- Allow time for adjustment to upright position in order to avoid the effects of postural hypertension.
- Ask or assist patient to move feet down to the floor.
- Retrieve assistive aids and hold them for patient to grasp with the dominant hand.
- Ask patient and, if assistance is needed to rise from the chair, offer support by placing arm under the patient's arm on the nondominant side until balance is obtained for walking.

PATIENT POSITION AND STABILIZATION

- The objectives in patient positioning and stabilization during treatment are to let the patient feel comfortable and secure while the clinician provides care in a position that provides adequate illumination, visibility, and accessibility.
- Extreme care is given to slightly raising the head of any patient with a swallowing defect or respiratory compromise; the patient may be unable to prevent aspiration of fluids or object placed in the mouth during treatment.

I. ADAPT CHAIR POSITION

- Start to tip the chair back SLOWLY, bringing the feet up first to provide balance so that the patient cannot fall.

- While tipping the chair back, place one hand on the patient's shoulder to offer assurance and support.
- Slowly advance the chair position in steps to allow the patient to adjust.
- A patient with a respiratory or cardiac complication is positioned with the chair back raised to a level that is comfortable for the patient. The patient can be asked, "How many pillows do you use at night?" and the chair can be adjusted accordingly.

II. BODY ADJUSTMENTS

- Patients with a spinal cord injury do a "push up" and patients with quadriplegia shift their weight every 20 minutes for 10–15 seconds to maintain good circulation in the tissues that do not have sensation, such as the buttocks.
- The procedure is a preventive measure for decubitus ulcers and is a particular consideration during long dental procedures.

III. SUPPORTIVE AND PROTECTIVE STABILIZATION

- Supportive stabilization, such as padding under flexed knees or bite block positioned to rest jaw muscles, can be used to facilitate patient comfort.
- Protective stabilization or medical immobilization techniques described below can help prevent injury to the patient and the dental practitioner, however, use of restraint is controversial and has the risk of causing injury or resulting in a lawsuit.[12]
- Protective stabilization is never used as a form of punishment.
- When protective support of any type is to be used, it is explained completely to the patient and/or the legal guardian and a signed informed consent is obtained.
- The least restrictive method of stabilization is selected for each patient and communication–based or desensitizing techniques are tried first.

A. Body Enclosure

- Although a small patient may be held by a parent, such positioning can be tiring for the parent, insecure, and may not provide good body mechanics for the clinician.
- *Pediwrap or papoose board:* Adjustable arm or leg immobilizer wraps with velcro closures or a padded board with wide fabric wraps around upper body, middle body and legs are available in adult and pediatric sizes, but not recommended unless the clinician has specialized training and informed consent has been obtained.

B. Head Stabilization

- *Arm of clinician:* From a working position at 12 o'clock (top of the patient's head), the nondominant arm is placed around the patient's head to stabilize it in position.

C. Oral Stabilization

A mouth prop can be used to assist the patient who has difficulty maintaining an open mouth. Training on technique for safe use of mouth props is required. Verbal encouragement of the patient continues throughout the appointment.

Ratchet Type (Molt's Mouth Prop)

- The most stable mouth prop is a sterilized prop that can be nearly closed for insertion between the teeth.
- It can be opened gradually to hold the jaws to the necessary position.
- The tips are covered with rubber tubing and are positioned over the maxillary and mandibular teeth on one side while the clinician treats the opposite side.

Bite Blocks

- Different types of rubber bite blocks are available; for example, **Figure 56-6** shows one that allows for placement of a suction tip.
- A long piece of dental floss is tied through the holes in a commercially available rubber mouth prop so that, in case of a sudden respiratory change, the prop can be quickly pulled out and breathing normalized.

Tongue Depressors

- A practical, disposable mouth prop can be made from three to six tongue depressors taped together.
- A folded gauze square is placed under the tape to provide a cushion, as shown in **Figure 56-7** along with an example of a prefabricated bite stick.

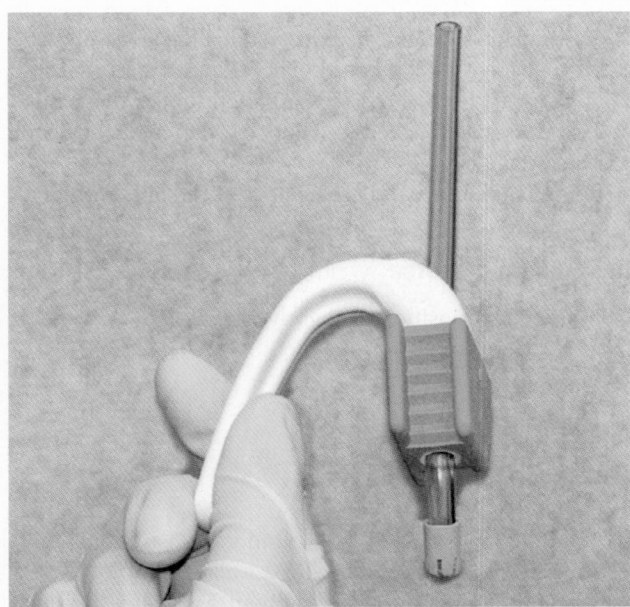

FIGURE 56-6 **Rubber Bite Block Mouth Prop With Saliva Ejector.**

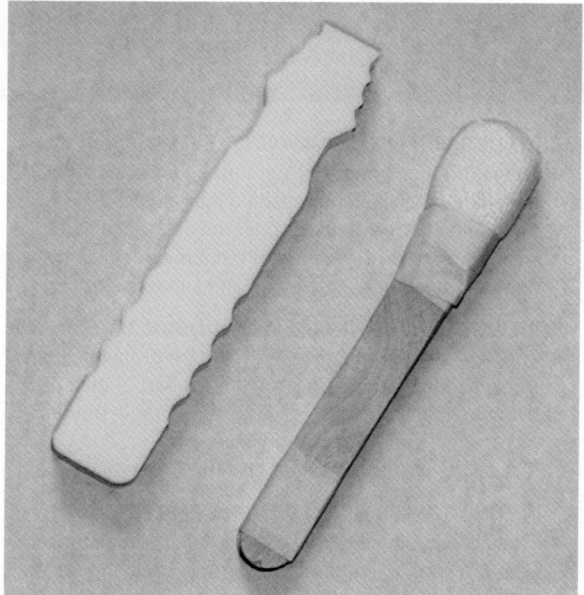

FIGURE 56-7 **Examples of Bite Sticks.** Left, a prefabricated model. Right, a self-made example made from tongue depressors taped together with a gauze pad for a comfortable biting surface.

D. Precautions for the Use of a Mouth Prop

- Patient and caregivers are informed of the risks and reassured that all stabilization devices are for comfort and to make the work easier and that they are in no way meant to hurt or punish.
- Mobile teeth could be knocked out and aspirated.
  - Loose primary teeth in young patient.
  - Mobile teeth in advanced periodontal infection.
- Fatigue of the patient's facial and masticatory muscles and temporomandibular joint.

INSTRUMENTATION

- With basic knowledge of methods for maintaining patient stability, adequate visibility of working area, secure instrument grasps and finger rests, and well-controlled strokes, instrumentation can be effectively accomplished.
- Patients who are hyperactive, lack muscular control, or have a mental impairment provide many challenges. The tasks of keeping the head and mouth positioned, the profuse saliva controlled, and the oversized or hyperactive tongue held back may seem insurmountable. Patience, a gentle but firm touch, and continuing experience are essential.

I. PREPARATION

A. Premedication

- Antibiotic coverage as indicated for susceptible patients, as described in Chapter 9 on page 131.
- Sedative for control of selected patients.

B. Biofilm Control Instruction Precedes Scaling

- Provide a clean mouth for professional instrumentation (conditioning).
- Disclose and present or review information on biofilm.
- Continue practice on biofilm removal methods selected for the particular patient.
- The patient and caregiver demonstrate correct technique.

C. Instruments

- Unbreakable mirrors are recommended for use with a patient subject to spasm or sudden closure.
- Use single-end sharp instruments to prevent accidents. When an unrestrained patient moves involuntarily, the nonworking end of an instrument can be a hazard.
- Use of an ultrasonic scaler is contraindicated for a patient at risk for aspiration and for patients who overreact to sensory stimuli, such as a patient with autism (page xx).

D. Technique Suggestions

- *Introduce each procedure and sound to prevent startling a patient:* Follow the basic instruction rule to "show, tell, then do."
- *Finger rests:* Firm, dependable finger rests are needed. Supplemental or reinforced rests can contribute to instrument stability. External finger and hand rests may be safer for the clinician.

II. PAIN AND ANXIETY CONTROL

While many special needs individuals can be treated easily in a dental clinic setting, some patients with behavioral or cognitive disabilities may need intervention beyond standard communication techniques and local anesthesia in order to receive dental care. Alternative methods of pain and anxiety control[13] for patients who are unable to cooperate during dental treatment include:

- Sedation—pharmacologically induced; three levels (minimum, moderate, and deep sedation); provided by trained dentist or anesthesiologist.
- General anesthesia: delivered in hospital, surgery centers, or dental offices; provided by trained anesthesiologists.

III. TREATMENT BY QUADRANTS

- For many patients, treatment by quadrants under local anesthesia is the procedure of choice.
- The occurrence of generalized heavy calculus deposits in disabled patients is not unusual due to factors related to the disabling condition.
- The objective of the clinical procedures is the complete removal of calculus and periodontal pocket debridement.

FOUR-HANDED DENTAL HYGIENE

- The use of a dental hygiene assistant during the appointment can enhance:
  - Efficiency
  - Patient management
  - Patient safety and comfort
  - Safety and comfort for clinician
  - Visibility during intraoral procedures
- Excess drooling, common with some disabilities, requires continuous suction to maintain a clear visual field for instrumentation and to decrease the risk of aspiration.
- A patient with impaired respiratory function, swallowing, or gag reflex is at risk for aspiration; attention to patient position and continuous suction to keep passageways clear are vital.
- When the patient's disorder involves orofacial muscles and nerves, the risk for splashing of aerosols into the eye is increased during dental hygiene care.

DISEASE PREVENTION AND CONTROL

I. PREVENTIVE PROGRAM COMPONENTS

- Education
- Dental biofilm control
- Fluorides
- Pit and fissure sealants
- Diet counseling
- Smoking cessation
- Regular professional examinations and treatment at intervals as recommended by the dentist and dental hygienist

II. COOPERATION

- Failure to perform daily personal oral hygiene can be due to:
  - Lack of knowledge and understanding about the need for biofilm removal and how it is accomplished.
  - Lack of motivation to carry out the necessary daily routines.
  - Lack of the necessary mental and/or physical coordination to carry out oral hygiene measures.
- Depending on the disability and level of function, the patient may need:
  - Complete assistance.
  - Partial assistance.
  - No assistance with daily biofilm removal.
- Assistance is provided by:
  - Parents, guardians, and other family members when living at home.
  - Aide or other caregiver responsible for the patient's care in a residence or long-term care setting.

BOX 56-3	Level of Function and Implications for Oral Self-Care

HIGH FUNCTION LEVEL: *ADL/IADL* LEVEL 0*
- The high-functioning, self-care group includes those capable of flossing and brushing their own teeth.
- Many patients, particularly children and those of all ages who are disabled mentally, need varying degrees of encouragement, motivation, and supervision.

MODERATE FUNCTIONING LEVEL: *ADL/IADL LEVELS 1 & 2*
- The moderate-functioning, partial-care group includes those capable of carrying out at least part of their oral hygiene needs but who require considerable training, assistance, and direct supervision.
- The assistance may be verbal, gestural, or hand-over-hand.

LOW FUNCTIONING LEVEL: *ADL/IADL LEVEL 3*
- The low-functioning, total-care group includes those who are unable to attend to their own care and are therefore dependent.
- Patients in this group may be bedridden and nonambulatory, although others may be confined to wheelchairs. With training, some may be able to attempt a part of their own care.

*Based on: ADL/IADL Measures of Patient Functioning in Table 23-3, page 343.

- There is a twofold responsibility to teach and supervise the patient and the patient's caregivers. Suggestions for in-service education are on page 869.

III. FUNCTIONING LEVELS

Functioning level refers to the daily living skills (bathing, toothbrushing, dressing, etc.) an individual can do alone, what range or degree of assistance is needed, or whether the person depends on others for complete care. Descriptions of the functioning levels are found in **Box 56-3** and in Table 23-3 on page 343.

IV. PREPARATION FOR INSTRUCTION

- To prepare for oral self-care instruction, the patient is asked basic planning questions such as those listed in **Box 56-4**.
- From the answers, an initial plan is developed and initiated on a trial-and-error basis.
- As the skills of the patient and caregiver improve, less biofilm is observed and recorded on succeeding appointments, and appropriate adaptations are made.
- The aim is complete daily biofilm control and with continuing reinforcement and motivation, progress can be made.
- Patient and caregiver attitudes, willingness and ability to participate, and acceptance of the recommended

BOX 56-4	Basic Planning Questions for a Patient With Disability

- What is the patient's functioning level?
- Is the patient capable to do all or part of the biofilm removal independently or will the patient require partial or total care?
- Is the patient involved in any community dental health programs (home, school, or day activity), and can the dentist and/or dental hygienist in such a program be contacted to coordinate the instruction given?
- What disabilities have the greatest influence on the extent of self-care possible and the anticipated success of the overall preventive program? Mental? Physical? Sensory? Learning? Oral?
- Which techniques and procedures will best fit the situation of the particular patient and the caregiver?
- How can the patient be helped to be as independent as possible?

procedures are taken into consideration when formulating or adapting the plan.

DENTAL BIOFILM REMOVAL

I. COMPONENTS

General procedures for instruction and methods for toothbrushing, biofilm removal on proximal tooth surfaces, and care of fixed and removable prostheses are provided for each patient. Individualized interventions are planned according to each patient's needs and abilities.

A. Provide Basic Information

Biofilm formation and disease development are described on a level at which the patient and caregiver can learn and be motivated.

B. Disclose and Show Biofilm

A graph that creates an ongoing record by which the patient and caregiver can watch progress of daily biofilm removal may help to motivate.

C. Toothbrushing

- Provide a soft toothbrush and ask the patient to remove the disclosed biofilm from the teeth. For the completely dependent patient, the parent will demonstrate. Alternative positions for the parent are described on page 869.
- Biofilm removal is more important than the specific technique used, as long as damage is not done to

the gingiva or teeth. A scrub-brush or circular Fones method may be appropriate and within the capability of certain patients, page 398 and Figure 27-8.

- Explain each step and demonstrate slowly.
- Adaptations for brush handles and other devices to promote or make possible a patient's independent performance are described on page 864.

D. Dentifrice

- A dentifrice containing fluoride is recommended for patients who can use a dentifrice.
- When a patient cannot control saliva, rinse, or expectorate, use of a dentifrice is contraindicated.
- A dentifrice may increase a gag reflex for certain patients.
- Dentifrice is not essential to biofilm removal, and another method of daily fluoride application may be more appropriate.
- When a parent or other caregiver is performing the brushing, the paste may limit visibility for thorough biofilm removal. When a paste is used, only a small amount is placed on the brush (pea size, Figure 49-7, page 771).
- The person who is severely disabled may be treated with a suction brush, as described in Chapter 57 on page 882 to help prevent aspiration.

E. Dental Floss

- If standard use of dental floss is not possible, the use of a floss holder described on page 866 can make flossing possible for certain patients, such as those with limited digital dexterity or the use of only one hand; the holder may also be useful for the caregiver.
- Methods for increasing the size of a toothbrush handle may be adapted for the handle of a floss holder.
- Some patients will need to use other interdental aids, described in Chapter 28 beginning on page 407.

II. EVALUATION

- Many patients and caregivers can learn with demonstration and practice how to examine the teeth and gingiva.
- The signs of healthy gingiva, especially color and absence of bleeding on brushing, can be noted.
- For selected patients, the thoroughness of brushing can be improved if a disclosing agent is used. The visible objective then is to remove all the color.
- Another system is to apply a disclosing agent after brushing to determine completion of biofilm removal. Then, any additional biofilm noted is brushed and removed.
- When a patient brushes first, followed by the caregiver, the disclosing agent might be applied by the caregiver so the task of removal can be completed. Because the

patient is encouraged to do as much as possible and is praised for whatever successes are accomplished, the biofilm disclosed for the caregiver to remove may be a factor of discouragement to the patient who really had done the very best to the extent of individual capability.

■ Another option is for the patient to do all the brushing and flossing once a day, and for the caregiver to do all the brushing and flossing at a different time.

SELF-CARE AIDS

■ Although a caregiver may be willing to brush the patient's teeth, as much as possible is carried out by the patient.

■ Benefits to the patient may include feelings of self-esteem and accomplishment when able to manage the important task of brushing, particularly with patients who have physical but no cognitive disability.

■ For patients whose main deterrent to personal self-care is related to grasp, manipulation, or control of a toothbrush, adaptations of the brush have been devised.[14–16]

■ Modifications to accommodate specific needs include enlarged handles, hand attachments, and elongated handles.

I. GENERAL PREREQUISITES FOR A SELF-CARE AID

■ Disinfectable
■ Durable. Can withstand exposure to water and saliva
■ Resistant to absorption of oral fluids
■ Replaceable
■ Inexpensive

II. TOOTHBRUSHING

A. For Patient With Fingers Permanently Fixed in a Fist

Insert the brush handle into the grasp.

B. For Patient Who Cannot Grasp and Hold

Objective: fasten the brush handle to the open hand.

■ Velcro strap around hand has a slit on the palm side into which the brush handle can be inserted. A vinyl pocket with an adjustable Velcro strap is commercially available. The toothbrush or floss aid handle fits into the pocket, as shown in **Figure 56-8A**. The patient can use the device to hold other objects, such as eating utensils.

■ Handle of fingernail brush attached to toothbrush by adhesive water-resistant tape, as shown in **Figure 56-8B**.

■ Wide rubber strap or a length of small-diameter rubber tubing attached through the hole in the toothbrush handle and tied adjacent to the brush head so the patient's hand can be slipped under the rubber and the brush can be held firmly, as shown in **Figure 56-8C**.

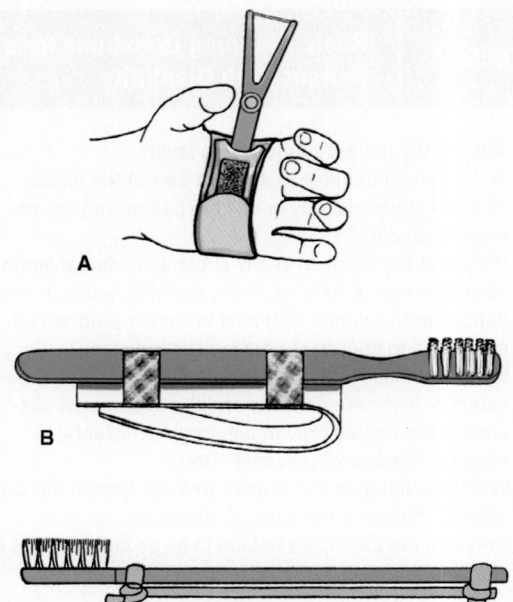

FIGURE 56-8 **Aids for Patient Who Cannot Grasp and Hold.** (A) Adjustable Velcro strap around hand has a pocket designed to hold the toothbrush handle or floss aid. (B) Handle of a fingernail brush attached to toothbrush by adhesive tape. (C) Rubber tubing attached firmly to toothbrush handle enables patient to hold brush across the palm of the hand. A floss holder also may be held by these methods.

C. For Patient With Limited Hand Closure (Unable to Manipulate Usual Toothbrush Handle or Floss Holder)

Objective: enlarge the diameter of the handle.

■ *Bicycle handle grip:* Insert toothbrush handle, as shown in **Figure 56-9A**.

■ Soft rubber ball or a styrofoam ball. Push brush handle into ball, as in **Figure 56-9B**. Styrofoam balls are available in various sizes from craft shops.

■ Juice or soda pop can. Place the rubber ball with toothbrush inside the can, as shown in **Figure 56-9C**.

■ *Quick-cure acrylic:* Obtain an impression of the hand grasp by having the patient grasp a cylinder of base plate wax. Then, fill the wax cylinder with quick-cure acrylic. Insert the toothbrush handle before the acrylic sets. The angle may be adjusted to set the brush head for the patient's convenient use. Polish the acrylic.

D. For Patient Unable to Lift Hand or Arm (With Limited Shoulder or Elbow Movement)

Objective: Lengthen the handle of the brush using a material that is strong or rigid enough to maintain the brush contact with sufficient lateral pressure to remove biofilm from the tooth surfaces.

■ Cylinder of wood with brush handle cemented inside.[17]

■ Two brushes. Cut the head from an old brush and fasten the handle to the end of the new brush handle (glue, tape, heat).

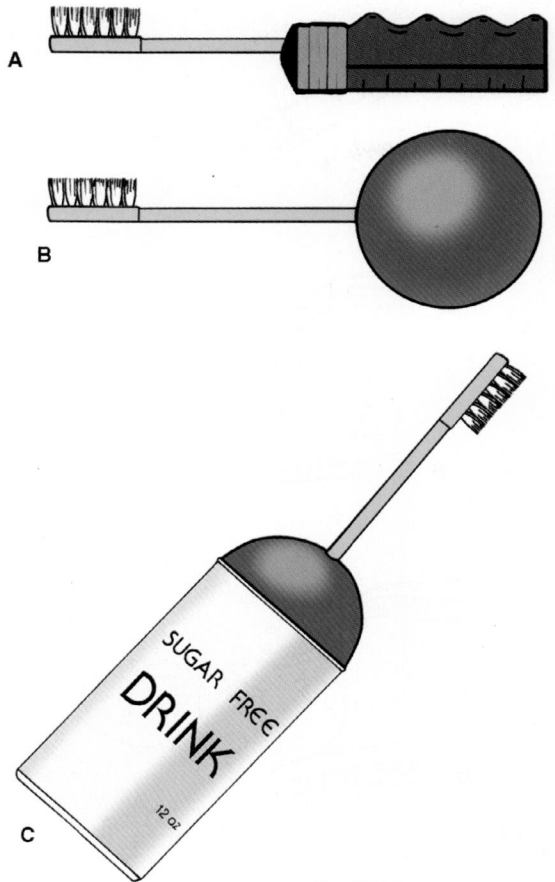

FIGURE 56-9 **Aids for Patient With Limited Grasp. (A)** Toothbrush inserted into a bicycle handle grip. **(B)** Toothbrush inserted into a soft rubber ball. **(C)** Toothbrush in soft rubber ball inserted into a juice or soda pop can provide a handle of appropriate diameter for patients with limited hand closure.

- Tongue depressors taped to the brush handle, then one or two other tongue depressors taped to overlap and provide an extension.
- Bicycle spoke, coat hanger, or other means for elongation fixed with a handle of acrylic resin. The metal tip may be heated and pushed into the toothbrush handle.[18,19] Use double or triple thickness to avoid flexibility.

E. For Patient Who Can Hold and Position the Toothbrush But Cannot Manipulate to Make Strokes for Biofilm Removal

Specially Designed Toothbrush
- A manual brush that brushes exposed tooth surfaces simultaneously, as shown in **Figure 56-10**.
- The brush with curved outer filaments and a short stiff center row of filaments.
- Research showed a similar reduction in debris and biofilm with this brush compared with a conventional brush.[20]

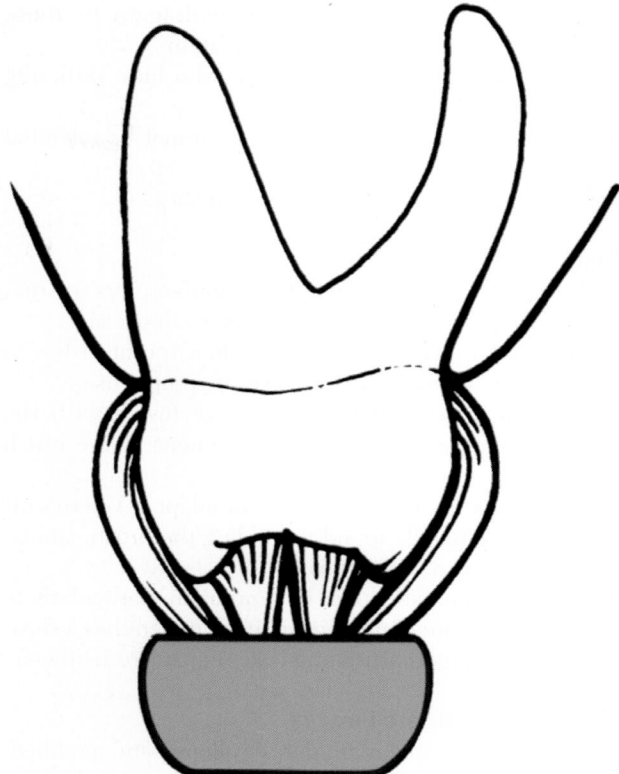

FIGURE 56-10 **Aid for Patient With a Brushing Problem.** A specially designed toothbrush is shown on the mesial of a maxillary second primary molar. Used with a back-and-forth motion, the filaments remove debris and dental biofilm simultaneously from the facial, lingual (palatal), and occlusal tooth surfaces.

- This type of brush can also aid those with hand tremors, such as with Parkinson's disease, by stabilizing brush placement in position.

Patient Moves Head Instead of Hand
Guide patient to learn to move the head up and down and from side to side while a conventional soft brush is held against the teeth.[19]

F. Use of a Power Toothbrush

- A power toothbrush can be a beneficial adjunct for many patients with disabilities and can motivate patients. This type of appliance can provide independence and more effective biofilm removal if patient has difficulty with a manual toothbrush.
- A power toothbrush can cause significant trauma if used incorrectly by, for example, a patient unable to hold the heavier weight of the power toothbrush or one lacking the comprehension for proper use.

Advantages and Disadvantages
- The extra size and weight of the handle may be advantageous for some patients or difficult for others with limited strength.

- The on/off mechanism may be difficult to use for those lacking finger strength and coordination.
- The larger handle can aid those who have difficulty grasping objects.
- The vibrations created during use cannot be tolerated by certain patients.
- Cost is higher than conventional brushes.

Suggestions for Use

- Patients are instructed to follow manufacturers' instructions for proper use as indicated on each package.
- Patients are instructed to bring their toothbrushes to dental appointments to demonstrate proper use.
- Care for a power toothbrush is reviewed with the patient including periodic replacement of the brush tip.
- A patient with limited grasp can adapt a Velcro cuff around the handle to aid in holding the brush, similar to those shown in **Figure 56-8**.
- Cross contamination can be a problem, particularly in group living situations. Ensure each patient has a separate marked toothbrush and is kept apart from others.

Other Power Oral Care Devices

- Power devices are continually developed and modified.
- Power-assisted flossers are available and may be an appropriate recommendation for use by certain patients.
- Dental professionals evaluate new products available and make appropriate suggestions for use with each individual patient.

III. USE OF FLOSS HOLDER

Careful instruction is provided and supervision given periodically to prevent tissue damage, as illustrated in **Figure 56-11**.

To avoid cutting the papilla when applied interproximally:

- Use a rest or fulcrum to prevent snapping through the contact.
- Pull the floss mesially (to clean the distal surface of a tooth) or push distally (to clean the mesial surface) to allow floss to be positioned on the side of the papilla.

IV. CLEANING REMOVABLE DENTAL PROSTHESES

- The details for cleaning removable prostheses are described in Chapter 31 on page 453.
- The same materials and procedures are recommended for the patient with a disability or another person who cares for the prosthesis.
- The sink is partially filled with water and/or a face cloth or small towel is placed in the sink to cushion and prevent damage if prosthesis is dropped.

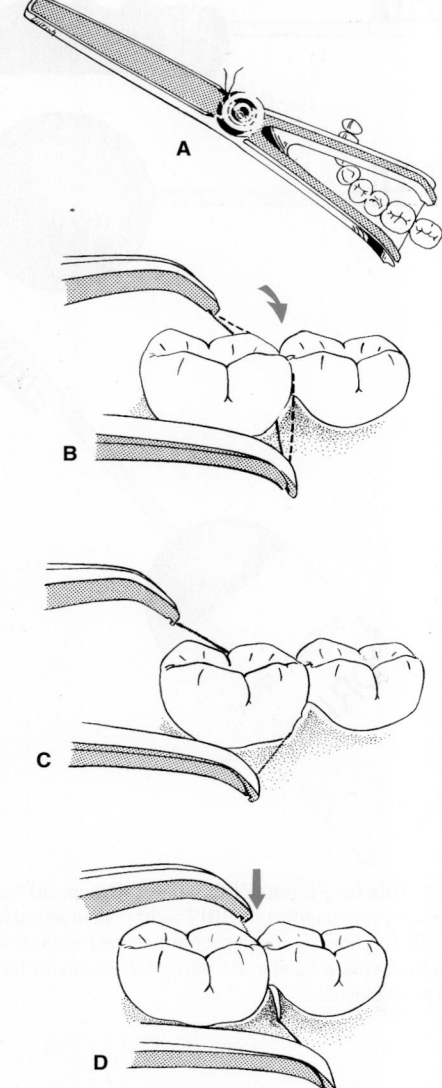

FIGURE 56-11 **Use of a Floss Holder. (A)** The floss is held over the proximal contact for insertion. A hand rest is maintained on the chin to prevent excess pressure. **(B)** As the floss is lowered gently and drawn through the contact area, the holder is pulled mesially when the floss is applied to the distal surface and pushed distally when the floss is applied to the mesial surface. **(C)** Floss is lowered slightly below the gingival margin. **(D)** Floss cut in the papilla when used incorrectly.

A. Grasp Problem

- For the patient with difficulty grasping or holding the brush, a denture brush handle may be adapted by any of the methods described for the regular toothbrush.
- A fingernail brush may be used instead of a standard denture brush provided all denture surfaces can be reached for biofilm removal.

B. One Hand

For the patient handicapped by hemiplegia or for the patient with use of two hands but who needs to grasp the

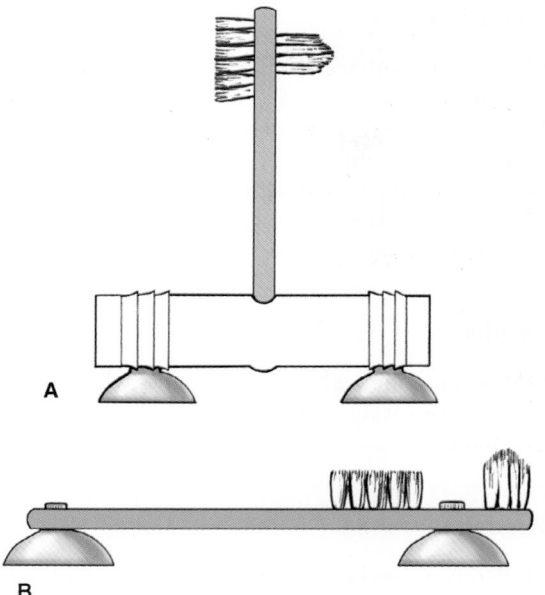

FIGURE 56-12 **Denture Brushes With Suction Cups. (A)** Denture brush in a commercially available mounting. **(B)** Suction cups attached directly to a denture brush. Either brush may be positioned in a sink to aid the person who has one hand or who needs to grasp the denture with two hands to prevent accidental dropping and breakage.

denture with two hands to prevent accidents, the following are recommended:

- Fingernail brush with suction cups.
- Denture brush in mounting that has suction cups. These are available commercially, as shown in **Figure 56-12A**.
- Denture brush with suction cups, as shown in **Figure 56-12B**, can attach low inside the sink bowl.

FLUORIDES

Selection of a multiple fluoride program for an individual patient depends on the caries risk status, and the concentration of fluoride in the water supply. A patient with a disability may be at increased risk for caries due to a decreased ability to cooperate and side effects of medications.

I. FLUORIDATION

- Water fluoridation has beneficial anticaries effects.
- Patient is encouraged to drink fluoridated water; bottled water may not have optimal fluoride level.

II. DIETARY SUPPLEMENTS

- When the fluoride level is below optimum in the community water supply, or the water intake by a child is low, a supplement is recommended, as shown in Table 35-1 on page 526.

- Fluoride can be prescribed in the form of a chewable tablet, lozenge, drops, or mouthwash to swallow after swishing depending on the masticatory function of the child.

III. PROFESSIONALLY APPLIED TOPICAL FLUORIDE

- Professionally applied topical fluoride is indicated based on a patient's risk for caries.
- Fluoride varnish is the agent of choice for children 6 years and under, and all disabled patients. The procedure for placing a fluoride varnish is described in Table 35-4 on page 531.

IV. SELF-APPLIED PROCEDURES

- Whether the individual with a disability is a child or an adult, a home fluoride program is indicated.
- After disease control techniques for flossing and toothbrushing have been completed before the patient retires, a mouthrinse, for the patient who can rinse; a gel applied by tray or toothbrush; or a chewable tablet, for the patient who can chew and who needs a fluoride supplement, may be advised.
- For a dependent, low-functioning person, brushing with a gel could be most applicable.
- Caregiver supervision and cooperation are essential and motivation of the parent or caregiver needs regular reinforcement by the dental team.

PIT AND FISSURE SEALANTS

- Pit and fissure sealants have been used for children with developmental disabilities with satisfactory results.[21]
- The principles for application are the same as those for all patients, as described in Chapter 36, starting on page 544.
- Use of a dental assistant can help maintain a dry field and enhance long-term sealant retention.
- The use of a rubber dam is particularly helpful for patients with excess saliva, hyperactivity of the tongue, or other management difficulties.
- When a severely disabled patient will be administered general anesthesia for restorative procedures, pit and fissure sealants are placed in all noncarious occlusal surfaces at that time.
- For all young patients, the sealant can be placed as soon after eruption as the tooth will hold a rubber dam.

DIET INSTRUCTION

- The patient and caregiver are given general dietary requirements for oral health and how to put the principles into daily practice is a distinct part of the total preventive program.

- Providing information related to diet and nutrition is applicable to patients with special needs as well as to all patients.
- A careful assessment of current eating habits, extent of knowledge, family customs, and economic factors as they relate to a patient's condition are considered before specific recommendations can be made.
- In an institutional setting, efforts can be directed to contact and work with the administrative personnel, teachers, dietitians, and aides.
- Coordination of biofilm control, snack selection, and availability, together with the fluoride program helps oral disease control.

I. FACTORS THAT INFLUENCE DIET HABITS

- For certain patients, diet selection and utilization center on problems of mastication; for others, the transport of food to the mouth is a challenge.
- The following partial list of issues is suggested to help during dietary analysis and counseling.
- Many of the issues are directly related to increases in biofilm accumulation and resultant dental caries and periodontal infections.

A. Masticatory or Feeding Issues

Problems with chewing and swallowing can lead to the use of a soft diet, often composed mainly of carbohydrates.

B. Overindulgence in Sucrose-Containing Foods

- Sweets are sometimes used as rewards or bribes by unsuspecting family members or teachers involved in behavior modification procedures in training programs.
- Nonambulatory or otherwise confined patients may have less access to between-meal foods and, therefore, may eat more regularly, as served.
- The confined person may have snacks and sweets readily available, which can lead to dental destruction.

C. Inability to Accomplish Personal Biofilm Control Measures

Problems of daily biofilm removal can be related to a physical disability, lack of assistance from a caregiver, or lack of knowledge, combined with a diet high in cariogenic foods, which leads to dental caries development.

D. Lack of Professional Care and Instruction

Many patients do not receive adequate professional care because of barriers to care such as those listed in **Table 56-2**.

E. Medications

- Medications with a side effect of xerostomia contribute to dental caries.
- Medications that diminish appetite as a side effect influence diet habits.
- Medications contained within a sucrose base designed to mask the flavor of the agent or to pacify the patient contribute to dental caries incidence.[22]

F. Obesity

Obesity is an issue with certain patients who suffer from inactivity, overeating, boredom, or lack of knowledge of proper food selection.

G. Food Preparation

- Difficulty of food preparation can be a major limitation to diet selection for adults with neuromuscular disorders.
- Wheelchair limitations, lack of muscular coordination, hemiplegia or paraplegia, and dependence on others for grocery shopping are examples of problems encountered.

II. DIET ASSESSMENT AND COUNSELING

A. Food Record

- A high-functioning patient may be able to keep a food diary, and participation is encouraged.
- The parent, advocate, or other caregiver can assist or, in the case of a low- or moderate-functioning person, may complete the entire diary.
- With the aid of the record and the information from the medical and dental histories, items for counseling can be selected.

B. Recommendations

- General procedures for assessment and counseling are described in Chapter 34 on page 507. Adaptations involve long-range planning for gradual modification of each patient's diet.
- The person who selects and prepares the food for the patient is involved in the planning. Sugarless snacks and sugarless rewards during behavior modification training are especially important to control.
- Parents need instruction as early as possible after a newborn is known to be developmentally disabled so that fluoride, diet, early personal hygiene, and the prevention of baby bottle caries can be coordinated into the daily program. The infant's early care includes an oral examination by the dentist and dental hygienist within 6 months of the eruption of the first tooth and no later than 12 months of age.

INSTRUCTION FOR CAREGIVER

- Individuals who need partial or total care present with varying degrees of ability to cooperate, depending on the type of disability.
- The size of the patient and whether the patient is ambulatory, bedridden, or in a wheelchair are among the factors that influence the technique for management.
- The instructions for the caregiver are given where the specific techniques can actually be demonstrated as they will be done at home.
- When the patient lies down with the head in the parent's lap, for example, a suitable couch is used, or chairs can be placed together.
- Time and repeated practice sessions may be needed for successful biofilm removal.

I. SELF-CARE AND ATTITUDE

- Whenever possible, instruction for the parents, family members, or other caregivers begins with their own personal oral care.
- Success comes when those who care for the patient have knowledge and understanding of the purposes and techniques, can demonstrate their own biofilm removal, and are motivated for self-care.

II. GENERAL SUGGESTIONS

A. Place

- The biofilm removal procedures are accomplished best when both the patient and the caregiver are comfortable and relaxed.
- A small bathroom may be the least desirable place because positioning the patient may be awkward, except when a standing position can be used.
- Good light, easy visibility of the teeth, and control of the head of the person with the disability are prerequisites.

B. Teaching Techniques for Biofilm Removal

- *Use of finger and hand rests:* The person performing the biofilm balances the toothbrush, dental floss, floss aid, or any other implement with a finger or hand rest on the side of the patient's face or chin. Such contact contributes to total patient control and to effective use of the biofilm removal device.
- *Use of a mouth prop:* For certain patients, biofilm removal is impossible without a mouth prop, and demonstration for insertion on both sides is needed. For home use, a rolled and moist washcloth may be appropriate.

III. POSITIONS

A. Caregiver Standing

With the caregiver standing from behind, the arm is brought around the patient's head and the chin is cupped while using the thumb and index finger to retract the lips and cheeks. The other hand applies the toothbrush, floss aid, or other device. This technique requires that the patient be able to bend the head back far enough for the parent to see the maxillary teeth. The procedure may be applicable for the following:

- Short patient standing in front of and backed up to the caregiver.
- Tall patient seated in a chair with the head tipped back to lean against the caregiver, or seated in a large chair or sofa with the head stabilized against the top of chair back.
- Patient in a wheelchair leaning back against the parent. Wheelchair brakes are set.

B. Caregiver Seated

- Patient seated on pillow on floor in front of parent, with back close to the chair and head turned back into parent's lap, as shown in **Figure 56-13A**. The caregiver may place his/her legs over the shoulders of the patient to restrain arms and body movements, as shown in **Figure 56-13B**.
- Caregiver is seated at the end of a sofa or couch, and patient is lying down with the head in parent's lap, as shown in **Figure 56-13C**.
- For a bedridden patient, the caregiver may sit at the patient's head and place the head in the lap. When body and arm movements need to be controlled, the caregiver can sit beside the patient, lean across the patient's chest, and hold the patient's arm against the body with the elbow. The hand of the restraining arm can hold the mouth prop, retract, or do whatever is necessary.

C. Two People

- In any of the positions previously mentioned, the parent may need the assistance of a second person to hold the hands and arms or otherwise restrain the patient.
- A small child may be placed across the laps of two persons seated facing each other. One stabilizes the head and brushes and flosses while the other person holds hands, arms, and legs as needed, as shown in **Figure 56-13D**.

GROUP IN-SERVICE EDUCATION

- In-service programs are provided for teachers, registered nurses, other health professionals, parents, and volunteers in school and community preventive programs. For example, all persons mentioned could be involved in the preparation of a program about classroom weekly rinsing with a fluoride mouthrinse. When a program is citywide and many dental hygienists are involved, in-service preparation for the dental hygienists themselves is necessary to provide coordination for the event.

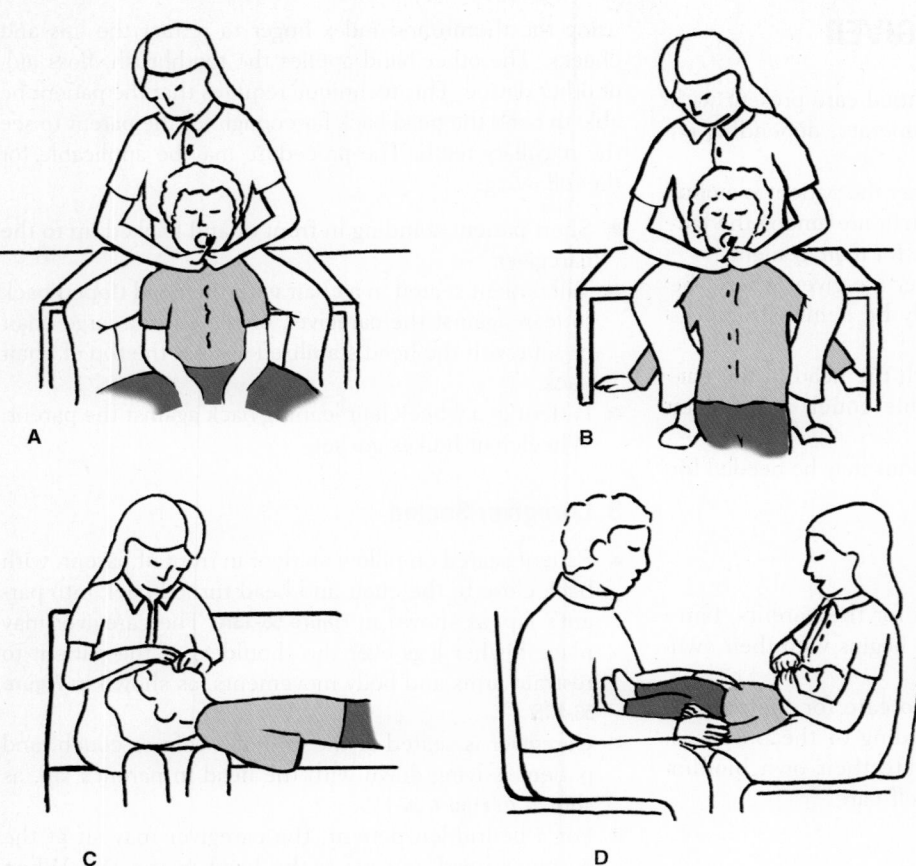

FIGURE 56-13 **Positions for Child or Disabled Patient During Biofilm Removal. (A)** Patient seated on floor with head turned back into the lap of the caregiver. **(B)** Patient's arms restrained by legs of caregiver. **(C)** Patient reclining on couch with head in lap of caregiver. **(D)** Two people participating with small child between. One holds patient for stabilization while the other holds the head for toothbrushing and flossing.

■ A special need exists for in-service instruction in oral health measures for caregivers in extended care institutions. Many patients in such facilities are unable to care for their own needs and may require total care, partial assistance, supervision, or regular reminders.

■ The dental hygienist is able to work with the caregivers to teach them appropriate techniques and to motivate them to incorporate oral care into the daily routine for each resident or patient.

■ The general suggestions outlined in the following sections pertain to preparation and content for in-service workshops for the oral care of long-term patients.

I. PREPARATION FOR AN IN-SERVICE PROGRAM

A. Planning

■ An in-service program needs careful planning. For many groups, time for an in-service is taken from an already busy work schedule. Nonmotivated participants require special considerations. A leading factor contributing to the success of a program is the genuine concern and enthusiasm of the program leader in motivating the participants.

■ Effective learning materials are clear and to the point, interestingly presented with appropriate visual aids, and stimulating for learning. Objectives are defined in writing and serve as a guide to preparation and evaluation.

■ Problems of the staff are recognized and addressed during the program. Some members may have negative oral health attitudes, minimal educational background, and poor personal oral health.

■ Initially, basic preparation includes learning about the functioning levels of the patient and assessing the procedures used for oral care. A survey of the biofilm control materials and devices available and in current use, methods for labeling or storing individual brushes, and the frequency of use is important.

B. Use of Clinic Records

■ HIPAA regulations may restrict a dental hygienist's access to individual patient records in an agency that requests an oral health presentation.

■ When a dental hygienist is employed regularly within an institution, a much more complete assessment can be made.

- If possible, clinic records and medical histories of patients are reviewed so that special general or oral health problems can be considered.
- The dental hygienist invited to the institution for the specific purpose of presenting the workshop needs to arrange a pre-workshop visit to observe and get to know the caregivers and the patients.

C. Gingival/Biofilm Index

- When the dental hygienist providing hands-on instruction for oral care, use of a gingival or biofilm index can provide a baseline of information from which progress can be evaluated.
- The caregivers could carry out the daily biofilm program and see the changes that take place by comparing survey results at a later date.
- Continuing participation and receiving feedback of successful biofilm removal can provide real motivation to caregivers.

II. PROGRAM CONTENT

An oral health in-service program will be more successful if the content presented is based on an assessment of specific needs identified by the institution, patients, and caregivers. Some topics that can be considered are as listed.

A. The Caregivers' Own Biofilm Control

- On the basis the premise that persons who are motivated to care for their own mouths have a clearer understanding of the effects and importance of oral care and give a higher priority to the time spent daily, an in-service education group needs to participate in a personal biofilm control program.
- A biofilm-free score, as described in Chapter 22 on pages 315 to 321, or another evaluation index can be used.
- A group may be willing to work in pairs and learn to evaluate and score each other, thereby learning the techniques to be applied to their patients.

B. Facts About Cause and Prevention of Oral Disease

- Basic information about biofilm, its formation, and how gingivitis and dental caries develop are important to most groups.
- The progress of disease from reversible gingivitis to severe periodontitis can be explained, as can the process of dental caries, which begins with a small white spot of demineralization and progresses to a diseased pulp.
- The concept of prevention through biofilm control, fluoride, dietary controls, sealants, and early treatment for restorations is carefully presented.
- Handout materials and colorful visual aids promote learning.

C. Oral Inspection

- *Oral mucosa:* Techniques demonstrated and practiced by the participants on each other include the use of a tongue depressor to retract, a disposable mouth mirror, and a light source to see the oral mucosa.
- *Tongue:* How to hold the tongue, using a sponge to lift and inspect all parts, can be shown.
- *Gingiva:* Color, size, and bleeding that occurs spontaneously or while brushing can be explained and demonstrated. When projection is possible, slides can be included for all aspects of the instructional material. When a camera is available for intraoral photography, "before" and "after" pictures of the patients can be shown. Changes effected by the biofilm control supervised by the caregivers are more meaningful than are pictures of strangers.
- *Biofilm:* Inspection for biofilm can be demonstrated when the disclosing agent is used before biofilm scoring and removal.
- *Denture-supporting mucosa:* Patients with dentures need the supporting tissues examined periodically by the dentist, but caregivers can notice changes during daily cleaning and massaging of the mucosa while the denture is out of the mouth for cleaning and call them to the dentists' attention at the next visit.
- *Dentures:* Sample dentures may be used to help the participants learn to examine each denture for cracks or sharp edges. Examination for deposits can be made by the patient and the caregivers and compared with the denture after it has been cleaned.

D. Techniques of Mouth Care and Disease Control

- Staff members can be trained to work in pairs.[23] Working in pairs is more efficient, particularly in the care of challenging patients.
- A plan for each patient can be worked out with the caregivers so that individual problems relative to dental caries prevention, gingival disease control, or complete or partial denture care can be solved.
- *Biofilm control:* Instruction includes positioning of the patient, application of disclosing agent, examination for biofilm on the teeth, toothbrush selection and technique, use of a mouth prop, and flossing with or without a floss aid. The use of a portable or bedside suction unit for removing debris from a patient's mouth can be practiced by a paired team.[23]
- *Fluoride application:* The objectives and techniques for brushing with a gel, swabbing with a mouthrinse, assisting the patient with a chewable tablet, or applying a gel tray can be included.
- *Denture care:* Procedures for care of dentures and of the mucosa under the denture are shown.
- *Saliva substitute:* Use of saliva substitute for dry mouth is demonstrated; instruction includes how to use a swab with saliva substitute to provide relief for certain patients (page 374).

E. Denture Marking Procedure

■ All dentures are marked for patient identification.
■ Most dentures are marked during processing.
■ The techniques for denture marking are outlined in Chapter 53 on page 819.

III. RECORDS

■ A record form to be completed for each patient is essential to evaluate the success of the in-service presentation.
■ During the instruction periods, the staff can learn how to complete the record and where to file the copies.
■ The form can be designed with spaces to record information obtained during the oral examination, the functioning level and degree of cooperation, the procedures needed for dental caries control, periodontal health, and/or denture care.
■ In addition, the instruction provided, the implements and materials used, the planned future instruction, the prognosis, and any other notes can be included. Successful techniques are described, and suggestions for future appointments can be made.

IV. FOLLOW-UP

■ After caregivers have tried their newly learned procedures, an opportunity to have questions answered is provided.
■ Direct observation by the dental hygienist of techniques performed with and for the patients, advice concerning oral problems of particular patients, and corrections when necessary can motivate and encourage both patient and caregiver.
■ Disclosing and recording the biofilm for comparison of scores before and after the program can show the progress being made.

V. CONTINUING EDUCATION

■ Individual instruction is provided for each new employee during the orientation period for that employee.
■ Periodic updating for all employees can be accomplished at regular intervals. Questions and problems can be discussed, and plans can be introduced for changing a certain procedure based on new research evidence.
■ A specific plan for scheduled oral health programs may be a requirement for licensure of a health-care facility.
■ Advanced education programs are available for extensive training in care of the disabled patient.

THE DENTAL HYGIENIST WITH A DISABILITY[24]

■ Disability is not necessarily an obstacle to dental hygiene licensure and provision of clinical care.
■ Adaptive technology, tax incentives for accessibility construction, and creative thinking can facilitate any necessary workplace modifications.
■ Additional dental hygiene roles, such as manager, advocate, or educator may provide employment opportunities for the dental hygienist with a disability.

DOCUMENTATION

In addition to the standard information recorded for a patient visit, documentation of care provided for a patient who has a disability includes:

■ Individualized information about the patient's condition or level of functioning that will affect modifications needed during dental hygiene care. Some suggestions for information needed are listed in **Box 56-5**.

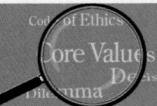 **Everyday Ethics**

When Mrs. Becker has her dental appointment, Lauren, the dental hygienist, must rush to finish the previous patient so she can have time to go to the storage closet in the basement and get the transfer board so Mrs. Becker can slide over to the dental chair from her wheelchair. Mrs. Becker has numerous medical and dental problems that she tends to complain about. She has been very difficult to motivate to perform daily biofilm control. Her current dental status indicates that she should be placed on more frequent 2- to 3-month maintenance appointments. Lauren feels overstressed to prepare for and treat Mrs. Becker in the time she is allowed for appointments. Lauren is considering ignoring the plan for more frequent maintenance visits and scheduling Mrs. Becker in 6 months to avoid another unpleasant experience for both of them.

Questions for Consideration

1. Which core values of dental hygiene ethics apply in this situation?
2. In terms of every patient's right to expect the best of care, how can Lauren fulfill her professional obligations of beneficence and fairness if Ms. Becker is not appointed at intervals appropriate for her oral health needs?
3. What are the legal implications related to standard of care if Lauren follows through with her plan to reduce the frequency of Mrs. Becker's maintenance visits?

BOX 56-5	Example Progress Note for Patient With a Disability

25-year-old male patient with Down's syndrome, who lives in an assisted-living group home, presents for routine 3-month periodontal maintenance appointment. No changes in medical history. The curved bristle toothbrush, introduced at his last appointment, is working quite well for him and his caregiver has affixed a rubber band to the handle in order to help stabilize the toothbrush in his hand. His biofilm index is now below 20%.

Worked with his caregiver to develop a personal "Daily Oral Care" list to identify all the steps and materials necessary for his daily oral care regimen. Caregiver will make up a large poster of the steps using pictures and will laminate and hang the poster by the bathroom sink in order to help the patient be more independent with his daily oral care regimen. Maintenance scaling and root planing completed. Used a "tell, show, do" approach to provide basic instructions for using a floss holder. First time efforts were clumsy, but patient is motivated to practice. Evaluate success at next visit scheduled in 3 months.

Signed: _____, RDH Date: _____.

■ Specific details related to patient management or communication strategies used during the dental hygiene appointment, and an indication of whether or not those strategies were successful.

■ Identification of self-care aids, modifications to standard oral hygiene instructions, and details of any recommendations or instructions provided for caregivers.

■ **Box 56-5** provides an example progress note.

Factors To Teach The Patient and Caregiver

■ Seek regular dental and medical examinations.

■ Learn about disability; know status, disease, names, and doses of medications including over-the-counter medications, and other changes in medical history.

■ Recognize the early warnings of complications of disease.

■ Recognize the side effects of treatments and medications.

■ Seek immediate medical attention for any complications.

■ Practice a healthy lifestyle, including healthy diet, daily exercise, no tobacco products, alcohol avoidance, attainment of ideal weight, and stress reduction. Accept assistance for smoking cessation.

■ Practice meticulous oral hygiene to prevent dental disease and adapt techniques as needed.

■ Ways to overcome barriers to dental care.

References

1. United States Department of Justice. Americans With Disabilities Act of 1990 as Amended in 2008 (P. L. 110–325) p. 7. [accessed 2010 Sept 7]. Available from: http://www.ada.gov/pubs/ada.htm
2. World Health Organization (WHO). International Classification of Functioning, Disability and Health (ICF). [Internet] Geneva: WHO. Endorsed 22 May, 2001. [cited 2010 Sept 7] Accessed from: http://www.who.int/classifications/icf/en/index.html
3. Glassman P. New models for improving oral health for people with special needs. *J Calif Dent Assoc.* 2005 Aug;33(8):625–33.
4. Johnson TL. Pilot study of dental hygienists' comfort and confidence levels and care planning for patients with disabilities. *J Dent Educ.* 2000 Dec;64(12):839–46.
5. Fiske J. The delivery of oral care services to elderly people living in noninstitutionalized setting. *J Public Health Dent.* 2000 Fall;60(4):321–5.
6. Glassman P, Henderson T, Helgeson M, Niessen L, Demby N, Miller C, Ceyerowita C, Ingraham R, Isman R, Noel D, Tellier R, Toto K. Oral Health for People with special needs: consensus statement on implications and recommendations for the dental profession. *J Calif Dent Assoc.* 2005 Aug;33(8):619–23.
7. Glassman P, Subar P. Creating and maintaining oral health for dependent people in institutional settings. *J Public Health Dent* 2010 Jun;70(Suppl 1):S40–8.
8. American Dental Hygienists' Association. *Direct access states.* Chicago: ADHA; 2010 Jun [cited 2011 Mar 1]. Available from: www.adha.org/governmental_affairs/downloads/direct_access.pdf
9. Meningaud JP, Pitak-Arnnop P, Chikhani L, Bertrand JC. Drooling of saliva: a review of the etiology and management options. *Oral Surg Oral Med Oral Pathol Oral Radiol Endod.* 2006 Jan;101(1):48–57.
10. Americans with Disabilities Act, [Internet]. 2010 ADA Standards for Accessible Design. Washington, DC: United States Department of Justice; 2010 Sep 15 [cited 2011 Mar 1]. Available from: http://www.ada.gov/2010ADAstandards_index.htm
11. Jaccarino J. The special needs patient in a wheelchair. *Dent Assist.* 2009 Mar–Apr;78(2):22–3, 46–51.
12. Romer M. Consent, restraint, and people with special needs: A review. *Spec Care Dentist.* 2009 Jan;29(1):58–66.
13. Glassman P, Caputo A, Dougherty N, Lyons R, Messieha Z, Miller C, Peltier B, Romer M; Special Care Dentistry Association. Special Care Dentistry Association consensus statement on sedation, anesthesia, and alternative techniques for people with special needs. *Spec Care Dentist.* 2009 Jan;29(1):2–8.
14. Price E. Toothbrush modifications for the handicapped. *Dent Hyg (Chic).* 1980 Oct;54(10):467–70.
15. Sroda R, Plezia RA. Oral hygiene devices for special patients. *Spec Care Dentist.* 1984 Nov–Dec;4(6):264–6.
16. Albertson D. Prevention and the handicapped child. *Dent Clin North Am.* 1974 Jul;18(3)595–608.
17. Duncan JL. Incorporating oral hygiene procedures in geriatric nursing homes. *Dent Hyg (Chic).* 1979 Nov;53(11):519–23.
18. Albertson D. Prevention and the handicapped child. *Dent Clin North Am.* 1974 Jul;18(3):595–608.
19. Ettinger RL, Pinkham JR. Oral hygiene and the handicapped child. *J Int Assoc Dent Child.* 1978 Jul;9(1):3–11.
20. Chava VK. An evaluation of the efficacy of a curved bristle and conventional toothbrush. A comparative clinical study. *J Periodontol.* 2000 May;71(5):785–9.
21. Richardson B, Smith DC, Hargreaves JA. A 5-year clinical evaluation of the effectiveness of a fissure sealant in mentally retarded Canadian children. *Community Dent Oral Epidemiol.* 1981 Aug; 9(4):170–4.
22. Neves BG, Farah A, Lucas E, de Sousa VP, Maia LC. Are paediatric medicines risk factors for dental caries and dental erosion? *Community Dent Health.* 2010 Mar;27(1):46–51.
23. Gertenrich RL, Hart RW. Utilization of the oral hygiene team in a mental health institution. *ASDC J Dent Child.* 1972 May–Jun; 39(3):174–7.
24. Smith DS. Challenges in dental hygiene employment for dental hygienists with disabilities. *Access.* 2010 Sep–Oct;24(8):35–7.

The Patient Who Is Homebound

CHARLOTTE J. WYCHE, RDH, MS

Chapter Outline

HOMEBOUND PATIENTS

In recent years, increased attention has been paid to the oral health needs of individuals who cannot access oral health services in a traditional dental practice setting. Patients of all age groups who are confined to hospitals, hospices, institutions, nursing homes, skilled nursing facilities, or private homes need special adaptations for oral care.

There are similarities in the limitations and needs of functionally dependent persons who reside in private homes and those who reside in institutions. Instruction in personal oral preventive procedures has particular significance for comfort and quality of life, as well as the systemic health of these individuals.

Key words and definitions related to caring for homebound patients are found in **Box 57-1**.

I. POTENTIAL HOMEBOUND PATIENTS

Potential homebound patients are listed in **Box 57-2**. A homebound patient may reside in:

- a private home and utilize home-based healthcare services.
- an institutionalized setting such as a group home, hospital, nursing home, or residential facility.

The individual who is homebound may:

- have limitation in one or more activities of daily living (ADL/IADL, Table 23-3, page 343).

BOX 57-1	**Key Words**

Homebound Patients

Advanced dental hygiene practitioner (ADHP): a dental hygienist with advanced education and certification in specialty areas who is licensed to provide a wide range of services including, but not limited to, diagnostic, preventive, restorative, and therapeutic services directly to the public; the model for this midlevel practitioner is similar to that of a nurse practitioner.

ADL/IADL (activities of daily living/instrumental activities of daily living): a measure of ability to carry out the basic tasks needed for self-care.

Ambulate: to walk or move about.

　Nonambulatory: inability to walk or move about freely.

Collaborative practice: an alternative oral care delivery model in which dental hygienists collaborate autonomously with members of interdisciplinary teams to provide dental hygiene services in a variety of nontraditional settings.

Coma: state of unconsciousness from which the patient cannot be aroused.

　Irreversible coma: brain death.

Comatose: pertaining to or affected with a coma.

Depression: temporary mental state or chronic disorder characterized by feelings of sadness and low self-esteem.

Disability: physical, mental, or functional impairment that restricts a major activity; may be partial or complete.

Frail elderly: medically and/or physically fragile, delicate, or weak older person; usually refers to those older than 80 years.

Functional dependence: inability to perform one or more activities of daily living (ADL) without help; the level of functional dependence is based on the level of assistance needed to perform ADL or the number of activities for which assistance is needed.

Hospice: an interdisciplinary program providing a continuum of home and inpatient palliative and supportive care to meet the physical, emotional, spiritual, social, and economic needs experienced by terminally ill individuals and their families during the final stages of illness and during dying and bereavement.

Interdisciplinary team: consists of specialists from many fields; combines expertise and resources to provide insight into all aspects of a given special area.

Nurse practitioner (NP): a licensed registered nurse who has had advanced preparation for practice that includes clinical experience in diagnosis and treatment of illness; NPs may work in collaborative practice with physicians or independently in private practice or nursing clinics; in some states NPs can prescribe medications.

Nursing home: a residential facility for persons with chronic illness or disability; often care for the frail elderly. Also called convalescent home or long-term care facility.

Oral health provider (OHP): a dental hygienist with advanced education and certification in specialty areas who is licensed as a mid-level care provider to provide expanded oral health services for underserved populations in the state of Minnesota.

Palliative: affording relief but not cure.

Polypharmacy: regular use of three or more drugs or medications; often an issue with elderly or medically compromised patients.

Sordes: foul matter that collects on the lips, teeth, and oral mucosa in low fevers; consists of debris, microorganisms, epithelial elements, and food particles; forms a crust.

Teledentistry: a model of healthcare delivery that uses Web-based technology to send electronic information such as patient history and digital radiographs, between on-site and off-site practitioners; this model can be used to support collaborative practice between dentists and dental hygienists who are caring for patients in nontraditional settings.

Terminally ill patient: a person who is experiencing the end stages of a life-threatening disease and for whom there is no longer hope of a cure.

Triage: screening and classification of individuals in order to make optimal use of treatment resources; sorting and allocating relative priority for patient treatment needs.

■ have an ASA classification of III or higher. See Table 23-1 on page 342.
■ Be functionally dependent on caregivers.

II. PATIENTS IN NURSING HOMES

United States federal regulations on dental services[1,2] require residential facilities that receive Medicaid or Medicare funding to contract with qualified dental personnel.

■ Medicare coverage does not include payment for dental services.

■ Medicaid-eligible residents are covered only for whatever dental services are included in the state plan; most state plans have limited coverage for adults.

　Under US federal guidelines, nursing homes are not required to cover the costs of dental care, but must help individuals residing in the facility to obtain the following:

■ Comprehensive assessment of dental status
■ Routine as well as emergency dental services
■ Transportation to dental appointments
■ Prompt referral to a dentist for lost or damaged dentures
■ Supplies related to oral health (e.g., toothbrush and dental floss) at no cost to the individual

BOX 57-2	Potential Homebound Patients

- Frail elderly
- Severely medically compromised
- Critically ill
- Physically disabled
- Developmentally disabled
- Chronically mentally ill
- Terminally ill

Regulations in each state regarding the provision of dental services for both Medicaid eligible and noneligible individuals vary greatly[2].

- Many states are silent on dental regulations or elaborate only briefly on federal guidelines.
- A few states provide guidelines in terms of frequency of examinations or spell out elements included in routine or emergency care.
- Some states require that facilities contract with a dentist to advise on policies and education.

National data[3] indicate that 62% of nursing homes provide dental and oral health services for their residents, but these data are inadequate to determine actual utilization of dental services by nursing home populations. However, regional studies[4,5] indicate that generally individuals residing in nursing homes:

- have poor oral health status,
- do not receive adequate daily oral care,
- cannot adequately access routine dental services.

III. COMMON ORAL PROBLEMS[6,7]

- Periodontal infections
- Lack of daily personal oral care
- Need for routine dental check-up
- Difficulty biting and chewing
- Losing weight/not eating because of oral problems
- Toothache/pain and abscess/swelling
- Trauma /fractured teeth
- Loose teeth
- Lost fillings/crowns
- Dental caries
- Loose, uncomfortable, or lost dentures

IV. SIGNIFICANCE OF ORAL HEALTH TO OVERALL HEALTH

- Systemic conditions can affect oral health status.
- Poor oral health can affect systemic conditions.
- Oral pain/discomfort can compromise nutritional status.

- Physical limitations can compromise daily personal oral care abilities.
- Oral health status and oral cleanliness can affect patient self-esteem, quality of life, and ability to communicate with family and caregivers.

V. BARRIERS TO ACCESS[4,8,9]

- Few on-site dental clinics in nursing homes or residential facilities
- Limited availability of general and specialty practitioners who provide home-based services
- Ageism or other negative attitudes of practitioners
- Cost
- Limited Medicaid coverage for adult dental services
- Nonpayment of Medicare for dental services
- Limited ambulation
- Nonavailability of transportation
- Fear
- Patient's health attitudes and beliefs
- Patient's daily pain or discomfort levels

VI. ELIMINATING BARRIERS

- Many services, including visiting nurses and personal/household assistance, are being delivered to homebound individuals by home health agencies.
- Midlevel allied health professionals, such as nurse practitioners, oversee programs that provide direct medical services for patients.
- New models for healthcare delivery use web-based communication tools to share electronic information, enhancing potential for collaboration between on-site and supervising health team members.
- Current public health programs in numerous states allow dental hygienists to provide care for certain underserved populations with broader supervision guidelines.
- A recent PEW Center report supports the creation of midlevel, direct access care providers to address access issues related to shortage of dentists, limited availability of safety net options for low-income populations, and need for care in non-traditional settings.[10]
- Several models currently being explored are based on utilization of dental hygienists who have received additional education and certification.[11,12]

DENTAL HYGIENE CARE AND INSTRUCTION

I. PORTABLE DELIVERY OF CARE

- For patients who cannot be transported to a dental treatment room, dental and dental hygiene services can be provided in a variety of surroundings using mobile equipment.

■ Dental hygiene procedures, provided within the limits of state practice acts, particularly lend themselves to care for the homebound because most dental hygiene treatment can be completed with manual instruments.

II. OBJECTIVES OF CARE

The objectives of dental hygiene care of homebound individuals will vary according to the patient's situation and needs. A dental hygienist providing care in a home-based setting may:

■ Provide intraoral/extraoral screening to triage patients who need treatment by a dentist.

■ Assist in preventing further complication of the patient's health status by identifying oral infections and other problems.

■ Provide routine screening to detect lesions that may be pathologic, particularly those that may be early cancer.

■ Provide dental hygiene treatment and education interventions to prevent dental caries and periodontal infections that require extensive treatment.

■ Encourage adequate daily personal oral care, whether performed by the patient or a caregiver.

■ Provide palliative care for the individual with a shortened life span.

■ Contribute to the patient's general well-being and quality of life.

III. PREPARATION FOR THE HOME VISIT

A. Understanding the Patient

When providing patient care in any situation, the rule is "know before you go." The following steps will help prepare for a homebound patient visit.

■ Review patient's medical history.
  ■ Provide form in advance for patient to complete and return.
  ■ Monitor medication lists carefully, especially when the patient takes multiple prescription or over-the-counter preparations.
  ■ Telephone before visit to clarify responses or ask questions.

■ Consider specific characteristics and special problems associated with the patient's age, chronic medical condition, medications, disability, or physical limitations.
    Chapters 48 through 68 review considerations for a variety of individuals with special needs.

■ Determine precautions that are necessary for the individual patient's care.

■ Arrange with dentist or attending physician when premedication or other prescription is required. Include arrangements for local anesthesia if necessary.

■ Arrange with patient or caregiver for items, such as extra towels or pillows, needed to support patient comfort during dental hygiene care.

B. Instruments and Equipment

■ Routine dental hygiene care can often be provided using manual instruments and without the need for powered equipment.

■ Several dental equipment companies, listed in **Box 57-3**, manufacture portable dental delivery units, suctions, X-ray units, and autoclaves.

■ Self-contained power-driven scalers can be transported and set up in the patient's home, but require the use of suction.

■ Additional equipment and supplies that can be transported by the clinician to the patient's residence are listed in **Box 57-4**. Covered plastic tubs or boxes, labeled for "clean" or "contaminated," are useful for carrying materials.

C. Appointment Time

■ Arrange the dental hygiene visit during a time when the patient is usually awake.

■ Consult with patient or caregivers to schedule as convenient a time as possible in relation to nursing care and mealtime schedule.

IV. APPROACH TO PATIENT

A. Communication

Because most patients who come to the dental office are active people with good general health, the adjustment to approaching a relatively helpless, disabled, or ill person is sometimes difficult.

■ Clinician empathy and understanding, as well as good interpersonal and communication skills can help the dental hygienist to project a caring attitude toward the patient.

■ An oversolicitous attitude may not contribute to the development of a cooperative patient relationship.

■ A direct approach with gentle firmness is most successful.

■ Direct communication with the patient is most appropriate; however, communication with a caregiver may be necessary.

B. Personal Factors

A patient who is comfortable with home-delivered care and aware of the difficulties under which the clinician is working may show more appreciation than the healthy patient who comes to the dental practice.

■ Establishment of rapport with the patient may depend on whether the patient has requested and anticipated the appointment or whether caregivers have insisted on and arranged the appointment.

■ Cooperation may depend on the patient's attitude toward the illness or disability.

BOX 57-3	**Commercial Sources for Portable Equipment**

DENTAL DELIVERY SYSTEMS

A-Dec, Inc.
Web site: *www.www.a-dec.com*
Toll Free Phone: (800) 547–1883

Aseptico
Web site: *www.aseptico.com*
Toll Free Phone: (866) 244–2954

ASI Medical, Inc.
Web site: *www.asimedical.net*
Toll Free Phone: (800) 566–9953

Bell Dental
Web site: *www.belldental.com*
Toll Free Phone: (800) 920–4478

DNTLworks Equipment Corporation
Web site: *www.dntlworks.com*
Toll Free Phone: (800) 847–0694

MDEC Mobile Equipment Corp.
Web site: *www.portabledentistry.com*
Toll Free Phone: (800) 321-MDEC

Safari Dental, Inc.
Web site: *www.safaridental.com*
Toll Free Phone: (800) 567–0013

HAND-HELD X-RAY SYSTEM

Aribex, Inc.
Web site: *www.aribex.com*
Toll Free Phone: (866) 340–5522

AUTOCLAVE

Alfa Medical
Web site: *www.statim-autoclave.com*
Toll Free Phone: USA: (800) 801–9934
Canada: (800) 247–6493

HEADLAMPS

Orascoptic
Web site: *www.orascoptic.com*
Toll Free Phone: (800) 369–3698

PeriOptix, Inc.
Web site: *www.perioptix.com*
Toll Free Phone: (888) 360–0033

SUCTION TOOTHBRUSHES

Sage Products, Inc.
Web site: *www.sageproducts.com*
Toll Free Phone: (800) 323–2220

Trademark Medical
Plak-Vac® suction toothbrush
Web site: *www.trademarkmedical.com*
Toll Free Phone: (800) 325–9044

- Prolonged illness, suffering, the effects of inactivity, and monotonous confinement can contribute to depression. Caring for the patient with depression is described in Chapter 63 on page 956.
- A homebound patient who is depressed requires extra attention to communication because that individual may:
  - have difficulty maintaining a cooperative attitude.
  - appear indifferent to personal appearance and general rules of personal hygiene
  - be noncompliant with the clinician's recommendations for improving oral health or preventing further complications.
  - have increased risk for dental disease because of effects of medications, poor oral hygiene, and high carbohydrate diet.[13,14]

C. Suggestions for General Procedure

- Request the caregiver to be present to assist as needed and to demonstrate current method of personal daily oral care.

- Prevent distraction by asking that other visitors remain out of the room during treatment.
- Introduce each step slowly to be sure patient knows what is being done. Do not make the patient feel rushed.
- Listen attentively; socializing is one of the best ways to establish rapport.
- Regardless of inconvenience of arrangements, plan two or more appointments when extensive scaling is required.
- Avoid tiring the patient.
- Observe tissue response.
- Provide encouragement in biofilm control procedures.

V. TREATMENT LOCATION

Because many homebound individuals can sit in a chair or wheelchair at least part of the day, only rarely must procedures be performed while the patient is in bed. For the patient in a chair, a kitchen or large bathroom may be

<table>
<tr>
<td>

BOX 57-4

</td>
<td>

Instruments and Equipment to Provide Dental Hygiene Care for Homebound Patients

</td>
</tr>
</table>

PERSONAL PROTECTIVE EQUIPMENT (PPE)
- Mask, protective eyewear, gloves, and gown

PATIENT EDUCATION/ORAL HYGIENE INSTRUCTION MATERIALS
- Toothbrushes
- A variety of interdental aids
- Hand mirror
- Examples of adaptive aids
- Written or printed patient education materials

STERILE INSTRUMENTS
- The clinician's selection of instruments and other items required for patient care
- Transported before treatment in the sealed packages in which they were sterilized
- Transported after use in special plastic containers labeled for contaminated instruments

DISPOSABLE ITEMS—PREPARED IN "SINGLE TREATMENT" PACKAGES THAT ARE CONVENIENT TO OPEN AND USE AT BEDSIDE
- Napkins
- Gauze sponges
- Cotton rolls and pellets
- Fluoride application trays
- Additional essential disposable items

COVERALL
- A large plastic drape (helpful if patient's coordination is limited during rinsing)

ADDITIONAL EQUIPMENT
- Emesis basin (kidney shaped basin facilitates the rinsing process)
- Portable headrest (attached to wheelchair or straight back chair to provide head support during treatment)

PHARMACEUTICALS
- Pretreatment mouthrinse
- Disclosing agent
- Topical fluoride preparation (varnish)

LIGHTING
- Adequate wattage to facilitate visibility
- Headlamp or reflector
- Photography spotlight or gooseneck lamp with narrow, concentrated beam

MISCELLANEOUS ITEMS—USUALLY AVAILABLE AT HOME
- Large towels (for covering pillows)
- Pillows (firm enough to assist in maintaining patients head in stationary position)
- Hospital bed (can be adjusted to position patient most effectively)
- Wheelchair or chair with high back for head support
- Container for prostheses
- Power toothbrush

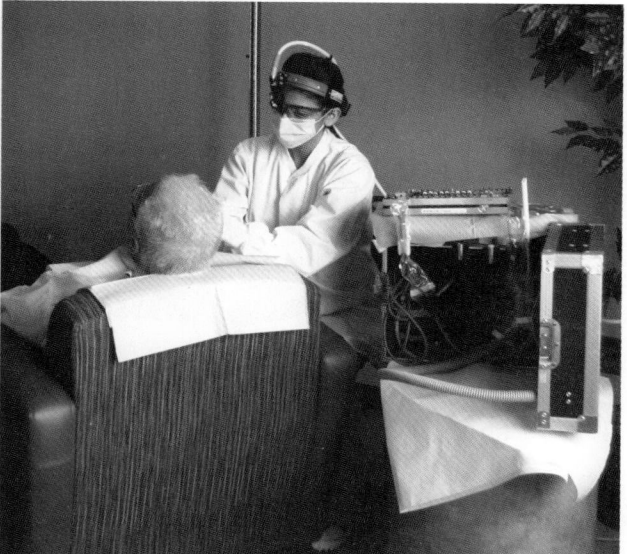

FIGURE 57-1 A dental hygiene student provides patient care using a headlamp and a portable dental unit that folds into a small suitcase-like container.

the most satisfactory treatment situation. Dental hygiene treatment is complicated by instability of the patient's head. Ingenuity is needed to arrange patient position to provide access for treatment as well as maintain comfort for both the patient and the clinician **(Figure 57-1)**.

A. Patient in Bed

- *Hospital bed:* Adjust to lift patient's head to desirable height.
- *Ordinary bed, sofa, or cushioned chair:* Use firm pillows to support and stabilize patient's head.
- *Small patient:* Positions for biofilm control described on page 869 and shown in Figure 56-13 (page 870) may be applicable during treatment.

B. Patient in Wheelchair

- A portable headrest can be attached to back of a plain chair or wheelchair (Figure 56-2, page 856).
- A straight chair or wheelchair can be backed against a wall to provide a stable headrest.
- A firm pillow can be inserted between the chair back and the patient's head to provide a cushioned resting surface.
- A chair or wheelchair can be moved into the patient's bathroom or kitchen to provide ready access to water and counter space.

VI. ADDITIONAL CONSIDERATIONS

- Use instruments directly from a sterile package or cassette.

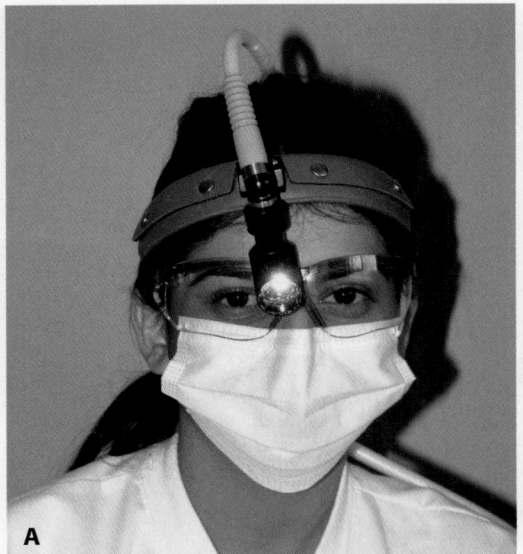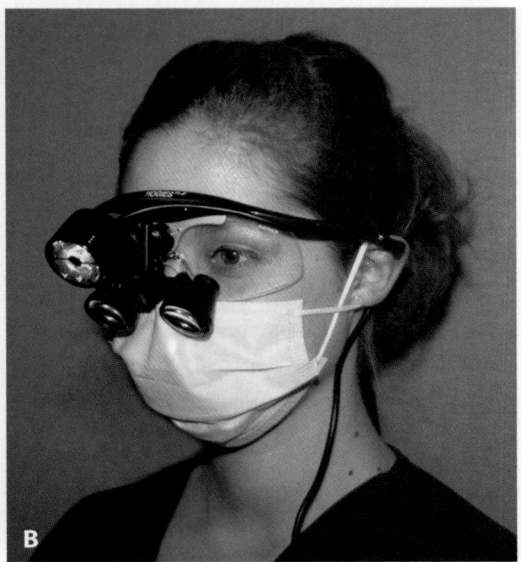

FIGURE 57-2 **(A)** Dental hygiene student wearing safety goggles and a headlamp. **(B)** Dental hygiene student wearing PeriOptix loupes with an attached LED headlamp. When using either system, the beam can be adjusted so that it is focused directly into the patient's oral cavity.

■ Place instrument packets and other supplies in a small tray on a bed or chair side table or on the bathroom/kitchen counter.
■ Provide adequate lighting.
  ■ Turn off overhead lighting to reduce shadows in the mouth.
  ■ A headlamp is usually the most convenient, efficient, concentrated form of light **(Figure 57-2)**.
  ■ A gooseneck-type floor lamp may be available in the patient's home or can be purchased as part of the clinician's mobile setup.

VII. ASSESSMENT AND CARE PLANNING

For the homebound patient, just as in any patient care setting, dental hygiene interventions are provided using the dental hygiene process of care.

■ Comprehensive patient assessment provides the basis for dental hygiene diagnoses.
■ The dental hygiene diagnosis provides the foundation for planning treatment and prevention strategies that meet individualized patient needs.
■ Follow-up appointments for maintenance and ongoing evaluation of the patient's oral condition determine whether treatment goals are met.

VIII. PROTOCOLS FOR PREVENTION

■ **Table 57-1** identifies special considerations for developing a personalized prevention plan for homebound individuals.
■ Strategies for preventing poor oral status for homebound patients can include training caregivers and consulting with members of interdisciplinary healthcare teams in addition to standard dental hygiene interventions.

THE UNCONSCIOUS PATIENT

■ Maintenance of oral cleanliness for the acutely ill or unconscious patient requires special procedures because of the complete helplessness of a patient who is not able to cooperate.
■ Methods need adaptation when the patient's head cannot be elevated.
■ When the patient's illness or injury involves the oral cavity, the advice and recommendations of the attending physician and/or oral surgeon are followed.
■ Personal oral care procedures for the unconscious patient are accomplished by the caregiver. The role of the dental hygienist is to train and motivate the caregiver to provide daily care.
■ Planning and conducting an oral health in-service program for nursing staff or other caregivers are described on page 869.

I. OBJECTIVES OF CARE

■ Observe the overall health of the oral tissues and provide routine screening to detect lesions that may be pathologic.
■ Prevent debris and microorganisms in the mouth from being aspirated and reduce risk for aspiration pneumonia in Chapter 65, page 991.
■ Minimize the possibility of oral infection.
■ Clean the mouth and provide comfort for the patient.
■ Relieve mouth dryness.

TABLE 57-1	PROTOCOLS FOR PREVENTION

Designing strategies to prevent problems related to poor oral status of homebound, unconscious, or hospice patients.

COMMON PROBLEMS	STRATEGIES FOR PLANNING DENTAL HYGIENE (based on assessment of individualized patient needs)
Need for Professional Oral Care	■ Provide complete intra-oral examination ■ Provide dental hygiene care ■ Triage patient needs and refer/facilitate access for dental treatment ■ Recognize and facilitate treatment for oral pain ■ Facilitate treatment for oral lesions ■ Facilitate reline/replacement of lost, broken, or poor-fitting dentures/prostheses
Inadequate Biofilm Removal	■ Educate regarding the role of biofilm in oral and systemic disease ■ Assess patient ADL levels, emotional status, and knowledge levels related to ability to perform self-care regimens ■ Provide oral hygiene aids or develop adaptive measures that facilitate self-care ■ Train caregivers, as necessary, to provide adequate daily oral cleansing
Increased Risk for Dental Caries	■ Identify/treat/prevent xerostomia ■ Provide for professional and/or home fluoride application ■ Provide dietary analysis ■ Educate about reducing intake of fermentable carbohydrates ■ Demonstrate daily oral self-care technique
Increased Risk for Periodontal Infections	■ Provide periodontal therapy ■ Provide regularly scheduled maintenance care ■ Educate regarding the effect of oral disease on systemic health ■ Provide oral hygiene aids or develop adaptive measures that facilitate self-care ■ Train caregivers, as necessary, to provide daily oral care
Oral Pain	■ Document and follow-up on patient complaints of oral pain ■ Provide oral examination to identify oral/mucosal lesions ■ Train caregivers, as necessary, to provide regular oral inspection and record observations
Trauma	■ Monitor patient for symptoms of abuse ■ Monitor/educate regarding potential for facial/oral trauma during a fall ■ Educate regarding protocols for oral injury emergency care
Xerostomia	■ Identify medications with a potential for causing xerostomia ■ Eliminate the use of oral products with alcohol, glycerin, or lemon ■ Educate regarding regular sips of water or ice chips to relieve dryness ■ Encourage use of over-the-counter saliva substitutes ■ Recommend use of non-sucrose-containing candies or gums
Inadequate Nutritional Intake	■ Identify oral pain or inadequate chewing function that may be affecting the patient's nutritional intake ■ Educate the patient or caregivers, as necessary, regarding oral status and potential for compromised nutritional status
Candidiasis (and other oral infections)	■ Educate regarding signs and symptoms of oral infections ■ Educate regarding effect of oral infections on systemic health ■ Train caregivers to provide oral inspection and record observations

II. INSTRUCTIONS FOR CAREGIVERS

A. Edentulous and Dentulous

■ Clean the mouth at least thrice a day to prevent dryness and sordes.

■ Sordes is a crustlike material that collects on the lips, teeth, and gingiva of a patient with a fever or dehydration in a chronic debilitating disease.

■ A soft toothbrush, swabs, or gauze sponges can be used to wipe the oral mucosa. Swabs and sponges are less effective and more time consuming than a toothbrush for removal of dental biofilm.[15]

■ A power toothbrush or a suction toothbrush may be more efficient and thorough.

■ Brush or wipe all surfaces of the lips, teeth, gingiva, tongue, and oral mucosa to remove biofilm.

■ A mouth prop can be placed in one side of the mouth while the other side is being retracted and brushed.

B. Removable Prosthesis

■ If dentures or other removable prostheses are present, remove them before providing oral care. Usual hospital policy requires removal of dentures when a patient is unconscious.
■ Procedure for removing dentures is described on page 456 in Box 31-3.
■ If the dentures are already removed, clean and mark them as described in Chapter 53 on page 819.
■ Store the dentures in water in a covered container. Instruct the caregiver to change the water or denture cleanser daily to prevent bacterial growth.[16]

C. Xerostomia

■ Swab oral mucosa using a saliva substitute as frequently as needed throughout the day and night.
■ Lemon and glycerin swabs are contraindicated due to the acidic effect of lemon on the demineralization of enamel[17] and the drying effect of glycerine.

III. TOOTHBRUSH WITH SUCTION ATTACHMENT

A. Description of Brush

When using a suction toothbrush (**Figure 57-3**), tubing is connected from the end of the hollow toothbrush handle to an aspirator outlet or portable suction unit.

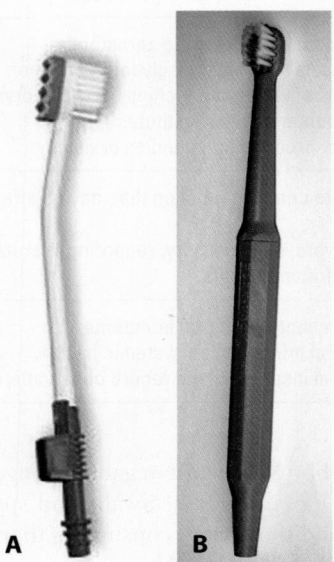

FIGURE 57-3 Commercial Suction Toothbrushes. Adapter on the hollow handle end attaches with tubing to portable or built-in hospital suction systems. **(A)** Single-use suction toothbrush (Sage Products, Inc., Cary, IL). **(B)** PlakVac® suction toothbrush (Trademark Medical®, St. Louis, MO).

BOX 57-5	Procedure for Use of Suction Toothbrush

■ Prepare the patient.
  □ Although not able to respond in a usual manner, the patient may be aware of what is going on.
  □ Tell patient that the teeth are going to be brushed, and thereafter maintain a one-way conversation despite patient's inability to respond verbally.
  □ Turn patient on the side and place a pillow at the back for support.
  □ Place a face towel over the bedding and an emesis basin under patient's chin.
■ Attach toothbrush to suction outlet and lay brush on towel near patient's mouth.
■ Place a rubber bite block on one side of the patient's mouth between the posterior teeth. Floss tied to the bite block is fastened to patient's gown with a safety pin.
■ Dip brush in nonalcoholic, fluoridated mouthrinse; do not use toothpaste.
■ Turn on suction.
■ Gently retract lip and carefully apply the appropriate toothbrushing procedures; apply suction over each tooth surface with particular care at each interproximal area. Remoisten brush frequently.
■ Move bite block to opposite side of mouth and continue brushing procedure.
■ After brushing, place brush in cup of clear water and allow water to be sucked through to clear and clean the tube.
■ Remove bite block, wipe patient's lips, and apply a water-based lubricant.
■ Rinse and disinfect toothbrush; sterilize bite block.

B. Procedure for Use of Brush

During caregiver training, the detailed procedure is outlined for hospital personnel and included in the nursing procedures manual. An abbreviated outline of the basic steps[18] is included in **Box 57-5**.

THE TERMINALLY ILL PATIENT

The role of the dental hygienist in the care of the terminally ill patient is to provide comfort care and to educate patients and their caregivers about the importance of daily oral care. The emphasis is on symptom relief and a clean oral environment, which may enhance the patient's sense of dignity and improve quality of life no matter how brief the life is to be.

■ Terminal illness is no excuse for neglect of oral cleanliness; daily personal oral hygiene care must be provided.
■ Hospice program caregivers are aware of oral care needs of their patients; however, in many programs standardized protocols are not followed.[19]

■ The major difference in providing dental hygiene care for a terminally ill patient is that the focus is on short-term palliative care rather than long-term preventive care.

I. OBJECTIVES OF CARE

■ Provide oral care that emphasizes patient comfort rather than only preventive or restorative aspects of care.

■ Provide relief of painful or aggravating symptoms of oral disease or lesions.

■ Prevent aspiration of debris and oral microorganisms and reduce risk for pneumonia.

■ Provide a "clean mouth" environment to reduce malodor and improve appearance, which may enhance personal interaction with caregivers and family members.

II. GENERAL MOUTHCARE CONSIDERATIONS

A. Cleanliness

■ Gentle but thorough daily cleaning of teeth, tongue, and oral mucosa is necessary.

■ Provide cleansing in any way the patient will allow.

■ Dentifrice or other oral products are not necessary, but can add a refreshing flavor that the patient may like.

B. Visual Inspection

Frequent inspection of the patient's mouth is necessary to identify oral lesions that can cause discomfort or lead to serious infection.

C. Oral Lesions

Mucosal soreness and ulceration, Candidiasis, glossitis, and xerostomia are frequently found on clinical examination of terminally ill patients.

■ *Candidiasis infection*
  ■ Oral cultures of *Candida albicans* have been found in as many as 79% of terminally ill patients.[20]
  ■ The infection can become life threatening in immunocompromised individuals.
  ■ Once recognized, Candidiasis infection is easily treated with antifungal medication.

■ *Xerostomia*
  ■ Xerostomia is common among terminally ill individuals owing to medications, dehydration, or mouth-breathing.[19,20]
  ■ Instruct patient or caregiver to moisten intraoral tissues and lips frequently using water, ice chips, or appropriate over-the-counter products as mentioned earlier in this chapter.
  ■ Avoid mouthrinses or other oral products that contain alcohol.

■ *Changes in oral mucosa*
  ■ Approximately 75% of hospice patients in one study had evidence of pathologic changes in the oral mucosa, and 42% reported soreness of the oral mucosa.[20]
  ■ Active oral lesions in the terminally ill may cause extreme discomfort when eating or talking as well as present an opportunity for development of secondary infections.
  ■ Daily examination of tissues is needed with follow-up for immediate care of developing lesions.

■ *Denture problems*
  ■ Because of severe weight loss, a denture may no longer fit. Chewing and talking are difficult. More than 70% of hospice patients who wore dentures reported having some kind of difficulty wearing their dentures.[20]
  ■ A more serious concern is development of intraoral lesions due to denture movement and accumulation of biofilm organisms on an unclean denture. Denture-induced lesions are described in Chapter 53 on page 817.
  ■ Several soft reline materials are available that, combined with proper daily oral and denture cleansing, may solve the problem for the duration of the patient's life.

DOCUMENTATION

Key concepts for documenting dental hygiene care for a homebound patient include:

■ Description of the patient's current health status and functional ability, particularly related to ability to provide self-care.

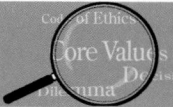

Everyday Ethics

Elena is 55 years old and is dying of esophageal cancer. She has been involved in an outpatient hospice program and receives all medical services in her home. Elena's daughter contacts the dental office of Dr. Gray and asks if someone can please come to the house and check her mother's teeth.

Sandy, the dental hygienist in the practice, offers to go and provide whatever "comfort care" she can for Elena.

Questions for Consideration
1. What legal and ethical concerns need to be addressed before going to Elena's home since care will be limited?
2. Reviewing the principle of justice, if Elena's homebound status prevents her from accessing dental care, what options can the dental team offer to her at this time?
3. Describe several "virtues" that can be exhibited by the dental team to benefit this patient.

BOX 57-6	Example of Components in a Progress Note: Bedside Oral Care Visit to Patient in a Nursing Home

Month, Day, Year

Routine nursing home visit for visual inspection and oral hygiene. Patient comfortable and alert; arm strength notably weakened since last visit and she can no longer support toothbrush for daily oral care. Nurse aide caregiver has been trying to assist. Excessive dental biofilm noted on facial surfaces of maxillary molars. Supervised caregiver in providing biofilm removal with soft child-sized toothbrush. Follow-up visit scheduled with patient and caregiver in 2 weeks.

Dental hygienists' signature_____

■ Indication of caregiver assistance in providing oral care.
■ Summary of oral health assessment data.
■ Specific recommendations/instructions for oral care techniques and adjunct oral hygiene aids.
■ Details of dental hygiene interventions/services provided.
■ Recommendations for follow-up care and/or education.
■ A sample progress note can be found in **Box 57-6**.

Factors To Teach The Patient

■ The contribution of good oral health to general health
■ How a clean mouth can contribute to wellness and quality of life factors
■ Need for prevention of dental caries by not using sugary snacks and sugar-sweetened beverages, especially between meals

Factors To Teach The Caregiver

■ How to care for the patient's natural teeth: toothbrushing, flossing, rinsing, and other personal needs
■ Removable denture care: cleaning daily, storage in a safe covered container when not in the mouth, changing solution for denture care daily
■ Selecting foods and snacks that are not cariogenic
■ How to use a suction toothbrush, power brush, or other device that can mean better oral care for the patient

References

1. Henry RG, Ceridan B. Delivering dental care to nursing home and homebound patients. *Dent Clin North Am.* 1994 Jul;38(3):537–51.
2. NH Regulations Plus [homepage on the Internet]. Minneapolis: University of Minnesota, Health Policy and Management, a division of the School of Public Health; © 2006 University of Minnesota Board of Regents. NH Regulations Plus: Dental Services; updated 2009 Dec 22 [cited 2010 Jan 1]; [about 10 screens]. Available from: http://www.hpm.umn.edu/nhregsplus/category_face_pages/category_dental_services.htm
3. U.S. Department of Health and Human Sevices. The national nursing home survey: 2004 overview (Series 13, number 167) DHHS Publication No. (PHS) 2009–1738. Hyattsville (MD): US Department of Health and Human Services, Center for Disease Control and Prevention, National Center for Health Statistics. 2009 June [cited 2010 Jan 1]. 3 p. Available from: http://www.cdc.gov/nchs/nnhs.htm
4. Smith BJ, Ghezzi EM, Manz MC, Markova CP. Perceptions of oral health adequacy and access in Michigan nursing facilities. *Gerodontology.* 2008 Jun;25(2):89–98.
5. Murray PE, Ede-Nichols D, Garcia-Godroy F. Oral health in Florida nursing homes. *Int J Dent Hyg.* 2006 Nov;4(4):198–203.
6. Simons D. Who will provide dental care for housebound people with oral problems? *Br Dent J.* 2003 Feb 8;194(3):13–8.
7. Gift HC, Cherry-Peppers G, Oldakowski RJ. Oral health status and related behaviours of US nursing home residents, 1995. *Gerodontology.* 1997;14(2):89–99.
8. Dolan TA, Atchison KA. Implications of access, utilization and need for oral health care by the non-institutionalized and institutionalized elderly on the dental delivery system. *J Dent Educ.* 1993 Dec;57(12): 876–87.
9. Strayer MS. Perceived barriers to oral health care among the homebound. *Spec Care Dentist.* 1995 May–June;15(3):113–8.
10. The PEW Center on the States, National Academy for State Health Policy, WK Kellogg Foundation. Help wanted: a policy maker's guide to new dental providers. Washington DC: The PEW Center on the States; 2009 May [cited 2010 March e]. pp. 18, 23–5. Available from: http://www.pewcenteronthestates.org/report_detail.aspx?id=52478
11. American Dental Hygienists' Association. Dental hygiene—focus on advancing the profession. Chicago: American Dental Hygienists' Association. 2005 June [cited 2010 Jan 1]. 22–23 pp. Available from: www.adha.org/downloads/ADHA_Focus_Report.pdf/
12. American Dental Hygienists' Association. The history of introducing a new provider in Minnesota. Chicago. American Dental Hygienists' Association. 2009 [cited 2010 Feb11]. 2 p. Available from : www.adha.org/downloads/MN_Mid-Level_History_and_Timeline.pdf
13. Little JW. Dental implications of mood disorders. *Gen Dent.* 2004 Sept–Oct;52(5):442–50.
14. Friedlander AH, Friedlander IK, Gallas M, Velasco E. Late-life depression: its oral health significance. *Int Dent J.* 2003 Feb;53(1):41–50.
15. Seto BG, Wolinsky LE, Tsutsui P, Avera C. Comparison of the plaque-removing efficacy of four nonbrushing oral hygiene devices. *Clin Prev Dent.* 1987 Mar–Apr;9(2):9–12.
16. DePaola LG, Minah GE. Isolation of pathogenic microorganisms from dentures and denture-soaking containers of myelosuppressed cancer patients. *J Prosthet Dent.* 1983 Jan;49(1):20–4.
17. Meurman JH, Sorvari R, Peittari A, Rytömaa I, Franssila S, Kroon L. Hospital mouth-cleaning aids may cause dental erosion. *Spec Care Dentist.* 1996 Nov–Dec;16(6):247–50.
18. Tronquet AA. Oral hygiene for hospital patients. *J Am Dent Assoc.* 1961 Aug;63:215–7.
19. Wyche CJ, Kerschbaum WE. Michigan hospice oral healthcare needs survey. *J Dent Hyg.* 1994 Jan–Feb;68(1):35–41.
20. Aldred MJ, Addy M, Bagg J, Finlay I. Oral health in the terminally ill: a cross-sectional pilot survey. *Spec Care Dentist.* 1991 Mar–Apr;11(2):59–62.

CHAPTER 58

The Patient With a Physical Impairment

CHARLOTTE J. WYCHE, RDH, MS

Chapter Outline

Many conditions related to the neuromuscular system, joints, or connective tissue have as a symptom, or leave as a chronic after-effect, loss of function in the form of a physical impairment. This chapter contains brief descriptions of selected diseases or conditions and describes modifications and adaptations needed by the patient during oral self-care, as well as by the dental hygienist during treatment appointments.

Box 58-1 lists key words and their definitions relating to physical impairments and disabilities. General suggestions that may be adapted to a variety of patients with disabilities are described in Chapter 56.

■ Communication to determine and support the patient's wishes in adapting patient care procedures is essential, particularly when the patient is unable to perform

---

BOX 58-1	Key Words

Physical Impairments

Akinesia: absence or loss of power of voluntary motion.

Ankylosis: immobility due to direct union between parts.

> **Bony ankylosis:** union of bone with bone or bone with tooth resulting in complete immobility; the periodontal ligament of an ankylosed tooth is completely obliterated.

Aphasia: defect in, or loss of power of, expression by speech, writing, or signs, or of comprehension of spoken or written language.

Apoptosis: cell death activated by a biochemical reaction; sometimes referred to as "programmed cell death"

Ataxia: failure of muscular coordination; irregularity of muscle action.

Atrophy: wasting; decrease in size; occurs when muscle fibers are not used or are deprived of their blood supply, or when the nerve connection is interrupted.

Bradykinesia: abnormal slowness of movements.

Cerebrovascular accident (CVA): a focal neurologic disorder caused by destruction of brain substance because of intracerebral hemorrhage, thrombosis, embolism, or vascular insufficiency; also called stroke.

Decubitus ulcer: ulcer that usually occurs over a bony prominence as a result of prolonged, excessive pressure from body weight; also called pressure sore or bed sore.

Demyelinate: destruction/removal of the myelin sheath of a nerve.

Diplopia: double vision; perception of two images of a single object.

Dysarthria: impairment of oral, lingual, or pharyngeal muscles that causes verbal clumsiness or impairment.

Dysphagia: difficulty in swallowing.

Hypercholesterolemia: excess of cholesterol in the blood.

Hypertriglyceridema: raised triglyceride blood level.

Ischemia: deficiency of blood caused by functional constriction or actual obstruction of a blood vessel.

Kyphosis: abnormally increased convexity in the curvature of the thoracic spine (viewed from the side).

Microcephaly: head that is small in relation to the rest of the body; contrast with macrocephaly, head that is large in relation to the rest of the body.

Myopathy: any disease of muscle.

Orthosis: orthopedic appliance or apparatus used to support, align, prevent, or correct deformities or to improve the function of a movable part of the body.

Pallidotomy: surgical excision or destruction of part of the globus pallidus in the basal ganglia to prevent symptoms

of Parkinsonism, including tremor, muscular rigidity, and bradykinesia.

Paralysis: a symptom of the loss or impairment of motor function in a body part caused by a lesion of the neural or muscular mechanism.

> **Diplegia:** paralysis of like parts on either side of the body.
>
> **Hemiplegia:** paralysis of one side of the body; usually caused by CVA or a brain lesion.
>
> **Paraplegia:** paralysis of the legs and in some cases the lower part of the body.
>
> **Quadriplegia:** paralysis of all four limbs from neck down; tetraplegia.
>
> **Triplegia:** paralysis of three limbs; hemiplegia with additional paralysis of one limb on the opposite side.

Paresis: slight or incomplete paralysis.

> **Hemiparesis:** slight or incomplete paralysis of one side of the body.

Paresthesia: abnormal sensation, such as burning, prickling, tingling.

Parkinsonism: a symptom complex comprising any combination of tremor, akinesia or bradykinesia, rigidity, loss of postural reflexes, and flexed posture. There are many causes of parkinsonism, one of which is Parkinson's disease.

Sclerosis: induration or hardening; especially hardening from inflammation and in disease of the interstitial substance.

Shunt: passage between two natural channels; to bypass or drain an area.

> **Ventriculoatrial shunt:** surgical creation of a communication between a cerebral ventricle and a cardiac atrium by means of a plastic tube; for relief of hydrocephalus.
>
> **Ventriculoperitoneal shunt:** communication between a cerebral ventricle and the peritoneum by means of a plastic tube; for relief of hydrocephalus.

Sialorrhea: excessive secretion of saliva.

Spinal shock: immediately after the injury, spinal shock causes a complete loss of reflex activity. The result is a flaccid paralysis below the level of injury that may last from several hours to 3 months.

TIA: transient ischemic attack; brief episode of cerebral ischemia that results in no permanent neurologic damage; symptoms are warning signals of impending CVA (stroke).

Visceral: pertaining to internal organs (digestive, respiratory, urogenital, endocrine, spleen, heart, and great vessels).

daily life activities independently and is dependent on others.
- Dental hygiene treatment modalities and oral care recommendations are adapted to the unique situations created by each disorder.
- Most patients with a physical impairment do not have an intellectual impairment.
- The oral cavity has added significance for those who have lost sensation in other areas of the body.

NEUROLOGICAL DISORDERS ASSOCIATED WITH PHYSICAL DISABILITY

Most of the disabling conditions described in this chapter are considered neurological disorders.

- A characteristic of many neurological disorders is the death of nerve cells in the central nervous system.[1]
- Disruption of sensory or motor neuron signals is the cause of partial or complete paralysis associated with neurological disorders.
- Acute ischemia or traumatic injury to the brain or spinal cord causes necrotic (immediate) death of nerve cells in the most severely affected areas and immediate/complete destruction of transmission of neurological signals.
- Apoptotic cell death, a slower, biochemical or metabolic destruction of the nerve cell, occurs in chronic or degenerative neurologic conditions as well as in areas not as severely affected in an acute neurologic injury.

I. ACUTE DISORDERS

- Acute neurological disorders can be caused when one or more neurons are injured by trauma or biological assault or when there is disruption of blood flow to an area of the brain.
- Complete or partial loss of motor ability, sensory perception, or cognitive function can result.
- Acute neurological disorders discussed in more detail in this chapter include spinal cord injury, stroke, Bell's palsy, and cerebral palsy.

II. DEGENERATIVE DISORDERS

- Degenerative neural disorders are a result of progressive destruction of nerve cells.
- Patients with these disorders typically become increasingly disabled and dependent on caregivers to help them with everyday activities and personal care as their disease progresses over time.
- Degenerative neural disorders discussed in this chapter include multiple sclerosis, amyotrophic lateral sclerosis (ALS), Parkinson's disease, post-polio syndrome, and myasthenia gravis.

III. DEVELOPMENTAL DISORDERS

- Developmental impairments have their onset early in life, around the time of birth or before a child is 18 years old.
- Depending on the disorder, either a stable or a progressive impairment can result.
- Developmental disorders highlighted in this chapter include cerebral palsy, muscular dystrophies, and myelomengocele.

OTHER CONDITIONS THAT LIMIT PHYSICAL ABILITY

Joint and connective tissue diseases can affect a patient's ability to provide oral self-care and require adaptations during delivery of dental hygiene care. Arthritis and scleroderma are discussed in sections of this chapter.

SPINAL CORD INJURY[2,3]

- The spinal cord extends down the middle of the back and carries both motor and sensory nerves that branch to send messages between the brain and specific areas of the body.
- External traumatic force can cause partial or complete loss of sensory and/or motor function related to the spinal cord level and the extent of the injury.

I. OCCURRENCE

- There are 450,000 people in the United States with spinal cord injury (SCI); approximately 100,000 new cases each year.
- More than one-third of trauma cases result from motor vehicle accidents; other causes are falls, diving accidents, violence, and combat injuries.
- The majority of these trauma cases involve young males between the ages of 16–30 years.

II. CHARACTERISTICS/EFFECTS OF SPINAL CORD INJURY

- The signs and symptoms of paralysis depend on the nature and level of injury to the spinal cord.
- There are 7 cervical (C), 12 thoracic (T), 5 lumbar (L), and 5 sacral (S) vertebrae, with paired spinal nerves extending from each; the areas of the body affected by injury at the different levels are illustrated in **Figure 58-1**.
- *Complete lesion*: A complete transection or compression of the spinal cord leaves no sensation or motor function below the level of the lesion.
- *Incomplete lesion*: Partial transection or injury of the spinal cord leaves some evidence of sensation or motor

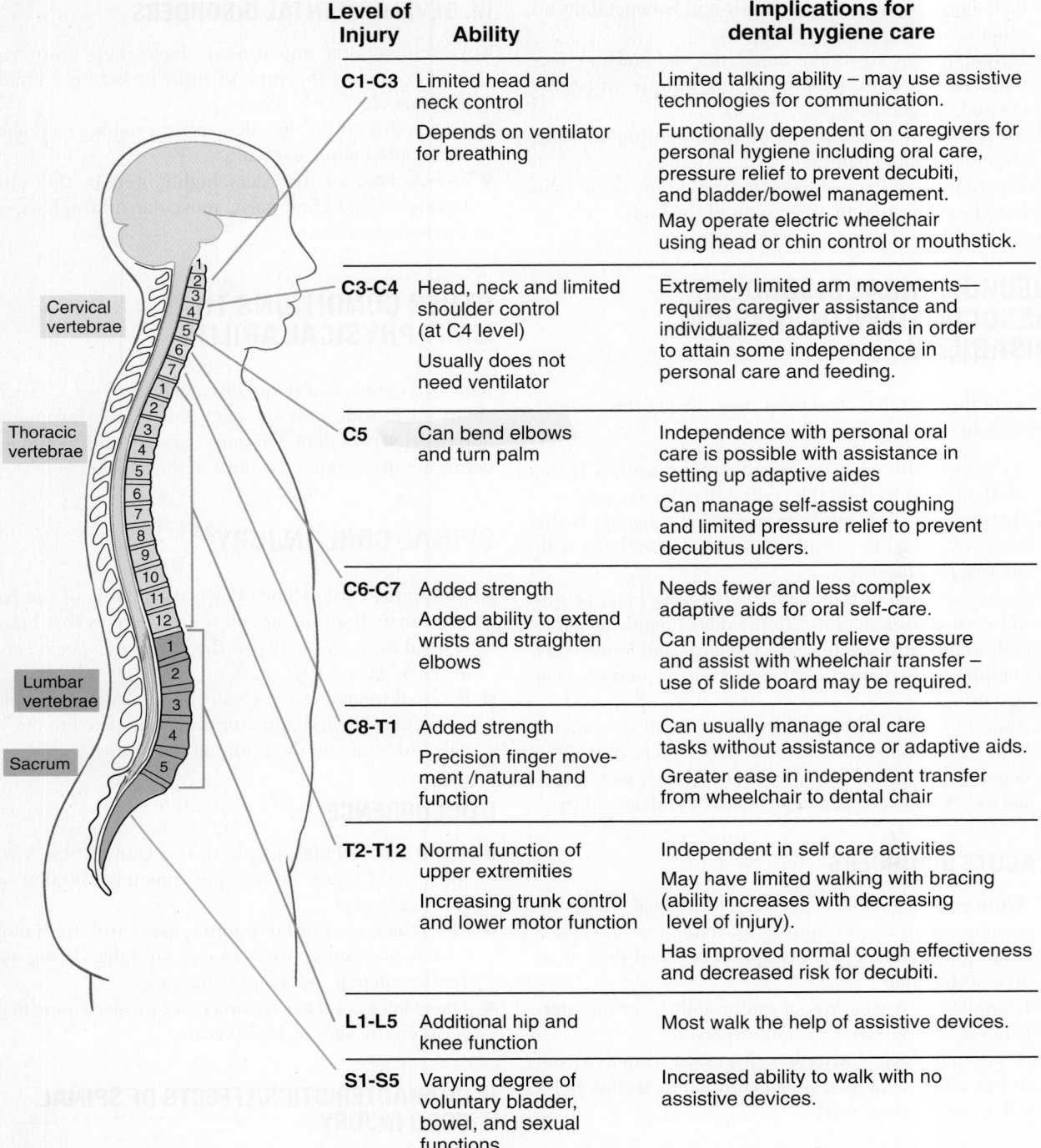

Level of Injury	Ability	Implications for dental hygiene care
C1-C3	Limited head and neck control	Limited talking ability – may use assistive technologies for communication.
	Depends on ventilator for breathing	Functionally dependent on caregivers for personal hygiene including oral care, pressure relief to prevent decubiti, and bladder/bowel management.
		May operate electric wheelchair using head or chin control or mouthstick.
C3-C4	Head, neck and limited shoulder control (at C4 level)	Extremely limited arm movements— requires caregiver assistance and individualized adaptive aids in order to attain some independence in personal care and feeding.
	Usually does not need ventilator	
C5	Can bend elbows and turn palm	Independence with personal oral care is possible with assistance in setting up adaptive aides
		Can manage self-assist coughing and limited pressure relief to prevent decubitus ulcers.
C6-C7	Added strength	Needs fewer and less complex adaptive aids for oral self-care.
	Added ability to extend wrists and straighten elbows	Can independently relieve pressure and assist with wheelchair transfer – use of slide board may be required.
C8-T1	Added strength	Can usually manage oral care tasks without assistance or adaptive aids.
	Precision finger movement /natural hand function	Greater ease in independent transfer from wheelchair to dental chair
T2-T12	Normal function of upper extremities	Independent in self care activities
	Increasing trunk control and lower motor function	May have limited walking with bracing (ability increases with decreasing level of injury).
		Has improved normal cough effectiveness and decreased risk for decubiti.
L1-L5	Additional hip and knee function	Most walk the help of assistive devices.
S1-S5	Varying degree of voluntary bladder, bowel, and sexual functions	Increased ability to walk with no assistive devices.

Cervical vertebrae

Thoracic vertebrae

Lumbar vertebrae

Sacrum

FIGURE 58-1 **Levels of Spinal Cord Injury.** On the left, the vertebrae are designated as C (cervical), T (thoracic), L (lumbar), and S (Sacral). The effects of spinal cord injury depend on the level of injury. (*Source:* The Spinal Cord Injury Information Network [internet] Birmingham: University of Alabama at Birmingham—Spinal Cord Injury Model System (UAB-SCIMS); c2008. SCI functional goals for specific levels of complete injury; [cited 2010 Aug 6]. Available from: http://www.spinalcord.uab.edu/show.asp?durki=30166.)

function below the level of the lesion. Some sensation and motor function may return within a few hours after injury, and maximum return may occur in 6–18 months.

■ The patient's condition is referred to by the letter C, T, L, or S followed by the specific vertebra number where the injury occurred.

■ The most severe disability occurs at a lesion level above C6, which refers to the sixth cervical vertebral level.

■ *Other possible effects:* Impairment of bladder and bowel control and sexual function; impairment of vasomotor and body temperature regulatory mechanisms.

III. POTENTIAL SECONDARY COMPLICATIONS

Patients with lesions at or above the T6 level are at greater risk for the complications described here.

A. Impaired Respiratory Function

■ Some quadriplegic patients are unable to elicit a functional cough and need assistance.

■ By placing manual pressure over the abdomen, below the diaphragm, after the patient has inhaled, the patient may be assisted while an attempt to cough is made.[4]

B. Tendency for Pressure Sores[5]

■ A pressure sore (*decubitus ulcer*) results from tissue anoxia or ischemia caused by pressure exerted on the skin and subcutaneous tissues by bony prominences and the object on which they rest, such as a mattress.

■ The cutaneous tissue becomes broken or destroyed, leading to destruction in the subcutaneous tissue.

■ The ulcer that forms may become infected by secondary bacterial invasion and be slow to heal; anemia and poor nutrition may also contribute.

C. Spasticity

■ As spinal shock subsides following a traumatic injury, muscle-reflex spasticity develops from a slight to a severe degree.

■ Stimuli, such as pressure sores, infections, and sensory irritation, may bring on a spasm.

D. Body Temperature

High-level quadriplegic patients are unable to regulate body temperature, requiring careful monitoring and intervention to warm or cool the patient as necessary.

E. Vulnerability to Infection

Complications related to elimination, urinary tract infections, renal stones, secondary infection of decubitus ulcers,

and respiratory infections occur more commonly in this population.

F. Cardiovascular Instability

■ Bradycardia and hypotension are common because of the loss of the sympathetic autonomic nervous system.

■ Deep vein thrombosis is another potentially serious complication.

G. Neurogenic Bladder and Bowel

Complications related to dysfunctions in emptying bladder and bowels require planning to avoid the complications of autonomic dysreflexia.

H. Autonomic Dysreflexia[6]

1. *Definition*
   ▨ Autonomic dysreflexia, or hyperreflexia, is a life-threatening *emergency* condition in which the blood pressure increases sharply.
   ▨ It may occur in patients with lesions at T6 or above.
   ▨ A variety of stimuli may precipitate dysreflexia, including irritation to the bowel or bladder distension.
2. *Symptoms*
   ▨ Increased blood pressure with slowed pulse rate. The blood pressure may rise to 300/160 mmHg.
   ▨ Pounding headache.
   ▨ Flushing, chills, perspiration, stuffy nose.
   ▨ Restlessness; increased spasticity.
3. *Prevention*
   ▨ Consult with physician if the patient has history of recurrent difficulties.
   ▨ Avoid abrupt changes in body position and maintain a semi-upright chair position.
   ▨ Monitor bladder outflow catheter tubing, outflow of urine into catheter bag, and bladder distention.
   ▨ Schedule appointments that allow the patient to maintain the regular schedule for the bowel elimination program at home.
4. *Emergency care*
   ▨ Position chair upright gradually.
   ▨ Do NOT recline the chair because increased blood pressure in the brain could result.
   ▨ Check bladder distention and straighten catheter if clamped.
   ▨ Manually relieve bowel impaction if necessary.
   ▨ Monitor the blood pressure and vital signs using a medical emergency report form (page 1063).
   ▨ Call for medical aid if blood pressure does not begin to drop within 2–3 minutes.

IV. MOUTH-HELD IMPLEMENTS

The patient with a high-level SCI who does not have strong function of hands and arms may use mouth-held appliances to perform many tasks and the teeth for holding objects. Optimum oral health and effective biofilm control has special significance because many functions cannot be accomplished by an edentulous mouth.

A. Uses

Fabrication of mouth-held appliances contributes to increased independence and makes possible such activities as operating an electric wheelchair, typing on a computer, or turning the pages of a book.

B. Criteria[7,8]

1. Does not harm the oral tissues.
   - Stabilization of occlusion with contact for all fully erupted teeth and the biting forces distributed to as many teeth as possible.
   - Is not traumatic to the periodontal supporting structures.
   - Does not prevent eruption of teeth.
2. Is comfortable and does not cause fatigue.
   - Patient can talk, swallow, and moisten the lips.
   - Orthosis can be inserted and removed by the patient.
   - Orthosis is adaptable for the various needs of the quadriplegic patient.
3. Can be cleaned and cared for easily.
4. Is relatively easy to construct; inexpensive.

V. DENTAL HYGIENE CARE

Factors to consider when planning dental hygiene care for the patient with an SCI:

- Impaired motor and sensory ability.
- Risk for secondary complications during treatment; autonomic dysreflexia and aspiration due to decreased respiratory function.
- Risk for pressure sores, potential for spasticity, poor control of body temperature.
- Use of mouth-held implements.

CEREBROVASCULAR ACCIDENT (STROKE)[9]

- Cerebrovascular accident (CVA) or stroke is a sudden loss of brain function resulting from interference of the blood supply to a part of the brain.
- CVA is the clinical manifestation of cerebrovascular disease.
- The patient is frequently disabled by changes in motor function, communication, and perception. Hemiplegia or hemiparesis is common.
- Stroke is the third leading cause of death, following heart disease and cancer, in the United States.

- The stroke may be severe and death can occur within minutes.
- The less severe attack leaves the patient with the symptoms and signs are as listed.

I. ETIOLOGIC FACTORS

Strokes can be caused by one of the following:

A. Thrombosis

- A clot within a blood vessel of the brain or neck closes or occludes the vessel and shuts off the oxygen supply to the portion of the brain supplied by that vessel, resulting in cerebral infarction.
- Cerebral thrombosis is the most common cause of stroke.

B. Intracerebral Embolism

- A blood vessel is blocked by a clot or other material carried through the circulation from another part of the body.
- Atherosclerotic plaque build-up in a blood vessel (atheroma) can become an embolism and increases the risk of stroke.
- Calcifications in the carotid artery may be observable in a panoramic radiograph and indicate an increased risk of CVA.

C. Ischemia

The blood flow decreases to an area of the brain, usually because of an atheromatous constriction of the arteries supplying the area.

D. Cerebral Hemorrhage

A cerebral blood vessel may rupture and bleed into the brain tissues.

E. Predisposing Factors

Patients with certain conditions have increased risk for having a stroke. Early diagnosis and treatment for control of the following predisposing factors are necessary in the prevention of stroke and its devastating effects.

- Atherosclerosis (in Chapter 66, page 1015).
- Hypertension, the greatest risk factor that leads to stroke (in Chapter 66, pages 1012 to 1014).
- Hypercholesterolemia, hypertriglyceridemia.
- Tobacco use, smoking.
- Cardiovascular disease (rheumatic heart disease, congestive heart failure, history of transient ischemic attacks (TIAs).
- Diabetes mellitus.
- Use of oral contraceptives (enhanced by hypertension, tobacco use, age over 35, and high estrogen levels).

■ Drug abuse (especially in adolescents and young adults).

II. SIGNS AND SYMPTOMS

The effects of a stroke depend on the location of the damage to the brain, as well as on the degree or extent of involvement.

A. Transient Ischemic Attack (TIA)

■ A brief event where the blood supply to a localized area of the brain is interrupted and the patient may have transient signs or symptoms of a stroke.
■ These "little strokes" may last a few minutes to an hour and may leave no permanent damage.
■ A history of transient attacks is a possible risk factor or warning for a stroke.

B. Acute Symptoms of a Stroke

Acute symptoms and emergency procedures are included in Table 69-4 (page 1077).

C. Residual or Chronic Effects

■ Approximately two thirds of those who survive have some degree of permanent disability.
■ Temporary or permanent loss of thought, memory, speech, sensation, or motion results.
■ The side of the brain affected influences the symptoms.
■ The side of the face and body affected is opposite that of the brain injury **(Figure 58-2)**.

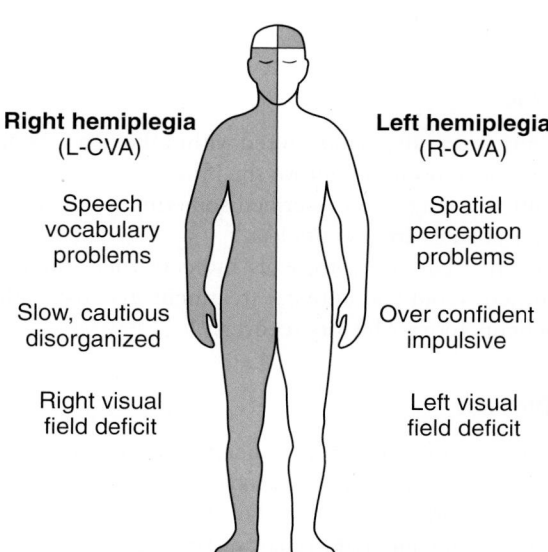

FIGURE 58-2 **Cerebrovascular Accident (Stroke).** Right hemiplegia is the result of left-sided brain damage; left hemiplegia results from right-sided brain damage.

Right hemiplegia (L-CVA)
Speech vocabulary problems
Slow, cautious disorganized
Right visual field deficit

Left hemiplegia (R-CVA)
Spatial perception problems
Over confident impulsive
Left visual field deficit

BOX 58-2	Description of Signs and Symptoms Following Stroke

■ **Paralysis:** hemiplegia (one side of the body) or portions, such as an arm, leg, or the face.
■ **Articulation:** difficulty of speech, which may be caused by involvement of the tongue, mouth, or throat, as well as aphasia by brain damage related to the speech centers, and the patient may have difficulty finding the right word.
■ **Salivation:** difficulty in control of saliva complicated by difficulty in swallowing; aspiration.
■ **Sensory:** loss in affected parts may result in superficial anesthesia, or the opposite may occur with resultant increased sensitivity to pain and touch.
■ **Visual impairment:** blurred vision, or diminished visual acuity.
■ **Mental function:** may be unaffected, but slowness, poor memory, and loss of initiative are common. Brain deterioration may occur over a period of time.
■ **Personal factors:** personality changes relate to emotional trauma, fear, discouragement, and dependency. Anxiety neuroses and periods of depression, which are common, may require assistance from a psychiatrist, psychologist, or social worker.

■ Persons with right hemiplegia have more difficulty with verbal communication and are more apt to be cautious, anxious, and disorganized.
■ Patients with left hemiplegia have difficulty with action requiring physical coordination and may respond impulsively with overconfidence.
■ Common signs and symptoms observed following a stroke are described in **Box 58-2**.

III. MEDICAL TREATMENT

A. Surgical

■ Treatment may include surgical correction of aneurysms, clots, or malformations.
■ Surgery, using a microscope, may include the removal of very small clots in the intracranial arteries or minute grafting to bypass blocked vessels and provide collateral circulation.

B. Physical and Occupational Therapy

Rehabilitation techniques are vital to the patient's functioning.

C. Drugs

Careful recording of the medical history includes the listing of medications. The patient may be taking a variety of drugs for some or all of the purposes found in **Box 58-3**.

- **Anticoagulant:** to thin the blood.
- **Antihypertensive:** to lower the blood pressure.
- **Thrombolytic:** to dissolve clots.
- **Vasodilator:** to relax the blood vessels of the brain.
- **Steroid:** to control brain swelling.
- **Antiepileptic:** to help to control seizures.

D. Disease Risk Detection

- Calcifications in the carotid artery are observable inferior and posterior to the inferior border of the mandible on a panoramic radiograph.[10] If present, the patient is referred for immediate medical evaluation.
- Radiation therapy is associated with an accelerated form of atherosclerosis formation and risk of stroke.[11]

IV. DENTAL HYGIENE CARE

Particular factors to consider when planning dental hygiene care for the patient with a stroke-related disability:

- Impaired motor and/or cognitive ability.
- Hemiplegia; particularly if the dominant hand is affected. For example, the patient who wears dentures requires a suction cup brush, illustrated in Figure 56-12 on page 867, to clean the dentures with one hand.
- Facial paralysis; decreased self-cleansing action of the tongue and lips; decreased control of saliva; risk for aerosol in eye during treatment.
- Medications for treatment of the condition; anticoagulant use is common following a stroke.

BELL'S PALSY (IDIOPATHIC TEMPORARY FACIAL PARALYSIS)

- Bell's palsy is paralysis of the facial muscles innervated by the facial or seventh cranial nerve.
- Although the cause is not known, various possible agents have been implicated, including:
  - Bacterial and viral infections; particularly herpes simplex
  - Injury, trauma from tooth removal or
  - Oral surgery such as the removal of a tumor in the parotid gland area.

I. OCCURRENCE

- Although relatively rare, the incidence increases with each decade of life.

- In younger age groups, women are more frequently affected than are men.
- After age 50 years, the disorder is more common in men.

II. CHARACTERISTICS[12]

A. Signs and Symptoms

Abrupt weakness or paralysis of facial muscles, usually without preceding pain, occurs on one side of the face.

- *Mouth:* The corner of the mouth droops, and salivation with drooling is uncontrollable.
- *Eye:* Eyelid on the affected side may not close; watering and drooping of the lower lid invites infection.
- When only the seventh nerve is affected, sensory responses are still intact.

B. Functional Problems

Speech and mastication may be impaired.

C. Prognosis

- A majority of patients experience a return to normal within a month with a spontaneous recovery.
- Others may have lasting residual effects or permanent paralysis.

III. MEDICAL TREATMENT

A. Palliative

- Eye protection such as an eye patch during sleep and eye lubrication drops during waking hours.
- Massaging the involved muscles provides some relief.
- Hot compresses.

B. Drugs

- Corticosteroids, administered within the first 72 hours, have been used to improve the prognosis.
- Antiviral drugs are prescribed sometimes, but the efficacy of such drugs is unclear.[13]
- Recent treatment protocols indicate that combining corticosteroid and antiviral treatment may have added benefits for satisfactory recovery.[14]

C. Surgical

- Surgical procedures have been used to improve the appearance, provide facial symmetry with voluntary motion, and provide control of the eye and the mouth.
- Surgery has included repair of the facial nerve, nerve transplantation and grafting, crossover nerve grafts from the uninvolved side of the face, muscle transfers, and free muscle grafts.

■ Prosthetic rehabilitation has been combined with surgical treatment.

IV. DENTAL HYGIENE CARE

Particular factors to consider when planning dental hygiene care for the patient with Bell's palsy:

■ Facial paralysis; decreased self-cleansing action of the tongue and lips; decreased control of saliva; risk for aerosol in eye during treatment.
■ Medications used for treatment of the condition.

MULTIPLE SCLEROSIS[15,16]

■ Multiple sclerosis is a genetically linked, chronic demyelinating disease of the central nervous system characterized by progressive disability with motor, sensory, cognitive, and emotional (depression, mania) changes.
■ Women are affected twice as frequently as are men.
■ Pathologically, the myelin sheath is destroyed within the white matter of the central nervous system.
■ The sheath degenerates in patches called *MS plaques* and is replaced by sclerotic tissue, which results in interference with the transmission of nerve impulses and frequent involvement of the spinal cord and optic nerves.
■ The direct cause of multiple sclerosis is not known.

I. OCCURRENCE

■ Prevalence is increasing; approximately 3 cases per 100,000 worldwide.
■ Usually adult onset; between 20 and 40 years of age, rarely before 15 or after 55 years.
■ Prevalence higher among Caucasians than other ethnic groups.
■ The disease is more prevalent in temperate climates.

II. CHARACTERISTICS

A. Initial Symptoms

■ Initial symptoms are often fluctuating, presenting with transient difficulty in coordination, tremor, fatigue, or weakness.
■ Transient tingling or paresthesia of the hands or feet may occur.
■ May have visual impairment with pain.
■ May have a sudden onset of severe illness with paralysis or marked weakness.

B. Course of Disease

■ *Relapses and remissions:* An attack may last several days or weeks and be followed by a symptom-free period. Physical impairment varies, but the condition worsens with each relapse.

■ *Longevity:* People with multiple sclerosis have a close to normal life span; approximately 80% have functional limitations after 15 years.

C. Risk Factors for Exacerbations

■ Infection.
  ■ Various types of infection, systemic or local, can stimulate a relapse.
  ■ Oral infections are no exception.
■ Pregnancy.
  ■ For certain patients, pregnancy may increase the risk and bring on an attack. Because the effect is more likely to be noticed during the first several months after delivery, fatigue and stress may be the direct precipitating effects.
  ■ Effects of multiple sclerosis on the pregnancy may be recognized. Possible side effects of medications on the developing fetus are considered because certain medications used may have to be discontinued if they are teratogenic.

D. Physical Symptoms

A wide variety signs and symptoms. Symptoms fluctuate, and several years may elapse between bouts of symptoms.

■ Fatigue.
■ Intermittent, unilateral facial numbness, pain, palsy or spasm.[15]
■ Involuntary motion of eyes (nystagmus); the individual may later become partially or completely blind.
■ Speech disorders; possible loss of speech in advanced stages.
■ Changes in muscular coordination and gait; loss of balance; spasms.
■ Paralysis of one or more extremities.
■ Autonomic derangements, such as urinary frequency and urgency; later urinary incontinence.
■ Susceptibility to infection, particularly upper respiratory.

III. CATEGORIES

■ *Relapsing-remitting:* acute episodes worsening with recovery and a stable course between relapses.
■ *Secondary progressive:* gradual neurologic deterioration with or without superimposed acute relapses in a patient who previously had relapsing-remitting multiple sclerosis.
■ *Primary progressive:* gradual, nearly continuous neurologic deterioration from the onset of symptoms.
■ *Progressive relapsing:* gradual neurologic deterioration from the onset of symptoms but with subsequent superimposed relapses (very uncommon).

IV. DIAGNOSIS AND TREATMENT

■ Diagnosis is based on history, clinical signs and symptoms, supplemented by radiographic and laboratory test findings; there is no single diagnostic procedure specific for MS.

■ Prompt diagnosis and early treatment within 6 months of onset is crucial to deter neurological damage.

A. Objectives of Treatment

■ *Disease course modification:* The goal of treatment is to prevent relapses and progressive worsening of the disease.
■ *Treat exacerbations.*
■ *Symptom relief:* Provide palliative treatment to manage symptoms, improve function, and safety.
■ *Psychological support:* The ramifications of having an incurable disease can be devastating. Understanding dental personnel can contribute in this area.

B. General Treatment Procedures

■ General hygiene care; adequate nutrition, rest, avoidance of strain and stress, and prevention of infections and injury.
■ Physical and occupational therapy; exercise, not strenuous exertion, is indicated.
■ Patient continues in a usual occupation as long as possible; activity is encouraged.
■ Psychotherapy or medication to address depression or psychological problems is indicated.

C. Medications

Medications used in the treatment of multiple sclerosis are listed in **Box 58-4**.

BOX 58-4	**Medications Used to Treat Multiple Sclerosis**

■ **Corticosteroids:** anti-inflammatory and immunomodulatory effects.
■ **Interferon beta (1a and 1b):** reduce or prevent severity and frequency of future exacerbations.
■ **Glatiramer acetate:** reduce or prevent relapse; useful for patients who become resistant to interferon-beta.
■ **Mitoxantrone:** anticancer medication found effective in reducing relapses and progression of multiple sclerosis.
■ **Natalizumab:** recent infusion medication approved for patients with relapsing forms of multiple sclerosis.
■ **Palliative medications:** For treatment of:
  ☐ Fatigue
  ☐ Spasticity, tremor
  ☐ Constipation
  ☐ Nausea, dizziness
  ☐ Pain
  ☐ Bladder dysfunction
  ☐ Urinary frequency
  ☐ Urinary tract infections
  ☐ Depression
  ☐ Erectile dysfunction

V. DENTAL HYGIENE CARE

Particular factors to consider when planning dental hygiene care for the patient with multiple sclerosis:

■ Impaired motor ability; changes to ability during relapses and remissions.
■ Effects of medications used for treatment of the condition.

AMYOTROPHIC LATERAL SCLEROSIS (ALS)[17]

ALS (often referred to as Lou Gehrig's Disease) is a progressive neurodegenerative disorder characterized by a progressive loss of motor neurons.

I. OCCURRENCE

■ Incidence is approximately 2–3 per 100,000 population
■ Men more often affected than women; Caucasians more frequently than other ethnic groups.
■ Onset usually occurs at middle age or later; only 5% of cases have onset before age 30 years.

II. DIAGNOSIS

■ There are no diagnostic tests for ALS.
■ Diagnosis is usually made after ruling out other disorders with similar symptoms.
■ Clinically diagnosed with both upper and lower neuron dysfunction, although variants include a pure upper motor and pure lower motor syndrome.[18]

III. ETIOLOGY AND PATHOGENESIS

■ Unknown cause
■ 90% of cases are sporadic
■ 5 to 10% are familial (predominantly autosomal dominant)
■ Average life expectancy is 3–5 years; but the range is broad and some live much longer.
■ Typically progressive degeneration of both upper and lower motor neurons with no periods of remission.
■ More areas of the body are affected over time; nearly all systems eventually become involved.
■ Respiratory failure is the usual cause of death.

IV. TWO FORMS OF ALS[19]

1. *Spinal form*
   ■ About 2/3 of patients.
   ■ Early symptoms include muscle weakness in upper and lower limbs and muscle wasting.
2. *Bulbar onset form*
   ■ Initially presents with dysarthria.
   ■ Sometimes dysphasia for solids or liquids is initial symptom.

- Facial weakness and wasting/spasticity of the tongue are common.
- Limb symptoms may develop simultaneously; or can happen later as the disease progresses.
- Sialorrhea (excessive secretion of saliva; drooling) develops in almost all who have the Bulbar onset form of the disease.

V. SYMPTOMS[20]

- Cramps and spasticity
- Weakness in extremities
- Increasing respiratory difficulty
- Difficulty swallowing and chewing
- Excessive saliva[20,21]
- Depression and anxiety
- Cognitive[22] and behavioral disorders that can affect compliance with recommendations.

VI. TREATMENT

- Only one current FDA approved treatment (Rilusole); only extends survival about 2 months.[18]
- Palliative treatment is provided by multidisciplinary teams.[23]
- Treatment focused on progressive management of symptoms.
- Sialorrhea managed with medications, but in later stages treatment can include radiation or Botox injection into salivary glands.[18]

VII. DENTAL HYGIENE CARE

Factors to consider when planning dental hygiene care for the patient with ALS:

- Increased motor impairment over time.
- Need for body stabilization and support.
- Risk for respiratory difficulties
- Effects of facial paralysis.
- Effects of treatment for sialorrhea.

PARKINSON'S DISEASE[24]

- Parkinson's disease is a progressive disorder of the central nervous system characterized by loss of postural stability, slowness of spontaneous movement, resting tremor, and muscular rigidity.
- It is also known as paralysis agitans and Parkinson's syndrome.
- Although the cause is not known, the basis for the specific group of symptoms is degeneration of certain neurons in the substantia nigra of the basal ganglia, where posture, support, and voluntary motion are controlled.
- In addition, a severe deficiency of dopamine, one of the substances that participates in nerve transmission, occurs.

I. OCCURRENCE

Parkinson's disease affects more than a million middle-aged and older persons in the United States, with a higher incidence in men than in women.

II. CHARACTERISTICS

- The signs and symptoms center around tremor, rigidity, and loss or impairment of motor function (akinesia).
- These factors also occur in other conditions, which are differentiated by a physician when a diagnosis is made.
- The disease progresses through stages; from mild/early to severe/advanced with increasing impairment of motor function.

A. General Manifestations

- Body posture bent, with bent head and general stiffness.
- Motion and responses slowed; difficulty in keeping balance and turning.
- Gait slow and shuffling.
- Speech monotonous and slow.
- Resting tremor of one or both hands is common; the tremor can be reduced or stopped when the person engages in a purposeful action such as toothbrushing.
- The fingers may be involved in a "pill-rolling" motion in which the thumb and index finger are rubbed together in a circular movement.
- Nonmotor symptoms include variations in blood pressure, cardiac dysrhythmias, excessive sweating, bowel and bladder dysfunction, and sleep disorders.
- Cognitive ability is seldom affected except in the advanced stages.
- Eventually, after 10 to 20 years, the person may become incapacitated and may require complete care.

B. Face and Oral Cavity

- Expression is fixed and masklike, with diminished eye blinking.
- Tremor or exaggerated movement in lips, tongue, and neck, and difficulty in swallowing.
- Excess salivation and drooling.

III. TREATMENT

- Maintenance of good general health is encouraged, including plenty of rest and nutritious meals.
- Professional physical therapy and occupational therapy have particular significance for a patient's well-being.
- Although no known cure exists for Parkinson's disease, symptomatic control can be accomplished, in part, by replenishing the dopamine shortage with levodopa in combination with other medications; side effects can include dizziness and confusion.

■ Surgical relief for symptoms has been accomplished using pallidotomy. The surgery alters the globus pallidus in the basal ganglia. The location of the basal ganglia in the brain is shown in **Figure 58-3**.

IV. DENTAL HYGIENE CARE

Particular factors to consider when planning dental hygiene care for the patient with Parkinson's disease:

■ Increased motor impairment over time; tremor and rigidity.
■ Rigid, uncontrolled facial muscles; poor control of eye, lips, tongue, and swallowing muscles.

MYASTHENIA GRAVIS[25,26]

Myasthenia gravis is an autoimmune neuromuscular disease characterized by weakness and fatigability of symmetrical voluntary muscles.

■ It is caused by an autoimmune process that results in a defect in nerve impulse transmission at the neuromuscular junctions.
■ In myasthenia gravis, the numbers of acetylcholine receptors in each neuromuscular junction are reduced markedly compared with the normal number of receptors.[27]

The patient with myasthenia gravis has a special significance for dental professionals because the facial and oral parts served by certain cranial nerves are involved early.

■ Muscles of the eyes, facial expression, mastication, and swallowing are affected.
■ In advanced severe forms of the disease, muscle involvement may be extensive and result in total paralysis.

I. OCCURRENCE

■ Prevalence of individuals with the condition is around 140 million in United States.
■ Peak age of onset for women is 20–40 years of age; for men peak onset is 50 or older.
■ Generally women are more affected than are men by a 3:2 ratio.

II. SIGNS AND SYMPTOMS

A. Early Signs

■ Weakness of eye movements with double vision (diplopia) and drooping eyelids (ptosis) may be the initial indicators.
■ In certain patients, the disease may not progress further.

B. Oral and Facial Problems

■ As the disease progresses, involvement of muscles of the face, mastication, and tongue lead to swallowing difficulties (dysphagia) and a lack of facial expression.
■ Disturbed speech and expression, with a weak voice that sounds tired and muffled, are typical.
■ A patient may support the chin with one hand to help during talking.
■ Because of the lack of facial expression, distress may be difficult for the patient to convey.

C. Progressive Involvement

■ When the muscles that are used during breathing become involved, serious respiratory complications can result.
■ Generalized fatigue is usually not so evident in the morning or immediately after rest. Weakness may increase as the day goes by, a factor pertinent to the time selected for dental and dental hygiene appointments.

D. Precipitating Factors

■ Individual reactions vary, but the more common predisposing or aggravating factors affecting the severity of muscular involvement include emotional excitement, surgical procedures, loss of sleep, alcoholic intake, and infections, including oral infection.
■ Treatment with immunosuppressive drugs makes the patient vulnerable to infection.
■ Myasthenic crisis is best avoided by elimination and prevention of infection and all precipitating factors.

III. TYPES OF CRISES

A. Myasthenic Crisis[28]

1. *Cause*
   ■ A myasthenic crisis may result from undermedication or increased severity of the disease, or it may be precipitated by one of the aggravating factors previously mentioned.
   ■ The relative deficiency of acetylcholine, which leads to the crisis symptoms, can usually be corrected by the administration of anticholinesterase by the physician.
2. *Symptoms and signs*
   ■ The inability to swallow, speak, or maintain a patent airway is sudden.
   ■ Marked weakness of respiratory and pharyngeal muscles leads to depression of respiration and obstruction.
   ■ The patient may also have double vision and drooping eyelids.
3. *Emergency care*
   ■ Suction.
   ■ Provide a patent airway.
   ■ Obtain medical assistance; transport to hospital emergency facility.

B. Cholinergic Crisis

1. Cause. The cholinergic crisis results from overmedication with anticholinesterase.
2. Symptoms and signs. Increased muscle weakness occurs within 30 to 60 minutes of taking the medication. Excessive pulmonary secretion, cramps, and diarrhea also are characteristic.
3. Treatment.
   - No further medication should be taken at that time.
   - Medical assistance is needed promptly.
   - When respiratory symptoms develop, urgent ventilation is required (page 1076).

IV. MEDICAL TREATMENT[26,27]

- Medical treatment may have two purposes: to influence the course of the disease and to induce disease remission.
- Anticholinesterase agents are used for most patients at intervals during the day. A sustained-release preparation may be used at bedtime, particularly for the patient who awakens with severe weakness.
- Therapy for attempting to induce remission can include surgical removal of the thymus gland, particularly if a tumor of the gland develops, and drug therapy is ineffective.
- Immunosuppressive medications include corticosteroids, azathioprine (when corticosteroids are contraindicated), and cyclosporin. Among the side effects of cyclosporin is gingival enlargement (page 253).

V. DENTAL HYGIENE CARE

Particular factors to consider when planning dental hygiene care for the patient with myasthenia gravis:

- Early, progressive involvement of orofacial muscles.
- Risk for myasthenic or cholinergic crisis.

POST-POLIO SYNDROME (PPS)[29]

I. DESCRIPTION

- Condition that affects adults, years after recovery from an initial attack of the poliomyelitis virus when they were children.
- Cause is unknown.
- Prevalence is currently unknown, but appears to be growing.
- Treatment focus is mainly palliative, with exercise often prescribed to strengthen specific muscle groups.
- Characterized by progressive muscle weakness, fatigue, muscle and joint pain and, potential muscle atrophy in muscles originally affected by the poliomyelitis as well as other muscles, including orofacial muscles.

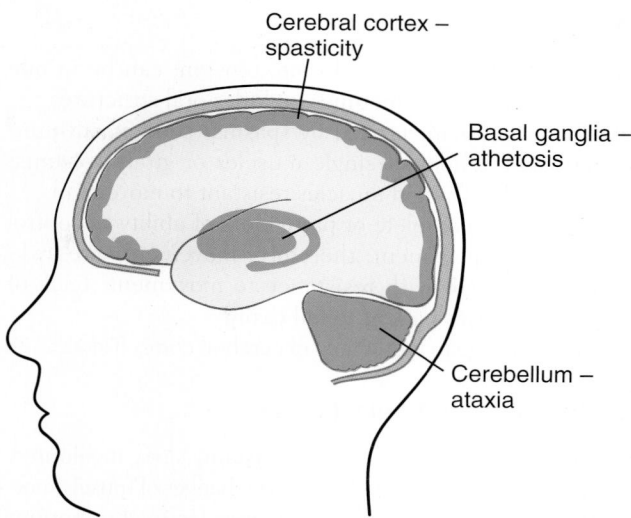

FIGURE 58-3 Cerebral Palsy. Shown are the major parts of the brain involved in each of the three major types of cerebral palsy: spastic, athetoid, and ataxic.

II. DENTAL HYGIENE CARE

Particular factors to consider when planning dental hygiene care for the patient with multiple sclerosis:

- Impaired motor ability.
- Weakness in respiratory and swallowing muscles.

CEREBRAL PALSY[30,31]

I. DESCRIPTION

- *Palsy* means impairment of the ability to control movement, and *cerebral palsy* means a condition in which injury to parts of the brain has occurred prenatally, natally, or postnatally and has resulted in paralysis or disruption of motor parts.
- Such a condition can occur at any age because of brain injury from a variety of causes.
- Cerebral palsy can be caused by anoxia during pregnancy or delivery, maternal infection during pregnancy (for example, rubella), blood type incompatibility, severe nutritional lack during pregnancy, or maternal diabetes endocrine imbalance.
- Later in infancy, infectious diseases, such as meningitis or encephalitis, lead poisoning, direct trauma from accidents, or battering (nonaccidental injury) may be implicated.
- Symptoms usually can be observed during the first year after birth but may not appear for several years.

II. CLASSIFICATIONS

Cerebral palsy is classified in four types according to associated motor impairment.

A. Spastic Palsy

- Muscles have increased tone, tension; can be in one limb or all four; sometimes includes oral structures.
- Condition characterized by spasms (sudden, involuntary contractions of single muscles or groups of muscles) and stiff, rigid muscles resistant to movement.
- Patient has complete or partial loss of ability to control muscular movement; therefore, movements are awkward and stiff with resistance to movement. Lack of control causes patient to fall easily.
- Brain damage to motor area of cerebral cortex (Figure 58-3).

B. Dyskinetic or Athetoid Palsy

- Condition characterized by constant, slow, involuntary writhing movements with frequent changes of muscle tone.
- Patient lacks ability to direct muscles in the motions desired.
- Grimacing, drooling, and speech defects are common.
- Factors influencing movements
  - Effort by patient to control muscle activity results in exaggerated muscle movement.
  - May be initiated and aggravated by stimuli outside body, such as sudden noises, bright lights, or quick movements by people or things in the area.
  - Intensity influenced by emotional factors. Patient is least in control in an emotionally charged environment, such as the dental office.
- Brain damage to basal ganglia (Figure 58-3).

C. Ataxic Palsy

- Loss of equilibrium, balance and depth perception; walk uncertain; has difficulty in sitting straight.
- Lack of coordination; needs time to execute changes.
- Involuntary muscle quivering may affect part or all of the body; placing gentle firm presser will help calm the tremor.
- Brain damage to cerebellum (Figure 58-3).

D. Combined Palsy

A combination of the three named types.

III. ACCOMPANYING CONDITIONS

A. Primitive Reflexes

- *Asymmetric tonic neck reflex:* When head is turned, same side extremities extend and stiffen, while opposite side extremities flex.
- *Tonic labyrinthine reflex:* If neck is extended back, extremities also extend and back is arched.
- *Startle reflex:* Any surprising stimuli can trigger uncontrolled body movement.

B. Seizures

Between 25% and 30% have seizures and undergo related drug therapy.

C. Sensory Disorders

Visual impairments and hearing loss and deafness are common.

D. Dysarthria

Speech may be slow and difficult to understand due to lack of control of mouth and throat muscles.

E. Cognitive Impairment

- Fewer than 50% of individuals with cerebral palsy also have significant cognitive impairment.
- More than 50% **do not** have intellectual or cognitive disabilities, therefore, an inability to communicate does not necessarily mean lack of comprehension.
- Of the 50% who are not significantly intellectually impaired, some may learn more slowly because of sensory impairments, perceptive-cognitive deficiencies, and speech difficulties.

IV. MEDICAL TREATMENT

- Surgical, orthopedic, and medical care, as well as speech, physical, and occupational therapy, may constitute a minimum of specialties involved in the care of a patient with cerebral palsy.
- Bracing to support the lower limbs and the use of cane, crutches, walker, or wheelchair all may help to increase function.
- Surgery may be needed for orthopedic deformities or for correcting eye or ear difficulties.
- Patients may use tranquilizers to reduce tension or aid in limiting problems associated with nerve damage. Other medication may include drugs for seizure control. Cerebral palsy has no cure.

V. ORAL CHARACTERISTICS

A. Disturbances of Musculature

- Facial grimacing, facial asymmetry, and abnormal function of muscles of mastication, swallowing, and speech are common.
- Inability to close lips contributes to increased drooling.
- Hyperactive bite and gag reflexes can present difficulties during dental and dental hygiene therapy, as well as during biofilm control at home.

B. Malocclusion

- The incidence of malocclusion is high; often a musculoskeletal abnormality rather than only misaligned teeth.
- Oral habits of mouthbreathing, tongue thrusting, and faulty swallowing contribute to open bite with protruding anterior teeth.

C. Attrition and Erosion

- Severe, constant, involuntary bruxism is common and can severely wear down tooth structure and restorations.
- Gastroesophageal reflux can cause erosion of oral tissues.

D. Oral Injury

Patients fall frequently, which can damage and fracture teeth and jaws.

E. Dental Caries

- The rate of dental caries may be higher, but the factors that operate for the patient with cerebral palsy are the same as the general population.
- Difficulties in maintaining biofilm control and problems of mastication can lead to the use of a soft diet, which increase risk for dental caries.

F. Periodontal Infections

- Periodontal or gingival infections are found in a high percentage of patients with cerebral palsy.
- *Phenytoin-induced gingival overgrowth:* When phenytoin is used for the prevention of seizures, the patient is susceptible to gingival enlargement. The condition and its prevention are described in Chapter 62 on page 945.
- *Risk factors for periodontal involvement:* Mechanical difficulties related to biofilm control, mouthbreathing, and increased food retention because of ineffective self-cleansing all lead to increased periodontal involvement and biofilm collection.
- Many patients with cerebral palsy have heavy calculus deposits.

VI. DENTAL HYGIENE CARE

Particular factors to consider when planning dental hygiene care for the patient with cerebral palsy:

- Impaired motor ability; uncontrolled movements, primitive reflex reactions.
- Involvement of muscles in head and neck.
- Need for body stabilization and support.
- Many with no cognitive or intellectual impairment.
- Numerous associated oral characteristics and predisposing factors for oral disease.

MUSCULAR DYSTROPHIES[32,33]

- The muscular dystrophies are genetic myopathies characterized by progressive severe weakness and loss of use of groups of muscles.

- The term *dystrophy* means degeneration and is associated with atrophy and dysfunction.
- The syndromes of muscular dystrophy have been separated by clinical and genetic means and range from mild (Becker type) with a later onset to more severe types (Duchenne, facioscapulohumeral).
- All types of muscular dystrophy are genetically inherited and the underlying pathologic processes do not differ.
- Generally, the diseases are limited to skeletal muscles, with cardiac muscle only rarely involved.
- All muscular dystrophies are rare. The two types described are the more common.

I. DUCHENNE MUSCULAR DYSTROPHY (PSEUDOHYPERTROPHIC)

A. Occurrence

- The Duchenne muscular dystrophy (DMD) type is primarily limited to males and transmitted by female carriers.
- Incidence is approximately 1 in 3,500 births.

B. Age of Onset

The condition is present at birth and becomes apparent during early childhood, usually between 2 and 5 years, but before 10 years.

C. Characteristics

- *Musculature:* Enlargement (pseudohypertrophy) of certain muscles, particularly the calves, is present in early years.
- *Weakness of hips:* Child falls frequently, has increasing difficulty in standing erect.
- *Lordosis:* With an abdominal protuberance.
- *Waddling:* Either walks on toes or flatfoot because of muscle contracture.
- *Precarious balance:* Patient arches back in attempt to find center of gravity; gait is slow because balance must be attained with each step.
- *Progressive muscular wasting:*
  - Eventual involvement of thighs, shoulders, trunk; weakness of respiratory muscles.
  - Inactivity is detrimental and increases the individual's helplessness and dependency.
- *Intellectual impairment:* A mild degree of mental impairment is noted in some persons with DMD.
- *Cardiac abnormalities:* Arrhythmia and cardiomyopathy are common.

D. Prognosis

- Disablement severe by puberty; child is confined to a wheelchair.
- Patients rarely live to reach their third decade.

II. FACIOSCAPULOHUMERAL MUSCULAR DYSTROPHY

A. Occurrence

■ Males and females are equally affected.
■ Incidence is approximately 1 in 20,000.

B. Age of Onset

■ Between 6 and 20 years, with an average at 13 years, after puberty.
■ Mild symptoms may appear at later ages.

C. Characteristics

■ Facial muscles involved, particularly involving the obicularis oris. The effect of gaping lips on oral tissues is similar to mouthbreathing.
■ Malocclusions and TMD problems have been noted.
■ Scapulae prominent; shoulder muscles weak; difficulty in raising the arms.
■ Difficulty in closing eyes completely.
■ Cardiac involvement is rare.

D. Prognosis

■ Progression is slower than that of the Duchenne type and progress may become arrested.
■ Most patients live a normal life span and become incapacitated late in life.

III. OTHER TYPES OF MUSCULAR DYSTROPHY[33]

Other, less common types of Muscular Dystrophy include:

■ *Becker:* Similar to Duchenne type, but more benign with a later onset (5–15 years).
■ *Emery–Dreifuss:* Onset between 5–30 years; generally benign, but severe cardiomyopathy and risk for sudden death is a feature.
■ *Limb-girdle:* Most severely affects muscles of the hips and shoulders; manifests in late childhood/early adolescence and ranges from rapidly to slowly progressive.
■ *Oculopharyngeal and myotonic dystrophies:* Each is relatively rare, has onset between 20–50 years of age, is slowly progressive, and features extensive involvement of orofacial muscles.

IV. MEDICAL TREATMENT

■ A specific treatment is not known. Symptoms may be relieved. The patient is encouraged to lead as full a life as possible and to keep active.
■ Prednisone may be prescribed along with other drugs to treat muscle weakness and cardiac symptoms.
■ Preventive treatment consists of prenatal diagnosis, carrier detection, and genetic counseling.

V. DENTAL HYGIENE CARE

Particular factors to consider when planning dental hygiene care for the patient with muscular dystrophy:

■ Impaired motor ability.
■ Potential need for body stabilization and support.
■ Some types involve orofacial muscles.

MYELOMENINGOCELE[34]

■ *Spina bifida* is a congenital defect or opening in the spinal column. A portion of the spinal membranes may protrude through the opening with or without spinal cord tissue.
■ When the spinal cord protrudes through the spina bifida, the condition is called *myelomeningocele*.
■ Anticipatory guidance prior to conception includes the use of multivitamins containing *folic acid*. A reduced risk of offspring with spina bifida and other neural tube defects has been shown when mothers received folic acid.[35]
■ Patients with spina bifida appear to be specifically at risk for latex hypersensitivity.[36,37] Proper precautions are found on page 69 in Chapter 5.

I. DESCRIPTION

■ Embryologically, a neural tube forms during the first month of pregnancy.
■ From the neural tube, the brain, brain stem, and spinal cord arise, and, eventually, the vertebrae form and enclose the spinal cord.
■ When a place in the spinal column fails to close, the result is an open defect in the spinal canal, which is called a spina bifida.

II. TYPES OF DEFORMITIES

A. Myelomeningocele

■ A myelomeningocele is a protrusion or outpouching of the spinal cord and its covering (meninges) through an opening in the bony spinal column.
■ Because part of the spinal cord and nerve roots protrude, flaccid paralysis of the legs and part of the trunk results, depending on the level of the protrusion (herniation).

B. Meningocele

■ A meningocele is a protrusion of the meninges through a defect in the skull or spinal column.
■ Because no neural elements are contained in the protrusion, paralysis is uncommon.

C. Spina Bifida

■ Spina bifida is a congenital cleft in the bony encasement of the spinal cord.

- When no outpouching of the meninges or spinal cord exists, the condition is called *spina bifida occulta*.
- Usually, spina bifida occulta has no symptoms.

III. PHYSICAL CHARACTERISTICS

Depending on the level of the myelomeningocele, some or all of the following signs and physical characteristics may be found.

A. Bony Deformities

Muscle imbalance from paralysis can cause dislocation of the hip, club foot, and spinal curvatures, such as humpback (kyphosis), curvature (scoliosis), or swayback (lordosis).

B. Loss of Sensation

Lack of skin sensitivity to pain, temperature, and other sensations can lead to problems of inadvertent burn or trauma unrecognized by the patient or caregiver or to pressure sores, described on page 889. Frequent position changes are necessary during dental hygiene care.

C. Bladder and Bowel Paralysis

The nerve supplies to the bladder and bowel are usually affected. Lack of bowel and bladder control requires continual attention. Kidney infection with loss of kidney function is one cause of shorter life expectancy.

D. Hydrocephalus

- A high percentage of children with myelomeningocele have hydrocephalus. Hydrocephalus is a condition characterized by an excessive accumulation of fluid in the brain. The fluid dilates the cerebral ventricles, causes compression of brain tissues, and separates the cranial bones as the head enlarges **(Figure 58-4)**.
- Development is slowed, and intellectual disability may be present.
- Many of these patients have seizures.

IV. MEDICAL TREATMENT

Surgical, orthopedic, and urologic treatment as well as physical and occupational therapy may constitute a minimum of specialties involved in the care of a patient with myelomeningocele.

A. Neurosurgery

- *Closure of the myelomeningocele.* Surgical closure helps to prevent infections that may otherwise enter into the spinal cord. Paralysis is not lessened by surgery.

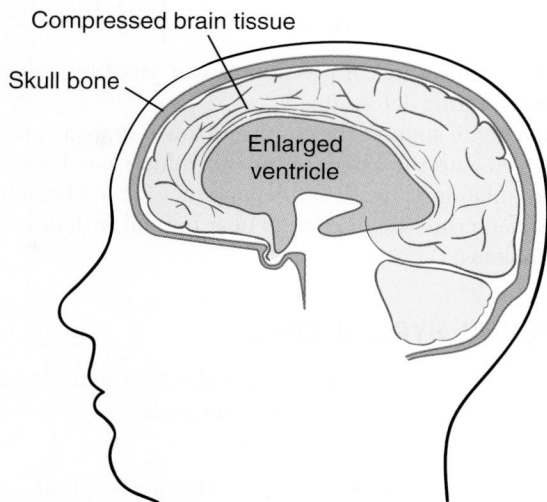

FIGURE 58-4 **Hydrocephalu.** The ventricle is enlarged because of the accumulation of fluid. Brain tissues are compressed.

- *Treatment of the hydrocephalus.* Permanent drainage systems may be accomplished in the form of a ventriculoatrial shunt between the cerebral ventricle and the atrium of the heart **(Figure 58-5)**. Sometimes, drainage by way of the abdomen in the form of a ventriculoperitoneal shunt is used.
- Individuals who have a cerebrospinal fluid shunt are at increased risk for transient infections. Need for premedication during dental treatment is established by medical consultation.[38]

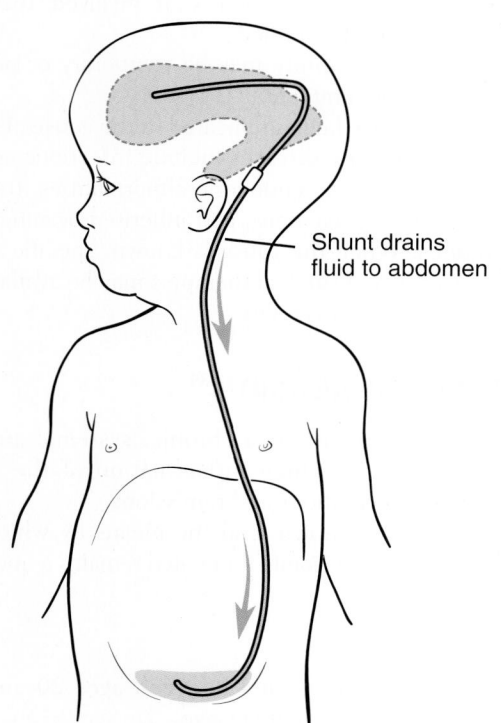

FIGURE 58-5 **Shunt for Hydrocephalus Treatment.** Fluid is drained by way of a ventriculoatrial or ventriculoperitoneal shunt.

B. Orthopedic Surgery

- Orthopedic surgical procedures can assist by reducing or correcting deformities.
- Bracing to support the trunk and lower limbs is used in accord with the extent of the individual's paralysis.
- Ambulation varies from dependency on a wheelchair, walker, crutches, or cane to near normal with only foot problems.

V. DENTAL HYGIENE CARE

Particular factors to consider when planning dental hygiene care for the patient with myelomeningoele:

- Impaired motor ability.
- Potential need for body stabilization and support.
- Increased risk for latex allergy and transient infections related to a cerebrospinal fluid shunt; medical evaluation determines need for premedication.

ARTHRITIS

Diseases of the joints, including arthritis, are among the most common causes of chronic illness in the United States. In addition to arthritis as a disease entity, arthritic manifestations are produced as part of various other chronic diseases. A person may suffer from more than one type at a time.

- Arthritis means inflammation in a joint. It may occur in an acute or chronic form and may be localized or generalized. When many joints are involved, the term *polyarthritis* may be applied.
- The resulting disability may be temporary or permanent, partial or complete.
- Factors that have been implicated in the cause of rheumatic and arthritic diseases include infectious agents, traumatic disorders, endocrine abnormalities, tumors, allergy and drug reactions, and inherited or congenital conditions. When the cause is known, specific medical, physical, and surgical therapies may be available to alleviate pain and disability.

I. RHEUMATOID ARTHRITIS[39]

- Rheumatoid arthritis is a chronic, systemic autoimmune disease in which inflammation of the joints occurs in exacerbations and remissions.
- The cause is unknown, and the means by which the inflammation in the joints is initiated remains a question.

A. Occurrence

- The onset usually occurs between ages 20 and 40, although it may occur at any age.
- More women than men are affected.
- It is rare in tropical countries.

B. Signs and Symptoms

- Joint pain and swelling. Rheumatoid arthritis is a polyarthritis with migratory pain, swelling, tenderness, and warmth in symmetrical joints. Fingers, hands, and knees are affected first.
- Morning stiffness and stiffness after periods of inactivity.
- Weakness, fatigue, loss of appetite and weight, anemia, low-grade fever.
- Subcutaneous nodules in elbows, wrists, or fingers in approximately 20% of the patients; nodules may appear in other body organs.
- A significant complication is temporomandibular joint involvement. There may be pain with jaw movements and difficulty in chewing. Ankylosis may develop but is not a common finding.
- Progressive deformity, with limited motion in the more severely involved joints and muscle atrophy adjacent to the joints.

C. Medical Treatment

- Without a specifically known cause, therapy is limited to an individualized program involving pain relief, physical and occupational therapy, and overall health maintenance with adequate nutrition.
- Drugs used in treatment include nonsteroidal anti-inflammatory drugs (NSAIDs), and drugs to aid in controlling the disease including methotrexate, gold compounds, azathioprine, and cyclosporin.[40]
- Selected patients are treated by joint replacement surgery.

D. Relationship to Periodontal Disease[41,42]

- Rheumatoid arthritis and periodontitis are both chronic inflammatory diseases. The pathogenesis of the two conditions show similarities.
- Indications are that the extent and severity of periodontal disease and rheumatoid arthritis are related.
- Medications used to manage one of these conditions may have implications for treatment of both.

II. JUVENILE RHEUMATOID ARTHRITIS

- Rheumatoid arthritis occurring in children under 16 years of age differs from the disease in adults. The onset is usually more acute, with prolonged fever and enlargement of the spleen and lymph nodes.
- The inflammation of many joints, particularly knees, wrists, and spine, may appear after a few weeks. The temporomandibular joint may be involved, with pain and limited oral opening.
- Many patients have complete remissions, some have increasing disability, and others have mild arthritic symptoms that continue for years. Children are encouraged to lead as normal a life as possible.

■ The long-term treatment program includes activity to maintain function and drugs to relieve pain.

III. DEGENERATIVE JOINT DISEASE[43]

■ Degenerative joint disease (DJD), or osteoarthritis as it is frequently called, affects the weight-bearing joints particularly. Because inflammation is not the basic joint problem, degenerative joint disease is a more accurate term.

■ No specific cause is known, but predisposing factors may include repeated trauma, obesity, age-related changes in the joint tissues, mechanical stresses to the weight-bearing joints, and genetic predisposition.

A. Occurrence

■ The onset occurs between 50 and 70 years of age, with the average onset 20 years later than that of rheumatoid arthritis.

■ As many as 85% of people over age 70 have evidence of degenerative joint disease.

B. Symptoms

At first insidious, with slight stiffness of a single joint, the eventual condition leads to much pain, deformity, and limitation of movement.

■ Hips, knees, fingers, and vertebrae affected most frequently.

■ Swelling rare; ankylosis does not occur.

■ Stiffness in the morning on rising and after periods of inactivity; diminishes with exercise.

■ Pain aggravated by temperature changes and bearing body weight.

■ Temporomandibular joint usually without pain or other clinical symptoms, although crepitation, clicking, or snapping may occur when the joints are exercised.

C. Medical Treatment

■ Moderate exercise, pain-relieving drug therapy, weight reduction for obese patients, physical therapy, and selected orthopedic surgical procedures comprise the general treatments available.

■ Total hip or knee joint replacement has proved satisfactory for many patients and has been used more widely for DJD than for rheumatoid arthritis.

■ Because of the susceptibility to infection at the interface of the bone and the prosthesis, prophylactic antibiotic premedication to prevent bacteremia is recommended for certain patients and procedures, as described in Chapter 9 on page 131.[44]

IV. DENTAL HYGIENE CARE

Particular factors to consider when planning dental hygiene care for the patient with arthritis:

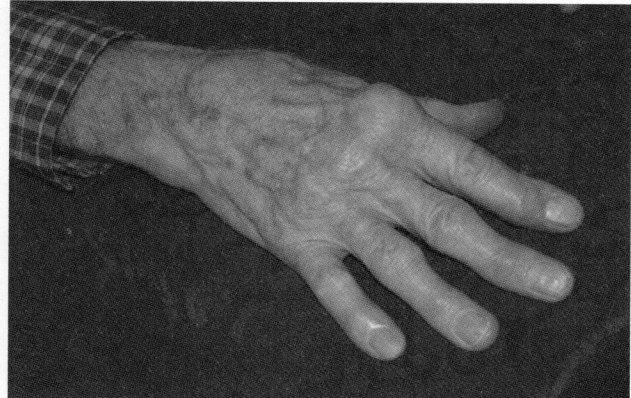

FIGURE 58-6 Adult hand compromised by degenerative joint disease. Pain and lack of ability to grasp the small handle of a toothbrush affect ability to hold and maneuver oral self-care implements.

■ Joint pain contributes to impaired motor function; affected areas and degree of impairment are considered for planning care. The effect of osteoarthritis on the hands of an older patient, which is considered when planning for self care, is pictured in **Figure 58-6**.

■ Joint replacement requires physician consultation regarding antibiotic premedication.

SCLERODERMA (PROGRESSIVE SYSTEMIC SCLEROSIS)[45,46]

■ Scleroderma is an autoimmune disease of connective tissue characterized by an overproduction of collagen.

■ The most striking physical symptom is the immobility and rigidity of the skin, but inflammation and sclerosis occur throughout the body. Thus, the disease has the full title of *progressive systemic sclerosis*.

■ The cause is not known, but collagen synthesis irregularities, associated immunologic disorders, and microvascular abnormalities have been implicated. Hereditary factors are not involved.

I. OCCURRENCE

■ Scleroderma usually has its onset between ages 30 and 50, but it may affect persons of any age, even infants.

■ It may develop over months or years and is between 2 and 5 times more common in females.

II. CHARACTERISTICS

■ Scleroderma may be localized and involve only the skin, or it may be generalized and involve all body organs.

■ The most notable changes are in the skin, gastrointestinal tract, kidneys, heart, muscles, and lungs.

■ Eventual death results from renal failure, cardiac failure, pulmonary insufficiency, or intestinal malabsorption.

■ Symptoms vary, and all individuals do not have all the symptoms and signs that follow.

A. General Manifestations

- *Joints:* pain, swelling, and stiffness of the fingers and knee joints.
- *Polyarthritis:* symmetrical polyarthritis, similar to rheumatoid arthritis.
- *Skin:* hard and fixed; ivory-white, yellow, or gray, sometimes with brown pigmentation in the late stages.
- *Face:* When affected, the face becomes masklike and expressionless.
- *Esophagus:* increasing dysmotility predisposes the patient to gastroesophageal reflux disease.
- Patients with scleroderma are sensitive to cold and dampness, stress, undue emotional tension, and fatigue.

B. Oral Characteristics

- *Lips:* thin, rigid, with oral stricture (microstomia) with limited opening capacity as well as difficulty in opening and closing.
- *Mucosa:* thin, pale, tender, rigid, with poor healing capacity.
- *Gingiva:* pale and unusually firm.
- *Teeth:* increased mobility.
- *Radiographic findings:* marked widening of the periodontal ligament spaces. This finding is sometimes considered pathognomonic for scleroderma.
- *Mastication:* difficult; temporomandibular joint movement is limited.
- *Tongue:* may be immobile; speech difficult.

III. MEDICAL TREATMENT

- Specific therapy is not known; medications that retard collagen deposition have not yet been determined to be effective for scleroderma.
- Treatment, therefore, has been directed at specific system complications, physical therapy, and attempts to maintain normal activities.

IV. DENTAL HYGIENE CARE

Particular factors to consider when planning dental hygiene care for the patient with scleroderma:

- Joint pain contributes to impaired motor function; affected areas and degree of impairment are considered for planning care.
- Involvement of orafacial tissues complicates dental hygiene treatment and oral self-care.

SUMMARY OF CONSIDERATIONS FOR DENTAL HYGIENE CARE

- Dental professionals are essential members of the interdisciplinary team providing care for a patient with a physical impairment.

- Early dental hygiene intervention and regular preventive care will aid in optimizing oral health status and minimizing oral problems.
- Knowledge and understanding of the specifics of a patient's particular condition will help the clinician become confident in managing adaptations needed during the dental hygiene appointment.
- Information provided in Chapter 56 and Chapter 57 is useful for planning dental hygiene care for a patient with a physical impairment, either in a dental clinic or in an alternative practice setting. General suggestions for the older adult patient in Chapter 52 may also prove useful.

I. PREPARATION FOR APPOINTMENTS

A. Information for appointment scheduling and providing a barrier-free environment is found on page 854.

B. Communication with patient or caregiver prior to appointment to assess specific needs will help the clinician to identify and prepare for modifications necessary to provide care based on the individual patient's needs.

C. Essential information, such as a completed health history and description of the patient's physical abilities and limitations, can be obtained by telephone.

D. On the basis of a generalized knowledge of the patient's specific disorder or conditions, specific questions may be asked about:

1. Abilities and limitations in performing activities of everyday living.
   - Specific information about assistance needed from caregivers.
   - Adaptive aids that the patient is currently using for oral self-care or other personal hygiene tasks.
2. Factors related to the best time of day for dental appointments.
   - Schedule of urinary/bowel management program for a patient with spinal cord injury.
   - The time of day when symptoms associated with the particular condition are most likely to be relieved or diminished.
3. Ability to communicate.
   - Methods used by the patient to communicate with healthcare providers or caregiver.
4. Special adaptations needed for the patient's comfort or safety during the appointment.
   - Blankets or increased air circulation if body temperature control is compromised.
   - Positioning and padding needed for stabilization.
   - Procedures for stress reduction.
5. Medications taken by the patient.
   - Factors related to the patient's condition that may place the patient at risk for xerostomia, increased bleeding.
   - Potential interactions with local anesthesia.

II. ADDITIONAL CONSIDERATIONS DURING CLINICAL CARE

A. Frequent, short appointments in a warm, quiet, comfortable atmosphere lessen patient fatigue and emotional stress.

B. Emergency care may be needed during the period of recovery, such as immediately following a stroke or traumatic spinal injury; non-emergency care is delayed until the patient is stabilized.

C. If the patient's condition involves partial or complete paralysis of facial muscles:

1. Decreased self-cleaning action of the tongue increases potential for collecting dental biofilm on oral surfaces.

2. Rinsing may be difficult or impossible.

3. When anesthesia is used, the affected check and lip may be at higher risk for biting injury until the anesthesia has worn off.

4. If the eyelid lacks natural ability to close for protection, care is taken to ensure that calculus, polishing agent, or other foreign material does not splash into the eye by assuring that protective eyewear and suction are used during treatment.

D. Potential effects from interactions with mediations taken for many disorders and conditions require particular care when administering anesthetics.

1. For example, epinephrine interaction with levadopa, often prescribed for Parkinson's disease, may cause the patient to experience an exaggerated effect on blood pressure and heart rate.

2. Dental hygiene care is complicated if the patient has a disorder that involves involuntary movement; for example, athetoid movements in a patient with cerebral palsy should not be interpreted as a lack of cooperation.

3. Danger for the patient and dental personnel result from the uncontrolled movement of the patient. Suggestions for body stabilization and use of mouth props are found in Chapter 56 on page 859.

4. Assistance throughout the appointments is necessary. Ask the patient or caregiver for suggestions for management.

5. Sedation through premedication may be possible.

III. ASSISTANCE FOR THE AMBULATORY PATIENT

Suggestions for how to aid patients who walk with one or more assistive aides such as braces, a cane, crutches, or a walker are found in Chapter 56 on page 859.

IV. WHEELCHAIR TRANSFER

- Most patients who use wheelchairs can readily be treated in a traditional clinical setting.
- Detailed information about wheelchair to dental chair transfer is available in Chapter 56 on page 857.

V. PATIENT POSITIONING AND BODY STABILIZATION

- Communication with patient or caregiver prior to appointment to assess specific needs related to body positioning and use of specific measures such as padding, warm coverings, or other supportive devices will help enhance clinician efficiency as well as patient comfort and safety.
- Slow and incremental adjustments of the patient chair during treatment will help maintain comfort and patient stability.
- Prevention of decubitus ulcers can be accomplished by appropriate positioning of the dental chair, the use of padding, and by periodic repositioning to prevent or reduce pressure. The patient is asked to provide direction for the correct, individualized procedures.
- Before dental hygiene treatment, the patient is asked about susceptibility to spasms and to describe the procedure to follow should one occur.
- Chapter 57 provides ideas for treatment adaptations that are used when the patient is bed-bound or if care is provided in a non-clinical setting such as a private home or nursing home facility.

VI. FOUR-HANDED DENTAL HYGIENE

- Use of a dental hygiene assistant when treating patients with a physical impairment is mandatory for certain patients and will enhance the clinician's efficiency as well as the patient's comfort and safety.
- Further discussion of four-handed dental hygiene is found in Chapter 56 on page 862.

VII. PERSONAL FACTORS THAT AFFECT SELF-CARE

- Depression from limitations or discouragement from the pain and pressure of treatment and rehabilitation can affect attitude toward oral self-care practices for the patient who has a physical impairment.
- Daily oral care can become a part of the daily personal hygiene routine accomplished as independently as the patient's ability allows. Physical and occupational therapists provide self-care training to enable as much independence as possible for personal care.
- Paralysis may make grasping and manipulating a toothbrush difficult or impossible; adaptive aids (described in Chapter 56 on page ___), a lightweight power driven toothbrush, or instruction for the caregiver are provided on the basis of patient ability and limitations.
- Hemiplegia, common after a stroke, can require the challenge of helping the patient develop dexterity in the non-dominant hand in order to manipulate biofilm removal implements.

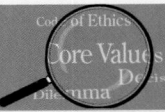

Everyday Ethics

John had an accident when diving into surf at the beach 2 years ago at age 18. He has a complete transection lesion at the C5 level. John came today for his biannual dental visit with his mother, who is his primary caregiver. Amy, the dental hygienist, was assisting in the wheelchair transfer into the dental chair. During the transfer, John's t-shirt was inadvertently lifted slightly, and Amy noticed obvious decubitus ulcers that showed signs of secondary infection. Amy continues to transfer him safely into the dental chair and then stops to consider what to do next. Dramatic images from a lecture in dental hygiene school flash through her mind. She will never forget those photographs of patients suffering from neglect.

Questions for Consideration

1. It is possible, although not clearly established in this scenario, that John is the victim of neglect. Is this an ethical issue or an ethical dilemma for Amy? What issues does Amy need to consider and what questions does she need to ask before she can proceed through the framework for making decisions about:
   - continuing today's appointment when she thinks that John's decubitus ulcers may be infected?
   - addressing the issue of potential neglect?
2. What does the core value of autonomy have to do with this scenario as Amy considers John's competency to make his own choices and treatment decisions vs. his dependence on his mother for care?
3. What additional core values (Table II-1 in Section II, Introduction, page 38) come into play as Amy contemplates how she can best advocate for her patient's safety and well-being?

DOCUMENTATION

Documentation in the permanent record for each appointment with a physically impaired patient includes a minimum of the following factors:

- Description of the patient's impairment level and ability to provide oral self-care, with changes/updates noted for each dental hygiene visit, particularly if the patient has a degenerative condition.
- Recommendations for adaptive aids and modifications to daily oral care regimens.
- Description of oral hygiene care instructions provided to the caregiver.

- Description of patient position modifications and other adaptations during patient care.
- An example progress note documenting an appointment for a patient with a physical disability is in **Box 58-5**.

Factors To Teach The Patient

- The need to communicate is key to successful dental treatment and oral health and is achieved by speaking openly about medical history, patient limitations, and adaptations needed for safe dental treatment and effective oral care.
- Daily, thorough biofilm removal is necessary to reduce the occurrence of oral disease.
- Regular maintenance appointments are needed to promote oral health.
- Why maintaining periodontal health can help maintain teeth that are necessary as abutments in order to tolerate a mouth-held adaptive aid.
- How to clean and maintain the mouth-held aid.

BOX 58-5	Example Progress Note: Patient With a Physical Impairment

Patient presents for routine 3 months maintenance appointment. Medical history includes diagnosis of Multiple Sclerosis two years ago. Patient is ambulatory with a walker and prefers no assistance at this time, but padding under knees helps her relax and enhances her comfort during treatment. Recent relapse has caused weakness in her dominant hand lessening her ability to maneuver a toothbrush and dental floss for complete biofilm removal during oral self-care. Instruction for using a power toothbrush and a floss holder was provided.

Signed: _____, RDH Date: _____.

References

1. Friedlander RM. Apoptosis and caspases in neurodegenerative diseases. *N Engl J Med.* 2003 Apr 3;348(14):1365–75.
2. Thornton JB, Sneed RC, Tomaselli CE, Boraz RA. Dental management of patients with spinal cord injury. *Compendium.* 1992 Feb;13(2):122, 124, 126 passim.
3. Yuen HK, Shotwell MS, Magruder KM, Slate EH, Salinas CF. Factors associated with oral problems among adults with spinal cord injury. *J Spinal Cord Med.* 2009;32(4):408–15.

4. Brown R, DiMarco A, Hoit J, Garshick E. Respiratory dysfunction and management in spinal cord injury. *Respir Care*. 2006 Aug; 51(8):853–68.

5. Remaley DT, Jaeblon T. Pressure ulcers in orthopaedics. *J Am Acad Orthop Surg*. 2010 Sept;18(9):568–75.

6. Furusawa K, Tokuhiro A, Sugiyama H, Ikeda A, Tajima F, Genda E, Uchida R, Tominaga T, Tanaka T, Magara A, Sumida M. Incidence of symptomatic autonomic dysreflexia varies according to the bowel and bladder management techniques in patients with spinal cord injury. *Spinal Cord [Internet]*. 2011 Jan;49(1):49–54. 2010 Aug 10 [Epub ahead of print, cited 2010 Oct 10]. Available from: http://www.nature.com

7. Smith R. Mouth stick design for the client with spinal cord injury. *Am J Occup Ther*. 1989 Apr;43(4):251–5.

8. Ruff JC. Selection criteria for static and dynamic mouthsticks. *Gen Dent*. 1990 Nov–Dec;38(6):414–16.

9. Little JW, Falace DA, Miller CS, Rhodus NL. Dental Management of the Medically Compromised Patient. 6th ed. St. Louis: Mosby; 2002. p. 423.

10. Uthman A, Al-Saffar A. Prevalence in digital panoramic radiographs of carotid area calcification among iraqi individuals with stroke-related disease. *Oral Surg Oral Med Oral Pathol Oral Radiol Endod*. 2008 Apr;105(4):e68.

11. Friedlander AH, Freymiller EG. Detection of radiation-accelerated atherosclerosis of the carotid artery by panoramic radiography. A new opportunity for dentists. *J Am Dent Assoc*. 2003 Oct;134(10):1361–5.

12. Dawidjan B. Idiopathic facial paralysis: a review and case study. *J Dent Hyg*. 2001 Fall;75(4):316–21.

13. Hazin R, Azizzadeh B, Bhatti MT. Medical and surgical management of facial nerve palsy. *Curr Opin Ophthalmol*. 2009 Nov;20(6):440–50.

14. de Almeida JR, Al Khabori M, Guyatt GH, Witterick IJ, Lin VY, Nedzelski JM, Chen JM. Combined corticosteroid and antiviral treatment for bell palsy: A systematic review and meta-analysis. *JAMA*. 2009 Sep 2;302(9):985–93.

15. Fischer DJ, Epstein JB, Klasser G. Multiple sclerosis: An update for oral health care providers. *Oral Surg Oral Med Oral Pathol Oral Radiol Endod*. 2009 Sep;108(3):318–27.

16. Rudick RA, Cohen JA, Weinstock-Guttman B, Kinkel RP, Ransohoff RM. Management of multiple sclerosis. *N Engl J Med*. 1997 Nov 27;337(22):1604–11.

17. The ALS Association. *Oral care for the patient with ALS: a guide for the caregiver*. Calabasas Hills, CA: The ALS Association; 2004. pp. 1–9. Available from: http://www.alsa.org/resources/fyi.cfm

18. Lomen-Hoerth C. Amyotrophic lateral sclerosis from bench to bedside. *Semin Neurol*. 2008 Apr;28(2):205–11.

19. Wijesekera LC, Leigh PN. Amyotrophic lateral sclerosis. *Orphanet J Rare Dis*. 2009 Feb 3;4:3.

20. Asher RS, Alfred T. Dental management of long-term amyotrophic lateral sclerosis: Case report. *Spec Care Dentist*. 1993 Nov–Dec;13(6):241–4.

21. Meningaud JP, Pitak-Arnnop P, Chikhani L, Bertrand JC. Drooling of saliva: A review of the etiology and management options. *Oral Surg Oral Med Oral Pathol Oral Radiol Endod*. 2006 Jan;101(1):48–57.

22. Mitsumoto H, Rabkin JG. Palliative care for patients with amyotrophic lateral sclerosis: "prepare for the worst and hope for the best". *JAMA*. 2007 Jul 11;298(2):207–16.

23. Houde SC, Mangolds V. Amyotrophic lateral sclerosis: A team approach to primary care. *Clin Excell Nurse Pract*. 1999 Nov;3(6):337–45.

24. Friedlander AH, Mahler M, Norman KM, Ettinger RL. Parkinson disease: systemic and orofacial manifestations, medical and dental management. *J Am Dent Assoc*. 2009 Jun;140(6):658–69.

25. Tolle L. Myasthenia gravis: a review for dental hygienists. *J Dent Hyg*. 2007 Winter;81(1):12.

26. Yarom N, Barnea E, Nissan J, Gorsky M. Dental management of patients with myasthenia gravis: a literature review. *Oral Surg Oral Med Oral Pathol Oral Radiol Endod*. 2005 Aug;100(2):158–63.

27. Drachman DB. Myasthenia gravis. *N Engl J Med*. 1994 Jun 23; 330(25):1797–810.

28. Appel SH. Myasthenia Gravis. In: Rakel RE, ed. *Conn's current therapy*. Philadelphia: W.B. Saunders Co.; 1998; p. 929.

29. National Institute of Neurological Disorders and Strokes (NINDS), National Institutes of Health (NIH). Post-Polio Syndrome Fact Sheet [Internet]. Office Communication and Public Liaison, NINDS, NIH; 2009 Dec 18. [cited February 9 2010]. Available from: http://www.ninds.nih.gov/disorders/post_polio/detail_post_polio.htm

30. National Institute of Dental and Craniofacial Research. Practical Oral Care for People with Cerebral Palsy. Bethesda: U.S. Department of Health and Human Services, National Institutes of Health, National Institute of Dental and Craniofacial Research (Pub. No. 04-5192); reprinted 2009 July [cited August 10, 2010]. Available from: https://www.nidcr.nih.gov.proxy.lib.umich.edu/OrderPublications/default.aspx

31. National Institute of Neurological Disorders and Stroke (NINDS). Cerebral Palsy: Hope Through Research [Internet]. Bethesda, MD: National Institute of Neurological Disorders and Stroke (NINDS), National Institutes of Health April 12, 2010 cited 4/13/2010]; [approximately 20 screens]. Available from: http://www.ninds.nih.gov.proxy.lib.umich.edu/disorders/cerebral_palsy/detail_cerebral_palsy.htm.

32. Bennett JC, Plum F, eds. *Cecil textbook of medicine*. 20th ed. Philadelphia: W.B. Saunders Co.; 1996. p. 2161.

33. Balasubramaniam R, Sollecito TP, Stoopler ET. Oral health considerations in muscular dystrophies. *Spec Care Dentist*. 2008 Nov–Dec;28(6):243–53.

34. Akar Z. Myelomeningocele. *Surg Neurol*. 1995 Feb;43(2):113–18.

35. Honein MA, Paulozzi LJ, Mathews TJ, Erickson JD, Wong LY. Impact of folic acid fortification of the US food supply on the occurrence of neural tube defects. *JAMA*. 2001 Jun 20;285(23):2981–6.

36. Engibous PJ, Kittle PE, Jones HL, Vance BJ. Latex allergy in patients with spina bifida. *Pediatr Dent*. 1993 Sep–Oct;15(5):364–6.

37. Nelson LP, Soporowski NJ, Shusterman S. Latex allergies in children with spina bifida: relevance for the pediatric dentist. *Pediatr Dent*. 1994 Jan–Feb;16(1):18–22.

38. Little JW, Falace DA, Miller CS, Rhodus NL. *Dental management of the medically compromised patient*. 6th ed. St. Louis: Mosby; 2002. p. DM 55, 435.

39. Treister N, Glick M. Rheumatoid arthritis: a review and suggested dental care considerations. *J Am Dent Assoc*. 1999 May;130(5):689–98.

40. Cash JM, Klippel JH. Second-line drug therapy for rheumatoid arthritis. *N Engl J Med*. 1994 May 12;330(19):1368–75.

41. Mercado FB, Marshall RI, Bartold PM. Inter-relationships between rheumatoid arthritis and periodontal disease. A review. *J Clin Periodontol*. 2003 Sep;30(9):761–72.

42. Dissick A, Redman RS, Jones M, Rangan BV, Reimold A, Griffiths GR, Mikuls TR, Amdur RL, Richards JS, Kerr GS. Association of periodontitis with rheumatoid arthritis: a pilot study. *J Periodontol*. 2010 Feb;81(2):223–30.

43. Neustadt DH. Osteoarthritis. In: Rakel RE, editor. *Conn's current therapy 1998*. Philadelphia: W.B. Saunders Co.; 1998; p. 995.

44. American Academy of Orthopaedic Surgeons. *Information statement: antibiotic prophylaxis for bacteremia in patients with joint replacement [Internet]*. Rosemont, IL: AAOS; February 2009 cited February 12, 2010]; [approximately 4 screens]. Available from: http://www.aaos.org/about/papers/advistmt/1033.asp.

45. Fischer DJ, Patton LL. Scleroderma: oral manifestations and treatment challenges. *Spec Care Dentist*. 2000 Nov–Dec;20(6):240–4.

46. Albilia JB, Lam DK, Blanas N, Clokie CM, Sandor GK. Small mouths ... big problems? A review of scleroderma and its oral health implications. *J Can Dent Assoc*. 2007 Nov;73(9):831–6.

The Patient With a Sensory Impairment

ESTHER M. WILKINS, BS, RDH, DMD

Chapter Outline

Successful management and treatment of any patient depends largely on the interpersonal communication between the patient and the clinician. When a patient has a vision or hearing impairment, communication assumes a different dimension. This chapter describes suggestions for adaptations for patients with hearing or visual problems. **Box 59-1** contains key words and definitions pertaining to sensory impairments.

AMERICANS WITH DISABILITIES ACT

- *Definition:* An individual with a disability is a person who has a physical or mental impairment that substantially limits a major life activity.
- The examples of physical and mental impairments provided with the Act include visual and hearing impairments.

- For the visually impaired, certain qualifications related to physical facilities are specified, such as the removal of physical barriers and the use of braille markers for elevators.
- The Act specifies that communications with individuals with hearing and vision impairments need to be as effective as communications with nondisabled people, and appropriate auxiliary aids are provided.
- Examples of auxiliary aids are such services and devices as qualified interpreters, assistive listening headsets, text telephone devices for deaf persons (TTYs), readers, taped texts, brailled materials, and large-print materials.
- Special skills used to counsel, motivate, and educate a patient with a sensory disability can be developed and practiced. Although visual modes of communication provide a primary method of communication with the deaf person, audible and "touch" approaches are essential for the person with visual disability.

BOX 59-1	Key Words

Sensory Disabilities

VISION

Astigmatism: impaired vision caused by irregularities in the curvature of the cornea or lens.

Blind spot: the area on the retina that marks the site of entrance of the optic nerve.

Blindness: no perception of visual stimuli; lack or loss of ability to see.

Legal blindness: less than 20/200 vision with corrective eyeglasses (see text).

Braille: a system of writing and printing by means of raised points representing letters; enables people with a visual disability to read by touch.

Cataract: clouding or opacity of the lens of an eye.

Color blindness: inability to distinguish between certain colors; most common is red/green confusion; color vision is a function of the cones of the retina.

Diplopia: double vision; perception of two images of a single object.

Glaucoma: group of diseases of the eye characterized by intraocular pressure from pathologic changes in the optic disc; person has visual-field defects.

Hyperopia: farsightedness; eyeball is shorter behind the retina; vision is better for distant objects than for near objects.

Myopia: nearsightedness; longer eyeball from front to back so the image is focused in front of the retina.

Nyctalopia: night blindness; may be hereditary or related to vitamin deficiency.

Ocular: pertaining to the eye.

Ophthalmologist: physician who specializes in diagnosing and prescribing treatment for defects, injuries, and diseases of the eye (obsolete term: oculist).

Ophthalmology: the branch of medicine that deals with the anatomy, diagnosis, pathology, and treatment of the eye.

Optician: technician who prepares and adapts lenses; fills prescriptions from an ophthalmologist.

Optometrist: a specialist in optometry, the measurement of visual acuity and the adaptation of lenses for correction of visual defects.

Retinitis: inflammation of the retina.

Retinopathy: noninflammatory disease of the retina; identified by the chronic disease of which it is a symptom; for example, diabetic retinopathy reflects the retinal manifestations of diabetes mellitus, including microaneurysms.

Retinopathy of prematurity: a condition peculiar to premature infants; characterized by opaque tissue behind the lens resulting from a high concentration of oxygen, which causes spasm of the retinal vessels, leads to retinal detachment, and arrests eye growth and development; prevented by keeping oxygen administration as low as possible and discontinuing the oxygen as soon as possible.

HEARING

Audiogram: graphic record of the findings of an audiometer.

Audiologist: certified allied health worker, often with advanced degrees; trained in the identification, diagnosis, measurement, and rehabilitation of hearing impairment.

Audiometer: instrument used to determine degree and type of hearing ability.

Aural: pertaining to the ear.

Decibel: unit for expressing the relative loudness of a sound; abbreviation, dB.

Hearing: the sense by which sounds are perceived; conversion of sound waves into nerve impulses, which are then interpreted by the brain.

Otitis: inflammation of the ear.

Otitis media: inflammation of the middle ear.

Otologist: physician specialist in otology, the branch of medicine dealing with the anatomy, physiology, pathology, and treatment of the ear.

Speechreading: recognizing spoken words by watching the speaker's lips, face, and gestures.

Tinnitus: noise in the ears, as ringing, buzzing, or roaring.

TTY: Text telephone device.

Tuning fork: instrument used to test for hearing loss; vibrations of the fork produce sound waves that can be heard in both ears by a person with normal hearing when the stem is placed on top of the head; sound is heard louder in an ear affected by conductive loss and softer in an ear affected by sensorineural loss.

Tympanic membrane: ear drum; vibrates when sound waves strike; transmits waves to nerve endings by way of ossicles in the middle ear and to cochlea in the inner ear.

Vertigo: sensation of rotation or movement of one's self (subjective vertigo) or of one's surroundings (objective vertigo); a subtype of dizziness, but not a synonym.

VISUAL IMPAIRMENT

- Limitations of sight cover a broad spectrum from the slightly affected to the completely blind with no perception of light.
- Loss of sight is a major physical deprivation. In many persons, blindness is secondary to a primary condition that may have been the cause of the blindness and in itself may be disabling.
- "Legal blindness" is defined as follows: having central vision (or acuity) of not more than 20/200 in the better eye with correction (glasses), or having peripheral fields (side vision) of no more than 20° diameter or 10° radius.
- Only approximately 3% of legally blind persons are totally blind. The term "legal blindness" is a legal term, not a medical one, but certification of the degree of severity of blindness is obtained from an ophthalmologist.

I. CAUSES OF BLINDNESS

A. Age-Related

■ The leading causes of blindness are diabetic retinopathy, age-related macular degeneration, senile cataracts, glaucoma, vascular disease, trauma, and infections.

B. Children

■ At least half of the blindness in children is of prenatal origin, particularly resulting from maternal infections (rubella, syphilis, toxoplasmosis).
■ Other causes are injuries, neoplasms, and retinopathy of prematurity (formerly called retrolental fibroplasia). The incidence of retinopathy of prematurity has increased as more premature babies survive.

II. PERSONAL FACTORS

■ Consider each patient in relation to individual aptitudes, interests, abilities, and potentialities, with sight as one factor involved.
■ The only common characteristic this group of patients has is difficulty in seeing.

A. Patient History

■ Assistance in completing the personal questionnaire may be needed.
■ Specific details of the patient's limitations are recorded so that adaptations can be made during the current and future appointments.

B. Child

1. *Learning ability*
   ■ Sensory defects may mask a child's intellectual capacity because responses may differ from other children.
   ■ Blind children may learn to speak later than sighted children and may start school when they are a year or two older.
   ■ A blind child may take longer than does the sighted child to cover the same amount of material; therefore, the educational level for the blind child may be different from that for the sighted child of the same chronologic age.
   ■ Blind children are deprived of the opportunity to learn by imitation.
2. *Personal factors*
   ■ Environment influences the child's adjustment, and parental attitude affects the blind child as it does the sighted child.
   ■ When the parent is overindulgent and protective, the child may be dependent, and emotionally less independent.

C. Adult

■ The adult who has always been blind or has been so since childhood has made adjustments and may be employed in a limited but useful occupation.
■ Many of those who become blind after adulthood experience an immediate natural reaction of depression and feeling of helplessness.
■ Loss of vision may be incipient; the reactions of shock and upheaval usually are less, but dread, worry, and anxiety may be experienced for years in anticipation.
■ When the individual begins to accept the disability, efforts for rehabilitation are made easier.
■ Independence and self-confidence are needed. The patient is helped to avoid helplessness.

III. DENTAL HYGIENE CARE: TOTALLY BLIND

A. Factors in Patient Care

■ A blind person can perceive a new experience readily if told about it in detail.
■ Because of the visual disability, the patient may tend to rely more on other senses and cultivate them.
■ A blind person tries to be neat and orderly. If something is put down, it needs to be found again.
■ A blind person learns to interpret and rely on tone of voice more than do persons with sight who can watch facial expressions.

B. Patient Reception and Seating

■ Lower chair before receiving the patient; move other dental equipment, such as the bracket tray and clinician's stool, from pathway.
■ Guide to dental chair. Patient holds arm and is led without being pushed or pulled **(Figure 59-1)**.
■ Provide forewarnings of potential hazards in the pathway.
■ The patient who has become familiar with the dental setting from previous appointments needs to be informed of changes to prevent embarrassment.
■ *Protective eyewear:* The patient may prefer to wear the personal glasses regularly worn. Many wear dark glasses.
■ When the dental hygienist leaves the treatment room during the appointment, explain absence; prevent embarrassment of patient speaking to someone who is not there; speak when reentering the room.

C. The Dog Guide

■ Do not distract a dog guide on duty by touching or speaking to it.
■ Ask the patient where the best place would be for the dog to stay during the appointment. The dogs are gentle, carefully trained animals, and may lie quietly in a corner of the treatment room as directed by the patient.

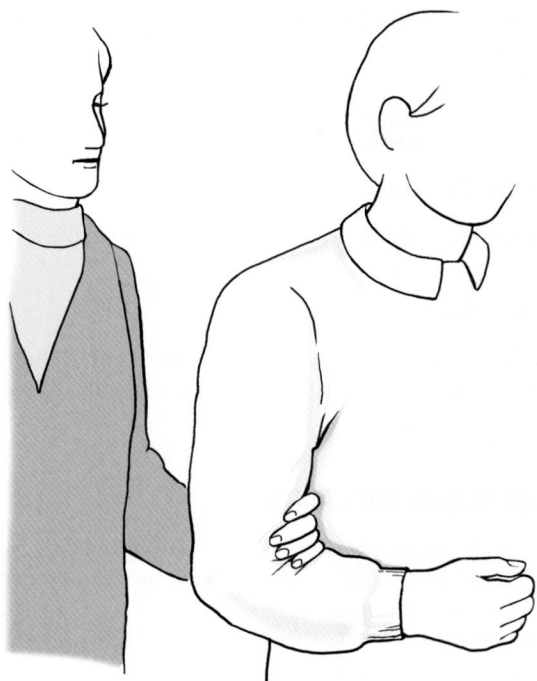

FIGURE 59-1 **Escorting a Blind Person.** The blind person holds the arm of the guide just above the elbow and walks beside and slightly behind. The guide verbally gives advance notice of approaching changes. The blind person can sense the body motion of the guide and anticipate changes.

D. Introduce Clinical Procedures

■ Describe each step in detail before proceeding. Explain instruments and materials, and how each will be applied. Mention flavors.

■ Permit patient to handle dull instruments, such as a mouth mirror. This applies particularly to a child patient who is not familiar with dental procedures.

■ Use other instruments of a similar size and shape when describing scalers or explorers because handling sharp instruments would be dangerous for the patient.

■ Prepare patient for power-driven instruments; avoid surprise applications of compressed air, water from syringe, or power-driven instruments.

■ Apply moving rubber cup to child's finger.

■ Speak before touching the patient. By maintaining contact of a finger on a tooth or through retraction while changing instruments, repeated orientation can be avoided.

■ Without evacuation, explain the water syringe and place rinsing cup in the patient's hand each time. Do not expect the patient to pick it up from unit.

E. Instructions for Patient

■ Give instructions clearly and concisely.

■ Demonstrate toothbrushing in the patient's mouth. Help learning by the feeling of the filament tips on and under the gingival margin and the feeling of clean teeth.

IV. DENTAL HYGIENE CARE: PARTIALLY SIGHTED

Persons with sight often underestimate how useful a little vision can be. Patience is needed to help a patient make full use of available vision, without oversolicitousness. Although many of the procedures described for the totally blind person can be applied to the partially sighted person, a few additional hints are suggested here.

■ Elderly patients with failing sight rarely admit such an impairment.

■ Sight failure in the older individual or lowered vision in a person of any age may be suspected from the patient's unusual squinting, blinking, or lack of continued attention.

■ Procedures can be adapted without mention of sight to the patient.

A. Patient Position

■ Adjust for patient comfort.

■ Tilting back a patient with glaucoma may increase pain and pressure in the eyes.

B. Light

■ Avoid glare of the dental light in the patient's eyes.

■ Sensitivity to light is characteristic of many eye conditions.

C. Patient Instruction

■ Position patient for best vision. For example, a patient with glaucoma has no peripheral vision; thus, instruction should be given directly from the front.

■ Do not expect a patient to see fine detail, such as that in a radiograph without enlargement or on a small model.

■ Work patiently and give instruction slowly. Patient may have slow visual accommodation.

HEARING IMPAIRMENT

■ When hearing is impaired to the extent that it has no practical value for the purpose of spoken communication, a person is considered deaf.

■ When hearing is defective but functional with or without a hearing aid, the terms "a person who is hard of hearing" or "a person with hearing loss" are used.

■ Terminology is changing and reflects the ways in which people prefer to identify themselves.

I. CAUSES OF HEARING IMPAIRMENT

■ The auditory system includes the anatomic parts from the outer ear to the termination of the auditory nerve in the brain.

- The cause of hearing loss may be associated with the outer, middle, or inner ear mechanisms, singly or in combinations. Many factors may contribute to deafness.
- Heredity, prenatal infection in the mother, especially rubella, and birth trauma are significant in the earliest years.
- Chronic inner ear infections, infectious diseases (meningitis), trauma, and toxic effects of drugs have all been implicated.
- *Newborn screening:* The spread of universal programs to identify hearing defects in newborns has been a significant contribution to healthcare.[1]

II. TYPES OF HEARING LOSS

A. Conductive Hearing Loss

Outer or middle ear involvement of the conduction pathways to the inner ear.

B. Sensorineural Hearing Loss

Damage to the sensory hair cells of the inner ear or the nerves that supply the inner ear.

C. Mixed Hearing Loss

Combination of conductive and sensorineural.

D. Central Hearing Loss

Damage of the nerves or nuclei of the central nervous system in the brain or the pathways to the brain.

III. CHARACTERISTICS SUGGESTING HEARING LOSS

- Partial deafness may not have been diagnosed, or certain patients, particularly elderly ones, may not admit hearing limitation. Clues to the identification of a hearing problem are suggested as follows.
  - Lack of attention; fails to respond to conversation.
  - Intentness; strained facial expression; stares at others.
  - Turns head to one side; hearing may be good on one side only.
  - Gives unexpected answer unrelated to question; does one thing when told to do another.
  - Frequently asks others to repeat what was said.
  - Unusual speech quality.

IV. HEARING AIDS

- A hearing aid is an electronic device that amplifies and shapes sound waves that enter the external auditory canal.
- Current hearing aids are more technically advanced and esthetic in their invisibility.

- Standards for the manufacture and distribution of hearing aids are set by the United States Food and Drug Administration. A medical evaluation is required along with extensive audiological testing.

A. In-the-Ear Model

The units are practically invisible and lightweight.

B. Canal Aid

This model fits entirely within the canal and is the most cosmetically acceptable of all types. It may take extra skill to remove and adjust.

V. COCHLEAR IMPLANTS

- A small electronic device that helps provide a sense of sound to a child or adult who is profoundly deaf or severely hard of hearing.
- The implant consists of an external portion that is behind the ear and a second part that is surgically placed under the skin.
- An implant does not restore normal hearing. It gives useful representations of sounds from the environment through a microphone and speech processor and sends them directly to the auditory nerve of the brain.

VI. MODES OF COMMUNICATION

A person with a hearing loss may learn a particular way of personal communication. Choices include speaking, speechreading, writing, manual, or a combination. Manual communication includes using sign language or "signing" and fingerspelling. *Always ask the patient which means of communication is preferred and how communication can be improved.*

A. American Sign Language (ASL)

The American manual alphabet is shown in **Figure 59-2**.[2] A few examples of signs are shown in **Figure 59-3**.

- ASL is a visual/gestural language with a unique grammar and syntax.
- Many deaf people who prefer this mode of communication grew up using ASL and consider themselves part of a cultural group.
- Other individuals who have become deaf in later years may learn sign language and use the signs in English word order.
- Some deaf people prefer to communicate using ASL in medical or dental situations. They can request the services of an ASL interpreter.
- Although a universal sign language has not been recognized, many countries have their own.

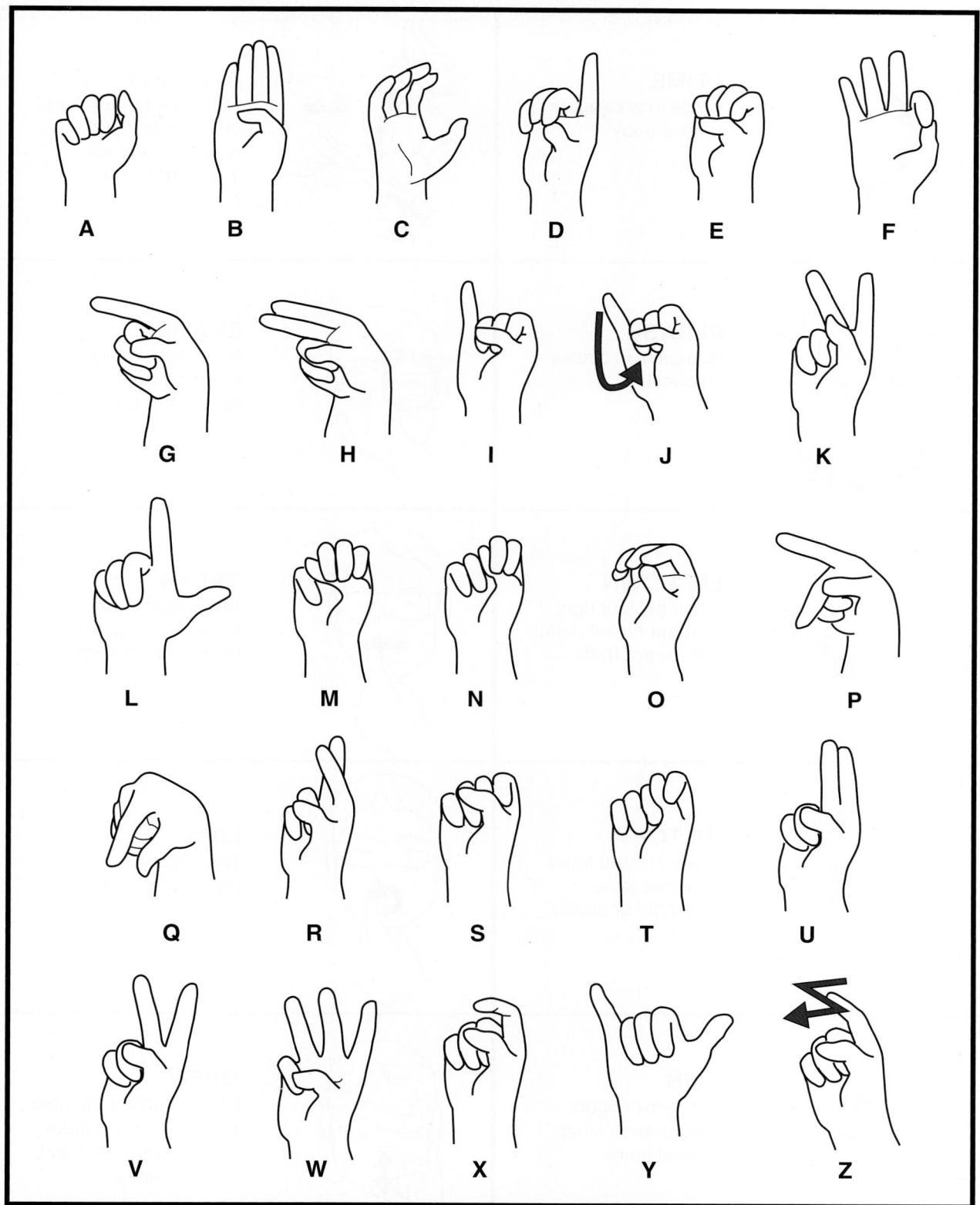

FIGURE 59-2 **American Manual Alphabet.** Fingerspelling is used in combination with signs and speechreading. (Reprinted with permission from Lane LG. *The Gallaudet survival guide to signing.* Washington: Gallaudet University Press; 1990.)

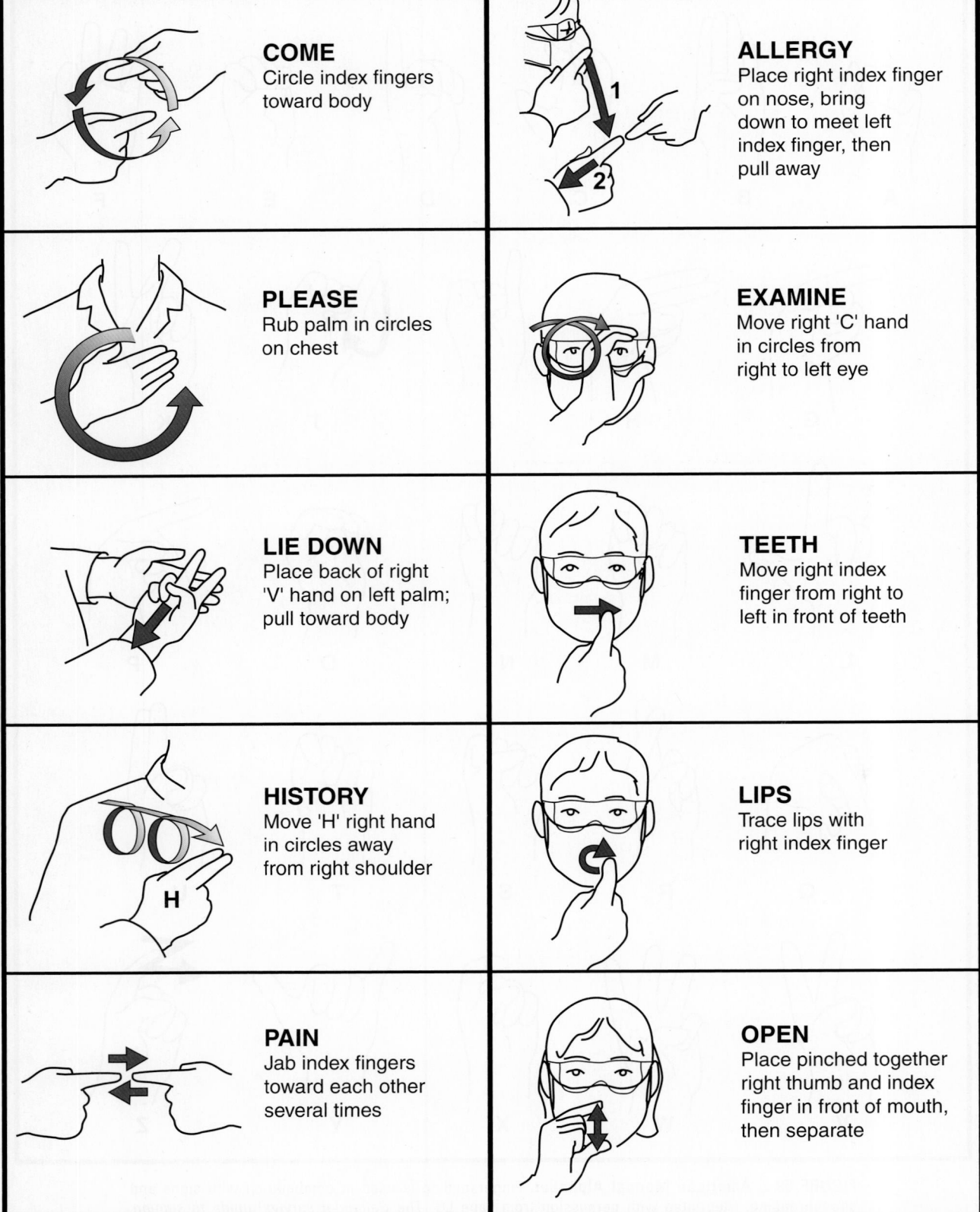

COME
Circle index fingers toward body

ALLERGY
Place right index finger on nose, bring down to meet left index finger, then pull away

PLEASE
Rub palm in circles on chest

EXAMINE
Move right 'C' hand in circles from right to left eye

LIE DOWN
Place back of right 'V' hand on left palm; pull toward body

TEETH
Move right index finger from right to left in front of teeth

HISTORY
Move 'H' right hand in circles away from right shoulder

LIPS
Trace lips with right index finger

PAIN
Jab index fingers toward each other several times

OPEN
Place pinched together right thumb and index finger in front of mouth, then separate

FIGURE 59-3 **Examples of Signing.** Selected words that may be used during a patient's dental appointment. (Adapted with permission from Lane LG. *The Gallaudet survival guide to signing.* Washington: Gallaudet University Press; 1990.) (*Continued*)

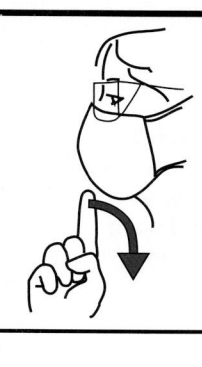

SWALLOW
Move extended right index finger from chin down throat

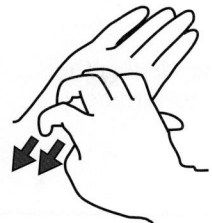

SCRAPE
Move fingertips of right hand on back of left hand in scraping motion

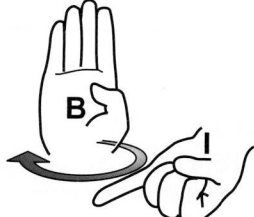

BACTERIA
Right 'B' hand circles on little finger of palm up 'I' hand

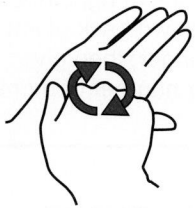

POLISH
Rub knuckles of right hand on back of left hand

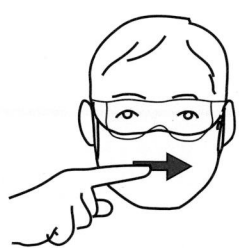

TOOTHBRUSH
Brush teeth with right index finger

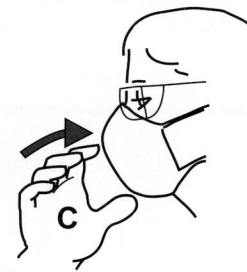

DRINK
Place thumb of right 'C' hand on chin and tip up to mouth

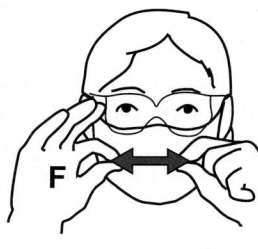

FLOSS
Hold imaginary floss between right 'F' hand and pinched together left thumb and index finger; move back and forth

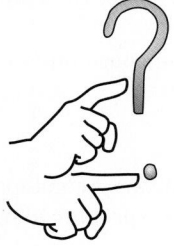

QUESTION
Draw question mark with index finger; place dot underneath

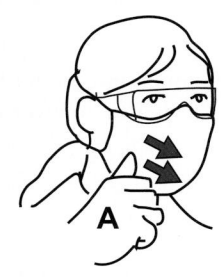

DAILY
Brush right 'A' hand forward on cheek twice

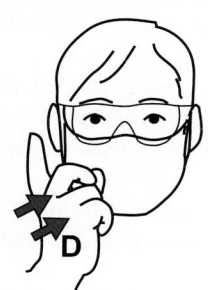

DENTIST
Tap right 'D' hand on corner of mouth twice

FIGURE 59-3 **Examples of Signing.** (*Continued*)

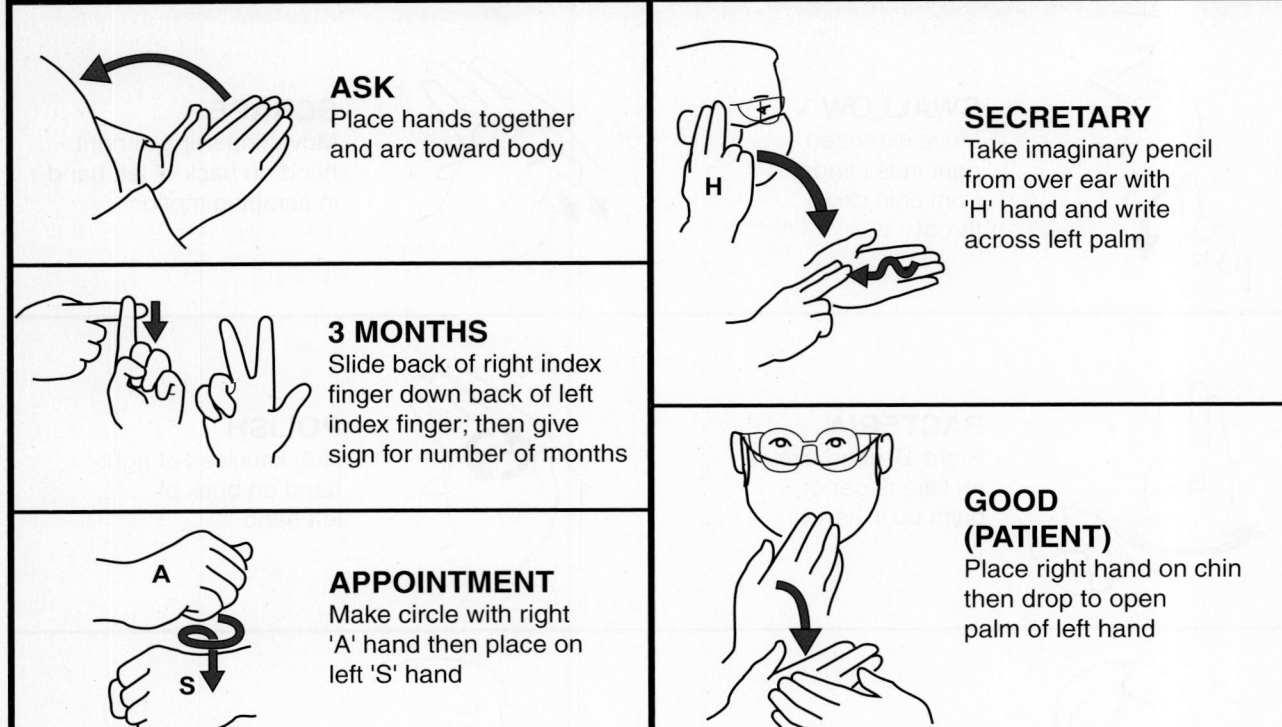

ASK
Place hands together and arc toward body

3 MONTHS
Slide back of right index finger down back of left index finger; then give sign for number of months

APPOINTMENT
Make circle with right 'A' hand then place on left 'S' hand

SECRETARY
Take imaginary pencil from over ear with 'H' hand and write across left palm

GOOD (PATIENT)
Place right hand on chin then drop to open palm of left hand

FIGURE 59-3 **Examples of Signing.** (*Continued*)

B. Fingerspelling

- Spelling "in the air" is often combined with sign language.
- When making an introduction, for example, the name may be fingerspelled.
- New words that enter the scientific language often do not have signs and are fingerspelled.

C. Oral Communication

Oral communication by a deaf person means a combination of some speech, residual hearing, and speechreading.

D. Speechreading

- Speechreading consists of recognizing spoken words by watching the lips, face, and gestures.
- Many of the mouth movements for spoken words have the same appearance as one or more other words, so speechreading may need to be combined with another method of communication.
- Speechreading is not a reliable means of communication for extended, complex discussions for most people with hearing loss.
- Speechreading is not a choice when clinician must wear a mask.

E. Writing

Writing may be an alternative when other methods are not satisfactory.

VII. DENTAL HYGIENE CARE

- Patients with hearing problems are of all ages; some have been deaf all their lives, and others lost their hearing later in life. Each has special problems.
- Determination of the mode of communication is an important step at the outset. Always ask the patient. An interpreter may be required.
- When the patient's preferred mode of communication is sign language and the clinician does not know sign language, or when the patient lip-reads but cannot read the clinician's lips because the clinician is wearing a mask, writing on a pad of paper may be the first choice.
- Some deaf individuals may not be fluent in the English language and will need the services of an interpreter for extensive communication such as review of an involved treatment plan.

A. Patient With Hearing Aid

- Be careful not to touch a hearing aid when it is turned on.
- Ask the patient to turn off or remove a hearing aid when a power-driven dental instrument, particularly a power-driven scaler, will be used. The noise can be amplified many times, much to the discomfort of the patient.

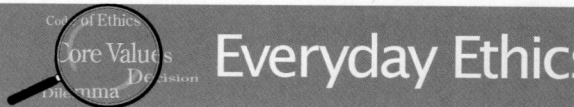
Everyday Ethics

Mr. Dolson was scheduled for 11:00 AM with Regan, the newest dental hygienist in the practice. He arrived about 15 minutes late, so Regan was ready and waiting to begin the maintenance appointment. She quickly escorted Mr. Dolson to the chair and began the oral examination without much talking. Mr. Dolson sensed that Regan was in a hurry but was uncertain of what to say. He wore a hearing aid but didn't always turn it on. He had been known to "blurt out" his thoughts rather loudly at times not realizing the volume or tone of his voice. "Tell me if I'm doing a good job with my brushing," began Mr. Dolson. Rather startled, Regan said "You're really not brushing well at all!" Mr. Dolson grew very quiet.

Questions for Consideration

1. Professionally and ethically, how would you describe the provider–patient relationship in this scenario? Which of the dental hygiene core values (Table II -1, in Section II Introduction, page 38) are illustrated here?

2. Was Regan's response to Mr. Dolson justified? Why or why not? Explain your rationale.

3. How can virtue ethics apply to a patient with special needs such as a hearing impairment or other loss of sensory functions? Go to Appendix II, page 1089, in the Canadian Dental Hygienists' Code of Ethics to read about "virtue ethics."

B. Patient With Partial Hearing Ability

- Speak clearly and distinctly. When it is necessary to talk, be sure to face the patient. With the dental light directed toward the patient's mouth, the clinician's face may be in the background.
- Eliminate interfering noises from the street outside or from saliva ejector suction.

C. Speechreader

- Be sure patient is looking; do not turn to side; speak directly.
- Speaker's face must be clearly visible so patient can read lips easily.
- Speak in normal tone; do not exaggerate words; slow the pace of speech; pause more frequently than usual.
- Do not raise voice; raising voice can distort lip movements and make lip reading more difficult.
- When the patient cannot understand, use alternate words to express the same thought; many letters and combinations of letters look the same on the lips; others are not visible at all.
- Keep calm; display of irritation or annoyance over difficulties in conversing can discourage or upset the patient.
- Write proper names or unusual words the patient fails to understand.
- When wearing a mask, certain gestures may be agreed upon in advance.

D. Sign Language

- All the points previously mentioned for the speechreader apply to patients who use sign language because lips are read along with signs.
- When a dental hygienist knows a few signs to use, a deaf patient will greatly appreciate them.

- Learning basic sign language and fingerspelling can provide healthcare workers with added skills and reduce stress for the deaf patient.

E. General Suggestions

- For written messages, use a clipboard with a marker-type pen attached and large paper, at least 8½ × 11 inches. Write clearly.
- Ask the patient if a gentle tap on the hand or arm is an appropriate way to get attention.
- Plan in advance for a signal the patient can give to show reaction or discomfort.
- Teach by demonstration; use mirror and show dental biofilm removal methods directly on teeth.
- Person with hearing loss always needs to have a written appointment card to ensure complete understanding.
- Use the state Telecommunication Relay Service (TRS) to call a deaf patient directly with appointment reminders.
- Use judgment in prolonging conversation with a deaf person. Certain patients are under tension and tire easily, whereas others enjoy the opportunity to communicate.

DOCUMENTATION

The permanent records for patients with sensory disabilities are completed at each appointment with changes in the patient's health history, medications, and oral examinations. In addition, progress notes concerning the following need to be emphasized with each individual appointment:

- Special needs and adjustments related to the individual physical problems and how the disability affects attaining optimum oral health.
- Frequency of appointments to allow for extra assistance that more professional care and attention will provide.
- A sample progress note may be read in **Box 59-2.**

BOX 59-2	Example Progress Note

Patient wearing very thick-lensed glasses, and walking with a cane appeared for 10:00 appointment. Nothing in the preliminary record had mentioned that Ms. Alton (new patient to the practice) had a vision problem. She had completed the health history questionnaire while in the reception area. Clara wrote: "I hastily scanned the questionnaire although handwriting was very difficult to read." Asked if she had a particular problem she said no, she had recently moved here and needed a dental hygienist to clean her teeth. Ms. Alton told me: "My niece is a dental hygienist where I used to live and she suggested that I find a dentist with a dental hygienist because dentists do not learn the high degree of skills that you girls do. Where did you go to school?" Most of our conversation was on that theme, and I finally completed an extra–intra oral exam and probing chart: some 3–4-mm depths with calculus in molar areas; she will ask her niece to mail the recent radiographs. Asked if she preferred to have anesthesia for scaling, she was surprised and said her niece never offered that so "I must not have needed it." Complete scaling mand left quad where the most calculus was found. Her vision seemed not to be a problem, but she preferred to keep her own glasses on rather than wear our eye-protection ones. Appt made for one week; will do biofilm review and continue scaling.

Signed: _____, RDH Date: _____

Factors To Teach The Patient

- Why it is important to provide complete information when the medical history is reviewed.
- New ways for better biofilm control.
- For the person with limited sight: why to avoid using toothpicks or other sharp objects to clean the teeth.
- Ways to prevent dental caries, especially for children and teenagers with limited sight.
- The importance of oral care for the dog guide.

References

1. Morton CC, Nance WE. Newborn hearing screening—a silent revolution. *N Engl J Med.* 2006 May;354(20):2151–64.
2. Lane LG. *The Gallaudet survival guide to signing.* Washington: Gallaudet University Press; 1990.

CHAPTER 60

The Patient With a Developmental or Behavioral Disorder

KAREN A. RAPOSA, RDH, MBA

Chapter Outline

More people with developmental disabilities are seeking dental care in private and community settings as the trend toward deinstitutionalization grows and emphasis on special training and education in local agencies and schools increases. Opportunities to contribute to the health and well-being of all patients are available in all dental care delivery environments.

- Developmental disabilities are a diverse group of severe chronic conditions that are due to mental and/or physical impairments.
- People with developmental disabilities have problems with major life activities such as language, mobility, learning, self-help, and independent living.
- Developmental disabilities begin anytime during development up to 22 years of age and usually last throughout a person's lifetime.[1]

This chapter includes mental disabilities with specific emphasis on Down syndrome and autism spectrum disorder (ASD), two of the major categories of mental disabilities that dental professionals encounter in standard dental settings. **Box 60-1** provides descriptive terminology and other key words and **Box 60-2** lists the major categories of disorders.[2]

AUTISM SPECTRUM DISORDER

Autism spectrum disorder is a complex developmental disorder marked by limitations in the ability to understand and communicate.

- Brain function is severely disordered; the way the brain uses or transmits information is affected.

BOX 60-1	Key Words

Intellectual Disorders

Autism spectrum disorder: a developmental disorder, generally evident before age 3, affecting verbal and nonverbal communications and social interaction.

Brachycephalic: having a short, wide head.

Comorbid: existing simultaneously with and usually independently of another medical condition; coexisting or additional disease processes. Comorbidity may affect ability to function or survive.

Coprolalia: involuntary utterance of vulgar or obscene words.

Dysgenesis: defective development; malformation.

Dysmorphism: abnormality in morphologic development.

Echolalia: echo reaction; the involuntary repetition of a word or sentence just spoken by another person.

Epicanthus: a vertical fold of skin on either side of the nose, sometimes covering the inner canthus; a normal characteristic in persons of certain races.

Hyperactivity: abnormally increased activity.

Development hyperactivity (hyperkinesis): characterized by constant motion, fidgetiness, excitability, impulsiveness, and a short attention span.

Intelligence quotient (IQ): numeric rating determined through psychologic testing that indicates the approximate relationship of a person's mental age (MA) to chronologic age (CA).

Macroglossia: very large tongue.

Microcephalus: abnormally small head size in relation to the rest of the body.

Mutism: inability or refusal to speak; deafness may prevent learning to speak.

Selective mutism: consistent failure to speak in specific social situations despite speaking in other situations.

Pathognomonic: characteristic or indicative of a particular disease or syndrome; especially one or more typical symptoms.

Pervasive: throughout entire individual, entire development is severely and markedly impaired, as in autism spectrum disorder.

Pica: persistent craving/eating of nonnutritive substances or unnatural articles of food.

Rumination: repeated regurgitation of food in the absence of any associated gastrointestinal illness.

Self-injury: act of deliberate harm to one's own body. Also called self-abuse, self-directed aggression, self-harm, self-inflicted injury, self-mutilation.

Stereotypic movement disorder: repetitive, nonfunctional motor behavior that interferes with normal activities and may result in bodily injury.

Tic: an involuntary, sudden, rapid, recurrent, nonrhythmic, stereotyped motor movement or vocal sound.

Ultrasonography: the location, measurement, or delineation of deep structures by measuring the reflection or transmission of ultrasonic waves. Used in examination of fetus to determine birth defects.

- Usually appears during early childhood and persists throughout life.
- Manifested by a range of impairments rather than by the presence or absence of a certain behavior or symptom.
- Variations of autism behaviors have been grouped by the American Psychiatric Association as related disorders under the broad heading *Pervasive Development Disorder (PDD)*, a general category of disorders marked by severe and pervasive impairment in several areas of development.
- The *DSM-IV-TR*[2] uses the terms PDD and ASD to describe five variations of autism behaviors. Major points that distinguish the differences between the categories are outlined in **Table 60-1**.[3]

I. CHARACTERISTICS

- Spectrum of symptoms ranging from mild to severe.
- Social, communication, and behavioral features are shown in **Box 60-3**. Not all individuals have the same degree of impairment; *any combination* of symptoms and behaviors *in any degree of severity* can be exhibited.[3]
- Characteristic features include the following:
  A. Problems with social interactions
  B. Problems with verbal and nonverbal communication

C. Ritualistic or compulsive behaviors
D. Atypical responses to the environment

II. PREVALENCE

- Prevalence has increased in recent years.
- Some increase in prevalence may be attributable to changes in diagnostic criteria and in the conditions being categorized under the PDD and ASD umbrella terms.
- Occurs in all racial, ethnic, and social groups worldwide.
- Frequency of occurrence is four times greater in males (usually the firstborn) than in females.

III. ETIOLOGY

- Exact cause is unknown.
- Related factors include genetics, viruses, chemicals, and inadequate oxygenation at birth.[4]

IV. INTERVENTIONS

There is no "cure," in the medical sense, for autism. Interventions based on the management of autism as a

BOX 60-2	Disorders Usually First Diagnosed in Infancy, Childhood, or Adolescence

INTELLECTUAL DISORDERS: disorders characterized by significantly subaverage intellectual functioning (IQ of approximately 70 or below) with onset before age 18, and concurrent deficits in adaptive functioning, and includes:

- Mild, moderate, severe, and profound classifications

LEARNING DISORDERS: disorders characterized by academic functioning substantially below the expected level for chronological age, measured IQ, and age-appropriate education, and includes:

- Reading disorder
- Mathematics disorder
- Disorder of written expression

MOTOR SKILLS DISORDERS: disorders characterized by motor coordination substantially below the level expected for chronological age and measured intelligence

- Developmental coordination disorder

COMMUNICATION DISORDERS: disorders characterized by difficulties in speech or language, and include

- Expressive language disorder
- Mixed receptive-expressive language disorder
- Phonological disorder
- Stuttering

PERVASIVE DEVELOPMENTAL DISORDERS: disorders characterized by severe deficits and pervasive impairment in multiple developmental areas, as reciprocal social interaction, communication, and the presence of stereotyped behavior, interests and activities, and includes

- autism disorder
- Rett disorder

- childhood disintegrative disorder
- Asperger disorder
- pervasive developmental disorder not otherwise specified

ATTENTION-DEFICIT and DISRUPTIVE BEHAVIOR DISORDERS: disorders characterized by prominent symptoms of inattention and/or hyperactivity-impulsivity, and includes

- Attention-deficit/hyperactivity disorder
- Conduct disorder
- Oppositional defiant disorder

FEEDING and EATING DISORDERS of INFANCY or EARLY CHILDHOOD: disorders characterized by persistent disturbances in feeding or eating, and includes

- Pica
- Rumination disorder
- Feeding disorder of infancy or early childhood

TIC DISORDERS: disorders that are inherent and neurological in nature, characterized by vocal and/or motor tics, and includes

- Chronic motor or vocal tic disorder
- Transient tic disorder

ELIMINATION DISORDERS: disorders characterized by repeated passage of body wastes into inappropriate places, and includes

- Enuresis
- Encopresis

OTHER DISORDERS not covered in previous sections

- Separation anxiety disorder
- Selective mutism
- Reactive attachment disorder of infancy or early childhood
- Stereotypic movement disorder

(Adapted with permission from American Psychiatric Association: DSM-IV-TR; 2000. 39–41 pp.)[2]

TABLE 60-1	PERVASIVE DEVELOPMENTAL DISORDER AND AUTISM SPECTRUM DISORDER
Autism Spectrum Disorder	- Impairments in verbal and nonverbal communication and social (aka: classic autism) interaction, and restrictive or repetitive patterns of behavior, interests, and activities. - Symptoms are usually measurable by 18 mo of age; formal diagnosis is usually made between ages 2–3 y, when delays in language development are apparent.
Asperger Disorder	- Characterized by impairments in social interactions and restricted interests and activities, without clinically significant delays in language, cognitive ability, or developmental age-appropriate skills.
Pervasive Developmental Disorder— Not Otherwise Specified	- Severe and pervasive impairment in specified behaviors, without meeting all of the criteria for a specific diagnosis (aka: atypical autism).
Rett Disorder (aka: Rett syndrome)	- Occurs only in girls, causing the development of autism-like (aka: Rett syndrome) symptoms after a period of seemingly normal development. - Purposeful use of hands is lost and replaced by repetitive hand movements beginning between ages 1–4 y. - In 1999, researchers identified a gene responsible for Rett syndrome.
Childhood Disintegrative Disorder	- Characterized by normal development for at least the first 2 y followed by a significant loss of previously acquired skills.

Modified with permission from Rapin I. Perspective: The Autistic-Spectrum Disorders. *N Engl J Med.* 2002 Aug; 347:302.

BOX 60-3	Characteristics of Autism

- Impairment in social interaction
  - A. Impairment in use of nonverbal behaviors (e.g., eye-to-eye gaze, facial expression, gestures)
  - B. Failure to develop peer relationships appropriate to developmental level
  - C. Lack of spontaneous seeking to share enjoyment, interests, or achievements with others
  - D. Lack of social or emotional reciprocity
- Impairment in communication
  - A. Delay or total lack of spoken language
  - B. Individuals with adequate speech: impairment in conversational abilities
  - C. Repetitive use of language
  - D. Lack of spontaneous make-believe play
- Restricted repetitive and stereotyped patterns of behavior
  - A. Preoccupation with stereotyped and restricted patterns of interest
  - B. Inflexible adherence to routines or rituals
  - C. Repetitive body movements and mannerisms
  - D. Persistent preoccupation with parts of objects
- Delays or abnormal functioning before age 3 years
  - A. Social interaction
  - B. Language as used in social communication
  - C. Symbolic or imaginative play

(*Source:* American Psychiatric Association. DSM-IV-TR; 2000. 70–74 pp.)[2]

brain-based disorder have changed treatments dramatically since it was first described by Dr. Leo Kanner.[5]

A. Pharmacological Treatments

- Purpose: relief of negative behavioral symptoms (such as aggression, self-injury, and other more difficult behaviors).
- Types of drugs: stimulants (such as methylphenidate, *Ritalin*), antidepressants, opiate blockers, and tranquilizers.
- *Risperidone*, an atypical antipsychotic medication, has been shown to be significantly more effective than placebo in improving behavior, representing the largest positive effect by a medication ever observed in children with autism.[6]
- Identification and medical management of comorbid, potentially treatable conditions (e.g., epilepsy seizures, allergies, gastrointestinal problems, or sleep disorders) can lead to quality-of-life improvements.

B. Behavioral Therapy Treatments

- Purpose: help people with autism lead more normal lives by decreasing symptoms and increasing their ability to respond.[7]

- Examples: special teachers in intensive structured programs directed toward individual instruction, applied behavior analysis, sensory integration, music therapy, occupational therapy, speech and language therapy, and auditory integration training.
- No one behaviorally based or educational approach is effective in alleviating symptoms in all cases of autism because of the spectrum nature of the condition and the many behavior combinations that can occur.[7]

C. Prognosis

- Life expectancy: normal.
- Social and communication deficits continue in some form throughout life; some of the negative behaviors may change or diminish over time with appropriate treatment.[7,8]

DOWN SYNDROME

- Unique group of individuals with a chromosomal abnormality: Down syndrome or trisomy 21 syndrome.
- Prenatal screening has contributed to lowering the incidence.[9]
- Parental age
  - A. Formerly, incidence of births with Down syndrome tended to increase with mother's age. More recently, mother's age has decreased.[10]
  - B. Evidence shows the father can be the source of the chromosomal abnormality.[11]

I. PHYSICAL CHARACTERISTICS

Patients with Down syndrome have a combination of characteristic abnormalities that is relatively constant. They tend to resemble one another.

- Stature: short with short neck.
  - A. Awkward, waddling gait.
  - B. General growth retardation.
- Head: microcephalus.
- Nose: short, underdeveloped.
- Hair: scanty.
- Eyes: oblique slant laterally.
  - A. Narrow opening between eyelids.
  - B. Epicanthic fold of skin continues from upper eyelid over the inner angle of the eye **(Figure 60-1)**.
  - C. Nearsightedness, eyes crossing inward, and cataracts are common.
- Hands
  - A. Fingers: stubby, short.
  - B. Palm: single, transverse palmar crease may be present **(Figure 60-2)**.

II. INTELLECTUAL ABILITY

- IQ usually under 70.
- Longer institutionalized person may have lower IQ score.

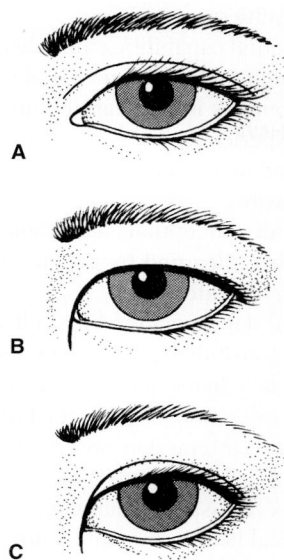

FIGURE 60-1 **Down Syndrome: Eye Characteristics. (A)** Absence of an epicanthic fold. **(B)** Epicanthic fold in Oriental populations. **(C)** Epicanthic fold of person with Down syndrome. (*Source:* Smith, GF and Berg, JM. Down's Anomaly, 2nd ed. Edinburgh: Churchill Livingstone; 1976).

- Socially, many children are more advanced and may appear to have higher intelligence.
- Many people with Down syndrome enjoy music and have a good sense of rhythm. Background music in office may help in gaining rapport.

III. PERSONAL CHARACTERISTICS

Typical characteristics listed here may suggest management approaches for dental and dental hygiene appointments.

- Like attention; require affection for feeling of security.
- Cheerful disposition; rarely irritable; easily amused.
- Sociable, observant; take initiative.

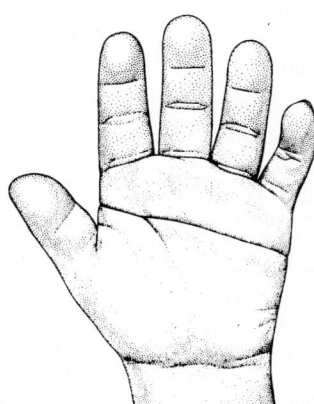

FIGURE 60-2 **Down Syndrome: Hand.** Short, stubby fingers with little finger curved inward are characteristic. An identifying feature is the single transverse palmar crease. (*Source:* Smith, GF and Berg, JM. Down's Anomaly, 2nd ed. Edinburgh: Churchill Livingstone; 1976).

- Tendency to imitate; mischievous.
- Periods of stubbornness; obstinate and determined to have their own way. Parental discipline is necessary. In the dental hygiene appointment, the initial approach can be important to continued control and cooperation.

IV. ORAL FINDINGS

- Lips
  - A. Habitually, the child with Down syndrome holds the mouth open with the tongue protruded.
  - B. Lips may be thickened, cracked, and dry, a result of bathing in saliva while the mouth is open.
- Mouthbreathing is common.
- Respiratory infections are frequent.
- Tongue and palate
  - A. Tongue may be deeply fissured and appear large.
  - B. The jaws and palate are narrow: tend to force the tongue into protrusion; may appear larger than it really is.
- Cleft lip, palate, or uvula: incidence greater than in general population.[12]
- Teeth
  - A. Delayed eruption: irregular in sequence of eruption.
  - B. Microdontia and congenitally missing teeth not uncommon.
  - C. Anomalies such as fused teeth, peg lateral.
- Occlusion
  - A. Angle's Class III and posterior crossbite are common and relate to the flat face and underdevelopment of the midfacial region.
  - B. Teeth may be spaced because certain anomalous teeth take less space.
- Periodontal infections[13]
  - A. Periodontal conditions are more severe in people with Down syndrome.
  - B. Bone loss and other effects of periodontal infection may be present.
  - C. Leukocyte function is altered by impaired chemotaxis and phagocytosis.[14]
  - D. Altered immune response contributes to the increased severity of periodontal infection.

V. HEALTH PROBLEMS SIGNIFICANT TO DENTAL HYGIENE CARE

- The mortality rate has been high during the early years because of high susceptibility to respiratory infections, leukemia, and congenital heart lesions.
- More recent improvements in child healthcare and immunizations have brought a longer life expectancy.
- Susceptibility to infection: defects in the body's immune defense mechanisms lead to greater susceptibility to various infections.
- Obstructive airway problems.[15]
  - A. Contributing factors: macroglossia, increased secretions, frequent respiratory infections, obesity, enlarged tonsils and adenoids.

B. Dental hygiene adaptations: chair position, fluid suctioning, gag reflex.
- Congenital heart lesions
  A. Antibiotic premedication will be needed for many patients.
  B. High incidence of mitral valve prolapse in this population.[16]
- Relation to Alzheimer's disease
  A. Adults with Down syndrome age prematurely.
  B. Many over the age of 40 develop an Alzheimer's-like dementia with pathologic brain changes similar to those of Alzheimer's disease.[17]
  C. Changes occur in memory, speech, gait, personality, and other characteristics. Alzheimer's disease is described in Chapter 52 on page 802.

INTELLECTUAL DISORDER

I. DEFINITION[18,19]

Intellectual disorder is sometimes referred to as a cognitive disorder or mental retardation and is characterized by:

- Significant limitations in intellectual functioning.
- Significant limitations in adaptive behavior as expressed in conceptual, social, and practical adaptive skills.
- Origination before age 18.

II. DIMENSIONS OF INTELLECTUAL DISABILITIES[19]

Five interrelated dimensions contribute to testing the individual's functioning ability.

- Intellectual abilities
  A. General mental capabilities include reasoning, planning, solving problems, thinking abstractly, comprehending complex ideas, learning quickly, and learning from experience.
  B. Represented by IQ scores.
- Adaptive behavior
  A. Collection of conceptual, social, and practical skills that have been learned by people in order to function in everyday life.
  B. Conceptual (language, reading, self-direction).
  C. Social (responsibility, self-esteem, law abiding).
  D. Practical (daily living activities, occupational skills).
- Participation, interactions, and social roles
  A. Participation (interaction observed by direct observation).
  B. Social roles (age-specific activity).
- Health (physical health, mental health, etiology)
  A. Physical and mental health and especially medications have definite influence on the assessment of intelligence and adaptive behavior.
  B. Etiology: related to four categories of risk factors **(Table 60-2)**.
- Context (environment, culture)
  A. Environmental: residence and surroundings that provide for learning and development.
  B. Fostering personal well-being, safety, in relation to all of the first four dimensions.

III. SUPPORTS[20]

- Supports are strategies and resources selected to improve the functioning of the individual.

TABLE 60-2	RISK FACTORS FOR INTELLECTUAL DISORDER			
TIMING	**BIOMEDICAL**	**SOCIAL**	**BEHAVIORAL**	**EDUCATIONAL**
Prenatal	Chromosomal disorders Single-gene disorders Syndromes Metabolic disorders Cerebral dysgenesis Maternal illnesses Parental age	Povery Maternal malnutrition Domestic violence Lack of access to prenatal care	Parental drug use Parental alcohol use Parental smoking Parental immaturity	Parental cognitive disorder without supports Lack of preparation for parenthood
Perinatal	Prematurity Birth injury Neonatal disorders	Lack of access to birth care	Parental rejection of caretaking Parental abandonment of child	Lack of medical referral of intervention services at discharge
Postnatal	Traumatic brain injury Malnutrition Meningoencephalitis Seizure disorders Fetal alcohol syndrome Congenital heart disease	Impaired child-caregiver Inadequate parenting skills Family poverty Chronic illness in the family Institutionalization	Child abuse and neglect Domestic violence Inadequate safety measures Social deprivation Difficult child behaviors	Impaired parenting Delayed diagnosis Inadequate early intervention services Inadequate special educational services Inadequate family support

Modified with permission from American Association on Mental Retardation: Mental Retardation, Definition, Classification, and Systems of Support. 10th ed. Washington, DC: AAMR; 2002. 127 p.

■ Purposes
  A. To promote development, education, interests, and personal well-being.
  B. To improve individual functioning and functional capabilities.
  C. To lessen the person's disorder by providing services and interventions that focus on prevention.
  D. To enhance personal outcomes related to independence, community participation, and personal well-being.
■ Types of supports
  A. Supported learning and education.
  B. Supported living.
  C. Supported health services.
  D. Supported employment.
■ Application of supports
  A. Needs of the individual determine supports.
  B. Health deficiencies can influence improvements expected from other supports.
■ Dental hygiene care provides support for the patient's
  A. freedom from oral discomfort and pain.
  B. learning self-care for daily oral biofilm removal.
  C. Improved quality of life.

IV. CLASSIFICATION OF INTELLECTUAL DISABILITIES

■ The levels of intellectual functioning are designated *mild, moderate, severe,* and *profound.*
■ Standardized intelligence tests are used to determine individual levels.
■ The intelligence quotient (IQ) expresses the test results.
■ The category of *"Unspecified"* is used when standard tests cannot be performed because of lack of cooperation, severe impairment, or infancy.

A. Mild

■ IQ approximate range 50 to 69 (adult mental age from 9 to under 12 years).
■ Adaptive behavior
  A. *Child*
    1. In special classes for the educable, child advances to a level of third to sixth grade.
    2. Practical skills can be learned.
  B. *Adult*
    1. Individual cares for personal hygiene and other necessities, with supports.
    2. Communication is good; attention span and memory are less than average.
    3. Activities that do not require involved planning or rapid implementation can be carried out satisfactorily.
    4. Most educable individuals can engage in semi-skilled or simple skilled work with guidance, and so maintain themselves.

B. Moderate

■ IQ approximate range 35 to 49 (adult mental age from 6 to under 9 years).
■ Adaptive behavior
  A. *Child*
    1. A marked developmental lag occurs in the early years; child can be trained in personal care and hygiene with support.
    2. Attends classes and learns simple habits and skills; does not learn to read and write.
    3. Speaks in short sentences; understands best when single-thought, short sentences are used.
    4. Participates well in group activities.
  B. *Adult*
    1. Attends to personal care, with support.
    2. Has relatively short attention span and memory.
    3. May have problems of coordination, but performs simple tasks and is conscientious about taking responsibility for errands and helpful duties.
    4. Not completely capable of self-maintenance; many do unskilled work with supervision and support.

C. Severe

■ IQ approximate range 20 to 34 (adult mental age from 3 to under 6 years).
■ Adaptive behavior
  A. *Child*
    1. Benefits from systematic habit training.
    2. May make attempts at personal care and dressing with support.
    3. Usually walks, uses some speech, and responds to directions.
  B. *Adult*
    1. Conforms to daily routine.
    2. May help with household and other small tasks in spite of limited attention span.
    3. Likely to need continuous support.

D. Profound

■ IQ under 20 (adult mental age below 3 years).
■ Adaptive behavior
  A. *Child*
    1. Delays occur in all phases of development.
    2. Close supervision and care are necessary.
  B. *Adult*
    1. Many remain inert and placid throughout early years; never learn to sit up.
    2. Results in severe limitation in self-care, continence, communication, and mobility.

V. ETIOLOGY

■ Intellectual disorder represents a more or less important symptom in well over 200 different conditions. Many of these are rare.

- Causes can be divided into factors occurring before birth, at or around birth, and after birth. A majority are prenatally related.
- Diagnosis can be complicated; many cases can only be identified as of unknown origin.

A. Importance of Etiology

- The cause may be treatable.
- Provide information for future functional support needs.
- Facilitate genetic counseling and family planning.
- Assist the individual for life planning.

B. Risk Factors

- Categories: biomedical, social, behavioral, and educational.
- Risk factors are listed in **Table 60-2** by categories and separated into the time of occurrence, namely prenatal, perinatal, and postnatal.[21]
- Several risk factors may interact over time and result in impaired functioning of the individual.

C. Determination of Etiology

- Search for all possible risk factors that lead to impaired functioning.
- Determine detailed three-generation family history.

VI. GENERAL CHARACTERISTICS

A. Physical Features

Because most individuals with an intellectual disorder are in the borderline and mild categories, no unusual physical characteristics are expected. There may be delayed growth and development.

- Facial or other characteristics may be pathognomonic for a particular condition or syndrome; for example, Down syndrome, described in this chapter.
- Skull anomalies include microcephalus (smaller), hydrocephalus (larger, contains fluid), spherical, conical, or otherwise asymmetrical shapes.
- Dysmorphic features, such as asymmetries of the face, malformations of the outer ear, anomalies of the eyes, or unusual shape of the nose, may become apparent as the child develops.

B. Oral Findings

A higher incidence of oral developmental malformations may be noted.

- Lips: increased thickness; lip biting is a self-injurious habit.

- Tooth anomalies: imperfect formation; delayed or irregular eruption patterns.
- Periodontal infections: common in individuals with intellectual disabilities: incidence influenced by supports (assisted oral care).
- Oral habits: increased clenching, bruxing, mouth-breathing, tongue thrusting.
- Dental caries
    A. Factors effective in dental caries control in special groups are the same as in the general population including fluorides and fluoridation, form and frequency of cariogenic foods consumed, and personal daily control of biofilm.
    B. Research has shown that when figures are separated for degree of intellectual disorder, the severely and profoundly affected patients have been shown to have significantly more carious lesions.[22]
    C. Literature reviews show much variation in results.[23]

VII. DENTAL HYGIENE CARE AND INSTRUCTION

- A patient with an intellectual disorder may have physical and sensory disabilities or systemic disease problems; therefore, information from various chapters in Section VIII of this book may be applied.
- Patients need basic dental hygiene care supports consisting of intensive daily personal biofilm removal and frequent maintenance supervision for the health of all oral tissues.
- Patience for repetition of instruction is needed.

DENTAL HYGIENE CARE

- Appointments for medical or dental health care may be frightening, difficult experiences for some patients with developmental or behavioral disorders, and most especially for patients with an ASD.
- Dental care may have been neglected due to problems with social interactions, language and communication problems, or difficult behaviors.
- Severity of symptoms dictates the appropriate setting for the delivery of dental care services for these patients.
- With some modifications to the treatment plan and implementation of appropriate behavior guidance techniques, patients with mild to moderate manifestations of the condition may be treated successfully in the general dental setting.
- Patients with more severe symptoms may require sedation, general anesthesia, or immobilization in a specialized setting.

I. ORAL HEALTH PROBLEMS

Except when a diagnosis of ASD has a comorbid diagnosis, no specific oral manifestation exists. Several factors can contribute to poor oral health.

A. Previous Dental Care

- Dental care may have been a low priority.
- Caregivers may no longer seek dental services if they have not found services that are available or appropriate in the past.
- Reasons for dental neglect
  A. Parental fear of embarrassment over resistant or possible aggressive/impulsive behaviors.
  B. Fear of discomfort.
  C. Fear of injury.
  D. Satisfactory quality of previous services may not have been achievable.

B. Dental Caries

- Feeding problems can lead to offering foods that will be accepted, without regard for nutrient content or caries prevention.
- Dietary selection may have been limited by needs for sameness, with the possibility of serving an excess of cariogenic foods.
- Sweet food rewards for behavior modification/guidance, repeated frequently over time, promote dental caries development.
- Aversion to certain food textures can lead to extreme diets that result in either entirely soft food selections or entirely hard crunchy/crispy food selections.
- Foods used in therapy sessions that may stimulate speech or help develop the muscles necessary for improved language are frequently cariogenic (i.e., chewy or sticky candy)

C. Oral Hygiene

- Daily oral care procedures may be inadequate for the uncooperative individual, even when delivered by an informed caregiver.
- Sensory issues may need to be overcome for the individual to be able to tolerate the mouth sensations that are a necessary part of routine home care.

II. DENTAL STAFF PREPARATION

- Learn how to work with the patient.
  A. Review medical, dental, and personal histories with the caregiver by telephone appointment in advance of the first office appointment.
  B. Discuss information with parent/caregiver, physician, psychiatrist, teacher, or other persons associated with the patient.
  C. Gather specific information about appropriate motivators and rewards that are safe and effective reinforcers for the individual.
- Provide the individual with photos of the office and staff before the first appointment.
- Make recommendations for practice sessions that can be conducted at home before the first appointment.
  A. Touch the teeth for a count of 10.
  B. Place a plastic mirror and flashlight in and out of the mouth.
  C. Follow commands such as "Hands on your tummy"…. "Feet out straight."
- Plan several short orientation and familiarization appointments initially with not more than a week between visits.
- Involve the same members of the dental team at each appointment to avoid distressing the patient and losing time for reorientation.

III. DENTAL HYGIENE CARE PLAN

- Plan four-handed dental hygiene for the resistant patient.
- Frequent appointments to include all phases of prevention:
  A. Dental biofilm control for the patient and the caregiver.
  B. Scaling.
  C. Fluoride therapy, including the use of fluoride varnish that can be especially helpful for patients unable to cooperate with biofilm control. Varnish application is an easy and simple procedure (page 527 in Chapter 35).
  D. Sealants.

IV. APPOINTMENT INTERVENTION

- Provide a predictable and consistent experience.
- Create a quiet environment free from sensory stimuli; patients with autism may have sensitivity to light, sounds, touch, and smell.
  A. Avoid loud, inconsistent background music, noisy dental equipment, and irrelevant conversations.
  B. Avoid unnecessary touching during treatment.
- Desensitization/practice
  A. Begin with orientation to the setting and each part of the equipment.
  B. If patient is not ready, instrumentation may not be included at the first appointment.
  C. Instruction takes the form of "tell–show–do" repeated many times. Patience and firmness are necessary elements.
  D. Have caregiver help condition the patient by giving a plastic mouth mirror and a few dental films to take home for practice in the mouth each day.

E. Use behavior guidance procedures when the patient is familiar with that method.
   1. Involve caregiver(s) while presenting preventive measures in a simple step-by-step manner.
   2. Provide reinforcing rewards immediately following each success.
   3. Use inedible rewards (stickers, picture cards, child-safe tokens, or toys) and explain rationale against cariogenic food rewards.
- Physical immobilization
   A. The least restrictive method of body stabilization is selected for each patient.
   B. The use of physical immobilization techniques during routine clinical procedures is currently considered inappropriate.
   C. Various body stabilization techniques for use in limited situations are described in Chapter 56 on page 859.
   D. Written informed parental/guardian consent and complete postprocedure documentation is provided if any type of physical body enclosure or body stabilization techniques are used during dental hygiene treatment.

V. BEHAVIOR SUPPORTS AND GUIDANCE

- Behavioral interventions are available to help patients who physically resist dental procedures learn to cooperate. Many resistant patients can cooperate more, and can learn these cooperative behaviors more quickly when:
   A. at least two or more active behavioral interventions are used.
   B. individualized tangible reinforcers are used and provided frequently.
   C. patients can be actively involved in the behavior intervention and are provided with choices when appropriate.
   D. the behavior intervention is practiced repetitively.[24]

BOX 60-4	Example Progress Note for a Patient With Autism Spectrum Disorder

Patient presented as a 10-year-old boy with a developmental age of approx 4 years old. Used three-four word simple sentences and caregivers presented with a picture board that showed the steps of the appointment. This helped the patient recognize how many more steps were needed to get to the end of the appointment. Patient needs to have his hands held to remind him not to touch and he finds comfort in holding a favorite rubber tube toy that he brought from home. Also loves to hear quiet singing and counting throughout the appointment. Was able to perform cursory "mirror only" exam and demonstrate proper brushing hand over hand with caregiver. Will reschedule for a 15-minute appointment in one week. Caregivers will practice increasing frequency and time of proper brushing and will practice counting teeth and applying prophy paste to one tooth per day.

Signed: _____, RDH Date: _____.

- The D-TERMINED Dental Program of Repetitive Tasking and Familiarization in Dentistry[25]
   A. A behavior guidance approach for dental professionals to use specifically for patients with ASD.
   B. D-TERMINED techniques have allowed many patients with ASD to receive appropriate dental treatment in standard practice environments without sedation.
   C. The D-TERMINED program involves:
      1. pretreatment assessment.
      2. familiarization visits.
      3. practicing and learning cooperation skills.

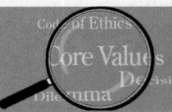 # Everyday Ethics

At the Caring Community Dental Health Clinic, the first and third Mondays of each month are reserved for special needs patients referred by health professionals in the local area. Adults and children with Down syndrome, ASD and other intellectual disabilities are scheduled frequently for dental hygiene appointments. With only one full-time and one part-time dental hygienist, more hygiene appointment time has been needed. Dental hygiene students from a nearby dental hygiene program have been invited to rotate through the clinic as a community practicum experience.

Questions for Consideration
1. Two days before a scheduled assignment, Ellie, a student, confides to her classmate, Julie, that she cannot participate in this field experience because she is too afraid of people with intellectual disabilities. Which core values are evident in this situation?
2. When arriving at the assignment, the students are greeted and oriented by the part-time hygienist, Ms. Gray. She advises the students, "Just get 'em in and get 'em out. They don't understand anything anyway and it's a waste of your time to try to talk to them for patient instruction." What are the ethical principles applicable to this situation?
3. How might the students handle these ethical issues using the "Steps in the Resolution of an Issue or Dilemma" in Chapter 1 on page 10 to determine an acceptable course of action?

D. Cooperation skills to be learned include:
1. positioning oneself in the dental chair.
2. sitting with legs straight and hands at side or on tummy.
3. making eye contact as instructions are given.
4. opening the mouth and remaining consistently open.
5. allowing instrumentation, and responding appropriately to instructions.

E. The Five "D" Steps for learning cooperation skills:
1. *Divide the skill into smaller parts:* the key for people with autism is to take each small step of a dental appointment one at a time, and master it before moving ahead.
2. *Demonstrate the skill:* use the tell–show–do technique.
3. *Drill the skill:* repeat/practice the skill many times until it becomes second nature.
4. *Delight the learner:* reward successful attainment of any small portion of the task with reinforcers.
5. *Delegate the repetition:* involve other members of the dental staff in reinforcing the skills, and have parents and caregivers rehearse/practice at home.

DOCUMENTATION

Factors to document include:
- Note chronological age versus developmental age.
- Note communication strengths and weaknesses.
- Note helpful behavioral supports and guidance techniques.
- Note treatment that was accomplished and modifications to treatment that were helpful.
- Note recommended home care oral hygiene and behavior practice skills.
- **Box 60-4** contains an example progress note for a patient with ASD.

Factors To Teach The Patient

If the patient is able to perform other self care skills independently and can expectorate, then proceed with instruction using language and methods appropriate to the intellectual level and abilities of each patient.

Explain:
- How to perform oral hygiene procedures at an appropriate skill level.
- What the disclosing agent shows and why the biofilm needs to be removed.
- Why assistance from others is an important supplement to the patient's own efforts.
- How to use and show their cooperation skills.

Factors To Teach The Caregiver

- Why complete oral examinations and oral hygiene care services at regular frequent intervals are necessary.
- Why a total preventive program is important; emphasize its significance.
- Individualized oral care techniques for each patient.
- Ways to provide assistance for patients with limited abilities, such as:
  A. How to stabilize the patient's head.
  B. How to retract the patient's lips to insert and adapt the toothbrush.
- How to incorporate behavior modification into oral care procedures.
- Emphasize the importance of repeating tell–show–do instructions often.

References

1. Department of Health and Human Services, Centers for Disease Control and Prevention [Internet]. Atlanta, Developmental Disabilities: Topic Home; [Cited 2010 Mar 29]. Available from: http://www.cdc.gov/ncbddd/dd/default.htm

2. American Psychiatric Association. *Diagnostic and statistical manual of mental disorders (DSM-IV-TR)*. Washington, DC: American Psychiatric Association; 2000. 39–41 pp.

3. Rapin I. Perspective: the autistic-spectrum disorders. *N Engl J Med*. 2002 Aug;347(5):302–3.

4. Muhle R, Trentecoste SV, Rapin I. The genetics of autism. *Pediatrics*. 2004 May;113(5):e472–86.

5. Kanner L. Early infantile autism. *J Pediatr*. 1944 Sep;25:211.

6. Pediatric Psychopharmacology Autism Network. Risperidone in children with autism and serious behavioral problems. *N Engl J Med*. 2002 Aug;347(5):314–21.

7. Longe JL. *The GALE encyclopedia of medicine*. 2nd ed. Vol. 1A–B. Detroit: Thomson Learning; 2002. 417–21 pp.

8. United States, National Institute of Child and Maternal Health. Autism questions and answers for health care professionals. Bethesda, MD: National Institute of Child Health and Human Development; Publication A0186: 2001.

9. Malone FD, Canick JA, Ball RH, Nyberg DA, Comstock CH, Bukowski R, Berkowitz RL, Gross SJ, Dugoff L, Craigo SD, Timor-Tritsch IE, Carr SR, Wolfe HM, Dukes K, Bianchi DW, Rudnicka AR, Hackshaw AK, Lambert-Messerlian G, Wald NJ, D'Alton ME. First-trimester or second-trimester screening, or both, for down's syndrome. *N Engl J Med*. 2005 Nov 10;353(19):2001–11.

10. Holmes LB. Decreasing age of mothers of infants with the down's syndrome. *N Engl J Med*. 1978 Jun 22;298:(25):1419–21.

11. Cohen FL. Paternal contributions to birth defects. *Nurs Clin North Am*. 1986 Mar;21(1):49–64.

12. Schendel SA, Gorlin RJ. Frequency of cleft uvula and submucous cleft palate in patients with down's syndrome. *J Dent Res*. 1974 Jul–Aug;53(4):840–3.

13. Sakellari D, Arapostathis KN, Konstantinidis A. Periodontal conditions and subgingival microflora in down syndrome patients. A case-control study. *J Clin Periodontol*. 2005 Jun;32(6):684–90.

14. Izumi Y, Sugiyama S, Shinozuka O, Yamazaki T, Ohyama T, Ishikawa I. Defective neutrophil chemotaxis in down's syndrome patients and its relationship to periodontal destruction. *J Periodontol*. 1989 May;60(5):238–42.

15. Jacobs IN, Gray RF, Todd NW. Upper airway obstruction in children with down syndrome. *Arch Otolaryngol Head Neck Surg*. 1996 Sep;122(9):945–50.

16. Barnett ML. Friedman D, Kastner T. The prevalence of mitral valve prolapse in patients with down's syndrome: implications for dental management. *Oral Surg Oral Med Oral Pathol*. 1988 Oct;66(4): 445–7.

17. Sigal MJ, Levine N. Down's syndrome and alzheimer's disease. *J Can Dent Assoc*. 1993 Oct;(10):328–5.

18. Department of Health and Human Services, Centers for Disease Control and Prevention [Internet]. Atlanta, Developmental Disabilities; [Cited 2010 Mar 29]. Available from: http://www.cdc.gov/ncbddd/dd/ddmr.htm

19. American Association on Mental Retardation: Mental Retardation. *Definition, Classification, and Systems of Supports*, 10th ed. Washington, DC: AAMR; 2002. 39–48 pp.

20. Ibid, pp. 145.

21. Ibid, p. 127.

22. Tesini DA. An annotated review of the literature of dental caries and periodontal disease in mentally retarded individuals. *Spec Care Dentist*. 1981 Mar–Apr;1(2):75–87.

23. Fung K, Allison PJ. A comparison of caries rates in non-institutionalized individuals with and without down syndrome. *Spec Care Dentist*. 2005 Nov–Dec;25(6):302–10.

24. Kemp F. Alternatives: a review of non-pharmacologic approaches to increasing the cooperation of patients with special needs to inherently unpleasant dental procedures. *Behav Anal Today*. 2005 June;6:88.

25. Tesini DA. *The D-TERMINED program of repetitive tasking and familiarization in dentistry: a behavior management approach*. Wellesley, MA: NLM Family Foundation; 2003.

CHAPTER 61

Family Abuse and Neglect

PAMELA S. RIDILLA, RDH, MS

Chapter Outline

Domestic violence is the abuse by one individual of another in an intimate relationship. The entire dental health team needs to be aware of the problem of family abuse and neglect as well as to identify and report suspected cases to authorities.

- Those most at risk for maltreatment are children, the elderly, persons with disabilities, and women.
- Family abuse may be categorized as physical violence, emotional abuse, sexual abuse, neglect, or financial exploitation.
- Abuse of women can include spouse abuse and dating violence.
- **Table 61-1** summarizes the major types of family maltreatment.

Identification:

- Abuse can be detected during the initial assessment of a patient, particularly during the extraoral and intraoral examination.
- Head and facial injuries, oral trauma, lesions, and abnormal pathology can lead to a suspicion of abuse and neglect.
- Patients may be seen in a dental office or clinic, whereas others may be taken to a hospital emergency department because serious bodily injuries have been inflicted.
- Key words associated with family abuse and neglect are defined in **Box 61-1**.

TABLE 61-1	MAJOR TYPES OF FAMILY MALTREATMENT
CATEGORY	**DESCRIPTION**
Physical Violence	Nonaccidental injuries on family members by parents, caregivers, spouses, or siblings.
Physical Neglect	Willful or unwillful failure of the caregiver or parents to provide the necessities to individuals in their care; abandonment; medical, dental, and deprivation neglect.
Sexual Violence	Nonconsensual or exploitive sexual contact, including sexual intercourse, oral sex, fondling, or pornographic activities on one family member by another.
Emotional Abuse	Mental anguish and despair caused by ridicule, intimidation, humiliation, name-calling, harassment, threats, and controlling behavior; isolation.

CHILD MALTREATMENT

- Any act or series of acts of abuse and neglect by a parent or other caregiver that results in harm, potential for harm, or threat of harm to a child under the age of 18.[1]
- Special needs children are more likely to be victims of abuse and neglect.
- Several thousands of children a year die as a result of severe physical damage, and others suffer permanent brain damage or physical deformities as well as emotional trauma. As much as 50–65% of child physical abuse involves injuries to the head, neck, or mouth.[2]
- Maltreatment is considered in the differential diagnosis for any injury involving a child.

I. DEFINITIONS

A. *Abuse.* The nonaccidental physical, emotional (psychological), or sexual acts against a child.[1]
B. *Neglect.* The intentional or unintentional failure to provide for a child's basic physical, emotional, educational, and medical/dental needs.[1]
C. *Dental neglect.* The willful failure of a parent or guardian to seek and follow through with treatment necessary to ensure a level of oral health essential for adequate function and freedom from pain and infection.[3]

II. GENERAL SIGNS OF ABUSE AND NEGLECT

Recognition of signs of suspected abuse is the first step toward protection of the child. As the child enters the treatment room, identifiable characteristics may be displayed that are suggestive of abuse or neglect.

A. Overall Appearance

- Clothing with long sleeves and long pants, even in warm weather, may suggest that bruises and lacerations are being covered.
- Uncleanliness and other signs of lack of care.
- Failure to thrive; malnutrition.
- Infestation of lice.
  A. Live bugs on the scalp.
  B. Bug bite marks on the scalp.

BOX 61-1	Key Words

Family Abuse and Neglect

Acute primary herpetic gingivostomatitis: clinical presentation of an initial HSV infection from HSV1 (oral) or HSV2 (genital) that can appear as multiple ulcerations on both keratinizing and gland-bearing mucosa.
Alopecia: baldness.
  Traumatic alopecia: an area of baldness on the head caused by pulling out the hair at the roots.
Cachexia: ill health, malnutrition, wasting (emaciating).
Condyloma acuminatum: multiple papillary or focal sessile-based lesions caused by the human papilloma virus (HPV6 or HPV11).
Differential diagnosis: identifying a disease by comparing the symptoms of two or more diseases that are similar.
Ecchymosis: discoloration on the skin that is blue-black with irregularly formed hemorrhagic areas. Color changes with time to yellow or greenish-brown.

Edema: swelling.
Forensic: pertaining to or used in legal proceedings.
Idiopathic thrombocytopenia purpura: hemorrhages on the skin caused by abnormal decrease in the number of blood platelets with unknown etiology.
Intimate relationship: marriage partners, partners living together, dating relationships, and former spouses, partners, and boyfriends/girlfriends.
Lichenification: area of skin that has thickened and hardened from continuous irritation.
Raccoon sign: bilateral periorbital ecchymosis, which can occur as a result of a basilar skull fracture.
Scale photography: a method of photography to record bite marks; the use of a metric scale placed directly above or below the injury to indicate scale; use of grid photographic film.

C. Nits or lice eggs on the shaft of the hair; appear as tiny silvery tear.

D. Drops that can be attached anywhere along the hair shaft from the scalp to the ends and that do not move or fall off.

B. Behavioral

In **Table 61-2**, categories of child abuse and neglect are separated into physical and behavioral indicators.

- May be very fearful and cry excessively or will show no fear at all.
- May appear unhappy and withdrawn.
- May not exhibit normal behavior consistent with the present age of the child.
- May act differently when the parent is present than when alone, which may provide clues to the type of relationship that exists.
- May exhibit evidence of developmental delays, including those of language or motor skills.

III. EXTRAORAL WOUNDS AND SIGNS OF TRAUMA

Abrasions and lacerations may be present at varying degrees of healing inconsistent with explanations given by the caregiver. Recognizing injuries to the head and neck and connecting them to suspected child maltreatment can save the lives of the children involved. Deliberate or inflicted injuries usually occur on both sides of the face, whereas accidental injuries usually occur only on one side. The common sites of deliberate injuries inflicted on children and accidental injuries on children are illustrated in **Figure 61-1**.

- Skull injuries; edema, combined with ecchymosis of varying stages.

- Bald spots (traumatic alopecia); caused by pulling the hair out by the roots.
- Raccoon sign: bilateral periorbital ecchymosis.
- Nose fractures or displacements.
- Lip bruises and lacerations; angular bruising, lichenification, or scarring, which can be caused from gags applied to the mouth.
- Marks on the skin that form a pattern of an object like a belt buckle or handprint.
- Human bite marks.

Table 61-3 lists possible conditions that can mimic lesions from child maltreatment.

IV. INTRAORAL SIGNS OF ABUSE

Care must be given to the assessment of intraoral traumatic injuries. Many injuries of the mouth in children can also be caused by accidental means.

- Lacerations of the tongue, buccal mucosa, or palate.
- Lingual and labial frenal tears.
- Teeth that are fractured, displaced, avulsed, or nonvital.
- Radiographic evidence of fractures in different degrees of healing.

V. SIGNS OF SEXUAL ABUSE

- Bruising or petechiae of the palate can indicate forced oral sex.
- Sexually transmitted genital lesions found intraorally.
  A. Condyloma acuminatum presents as a focal sessile-based lesion and also as a multiple papillary lesion. When present, it is necessary to look for other signs of oral sexual abuse because condyloma acuminatum can also occur with contact to verruca vulgaris or from self-inoculation.

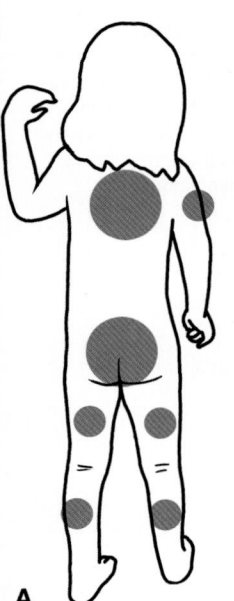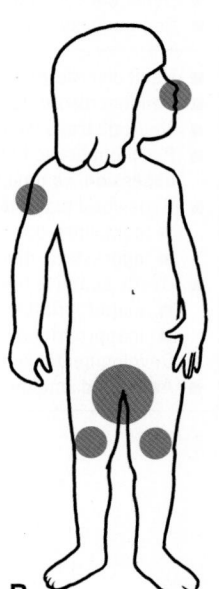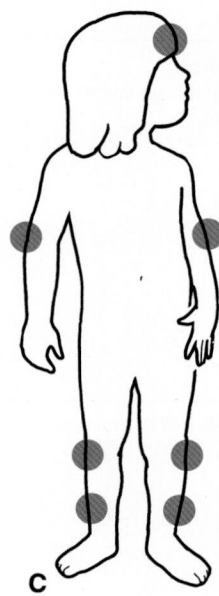

A   **B**   **C**

FIGURE 61-1 **Common Sites of Children's Injuries. (A)** and **(B)** Common sites of inflicted or deliberate injuries. **(C)** Common sites of accidental injuries.

TABLE 61-2	PHYSICAL AND BEHAVIORAL INDICATORS OF CHILD ABUSE AND NEGLECT

TYPE OF CHILD ABUSE AND NEGLECT	PHYSICAL INDICATORS	BEHAVIORAL INDICATORS

Physical Abuse	Unexplained bruises and welts:
	■ face, lips, mouth
	■ torso, back, buttocks, thighs
	■ various stages of healing
	■ clustered, regular patterns
	■ reflecting shape of article used to inflict (e.g., buckle)
	■ on several different areas
	■ regular appearance after absence, weekend, vacation
	Unexplained burns:
	■ cigarette, cigar burns, esp. on soles, palms, back, buttocks
	■ immersion burns (sock or glove-like, circular, on buttocks or genitalia)
	■ patterned: electric burner, iron
	■ rope burns on arms, legs, or torso
	Unexplained fractures:
	■ skull, nose, facial structures
	■ in various stages of healing
	■ multiple or spiral fractures
	Unexplained laceration or abrasion:
	■ to mouth, lips, gingiva, eyes
	■ to external genitalia
		■ Wary of adult contacts
		■ Apprehensive when others cry
		■ Behavioral extremes:
		  ■ aggressive
		  ■ withdrawn
		■ Frightened of parents
		■ Afraid to go home
		■ Reports injury by parents

Physical Neglect	■ Constant hunger, poor hygiene, inappropriate dress ■ Consistent lack of supervision, esp., in dangerous situations or for long periods ■ Unattended physical problems or medical/dental needs ■ Abandonment	■ Begging, stealing food ■ Extended stays at school, early arrival, late departure ■ Constant fatigue, falling asleep in class ■ Alcohol or drug abuse ■ Delinquency (e.g., thefts) ■ Says there is no caretaker
Sexual Abuse	■ Difficulty in walking or sitting ■ Torn, stained, bloody underwear ■ Pain or itching in genital area ■ Bruises or bleeding on external genitalia, vaginal, or anal areas ■ Venereal disease, esp. in pre-teen ■ Pregnancy	■ Unwilling to change for physical education ■ Withdrawal, fantasy or infantile behavior ■ Bizarre, sophisticated sexual knowledge or behavior ■ Poor peer relationship ■ Delinquency; runaways ■ Reports sexual assault by caretaker

Emotional Maltreatment	■ Speech disorders
	■ Lags in physical development
	■ Failure to thrive
		■ Habit disorders (sucking, biting, rocking, etc.)
		■ Conduct disorders (antisocial, destructive)
		■ Neurotic traits (sleep disorders, inhibited play)
		■ Psychoneurotic behaviors (hysteria, phobia, obsession, compulsion, hypochondria)
		■ Behavioral extremes:
		  ■ compliant, passive
		  ■ aggressive, demanding
		■ Overly adaptive behavior:
		  ■ inappropriately adult
		  ■ inappropriately infantile
		■ Developmental lags (physical or mental)
		■ Attempted suicide

© 1992 by Lynn Douglas Mouden, DDS, MPH; Little Rock, AR used by permission.

TABLE 61-3	CONDITIONS THAT CAN MIMIC ABUSE
APPEARANCE	**POSSIBLE CONDITIONS**
Bruising	Accidental injuries Idiopathic thrombocytopenia purpura Hemophilia
Burns/Red Lesions	Port-wine stain Accidental burns
Skin Lesions	Bullous impetigo Birthmarks

B. Primary herpetic gingivostomatitis can occur as a primary infection of herpes simplex virus type 2 (HSV2), which is a genital infection transmitted through oral sex.
■ Exhibits difficulty in walking or sitting.
■ Extreme fear of the oral examination.
■ Pregnancy, especially in the early adolescent years.

VI. INTRAORAL SIGNS OF NEGLECT

Failure of the caregiver, who is responsible for a child, to seek dental care for that child can be considered intentional or unintentional neglect. Neglect becomes intentional when the caregiver is negligent in following through with the recommended treatment.

A. Signs of Oral Neglect

■ Signs of lack of personal daily care.
■ Untreated disease, including rampant dental caries, pain, gingival inflammation, and bleeding.
■ Lack of regularity of dental care; appointments may have been made primarily for tooth or mouth pain.

B. Responsibilities of Dental Professionals

■ Provide education to the caregivers and age-appropriate children in the required personal oral health care and disease prevention procedures.
■ Inform the caregiver of the total treatment plan necessary to control oral diseases.
■ Provide information about access to care, financial aid, and transportation, when needed.

VII. PARENTAL ATTITUDE

A. Reasons for Dental Neglect: Parental Factors Involved

■ Oral healthcare considered a low priority.
■ Lack of education concerning the significance of oral healthcare and the relation to general health.
■ Limited finances.

■ Family isolation: access to care.
■ Religious beliefs.

B. General Attitudes of Abusers

■ Disinterest or denial in relationship to the child; may be critical, scolding, or belittling in front of others, including dental personnel.
■ Lack of interest in proposed dental and dental hygiene treatment plan, with a tendency to want only pain relief for the child. Such an attitude may not be shown toward other children in the family.
■ Unavailable for consultation. Does not usually accompany the child for dental appointments, but sends the child with another sibling.
■ Provides inconsistent information about the sources and causes of damaged teeth, bruises, or other signs of trauma.

C. Contributing Factors to Abusive Parents

■ Immature and unprepared for accepting the responsibilities of parenthood.
■ May have been abused by their parents.
■ Unable to handle daily stresses of financial difficulties, work stress, job loss, marital conflicts.
■ Drug use and alcoholism are sometimes involved.

ELDER MALTREATMENT

I. GENERAL CONSIDERATIONS

■ Elder abuse is much more than physical injury or neglect inflicted at the hands of a caretaker.
■ Mistreatment occurs in institutional settings as well as in family home environments.
■ Harm to the elder can occur through intentional (active) infliction or by unintentional (passive) neglect.[4]
■ It is consistently reported that family members are the primary elder abusers.[5]
■ The dental team, as in child abuse, can be a key source for the gathering of information to prove or disprove abuse of the elder patient.

II. DEFINITIONS

A. *Physical abuse.* The intentional use of force that results in bodily injury, pain, or anguish.
B. *Physical neglect.* The failure to provide basic necessities such as food, clothing, water, shelter, medicine, dental care, and personal hygiene. This type of neglect can be intentional or unintentional due to the caregiver's lack of ability to provide such care.
C. *Psychological abuse.* Mental anguish and despair caused by ridicule, name-calling, humiliation, harassment, manipulation, threats, and controlling behavior.

D. *Psychological neglect.* Nonverbal anguish caused by the lack of communication and isolation.

E. *Financial abuse.* Improper, illegal, or unethical exploitation of resources or assets.

F. *Sexual abuse.* Sexual contact with an elder who is unable to consent or otherwise nonconsensual sexual contact or exploitation.

G. *Self-neglect.* This can occur owing to depression from a loss of a loved one. The elder may feel unable to continue living.

III. GENERAL SIGNS OF ABUSE AND NEGLECT

When assessing for the possibility of abuse it is necessary to have a working knowledge of lesions that are related to aging, health problems, or medications. Taking a thorough history and comparing it with lesions present will help determine an appropriate differential diagnosis.

- Appears withdrawn, anxious, and shy and has low self-esteem.
- Gives an illogical explanation of how an injury occurred.
- Depression and hostility may be evident.
- May seem to dodge a motion of another person as if expecting to be hit.
- Overly eager to please and to be compliant.

IV. PHYSICAL SIGNS OF ABUSE AND NEGLECT

- Bruises in various degrees of healing or in areas of restraint like the legs or wrists.
- Traumatic alopecia.
- Human bite marks.
- Dislocations or sprains accompanied by fingertip pattern.
- Poor personal hygiene.
- Inadequate clothing for the season.
- Scratches or burns.
- Patterned marks and bruising indicating object used to inflict injury such as belt buckle, ropes, or a hand.
- Cachexia.

V. EXTRAORAL SIGNS OF ABUSE AND NEGLECT

- Lip trauma.
- Bruising of facial tissues.
- Eye injuries.
- Fractured or bruised mandible.
- Temporomandibular joint pain.

VI. INTRAORAL SIGNS OF ABUSE AND NEGLECT

- Fractured, displaced, or avulsed teeth.
- Bruising of the edentulous ridge. May indicate forced oral sex.
- Sexually transmitted disease lesions such as condyloma acuminatum and primary herpetic gingivostomatitis.

- Lesions or sore areas in the mouth from ill-fitting dentures: epulis fissuratum, atrophic candidiasis. (Lesions that occur under dentures are described in Chapter 53 on pages 817–818.)
- Fractured denture.
- Poor oral hygiene.
- Rampant dental caries.
- Untreated periodontal disease.

INTIMATE PARTNER ABUSE AND VIOLENCE

Spouse or partner abuse is another type of abuse that can be detected in the dental setting. The dental team is in a good position to examine and evaluate the oral areas of injury to a battered partner. The majority of intimate partner violence cases have female victims. Such abuse often goes unreported.

I. SIGNS AND ATTITUDES OF THE ABUSED

- Many of the same injuries listed for the elder person are also evident with partner abuse. They involve most frequently the face, eyes, and neck.
- Battered partner may be very reluctant to admit abuse because of threats of more serious harm.
- Abused may deny the abuse, defend the abuser, or provide excuses.
- Types of abuse are physical, sexual, emotional, psychological, and economic deprivation.

II. DENTAL HYGIENIST'S APPROACH

- Provide support; encourage open communication; be a source of reassurance.
- Discuss clinical findings in a nonjudgmental manner.
- Respect and maintain confidentiality; talk in a private setting (door closed to treatment room).
- Provide references for counseling; telephone numbers; community services.
- Respect patient's autonomy; ask about plans for future safety.
- Prepare to share your findings with authorities when called to provide evidence.
- When it is known that the interview will be used in a legal setting, a witness needs to be present.
- Document clinical findings, including extra/intraoral photographs of injuries.

III. DISCUSSION OF FINDINGS

- The decision must be made by the dental team whether or not to discuss the suspicion of abuse with the caregiver.
- If the decision is made to confront the parent or caregiver, the professional must never accuse anyone and must refrain from being judgmental.

■ The legal obligation to report a suspected case of abuse can be explained.

REPORTING MALTREATMENT

I. PROPER TRAINING

■ Training in the recognition and reporting of abuse and neglect need to be implemented in every dental practice. Abusers may avoid the same physician but return to the same dentist.[6]

■ Many state governing boards require completion of continuing education courses on abuse and neglect before licensure and relicensure to practice dentistry and dental hygiene.

■ "Prevent Abuse and Neglect through Dental Awareness" (P.A.N.D.A.) is a program for proper training of dental personnel. The coalition, founded in 1992 by the Missouri Department of Health in conjunction with Delta Dental of Missouri and the Missouri Dental Association, is a public–private partnership committed to the education of all dental professionals in the recognition and reporting of suspected cases of child abuse and neglect. Since its inception, nearly all of the United States and several international coalitions have replicated the program.[7]

■ "Ask, Validate, Document, Refer (AVDR) Tutorial for Dentists" is an interactive tutorial program that utilizes a case study to demonstrate the AVDR steps in response to domestic violence. The four-step process is: *asking* the patient about the abuse, *validating* messages that acknowledge that battering is wrong, *documenting* the signs, symptoms, and disclosures, and *referring* victims to specialists and community resources.[8]

■ Project RADAR is a provider-focused initiative to promote the assessment and prevention of intimate partner violence in the healthcare setting. The RADAR initiative seeks to enable health care providers to recognize and respond to intimate partner violence (IPV) by providing them access to: "Best Practices" policies, guidelines, and assessment tools; training programs and specialty-specific curricula; awareness and educational materials; and information on the latest research/data related to IPV. RADAR is an acronym for: *Routinely* inquire about current and past violence; *Ask* direct questions; *Document* findings; *Assess* safety; and *Review* options and referrals.[9]

II. REPORTING LAWS

■ Reporting laws vary from state to state.

■ Each state has laws regarding the reporting of abuse and neglect to the proper authorities. It is imperative to research the laws for the state and have them available for reference in the office.

■ Each dental practice needs a written protocol for the documentation and reporting of abuse and neglect.

III. REPORTABLE REQUIRED INFORMATION

All states mandate healthcare workers to report suspected violence, abuse, and neglect of children to child protective services agencies. When reporting suspected child maltreatment, it is necessary to have the following information available:

■ Name and address of the child and parents or other persons having custody of the child.

■ Child's age.

■ Names of siblings if there are any.

■ Nature of the child's condition, including evidence of previous injuries.

■ Any information that might be helpful in establishing the cause of abuse or neglect and the identity of the person believed to have caused such abuse or neglect.

In most states, healthcare workers are legally required to report suspected maltreatment of elders and adults with disabilities. However, healthcare workers are required by law to report suspected intimate partner violence in only a few states.

FORENSIC DENTISTRY

Forensic dentistry is that aspect of dental science that relates and applies dental facts to legal problems. Forensic dentistry encompasses dental identification, malpractice litigation, legislation, peer review, and dental licensure.

I. USE OF FORENSICS IN ABUSE CASES

There are instances when it becomes necessary to request the aid of a forensic odontologist to determine if a particular injury, usually a bite mark, is a result of abuse by a particular suspect.

■ Many times the abuser will state that the bite mark occurred from a sibling squabble, an animal bite, or the child biting himself or herself.

■ When photographs have been obtained and the history of the injury does not match the location of the marks, a bite mark analysis can be requested of the forensic odontologist.

■ Impressions and a bite registration are taken from the suspect/caregiver. A careful analysis will determine if the bite came from that suspect.

■ The information can then be taken into the legal process involved with prosecuting a child abuser.

II. OTHER USES OF FORENSICS

■ Forensic procedures are utilized in the identification of victims of a disaster.

■ Forensic teams include dentists, dental hygienists, and assistants with special training in the process of identifying remains by comparing the dentition of the remains with dental records.

■ Team members are assigned a task, and the team works together to check and double check results so the families of the victims can have closure regarding the loss of a loved one.

DOCUMENTATION

I. PURPOSES OF THOROUGH AND ACCURATE DOCUMENTATION

■ For future reference and comparison.

■ To provide authorities meticulous information to support an investigation.

■ To protect the abused patient from harmful circumstances or even death. A second person needs to be present to witness the examination and interview.

II. CONTENT OF THE RECORD

■ Obtain thorough histories of the injury from both the caregiver and the patient. Identify inconsistencies.

■ Document the date, time, and place of the examination.

■ Record all observable facts.

■ Record questions asked to the abused patient and document all answers in the patient's exact words as closely as possible.

■ Document all lesions, giving descriptive location, size, shape, and color. Pay close attention to ecchymoses of varying colors and injuries that appear bilaterally.

■ Use diagrams showing the location, size, and description.

■ Photographs and radiographs can also be used to supplement findings. Photographs must have patient consent

BOX 61-2	Example Progress Note

Patient came into the office for an emergency visit because of pain in mandibular right second premolar area. She complained of recent headaches and pain in right TMJ area. She presented with multiple contusions on right side of face above inferior border of mandible and right buccal mucosa. Bruises are in various stages of healing; red, purple, and greenish yellow. Bruises are oval shaped about 2–5 cm in size. On questioning her about the bruises, she stated that "my boyfriend slapped me recently, but he has been under a lot of pressure lately and he didn't mean to bruise me". Patient seemed nervous and agitated. Panoramic radiograph revealed a simple fracture on the body of the mandible below right second premolar area. Intraoral photographs were taken of contusions. Reassured patient that she did not deserve the abuse and provided her with the National Domestic Violence Hotline number. Patient was referred to oral surgeon for evaluation of fractured mandible.

Signed: _____, RDH Date: _____.

and could be released only with consent. There may be special provisions by law that allow the taking and releasing of photographs without consent if the healthcare provider is required by law to report suspected abuse.

■ Scale photography would be necessary for bite marks so further analysis can be done.

■ Use the words *suspected abuse* if the patient denies abuse.

■ **Box 61-2** provides a sample Progress Note.

Everyday Ethics

Sarah, a young, usually vivacious patient in Dr. Stuart's practice for about 2 years, presents for a maintenance appointment with Amy, the dental hygienist. Since her previous appointment, Sarah had had a big wedding. Amy was expecting to hear about it and maybe even see pictures.

When Sarah came into the treatment room, she seemed very quiet and avoided eye contact with Amy. On completion of Sarah's oral assessment, the following was noted: Class II mobility on teeth numbers 6, 7, and 8; distoincisal edge fractures on 7 and 8; a 4-mm scar on the vermilion border of the upper lip. Sarah explained that she slipped and fell on a wet kitchen floor. She could not remember how she got the scar, which was not present 6 months ago. Amy is not sure that Sarah is telling the truth. She suspects Sarah may be in an abusive relationship with her new husband. There is not enough time to have a long discussion with Sarah or with Dr. Stuart, who is in the middle of a crown preparation procedure.

Questions for Consideration

1. Which of the dental hygiene Core Values (Table II-1, page 38) have application in this case? Explain the relationship of each dental hygiene Core Value you select.

2. Is this an ethical issue or an ethical dilemma for Amy? Why? Using the four-step framework in making ethical decisions in Chapter 1 on page 10, develop a course of action that would assist Amy in resolving the issue.

3. How would Amy incorporate her suspicions about Sarah into her discussion of the oral assessment with Dr. Stuart?

Factors To Teach The Patient

Factors to Teach the Abused or Neglected Child

- The value of oral hygiene with age-appropriate materials.
- What the dental biofilm is on teeth, using disclosing agent.
- How to use the new toothbrush the child just received from the dental hygienist.
- Why it is especially important to brush the teeth and tongue just before going to sleep.

Factors to Teach the Abused Elder or Intimate Partner

- Where help can be obtained: emergency assistance including phone numbers and referrals.
- The tendency for the maltreatment to increase in severity and frequency over time.
- Battering is a choice. It is used to gain power and control over another individual.

References

1. Leeb RT, Paulozzi LJ, Melanson C, Simon TR, Arias I. *Child maltreatment surveillance: uniform definitions for public health and recommended data elements, version 1.0.* Atlanta, GA: Center for Disease Control and Prevention; 2008 Jan. 19 p.
2. Senn DR, McDowell JD, Alder ME. Dentistry's role in the recognition and reporting of domestic violence, abuse, and neglect. *Dent Clin North Am.* 2001 Apr;45(2):343–63.
3. American Academy of Pediatric Dentistry. Guideline on oral and dental aspects of child abuse and neglect. *Pediatr Dent.* 2008–2009;30(7 Suppl):86–9.
4. Lloyd JD. *Family violence.* San Diego, CA: Greenhaven Press, Inc.; 2001. 34 p.
5. Cowen HJ, Cowen PS. Elder mistreatment: dental assessment and intervention. *Spec Care Dentist.* 2002 Jan–Feb;22(1):23–32.
6. Nelms AP, Gutmann ME, Solomon ES, Dewald JP, Campbell PR. What victims of domestic violence need from the dental profession. *J Dent Educ.* 2009 Apr;73(4):490–8.
7. Oertling KM. Prevent Abuse and Neglect through Dental Awareness (P.A.N.D.A.). *LDA J.* 2003 Spring;62(1):16–17.
8. Hsieh NK, Herzig K, Gansky SA, Danley D, Gerbert B. Changing dentists' knowledge, attitudes and behavior regarding domestic violence through an interactive multimedia tutorial. *J Am Dent Assoc.* 2006 May;137(5):596–603.
9. VDH. Project RADAR [Internet]. Virginia: Virginia Department of Health, Division of Injury and Violence Prevention; c2009 [cited 2010 Oct 3]. Available from: http://www.vahealth.org/Injury/projectradarva/index.htm

The Patient With a Seizure Disorder

ESTHER M. WILKINS, BS, RDH, DMD

KATHRYN RAGALIS DAVIS, RDH, MS, DMD

Chapter Outline

A seizure is a paroxysmal event that results from abnormal brain activity. A seizure may involve loss of consciousness or awareness with or without convulsive movements or spasms. Epilepsy is a term to describe a group of functional disorders of the brain that are characterized by recurrent seizures. Seizures are a symptom of epilepsy.

■ The patient's medical history may reveal a susceptibility to seizures. A complete evaluation is required in all cases.

■ Treatment modalities of epilepsy and a seizure itself may affect the oral tissues and dental and dental hygiene treatment.

■ Dental personnel need to be aware of the issues associated with seizures, know how to evaluate the patient, and how to apply emergency measures in and out of the dental office.

■ Care of the oral cavity is important for its relationship both to general health and to oral accidents that may occur during a seizure.

■ All patients are advised by their physicians to live a moderate lifestyle and to pay strict attention to general health.

■ Occupation and lifestyle may be limited for patients who have recurrent seizures. A person susceptible to seizures cannot participate in activities that may precipitate a seizure or that provide hazards in the event of a seizure. Such limitations may lead to loss of driving privileges or loss of work and may lead to depression.

■ Box 62-1 contains key words used in this chapter.

BOX 62-1	**Key Words**

Seizures

Absence: a generalized seizure of sudden onset characterized by a brief period of unconsciousness. Formerly called **petit mal.**

Anticonvulsant: a drug that inhibits or suppresses convulsions.

Antiepileptic: a remedy for epilepsy.

Ataxia: failure of muscular coordination; irregularity of muscular action.

Atonic: relaxed; without normal tone or tension.

Aura: warning sensation felt by some people immediately preceding a seizure; may be flashes of light, dizziness, peculiar taste, or a sensation of prickling or tingling.

Automatism: involuntary motor activity, such as lip smacking or repeated swallowing.

Autonomic symptoms: pallor, flushing, sweating, pupillary dilation, cardiac arrhythmia, incontinence.

Clonic: alternate contraction and relaxation of muscle; **clonic phase** is the convulsion phase of a seizure.

Consciousness: degree of awareness and/or responsiveness of a person to externally applied stimuli.

Convulsion: violent spasm.

Cryptogenic: a disorder for which the cause is hidden or occult.

Diplopia: perception of two images of a single object; double vision.

Dyspepsia: impairment of the power or function of digestion.

Electroencephalography: the recording of changes in electric potentials in various areas of the brain by means of electrodes placed on the scalp or on/in the brain itself and connected to a vacuum-tube radio amplifier that amplifies the impulses more than a million times; the impulses move an electromagnetic pen that records the brain waves; a clinical test used for partial diagnosis of epilepsy.

Facies: expression or appearance of the face.

Grand mal: former name for a generalized or major seizure as contrasted with **petit mal,** a minor or relatively mild seizure.

Hirsutism: abnormal hairiness;

Hypertrichosis: excessive growth of hair.

Ictal: pertaining to or resulting from a stroke or a seizure.

Myoclonus: isolated or repetitive shock-like contractions of a muscle or group of muscles; adj., myoclonic.

Paresthesia: an abnormal sensation, such as burning, prickling, or tingling.

Paroxysm: sharp spasm or convulsion; sudden recurrence or intensification of symptoms.

Petit mal: attack or brief impairment of consciousness often associated with flickering of the eyelids and mild twitching of the mouth.

Prodrome: a premonitory symptom; a symptom indicating the onset of a disease or condition; adj., prodromal.

Psychic: pertaining to the mind or psyche.

Refractory epilepsy: not readily yielding to basic treatment; usually with a single antiepileptic drug.

Seizure: paroxysmal spell of transitory alteration in consciousness, motor activity, or sensory phenomenon; convulsion.

Spasm: sudden involuntary contraction of a muscle or group of muscles; may be tonic or clonic; may vary from small twitches to severe convulsions.

Status epilepticus: rapid succession of epileptic spasms without intervals of consciousness; life threatening; emergency care urgent.

Teratogenesis: production of deformity in the developing embryo.

Tonic: state of continuous, unremitting action of muscular contraction; patient appears stiff.

Tonic–clonic: in a seizure, a sudden sharp tonic contraction of muscles followed by clonic convulsive movements.

SEIZURES

I. SEIZURE DEFINITION

- A sudden paroxysmal electrical discharge of neurons in the brain.
- Results from a transient, uncontrolled alteration in brain function.
- Seizures are usually unprovoked, unpredictable, and involuntary.
- A seizure begins with an abrupt onset of symptoms that may be of a motor, sensory, cognitive, or emotional nature, depending on which brain cells are involved.
- As a seizure progresses, it may or may not cause loss of consciousness or awareness, tonic and/or clonic movements, incontinence, or tongue biting.
- Length of a seizure is uncontrollable.
- Other terms: convulsion, fit, spell, ictus.

II. CLASSIFICATION

The epileptic syndromes are complex. Diagnosis is made from the following:

- Clinical signs and symptoms
- History
- Electroencephalography (EEG)
- Functional neuroimaging

The syndromes have been classified by the following:

- Age-related onset
- Symptoms (vary with the type of seizure)
- Anatomic localization in the brain (temporal, frontal, parietal, or occipital lobes)

BOX 62-2	International Classification of Seizures

Partial Seizures (Seizures Beginning Locally)
Simple Partial Seizures (without loss of consciousness)
- With motor signs
- With somatosensory or special sensory symptoms
- With autonomic symptoms
- With psychic symptoms

Complex Partial Seizures
- Simple partial onset followed by impairment of consciousness
- With impairment of consciousness at onset

Partial Seizures Evolving to Generalized Tonic–Clonic Convulsions (Secondarily Generalized)

Generalized Seizures (Bilaterally Symmetrical, without Local Onset)
Nonconvulsive Seizures
- Absence seizures
- Atypical absence seizures
- Myoclonic seizures
- Atonic seizures

Convulsive Seizures
- Tonic–clonic seizures
- Tonic seizures
- Clonic seizures

Unclassified Epileptic Seizures

Source: Reprinted with permission from International League Against Epilepsy, Commission on Classification and Terminology. Proposal for revised clinical and electroencephalographic classification of epileptic seizures. *Epilepsia.* 1981 Aug;22(4):489–501.

III. TYPES OF SEIZURES[1,2]

- The two basic types of seizures are *generalized* and *partial.*
- The international classification of seizures is outlined in Box 62-2.
- A seizure of focal origin that involves only a part of the brain is called a partial seizure.
- A generalized seizure affects the entire brain at the same time.

IV. ETIOLOGY

In addition to epilepsy, seizures can be a symptom of many different conditions. The causes can be divided into primary and secondary.

A. Primary (Idiopathic)

Genetic predisposition to seizures or to other neurologic abnormalities for which seizure may be a symptom.

B. Secondary (Symptomatic)

Seizures can arise during many neurologic and nonneurologic medical conditions, such as:

- Congenital conditions, such as maternal infection (rubella); toxemia of pregnancy
- Perinatal injuries
- Brain tumor
- Cerebrovascular disease (stroke)
- Trauma (head injury)
- Infection (meningitis, encephalitis, opportunistic infections of AIDS)
- Degenerative brain disease
- Metabolic and toxic disorders, including alcoholism and other drug addictions; seizures are common during drug withdrawal
- Complication of cancer

V. PROGNOSIS[3]

- Prognosis for seizure control is good.
- Approximately 75% of patients become seizure-free.
- Seizure disorders tend to be stable, and do not worsen over time.

VI. IMPLICATIONS

Owing to a possibility of severe injury, accidents, or embarrassment, patients who experience recurrent seizures may choose to avoid or be legally restricted from participating in certain activities. These may include:

- *Vocation:* occupations that involve use of machinery or require physical activity may not be an option.
- *Licenses:* certain licenses, such as driver's license, may be restricted until the patient is deemed to be seizure-free.
- *Independent living:* living alone may not be advised due to health risks.

CLINICAL MANIFESTATIONS[4]

I. PRECIPITATING FACTORS

A patient may have factors that precipitate a seizure. The patient or a caregiver may provide helpful information to prepare healthcare personnel to handle an emergency. Possible precipitating factors include the following:

- Psychological stress; apprehension
- Fatigue; sleep deprivation
- Sensory stimuli, such as flashing lights, noises, peculiar odors
- Use or withdrawal of alcohol or other addictive drugs

II. AURA

- Not all patients have a warning, or aura, before a seizure.

- A patient with a warning may seek a safe place to sit or lie down in privacy.
- In the dental environment, the patient can inform the personnel so that procedures can be terminated and brief preparations can be made.
- The aura may be a special sensory stimulus, a sensation of numbness, tingling, or twitching or stiffness of certain muscles.

III. THE SEIZURE

The following are some of the clinical manifestations that may or may not occur during several types of seizures. A patient may experience only one type of seizure or differing types.

A. Partial (More Common in Adults)

1. *Simple*
   - Cessation of ongoing activity.
   - Staring spell; dizziness.
   - Jerking of muscles around the mouth.
   - No loss of consciousness.
2. *Complex*
   - Trance-like state with confusion lasts usually for a few minutes to hours.
   - Consciousness is impaired to varying degrees.
   - Patient may manifest purposeless movements or actions followed by confusion, incoherent speech, ill humor, unpleasant temper; does not remember what happened during the attack.

B. Generalized

1. *Absence (Petite Mal) Seizure*
   - Loss of consciousness begins and ends abruptly in about 5 to 30 seconds.
   - Most common in children, and might lead to learning difficulties if not identified.
   - Patient has blank stare, usually does not fall, posture becomes fixed, may drop whatever is being held.
   - May become pale.
   - May have rhythmic twitching of eyelids, eyebrows, head, or chewing movements.
   - Attack ends as abruptly as it begins. Patient quickly returns to full awareness, resumes activities, unaware of what occurred.
2. *Tonic–Clonic (Grand Mal) Seizure*
   - Muscles of the chest and pharynx may contract at the same time, forcing air out and a sound known as the "epileptic cry."
   - Loss of consciousness is sudden and complete, the patient becomes stiff and falls or may slide out of the dental chair.
   - Musculature contraction: tonic phase tension with rigidity, clonic movements follow with intermittent muscular contraction and relaxation.

- Skin color turns pale to bluish, breathing is shallow or stops briefly.
- Possible loss of bladder, and rarely, bowel control. Tongue may be bitten.
- Incident usually lasts 1 to 3 minutes.
- Respiration returns.
- Saliva, which previously could not be swallowed, may become mixed with air and appear as foam.
- Patient begins to recover, may be confused, tired, complain of muscle soreness or injury; falls into a deep sleep.
- Phases of seizure may be called preictal, ictal, and postictal.
- Grand mal seizure may continue without recovery and progress to *status epilepticus*.

TREATMENT

I. MEDICATIONS

Antiepileptic drug therapy is one method used to control seizures.

A. Choices

- Patients may be on one antiepileptic drug or a combination of several.
- Choice of therapy is related to type of seizure disorder and possibly to desired side effect or elimination of an undesirable side effect.
- Frequently prescribed medications are listed in **Table 62-1**.

B. Side Effects

1. *Each* medication has side effects that a patient may experience to varying degrees. Clinicians learn the use, side effects, and mode of action.
2. *Side Effects may Include the Following:*
   - Allergic reaction, rash
   - Fatigue, drowsiness, weakness, ataxia, headache, slurred speech
   - Nausea, vomiting
   - Memory loss; behavioral and cognitive deficits
   - Damage to liver, interactions of medications processed in liver
   - Leukopenia: delayed healing and infection
   - Thrombocytopenia or decreased platelet aggregation: increased bleeding, petechiae
   - Osteoporosis
   - Increased or unknown risk of birth defects
   - Hirsutism; hypertrichosis
   - Oral change of *gingival enlargement* most common with phenytoin
   - Numerous drug interactions, including other antiepileptic drugs, acetaminophen, nonsteroidal anti-inflammatory drugs, erythromycins, and reduction in efficacy of *oral contraceptives*.

TABLE 62-1	ANTIEPILEPTIC MEDICATIONS

GENERIC NAME	BRAND NAME
Older Medications	
Carbamazepine	Tegretol, Carbatrol
Phenytoin	Dilantin
Valproic acid/valproate	Depakote
Phenobarbital	Luminal
Primidone	Mysoline
Ethosuximide	Zarontin
Clonazepam	Klonopin
Clorazepate	Tranxene
Newer Medications	
Felbamate	Felbatol
Gabapentin	Neurontin
Lamotrigine	Lamictal
Topiramate	Topamax
Tiagabine	Gabitril
Levetiracetam	Keppra
Oxcarbazepine	Trileptal
Zonisamide	Zonegran

3. *Elderly and Children*
- Both are more sensitive to side effects of weakness, unsteadiness, cognitive alterations.
- Elderly more likely to be on other medications with possible drug interactions and more likely to forget to take medications.

C. Precaution: Herbal Supplements

- Certain over-the-counter herbal supplements are used as a self-medication to help prevent seizures. These supplements may interfere with the prescribed antiepileptic drug and cause serious complications.
- Patients must inform their physician and dental team when using.
- Herbal supplements may also affect dental treatment, for example, with the side effect of increased bleeding.

II. SURGERY[5]

A variety of surgical interventions are available and indicated when epilepsy is refractory to traditional antiepileptic drug therapy. Treatments have been made possible through the advances in identifying the epileptogenic area with magnetic resonance imaging, electroencephalographic studies, tomography, neuropsychological testing, and other analyses. Surgical options include:

- *Resection* of the epileptogenic area in the brain.
- If total resection leads to unacceptable deficits, *multiple subpial transections,* which are a series of small parallel slices, are removed,
- *Gamma-knife radiosurgery* involves delivery of a focused dose of radiation to the epileptogenic area in the brain. This technique reduces risk of infection, bleeding, and hospitalization.

III. VAGUS NERVE STIMULATION[6]

- Some patients are treated with an implantable vagus nerve stimulator.
- A pacemaker-like device is implanted in the upper left chest and delivers an intermittent signal to the vagus nerve.
  A. It may cause voice alteration, swallowing difficulty, and neck and throat pain during stimulation.
  B. Certain dental instruments, such as the diathermy devices for electrosurgery and electric pulp testing, may interfere with implantable devices and must not be used.

IV. KETOGENIC DIET

- The goal of the ketogenic diet is to induce fat metabolism and maintain ketosis.
- It is initiated after a starvation period, which induces fat metabolism and the production of ketones.
- When food is reintroduced, it is mainly fat and low proteins with nearly no carbohydrates.
- The diet has been shown to be an effective treatment for patients with epilepsy, particularly children.

ORAL FINDINGS

Epilepsy in itself produces no oral changes. Specific changes relate to side effects of antiepileptic drugs or other therapy, results of oral accidents during a seizure, or side effects of the epilepsy, such as depression leading to poor oral hygiene and neglect.

I. EFFECTS OF ACCIDENTS DURING SEIZURES

A. Scars of Lips and Tongue

- Oral tissues, particularly tongue, cheek, or lip, may be bitten.
- Scars may be observed during the extraoral/intraoral examination, and the cause may be differentiated from other types of healed wounds.

B. Fractured Teeth

- Teeth may be clamped and bruxing may be forceful enough to fracture teeth.
- Fractured teeth may be sharp and lacerate tissue and should be smoothed or restored.
- Fractures may extend into pulp of a tooth, allowing bacterial infection, which requires treatment with root canal therapy or extraction.

II. GINGIVAL OVERGROWTH/GINGIVAL HYPERPLASIA

- Gingival overgrowth occurs in 25% to 50% of persons using phenytoin for treatment.[7]
- Other antiepileptic drugs also induce gingival overgrowth less frequently.[8]
- Phenytoin and the other antiepileptic drugs have been used in the treatment of many conditions other than epilepsy, including stuttering, headaches, neuromuscular disturbances, and cardiac conditions; therefore their use does not lead to an assumption that the patient has epilepsy.
- When related to phenytoin use, gingival enlargement may also be called Dilantin hyperplasia, diphenylhydantoin-induced hyperplasia, diphenylhydantoin gingival hyperplasia, Dilantin-induced gingival fibrosis, and phenytoin-induced hyperplasia.

A. Mechanism

- Phenytoin may cause fibroblasts and osteoblasts to deposit excessive extracellular matrix, causing gingival overgrowth.
- Tissue color and texture are generally within normal limits with lobular shape.
- Local irritants such as biofilm or ill-fitting appliances make response more excessive.
- Meticulous oral hygiene has been found to reduce the occurrence and severity of gingival overgrowth.

B. Occurrence[9]

- Incidence is greater in younger patients than in older patients just beginning therapy.
- The gingiva may start to enlarge within a few weeks or even after a few years following the initial administration of the drug.
- The size of the dose and the length of treatment are not necessarily factors in the incidence or nature of the gingival enlargement.
- The anterior gingiva are usually more affected than are the posterior, and the maxillary more than the mandibular.
- Facial and proximal areas are usually more affected than lingual and palatal areas.
- Although rare, an overgrowth of tissue may occur in an edentulous area and is usually associated with trauma,

irritation from a denture, the presence of retained roots, or unerupted teeth.[10,11]
- Overgrowth of tissue surrounding dental implants can occur.[12]

C. Effects[13]

- Poses dental biofilm control problem
- May affect mastication
- May alter tooth eruption
- May interfere with speech
- May cause serious esthetic concerns

D. Tissue Characteristics

- *Early Clinical Features:* The overgrowth appears as a painless enlargement of interdental papillae with signs of inflammation. Eventually, the tissue becomes fibrotic, pink, and stippled, with a mulberry- or cauliflower-like appearance, as in **Figure 62-1B**.
- *Advanced Lesion:* The tissue increases in size, extends to include the marginal gingiva, and covers a large

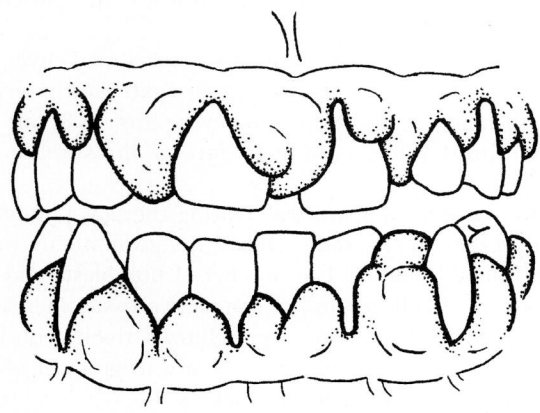

A

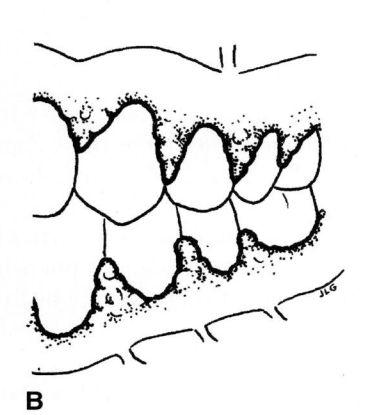

B

FIGURE 62-1 **Phenytoin-Induced Gingival Enlargement. (A)** Papillary enlargement with cleft-like grooves. Note the effect of the pressure of the fibrotic tissue on the position of teeth. Maxillary incisors and the mandibular left canine have been wedged away from normal positions. **(B)** Mulberry-like shape of interdental papillae.

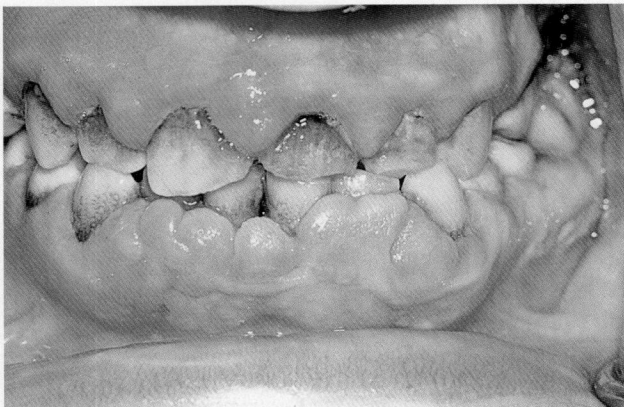

FIGURE 62-2 Severe Phenytoin-Induced Gingival Enlargement.
Note extent of gingival overgrowth on lower left between canine and lateral incisor and presence of local irritants of biofilm, calculus, and stain. (*Source:* Reprinted with permission from Langlais RP, Miller CS. *Color atlas of common oral diseases.* 3rd ed. Philadelphia: Lippincott Williams & Wilkins; 2003. Section 5, Intraoral findings by color changes; 81 p.)

portion of the anatomic crown. Often, cleft-like grooves occur between the lobules, as shown in **Figure 62-1A**.

- *Severe Lesion*: Large, bulbous gingiva may cover the enamel, tend to wedge the teeth apart, and interfere with mastication. Note the severe growth about the mandibular left canine to lateral incisor area in **Figure 62-2**.
- *Microscopic Appearance*: During therapy, phenytoin is present in the saliva, blood, gingival sulcus fluid, and dental biofilm. The number of fibroblasts and the amount of collagen in the connective tissue increases. The stratified squamous epithelium is thick, with long rete ridges. Inflammatory cells are in greatest abundance near the base of the pockets.

E. Complicating Factors

1. *Dental Biofilm and Gingivitis*
   - Biofilm appears to be the most important determinant of the severity of phenytoin-induced gingival enlargement.[14]
   - Adequate biofilm control, particularly if started before the administration of phenytoin, helps control the extent of gingival overgrowth.
2. *Contributing Factors*
   - Mouth breathing.
   - Overhanging and other defective restorations.
   - Large carious lesions.
   - Calculus and other biofilm-retaining factors encourage gingival overgrowth.
   - Treatment must include removal of these factors by recontouring overhangs, placing or replacing restorations, and removing calculus.

F. Treatment[15]

There are varying modes to treat gingival enlargement based on the medication used and the clinical presentation of the lesion. **Figure 62-3** is a decision tree to help determine the type of treatment indicated.

1. *Change in Drug Prescription*
   - Since the medication is the cause, the physician could be approached concerning the possibility of changing the prescription to a different drug with a lower chance of causing gingival enlargement.
   - If possible, such a change should be made just prior to a surgical removal procedure that may be planned.
2. *Nonsurgical Treatment*
   - Scaling with a concentrated program of biofilm control may help early lesions regress.
   - Once the tissue has become fibrotic; however, shrinkage cannot be expected.
   - A program of prevention and control should be started prior to, or simultaneously with, the initial administration of the medication.
   - Chlorhexidine gluconate rinses have been used with some success to prevent return of gingival enlargement caused by another medication.[16,17]
   - A positive pressure appliance has been used with some success to reduce gingival enlargement.[18]
3. *Surgical Removal*
   - If a sufficient band of attached gingiva exists, one surgical procedure that has been used for tissue removal has been *gingivectomy.*
   - A *periodontal flap* procedure may be the choice for healing and esthetics.
   - Prior to surgery, a regulated program of biofilm control should be introduced and continued after surgical dressings have been removed.
   - For the patient with epilepsy, general health has special significance, and oral health contributes to general health.
   - For the patient with drug-induced gingival enlargement, emphasis in appointments is on a rigid oral hygiene program if the gingival overgrowth is to be kept to a minimum.

G. Differential Diagnosis of Medications Causing Gingival Enlargement[19]

Numerous medications may cause gingival enlargement, including:

- Antiepileptic medications, especially phenytoin and to a lesser extent ethosuximide, valproic acid, and primidone.
- Calcium channel blocking agents used for the treatment of hypertension and other diseases.
- Immunosuppressant cyclosporin used frequently with organ transplant patients. Tacrolimus may be a substitute with less occurrence of gingival overgrowth.

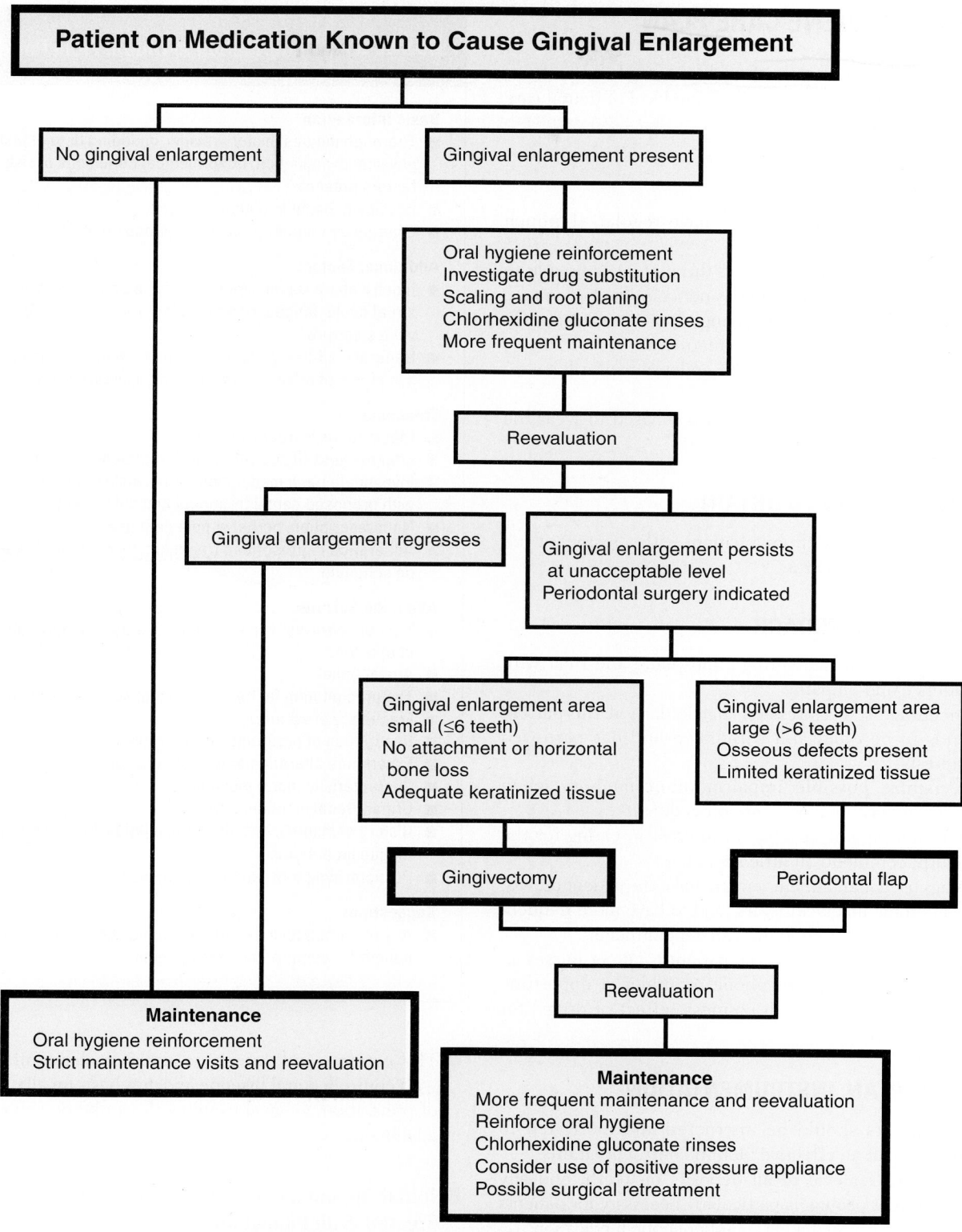

FIGURE 62-3 **Decision Tree of Treatment for Gingival Enlargement.** (*Source:* Adapted with permission from Camargo PM, Melnick PR, Pirih FQ, Lagos R, Takei HH. Treatment of drug-induced gingival enlargement: aesthetic and functional considerations. *Periodontol 2000.* 2001;27:131–8.)

DENTAL HYGIENE CARE PLAN

The majority of patients with epilepsy or a history of seizure can and should receive the same level of dental care as the general population.

I. PATIENT HISTORY

- Most patients with epilepsy have regular, thorough medical examinations.
- The physician is contacted if the patient is unable to provide needed information, is noncompliant, if seizure activity has increased or changed, or if treatment for epilepsy is impacting dental treatment.
- A well-controlled patient with epilepsy may still have a seizure.
- When seizure-prone, a person is advised to wear the Medical Alert jewelry (page 1059).

II. INFORMATION TO OBTAIN

Information to obtain from a patient with a history of seizures is listed in **Box 62-3**.

III. PATIENT APPROACH

- Provide a calm, reassuring atmosphere and treat with patience and empathy.
- Encourage self-expression, particularly if the patient tends to be quiet and withdrawn and has narrowed interests.
- Recognize possible impairment of memory when reviewing personal oral care procedures.
- Help the patient develop an interest in caring for the mouth; commend all little successes.
- Drugs used in treatment tend to make the patient drowsy, and chronic illness sufferers tend to have more frequent health issues that interfere with appointments.
- Be understanding when the patient is late or misses an appointment; plan telephone reminder at opportune time; do not mistake drowsiness (effect of drugs) for inattentiveness.

IV. CARE PLAN: INSTRUMENTATION

- All patients should be instructed and motivated to comply with an effective biofilm control program.
- Complete removal of all deposits on teeth, and any needed root planing is particularly necessary for patients who plan to or are taking an antiepileptic medication.
- Options for treatment of gingival enlargement are found in **Figure 62-3**.

A. Prior to and at the Start of Phenytoin Therapy

- A rigorous biofilm control program and complete scaling are introduced in preparation for phenytoin therapy.

BOX 62-3　Information to Obtain From Patient

Basic Information
- Thorough medical history review, including date of last physical examination, other medical conditions or risk factors present
- Physician: name and phone number
- Emergency contact person and phone number

Additional Factors
- Inquire about recent illness, stress, alcohol use, menstrual cycle, fatigue, or pain as factors that may provoke a seizure.
- General well-being; refer for evaluation for any signs or symptoms of other conditions such as depression.

Treatment
- Medications, surgery, or diet
- Effectiveness of seizure control treatment
- Investigate each medication for possible interaction with proposed dental treatment and side effects
- Nonprescription, herbal supplement use
- Adherence to prescribed treatment; medications taken on schedule

About the Seizures
- Type of seizure(s) experienced, severity, and duration of episodes
- Age at onset
- The precipitating factors or cause of seizure if known
- Frequency of seizures
- Description of prodrome, aura if known
- Experience alteration or loss of consciousness
- Characteristic motor movements
- Urinary/fecal incontinence
- History of injuries, including oral injuries, broken teeth, tongue lacerations
- Postictal symptoms such as confusion

Suggestions
- Any other helpful information that may be provided by patient for comfort and management

---

- The patient (and caregivers) must understand that, with controlled oral hygiene and emphasis on all phases of prevention, gingival overgrowth can be prevented to a large degree.

B. Initial Appointment Series for the Patient Treated With Phenytoin

Weekly appointments for complete biofilm control instruction and scaling are planned with the following objectives:

1. *Slight or Mild Gingival Overgrowth*
   - Nonsurgical treatment, including frequent thorough scalings, can be expected to lead to tissue reduction,

provided the patient cooperates in daily biofilm control.

  - Frequent maintenance appointments can contribute to function and comfort with minimum periodontal involvement.

2. *Moderate Gingival Overgrowth*
  - After the initial series of weekly biofilm instruction and scalings, reevaluation of the tissue can determine whether further procedures are needed.
  - An optimum level of oral health may be attained by changing the medication to another antiepileptic drug, using surgical pocket removal, and continuing frequent maintenance appointments.

3. *Severe Fibrotic Overgrowth*
  - Initial scaling and biofilm control are carried out to prepare the mouth for surgical pocket removal.
  - Plans for changing the drug or altering the dose should be discussed with the patient's physician.

C. Maintenance Appointment Intervals

- Frequent appointments on a 1-, 2-, or 3-month plan are indicated, depending on the severity of the gingival enlargement and the ability and motivation of the patient to maintain the oral health.
- Most patients need continuing assistance and supervision, and their response is influenced by the instruction and devotion of the dental personnel.

V. CARE PLAN: PREVENTION

- Daily biofilm removal and fluoride therapy, the use of pit and fissure sealants, and dietary control all have a vital part in the care of the patient with a seizure disorder.
- Initiation of preventive measures as soon as possible after the disorder has been diagnosed can contribute to the total health and well-being of the patient.

EMERGENCY CARE

I. OBJECTIVES

A. To prevent body injury and accidents related to the oral structures, such as:
  - Tongue bite
  - Broken or dislocated teeth
  - Dislocated or fractured jaw
  - Broken fixed or removable dentures
B. To ensure adequate ventilation.

II. DIFFERENTIAL DIAGNOSIS OF SEIZURE[20]

- Syncope
- Migraine headache
- Transient ischemic attack
- Cerebrovascular accident, stroke
- Sleep disorder such as narcolepsy
- Movement disorders such as dyskinesia, common, for example, in patients with cerebral palsy or multiple sclerosis
- Overdose of local anesthetic
- Hypoglycemia or insulin overdose in a patient with diabetes
- Hyperventilation

III. PREPARATION FOR APPOINTMENT

When the patient's medical history indicates susceptibility to seizures, precautions may prevent complications should a seizure occur.

- Place emergency materials in a convenient location.
- Have patient remove dentures for duration of appointment.
- Provide a calm and reassuring atmosphere.
- Have other dental personnel available in case of an emergency.

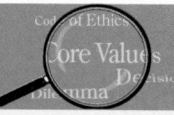

Everyday Ethics

Lillian, the dental hygienist, just finished treating her last patient of the day. Diana, the patient, is a very pleasant woman with excellent oral health and a history of a car accident with concussion over a month ago. She has no other medical findings. While passing the window, Lillian notices that Diana has collapsed in the parking lot and is convulsing. She calls for assistance from the dentist and assistant, and they rush out. By the time they reach Diana, she is getting to her feet and says she just tripped and fell.

Individuals with seizures may have their driver's license revoked because of the potential for serious automobile accidents that may occur during a seizure. Diana is about to get into her car to drive home.

Questions for Consideration

1. Which of the dental hygiene ethical core values have application in this scenario?
2. Given the patient's medical history, will this information be documented in Diana's dental record, remain confidential, or be otherwise handled? To evaluate one's responsibilities towards self, one's patients, and others, read over, in the Codes of Ethics (Appendices I, II, and III (starting page 1085) professional responsibilities to help Lillian decide the correct procedure.
3. Describe the rights of the patient and the professional duties of the dental hygienist having witnessed the incident.

IV. EMERGENCY PROCEDURE

The dental clinic or office team has assigned responsibilities during any emergency. Initiation of procedures for seizure emergency follows preplanned routines.

A. Make no attempt to stop the convulsion or to restrain the patient.
B. Terminate clinical procedure; call for assistance.
C. Protect the patient from injury.
   1. Position patient: lower chair and tilt to supine; raise feet.
   2. Keep patient from falling out of dental chair.
   3. Push aside sharp objects, movable equipment, and instrument trays.
   4. Loosen tight belt, collar, necktie.
   5. Do *not* place (or force) anything between the teeth.
   6. Establish airway; check for breathing obstruction; provide basic life support when indicated. Place on side recovery position. Use high-speed suction with wide tip to remove vomit.
   7. Monitor vital signs.
   8. Stay beside the patient to prevent personal injury and reassure.
   9. Check for level of consciousness and determine if emergency medical assistance is required.
   10. When seizure in still occurring or has recurred within 5 minutes, activate emergency medical system.

V. POSTICTAL PHASE

- Complete the record of emergency, as described in Figure 69-1 (page 1064).
- Allow the patient to rest.
- Talk to the patient in a low, reassuring tone. Ask onlookers to leave the patient in privacy.
- Check oral cavity for trauma to teeth or tissues. Palliative care can be administered. When a tooth is broken, the piece must be located so that aspiration can be prevented.
- Contact the patient's family/friend to accompany the patient if requested.

VI. STATUS EPILEPTICUS

- Status epilepticus is defined as one or more seizures lasting more than 30 minutes.
- The prolonged seizure may not end spontaneously; brain injury may occur and result in long-term morbidity or death.
- Generally, a seizure lasting more than 5 minutes should be considered to progress to status epilepticus unless emergency intervention is taken.
- Emergency medical assistance must be sought immediately, and the patient must be transported to an emergency department.
- Basic life support and intravenous lorazepam or diazepam are given.

BOX 62-4	**Example Progress Note**

Appointment for final scaling and planing Quadrant 4 with review of other quadrants. Took time to discuss poor response and made a "plaque score" with disclosing agent to show Josh how much biofilm he was leaving. Gave him another new toothbrush and watched how it was being applied.

   Made suggestions: he just hasn't spent time enough; I explained halitosis and in his business, he sees a lot of people. He has a powered brush—when asked why he doesn't use it more, his only answer was "it isn't handy. I'll bring it down and keep it nearer the sink. And hope my little boy doesn't climb up and play with it." My suggestion was to have one of his own for the child, and suggested a brand name for him to find in his drug store. "Brush yours when he is brushing. Set him a good example." He smiled at that.

Signed:_____, RDH Date:_____

DOCUMENTATION

The patient who is subject to seizures will need complete permanent records that show the following:

- All the same as for all patients: initially, the complete health history, vital signs, radiographs, findings of the extra- and intraoral examination; periodontal history, charting, and tissue description; dental caries history, charting, and current demineralization and carious lesions.
- Progress notes for each appointment with abbreviated history and current clinical findings.
- Information about the need for understanding the type of seizure; the treatment that is used; how to handle in an emergency.
- A sample progress note may be reviewed in **Box 62-4.**

Factors To Teach The Patient

- Relationship of systemic health to oral health.
- Importance of careful daily care of mouth.
- Need for providing complete medical history information for dental appointments.
- Antiepileptic medication side effects, including gingival enlargement and how to minimize its growth.
- Seek immediate care if any oral change or injury is suspected.

References

1. International League Against Epilepsy, Commission on Classification and Terminology. Proposal for revised clinical and electroencephalographic classification of epileptic seizures. *Epilepsia.* 1981 Aug;22(4):489–501.

2. International League Against Epilepsy, Commission on Classification and Terminology. Proposal for revised classification of epilepsies and epileptic syndromes. *Epilepsia.* 1989 Jul–Aug;30(4):389–99.

3. Brodie M, de Boer HM, Johannessen SI. Epidemiology. *Epilepsia.* 2003;44(6 Suppl):17.

4. Malamed SF, Robbins KS. *Handbook of medical emergencies in the dental office.* 5th ed. St. Louis: Mosby; 2000. Chapter 21, Seizures; pp. 279–97.

5. Nguyen DK, Spencer SS. Recent advances in the treatment of epilepsy. *Arch Neurol.* 2003 Jul;60(7):929–35.

6. Roberts HW. The effect of electrical dental equipment on a vagus nerve stimulator's function. *J Am Dent Assoc.* 2002 Dec;133(12):1657–64.

7. Angelopolous AP, Goaz PW. Incidence of diphenylhydantoin gingival hyperplasia. *Oral Surg Oral Med Oral Pathol.* 1972 Dec;34(6):898–906.

8. Rees TD, Levine RA. Systemic drugs as a risk factor for periodontal disease initiation and progression. *Compendium.* 1995 Jan;16(1):20, 22, 26.

9. Hassell TM (ed). *Epilepsy and the oral manifestations of phenytoin therapy.* London: Karger; 1981, pp. 116–27. (Huysmans MC, Lussi A, Weber HP, editors. Monographs in Oral Science; vol 9).

10. Bredfeldt GW. Phenytoin-induced hyperplasia found in edentulous patients. *J Am Dent Assoc.* 1992 Jun;123(6):61–4.

11. McCord JF, Sloan P, Hussey DJ. Phenytoin hyperplasia occurring under complete dentures: a clinical report. *J Prosthet Dent.* 1992 Oct;68(4):569–72.

12. Chee WW, Jansen CE. Phenytoin hyperplasia occurring in relation to titanium implants: a clinical report. *Int J Oral Maxillofac Implants.* 1994 Jan–Feb;9(1):107–9.

13. Camargo PM, Melnick PR, Pirih FQ, Lagos R, Takei HH. Treatment of drug-induced gingival enlargement: aesthetic and functional considerations. *Periodontology 2000.* 2001;27:131–8.

14. Majola MP, McFadyen ML, Connolly C, Nair YP, Govender M, Laher MH. Factors influencing phenytoin-induced gingival enlargement. *J Clin Periodontol.* 2000 Jul;27(7):506–12.

15. Newman MG, Takei HH, Carranza FA (eds). *Carranza's clinical periodontology.* 9th ed. Philadelphia: Saunders; 2002. Camargo PM, Carranza FA. Treatment options; pp. 756–9.

16. Saravia ME, Svirsky JA, Friedman R. Chlorhexidine as an oral hygiene adjunct for cyclosporine-induced gingival hyperplasia. *ASDC J Dent Child.* 1990 Sep–Oct;57(5):366–70.

17. Pilatti GL, Sampaio JE. The influence of chlorhexidine on the severity of cyclosporin A–induced gingival overgrowth. *J Periodontol.* 1997 Sep;68(9):900–4.

18. Zaiman R. The use of positive pressure mouthpiece as a new therapy for Dilantin gingival hyperplasia. *Chron Omaha Dent Soc.* 1968 Apr;31(8):244–5.

19. Jaiarj N. Drug-induced gingival overgrowth. *J Mass Dent Soc.* 2003 Fall;52(3):16–20.

20. Shneker BF, Fountain NB. Epilepsy. *Dis Mon.* 2003 Jul;49(7):426–78.

The Patient With a Psychiatric Disorder

ESTHER M. WILKINS, BS, RDH, DMD
JANET H. TOWLE, RN, RDH, BS, MED

Chapter Outline

A psychiatric or mental disorder is a complex, clinically significant behavioral or psychological syndrome or pattern that is associated with present distress or disability. The causes may be related to behavioral, psychologic, or biologic dysfunction in the individual.[1]

- A classification of mental disorders does not classify people, but rather it is the disorders that people have that are classified. For example, the patient should be referred to as "an individual with schizophrenia," not as "a schizophrenic."[1]
- With the discovery and official approval of new psychotropic drugs for more effective therapy, and with the current policies of deinstitutionalization, more individuals with mental disorders are seeking dental and dental hygiene care in dental offices and clinics.

- Care for a person with a psychiatric illness, or for one who may be undergoing an emotional crisis, presents increased challenges for health professionals.
- The American Psychiatric Association has classified more than 200 types of mental disorders in the document *Diagnostic and Statistical Manual of Mental Disorders (DSM-IV-TR)*. The *DSM* is in accord with the *International Classification of Diseases (ICD)* published by the World Health Organization.[2] Each disorder has characteristic signs and symptoms. Terminology related to the disorders is listed and defined in **Box 63-1**.
- This chapter includes descriptions of frequently encountered psychiatric disorders, namely, schizophrenia, mood disorders, anxiety disorders, and eating disorders. Other disorders are described elsewhere in the text, for example, alcoholism (in Chapter 64),

BOX 63-1	Key Words

Mental Disorders

Affect: emotion or feeling; tone of reaction to persons and events

Agitation: excessive motor activity, usually not purposeful and associated with internal tension.

Anxiolytic medication: ability to relieve anxiety or emotional tension, also called antianxiety agent.

Bradykinesia: abnormal slowness of movement; sluggish physical and mental responses.

Catatonia: no voluntary movement; physical rigidity; fixed position may be maintained for hours.

Cognitive: mental process of comprehension, judgment, memory.

Decompensate: appearance or exacerbation of a mental disorder.

Delusion: false belief firmly held though contradicted by social reality.

Dementia: loss of cognitive and intellectual functions sufficiently severe to interfere with social and occupational functioning.

Dysarthria: impairment in uttering words due to diseases that affect oral and pharyngeal muscles.

Electroconvulsive therapy (ECT): electroshock therapy; a form of somatic therapy in which an electric current is used to produce convulsions; primarily used to treat depression.

Euphoria: feeling of well-being; in psychiatry, abnormal or exaggerated sense of well-being.

Hallucination: false sensory perception in the absence of an actual external stimulus.

Illusion: a mental impression derived from misinterpretation of an actual sensory stimulus; a false perception.

Insomnia: wakefulness; inability to sleep in the absence of noise or other disturbance.

Lanugo: fine, downy hair.

Neurosis: a mental disorder that usually involves the use of unconscious defense mechanisms as a means of coping; individual is not out of touch with reality.

Noncompliance: failure to carry out prescribed healthcare plan, for example, failure to take medications as prescribed.

Paranoia: mental disorder characterized by delusions of persecution.

Perimylolysis: erosion of enamel and dentin as a result of chemical and mechanical effects.

Phobia: persistent, unrealistic pathologic fear or dread out of proportion to the stimulus from a particular object or situation.

Prodrome: a premonitory symptom; a symptom indicating the onset of disease.

Psychosis: a significant major mental disorder that so greatly impairs perception, thinking, emotional response, and/or personal orientation that the individual loses touch with reality.

Psychotherapy: treatment of emotional, behavioral, personality, and psychiatric disorders by means of individual or group verbal or nonverbal communication with the patient.

Psychotropic medication: a medication that alters the mind; the major categories are antipsychotic, antianxiety, antidepressant, and antimanic agents.

Tardive dyskinesia: involuntary movements of the mouth, lips, tongue, and jaws, usually associated with long-term use of antipsychotic medication.

Alzheimer's disease (Chapter 52), and dementia due to Parkinson's disease (Chapter 58).

Knowledge of the types of mental disorders and their signs and symptoms can help the clinician recognize a patient's needs and understand a patient's behaviors. Confidence and trust by the patient are essential for communication and the patient's acceptance of clinical care.

Principles of informed consent are applied for patients of all ages with mental disorders. Many patients with mental disorders are capable of signing their own consent form. Information for obtaining informed consent is described in Chapter 24 on page 358.

SCHIZOPHRENIA

- Schizophrenia is a complex, chronic mental disorder. Disturbances in feeling, thinking, and behavior significantly impair function to a level below normal for the individual.

- Schizophrenia is a major psychotic illness in which the individual may be out of touch with reality.
- Symptoms include delusions, hallucinations, disorganized thinking, and incoherence.
- The onset is usually between the ages of 15 and 24 in males, and 25 and 35 in women.
- The onset can be gradual or abrupt. Most people have a slow-developing prodromal phase in which there is a gradual appearance of the signs and symptoms.
- Some patients remain chronically ill, whereas others have periods of remission and recurrence.
- Although the cause is not understood, genetic factors can make an individual more vulnerable.

I. SYMPTOMS OF SCHIZOPHRENIA

Phases of the disease are described as *prodromal, active,* and *residual*. Prodromal symptoms may appear as signs of deterioration for as long as 1 year before the active phase. **Box 63-2** shows the symptoms of each phase.

Active-phase symptoms are *positive,* those that reflect unusual, exaggerated behavior, or *negative,* those that show the absence of behavior that might be expected normally.

Rates of alcohol and other drug abuse are high among patients with schizophrenia. Many patients diagnosed with schizophrenia also qualify for a diagnosis of alcohol abuse. Drug and alcohol abuse can aggravate psychiatric symptoms and lead to poor treatment compliance, increased hospitalization, homelessness, and suicide.[3]

II. TREATMENT OF SCHIZOPHRENIA

The response to initial treatment can be a predictor of the long-term prognosis. The prognosis has generally been considered guarded to poor. Evidence shows that although deterioration may occur during the early years, the condition may stabilize with treatment during middle age.

A. Pharmacotherapy[4,5]

- The objectives of treatment are to reduce or alleviate the delusions, hallucinations, and other symptoms (Box 63-2) and to enable the patient to function in daily living.

BOX 63-2	Symptoms of Schizophrenia

PRODROMAL AND RESIDUAL SYMPTOMS
- Marked social isolation or withdrawal
- Marked impairment in role functioning (as wage earner, student, homemaker)
- Markedly peculiar behavior
- Marked impairment in personal hygiene
- Blunted or inappropriate affect
- Digressive, vague speech or lack of speech
- Odd beliefs or magical thinking
- Unusual perceptual experiences
- Marked lack of initiative, interests, or energy

ACTIVE-PHASE SYMPTOMS
Positive Symptoms
- Delusions
- Hallucinations
- Disorganized speech
- Disorganized or bizarre behavior
- Catatonia

Negative Symptoms
- Flat affect
- Lack of voluntary action
- Speechlessness
- No pleasure from events that usually give pleasure
- Inability to perform goal-directed activities.

Source: American Psychiatric Association. *DSM-IV-TR.* Washington: APA; 2000. p. 312.

- The use of antipsychotic medications has improved the outcomes of treatment and led to the process of deinstitutionalization.
- Schizophrenia is associated with an excess of dopamine at specific synapses in the brain.
- Conventional antipsychotic drugs are used to block dopamine receptors and are effective against positive symptoms with less effect on negative symptoms.
  - Phenothiazines (chlorpromazine [Thorazine™])
  - Butyrophenones (haloperidol [Haldol™])
  - Thioxanthenes (thiothixene [Navane™])
- Atypical drugs generally have fewer motor side effects and are effective against negative symptoms.
  - Dibenzodiazepines (clozapine [Clozaril™])
  - Benzisoxazoles (risperidone [Risperdal™])
  - Olanzapine, quetiapine, ziprasidone, and others.

B. Adverse Effects of Medications

- Careful monitoring is essential because side effects can be severe.
- For example, weekly white blood cell counts are needed during the first 6 months of clozapine therapy, and routinely thereafter, because of the high risk of agranulocytosis.[5]
- Table 63-1 lists a few of the many side effects of antipsychotic medications, with suggestions for appointment adaptations.

C. Maintenance

- After an acute episode, the dosage is adjusted for the remission period.
- A minimal effective dose is important to reduce adverse reactions, particularly the risk of tardive dyskinesia.
- Noncompliance in continuing medication is a common cause of psychotic relapse and rehospitalization.[4]

D. Psychosocial Therapy

- Psychosocial therapy is integrated with pharmacotherapy.
- Objectives are meant to ensure compliance with the use of prescribed medications and to give general support in dealing with the illness.
- Long-term treatment for psychosocial and vocational recovery after an acute psychotic episode is enhanced when family and all those close to the patient are included.
- Psychotherapy may include a variety of vocational rehabilitation efforts and training in social skills.

III. DENTAL HYGIENE CARE

A. Oral Implications[6,7]

- Overall degeneration of health factors may have occurred because of neglect of diet, exercise, sleep,

TABLE 63-1	EFFECTS OF ANTIPSYCHOTIC MEDICATION
SIDE EFFECTS	**IMPLICATIONS FOR APPOINTMENT**
Dystonia Muscle contractions	Laryngeal spasm; coughing Unable to turn head
Dysarthria Difficult speech	Communication difficulty
Parkinson-like syndrome Shuffling gait Muscular rigidity Resting tremor (pill rolling) Facial grimacing Bradykinesia	Cooperation may be difficult Patient positioning Instrument positioning; retraction
Akathisia Restlessness, pacing	Plan short appointments
Akinesia Loss of voluntary movement Lethargy, fatigue feelings	Adjust patient position
Tardive dyskinesia Involuntary mouth and jaw movements	Difficulty in instrumentation Wearing dentures difficult or impossible Muscle fatigue; may need mouth prop
Anticholinergic effects Xerostomia Blurred vision	Dental caries prevention Fluoride dentifrice; saliva substitute Difficulty seeing visual aids
Cardiovascular Postural hypotension Tachycardia, palpitations	Have patient sit up slowly and wait before standing Monitor vital signs
Sedation Drowsiness	Interfere with patient's daily routine Patient may be late; needs reminders
Blood Reduced leukocytes Agranulocytosis	Increased susceptibility to infection Oral candidiasis may be present

general cleanliness, personal grooming, and oral care.

- Concurrent alcohol and/or other drug abuse, as well as smoking, can influence dental and periodontal health.
- Xerostomia can lead to an increase in rampant dental caries.

B. Appointment Planning

- Elective dental and dental hygiene treatment is not carried out during an acute exacerbation.
- Treatment is undertaken when the patient's symptoms are reasonably controlled by medications.

- If the patient decompensates during a dental or dental hygiene appointment, immediate referral is needed.
- Telephone numbers of the patient's physicians are kept in an easily accessible location for quick referrals.

C. Appointment Interventions

- Because schizophrenia is often a lifelong disorder, planning for future oral health is essential.
- Review medical and medication history; analyze drugs for possible side effects that require appointment modifications **(Table 63-1)**.
- Review consultation notes from the mental health physician relative to medications, alcohol or other substance use, and medicolegal competence for informed consent.
- Plan a simple routine. For a series of appointments and maintenance, use a familiar, organized routine that is comfortable for the patient.
- Decrease stimulation; create a restful atmosphere; if background music is present, keep it low and soft.
- Provide instruction in oral care.
  - Help the patient to improve the level of personal oral care on a daily basis.
  - When applicable, evaluate the patient's personal caregiver for attitude and knowledge and provide information and instruction.
- Use a mouth prop to assist the patient with tardive dyskinesia. The patient does not have control of mouth movements and can appreciate stability.

MOOD DISORDERS

The primary mood disorders are *major depressive disorder* and *bipolar disorder*. A major depressive disorder is unipolar, whereas a bipolar disorder is marked by severe mood swings from depression to elation (mania). Both unipolar and bipolar disorders are characterized by periods of remission and recurrence.

- Depression is among the most common of the many psychiatric illnesses, yet it may not always be recognized and treated.
- Depression occurs at any age.
- Onset for major depression is usually the mid-20s and is more common in women than men.
- Bipolar disorder begins about age 20 and is equally common in men and women.
- Minor forms of depression are more common in the elderly, especially those who are chronically ill or are cognitively intact and reside in nursing homes.[8]
- Depression is a disturbance marked by apathy, fear, sadness, and loss of mobility and energy.
- Transient depressed moods occur in the lives of most people. Sadness over unforeseen tragic events, illnesses, death, or disappointments in career or other life plans can cause depressed feelings.

BOX 63-3	Characteristics of a Major Depressive Episode

- Depressed mood
- Markedly diminished interest or pleasure in all or almost all activities
- Significant weight loss or gain
- Insomnia or hypersomnia
- Psychomotor agitation or retardation
- Fatigue or loss of energy
- Feelings of worthlessness or excessive guilt
- Diminished ability to concentrate; indecisiveness
- Recurrent thoughts of death or suicide

Source: Adapted with permission from American Psychiatric Association. *DSM-IV-TR.* Washington: APA; 2000. 356 p.

- Transient depressed moods usually can be overcome in time and need to be differentiated from depression as a major depressive illness.

MAJOR DEPRESSIVE DISORDER

I. CHARACTERISTICS OF A MAJOR DEPRESSIVE EPISODE

- Characteristics of a major depressive episode are listed in Box 63-3. Both thought disorders and physical signs are involved. Depression increases the risk of suicide.
- The manifestations of depression can vary considerably among patients and between age groups.
- Some individuals experience only one episode of major depression in their entire lives.
- For children, depression interferes with interrelations with other children and with motivations to learn and play.
- The adolescent may demonstrate with substance abuse, antisocial behavior, school difficulties, and/or poor hygiene.[9]
- Depressed adults may lack motivation and initiative and may find interactions with people at work or in social settings difficult.
- Elderly depressed individuals can feel isolated because of the many losses in their lives. In addition, their lives may be influenced by physical and mental changes associated with aging.

II. TREATMENT OF DEPRESSION

Antidepression medications are the primary treatment for individuals with depression. In addition, treatment may include lifestyle changes, correction of sleep disorders, new diet and eating patterns, and exercise, along with counseling and practical psychotherapy.

Hospitalization may be indicated when potential danger of suicide or harm to others exists. Severe health problems can be related to self-neglect with excessive weight loss.

A. Psychopharmacotherapy[10,11,12]

Antidepressive medications are indicated for major depression and the depressive stage of bipolar disorder. For a patient with a substance-induced mood disorder, antidepressant or mood-stabilizing therapy is withheld for at least 30 days to confirm medical diagnosis of primary mood disorder.

Each drug has characteristic adverse reactions. Xerostomia is the major oral problem.

- SSRIs (selective serotonin re-uptake inhibitors)
  - Often the initial therapy for depressive illness
  - *Advantages:* tolerability better than earlier drugs; better compliance; safety in overdose
  - *Specific products:* fluoxetine (Prozac™), sertraline (Zoloft™), paroxetine (Paxil™), fluvoxamine (Luvox™)
- SNRIs (serotonin and noradrenergic re-uptake inhibitors)
- Tricyclic and heterocyclic antidepressants
  - Not used for initial treatment; higher risk of overdose
  - Xerostomia often a serious side effect
- *MAOIs (monoamine oxidase inhibitors):* certain foods and other drugs to be avoided to prevent hypertensive crisis
- Number of atypical antidepressant medications is increasing.

B. Psychotherapy/Cognitive Behavior Therapy

Patients with lesser degrees of depression may benefit from psychotherapy alone. Therapy and pharmacotherapy lend support to each other. Improvement in work performance and social adjustment with increased compliance in carrying out basic personal health needs, including oral hygiene, can be noted.

C. Electroconvulsive Therapy: Indications

- Patient for whom antidepressant medications are contraindicated
- Patient who is nonresponsive to optimal pharmacotherapy
- Patient with major depression who also has delusions
- Patient with overwhelming suicidal preoccupation or substantially diminished food intake
- The need for an immediate response (such as for a catatonic patient)

III. DENTAL HYGIENE CARE

The patient with a major depressive disorder and the patient with the depressive phase of bipolar disorder have the same general characteristics as those described in this section.

A. Personal Factors

■ The symptoms of the depressed individual not controlled by medication are listed in Box 63-3 and can be considered in preparation for dental hygiene care.

■ By appearance and facial expression, the patient may appear to be pessimistic and show feelings of sadness and gloom. Inattentiveness, memory impairment, and diminished motivation are typical.

■ The medicated patient may demonstrate symptoms of the side effects of medication.

■ When food and alcoholic beverages are used as coping mechanisms, weight gain may be considerable. Food choices frequently include many sweets, which contribute to dental and periodontal breakdown. Oral problems related to substance abuse are described in Chapter 64 pages 981 to 983.

B. Oral Health Implications[13]

■ *Side effects of medications:* xerostomia, which leads to high risk of enamel and root caries and to problems of denture retention.

■ Omission of general health habits and neglect of oral care make the person susceptible to various infections and illnesses.

■ Loss of taste perception can contribute to a diet high in cariogenic foods with high levels of sucrose.

C. Appointment Interventions[8,13,14]

1. **Assessment**
   ■ Monitor the medical and medications histories closely; note side effects and contraindications for new drug therapies.
   ■ Review consultations with medical/psychiatric specialists caring for the patient.
   ■ *Intraoral/extraoral examination:* Check for signs of xerostomia.

2. **Approach**
   ■ Provide positive reinforcement and reassurance. Avoid negative guilt-inducing words. Depressed patients may needlessly blame themselves.
   ■ Show genuine interest, but avoid attempts to cheer the patient by joking or laughing or making such remarks as, "Let's see you smile now."

3. **Preventive Instruction**
   ■ *Dental biofilm control:* Teach patient and caregivers the need for daily measures to preserve the teeth and periodontal tissues.
   ■ *Xerostomia*
      ■ Home fluoride custom tray daily
      ■ Saliva substitute containing fluoride
      ■ Alcohol-free, over-the-counter fluoride rinse or brush-on gel

4. **Implementation of Care Plan**
   ■ Adjust dental light carefully and provide tinted protective eyewear for the patient with photosensitivity, a side effect of certain medications.
   ■ Use local anesthesia. Anxious and depressed patients can be sensitive and may need profound anesthesia.
   ■ Provide fluoride treatment after instrumentation.
   ■ Use care to prevent postural hypotension. Sit the patient up slowly from a reclined position and have the patient remain seated a few moments before standing.

BIPOLAR DISORDER

Bipolar disorder is a major mood disorder in which episodes of varying degrees of mania (elation) and depression occur. It was formerly called "manic-depressive" disorder. When untreated, periods of elation can average 6 months in duration, whereas periods of depression may last longer. A return to normal behavior between episodes is usual.

I. PHASES AND SYMPTOMS

A. Depressive Phase

The characteristics for a major depressive episode (Box 63-3) and for a depressed episode of bipolar disorder are similar.

B. Manic Phase

Mania is characterized by excessive elation, hyperactivity, and accelerated thinking and speaking. A severe manic episode causes marked impairment in occupational and social functioning. Characteristics of a manic episode are listed in Box 63-4.

BOX 63-4	Characteristics of Manic Episode

■ Inflated self-esteem or grandiosity
■ Decreased need for sleep
■ More talkative than usual or pressure to keep talking
■ Flight of ideas
■ Distractibility (that is, attention easily drawn to unimportant or irrelevant external stimuli)
■ Increase in goal-directed activity (socially, at work or school, or sexually) or psychomotor agitation
■ Excessive involvement in pleasurable activities that have a high potential for painful consequences (for example, engages in unrestrained buying sprees, sexual indiscretions, or foolish business investments)

Source: Adapted with permission from American Psychiatric Association. *DSM-IV-TR.* Washington: APA; 2000. 362 p.

II. TREATMENT OF BIPOLAR DISORDER

Both pharmacotherapy and psychosocial therapy are used during all phases of the disease. Initially, hospitalization may be needed to protect the individual from harm to self or others.

A. Pharmacotherapy[10,15,16]

Treatment requires a three-pronged approach.

- Acute manic phase; to stabilize the patient's mood, use
  - Sedation with a high-potency benzodiazepine to control acute agitation
  - *Anticonvulsants:* valproic acid and its derivatives, safe and effective against mania
  - *Antipsychotics:* olazapine and risperidone, control acute agitation
  - *Lithium carbonate:* mood stabilizer
- Antidepressant therapy during periods of moderate to severe depression. Treatment for the depressive phase is described under major depression on page 956.
- *Maintenance therapy:* to obtain long-term mood stabilization and prevent the occurrence of both manic and depressive episodes, use
  - Lithium carbonate
    1. Possible side effects include gastrointestinal irritation, fine hand tremor, thirst, polyuria, and muscular weakness. Prolonged use may lead to renal tube damage and hypothyroidism.
    2. Frequent monitoring is important to guard against lithium toxicity, which can occur with long-term drug use.
  - *Anticonvulsants:* valproic acid and its derivatives; fewer side effects than lithium.

B. Psychosocial Interventions[16]

- Provide education to the patient and the family about the disease.
- Encourage adherence to drug regimens.
- Recognize early warning signs of an approaching high or low mood.
- Develop practical techniques for dealing with stress.

III. DENTAL HYGIENE CARE

A. Personal Factors

- Characteristics of an individual during a manic episode can be studied in **Box 63-4**.
- During the manic phase, the patient is overactive, restless, and in constant motion, and may behave in an aggressive, fearless manner.
- Many patients talk quickly, jump from thought to thought, and have a short attention span. A tendency to argue and become irritable may be apparent if pressured in any way.

B. Oral Health Implications[16]

- Oral hygiene needs are often unmet. At a high risk for both dental caries and periodontal disease.
- Patient unlikely to report injury or illness; a complete oral assessment can be especially significant.
- Gingival tissues may appear abraded and lacerated because of overeager grandiose brushing motions.
- Xerostomia from long-term use of medications will require use of a saliva substitute. A complete preventive program with daily fluoride therapy and an anticariogenic diet is indicated.
- Lithium may cause dysgeusia and impart a metallic taste in the mouth.
- Other possible adverse reactions to medications include stomatitis and glossitis, loss of taste acuity.

C. Appointment Interventions

Lithium medication and other treatments usually provide control for the nonhospitalized patient. The need for protecting the patient and others from overactive behavior may not be experienced in the private clinical setting because elective dental and dental hygiene appointments usually are postponed until the patient is under medical control.

- Carefully review medical and medication history; consult with patient's physician/psychiatrist as needed.
- Simplify the surroundings; provide a comfortable uncluttered environment.
- Do not rush the patient.
- When applicable, help the patient's caregiver to learn procedures for dental caries prevention and periodontal health.
- Three- to four-month maintenance appointments may be needed.
- Patient instruction may be difficult due to a short attention span. Use direct, simple instructions.

POSTPARTUM MOOD DISTURBANCES[17]

- The puerperium is the 6-week period after childbirth when the body undergoes physical and physiologic changes.
- During the entire postpartum period, many physiologic and psychologic stresses are related to the changes taking place in the mother's life.
- Degrees of emotional reactions are evident and range from postpartum blues to psychosis.
- Postpartum psychosis is considered a major psychiatric emergency.

I. POSTPARTUM BLUES

A period of nonpsychotic depression for a few days after giving birth is not uncommon. There may be crying, irritability, and mood shifts.

II. POSTPARTUM DEPRESSION

A moderate to severe depression may begin by the second to third week postpartum. Symptoms include excessive fatigue, insomnia, loss of appetite, and loss of interest and enthusiasm.

III. POSTPARTUM PSYCHOSIS

Postpartum or puerperal psychosis is a mood disorder. It may be of a depressive or manic type.

A. Risk Factors

- Preexisting mental illness, such as bipolar disorder or schizophrenia
- Stress
- Conflicts about motherhood, such as unwanted pregnancy; fears about mothering; and marital problems

B. Symptoms

- *Early.* Complaints of insomnia, restlessness, tearfulness, fatigue, and emotional unsteadiness
- *Progressive.* Confusion, irrationality, delirium, and obsessive concerns about the baby. Thoughts of bringing harm to the baby or oneself are not unusual

C. Treatment

Without treatment, risk of suicide, infanticide, or both exists. A favorable outcome can be expected with appropriate treatment, family support, and no preexisting illness.

- *Medical care.* Treat for other (organic) illnesses.
- *Suicidal precautions.* Do not leave baby alone with mother.
- *Pharmacotherapy.* In accord with symptoms of depression.
- *Psychotherapy.* Individual and marital. Arrangements for assistance at home must be made before hospital release.
- *Extended treatment.* Counseling in infant care with observation for emergence of a major mood disorder.

ANXIETY DISORDERS

Anxiety is experienced as apprehension, tension, or dread that results from the anticipation of danger, the source of which is unknown or unrecognized. Anxiety is the result of feeling a threat to the person's being, self-esteem, or identity. Fear, on the other hand, is an emotional or physiologic response to a recognized source of danger.

In normal life, some mild anxiety provides an effective stimulus to improved performance. As a psychiatric symptom, anxiety can be excessive, irrational, and beyond the control of the individual.

BOX 63-5	Symptoms of Panic Attack

- Shortness of breath
- Dizziness, unsteady feelings, or faintness
- Palpitations or accelerated heart rate
- Trembling or shaking
- Sweating (clammy hands)
- Choking
- Nausea or abdominal stress
- Numbness or tingling sensations
- Flushes (hot flashes) or chills
- Chest pain or discomfort
- Fear of dying
- Fear of going crazy or losing control

Source: Adapted with permission from American Psychiatric Association. *DSM-IV-TR.* Washington: APA; 2000. 432 p.

I. TYPES AND SYMPTOMS OF ANXIETY DISORDERS[18]

The most common anxiety disorders are described in this section. The disorders have symptoms of fear, excess worry, and avoidance behavior that are revealed in a variety of ways and degrees of severity. The anxiety disorders also can produce varying degrees of occupational and social dysfunction. Certain patients may have secondary problems of alcohol and other substance abuse. The abuse may be the result of an attempt at self-medication.

A. Panic Attack

- The symptoms that may occur in a panic attack are listed in **Box 63-5**.
- The panic attack itself is a symptom in several of the anxiety disorders.
- *An overwhelming sense of impending doom is the cardinal symptom of the attack.*
- A panic attack may be unexpected (uncued) or "situationally bound" (cued). A situationally bound panic attack invariably results from exposure to a specific trigger.
- Such triggers are characteristic of social and specific phobias that are described in this section.

B. Panic Disorder

- Panic disorder is characterized by recurrent panic attacks that are usually unexpected.
- Panic disorder may occur alone or with agoraphobia.
- Agoraphobia is the fear of being in places or situations from which escape might be difficult or embarrassing or in which help might not be available in the event of a panic attack. The fear is of open spaces, of crowds, or

of going outside the home alone and away from a safe place.

■ Studies indicate that between 8 to 33% of people with panic disorder have mitral valve prolapse.[19]

C. Posttraumatic Stress Disorder

■ An initiating traumatic event has occurred outside the range of usual human experience.

■ It may be destruction to the home or family or may result from a manmade disaster, such as war, imprisonment, torture, rape, or other exposure associated with intense horror, fear, or serious threat to life.

■ A child may have stress disorder brought on by physical or sexual abuse.

■ Flashbacks of the traumatic experience and the attendant terror may be precipitated by a stimulus that can be readily associated with the original event.

■ Through dreams or recollections, the patient may have the feeling of reliving the event.

■ Symptoms of depression or panic attacks may be evident in an acute episode.

D. Generalized Anxiety Disorder

■ There is persistent, pervasive anxiety and excessive worry but they are not associated with life-threatening fears or "attacks."

■ It may be complicated by depression, alcohol abuse, or anxiety related to a general medical condition.

II. TREATMENT OF ANXIETY DISORDERS[20]

A. Basic Therapeutic Approach

■ Eliminate the intake of caffeine, alcohol, and other drugs of abuse. Anxiety disorders are frequently complicated by alcohol abuse.

■ Diagnose and treat other medical and psychiatric problems. Anxiety disorders may emerge with depression.

■ *Exercise.* Participation in vigorous aerobics or an active sport helps to eliminate physical and psychologic symptoms and enhances the patient's sense of control.

B. Cognitive-Behavioral Therapy

A skilled behavioral therapist is needed. Relaxation, biofeedback, and other behavioral therapies have shown selective successes. The support of family and friends can be significant.

C. Pharmacotherapy

■ As few medications as possible are indicated.

■ Treatment can best be focused on the patient's sleeping habits, physical activity, and attainment of personal control in general.

■ Determination of a patient's specific problem is essential because treatment for each disorder is different.

■ When treatment is indicated, antianxiety and antidepressant medications are the drugs of choice.

■ **Antianxiety Medications:** Benzodiazepines
  ■ *Objectives:* reduce tension and relieve anxiety; induce sleep
  ■ *Prescription:* short-term basis for immediate need only; gradual discontinuance to prevent withdrawal symptoms
  ■ *Possible side effects:* confusion, dizziness, muscle weakness, difficulty in speaking, skin rash
  ■ *Adverse effects:* potential for addiction, withdrawal symptoms, diminished alertness (drowsiness), impaired eye-hand coordination, xerostomia

■ *Antidepressant medication.* Antidepressants are effective in the treatment of panic attack and disorder, posttraumatic stress disorder, and generalized anxiety disorder.

III. DENTAL HYGIENE CARE

A. Personal Factors

Each anxiety disorder has its own specific characteristics. Individuals suffering from an anxiety disorder maintain contact with reality and may be aware of the type of their disorder. Relationships with other people can be strained.

Physical complaints, such as rapid heartbeat, hyperventilation, tightness in the throat, and constant fatigue, are common.

B. Oral Implications

■ Hypersensitivity of the teeth, related to patient's general tenseness and irritability, may be present.

■ Xerostomia related to medications can cause severe problems for dental caries. Candy or cariogenic beverages used to allay dry mouth lead to enamel and root caries.

■ Oral cleanliness may not be present, even in a patient with an obsession for cleanliness. The opposite may be true, however, and a patient may perform such excessive, vigorous toothbrushing that gingival and dental abrasion result.

C. Appointment Interventions[20]

■ Review medical history and medications carefully.

■ Help the patient to feel in control. Patient may appear very nervous, jumpy, and tense. Accept the patient without judgment or criticism. Attempting to change behavior could cause symptoms of panic attack.

■ Explain each step to the patient and keep communication as open as possible. When the patient must remain still, such as during sealant placement, explain and then distract the patient's attention from the procedure.

■ Effective pain control is needed. Use local anesthesia for instrumentation. Provide gentle, painless injections.

- Appointments are best scheduled in the morning; eliminate unnecessary waiting in the reception area; length of appointment can be minimized and planned to prevent stress.
- Be alert to symptoms of panic attack **(Box 63-5)**, such as sweating or hyperventilation. Allow the patient to sit up and enjoy short breaks.

EATING DISORDERS

Anorexia nervosa, bulimia nervosa, and bulimarexia (a combination of the two) are examples of serious eating disorders. They occur primarily in adolescent girls and young adult women, but men and people of other age groups may be involved. The incidence and awareness of the conditions have increased possibly because of better recognition and diagnosis.

- Recognition of the oral manifestations can lead to detection of the patient's problem.
- Referral and medical evaluation may be lifesaving because serious medical problems may exist and psychiatric therapy may be indicated.
- Because of patient resistance and denial, however, referral for help may be difficult or impossible.
- An interdisciplinary team approach for successful rehabilitation of an individual with an eating disorder involves, at the least, medical, psychiatric, nutritional, dental, and dental hygiene professionals.
- Dental and dental hygiene care may need to be postponed until the eating disorder is under control. For other patients, definitive dental care can provide the patient with confidence and encouragement through improved esthetics and relief from tooth sensitivity.

ANOREXIA NERVOSA[21–23]

The syndrome anorexia nervosa is characterized by a refusal of the individual to maintain body weight over the minimal normal weight for age and height. The aversion to eating results in life-threatening weight loss.

- Anorexia involves self-imposed starvation that results from an obsessive desire to be thin and a marked fear of gaining weight.
- Perceptual disturbances relative to body image are present **(Figure 63-1)**.
- The course of the disease may continue until hospitalization is necessary to prevent death.

I. SIGNS AND SYMPTOMS

The characteristics of anorexia nervosa are listed in **Box 63-6**. The two types are defined in the box. There is an increased incidence of major depression or a family history of major depression or bipolar disorder in anorectic individuals.

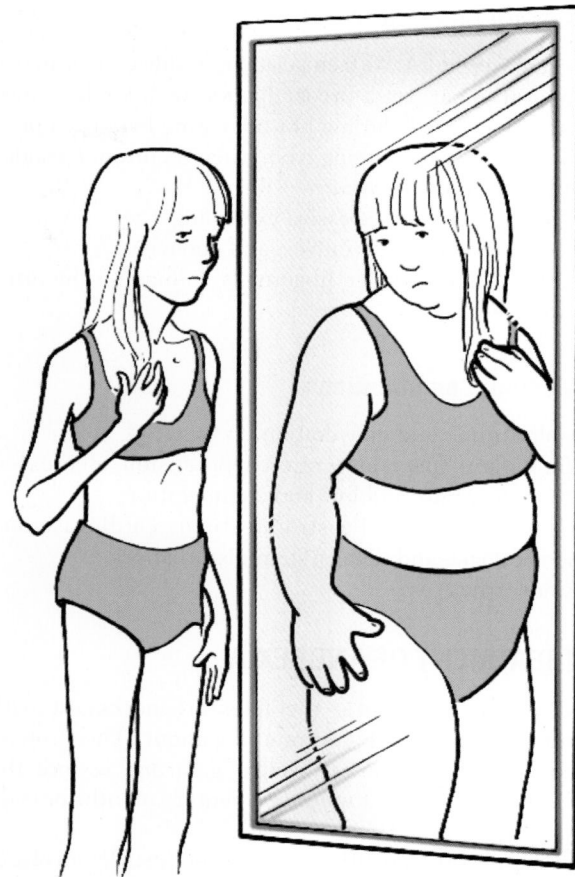

FIGURE 63-1 **Anorexia Nervosa.** The person with anorexia typically has a distorted body self-image. Although small and waiflike in real life, the mirror image appears as an overweight individual.

BOX 63-6	**Characteristics of Anorexia Nervosa**

- Refusal to maintain body weight over a minimally normal weight for age and height
- Intense fear of gaining weight or becoming fat, even though underweight
- Disturbance in the way in which one's body weight or shape is experienced
- Denies the seriousness of the current low body weight
- In females, absence of menstrual cycles when otherwise expected to occur

TYPES

Restricting type: does not regularly engage in binge-eating or purging behavior (i.e., self-induced vomiting or misuse of laxatives, diuretics, or enemas).

Binge-eating/purging type: regularly engages in binge-eating or purging behavior (i.e., self-induced vomiting or the misuse of laxatives, diuretics, or enemas).

Source: Adapted with permission from American Psychiatric Association. *DSM-IV-TR.* Washington: APA; 2000. 589 p.

A. General Characteristics

- Severe weight loss with emaciation; "waiflike" appearance
- Refusal to eat, yet a preoccupation with food; strange habits, such as hoarding but not eating food (except in the binge-eating/purging type, when recurrent episodes of binge eating do occur)
- Hyperactivity and excessive exercising
- Abuse of diuretics, laxatives, and enemas
- Dry, flaky skin, brittle fingernails; lanugo on the arms and face

B. Medical Complications

- Malnutrition and dehydration
- *Vital signs:* low pulse rate, hypotension, decreased respiratory rate, and low body temperature
- *Metabolic changes:* gastrointestinal, cardiovascular, hematologic, and renal system disturbances
- Amenorrhea

II. TREATMENT OF ANOREXIA

Medical and psychiatric therapies are necessary, with hospitalization for the severely ill patient. The primary objectives are to promote weight gain and restore the nutritional status. Treatment may require months or even years.

Pharmacotherapeutic agents are not usually involved, although the patient may be taking antidepressants, tranquilizers, antipsychotics, or antianxiety medication. Vitamin supplements may have been prescribed.

Psychotherapy varies and involves individual behavior modification, as well as group and family therapies. Professional therapists can help the individual to discover the underlying causes of the problems and the sources of the anorectic and bulimic behaviors.

III. DENTAL HYGIENE CARE

A. Personal Factors

- The individual with anorexia is frequently engaged in excessive exercise and preoccupied with food and weight loss.
- Depression may be apparent and shown by crying spells, sleep disturbances, and even thoughts of suicide.
- Frequently the person is a high achiever and highly motivated scholastically, but may be socially isolated and withdrawn.

B. Oral Implications

- Xerostomia from medications, leading to enamel and cervical root caries.
- Perimylolysis and other findings of bulimia can be noted in the binge-eating/purging type of anorexia.

C. Appointment Interventions

- Present a nonthreatening demeanor. Develop rapport through mutual respect and a trusting relationship.
- Recognize that denial of anorexia is common.
- Be aware that answers to medical and personal history questions concerning diet, medications, use of laxatives and diuretics, and weight and weight loss may provide strong suspicions of anorexia or bulimarexia.
- Assess the nutritional status through use of a dietary assessment.
- Record vital signs.
- Introduce a concentrated preventive program. Apply significant points itemized for bulimia.

BULIMIA NERVOSA[22-24]

- Bulimia nervosa is a psychiatric compulsive disorder marked by recurrent episodes of uncontrollable binge eating.
- The two types of bulimic individuals are known as the purging type and the nonpurging type (Box 63-7).
- Because of the fear of becoming overweight, self-induced vomiting after eating or the use of laxatives or diuretics is characteristic of the purging type.
- The nonpurging type uses strict dieting, fasting, and/or vigorous exercise.

BOX 63-7	Characteristics of Bulimia Nervosa

- Recurrent episodes of binge eating. An episode of binge eating is characterized by both of the following:
  - ☐ Eating, within any 2-hour period, an amount of food that is definitely larger than most people would eat in a similar period of time.
  - ☐ A sense of lack of control over eating during the episode, for example, a feeling that one cannot stop eating or control what or how much one is eating.
- Recurrent inappropriate behavior to prevent weight gain, such as self-induced vomiting; misuse of laxatives, diuretics, enemas; fasting; or excessive exercise.
- Self-evaluation is unduly influenced by body shape and weight.

TYPES

Purging type: regularly engages in self-induced vomiting or the misuse of laxatives, diuretics, or enemas.

Nonpurging type: uses inappropriate compensatory behaviors such as fasting or excessive exercise, but does not engage in self-induced vomiting or the misuse of laxatives, diuretics, or enemas.

Source: Adapted with permission from American Psychiatric Association. *DSM-IV-TR.* Washington: APA; 2000. 594 p.

The individual with bulimarexia has bulimic-type anorexia and shows symptoms of both anorexia and bulimia. All of these individuals are concerned with body weight and shape.

I. SIGNS AND SYMPTOMS

The characteristics of a person with bulimia nervosa are listed in **Box 63-7**. The illness may last many years and may alternate with periods of normal eating or periods of fasting.

A. General Characteristics

- Normal body weight or slightly overweight is typical, in contrast to the thin anorectic person.
- Food consumed during a binge may include cariogenic items with a high caloric content, a sweet taste, and a texture that allows rapid eating. Often, favorite foods are selected.
- Drug and/or alcohol abuse by the patient or in the family history is not uncommon.

B. Medical Complications

- Problems include dehydration, electrolyte imbalance, protein malnutrition, and cardiac arrhythmia.
- Self-medications include abuse of laxatives and diuretics, which contribute to gastrointestinal disturbances.
- Amenorrhea when the person also has a history of anorexia nervosa.
- Complications of drug and alcohol abuse.

II. TREATMENT OF BULIMIA

- Cognitive behavioral therapy is considered the treatment of choice for bulimia nervosa.
- Treatment focuses on modifying dysfunctional beliefs about body shape and weight.
- Antidepressants have been demonstrated effective in reducing binge eating and purging.[25]

III. DENTAL HYGIENE CARE

A. Personal Factors

- The individual with bulimia nervosa tends to be socially extroverted and more outgoing in contrast to the person with anorexia.
- The patient is well aware that the eating habits are abnormal, and as a result may suffer low self-esteem and guilt feeling.

B. Oral Findings[22,23]

- *Perimylolysis.* Perimylolysis is the chemical erosion of the tooth surfaces by acid from the regurgitation of stomach contents. After vomiting, acid is retained by the tongue papillae and provides longer contact with the palatal surfaces of maxillary teeth.
- Because of perimylolysis, the earliest evidence of bulimia may be on the smooth palatal surfaces of the teeth. The lingual surfaces of the maxillary anterior teeth appear translucent and glasslike. With time, the erosion extends over the occlusal and incisal surfaces. The mandibular teeth are protected in part by the tongue, lips, and cheeks.
- *Restorations.* Restorations may appear raised because of erosion of the enamel around the margins.
- *Dental Caries.* An increase in caries incidence is found, particularly in cervical caries. Demineralization results from the pH changes in the saliva, from xerostomia, and from the large quantities of cariogenic foods ingested during binges.
- *Saliva.* The decrease in quantity, quality, and pH of the saliva limits its buffering and lubricating properties. Dehydration of the oral soft tissues occurs.
- *Xerostomia.* Body fluid is lost from vomiting and the use of diuretics. Xerostomia is also a side effect of antidepressant medication prescribed for certain patients with bulimia and anorexia.
- *Hypersensitive Teeth.* The loss of enamel and the exposure of dentin results in sensitivity, which can be especially noticeable for the maxillary anterior teeth.
- *Trauma*
  - The soft palate can be traumatized by fingers, comb, pencils, or toothbrush used to induce vomiting. The same implement may injure the mouth at the commissures.
  - Pharyngeal trauma is caused by a large food bolus that is swallowed or regurgitated.
  - Callous formation or scars on fingers or knuckles used for self-induced vomiting may be seen.
- *Parotid Gland.* Enlargement may occur for 2 to 6 days after a binge. A cause for the enlargement is not known. The degree of enlargement increases with the frequency of vomiting. The gland functions normally and is not sensitive to palpation.
- *Bruxism.* Tooth wear is related to stress and tension.
- *Taste.* Taste perception is impaired.

C. Appointment Interventions

- Patient instruction in cause and prevention of perimylolysis and dental caries is as follows:
  - Reduce use of cariogenic foods; provide list of suggestions for substituting sugar-free products.
  - Improve personal oral care. Show use of appropriate brushing and flossing with additional interdental aids if required for biofilm removal. Clean the tongue (in Chapter 27, page 402).
- Do not brush after vomiting. Demineralization of the tooth surface by the acid from the stomach starts immediately on contact. Brushing may abrade the demineralized areas.

- Remineralization can be helped by an alkaline rinse of sodium bicarbonate or magnesium hydroxide solution to neutralize the acid. A 0.05% neutral sodium fluoride rinse could also be used.
- Fluoride therapy to reduce dental hypersensitivity and build resistance of teeth to acid demineralization is as follows:
  - Use fluoride dentifrice with several brushings daily.
  - Use neutral pH sodium fluoride mouthrinse (0.05%) daily.
  - Use custom-fitted tray for daily home application (1.1 neutral sodium fluoride gel).
- To reduce problems caused by xerostomia:
  - Advise sugar-free mints or chewing gum if patient uses them to stimulate saliva flow.
  - Recommend saliva substitutes containing fluoride.
- To reduce problems caused by hypersensitive teeth:
  - Use sugar substitute and acid -free foods and other products.
  - Use fluoride dentifrice, mouthrinse, varnish and gel tray to ease the sensitivity. Additional suggestions can be found in Chapter 35 on page 684.

PSYCHIATRIC EMERGENCIES

I. PSYCHIATRIC EMERGENCY

A psychiatric emergency in a dental clinic or private dental practice would be rare. The most common causes of emergency include panic attack, atypical drug reaction, and schizophrenic or manic decompensation.[26]

II. RISK PATIENTS FOR EMERGENCIES

- Patient with a significant psychiatric history
- Patient with a known substance abuse history
- Patient new to the clinic or office; not known by the practitioners

III. PREVENTION OF EMERGENCIES

- Prepare a complete history; collect as much information as possible; consult with the patient's physician and psychiatrist.
- Be alert to risks and characteristic symptoms of each disorder.
- Apply all the principles of stress management.
- Know the patient's medications and when they are taken. Request that patient (or caregiver if accompanied) have readily available any necessary medication that may be effective in an emergency.
- Develop rapport with each patient; avoid confronting the patient and present a nonthreatening demeanor.

IV. PREPARATION FOR AN EMERGENCY

- Attend to surroundings, such as door access, objects in the room.
- Arrange for colleagues to be aware of the possible needs of a special patient appointment; plan for an assistant to participate in clinical procedures.
- Review characteristics of specific emergencies; have necessary equipment ready.

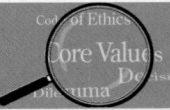 Everyday Ethics

Samuel, age 28, suffers from panic disorder and generally requests short appointments because he becomes very anxious while receiving dental care. Even with a moderate amount of generalized deposits, Ginny, the dental hygienist, usually schedules two visits to complete the treatment.

    During his visit today, Samuel appears in an almost dreamlike state. He was asked by the receptionist at the check-in about any new medications, but he stated that only a sleep aid was added to his pills, which he takes at night. Ginny suspects the patient may have taken his medication incorrectly and is concerned that Samuel is driving himself home after the appointment.

Questions for Consideration

1. Without breaching confidentiality, what ethical or other responsibility does Ginny have in verifying the type and amount of medication Samuel took and how does that influence the current day's dental hygiene appointment procedures?
2. Which of the dental hygiene core values (Table II-1, Section II Introduction, page 38) are evidenced in this scenario? Describe each in terms of the concern Ginny shows relative to Samuel's "competency" at driving himself home after the appointment as well as management during the appointment.
3. Is this an ethical dilemma or issue for Ginny? Using the questions in Table V-1 in Section V Introduction (page 362), suggest several alternative procedures that Ginny can follow during this appointment.

BOX 63-8 | **Example Progress Note**

Betty came for her maintenance scheduled 3 weeks late because of new baby; walked in saying she was having a "bad day." Rev health history she reported that she had had a tough relapse of her postpartum depression two weeks ago, but the baby was doing fine; same meds; blood pressure 140/75; oral exam with probing; lack of the meticulous care she had been in habit of; said "no anesthesia today, I need to leave early for a lunch date." Discussed her personal daily care and scaled right max and mand. quads. She seemed very nervous and jumpy during the scaling. Second appt planned for 2 weeks.

Signed: _____, RDH Date: _____

 **Factors To Teach The Patient**

- The significance of personal daily care of the oral cavity
- How medications cause dry mouth and how the incidence of carious lesions can result
- The importance of avoiding candies and drinks containing sugar to prevent dental caries
- The use of saliva substitutes to make a dry mouth more comfortable
- For the patient with bulimia or the binge-eating/purging type of anorexia:
  - ☐ The causes and effects of enamel erosion; the high acidity of the vomitus from the stomach
  - ☐ How to rinse after vomiting but not brush immediately; demineralization begins promptly after the acid from the stomach reaches the teeth. Brushing can cause abrasion of the demineralizing enamel.
- The need for multiple fluoride applications through use of home dentifrice, rinse and brush-on gel, as well as professional application of varnish or gel-tray at regular dental hygiene appointments

---

- Keep names of the patient's case worker, psychiatrist, and responsible family member in the record in a prominent position for ready reference.

V. INTERVENTION

- Stay with the patient; request colleague to contact patient's case worker, psychiatrist, or other responsible person.
- Maintain a calm, serene manner; talk quietly but firmly.
- Move the patient to a quiet, less stimulating environment. The dental equipment and environment may have contributed to the patient's disturbance.
- Assist with medication when indicated.
- Other general emergencies: refer to Tables 69-4 and 69-5 (pages 1076 to 1081).

DOCUMENTATION

The patient with a psychiatric disorder needs carefully prepared complete health history with details of the medical problem and medication history at the initial appointment and follow-up with progress notes at each succeeding appointment to review all procedures and medications for changes. The following list suggests the minimum of information to enclose in the permanent record:

- Resources for assistance in a very convenient place in the event of need to contact: Telephones, emails, and working addresses for physicians, psychiatrist, family, emergency sources
- Progress notes for each appointment and other contacts to update all personal data and treatment
- Contacts and correspondence with specialists and others
- A sample progress note may be reviewed in **Box 63-8**.

References

1. American Psychiatric Association. *Diagnostic and statistical manual of mental disorders.* 4th ed. Text revision (DSM-IV-TR). Washington: American Psychiatric Association; 2000. p. xxxi.
2. World Health Organization. *International classification of diseases (ICD-10).* Geneva: World Health Organization; 1993.
3. Selzer JA, Lieberman JA. Schizophrenia and substance abuse. *Psychiatr Clin North Am.* 1993 Jun;16(2):401–12.
4. Kane JM. Drug therapy: schizophrenia. *N Engl J Med.* 1996 Jan; 334(1):34–41.
5. Friedlander AH, Marder SR. The psychopathology, medical management and dental implications of schizophrenia. *J Am Dent Assoc.* 2002 May;133(5):603–10.
6. Steifel DJ, Truelove EL, Menard TW, Anderson VK, Doyle PE, Mandel LS. A comparison of the oral health of persons with and without chronic mental illness in community settings. *Spec Care Dentist.* 1990 Jan–Feb;10(1):6–12.
7. Friedlander AH, Liberman RP. Oral health care for the patient with schizophrenia. *Spec Care Dentist.* 1991 Sep–Oct;11(5):179–83.
8. Friedlander AH, Friedlander IK, Gallas M, Velasco E. Late-life depression: its oral health significance. *Int Dent J.* 2003 Feb; 53(1):41–50.
9. Friedlander AH, Friedlander IK, Yagiela JA, Eth S. Dental management of the child and adolescent with a major depression. *ASDC J Dent Child.* 1993 Mar–Apr;60(2):125–31.
10. Friedlander AH, Mahler ME. Major depressive disorder. Psychopathology, medical management and dental implications. *J Am Dent Assoc.* 2001 May;132(5):629–38.
11. Potter WZ, Rudorfer MV, Manji H. The pharmacologic treatment of depression. *N Engl J Med.* 1991 Aug;325(9):633–42.
12. Little JW. Dental implications of mood disorders. *Gen Dent.* 2004 Sep–Oct;52(5):442–50.
13. Friedlander AH, West LJ. Dental management of the patient with major depression. *Oral Surg Oral Med Oral Pathol.* 1991 May; 71(5):573–8.
14. Friedlander AH, Kawakami KK, Ganzell S, Fitten LJ. Dental management of the geriatric patient with major depression. *Spec Care Dentist.* 1993 Nov–Dec;13(6):249–53.
15. Clark DB. Dental care for the patient with bipolar disorder. *J Can Dent Assoc.* 2003 Jan;69(1):20–4.

16. Friedlander AH, Friedlander IK, Marder SR. Bipolar I disorder: psychophysiology, medical management and dental implications. *J Am Dent Assoc.* 2002 Sep;133(9):1209–17.

17. Nonacs R, Cohen LS. Postpartum psychiatric syndromes. In: Sadock BJ, Saddock VA, editors. *Kaplan and Sadock's comprehensive textbook of psychiatry.* Volume 1. 7th ed. Philadelphia: Lippincott Williams & Wilkins; 2000. pp. 1276–82.

18. Katon W, Geyman JP. Anxiety disorders. In: Rakel RE. *Textbook of family practice.* 6th ed. Philadelphia: Saunders; 2002. pp. 1438–9.

19. Friedlander AH, Marder SR, Sung EC, Child JS. Panic disorder: psychopathology, medical management and dental implications. *J Am Dent Assoc.* 2004 Jun;135(6):771–8.

20. Katon. op. cit., pp. 1445–50.

21. American Psychiatric Association. op. cit., pp. 583–9.

22. Little JW. Eating disorders: dental implications. *Oral Surg Oral Med Oral Pathol Oral Radiol Endod.* 2002 Feb;93(2):138–43.

23. Studen-Pavlovich D, Elliott MA. Eating disorders in women's oral health. *Dent Clin North Am.* 2001 Jul;45(3):491–511.

24. American Psychiatric Association. op. cit., pp. 589–94.

25. Goldman L, Ausiello D, editors. *Cecil textbook of medicine.* 22nd ed. Philadelphia: Saunders; c2004. West DS. The eating disorders; p. 1338.

26. Storrie-Lombardi MC, Storrie-Lombardi IJ, Margon C, Stiefel DJ, editors. *Dental treatment of the patient with a major psychiatric disorder. A self-instructional series in rehabilitation dentistry.* Seattle: University of Washington School of Dentistry; 1987. p. 36.

CHAPTER 64

The Patient With a Substance-Related Disorder

ERNESTINE R. DANIELS , RDH, BS
JANICE A. ARRUDA , RDH, MPH

Chapter Outline

People who are dependent on alcohol are more likely than the general population to use other drugs, and people with drug dependence are more likely to drink alcohol. For these reasons drug and alcohol dependence often go hand in hand.[1]

■ Drug use varies from recreational use to addiction. People from various stages of drug use appear as patients needing dental and dental hygiene care. Patients who use drugs recreationally may "pre-medicate" themselves when a stressful situation such as a dental appointment is anticipated. Daily drug use varies, therefore questions at each appointment are required to determine clinical procedure and prevent complications.

■ There is no classic cultural, socioeconomic, or educational profile for a substance abuser. A patient's medical and dental history does not always provide the information necessary to determine whether the patient uses substances at all, or the level of dependency.

■ It is a professional responsibility of the dental hygienist to view chemical dependency as an illness and to be aware of the characteristics that suggest possible substance use. The knowledge will enable the dental hygienist to address the issues of an appropriate dental hygiene care plan for the chemically dependent patient.

■ Key words and terminology to describe the use and abuse of drugs are defined in **Box 64-1**.

ALCOHOL-RELATED DISORDERS

■ Alcohol use is common in a large percentage of the population and varies from social drinking to alcoholism.

■ Physical dependence and tolerance are both present in an individual suffering from alcoholism.

■ Alcohol used for consumption purposes is ethyl alcohol or ethanol. Other alcohols are methyl, an industrial solvent, and isopropyl, used for rubbing alcohol.

BOX 64-1	Key Words

Alcoholism and Drug Abuse

Abstinence: refrain from use; complete abstinence from alcohol is the objective of a recovering alcoholic.

Abuse: substance abuse with respect to alcohol abuse involves persistent patterns of heavy alcohol intake associated with health consequences and/or impairment in social functioning.

Acne rosacea: facial skin condition usually characterized by a flushed appearance; often accompanied by puffiness and a "spider-web" effect of broken capillaries.

Addiction: habitual psychologic and physiologic dependence on a substance or practice that is beyond voluntary control.

Alcohol intoxication: results from recent ingestion of excessive amounts of alcohol. It is characterized by behavioral changes that alter the usual behavior of the individual.

Alcoholism: a chronic progressive behavioral disorder characterized by a strong urge to consume ethanol and the inability to limit the amount despite adverse consequences.

Amnesia: impairment of long and/or short-term memory.

Anterograde amnesia: difficulty in recalling new information.

Retrograde amnesia: difficulty in remembering old information.

Analgesia: loss of sensibility to pain without loss of consciousness.

Antabuse: brand name of the generic drug disulfiram; used to deter consumption of alcohol by persons being treated for alcohol dependency by inducing vomiting.

Blackout: temporary amnesia occurring during periods of intensive drinking; person is not unconscious.

Delirium: extreme mental and usually motor excitement marked by a rapid succession of confused and unconnected ideas; often with illusions and hallucinations; may be accompanied by tremors.

Delirium Tremens: "DTs"; a serious acute condition associated with the last stages of alcohol withdrawal.

Dementia: condition of deteriorated mentality characterized by a marked decline of intellectual functioning.

Dependence: drug or substance dependence; with respect to alcohol refers to a physical and psychological dependence on alcohol that results in impaired ability to control drinking behavior; dependence is differentiated from abuse by manifestations of craving tolerance and physical dependence, as well as an inability to exercise restraint over drinking.

Chemical dependence: the interaction between a drug and the individual when there is a compulsion to take the drug to obtain its effects and/or to avoid the discomforts of withdrawal.

Physical dependence: when a drug becomes necessary for continued body functioning. An altered physiologic state has developed from repeatedly increasing drug concentrations.

Polysubstance dependence: addiction to at least three categories of psychoactive substances (not including nicotine or caffeine) but in which no single psychoactive substance predominates.

Psychologic dependence: refers to the state of mind in which the individual believes the drug is required for maintaining well-being.

Detoxification: treatment designed to assist in recovery from the toxic effects of a drug; involves withdrawal and may include pharmacologic and/or nonpharmacologic treatment with psychotherapy and counseling.

Drug: a chemical substance used for diagnosis, prevention, or treatment of disease. Drugs are classified by biochemical action, physiological effect, or organ system involved.

Euphoria: feeling of well-being, elation; without fear or worry.

Hallucination: a sensory impression (sight, sound, touch, smell, or taste) that has no basis in external stimulation; may have psychological causes, or may result from the use of drugs, (including alcohol), a brain tumor, senility, or exhaustion.

Hyperthermia: greatly increased temperature.

Illicit: illegal; not authorized, not sanctioned by law.

Maladaptive patterns of abuse: a maladaptive behavior is a behavior or trait that is not adaptive—it is counterproductive to the individual. Maladaptivity is frequently used as an indicator of abnormality or mental dysfunction, since its assessment is relatively free from subjectivity.

Micrognathia: abnormal smallness of the jaws, especially of the mandible.

Nystagmus: involuntary, rapid, rhythmic movements of the eyeball.

Alcoholism and Drug Abuse (Continued)

Opiate antagonist: Examples include naltrexone and naloxone that have a high affinity for opiate receptors but do not activate them. These drugs block the effect of exogenously administered opioids (e.g., morphine, heroin, and methadone) or of endogenously released endorphins.

Opioid: any synthetic narcotic that has opiate-like activities but is not derived from opium.

Psychotropic drug: a drug capable of modifying mental activity; used in the treatment of mental illness.

Recovering alcoholic: a person afflicted with the disease of alcoholism who is abstaining from the use of alcohol; recovering alcoholics prefer the term "recovering" to reformed, cured, or recovered because recovering implies an ongoing process.

Saddlenose deformity: a collapse of the nasal bridge.

Substance abuse: The regular use of a drug for other than its accepted medical purpose or in dosages greater than those that are considered appropriate.

Tolerance: ability to endure without effect or injury. Increased amount of the drug is needed to achieve the same effect.

Drug tolerance: the need for higher and higher dosages of a drug to achieve the same effect.

Withdrawal syndrome: a group of signs and symptoms, both physiologic and psychologic, that occurs on abrupt discontinuation of drug use.

I. CLINICAL PATTERN OF ALCOHOL USE

- Abstinence and low-risk use.
- Increased consumption.
- Moderate alcohol use: two drinks per day for men and one drink per day for women is not considered harmful for the average adult.[2] The individual is able to function appropriately in work, family, and social situations.
- Unhealthy alcohol use: early-stage problems such as hypertension, depression, insomnia, heartburn, and absenteeism develop.[3]
- Alcohol dependency and alcoholism develop after periods of unhealthy alcohol use followed by pathologic abuse.[4]
- Alcohol content of a standard drink of various alcoholic beverages is shown in **Box 64-2**.
- The spectrum of alcohol use is illustrated in **Figure 64-1**.

A. Effects of Alcohol Intoxication

- Behavioral changes: aggressiveness, mood instability, impaired judgment; impaired social or occupational functioning; impaired attention and memory; stupor or coma.
- Physical characteristics: slurred speech, lack of coordination, unsteady gait, and nystagmus.

BOX 64-2	A Standard Drink

0.5 oz (15 g) of alcohol
12 oz (355 ml) of beer or wine cooler
5 oz (148 ml) of wine
1.5 oz (44 ml) of 80-proof distilled spirits

Data from NIAAA. 10th special report to the U.S. Congress on alcohol and health. Rockville (MD): NIAAA; 2000 Jun. p. 4.

- Complications: irresponsible actions in work and family settings.
- Accidents with resultant bruises, fractures, or brain trauma.
- Suicide.

B. Consequences of Underage Drinking[5]

- Drinking and driving.
- Suicide.
- Sexual assault.
- High-risk sex.
- Alcohol-induced mental impairment.

C. Signs of Alcoholism[6]

Alcoholism, also known as alcohol dependence, includes four main symptoms:

- *Craving*: A strong need or compulsion to drink.
- *Loss of control*: The inability to limit one's drinking on any given occasion.
- *Physical dependence*: Withdrawal symptoms, such as nausea, sweating, shakiness, and anxiousness, when alcohol use is stopped after a period of heavy drinking.
- *Tolerance*: The need to drink greater amounts of alcohol in order to get intoxicated. Other signs include amnesia and binge drinking.

II. ETIOLOGY

A. Genetics

- The Collaborative Study on the Genetics of Alcoholism (COGA), has successfully identified GABRA2 and CHRM2 as two genes involved in the predisposition to alcohol dependence.[7]
- A defective allele (variant) of the gene ALDH2 substantially (although not completely) protects carriers from developing alcoholism by making them ill after drinking alcohol.[8]

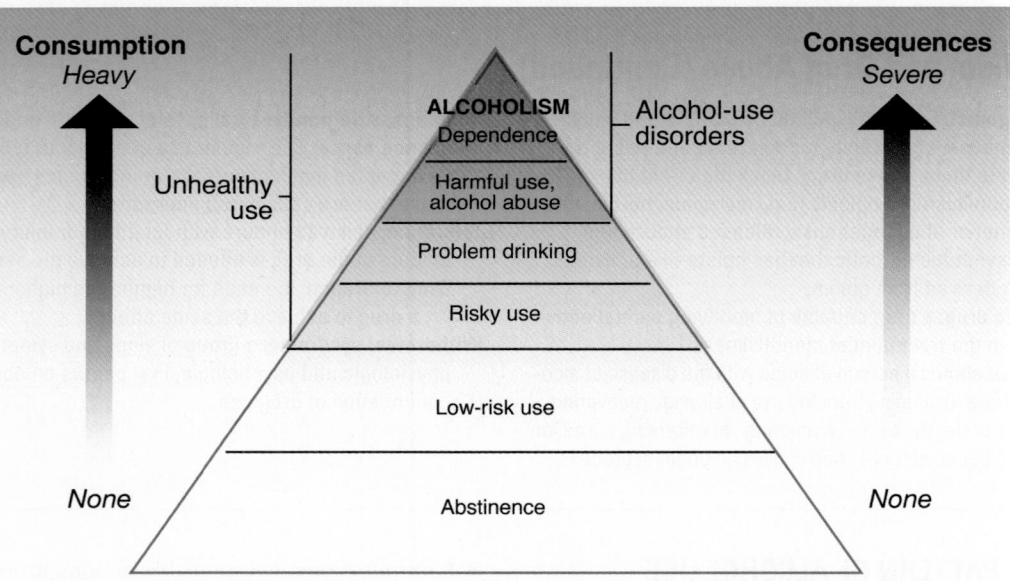

FIGURE 64-1 **The Spectrum of Alcohol Use.** As clinicians, the shaded categories in the upper portions of the pyramid are of primary concern while treating patients. These categories reflect unhealthy alcohol use. (Source: Saitz R. Clinical practice. Unhealthy alcohol use. N Engl J Med. 2005 Feb 10;352(6)596–607.)

B. Biopsychosocial

Children of alcohol-dependent parents are exposed to a higher level of multiple risk factors that lead to alcohol-related problems:

- Mental and behavioral disorders and adverse family environments.
- Decreased sensitivity to intoxication effects of alcohol.
- Increased sensitivity of reduced anxiety.

C. Environmental

- Psychologic stress, family, peers, and social forces.
- Current lifestyle, culture, advertisements, and economics.
- Motivational factors: both emotional (stress reduction, mood enhancement, social rewards) and cognitive (conscious and unconscious beliefs about alcohol) may play a role in an individual's decision to drink.

METABOLISM OF ALCOHOL[9]

I. INGESTION AND ABSORPTION

- Upon intake, alcohol is absorbed promptly from the stomach and small intestine into the bloodstream.
- Transported to liver for metabolism.

II. LIVER METABOLISM

- More than 90% of ingested alcohol is converted into acetaldehyde, then acetone, and finally into carbon dioxide and water by action of various liver enzymes.

- High acetaldehyde levels and chronic alcohol consumption impair liver function and lead to liver damage.

III. DIFFUSION

- Within 5 minutes after ingestion, alcohol can be detected in the blood.
- Alcohol is quickly diffused into all cells and intercellular fluid of the body.
- Less than 10% is excreted directly through the lungs, skin, and kidney (breath, sweat, and urine).
- A person's alcohol level can be determined by several tests of the blood, urine, saliva, or water vapor in the breath.

IV. BLOOD ALCOHOL CONCENTRATION (BAC)[10]

- In the United States, law enforcement agencies primarily test the BAC of automobile drivers using the breath test. The results are then converted to equivalent blood alcohol concentrations.
- A BAC of 0.08% has been established as the legal level of intoxification.
  - The amount of alcohol by weight, in a set volume of blood.
  - Measured in milligrams per deciliter (mg/dl).
  - A BAC of 0.10% is equivalent of 0.10 g of alcohol per 100 ml of blood.
- The tolerance level varies among individuals. The inexperienced drinker may lose self-control and become nauseated with low levels of alcohol. The experienced drinker tolerates a higher level of alcohol without nausea.

TABLE 64-1	EFFECTS OF BLOOD ALCOHOL CONCENTRATIONS AT VARIOUS LEVELS
DOSE	**EFFECT**
50 mg/dl	Sedation, tranquility, fine motor coordination reduced, unsteadiness on standing.
50–100 mg/dl	Reduced anxiety, alertness, and critical judgment; enhanced self-esteem, slowed reaction time, and impulsive risk-taking behavior.
100–300 mg/dl	Slowed reaction time, slurred speech, staggering; mood swings, memory deficits, blackouts; increased aggressive behavior.
300–400 mg/dl	Labored breathing, nystagmus, lowered blood pressure and body temperature; loss of consciousness.
400–500 mg/dl	Depressed respiration, alcoholic coma, possibly fatal.

Source: NIAA. 8th special report to the U.S. Congress on alcohol and health. Rockville (MD): NIAA; 1993 Sep. p. 89.
Noel BK. Methamphetamine abuse: oral implications and care. *RDH.* 2010 Feb; 30(2):75.

- BAC measurement reflects a person's drinking rate and rate of metabolism.
- Alcohol is metabolized more slowly than it is absorbed. The BAC increases when alcohol is consumed faster than previous drinks are metabolized.
- The rate at which the body will absorb and metabolize alcohol is based on factors such as age, gender, percentage of fatty tissue in the body, and whether food is also being metabolized.
- Ethanol is a powerful depressant of the central nervous system. In low doses, alcohol can act as a disinhibitor and as a relaxant. Euphoria may be produced.
- In high doses, alcohol can produce analgesic effects with reduction of anxiety generally accompanied by reduced alertness and reduced judgment.
- The characteristic effects exhibited at various levels can be seen in **Table 64-1**.

HEALTH HAZARDS

Prolonged alcohol use causes many serious medical disorders. The alcohol-dependent person is most seriously afflicted, but even unhealthy alcohol use may have complications. Alcohol-related illnesses may involve any body system. A few are mentioned here.

I. LIVER DISEASE

Chronic alcohol abuse is the most frequent cause of morbidity and mortality from liver diseases. Alcoholic liver disease (ALD) includes the following conditions:[11]

- Fatty liver with degeneration: early stages are reversible with abstinence.
- Alcoholic hepatitis: inflammation of the liver.
- Early fibrosis: healthy cells replaced by scar tissue.
- Cirrhosis: scarring of the liver with irreversible damage.
- Individuals with hepatitis C virus are more susceptible to ALD.[12]

II. IMMUNITY AND INFECTION

- Those who abuse alcohol have diminished immune response: suppression of immune system defense and disturbed function of neutrophils.
- Risk for many bacterial infections is increased, particularly pulmonary diseases (pneumonia, tuberculosis) and viral infections (hepatitis B and C).

III. DIGESTIVE SYSTEM

- Alcohol ingestion alters the stomach mucosa, stimulates gastric acid secretion, and affects gastric function.
- Lesions that bleed may develop with desquamation of the stomach lining (acute gastritis).
- Injury to small intestines: diarrhea, weight loss, and vitamin deficiencies.

IV. NUTRITIONAL DEFICIENCIES

- Alcohol provides an excess of caloric intake. With the intake of large quantities of alcohol, the individual loses interest in regular mealtime nutritious food, which leads to many deficiencies.
- Deficiencies result from malabsorption of vitamins and essential nutrients.
- Secondary malnutrition develops from direct effects of alcohol on the gastrointestinal tract, malabsorption and maldigestion occur after cellular changes in the intestinal wall.

V. CARDIOVASCULAR DISEASES

- Risk for cardiomyopathy, coronary artery disease, hypertension, arrhythmias, and hemorrhagic stroke.
- Decreased risk for heart attack and stroke is associated with light to moderate alcohol use.[13]
- Heavy consumption increases the death rate from cardiovascular disease.
- Associated with early coronary calcification in young adults.[14]

VI. NEOPLASMS

- Alcohol use increases the risk for many types of cancers, notably of the alimentary and respiratory tracts.[15]
- Alcohol combined with tobacco use has long been associated with increased neoplasms of the oral cavity, pharynx, and larynx.

VII. NERVOUS SYSTEM

A. Central and Peripheral

- Early changes affect intellectual actions, judgment, and learning ability.
- Long-term alcohol abuse combined with malnutrition can lead to damage of both central and peripheral nervous systems.
- Prolonged and heavy alcohol consumption leads to chronic brain damage.

B. Wernicke–Korsakoff's Syndrome[16]

Brain disorder of the cerebellum is the result of a thiamine deficiency associated with chronic alcohol consumption. Two syndromes are involved as follows:

- *Wernicke's encephalopathy:* symptoms of mental confusion, ocular, and gait disturbances.
- *Korsakoff's psychosis:* persistent knowledge and memory problems characterized by forgetfulness, easy frustration, lack of muscle coordination, and retrograde and anterograde amnesia.

VIII. REPRODUCTIVE SYSTEM

- Alcohol affects every branch of the endocrine system, directly and indirectly, through the body's organization of the endocrine hormones.
- Female: menstrual disturbances, failure to ovulate, and early menopause.
- Male: testicular atrophy, suppression of testosterone, loss of mature sperm cells, feminization, and failure of gonadal function.

FETAL ALCOHOL SYNDROME (FAS)

- The significant incidence and prevalence of fetal alcohol syndrome (FAS) defines the need for dental professionals to recognize symptoms of FAS.
- Patients with FAS have orofacial characteristics and various pychological and physical symptoms that may affect a dental hygiene treatment plan.
- The offspring of women who use alcohol to excess during pregnancy, have an increased risk for developmental disorders that range from subtle to lifelong serious effects.[17]

I. ALCOHOL USE DURING PREGNANCY[18]

- There is no safe amount of alcohol use during pregnancy.
  - The amount of alcohol required to produce adverse fetal consequences is unknown.
  - Complete abstinence is safest to prevent FAS.
- Prenatal alcohol exposure is cited as the leading preventable cause of birth defects.
- **Box 64-3** contains terminology abbreviations for FAS.

BOX 64-3 | **Fetal Alcohol Syndrome Terminology Abbreviations**

FAS — **Fetal Alcohol Syndrome**: A characteristic pattern of abnormal growth and development resulting from maternal consumption of alcohol during pregnancy.

FASD — **Fetal Alcohol Spectrum Disorders**: An umbrella term describing the range of effects that can occur in an individual whose mother drank alcohol while pregnant.

FAE — **Fetal Alcohol Effects**: All of the diagnostic features of FAS but at mild or severe levels.

ARND — **Alcohol-Related Neurodevelopment Disorder**: Characterized by learning difficulties, poor school performance, poor impulse control, mathematical skills, memory, attention, and/or poor judgment.

ARBD — **Alcohol-Related Birth Defects**: *Health problems related to organ malformation*
- Cardiac, hepatic, muscular, skeletal, and renal.
- Vision or hearing defects.
- Immune system may be compromised leading to susceptibility to infection.

Source: NIAA. Alcohol-related birth defects: an update. *Alcohol Res Health.* 2001;25(3):154.

A. No Placental Barrier

- Alcohol passes freely across the placenta.
- Increased incidence of spontaneous abortions and stillbirths associated with alcohol consumption.
- Severe effects result in FAS and fetal alcohol syndrome disorders (FASD).

B. Other Factors

- Other poor health habits often accompany the use of alcohol, including inadequate diet and use of tobacco.
- The use of prescription or illicit drugs with alcohol can result in abnormalities.

II. DIAGNOSTIC CRITERIA FOR FETAL ALCOHOL SYNDROME[19]

- Prenatal and postnatal growth retardation.
- Facial dysmorphology shown in **Figure 64-2**.
- Other possible facial characteristics of FAS:
  - Midface: flattened, depressed; underdeveloped maxilla.
  - Nose: short, upturned, with sunken nasal bridge.
  - Micrognathia.
  - Ears: anomalies of shape and position.
- Central nervous system (CNS) involvement.[20]
- Structural: reduction in size of corpus callosum, cerebellum, or basal ganglia.

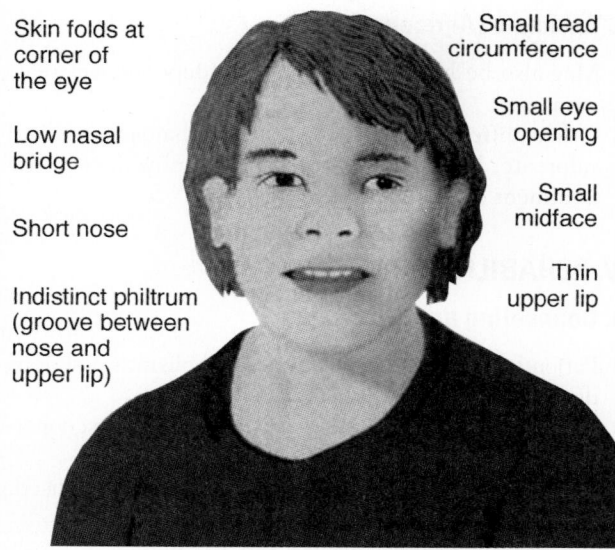

Skin folds at corner of the eye

Low nasal bridge

Short nose

Indistinct philtrum (groove between nose and upper lip)

Small head circumference

Small eye opening

Small midface

Thin upper lip

FIGURE 64-2 **Facial Features of Fetal Alcohol Syndrome.** A pattern of abnormal facial features that may be seen in cases of prenatal alcohol exposure. (Reprinted from The United States Department of Health and Human Services, National Institute on Alcohol Abuse and Alcoholism. Alcohol alert number 63: alcohol and the developing brain. Bethesda (MD): Department of Health and Human Services; 2004 Oct. p 5.)

- Neurological: can include seizures.
- Functional:
    - Cognitive or developmental deficits: verbal or visual spatial learning.
    - Executive function: abstract mental thoughts, plans, organization.
    - Motor functions: poor coordination, abnormal gait.
    - Attention or hyperactivity problems.
    - Social skills, behavioral dysfunction.

ALCOHOL WITHDRAWAL SYNDROME[21]

Withdrawal consists of the disturbances that occur after abrupt cessation of alcohol intake in the alcohol-dependent person. Withdrawal signs appear within a few hours after drinking has stopped. Even a relative decline in blood concentration can precipitate the syndrome.

I. PREDISPOSING FACTORS

- Malnutrition, fatigue, depression, and physical illnesses aggravate withdrawal symptoms.

II. SIGNS AND SYMPTOMS

- Tremor of hands, tongue, and eyelids.
- Nervousness and irritation; anxiety.
- Malaise, weakness, and headache.
- Dry mouth.
- Autonomic hyperactivity: sweating, rapid pulse rate, and elevated blood pressure.

- Transient visual, tactile, or auditory hallucinations.
- Insomnia.
- Grand mal seizures.
- Nausea or vomiting.

III. COMPLICATIONS

A. Alcohol Withdrawal Delirium (Delirium Tremens, "DTs")

- May occur within 1 week of cessation of heavy alcohol intake.
- Features: marked autonomic hyperactivity: rapid heartbeat and sweating.
- Vivid hallucinations (visual, auditory, tactile).
- Delusions and agitated behavior; tremor.
- Confusion and disorientation.

B. Alcohol Hallucinosis

- Auditory and visual hallucinations develop within 48 hours after the abrupt stop or reduction of heavy alcohol intake of long-standing dependency.
- Symptoms: may last weeks or months.
- Impairment is severe with schizophrenic symptoms, although schizophrenia is not a predisposing factor.
- Delirium is not present.

TREATMENT FOR ALCOHOLISM

- The overall objective of treatment is to help the person achieve and maintain total abstinence. An alcohol-dependent person can never drink even small amounts of alcohol without an eventual return to dependency.
- Treatment includes a combination of medical and psychiatric therapy with self-help.
- Patients are encouraged not to take other psychoactive drugs, including minor tranquilizers and caffeine.

I. EARLY INTERVENTION

When problem drinkers who are not yet dependent can be identified, counseling may help to reduce and perhaps eliminate the use of alcohol.

II. DETOXIFICATION

The term detoxification applies to the management of acute intoxication and the withdrawal syndrome. A variety of treatments may be involved.

A. Treatment for Immediate Emergencies

- Accident or medical emergency other than withdrawal symptoms.
- Fractures, head injury, internal bleeding, or other problems may require initial attention.

- Alcohol dependency may be revealed after hospital admittance for other causes.

B. Removal from Source of Alcohol: Abstinence

- Advantages of hospitalization: supervision is available.
- No access to sources of alcohol.

C. Goals of Therapy

- Treat medical complications.
- Restore general physical health: rest, sleep, and exercise.
- Treat nutritional deficiencies: proper diet.

D. Relief from Acute Withdrawal Signs

- Tranquilizers may be prescribed for short-term use.
- Vitamins, particularly thiamine, are usually administered.

III. PHARMACOTHERAPY[22]

A. Medications Used in Alcoholism Treatment

Agents for withdrawal management include:

- Alcohol-sensitizing agents (cause aversive reactions in combination with alcohol).
- Anticraving agents (decrease desire for and consumption of alcohol).
- Amethystic agents (reverse the acute intoxicating and depressant effects of alcohol).
- Medications for treatment of coexisting psychiatric disorders, such as depression and anxiety.

B. Disulfiram (Antabuse): Alcohol-Sensitizing Agent

- Interferes with the metabolism of alcohol by acting on the enzyme that converts acetaldehyde to acetone in the liver.
- Effect: acetaldehyde accumulates in the tissues.
- Alcohol and disulfiram taken at the same time result in nausea, vomiting, and hypotension.
- Drug acts as a deterrent to provide an adjunct to comprehensive therapy in selected patients.

C. Naltrexone (ReVia): Anticraving Agent

- Interferes with neurotransmitter systems that produce pleasurable effects.
- The effect of taking alcohol with an "opiate antagonist": no experience of a rewarded high or feelings of euphoria.

D. Acamprosate

- Affects certain chemical messengers (neurotransmitters) in the brain.
- Reduces the risk of heavy drinking; doubles the likelihood that patients will achieve abstinence.

E. Toirimate (Anticonvulsant)

- May also be beneficial for cocaine dependence treatment.
- Other anticonvulsants, including carbamazepine and valproate, have also shown some effectiveness in the treatment of alcohol use disorders.

IV. REHABILITATION

A. Counseling and Education

- Patients need to recognize that alcoholism is a serious disease and be agreeable to accept help.
- Family and work associates may be recruited to cooperate with the program.
- Behavioral therapy and psychotherapy have been used.

B. Group Therapy

- *Alcoholics Anonymous (AA)*: a fellowship of men and women who help themselves and others to recover from alcoholism; can provide help for motivated individuals.
- Some patients prefer treatment through special clinics and centers.
- *Al-Anon*: a separate program for parents, adult children, siblings, and spouses, as well as other persons concerned with the alcoholic patient in recovery.
- *Alateen*: a program for teenage children.

C. Psychiatric Treatment

- An increased frequency of schizophrenia, psychoneurosis, sociopathy, and manic-depressive diseases is being recognized among alcohol-dependent people.

D. Aftercare Services

- Recovery takes a long time; extended treatment required.
- Relapse more likely when a recovering alcoholic leaves a treatment system too early.
- Typical follow-up includes weekly aftercare group meetings for 9 to 12 months.

PRESCRIPTION AND STREET DRUGS

- Drug abuse: habitual use of drugs not needed for therapeutic purposes.
- Prescription drug abuse: taking prescription medication that is not prescribed for that person using a prescription for reasons or in dosages other than prescribed.
- Drugs interfere with the function of the brain and create long-term effects on brain metabolism and activity.
- Dependency develops after periods of drug use followed by pathologic abuse.

BOX 64-4	Criteria for Substance Dependence

A maladaptive pattern of substance use, leading to clinically significant impairment or distress, as manifested by three (or more) of the following, occurring at any time in the same 12-month period:

1. Tolerance as defined by either of the following:
   ☐ A need for markedly increased amounts of the substance to achieve intoxication or desired effect.
   ☐ Markedly diminished effect with continued use of the same amount of the substance.
2. Withdrawal, as manifested by either of the following:
   ☐ The characteristic withdrawal syndrome for the substance.
   ☐ The same (or a closely related) substance is taken to relieve or avoid withdrawal symptoms.
3. The substance is often taken in larger amounts or over a longer period than was intended.
4. There is a persistent desire or unsuccessful efforts to cut down or control substance use.
5. A great deal of time is spent in activities necessary to obtain the substance (e.g., visiting multiple doctors or driving long distances), use the substance (e.g., chain smoking), or recover from its effects.
6. Important social, occupational, or recreational activities are given up or reduced because of the substance use.
7. The substance use is continued despite knowledge of having a persistent or recurrent physical or psychological problem that is likely to have been caused or exacerbated by the substance (e.g., current cocaine use despite recognition of cocaine-induced depression, or continued drinking despite recognition that an ulcer was made worse by alcohol consumption).

Source: American Psychiatric Association. DSM-IV-TR. Washington: APA; 2000.

- An increase in the amount and frequency of a drug is needed to alleviate withdrawal responses; the withdrawal symptoms become more severe and require a greater intake of the drug.
- Brain circuitry becomes altered with this cyclic process and the voluntary use of drugs becomes drug addiction: a compulsive craving for drugs, seeking, and use.
- Substance dependency is manifested by selected criteria from those listed in **Box 64-4**.

MOST COMMON DRUGS OF ABUSE

The most common drugs of abuse are alcohol and those found in the categories in this section.[23] Examples of the substance names in each category and the commercial and street names are listed in **Table 64-2**.

I. CANNABINOIDS

- Organic substances present in the plants of *Cannabis sativa* that have a variety of pharmacologic properties.
- Upper leaves, tops, and stems are cut, dried, and rolled into cigarettes (*marijuana*).
- Dried exudate that seeps from the tops and undersides of cannabis leaves (*hashish oil*).

II. DEPRESSANTS

- An agent (such as a sedative or anesthetic) that reduces nervous or functional activity.
- Examples are *downers, sleeping pills, ludes, rophies.*

III. DISSOCIATIVE ANESTHETICS

- A form of general anesthesia that promotes dissociation from the environment but not necessarily complete unconsciousness. Sometimes used for short diagnostic or surgical procedures.
- Street names: *angel dust, Special K.*

IV. HALLUCINOGENS

- Chemical substances that produce mind-altering or mental perception-altering properties.
- A popular example is *LSD* (lysergic acid diethylamide).
- A disorder associated with the use of these substances can produce hallucinogen persisting perception disorder, commonly known as "flashbacks."
- *MDMA* (3–4 dimethoxymethamphetamine) or *Ecstasy*, a popular drug among teens and young adults, widely used at nightclubs and bars (a club drug).
- *MDMA* is classified as a stimulant, but is known for its hallucinogenic effects.

V. OPIOIDS AND MORPHINE DERIVATIVES

- Narcotic substances made from the Asian poppy or produced as synthetic drugs with the effects of opium: they result in analgesic and euphoric effects.
- Opioids are prescribed as analgesics, anesthetics, antidiarrheal agents, and cough suppressants.
- *Heroin* is one of the most commonly abused drugs of this class: it can be injected, smoked, or snorted.

VI. STIMULANTS

- A class of drugs that enhances brain activity.
  A. Stimulants cause an increase in mental alertness, attention, and energy; they improve motor skills and elicit a general sense of well being.
  B. Stimulants increase cardiac and respiratory function and speed up metabolism.

TABLE 64-2	MOST COMMONLY ABUSED STREET DRUGS		

DRUG CATEGORY AND DEA SCHEDULE	STREET NAMES AND COMMERCIAL NAME	HOW ADMINISTERED*	INTOXICATION EFFECTS
Depressants:			
Barbiturates, II, III, V	Barbs, reds, red birds, phennies, tooies, yellows, yellow jackets; *Amytal, Nembutal, Seconal, Phenobarbital*	Injected, swallowed	Reduced pain and anxiety; feeling of well-being; lowered inhibitions; slowed pulse, breathing; lowered blood pressure; poor concentration
Benzodiazepines, IV [other than flunitrazepam]	Candy, downers, sleeping pills, tranks; *Ativan, Halcion, Librium, Valium, Xanax*	Swallowed	Sedation, drowsiness; also, for barbiturates
Flunitrazepam[†,‡], IV	Forget-me pill, Mexican Valium, R2, Roche, roofies, roofinol, rope, rophies; *Rohypnol*	Swallowed, snorted	Sedation, drowsiness/dizziness increased heart rate and blood pressure, impaired motor function/memory loss
Dissociative Anesthetics:			
Ketamine, III	cat Valium, K, Special K, vitamin K; *Ketalar SV*	Injected, snorted, smoked	At high doses, delirium, depression, respiratory depression and arrest pain relief, euphoria, drowsiness
Opioids and Morphine Derivatives:			
Codeine, II, III, IV	Captain Cody, Cody, schoolboy; (with glutethimide) doors & fours, loads, pancakes and syrup; *Empirin with Codeine, Fiorinal with Codeine, Robitussin A-C, Tylenol with Codeine*	Injected, swallowed	Less analgesia, sedation, and respiratory depression than morphine
Fentanyl, II	Apache, China girl, China white, dance fever, friend, goodfella, jackpot, murder 8, TNT, Tango and Cash; *Actiq, Duragesic, Sublimaze*	Injected, smoked, snorted	
Morphine, II	M, Miss Emma, monkey, white stuff; *Roxanol, Duramorph*	Injected, swallowed, smoked	
Opium, II, III	big O, black stuff, block, gum, hop; *laudanum, paregoric;*	Swallowed, smoked	
Other opioid pain relievers (oxycodone, meperidine, Hydromorphone, Hydrocodone, Propoxyphene), II, III, IV	oxy 80s, oxycotton, oxycet, hillbilly heroin, percs; *Tylox, OxyContin, Percodan, Percocet* demmies, pain killer *Demerol, meperidine hydrochloride* juice, dillies *Dilaudid, Vicodin, Lortab, Lorcet; Darvon, Darvocet*	Swallowed, injected, suppositories, chewed, crushed, snorted	
Stimulants:			
Amphetamines, II	Bennies, black beauties, crosses, hearts, LA turnaround, speed, truck drivers, uppers; *Biphetamine, Dexedrine*	Injected, swallowed, smoked, snorted	Increased heart rate, blood pressure, metabolism; feelings of exhilaration, energy, increased mental alertness
Cocaine, II	Blow, bump, C, candy, Charlie, coke, crack, flake, rock, snow, toot; *Cocaine hydrochloride*	Injected, smoked, snorted	Rapid breathing; hallucinations; also, for amphetamines

(continued)

TABLE 64-2	MOST COMMONLY ABUSED STREET DRUGS (*Continued*)		
DRUG CATEGORY AND DEA SCHEDULE	**STREET NAMES AND COMMERCIAL NAME**	**HOW ADMINISTERED***	**INTOXICATION EFFECTS**
Methamphetamine, II	Chalk, crank, crystal, fire, glass, go fast, ice, meth, speed; *Desoxyn*	Injected, swallowed, smoked, snorted	Aggression, violence, psychotic behavior; also for methylphenidate
Methylphenidate, II	JIF, MPH, R-ball, Skippy, the smart drug, vitamin R; *Ritalin*	Injected, swallowed, snorted	Increase or decrease in blood pressure, psychotic episodes
Other Compounds			
Anabolic steroids	Roids, juice; *Anadrol, Oxandrin, Durabolin, Depo-Testosterone, Equipoise*	Injected, swallowed, applied to skin	No intoxication effects

*Taking drugs by injection can increase the risk of infection through needle contamination with staphylococci, HIV, hepatitis, and other organisms.
†Associated with sexual assaults.
‡Not available by prescription in the United States.
Source: National Institute on Drug Abuse: the science of drug abuse and addiction [Internet]. Commonly abused drugs; [cited 2011 Jan 11]; [about 4 screens]. Available from: http://www.drugabuse.gov/DrugPages/DrugsofAbuse.html

■ *Cocaine hydrochloride powder* can be "snorted" through the nostrils; or, when mixed with water, can be injected intravenously.
  ■ *Crack cocaine* is a cocaine alkaloid in the form of a small rock.
  ■ *Crack* is cocaine that has been processed from cocaine hydrochloride to a free base for smoking. It is easily vaporized and inhaled and exhibits an extremely rapid onset of effects.
■ *Methamphetamine* (*meth, speed*) is taken orally, intranasally (snorting the powder), by intravenous injection, or by smoking. Meth users are resistant to local anesthesia.[24]
■ *Ice*, a very pure form of methamphetamine (seen as crystals under a high magnification), produces an immediate and powerful stimulant when smoked.

VII. OTHER COMPOUNDS

A. Steroids

■ Used to build muscles and increased performance.
■ May produce a feeling of well-being or euphoria; followed by lack of energy and irritability.
■ More severe symptoms include depression and liver disease.

B. Inhalants

■ A breathable chemical vapor that produces psychoactive effects.
■ Available in a wide variety of commercial products: paint thinners, gasoline, and glue.

Methods for Application

■ A substance-soaked cloth is applied to the nose and mouth and vapors are breathed in.
■ Substance can also be placed in a paper or plastic bag and inhaled.

Effects

■ All capable of producing intoxication, abuse, and dependence.
■ Intoxication is characterized by a mild euphoria and a change in perception of time.
■ Causes relaxation of the smooth muscle and a decrease in oxygen-carrying capacity of the blood.
■ Toxic reactions: vomiting, headache, hypotension, and dizziness.

MEDICAL EFFECTS OF DRUG ABUSE

I. CARDIOVASCULAR EFFECTS

There is a connection between the abuse of most addictive drugs and adverse cardiovascular effects that may range from arrhythmias to heart attacks. Cocaine in particular can:

■ Increase blood pressure.
■ Cause vasoconstriction.
■ Alter electroactivity of the heart.
■ Promote a cardiac stimulant effect.
■ Induce angina; precipitate myocardial infarction.
■ Cause a variety of arrhythmias and palpitations including sudden cardiac death.[25]

■ Contribute to early subclinical atherosclerotic cardio-vascular disease.[26]

II. NEUROLOGICAL EFFECTS

■ Drug use can cause changes in the brain leading to:
  ▪ Memory lapses and decision or attention problems.
  ▪ Euphoric effects.
  ▪ Seizures, stroke, or intracerebral hemorrhage.[27,28]
  ▪ Depression, paranoia, aggression, or hallucinations.
■ Substance-induced disorders can include:
  ▪ Amnesia, delirium, or dementia.
  ▪ Mood or anxiety disorders.
  ▪ Sleep disorders.

III. GASTROINTESTINAL EFFECTS

■ Cocaine in particular has been associated with gas-trointestinal complications and abdominal pain. The possibility of life-threatening hemorrhage has been reported with cocaine use.[29,30]
■ Cocaine that is ingested can cause severe bowel gan-grene due to reduced blood flow.
■ Many drugs of abuse have been known to cause nausea and vomiting soon after use.

IV. KIDNEY DAMAGE

■ Chronic drug use causes toxicity to several organs including the kidney.
■ Drugs affect renal function either through the toxic effects of the drug, or by a reduction in kidney func-tion.
■ Pain medications, alcohol, antibiotics, and illegal drugs can all cause kidney damage if not used properly.
■ Toluene can affect the liver and kidneys severely.[31]

V. LIVER DAMAGE[32]

■ The liver detoxifies drugs, chemicals, and alcohol that are ingested.
■ Changes in liver function due to drug abuse decrease the metabolism of drugs: when not able to break down properly, the drug can remain at a toxic level.
■ Chronic abuse of heroin, inhalants, and steroids may cause significant liver damage.
■ The consumption of alcohol and cocaine together com-pound the danger each drug poses.
  ▪ The liver combines cocaine and alcohol to form a third substance: cocaethylene.[33]
  ▪ Cocaethylene intensifies cocaine's euphoric effects, potentially increases the risk of sudden death.

VI. MUSCULOSKELETAL EFFECTS[34]

■ Rising levels of testosterone and other sex hormones trigger the growth spurt that occurs during puberty; when the hormones reach a certain level, they signal the bones to stop growing.
■ Steroid use during childhood or adolescence can result in artificially high hormone levels; bone growth culmi-nates earlier than usual which results in a short stature.
■ Other drugs may cause severe muscle cramping and overall weakness.

VII. RESPIRATORY EFFECTS

■ Drug abuse can lead to a variety of respiratory problems.
■ The use of smoking tobacco, marijuana, and inhalants all damage sensitive lung tissue.
■ A compromised respiratory system can result in a reduced respiration rate, asthma, bronchitis, emphy-sema, and lung cancer.

VIII. PRENATAL EFFECTS

■ Prenatal drug abuse may result in:
  ▪ Miscarriage.
  ▪ Premature birth.
  ▪ Low birth weight.
■ Inhalant abuse by expectant women can result in Fetal Solvent Syndrome with abnormalities similar to those occurring in FAS[35]

IX. INFECTIONS[36]

■ Drug users are at risk for acquiring a large range of infections.
■ Common bacterial infections among drug users:
  ▪ Skin and soft tissue: abscesses and cellulitis located at injection sites.
  ▪ Musculoskeletal infections, septic arthritis, and osteo-myelitis, a local extension of soft tissue infection.
■ Immunosuppression results from poor nutrition and human immunodeficiency virus (HIV), and increases the risk for:
  ▪ Infective endocarditis.
  ▪ Pulmonary tuberculosis (increased in crowded living quarters, crack houses, and homeless shelters).
  ▪ Respiratory tract infections, including community-acquired pneumonia.
■ Role in disease transmission between drug users and their partners
  ▪ Major mode for transmission of HIV, and other sexu-ally transmitted diseases, and viral hepatitis.
  ▪ Bloodborne diseases by way of shared needles and other paraphernalia.
  ▪ Transmission through drugs, drug adulterants, or unique drug preparations.
  ▪ Poor hygiene may exacerbate the risk of infection with commensal flora.
■ Prevention
  ▪ Eliminate drug use.
  ▪ Utilize risk-reducing strategies.

- Medically supervised injection facilities; needle exchange programs.
- Street-based education programs aimed at the use of sterile injection practices.
- Clean the injection site with alcohol and the drug paraphernalia with bleach.
- Avoid contamination by sharing needles.
- Avoid the use of dangerous injection sites such as the neck and groin.
- Reduce high-risk behavior such as unprotected sex and sex with multiple partners.
- Administer vaccinations and routinely screen for tuberculosis, HIV, and other sexually transmitted diseases. This can help to reduce disease transmission and prevent bacterial infections.

TREATMENT METHODS

- Drug addiction is a treatable disorder.
- Treatment is tailored to the individual needs of the patient and may involve behavioral changes and medications.
- Medications help to suppress the need to crave drugs and withdrawal symptoms.
- The principles that characterize the most effective drug abuse treatment can be found in **Box 64-5**.

I. BEHAVIORAL CHANGES

- Counseling
- Support groups
- Psychotherapy
- Family therapy

II. MEDICATIONS

The primary medically assisted withdrawal method for narcotic addiction is to switch the patient to a comparable drug with milder withdrawal symptoms, and then gradually taper off the substitute medication. Some patients, however, cannot continue to abstain from opiates and are therefore given a maintenance therapy. The following drugs are used in maintenance therapy:

A. Methadone

- Suppresses withdrawal symptoms and drug craving, associated with narcotic addiction.
- In methadone maintenance programs, a daily dose (usually a minimum of 60 mg) is administered.

B. LAAM (Levo-Alpha-Acetyl-Methadol)

- Suppresses withdrawal symptoms and drug cravings.
- Administered three times per week only.

BOX 64-5	**Principles of Drug Addiction Treatment**

Nearly three decades of scientific research has yielded 13 fundamental principles that characterize effective drug abuse treatment.

1. No single treatment is appropriate for all individuals.
2. Treatment needs are readily available.
3. Addresses drug use and associated medical, physiological, social, vocational, and legal problems.
4. Medical, social, and legal services; family therapy; and vocational rehabilitation are available.
5. Remaining in treatment for an adequate period of time.
6. Individual, group counseling, and other behavioral therapies are essential.
7. Treatment medications for many patients are an important element especially when combined with counseling.
8. Addicted or drug-abusing individuals with coexisting mental disorders need to have both disorders treated in an integrated way.
9. Medical detoxification is only the first stage of effective addiction treatment.
10. Treatment does not need to be voluntary to be effective.
11. Possible drug use during treatment needs to be monitored continually. (urinalysis)
12. Provide infectious disease assessment and counseling. (HIV/AIDS, Hepatitis B, and C.)
13. Recovery can be a long time process and relapses often occur during treatment.

Source: National Institute on Drug Abuse. Principles of drug addiction treatment: a research-based guide. NIH Publication No. 00-4180. Bethesda (MD): NIDA; 1999 Oct. Rep 2000 Jul.

C. Naltrexone

- Competes with opioids at the opioid receptor sites, therefore blocking the effects of heroin.
- Does not eliminate drug craving so is not the preferred treatment for those addicted.
- This drug works best with highly motivated patients.

D. Phenobarbital or Diazepam

- Longer-acting sedatives used to treat sedative withdrawal symptoms.
- The dose is reduced gradually until there are no signs of withdrawal.

DENTAL HYGIENE PROCESS OF CARE

Millions of people in the United States meet the diagnostic criteria for alcoholism and drug abuse. Dental professionals often have the first opportunity to treat early signs and symptoms of oral complications for the substance abuser. It is necessary to recognize the characteristics of each patient before treatment since it is rare that a patient will disclose information about an addiction.[37]

- Many drug dependent people continue to maintain home, work, and social relationships, at least initially, and for a span of years.
- The spectrum of substance use found in dental and dental hygiene patients varies from abstinence to alcohol and drug dependence.
- Many patients with an alcohol use disorder may use psychoactive drugs such as cocaine, heroin, amphetamines, marijuana, and assorted sedatives or hypnotics.
- Identification of the abstainer or "teetotaler" is particularly essential to recognize because the patient may be a recovering alcoholic or other substance abuser.

I. ASSESSMENT

A. Patient History

Carefully prepared personal, medical, and dental histories are needed to provide information for comprehensive patient care. A reluctance of the patient to reveal symptoms of alcoholism presents a danger because of alcohol's effect on oral and systemic health and an enhanced risk of medically related adverse events and drug interactions.[38]

- Many patients with a drug abuse problem are in denial, which makes their medical history less reliable.
- The medical history is updated with an interview at each maintenance appointment.
- Patients that abuse drugs may have many general health-related problems.
- Precautions, modifications, or adaptations may be needed to prevent an emergency situation.
- Other conditions may be identified that may signify further diagnosis, treatment, or referral.

B. The Interview

Effective Communication

- Keep the lines of communication open; refrain from using comments that will place the patient on the defensive.
- Remain empathetic, respectful, and nonjudgmental; patients may be far more likely to respond to questions.
- Discuss the effects of drug use on physical, psychosocial, and economic well-being at a level appropriate for patient understanding.

Obtain Patient Confidence

- Patients may hesitate to reveal personal information about substance use because of the social stigma attached to users.
- Patients need to understand the information is required as a health-safety measure.

BOX 64-6	CAGE Questionnaire and Scoring

Questionnaire

C Have you ever felt you ought to **C**ut down on your drinking or drug use?

A Have people **A**nnoyed you by criticizing your drinking or drug use?

G Have you ever felt **G**uilty about your drinking or drug use?

E Have you ever had a drink or used drugs first thing in the morning (**E**ye-Opener) to steady your nerves or to get rid of a hangover or to get your day started?

Scoring

- Each positive response receives one point.
- A score of 2 or more is considered probable for alcoholism.
- The predictive value of two positive responses is 30–60%.
- Three positive responses is 60–75%.
- Four positive responses is higher than 90.*

*Refer all patients with test results that suggest alcohol dependence to their primary care physician for a more in-depth evaluation. Adapted with permission from Schorling JB, Buchsbaum DG. Screening for alcohol and drug abuse. *Med Clin North Am.* 1997;81:845–65.

- The patient needs to be assured that personal information will remain confidential.

C. Screening

- Dental providers who believe that a patient may be currently (or in the past) abusing alcohol or may be alcohol and/or drug dependent can screen for the illness using the CAGE questionnaire as shown in **Box 64-6**.[39]

This instrument is most effective when used during a routine medical history.

- It consists of four selected questions that may not provide a positive diagnosis, but research has shown that they can alert the interviewer and provide a high index of suspicion.
- One positive reply can be followed by additional questions as suggested in **Box 64-7**.

D. The Older Adult Patient[40]

- The number of older adult alcohol consumers is ever increasing; some of these are alcoholics.
- The potential for substance abuse in the older adult is high because of the number and variety of medications used.
- Physiological changes associated with aging permit the harmful effects of alcohol consumption to arise at lower levels than with a younger person.
- Excessive use of alcohol exacerbates medical and emotional problems and predisposes the person to drug reactions with medications used to control other illnesses.

BOX 64-7	**Additional Information to Obtain From a Patient Suspected of Drug Use**

- Last recall of any drinking or drug use.
- Pattern of substance use: consumption, frequency, or amount on a given day.
- The number of days per week and the amount on a given occasion.
- Any instances of five or more drinks at a time.
- Systemic conditions related to substance abuse related diseases.
- Accidents or hospital admittances due to substance abuse.
- Types of medications including prescribed, over-the-counter, and illicit drugs.
- Prescription drugs from multiple doctors.
- Taking prescription medications for reasons other than the intended use, such as to relieve stress.
- Taking or buying prescriptions intended for another.

Source: Trachtenberg AI, Fleming MF. National Institute on Drug Abuse archives [Internet]. Diagnosis and treatment of drug abuse in family practice; 8p. Bethesda (MD): National Institute on Drug Abuse; [cited 2006 Feb]; Available from: http://archives.drugabuse.gov/Diagnosis-Treatment/diagnosis.html.

- Memory lapses can upset routine prescription drug use.
- Use of over-the-counter medications and alcohol, combined with prescribed medications, can increase potential health risks associated with substance abuse.

E. Vital Signs

- Record in patient record.
- Blood pressure frequently is increased when alcohol and other drugs are used; fluctuations can be particularly significant.

F. Clinical Examination[41]

- Information in the patient history may not reveal accurately the extent of a patient's drug use.
- Clinical observations along with the medical history may provide a high degree of suspicion.
- Oral manifestations associated with particular drugs can be found in **Box 64-8**.
- The characteristics below have been observed frequently with alcohol and other drug use. When present, they assist in patient evaluation and dental hygiene care planning.

G. Extraoral Examination

Alcohol Signs

- *Breath and body odor of alcohol and of tobacco*: Many alcohol users are also heavy tobacco users.

BOX 64-8	**Oral Manifestations of Particular Drugs**

A. **"Meth mouth"**: key ingredients used in meth manufacturing are all corrosive.[42,43]
  - Meth smoker swirls heated, vaporized substances in the mouth.
  - Oral mucosa is irritated and burned, creating sores and leading to infection.
  - Chronic meth smoker: teeth decayed to the gingiva.
  - Snorting meth also causes chemical damage to teeth.
  - Symptoms: xerostomia, dryness of the mouth from a lack of normal secretions.
  - Rampant dental caries between teeth and at the gingival margin.
  - Cracked teeth caused from grinding and clenching.
  - Enamel erosion: corrosive acids in ingredients.
  - Periodontal infection: reduced blood supply and tissue breakdown.
B. **Cocaine abuse**[44–47]
  - Perforation of the nasal septum and/or perforation of the palate **(Figure 61-4)**.
  - Saddlenose deformity.
  - Erosive carious lesions.
  - Rapid gingival recession and mucosal ulcerations.
  - Trismus.
C. **"Speed" and "ecstasy," amphetamine-based drugs.**[48–50]
  - Xerostomia.
  - Tooth wear associated with chewing and grinding.
  - Temporomandibular joint tenderness.
  - Bruxism leading to trismus.
  - Rampant dental caries.
D. **Cannabis abusers generally have poorer oral health than nonabusers.**[51]
  - Increased dental caries.
  - Increased periodontal infections.
  - Dysplastic changes: a premalignant stage in cellular structures.
  - Premalignant lesions of the oral mucosa.
  - Leukoplakia.
  - Increased oral infections due to immunosuppressive effects.

- *Tremor of hands, tongue, eyelids.* Signs of withdrawal.
- *Skin:* Redness of forehead, cheeks, dilated blood vessels that produce spider petechiae on the nose; may worsen pre-existing acne rosacea.
- *Face color:* Light yellowish brown may indicate jaundice from liver disease.
- *Eyes:* Red, baggy eyes or puffy facial features; bloated appearance.
- *Evidences of trauma:* Facial injuries related to falls when intoxicated. Alcohol abusers are especially prone to traumatic accidents.
- *Lips:* Angular cheilitis related to poor nutrition.
- *Parotid glands:* Swelling.

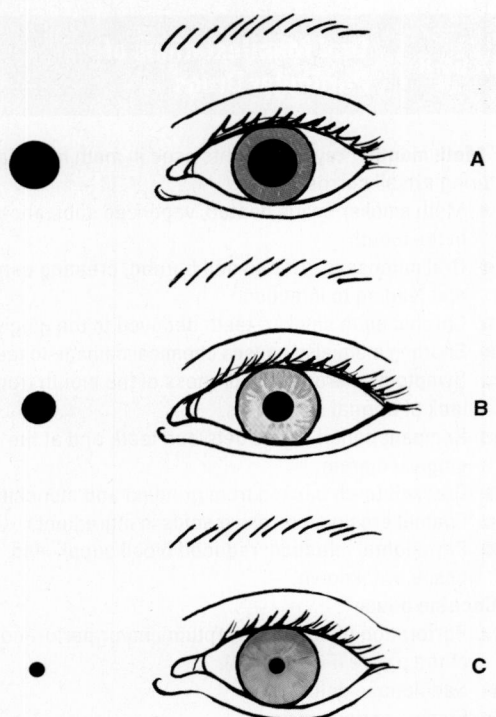

FIGURE 64-3 **Examination of the Pupils. (A)** Dilated; occurs in shock, heart failure, other emergencies, and in the use of hallucinogens and amphetamines. **(B)** Normal. **(C)** Pinpoint; occurs in the use of morphine and related drugs, heroin, barbiturates. (*Source: The American National Red Cross: Standard First Aid and Personal Safety.*)

Personal Appearance
- Lack of interest in proper dress and personal hygiene.
- Wears long sleeves to cover needle marks.
- Small blood stains on clothes from previous injections.
- Dramatic weight loss.

Eyes
- Wears sunglasses to conceal dilated or constricted pupils and eye redness, or to avoid bright light because of eye sensitivity.
- Pupils dilated (amphetamine, LSD, cocaine, marijuana).
- Pupils constricted (heroin, morphine, methadone), as shown in **Figure 64-3**.
- Red, inflamed, bloodshot (marijuana).

Arms
- Needle marks may be noted when determining blood pressure.

Behavior
- Sneezing, itching.
- Tendency to gaze into space; moodiness.
- Drowsiness, yawning; may sleep long hours.
- Appearance of intoxication without the odor of alcohol. Slurred speech.
- Changes in habits, attitudes, and efficiency. Irregular attendance at appointments by one who was previously prompt.

- Possession of pills, capsules.
- Hallucinations or convulsions indicate need for immediate emergency care.

H. Intraoral Examination

Mucosa, Lips, Tongue
- Dry; drug-induced xerostomia, soft tissue abnormalities.
- Tongue coated; glossitis related to nutritional deficiencies.

Gingiva
- Generalized poor oral hygiene; heavy biofilm not unusual.
- Calculus deposits may be generalized, depending on patient neglect.
- Moderate to severe gingival inflammation.
- Gingiva that bleeds spontaneously or on probing.
- Gingival lesions resulting from the direct application of cocaine.[52]
- Higher incidence of periodontal infections than peers.

Palate
- Perforation of palate due to chronic cocaine snorting **(Figure 64-4)**.

Teeth
- Chipped and fractured from falls and injuries; stained from tobacco use.
- Attrition secondary to bruxism.
- Erosion secondary to frequent vomiting, wine consumption,[53] and meth mouth.[54]
- Removable or fixed partial dentures: chipped or broken, may require frequent repairs.

Dental Caries
- Increased risk factors: poor diet, lack of dental care, accumulation of biofilm, and xerostomia.
- Diet high in cariogenic substances.

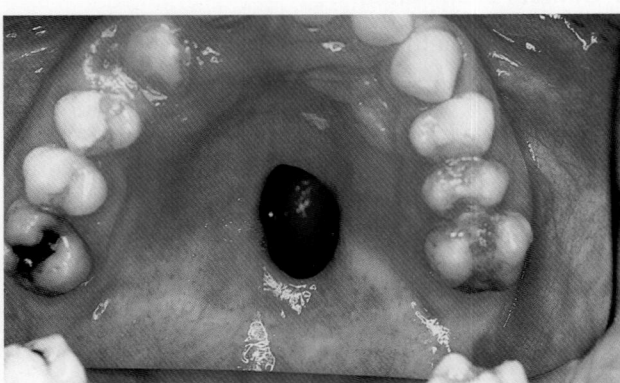

FIGURE 64-4 **Nasopalatal Defect.** The problems due to chronic cocaine snorting began to manifest themselves as nosebleeds followed by recurring sinus infections. Within 4 months, the patient discovered a pinhole in his palate. Each time he tried to swallow liquid it came out of his nose. (Photo courtesy of Peter Villa, DDS, FRDC©.)

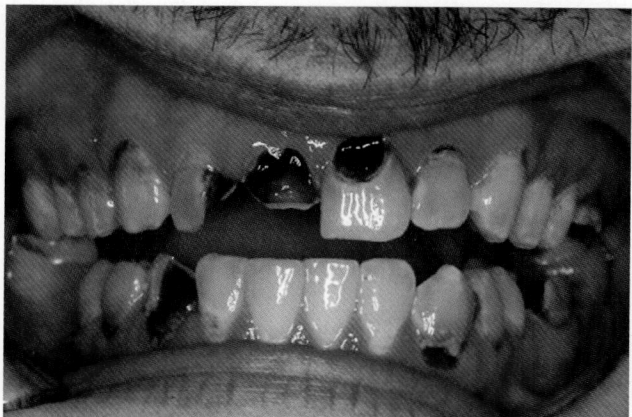

FIGURE 64-5 **Case Report.** Rampant dental caries due to meth-amphetamine use in a 24-year-old patient who presented for treatment after serving time in prison and going to rehab; patient started using meth at age 16, initially snorting the powder and progressed to smoking the drug. Although some teeth could have been saved, the patient chose to have all remaining teeth extracted in order to receive full dentures. (Photo courtesy of Brett H. Kessler, DDS (Kessler BH, Dinnen M. Methamphetamine: oral effects and treatment. Inside Dent. 2010 Feb;6(2):44–6).

- Root caries if gingival recession is evident.
- Open rampant carious lesions: abuse of Meth, diet of sweets, alcohol and soda pop as shown in **Figure 64-5**[54]
- Tooth loss.

Minimal Professional Care
- Substance abuse patients tend to delay dental and dental hygiene care.
- Any available money is used in the purchase of drugs.
- Dental care is used on an emergency basis to alleviate any pain or discomfort, and to obtain prescriptions for drugs.

II. DENTAL HYGIENE DIAGNOSIS

Examples of dental hygiene diagnosis for drug users are suggested as follows:

- **Rampant caries** related to the changes in the addicted patient's lifestyle including diet (multiple daily exposures to sucrose-containing foods and beverages) and neglect of daily care of the oral cavity (lack of biofilm removal and use of fluoride dentifrice and other fluoride sources).
- **Xerostomia** related to methamphetamine use (many drugs have dry mouth as a side effect).

III. PLANNING

- Develop strategies to meet the individual needs of the patient as identified for the dental hygiene diagnosis.
- Priorities and goals are determined by the immediacy of the condition, severity of the problem.

- Examples of interventions to reduce, eliminate, or prevent rampant caries due to drug uses:
  - A. Use of fluoride toothpaste and fluoride mouthrinse without alcohol.
  - B. Apply fluoride applications such as fluoride varnish in office or custom trays for at home use.
  - C. Do not administer local anesthetic for any procedure if unsure whether the patient has taken meth within the last 24 hours – as meth users are resistant to local anesthesia.

IV. IMPLEMENTATION

The clinical procedures for dental hygiene care are greatly influenced by the many health problems that can result from drug use.

A. Preparation for Treatment

- Consult with patient's physician to determine whether prophylactic antibiotic premedication is indicated.
- Precaution is needed for potential drug interactions between specific drugs.
- Preprocedural rinse, antibacterial agents, and oral hygiene products that contain alcohol are to be avoided for all patients suffering from an alcohol use problem. The minutest amount of alcohol ingested by a patient being treated with disulfiram can cause an emergency.

B. Scaling and Debridement

- Use of anesthesia: drug interactions, use of epinephrine, and choice of nitrousoxide/oxygen versus local anesthesia is reviewed and discussed with the patients' physician.
- Contraindications for use of nitrous oxide/oxygen may be found in Chapter 37 on page 558, and medical considerations for local anesthesia with or without epinephrine are in Chapter 37 on page 566.

C. Power-Driven Instruments

- Patients at an increased risk for infection can be susceptible to complications resulting from aerosols or contaminated water lines in power-driven instruments.
- Use ultrasonic scalers and air-powder stain-removal devices with caution to prevent inhalation of oral microorganisms by the patient.
- High-powered suction is essential.
- Patients with immunosuppression resulting from poor nutrition and HIV are more susceptible to lung infections caused by bacteria taken into the lungs from the oral cavity.
- Take extreme care with patients having respiratory and pulmonary problems, hepatitis, tuberculosis, and diabetes.

D. Response to Therapy

The usual oral tissue response expected following periodontal instrumentation may be limited by the changes in the patient's tissues such as:

- Prolonged bleeding time; impaired clotting mechanism from chronic liver disease.
- Resistance to local anesthetic.
- Impaired healing.
- Interference with collagen formation and deposition.
- Decreased immune system function.
- Increased susceptibility to post-care infection.

E. Dental Biofilm Control

- Maintaining oral health and cleanliness is essential for the prevention of infections.
- Motivation may be difficult because many patients with substance abuse problems are preoccupied with drugs and place less priority on personal hygiene.
- A preventive oral care program for a recovering substance abuse patient is a necessary part of the total rehabilitation process.

F. Diet and Nutrition

Relation of Diet to Alcoholism and Other Drugs[55]

- Alcoholic beverages contain calories; a day's allotment of calories may be ingested when alcohol is used in excess.
- Too few of the essential nutrients such minerals as, proteins, and vitamins are ingested when there is a preoccupation with alcohol and other drugs.
- Deficiencies in proteins and vitamins, in particular vitamin A, may contribute to liver disease and other disorders related to drug use.

Instruction

- Review dietary assessment.
- Provide information about basic dietary needs.
- Encourage use of foods from the MyPlate guide as shown on page 499.

V. EVALUATION

- Develop maintenance program to prevent progression of reoccurrence of disease.
- Evaluate treatment plans and goals with patient.
- Make changes according to the patient's progress.

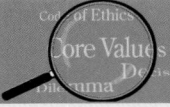

Everyday Ethics

Christy's first patient in the morning is Mr. Phillips who is 20 minutes late for this appointment. Mr. Phillips has missed two consecutive appointments for his routine maintenance care program. As he is being seated, he states that he wants Christy to "*hurry up and clean my teeth*". He smells of smoke and appears quite agitated. Christy starts by taking his blood pressure, which she notes is slightly higher than the one from his previous assessment about a year ago. Sensing Mr. Phillip's strange behavior, Christy calls in Dr. Franks to examine the patient before she begins treatment. The receptionist also alerts Dr. Franks that Mr. Phillips refused to update his medical history today. Dr Franks comes in and greets Mr. Phillips, then turns to Christy and asks to look at his last health history. Noting that information and the new blood pressure reading, Dr. Franks calmly begins to question Mr. Phillips about his medical history, including the CAGE questionnaire.

Dr. Franks notices a strong odor of alcohol on Mr. Phillips breath and he realizes that Mr. Phillips just answered positive to three CAGE questions. Dr. Franks informs the patient that, because he is concerned about his health, he is referring Mr. Phillips to his medical doctor for a complete physical checkup. He requests that the patient stop by the receptionist to reschedule his appointment for further treatment. Mr. Phillips becomes very aggressive and verbally abuses the staff before storming out of Dr. Frank's office without making an appointment. Dr. Frank sadly says, "Maybe we just cannot see this patient any more if he is going to act that way and get my staff all upset."

Questions for Consideration

1. Does the decision to postpone treatment for today violate Mr. Phillip's rights? Why or why not?
2. If Dr. Frank decides to terminate his practitioner–client relationship with Mr. Phillips could this be considered "abandonment"? Answer the questions provided in the Questions to Ask column of Table V-I on page 362 to determine at least one other ethical alternative action that Christy might recommend for Dr Frank to take.
3. How might each of the professional issues listed in Table VI-1, page 553 apply to a decision whether or not to terminate the patient–client relationship with Mr. Phillips?

■ Evaluate to determine the frequency of maintenance appointment.

RISK MANAGEMENT

A major problem facing health care is the abuse of prescription drugs and diversion of medication. Prescription drugs may become a very valuable product for drug traffickers. The theft of prescription pads and medication occurs in a variety of ways. Healthcare professionals need to safeguard against becoming an easy target for drug diversion.[56]

To avoid prescription pad theft and abuse, certain risk management principles need to strictly observed, including the following:

■ Secure inventory of prescription pads in locked area.
■ Number the prescription pads; keep count of all prescription pads by having a staff member appointed to document a weekly inventory count.
■ Do not leave prescription pads in dental treatment rooms or at workstations.
■ Omit the Drug Enforcement Administration (DEA) number on preprinted prescription pads.
■ Do not give DEA number to anyone in the office or family members.
■ Write out the quantity (in words not a number) of doses on the prescription and indicate "No Refills." Never add extra doses: only minimum number that may be needed.
■ The dentist cannot allow anyone besides her/himself to sign a prescription.
■ Know employees; conduct a pre-employment criminal background investigation and pre-employment drug screening for potential employees; include a policy for random drug testing in the office policy manual.

■ Dental hygienists, dental assistants, and front office staff can query prescription monitoring programs (PMPs), which are statewide electronic databases of data about controlled substances dispensed.
■ Establish an office policy to ensure that all risk management principles are met and understood by the entire dental team, reviewed frequently, and included for instruction of all new employees.[57]

DOCUMENTATION

■ Patient record medical alert box for possible substance abuse alerts dental personnel to:
  ▨ use a non-alcoholic mouthwash.
  ▨ review score of CAGE questionnaire.
  ▨ avoid using local anesthetic with vasoconstrictors if patient is identified as an active user or has a positive CAGE score.
  ▨ possible aggressive behavior.
■ Key concepts: documentation for sign/symptoms of early identification of substance abuse. Include in the permanent record:
  ▨ *Oral examination*: with attention to ulcerations, infections, or xerostomia.
  ▨ *Dental examination*: especially cervical dental caries.
  ▨ *Periodontal examination*: noticing rapid changes in periodontal status.
  ▨ *Patient education*: regarding relapse of previously good oral hygiene.
  ▨ *Psychological reactions and/or aggressive behavior*.
■ Example of Progress Note for the substance abuse patient is shown in **Box 64-9**.

BOX 64-9	**Example Progress Note for a Patient With Substance Abuse**

Patient present for 3-month maintenance appointment. Reviewed medical and dental history, patient reports he cannot eat due to pain on inside lower left area. BP 146/90, pulse 98 bpm, changes in intra/extra oral exam: a cluster of ulcerations observed on mandibular left buccal fold. Score of 3 on OHI-S Index. Reviewed modified bass technique, encouraged patient to increase flossing 2 × daily. Recommended toothpaste for dry mouth and a non-alcoholic anesthetic mouthrinse for oral ulcerations. Referred patient for medical consult to discuss possible hypertension. No scaling performed, reappoint patient in two weeks to continue treatment, assess oral tissues, and reinforce changes in patient's personal oral hygiene care.

Signed: _____, RDH Date: _____

Factors To Teach The Patient

■ Drug abuse is a great risk to overall health.
■ Risk of oral cancer is increased by the use of alcohol, tobacco, and marijuana.
■ Need for routine oral screening at least twice a year for signs of early cancer.
■ Drinking alcohol and using other drugs (prescription or over-the-counter), can lead to medical emergencies. Always check each drug and its actions before using it in combination with alcohol or in combination with another drug.
■ Commercial antibacterial and fluoride mouthrinse may contain up to 30% alcohol. Labels must be read carefully. Keep mouthrinse bottles out of reach of children.
■ Alcohol and other drugs readily enter the breast milk and are transmitted to the infant during nursing.
■ Illicit drug use during pregnancy can pose serious risks for unborn babies.

References

1. National Institute on Alcohol Abuse and Alcoholism. *Alcohol alert number 76: alcohol and other drugs.* Bethesda (MD): Department of Health and Human Services (US); 2008 Jul.
2. United States Department of Health and Human Services; Secretary of Health and Human Services. Alcohol and health: 10th special report to the U.S. Congress on alcohol and health. Rockville (MD): NIAAA; 2000 Jun. p. 4.
3. Saitz R. Unhealthy alcohol use. *N Engl J Med.* 2005 Feb 10;352(6): 596–607.
4. American Psychiatric Association. *Diagnostic and statistical manual of mental disorders (DSM-IV-TR).* Washington: American Psychiatric Association; 2000. Substance-related disorders; p. 199.
5. National Institute on Alcohol Abuse and Alcoholism. *Alcohol alert number 59: underage drinking: a major public health challenge.* Bethesda (MD): Department of Health and Human Services (US); 2003 Apr.
6. National Institute on Alcohol Abuse and Alcoholism. *Alcoholism, getting the facts.* Bethesda (MD): Department of Health and Human Services (US); 2004. pp. 2–4. NIH Publication No. 96-4153.
7. Dick DM, Jones K, Saccone N, Hinrichs A, Wang JC, Goate A, Bierut L, Almasy L, Schuckit M, Hesselbrock V, Tischfield J, Foround T, Edenberg H, Porjesz B, Begleiter H. Endophenotypes successfully lead to gene identification: Results from the collaborative study on the genetics of alcoholism. *Behav Genet.* 2006 Jan;36(1):112–26.
8. United States Department of Health and Human Services. op.cit., pp. 169–190.
9. United States Department of Health and Human Services. op.cit., p. 384.
10. Hingson R, Winter M. Epidemiology and consequences of drinking and driving. *Alcohol Res Health.* 2003 Dec;27(1):63–78.
11. National Institute on Alcohol Abuse and Alcoholism. *Alcohol alert number 64: alcoholic liver disease.* Bethesda (MD): Department of Health and Human Services (US); 2005 Jan.
12. Schiff ER, Ozden N. Hepatitis C and alcohol. *Alcohol Res Health.* 2003 Mar;27(3):232–9.
13. United States Department of Health and Human Services. op.cit., p. 240.
14. Pletcher MJ, Varosy P, Kiefe CI, Lewis CE, Sidney S, Hulley SB. Alcohol consumption, binge drinking and early coronary calcification: findings from the Coronary Artery Risk Development in Young Adults (CARDIA) Study. *Am J Epidemiol.* 2005 Mar;161(5):423–33.
15. Lieber CS. Medical disorders of alcoholism. *N Engl J Med.* 1995 Oct;333(16):1058–65.
16. National Institute on Alcohol Abuse and Alcoholism. *Alcohol alert number 63: alcohol's damaging effect on the brain.* Bethesda, (MD): Department of Health and Human Services (US); 2004 Oct. p. 3.
17. Itthagarum A, Nair RG, Epstein JB, King NM. Fetal alcohol syndrome: case report and review of the literature. *Oral Surg Oral Med Oral Pathol Oral Radiol Endod.* 2007 Mar;103(3):e20–5.
18. National Institute on Alcohol Abuse and Alcoholism. *Alcohol alert number 50: fetal alcohol exposure and the brain.* Bethesda, (MD): Department of Health and Human Services (US); 2000 Dec. pp. 1–4.
19. Bertrand J, Floyd RL, Weber MK, O'Connor M, Riley EP, Johnson KA, Cohen DE, National Task Force on FAS/FAE. *Fetal alcohol syndrome: guidelines for referral and diagnosis.* Atlanta (GA): Centers for Disease Control and Prevention; 2004. p. 1–37.
20. American Psychiatric Association. op.cit., pp. 215–70.
21. American Psychiatric Association. op.cit., pp. 215–6.
22. United States Department of Health and Human Services. op.cit., p. 451
23. National Institute On Drug Abuse (US). Methamphetamine abuse and addiction. NIH Publication Number 06-4210. Bethesda (MD): National Institute on Drug Abuse. 1998 Apr; Rev 2006 Sep. 8 p.
24. Noel BK. Methamphetamine abuse: oral implications and care. February 2010 RDH 2010 Feb;30(2):75.
25. American Psychiatric Association. op.cit., p. 248.
26. Lai S, Lima JA, Lai H, Vlahov D, Celentano D, Tong W, Bartlett JG, Margolick J, Fishman EK. Human immunodeficiency virus 1 infection, cocaine, and coronary calcification. *Arch Intern Med.* 2005 Mar 28;165(6):690–5.
27. Ohta K, Mori M, Yoritaka A, Okamoto K, Kishida S. Delayed ischemic stroke associated with methamphetamine use. *J Emerg Med.* 2005 Feb;28(2):165–7.
28. McGee SM, McGee DN, McGee MB. Spontaneous intracerebral hemorrhage related to methamphetamine abuse: Autopsy findings and clinical correlation. *Am J Forensic Med Pathol.* 2004 Dec;25(4):334–7.
29. Bellows CF, Raafat AM. The surgical abdomen associated with cocaine abuse. *J Emerg Med.* 2002 Nov;23(4):383–6.
30. Devitt E, Carroll R, Donnelly C, Bergin C. An unusual cause of abdominal pain. *Ir Med J.* 2005 Mar;98(3):88–9.
31. Voss JU, Roller M, Brinkmann E, Mangelsdorf I. Nephrotoxicity of organic solvents: biomarkers for early detection. *Int Arch Occup Environ Health.* 2005 Jul;78(6):475–85.
32. United States Department of Health and Human Services. op.cit., pp. 197–205.
33. National Institute On Drug Abuse (US). NIDA infofacts: cocaine. Bethesda (MD): National Institute on Drug Abuse. Rev 2010 Mar. 5 p.
34. United States Department of Health and Human Services. op.cit., pp. 258–66.
35. Anderson CE, Loomis GA. Recognition and prevention of inhalant abuse. *Amer Fam Physician.* 2003 Sep 1;68(5):869–74.
36. Gordon RJ, Lowy FD. Bacterial infections in drug users. *N Engl J Med.* 2005 Nov;353(18):1945–54.
37. National Institute on Alcohol Abuse and Alcoholism. *Alcoholism, getting the facts.* Bethesda (MD): National Institute on Drug Abuse; 2004. p. 2–4. NIH Publication No. 96-4153.
38. United States Department of Health and Human Services. op.cit., p. 430.
39. Schorling JB, Buchsbaum DG. Screening for alcohol and drug abuse. *Med Clin North Am.* 1977;81:845–65.
40. Friedlander AH, Norman DC. Geriatric alcoholism: pathophysiology and dental implications. *J Am Dent Assoc.* 2006 Mar;137(3):330–8.
41. Friedlander AH, Marder SR, Pisegna JR, Yagiela JA. Alcohol use and dependence: psychopathology, medical management, and dental implications. *J Am Dent Assoc.* 2003 Jun;134(6):731–40.
42. Rhodus NL, Little JW. Methamphetamine abuse and "meth mouth." *Northwest Dent.* 2005 Sep-Oct;84(5):29, 31, 33–7.
43. National Institute on Drug Abuse: the science of drug abuse and addiction [Internet]. Bethesda (MD): NIDA: [cited 2011 Jan 11]. Commonly abused drugs; [cited 2011 Jan 11]; [about 4 screens]. Available from: http://www.drugabuse.gov/DrugPages/DrugsofAbuse.html
44. Vilela RJ, Langford C, McCullagh L, Kass ES. Cocaine-induced oronasal fistulas with external nasal erosion but without palate involvement. *Ear Nose Throat J.* 2002 Aug;81(8):562–3.
45. Villa PD. Midfacial complications of prolonged cocaine snorting. *J Can Dent Assoc.* 1999 Apr;65(4):218–23.
46. Driscoll SE. A pattern of erosive carious lesions from cocaine use. *J Mass Dent Soc.* 2003 Fall;52(3):12–4.
47. Kapila YL, Kashani H. Cocaine-associated rapid gingival recession and dental erosion. A case report. *J Periodontol.* 1997 May;68(5):485–8.
48. Shaner JW. Caries associated with methamphetamine abuse. *J Mich Dent Assoc.* 2002 Sep;84(9):42–7.
49. Richards JR, Brofeldt BT. Patterns of tooth wear associated with methamphetamine use. *J Periodontol.* 2000 Aug;71(8):1371–4.
50. McGrath C, Chan B. Oral health sensations associated with illicit drug abuse. *Br Dent J.* 2005 Feb 12;198(3):159–62.
51. Cho CM, Hirsh R, Johnstone S. General and oral health implications of cannabis use. *Aust Dent J.* 2005 Jun;50(2):70–4.
52. Yukna RA. Cocaine periodontitis. *Int J Periodontics Restorative Dent.* 1991;11(1):72–9.
53. Mandel L. Dental erosion due to wine consumption. *J Am Dent Assoc.* 2005 Jan;136(1):71–5.
54. Kessler BH, Dinnen M. Methamphetamine: oral effects and treatment. *Inside Dent.* 2010 Feb;6(2):44–6.
55. Lieber CS. Relationships between nutrition, alcohol use, and liver disease. *Alcohol Res Health.* 2003 Mar;27(3):220–31.
56. Rapp C. *Risk management for the medical practice.* Jacksonville (FL): First Professionals Insurance Co.; 2009.
57. Denisco RC, Kenna GA, O'Neil MG, Kulich RJ, Moore PA, Kane WT, Mehta NR, Hersh EV, Katz NP. Prevention of prescription opioid abuse. The role of the dentist. *J Am Dent Assoc.* 2011 Jul;142(7):800–10.

CHAPTER 65

The Patient With a Respiratory Disease

JANET B. SELWITZ-SEGAL, RDH, CDA, MS

Chapter Outline

Patients with respiratory diseases have increased risks for complications due to decreased breathing function and drug interactions. By understanding the cause and symptoms of the respiratory condition and the need to modify dental hygiene services, the prevention of an acute episode and a safe dental hygiene appointment can be facilitated.

■ *Tobacco cessation:* Many respiratory diseases are caused or aggravated by use of tobacco products. Dental hygienists have a unique opportunity to educate their patients about this health hazard.

■ *Emergency treatment:* Patients with respiratory distress may need emergency treatment for which dental hygienists are prepared to prevent or treat when necessary. Signs and symptoms and medical emergency procedures for local anesthesia reactions, respiratory failure, airway obstruction, asthma attack, hyperventilation, anaphylaxis, and allergic reactions are found in Table 69-4 (pages 1076 to 1078).

BOX 65-1	Key Words

Respiration and Respiratory Diseases

Acute: (of a disease or disease symptom) beginning abruptly with marked intensity or sharpness, then subsiding after a relatively short time; opposite of **chronic**.

Analgesic: relieving pain.

Allergen: see **antigen**.

Anaphylaxis: an exaggerated life-threatening hypersensitivity reaction to a previously encountered allergen.

Antigen: any substance that is capable of inducing a specific immune response and of reacting with the products of that response; that is, with specific antibody or specifically sensitized T-lymphocytes or both. When used to describe an allergic response, these antigens are called **allergens**.

Antipyretic: pertaining to a substance or procedure that reduces fever.

Atopy: hereditary tendency to experience immediate allergic reactions (allergic asthma).

Atopic: adj.

Bronchodilator: a drug that relaxes contractions of the smooth muscle of the bronchioles to improve ventilation of the lungs.

Chronic: (of a disease or disorder) developing slowly and persisting for a long period, often for the remainder of a person's lifetime; opposite of **acute.**

Comorbid: medical condition(s) existing simultaneously but independently with another condition.

Communicable disease: (contagious) any disease transmitted from one person or animal to another. *Direct:* from excreta or other bodily discharges. *Indirect:* from substances or inanimate objects (contaminated drinking glasses, water, insects, or toys).

Coryza: profuse discharge from mucous membrane of the nose.

Dysphagia: difficulty in swallowing. Do not confuse with **dysphasia:** loss of ability to understand language as a result of injury or disease to the brain.

Dyspnea: labored or difficult breathing.

Edema: abnormal accumulation of fluids in the intercellular spaces of tissues causing swelling.

Exacerbation: increase in severity of a disease or any of its symptoms.

Expiration: Release of air from the lungs through the nose or mouth. see **inspiration**

Gastroesophageal reflux: backflow of stomach contents into the esophagus where gastric juices produce a burning sensation.

Goblet cell: specialized epithelial cell that secretes mucus.

Hemoptysis: spitting of blood from lesion in the larynx, trachea, or lower respiratory tract.

Hyperventilation: greater rate and volume of breathing than metabolically necessary for pulmonary gas exchange, which may lead to dizziness and possible syncope.

Hypoxia: diminished availability of oxygen to the body tissues characterized by tachycardia, hypertension, peripheral vasoconstriction, and mental confusion.

Inspiration: Inhaling air into the lungs. See **expiration.**

Malaise: a vague uneasy feeling of body weakness, often marking the onset of, and persisting throughout, a disease.

Mast cell: constituent of connective tissue; releases substances in response to injury or infection.

Mediator: intermediary substance that effects a change.

Morbidity: relating to disease. See **comorbid.**

Mortality: relating to death.

Mucus: (n.) viscous, slippery secretion of mucous membranes and glands. Contains mucin, white blood cells, inorganic salts, and exfoliated cells.

Mucous: adj.

Myalgia: muscle pain accompanied by malaise.

Mycoplasm: bacteria without a cell wall, more resistant to antibiotics.

Nosocomial: pertaining to, or originating in, a healthcare facility.

Nosocomial pneumonia: pneumonia contracted during confinement in a healthcare facility.

Orthopnea: ability to breathe easily only in an upright position.

Otalgia: pain in the ears.

Pathophysiology: disruption of bodily functions due to disease.

Pleura: delicate membrane enclosing the lungs.

Pleurisy: inflammation of the pleura; may be caused by infection, injury, or tumor, or a complication of lung diseases. Pleuritic: adj.

Pneumothorax: collection of air or gas causing the lungs to collapse.

Pulmonary hypertension: condition of abnormally high pressure within the pulmonary circulation.

Spirometer: instrument for measuring volume of air entering and leaving the lungs to determine lung function and breathing capacity.

Sputum: matter expectorated (coughed up) from the respiratory system, especially the lungs in a diseased state, composed chiefly of mucus and may contain pus, blood, or microorganisms.

Tachycardia: abnormally high heart rate (greater than 100 beats per minute) for an adult.

Tachypnea: abnormally high respiration rate (greater than 20 breaths per minute) for an adult.

Tracheostomy: direct opening into the trachea through the neck to facilitate breathing or removal of secretions.

Wheeze: breathe with difficulty, usually with a whistling sound.

■ *Oral–systemic link:* Scientific evidence shows that dental biofilm and microorganisms from periodontal infections can contribute to the initiation and/or progression of certain infections in the respiratory system.[1] Dedication of the dental hygienist to the prevention and control of periodontal infections will have a major influence on the overall health of the patient.

■ **Box 65-1** defines key words related to respiration and respiratory diseases and **Box 65-2** lists key abbreviations related to tuberculosis.

BOX 65-2	Key Abbreviations

Tuberculosis

AFB: acid-fast bacilli
HIV: human immunodeficiency virus
IGRA: interferon-gamma release assay
LTBI: latent tuberculosis infection
MEDICATIONS:
- **EMB:** ethambutol
- **INH:** isoniazid
- **PZA:** pyrazinamide
- **RIF:** rifampin

MEDICATION RESISTANCE:
- **MDR-TB:** multidrug-resistant tuberculosis
- **XDR-TB:** extensively drug-resistant tuberculosis

PPD: purified protein derivative
TB: tuberculosis
TST: tuberculin skin test

THE RESPIRATORY SYSTEM

I. ANATOMY[2]

Structures: sinuses, nasal cavity, larynx, pharynx, trachea, bronchi, lungs, and pleura (**Figure 65-1A**).

II. PHYSIOLOGY

The respiratory tract from nasal cavity to lungs serves as a passageway for air exchange (**Figure 65-1A**).

- *Inhaled fresh air:* warmed and filtered in the nasal cavity, enters the lungs.
- *Exhaled air:* with carbon dioxide, leaves the body.
- *Gas exchange:* at the cellular level, occurs in the alveoli at the ends of the bronchioles, as shown in **Figure 65-1B**.
- *Cardiovascular system:* functions with the respiratory system to pump oxygenated blood from the lungs to every cell in the body and deoxygenated blood back to the lungs for exhalation.

III. FUNCTION OF THE RESPIRATORY MUCOSA

Figure 65-2 shows ciliated epithelial cells and mucus-secreting goblet cells that line the respiratory tract to make up the respiratory mucosa.

- Mucus secreted from goblet cells moistens inspired air, prevents delicate alveolar walls from becoming dry, and traps dust and other airborne particles.
- Cilia assist in removing foreign material and contaminated mucus by a constant beating and wavelike motion that propels this material back into the larger bronchi and trachea where it can be coughed up and expectorated or swallowed.
- Lack of function results when the inflammatory process (of asthma and chronic bronchitis) initiates an overabundance of mucus. Congestion is created, preventing the cilia from assisting with normal breathing.

IV. RESPIRATORY ASSESSMENT

Respiratory disease assessment includes several objective measures.

A. *Vital Signs*
- Determination of five vital signs—*body temperature, pulse, respiratory rate, blood pressure, and smoking status* is considered standard procedure in dental patient care.
- Methods for determination of vital signs are described in Chapter 10 on pages 135 to 143.

B. *Spirometry*
- Medical test that measures various aspects of breathing and lung function.
- Used to diagnose and monitor many lower respiratory tract diseases.
- Performed with a spirometer, a device that registers the amount of air a person inhales or exhales and the rate at which air is moved in and out of the lungs.
- **Figure 65-3** shows the use of a spirometer to evaluate lung function.

C. *Pulse oximetry*[3]
- Medical test that measures blood oxygen saturation levels.
- Performed with a pulse oximeter.
- Color of blood varies depending upon the amount of oxygen it contains. Pulse oximeter emits a light through the finger to calculate the percentage of oxygen.
- Any finger (excluding the thumb) can be used. Nail polish or skin callous may interfere with reading.
- Intended only as an adjunct in patient assessment along with other methods of assessing clinical signs and symptoms.
- Healthy patients have an oxygen saturation of 97–100%.
- Saturation of 91% or below signifies poor oxygen exchange.
- **Figure 65-4** shows the use of a pulse oximeter to measure blood oxygen saturation levels.

D. *Chest radiography (imaging)*
- Indicates presence of pathological density (radiopacity) in the lungs.
- *Standard chest radiograph:* shows a two-dimensional view of lung tissues.
- *CAT or CT scan* (computed or computerized axial tomography radiograph): shows a three-dimensional cross section of lung tissues.

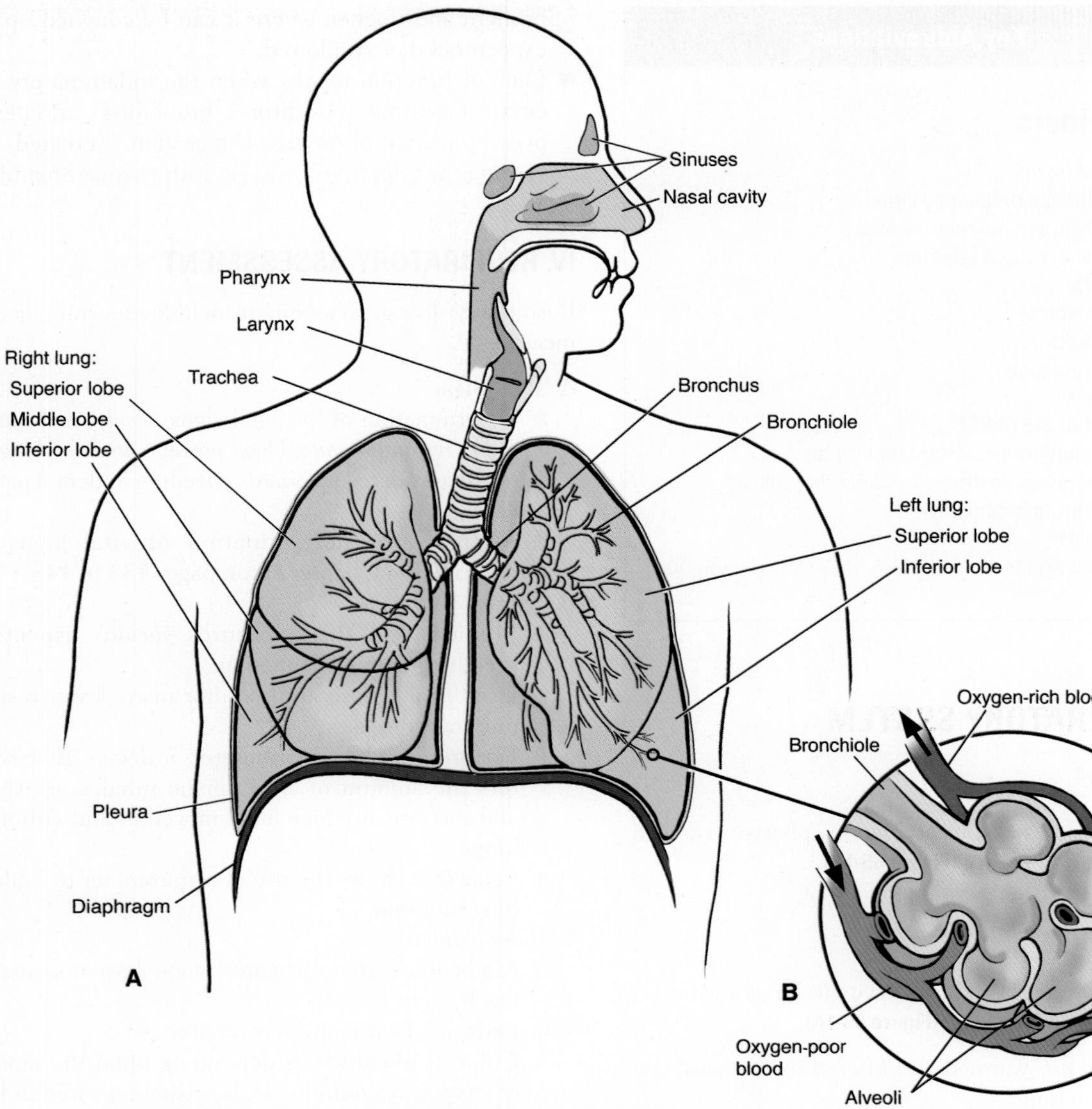

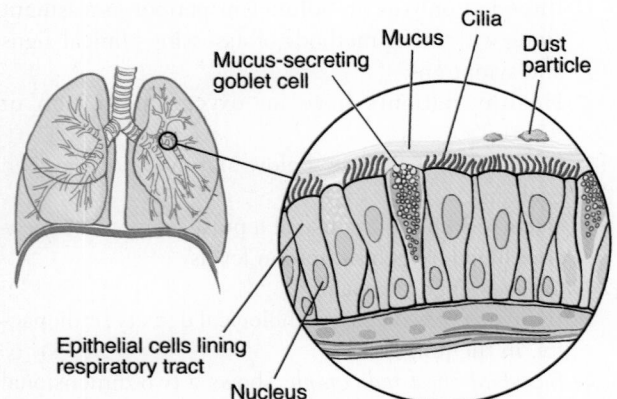

FIGURE 65-1 **Structures of the Respiratory System. (A)** Structures. The major anatomic structures of the respiratory system are shown. Each bronchus branches out to the bronchioles. **(B)** Gas exchange. Exchange of oxygen and carbon dioxide occurs in the alveoli of the bronchioles.

FIGURE 65-2 **Lining of the Respiratory Mucosa.** Ciliated epithelial cells and mucus secreted by goblet cells help to remove foreign objects (dust particles). The material is coughed up and either expectorated or swallowed.

E. *Blood gas analysis*
   - Blood test to determine acid/base balance, alveolar ventilation, arterial oxygen saturation, and carbon dioxide elimination.
F. *Cytology (body cells and fluids) and hematology evaluation*
   - Examination of body cells, blood, and other fluids to determine the presence of microorganisms that cause respiratory diseases.
   - Samples are taken from sputum, pleural cavity fluid, bronchial biopsy, or blood.

V. CLASSIFICATION

Classification of respiratory diseases is shown in **Table 65-1**.

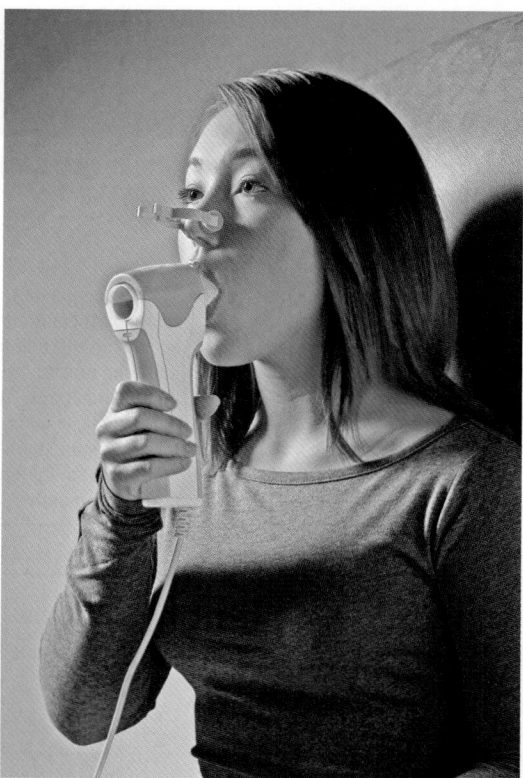

FIGURE 65-3 **Use of a Spirometer to Evaluate Lung Function.** Person being tested takes in a full breath, seals their lips over the mouthpiece of the spirometer, and then blows out as hard and as fast as possible for at least 6 seconds. Nose clips may be applied to ensure no air escapes through the nose. (Courtesy of Midmark Diagnostics, Versailles, Ohio).

TABLE 65-1	CLASSIFICATION OF RESPIRATORY DISEASES	
LOCATION/ STRUCTURES	**ACUTE**	**CHRONIC**
Upper Respiratory Tract: Diseases of the Nose, Sinuses, Pharynx, Larynx	Rhinitis (common cold) Sinusitis Pharyngitis/ tonsillitis Influenza (flu) ■ Seasonal ■ Viral	Allergic rhinitis (hay fever)
Lower Respiratory Tract: Diseases of the Trachea, Lungs	Acute bronchitis Pneumonia	Tuberculosis (TB) Asthma Chronic obstructive pulmonary disease (COPD) ■ Chronic bronchitis ■ Emphysema Cystic fibrosis

■ Signs and symptoms, etiology, medical treatment, and clinical evaluation assessment are summarized in **Table 65-2**.

I. MODES OF TRANSMISSION[4]

■ Inhalation of airborne droplets.
■ Indirectly by contaminated hands or articles freshly soiled with discharge of nose or throat of infected person.

II. DENTAL HYGIENE CARE

A. Disease Prevention

■ All healthcare professionals are expected to obtain immunizations for seasonal viral influenza.
■ Observe standard precautions including respiratory hygiene and cough etiquette as shown in **Table 65-3** to prevent transmission of pathogens from patient to clinician and to prevent healthcare-associated infections to the patient.[5]

B. Appointment Management[6]

■ Delay treatment until patient is no longer infectious.
■ Noninfectivity is determined by temperature return to normal and regression of oral lesions such as erythematous lesions of the soft palate and erythema multiforme.

C. Bacterial Resistance to Antibiotics[7]

■ Bacteria may become resistant to antibiotics within 14 days.
■ For patients currently prescribed an antibiotic for a nondental condition (such as acute bacterial bronchitis or sinus infection): a different category of antibiotic will be necessary to treat an odontogenic (dental origin) infection.

UPPER RESPIRATORY DISEASES

The more common disorders of the upper respiratory tract are caused by infections or allergic reactions that result in inflammation.

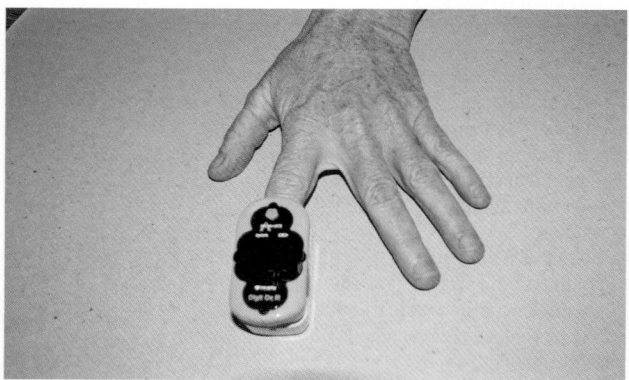

FIGURE 65-4 **Use of a Pulse Oximeter to Measure Blood Oxygen Saturation Level.** Color of blood varies depending on the amount of oxygen it contains. The pulse oximeter clips on any finger (except the thumb) and emits a light through the finger to calculate the percentage of oxygen in the blood. Nail polish and skin callous may interfere with reading.

TABLE 65-2	SUMMARY OF UPPER RESPIRATORY DISEASES: SIGNS/SYMPTOMS, ETIOLOGY, MEDICAL MANAGEMENT, AND DENTAL HYGIENE CARE- CLINICAL EVALUATION ASSESSMENT

SIGNS/SYMPTOMS	ETIOLOGY	MEDICAL MANAGEMENT	CLINICAL EVALUATION ASSESSMENT
Upper Respiratory Infections—Infectious Rhinitis (Common Cold)			
■ Sneezing ■ Nasal congestion ■ Nasal discharge (Coryza) ■ Headache ■ Watering of the eyes	■ Viral	■ Analgesic for sore throat, muscle ache ■ Anticholinergic agent to decrease nasal discharge ■ Oral decongestant to decrease nasal congestion ■ Antihistamine for itching, sneezing, "runny nose" ■ Fluids	■ May observe small round erythematous lesions on soft palate, enlarged tonsils, erythema multiforme, acute ulcerative gingivitis ■ Decongestants and mouth breathing may cause dry mouth
Allergic Rhinitis (Hay Fever)			
■ Watering, burning eyes ■ Sneezing ■ Nasal congestion	■ Seasonal triggers (grass, trees, pollen) or perennial triggers (dust mites, mold spores, animal dander) result in IgE-mediated hypersensitivity reactions	■ Avoidance of the allergen ■ Pharmacotherapy medication: antihistamines, decongestants ■ Immunotherapy: allergy injections increase tolerance to allergens and reduce symptoms	■ Dry mouth ■ Oral candidiasis from long-term use of topical corticosteroids
Sinusitis			
■ Nasal obstruction ■ Fever, chills ■ Constant mid-face head pain, more severe when lying down ■ Palpation over sinus area: tenderness, swelling	■ Bacterial infection of the epithelial lining of the sinus ■ Triggers include upper respiratory infections, dental infections, direct trauma	■ Antibiotics ■ Decongestants ■ Fluids	■ Dry mouth ■ Sinus congestion creates pressure on nearby maxillary molar roots and may cause symptoms of toothache; *important to determine if pain originates from tooth or sinus infection*
Pharyngitis/Tonsillitis			
■ Sore throat	■ Mostly viral ■ Rarely bacterial: Group A beta-hemolytic streptococcus (GABHS) infection	■ Viral: treat symptoms ■ Bacterial: antibiotics ■ Patient is no longer infective after 1 day on antibiotics	■ Enlarged tonsils ■ Erythematous tissues
Influenza (Flu)			
■ Chills, fever ■ Headache, coryza, ■ Sore throat ■ Nonproductive dry cough ■ Myalgia, malaise	■ Viral ■ Mode of transmission: airborne (coughing, sneezing) or direct (contact with contaminated surface) ■ Diagnostic testing is required to distinguish between types of influenza viruses.	■ Bed rest, fluids ■ Analgesics, antivirals ■ (amantadine, rimantadine, zanamivir, oseltamivir) ■ Monitor for secondary bacterial infection ■ Prevent with vaccine ■ For information on infection control, vaccinations, prevention, treatment, and updates, see: www.cdc.gov/flu/professionals	■ Dry mouth

Source: Desai S, Scannapieco FA, Lepore M, Anolik R, Glick M. Chapter 12: Diseases of the respiratory tract. In: Greenberg MS, Glick M, Ship JA. *Burket's oral medicine.* 11th ed. Hamilton, (Canada): BC Decker Inc.; 2008. pp. 297–322; Terezhalmy GT, Molinari JA. Chapter 4: Tuberculosis and other respiratory infections. In: Molinari JA, Harte JA. *Cottone's practical infection control in dentistry.* 3rd ed. Philadelphia: Lippincott Williams & Wilkins; 2010. pp. 45–62.

TABLE 65-3	RESPIRATORY HYGIENE AND COUGH ETIQUETTE IN HEALTHCARE SETTINGS[5]
To prevent transmission of *all* respiratory infections in healthcare settings, incorporate the following infection control practices as one component of Standard Precautions:	
1. **Visual Alerts**	■ Post visual alerts: symptoms of respiratory infection and respiratory hygiene and cough etiquette.
2. **Respiratory Hygiene and Cough Etiquette**	■ Use tissue to cover coughs and sneezes and discard in no-touch receptacle. ■ Perform hand hygiene (handwashing with non-antimicrobial soap and water, alcohol-based rub, or antiseptic hand wash) after contact with respiratory secretions or contaminated objects.
3. **Masking and Separation of Persons With Respiratory Symptoms**	■ Offer masks to persons who are coughing and encourage coughing persons to sit at least three feet away from others in common waiting areas.
4. **Droplet Precautions**	■ Observe Droplet Precautions (wearing a surgical or procedure mask for close contact) in addition to Standard Precautions when examining a patient with symptoms of a respiratory infection, particularly when a fever is present.

TABLE 65-4	COMPARISON OF ACUTE VIRAL AND BACTERIAL BRONCHITIS	
ITEM	**VIRAL**	**BACTERIAL**
Occurrence	■ Most prevalent	■ Least prevalent
Medical Treatment	■ Supportive: bed rest, fluids ■ May need inhaled bronchodilators and/or cough suppressant	■ Antibiotics: amoxicillin, macrolides, cephalosporin

LOWER RESPIRATORY TRACT DISEASES

■ Diseases of the lower respiratory tract are listed in **Table 65-1**.

ACUTE BRONCHITIS[8]

■ Acute bronchitis: an acute respiratory infection that involves large airways (trachea, bronchi).
■ Primary symptom: cough with or without phlegm, may last up to three weeks.
■ Differentiated from pneumonia: no significant findings on chest radiography.
■ A comparison of acute viral and bacterial bronchitis is shown in **Table 65-4**.

PNEUMONIA

Pneumonia, an infection and subsequent inflammation of the lungs, is caused by viruses, bacteria, fungi, mycoplasma, or parasites. The respiratory tract of a healthy person is able to defend against organisms aspirated into the lungs. However, with diminished salivary flow, decreased cough reflex, swallowing disorders, poor ability to perform good oral hygiene, or other physical disabilities, there is an increased risk of aspiration and respiratory infection.[9]

I. ETIOLOGY

A. Viral and Bacterial

■ Comparison of viral and bacterial pneumonias shown in **Table 65-5**.

B. Fungal

■ Etiologic agent of *pneumocystis* pneumonia (PCP) is *Pneumocystis jirovecii* (yee-row-vetsee).
■ Susceptibility is enhanced by chronic debilitating disease in which immune mechanisms are impaired, such as in HIV/AIDS.

II. CATEGORIES AND ROLE OF ORAL BACTERIA[1,9]

Pneumonia is often categorized by location and/or procedure.

A. Community-Acquired Pneumonia (CAP)

■ Infection occurring in any individual in the community (not in a healthcare facility).
■ Person-to-person transmission.

B. Healthcare-Associated (Nosocomial) Pneumonia (HCAP)

■ Infection occurring 48–72 hours after admission to a healthcare facility.
■ Main cause of death in hospitalized patients.
■ Bacteria in periodontal pockets may serve as a reservoir for lung infection, especially in institutional settings. Bacteria from oral biofilm are released into saliva and can be aspirated into the lungs.

TABLE 65-5	COMPARISON OF VIRAL AND BACTERIAL PNEUMONIAS	
ITEM	**VIRAL**	**BACTERIAL**
Occurrence	■ Most prevalent	■ Least prevalent
Causative Agent	■ Virus	Bacteria **NOSOCOMIAL** *Aerobic gram-negative bacilli* Example: *Pseudomonas aeruginosa* *Escherichia coli* *Klebsiella pneumoniae* *Gram-positive cocci* Example: *Staphylococcus aureus* Methicillin-resistant *S. aureus* (MRSA) **COMMUNITY-ACQUIRED** *Gram-negative* Example: *Haemophilus influenzae* *Gram-positive cocci* Example: *Streptococcus pneumonia*
Signs and Symptoms	■ Mild symptoms ■ Cough, sputum ■ Mild fever ■ Dyspnea	■ Sudden onset ■ Cough, purulent sputum ■ High fever ■ Dyspnea, tachypnea ■ Pleuritic chest pain
Diagnosis	■ Patient history ■ Physical findings ■ Chest radiography	■ Patient history ■ Physical findings ■ Chest radiography ■ Sputum sample
Medical Treatment	■ Supportive: Bed rest, fluids	■ Antibiotics

Source: Desai S, Scannapieco FA, Lepore M, Anolik R, Glick M. Chapter 12: Diseases of the respiratory tract. In: Greenberg MS, Glick M, Ship JA. *Burket's oral medicine.* 11th ed. Hamilton, (Canada): BC Decker Inc.; 2008. pp. 297–322; Heymann DL. ed. *Control of communicable diseases manual.* 19th ed. Washington, D.C.: American Public Health Association; 2008. Pneumonia pp. 471–84.

■ While a direct causal relationship between periodontitis and pneumonia has not been established, poor oral health, dependence on others to perform daily oral hygiene, oral colonization of periodontal and respiratory pathogens, all influenced by periodontitis, are associated with nosocomial pneumonia.
■ *Nursing home–acquired pneumonia (NHAP)*
  A. Due to dysphagia from decrease in saliva, cough reflex, and/or swallowing disorders, aspiration of saliva can be the main route of bacteria into the lungs and may lead to aspiration pneumonia.

■ *Hospital-acquired pneumonia (HAP)*
  A. Ventilator-associated pneumonia (VAP): mechanically ventilated patients in the immediate care unit with no ability to clear oral secretions by swallowing or coughing.
  B. Non-ventilator-associated pneumonia (non-VAP): biofilm forms on endotracheal tubes, catheters.

III. MEDICAL MANAGEMENT

■ *Viral:* supportive treatment of bed rest and fluids.
■ *Bacterial:* antibiotic therapy.
■ *Fungal:* sulfa drugs.

IV. DENTAL HYGIENE CARE

Control of oral disease and periodontal disease in particular for patients in nursing homes and hospitals will help prevent aspiration pneumonia.

TUBERCULOSIS (TB)

■ Tuberculosis is a chronic, infectious, and communicable disease with worldwide public health significance as a cause of disability and death, especially in developing countries.
■ Groups at high risk for exposure to TB include those who:
  A. have close contact with people infected with TB.
  B. reside and work in institutional settings (prisons, nursing homes).
  C. are from countries that have a high TB incidence/prevalence.
  D. provide medical/dental care for any of the aforementioned high-risk groups.
■ After locating and curing active TB cases, locating and treating contacts of TB patients (especially pediatric and HIV contacts) is the highest public health priority.
■ **Box 65-2** lists key abbreviations related to TB.

I. ETIOLOGY

Mycobacterium tuberculosis, a rod-shaped bacterium (tubercle bacillus), is the most common causative agent.

II. TRANSMISSION

■ Tubercle bacilli travel in airborne droplet nuclei in infected saliva or mucus from persons with pulmonary or laryngeal TB during forceful expirations (coughing, sneezing, talking, singing).
■ Inhalation and other modes of transmission are described in Chapter 4, page 44.

III. DISEASE DEVELOPMENT

■ Inhaled tubercle bacilli travel to the lung alveoli where local infection begins.

- While TB can affect any organ or tissue, *M. tuberculosis* is an aerobe and survives best in an environment of high oxygen tension, such as the lungs.
- Latent tuberculosis infection (LTBI) and tuberculosis (TB disease).
  A. Within 2–10 weeks following exposure, immune response will limit further growth of *M. tuberculosis*, although not all bacilli will be eliminated.
  B. At this stage, the infected person is categorized as having LTBI.
  C. Approximately 5–10% of people infected with *M. tuberculosis* and not treated for LTBI will develop TB disease during their lifetime.
  D. Comparison of LBTI and active TB disease including signs/symptoms, diagnosis, and medical treatment with TB drugs is shown in **Table 65-6**.

IV. DIAGNOSIS

A. Latent Tuberculosis Infection (LTBI)

Two tests are available to determine exposure to *M. tuberculosis*.

- Tuberculin skin test (TST).
  A. Also known as Mantoux test, purified protein derivative (PPD) test.
  B. PPD is injected under the skin on the forearm. After 72 hours, the circumference of induration (hard swelling) is measured to determine exposure.
  C. A negative TST does not exclude TB disease in a person with signs and symptoms of TB disease.
- Interferon-gamma release assay (IGRA).
  A. Blood test to determine exposure to *M. tuberculosis*.

TABLE 65-6	COMPARISON OF LATENT TB INFECTION (LTBI) AND ACTIVE TB DISEASE: SIGNS/ SYMPTOMS, DIAGNOSIS, AND MEDICAL MANAGEMENT WITH TB DRUGS	
ITEM	**LATENT TUBERCULOSIS INFECTION (LTBI)**	**ACTIVE TB DISEASE**
Signs and Symptoms of Pulmonary Tuberculosis	None	*Early Onset:* Low-grade fever Non-productive cough lasting 3 wk or longer Fatigue Unexplained weight loss Sweating at night *Later Onset:* Fever Chills Persistent cough with purulent sputum Hemoptysis Hoarseness (associated with pharyngeal TB) Chest pain Dyspnea
Wellness of Patient	Does not feel sick	Usually feels sick
Infectivity	Does not infect others	May infect others
Tuberculin Skin Test (TST, PPD, or Mantoux)	Positive	May be positive
IGRA Blood Test	Positive	Positive
Sputum Sample for AFB (Acid-Fast Bacilli) and Culture	Negative	May be positive
Chest Radiograph	Normal	Abnormal
Medical Management for Adults: Commonly Prescribed TB Drugs	**Isoniazid (INH)** taken daily for 9 mo (twice weekly if directly observed therapy is available). **OR Rifampin (RIF)** taken daily for 4 months	Various combinations of drugs taken daily for a minimum of 6 mo Drugs commonly prescribed: **Isoniazid (INH)** **Rifampin (RIF)** **Ethambutol (EMB)** **Pyrazinamide (PZA)**

Source: Molinari JA, Harte JA. *Cottone's practical infection control in dentistry.* 3rd ed. Philadelphia: Wolters Kluwer/ Lippincott Williams & Wilkins; 2010, Chapter 4, Tuberculosis and other respiratory infections; pp. 45–62; Heymann DL. ed. *Control of communicable diseases manual.* 19th ed. Washington, DC: American Public Health Association; 2008. Tuberculosis; pp. 639–58; Little JW, Falace DA, Miller CS, Rhodus NL. *Dental management of the medically compromised patient.* 7th ed. St. Louis: Mosby Elsevier; 2008. Chapter 9, Tuberculosis; pp. 115–23.

B. IGRA blood test, as with TST, cannot differentiate LTBI from active TB disease. Laboratory sputum smear and culture is required.

B. Active TB Disease

When tests to determine exposure to *M. tuberculosis* are positive, further examination is required to rule out active TB disease.

- Chest radiograph.
- Physical examination and evaluation of signs and symptoms.
- *Preliminary diagnosis*: Perform microscopic examination of sputum smears for acid-fast bacilli (AFB).
  A. The waxy cell wall of tubercle bacilli does not absorb the traditional water-soluble Gram stain and cannot be identified. B. However, when treated with an acid stain, the organisms appear pink, and are named acid-fast bacilli.
- *Definitive diagnosis*: When acid-fast bacilli are seen on a stained smear of sputum, or other clinical specimen, a diagnosis of TB disease is *suspected*. However, the diagnosis is *not confirmed* until a laboratory culture is grown and identified as *M. tuberculosis*.

V. MEDICAL MANAGEMENT

A. Commonly Prescribed Drugs

Commonly Prescribed TB drugs are Included in **Table 65-6**.

B. Directly Observed Therapy

Observing the patient swallow anti-tuberculosis drugs is recommended for all LTBI and TB disease patients and will result in:

- High medication compliance.
- Prevention of multidrug-resistant bacterial development.
- Prevention of multidrug-resistant TB disease, which is more severe and difficult to treat.

C. Drug Resistance[10]

TB bacteria can become resistant (drugs are no longer effective in killing the bacteria). This can occur when patients do not complete their full course of treatment, when incorrect treatment is prescribed, or if drugs are not available.

- Multidrug-resistant TB (MDR-TB).
  A. TB bacterial resistance to at least two of the first-line (most preferred) drugs, isoniazid and rifampin.
- Extensively drug-resistant TB (XDR-TB).
  A. TB bacterial resistance to isoniazid, rifampin, fluoroquinolone, and at least one of three injectable second-line drugs.

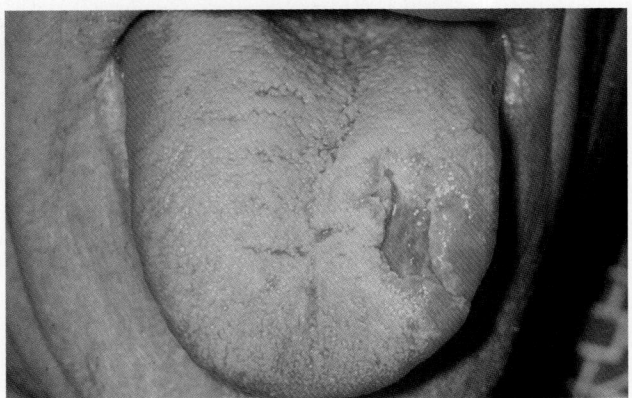

FIGURE 65-5 Oral Ulcer Caused by *Mycobacterium tuberculosis*. The classic oral mucosal lesion is a painful, deep, irregular ulcer on the dorsum of the tongue. (Courtesy of the United States Department of Veteran's Affairs. From DeLong L and Burkhart N. *General and oral pathology for dental hygienists*. Baltimore, Maryland: Lippincott Williams & Wilkins; 2008.)

VI. ORAL MANIFESTATIONS

- TB infrequently appears in the oral cavity from pulmonary organisms in infected sputum brought to the mouth by coughing.
- Classic mucosal lesion: painful, deep, irregular ulcer on dorsum of the tongue as seen in **Figure 65-5**.
- Lesions can also occur on palate, lips, buccal mucosa, and gingiva.
- A biopsy and laboratory culture of an oral lesion that reveals *M. tuberculosis* confirms a diagnosis of TB.
- Glandular swelling: cervical or submandibular lymph nodes infected with TB. Nodes may become enlarged.

VII. DENTAL HYGIENE CARE

A. Implementation of Infection Control Measures

- Update medical history.
- Recognize signs and symptoms of TB as shown in **Table 65-6**.
- Follow CDC guidelines in Appendix IV, (page 1096) for infection control and prevention of transmission of TB in healthcare settings.
- Create and routinely update written office/clinic protocols for:
  A. educating and training staff.
  B. instrument reprocessing and operatory cleanup.
  C. identifying, managing, and referring patients with active TB disease.
  D. assessing, managing, and investigating dental staff with positive tuberculin skin test (TST, PPD).

B. Management of Patients With Symptoms or History of TB[11]

Potential infectivity dictates decisions regarding whether to treat a patient or refer to a physician for medical clearance.

- Active TB disease and sputum-positive TB

A. Do not treat in the dental office or any outpatient facility.

B. Treatment needs to be performed in a hospital with appropriate isolation, sterilization, and engineering controls.

■ History of TB

A. Use caution, obtain history of disease, treatment duration, and discuss signs and symptoms of disease.

B. Consult with physician before treatment.

C. Also consult with physician if adequate treatment time/appropriate medical follow-up is unclear or patient presents with signs or symptoms of relapse.

D. Treatment is permitted when patient is free of clinically active disease.

■ Recent conversion to positive tuberculin skin test or blood test.

A. Treatment is permitted after:

1. evaluation by physician to rule out active TB disease

2. verification by physician of receiving isoniazid for 6 months to 1 year to prevent active TB disease.

■ Signs and symptoms of TB

A. Postpone treatment and refer to physician.

ASTHMA[12]

Asthma is a chronic respiratory disease consisting of recurrent episodes of dyspnea, coughing, and wheezing leading to bronchial inflammation and muscle constriction.

I. ETIOLOGY

The exact cause of asthma is not completely understood. The following types are based on pathophysiology.

A. Extrinsic (Allergic or Atopic): Allergic Triggers From Outside the Body

■ Most common type of asthma.

■ Exaggerated inflammatory response triggered by inhalation of an environmental allergen (dust, pollen, tobacco smoke, mold, dust mites, or animal dander).

■ Allergic stimulus leads to activation of airway epithelial mast cells.

■ Steps in an IgE-mediated hypersensitivity reaction are shown in **Figure 65-6**.

B. Intrinsic (Non-Allergic): Non-Allergic Triggers From Within the Body

■ Triggers: emotional stress, gastroesophageal reflux disease (GERD).

■ Trigger may be unidentified.

■ Usually seen in adults.

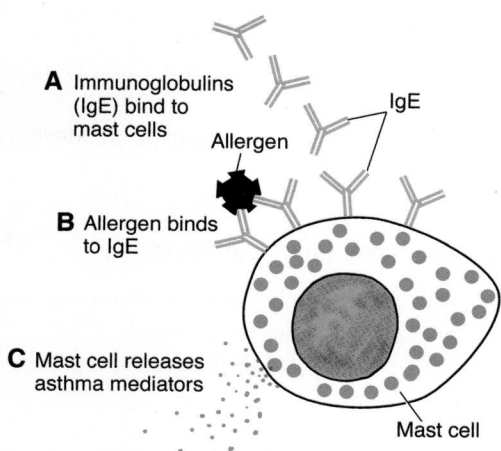

FIGURE 65-6 How Do Allergens Trigger Asthma? Steps in an IgE-mediated hypersensitivity reaction. **(A)** Initial exposure. On initial exposure to an allergen (dust, pollen), immunoglobulins (IgE) are produced and bind to mast cells. **(B)** Subsequent exposure. On subsequent exposures, allergen binds to IgE on the mast cell. **(C)** Mast cells respond by releasing asthma mediators (histamines, leukotrienes, prostaglandins). The asthma mediators cause bronchoconstriction, vasodilation, and mucus production, resulting in coughing, wheezing, and dyspnea.

C. Drug- or Food-Induced (Non-Allergenic, Non-Atopic)

■ Aspirin.

■ Nonsteroidal anti-inflammatory drugs (NSAIDS).

■ Beta-blockers.

■ Food substances: nuts, shellfish, milk, strawberries.

■ Tartrazine (yellow food dye).

■ Metabisulfite preservative in food (wine, beer, shrimp, dried fruit).

■ Metabisulfite preservative in drugs (local anesthetic with epinephrine).

D. Exercise-Induced

■ Vigorous physical activity: usually affects young people due to their level of activity.

■ Thermal changes during inhalation of cold air may provoke mucosal irritation and airway hyperactivity.

E. Infection-Induced

■ Lung infections caused by viruses, bacteria, or fungi may provoke asthmatic symptoms.

■ Treatment of the infection improves breathing.

II. ATOPIC (ALLERGIC) ASTHMA

Atopic asthma is one type of immunoglobulin E (IgE)–mediated hypersensitivity reaction.

A. Immunoglobulin E (IgE)

■ One of the five types of antibodies produced by the body.

■ Provides the primary defense against environmental allergens (pollen, tobacco smoke, and food substances).

B. Normal Inflammatory Reaction

- IgE breaks down the allergens and removes them from the body.
- Normally, such activity does not produce noticeable symptoms.

C. Asthmatic Hypersensitivity Reaction

- People with asthma are believed to "hyperreact" and produce more IgE antibodies than normal.
- The results can be symptoms of asthma: wheezing, coughing, dyspnea.

D. How Do Allergens Trigger Asthma?

Steps in an IgE-mediated hypersensitivity reaction (**Figure 65-6**):

1. On initial exposure to an allergen (dust, pollen, food), immunoglobulins (IgE) are produced and bind to mast cells **(Figure 65-6A)**.
2. On subsequent exposures, the antigen binds to the IgE on the mast cell **(Figure 65-6B)**.
3. Mast cells release asthma mediators such as histamines, leukotrienes, and prostaglandins **(Figure 65-6C)**.
4. Asthma mediators cause bronchoconstriction, vasodilation, and mucus production. The result is wheezing, coughing, and dyspnea.

E. Summary of IgE-Mediated Hypersentitivity Reactions

- Local anaphylaxis.
  A. *Allergen binds to mast cell in nasal cavity:* results in allergic rhinitis (hay fever).
  B. *Allergen binds to mast cell in bronchiole:* results in asthma.
- Systemic anaphylaxis.
  A. *Allergen (penicillin, bee venom, food substance) binds to mast cells throughout the body:* results in anaphylaxis (anaphylactic shock).

III. ASTHMA ATTACK

A. Recognize Signs and Symptoms of Severe or Worsening Asthma Attack

- Chest tightness, sense of suffocation.
- Ineffectiveness of bronchodilator to relieve dyspnea.
- Wheezing, cough.
- Flushed appearance, sweating.
- Confusion due to lack of oxygen.
- Dilated pupils.
- Inability to complete a sentence in one breath.
- Tachypnea.
- Tachycardia.

B. Prepare for Possible Emergency Care

- Recognize signs and symptoms.
- Stop dental hygiene treatment.
- Rule out foreign body obstruction.
- Assist with patient's own bronchodilator inhaler.
- Administer supplemental oxygen by nasal cannula.
- Assist with the administration of subcutaneous injection or inhalation of epinephrine.
- Monitor vital signs.
- Call EMS and initiate emergency procedures listed in Chapter 69, page 1077.

IV. MEDICAL MANAGEMENT[13]

A. Diagnosis

Conduct physical examination and lung function assessment (spirometry).

B. Achieve and Maintain Asthma Control

- *Assess and monitor asthma severity and asthma control:*

  The National Asthma Education and Prevention Program (NAEPP) classification is based on four levels of severity and frequency of symptoms as well as pulmonary function assessment (spirometry).
  A. Intermittent.
  B. Persistent–mild.
  C. Persistent–moderate.
  D. Persistent–severe.
- *Education:* Patients are advised to have a written control plan from the physician explaining the process of disease, treatment options, and how to treat exacerbations (worsening of symptoms).
- *Control of environmental factors* (pollutants and allergens) and *comorbid conditions that affect asthma* (GERD, obesity, obstructive sleep apnea, rhinitis/sinusitis, stress/depression).
- *Medications:*
  A. There are two main types:
    1. Long-term control medications
    2. Quick-relief medications
  B. Categories and examples of asthma medications are shown in **Table 65-7**.
  C. People with asthma are advised to get seasonal and H1N1 influenza vaccinations and may also benefit from immunotherapy (allergy injections).
- *Potentially harmful drugs to avoid*
  A. Asthma attack triggers:
    1. Aspirin-containing medications (use acetaminophen).
    2. Sulfite-containing local anesthetic solution, such as epinephrine.
    3. Nonsteroidal anti-inflammatory drugs (NSAIDS).
  B. Drugs that decrease respiratory function:
    1. Narcotics and barbiturates.

TABLE 65-7	TYPES, CATEGORIES AND EXAMPLES OF ASTHMA MEDICATIONS	
TYPE	**CATEGORY**	**EXAMPLE**
Long-Term Control: Mediation Used Daily to Achieve Control of Persistent Asthma	**Corticosteroids** ■ Anti-inflammatory ■ Decreases airway hyper-responsiveness *Preferred*: inhaled corticosteroid (ICS) for all levels of persistent asthma: oral systemic corticosteroid for severe, persistent asthma	Beclomethasone (Vanceril®) Prednisone
	Mast cell stabilizers *Alternative:* for mild persistent asthma.	Cromolyn sodium (Intal®)
	Immunomodulators ■ Prevents binding of IgE to basophils and mast cells *Alternative:* for severe persistent asthma with sensitivity to allergens	Omalizumab
	Leukotriene receptor antagonist (LTRA) **–also known as leukotriene modifiers** ■ Interferes with leukotriene mediators that are released from mast cells, eosinophils, and basophils. *Alternative:* for mild persistent asthma	Montelukast (Singulair®) (Zafirlukast)
	Long-acting beta 2-agonists (LABA) ■ Inhaled bronchodilator with 12-h duration ■ Used in combination with other medications	Salmeterol, Formoterol
	Methylxanthines ■ Bronchodilator to relax smooth muscle *Alternative:* for mild persistent asthma	Sustained-release theophylline (Theolair,Theo24®)
Short-Term Control: Quick Relief Medication	**Short-acting beta 2-agonists (SABA)** ■ Bronchodilator to relax smooth muscle *Preferred*: for relief of acute symptoms	Albuterol (Ventolin®) levalbuterol pirbuterol
	Anticholinergics ■ Used in hospital emergency room and in inhalers	
	Systemic corticosteroids ■ For exacerbations used with SABAs to speed recovery and prevent re-occurrence of exacerbations	
Combination Medication	■ Combines anti-inflammatory medication with bronchodilator medication	Advair Discus (fluticasone and salmeterol)

C. Harmful drug-to-drug interactions:
1. Avoid macrolide antibiotics (such as erythromycin) if patient takes theophylline.
2. Erythromycin inhibits metabolism of theophylline, which can result in an increase in serum level and possible overdose.
3. Discontinue cimetidine 24 hours before intravenous sedation in patients taking theophylline.

V. ORAL MANIFESTATIONS

■ Beta-2 agonist inhalers:
 A. cause a decrease in salivary flow and dental biofilm pH.
 B. are associated with xerostomia and a possible increase in caries and gingivitis in patients with less than ideal dental hygiene.

■ Increase in gastroesophageal reflux disease (GERD) with use of beta-2 agonists and theophylline, which may contribute to enamel erosion.
■ Oral candidiasis may occur with high dosage or frequency of inhaled corticosteroids. Occurrence may decrease with use of a "spacer" or aerosol-holding chamber attached to metered-dose inhaler and rinsing mouth with water after each use.

VI. DENTAL HYGIENE CARE

Dental hygienists play a leading role in the treatment of patients with asthma. **Table 65-8** summarizes dental hygiene care before, during, and after treatment.[14]

TABLE 65-8	DENTAL HYGIENE CARE FOR THE PATIENT WITH ASTHMA

TIME	DENTAL HYGIENE CARE

Before Treatment	■ Remind the patient to bring inhaler (rescue drug) and/or other medications.
	■ Assess risk level: Review medical history, frequency/severity of acute episodes, and triggering agents.
	
	Questions to ask: In the past 2 wk, how many times have you:
	   a. had problems with coughing, wheezing, shortness of breath, or chest tightness during the day?
	   b. awakened at night from sleep because of coughing or other asthma symptoms?
	   c. awakened in the morning with asthma symptoms?
	   d. had asthma symptoms that did not improve within 15 minutes of using inhaled medication?
	   e. had symptoms while exercising or playing?
	■ Evaluate current symptoms: Reappoint if symptoms are not well controlled.
	■ Review current medications. See **Table 65-7** for commonly prescribed asthma medications.
	■ Ask if all prescription medication has been taken.
	■ Schedule morning appointments for patients with nocturnal asthma (symptoms worsen at night).
	■ Have bronchodilator and oxygen available. May use patient's bronchodilator as a preventive measure before the appointment.
	■ Obtain a medical consultation for patients with unstable or severe acute asthma or if on corticosteroid to determine necessity of steroid replacement and/or antibiotics to prevent infection.
	■ Provide a stress-free environment.

During Treatment	■ Prevent triggering a hypersensitive airway by properly placing cotton rolls, fluoride trays, and suction tip. ■ Use local anesthetic without sulfites. ■ Fluoride treatment for all patients with asthma especially those using beta-2 agonists. ■ If asthma attack occurs, stop treatment, rule out foreign body obstruction, initiate emergency procedures shown on (page 1077).
After Treatment	■ Home care instructions: advise patient to rinse mouth with water after using inhaler to decrease oral candidiasis. ■ Analgesic drug of choice is acetominophen (aspirin or NSAIDs may trigger attack).

CHRONIC OBSTRUCTIVE PULMONARY DISEASE (COPD)

■ The term "COPD" is used to describe pulmonary disorders that obstruct airflow.

■ Two of the most common diseases are chronic bronchitis and emphysema.

■ The primary etiology is inhaling tobacco smoke with occupational and environmental pollutants as contributing factors.

■ Tobacco use accounts for 80–90% of COPD mortality in men and women.[15]

■ Motivating a patient with COPD to begin a tobacco cessation program can be one of the most rewarding aspects of dental hygiene practice.

I. CHRONIC BRONCHITIS

A. Etiology

Chronic bronchitis is defined as excessive respiratory tract mucus production sufficient to cause a cough with expectoration (coughing up mucus) for at least 3 months of the year for 2 or more years.

■ Obstruction caused by narrowing of small airways, increased sputum (phlegm), and mucus plugging.

■ Difficulty breathing present on *inspiration* (breathing in) and *expiration* (breathing out).

B. Signs and Symptoms

■ Chronic cough.
■ Copious sputum.
■ Chest radiograph abnormalities.
■ Sedentary, overweight, cyanotic, edematous, breathless, leading to the term "blue bloater".

II. EMPHYSEMA

A. Etiology

Emphysema is defined as a distension (widening) of the air spaces distal to terminal bronchioles due to destruction of alveolar walls (septa).

■ Smoke injures alveolar epithelium destroying alveolar walls and creating large air spaces.

■ Difficulty breathing only on *expiration*.

B. Signs and Symptoms

■ Difficulty in breathing on exertion.
■ Minimal, nonproductive cough (dry, no mucus).
■ Barrel chest (enlarged chest walls) due to increased use of respiratory chest muscles.
■ Weight loss.
■ Chest radiograph abnormalities.
■ Purses lips to forcibly expel air, leading to the term "pink puffer."

III. MEDICAL MANAGEMENT

There is no cure for COPD. To decrease exacerbations, patients are encouraged to stop smoking, eliminate exposure to environmental pollutants, have adequate nutrition, drink water, and exercise regularly. The four areas of medical intervention strategies are:[16]

A. Assess and Monitor Disease

- Confirm diagnosis with spirometry and determine severity.
- COPD is classified into five stages: at risk, mild, moderate, severe, and very severe.
    - A. *At-risk* stage is defined by normal spirometry but patients have chronic symptoms of cough and sputum production.
    - B. *Mild, moderate, and severe* COPD has evidence of increasing airway obstruction on spirometry in each progressive stage.
    - C. *Very severe* COPD is defined by severe airway obstruction with chronic respiratory failure. At this stage, quality of life is significantly impaired and exacerbations may be life threatening.

B. Reduce Risk Factors

- Tobacco cessation.
- Reduction of exposure to environmental indoor/outdoor pollutants.

    Examples: Ozone and industrial air pollution, automobile emissions, household cleaning products.

C. Manage Stable COPD

- Relief of symptoms: aerosol bronchodilators, inhaled corticosteroids, and other medications similar to those used to treat asthma.
- Pneumonia and seasonal/H1N1 influenza vaccinations.
- Antibiotics for infectious exacerbations.
- Pulmonary rehabilitation including a structured exercise program to relieve symptoms and improve quality of life.
- Surgery:
    - A. In severe emphysema, the removal of part of one or both lungs may result in more space for the remaining lungs to function.
    - B. Lung transplant.
- Oxygen therapy: A patient who uses oxygen to improve breathing function may hold a portable unit during treatment as shown in **Figure 65-7**.
    - A. Types: *Continuous flow:* oxygen flows at a determined rate of liters per minute.
    - B. *On demand:* oxygen flows during inhalation only, extending the period of time between oxygen tank refills.

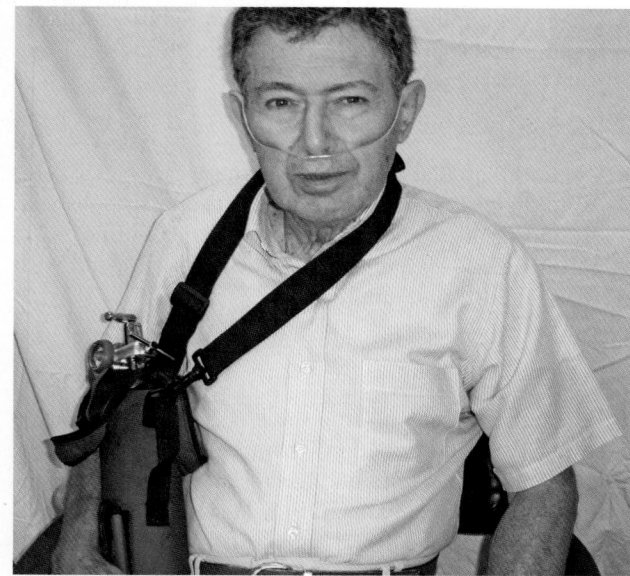

FIGURE 65-7 Use of a Portable Oxygen Tank. A patient who uses oxygen to improve breathing function may hold a portable unit during treatment. (Picture courtesy of Anne MacNeil Photography).

- C. Precautions: Oxygen promotes rapid burning. Keep away from heat, flame, or other ignition source (cigarettes, Bunsen burner).

D. Prevent and Manage Exacerbations

- Infections, inhalation of irritants, and non-adherence to management programs lead to exacerbations.

IV. ORAL MANIFESTATIONS[17]

- Similar to patients with asthma as shown on (page 999).
- Patients who use any form of tobacco have an increased risk of the following oral conditions:
    - A. Oral cancer.
    - B. Nicotine stomatitis.
    - C. Halitosis.
    - D. Periodontal infections.
    - E. Extrinsic tooth stain.

V. DENTAL HYGIENE CARE

A. Before Treatment

- Precautions are needed when concurrent cardiovascular disease is present. Emergency procedures are outlined in Chapter 69, page 1078.
- Assess severity of COPD and breathing difficulty.
- Treatment may be performed on stable patients with adequate breathing.
- Identify patients who may experience exacerbation of symptoms under emotional stress.
- Monitor blood pressure.
- Appointment length may need to be modified.

■ Chair positioning: upright or semi-upright to facilitate breathing as shown in Chapter 7, page 90.

B. During Treatment

■ Use antimicrobial preprocedural rinse.
■ Avoid the use of power-driven scalers and air polishers.
■ Administer local anesthesia without epinephrine.
■ Nitrous oxide–oxygen inhalation sedation: avoid with severe COPD and emphysema.

C. Patient Education

■ Encourage patients to stop smoking. Tobacco cessation strategies are described in Chapter 33, page 489.
■ Promote oral care and oral health knowledge in prevention and treatment of COPD. Periodontal infection, inadequate personal oral care, and lack of oral health knowledge are associated with increased risk of COPD.[18]
■ Discuss oral–systemic link between periodontitis and COPD.
■ Teach and promote oral cancer self-examination.
■ Schedule frequent periodontal and maintenance visits.

CYSTIC FIBROSIS (CF)

Cystic fibrosis is an autosomal recessive gene disorder meaning both parents must carry the genetic mutation for the disease to be transmitted to their children.

■ CF is progressive and ultimately fatal.
■ With improved multifaceted healthcare, many people now live beyond 30–40 years of age.[19]
■ Clinical signs and symptoms are shown in **Box 65-3**.

I. DISEASE CHARACTERISTICS

The gene disorder affects salt and water in epithelial cells of the respiratory tract and exocrine glands (respiratory, pancreas, gastrointestinal) and results in thickened secretions. Main systems affected are:

A. Respiratory Tract

Airways are filled with phlegm, similar to pus, leading to:

■ chronic sinusitis.
■ opportunistic bacterial lung infection:
  Both are difficult to eradicate, even with antibiotics, due to the ability of *Pseudomonas aeruginosa* to form biofilm.[20]

B. Pancreas and Intestinal Tract

■ Thick mucus clogs pancreatic ducts.
■ Clogged ducts prevent the release of pancreatic enzymes into the intestinal tract.
■ Without enzymes, food is not properly digested or absorbed.

BOX 65-3	**Clinical Signs and Symptoms of Cystic Fibrosis (CF)**

Early-Stage
■ In infancy, failure to thrive
■ Persistent cough and wheezing
■ Recurrent pneumonia
■ Excessive appetite but poor weight gain
■ Salty skin or sweat
■ Bulky, foul-smelling stools (undigested lipids)

Late-Stage With Pulmonary Involvement
■ Tachypnea (rapid breathing)
■ Sustained chronic cough with mucus production and vomiting
■ Barrel chest
■ Cyanosis and digital (finger) clubbing
■ Exertional dyspnea with decreased exercise capacity
■ Pneumothorax
■ Right heart failure secondary to pulmonary hypertension

Adapted with permission from McArdle WD, Katch FI, Katch VL. *Exercise physiology.* 7th ed. Baltimore: Wolters Kluwer/Lippincott Williams & Wilkins; 2010. 914 p.

II. MEDICAL MANAGEMENT

Patients are encouraged to have regular physical activity and to adjust their diet to include pancreatic enzyme supplements, fat-soluble vitamins, liquids with high salt intake, and caloric supplementation. Comprehensive medical care includes:[21]

A. Antibiotics including inhalation solution: Tobramycin® nebulizer.
B. Bronchodilators and anti-inflammatory agents.
C. Chest physiotherapy.
  ■ Postural drainage: patient is placed in various body positions to allow mucus to drain from the airway.
  ■ Percussion (tapping): to loosen secretions.

III. DENTAL HYGIENE CARE

A. Oral manifestations:
  ■ No specific oral lesions related specifically to CF.
  ■ Gingivitis associated with dry mouth.
B. To facilitate breathing:
  ■ adapt chair positioning.
  ■ avoid use of rubber dam.

SUMMARY GUIDELINES FOR DENTAL HYGIENE CARE

Summary guidelines for dental hygiene care for a patient with a respiratory disease are shown in **Table 65-9**.

TABLE 65-9	SUMMARY GUIDELINES FOR ORAL HYGIENE CARE FOR PATIENTS WITH A RESPIRATORY DISEASE
ITEM	**DENTAL HYGIENE CARE**
Medical Consultation Required When:	■ Signs or symptoms suggest respiratory disease. Examples: Cough/dyspnea at rest, hemoptysis, sputum, wheeze, chest pain, oxygen saturation level of 91% or lower as determined by pulse oximetry, or positive tuberculosis skin test (TST, PPD, Mantoux) ■ The clinician is uncertain of the patient's medical status, severity of disease, or level of control. ■ Patients with systemic conditions have not seen their physicians within the past year. ■ Patients have American Society of Anesthesiologists (ASA) risk status class III or higher as shown in Chapter 23, page 342. ■ Patients have taken corticosteroids within the past 12 mo. ■ Patients unsure of medications and dosages.
Stress Reduction Protocol	■ Prevent asthma attack; helpful for patients with COPD. ■ Short morning appointments. ■ Avoid precipitating factors.
Chair Position	■ Semi reclined or upright position may make breathing easier.

Anxiety and Pain Control	■ Local anesthetic: avoid epinephrine for patients with asthma/COPD.
	■ Nitrous oxide–oxygen may be contraindicated:
	  ■ For patients with upper respiratory infection or moderate/severe COPD.
	  ■ With upper respiratory tract obstruction or infection if nose breathing would be difficult or breathing apparatus cannot be sterilized or replaced.
	■ Be prepared to handle an emergency.

Analgesia	■ Avoid aspirin, aspirin-containing analgesics, and other NSAIDs as 10% of patients with asthma have aspirin-induced asthma.
Antibiotics	■ Patients with extrinsic asthma may have allergy to antibiotics.
Infection Control	■ Standard precautions including respiratory hygiene and cough etiquette.
Emergency Protocol	■ Recognize symptoms of respiratory distress. ■ Terminate treatment. ■ Emergency protocol is shown in Chapter 69, page 1076.
Use of Equipment That Produces Aerosols	■ Ultrasonic, sonic scalers, and polishing contraindicated. Septic material and microorganisms from biofilm and periodontal pockets can be aspirated into the lungs. For additional contraindications, see Chapter 39, page 624.

Adapted with permission from Bricker SL, Langlais RP, Miller CS. *Oral diagnosis, oral medicine, and treatment planning.* 2nd ed. Shelton, (CT): People's Medical Publishing House; 2002; Chapter 9, Respiratory system; pp.165–91.

DOCUMENTATION

Include in the patient's permanent record:
■ Alerts for dental personnel to the possibility of disease transmission or a medical emergency due to medical condition or allergy.
■ *Paper records:* to protect patient confidentiality, place the medical alert box inside front cover.
■ *Electronic records:* insert in a prominent area.
■ Box 65-4 shows an example of a medical alert box.
■ *Medical consultation:* file written reports and document telephone conversations.

■ *Patient's current health status:* especially related to signs and symptoms of respiratory disease, known allergies, current medications.

BOX 65-4	Example of Medical Alert Box
Medical Alert: Asthma Medical Alert: XDR-TB	

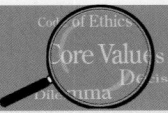

Everyday Ethics

On a beautiful spring day, Lana Thomas arrived for her 3-month preventive maintenance visit. Vicki, the dental hygienist, noticed a labored breathing pattern as they walked down the hall to the dental hygiene treatment room. She rechecked the patient history before beginning the intraoral assessment but found the information unremarkable.

Lana offered that she was taking an OTC product for seasonal allergies but it didn't seem to be helping with her nasal and chest congestion. The patient also requested that she not be placed so far back in the dental chair because it was difficult for her to breathe. Vicki began to reconsider her plan to use the ultrasonic scaler given the patient's current condition.

Questions for Consideration

1. What are the ethical responsibilities of a primary health-care, clinical dental hygienist when a patient presents with symptoms such as those of Lana Thomas?
2. How does each of the dental hygiene core values listed in Table II-1, page 38, have an application as Vicki prepares her care plan for the immediate appointment?
3. Take partners and plan a conversation between Vicki and Lana as Vicki explains:
   a. the procedures they will follow for this appointment,
   b. the need for medical clearance from Lana's physician for using anesthesia and other treatments, and
   c. the special care Lana will need for her daily care because of the oral–systemic relationship that exists.

- *Vital signs:* including pulse oximetry.
- *Oral examination:* with attention to oral cancer screening and periodontal evaluation.
- *Patient education:* especially issues about dry mouth, tobacco cessation, and medication compliance.
- *Changes in respiratory signs and symptoms during treatment and interventions performed.*
- A sample Progress Note for a patient with a positive tuberculin skin test is shown in **Box 65-5**.

Factors To Teach The Patient

- Attention to respiratory hygiene and cough etiquette.
- The need for frequent hand washing to help prevent transmission of respiratory disease.
- The need for thorough daily cleaning and drying of toothbrushes to help prevent spread of infections.
- How using a new toothbrush and cleaning dentures/orthodontic appliances after bacterial infections can decrease possibility of reinfection.
- For elderly patients and those with chronic respiratory or cardiovascular disease, diabetes, or immunosuppressed conditions, the need for pneumonia and seasonal/H1N1 influenza immunization.
- To improve compliance in taking all prescribed medications, maintain a medication list and use pill containers that open easily and are labeled with large type.
- Options to combat medication-induced dry mouth.

BOX 65-5	**Sample Progress Note for a Patient With a Positive Tuberculin Skin Test (TST)**

Sign _____, RHD ____ Date

Called office of Dr. Roberts to obtain medical clearance for Amanda Benjamin, a nurse at Community Hospital, who reported that she had a positive TST test 1 year ago. Spoke with Jennifer, office manager. She will send a written report.

Sign _____, RHD ____ Date

Received medical clearance from Dr. Roberts.
Summary: Chest radiograph-negative
    Sputum smear and culture-negative
    Signs and symptoms-none
    No signs of active TB disease
    Successfully completed regimen of isoniazid for
      9 months
    May receive all needed dental treatment.

Sign _____, RHD ____ Date

References

1. Raghavendran K, Mylotte JM, Scannapieco FA. Nursing home-associated pneumonia, hospital-acquired pneumonia and ventilator-associated pneumonia: the contribution of dental biofilms and periodontal inflammation. *Periodontol 2000.* 2007;44:164–77.
2. Underwood JC. ed. *General and systematic pathology.* 3rd ed. New York: Churchill Livingstone; 2000. Chapter 14, Respiratory tract; pp. 323–58.
3. Little JW, Falace DA, Miller CS, Rhodus NL. *Dental management of the medically compromised patient.* 7th ed. St. Louis: Mosby Elsevier; 2008. Chapter 7, Pulmonary disease; pp. 92–105.
4. Heymann DL. ed. *Control of communicable diseases manual.* 19th ed. Washington: American Public Health Association; 2008. Respiratory Diseases, Acute Viral; pp. 515–20.

5. CDC Healthcare Infection Control Practices Advisory Committee. CDC: Your Online Source for Credible Health Information [Internet]. Atlanta: Centers for Disease Control and Prevention; [updated 2010 Nov 1]. Respiratory hygiene/cough etiquette in healthcare settings; [updated 2009 Aug 1, cited 2010 Apr 18]; [about 2 screens]. Available from: http://www.cdc.gov/flu/professionals/infectioncontrol/resphygiene.htm

6. Bricker SL, Langlais RP, Miller CS. *Oral diagnosis, oral medicine, and treatment planning*. 2nd ed. Shelton (CT): People's Medical Publishing House; 2002. Chapter 9, Respiratory system; pp. 165–91.

7. Greenberg MS, Glick M, Ship JA. *Burket's oral medicine*. 11th ed. Hamilton (Canada): BC Decker Inc.; 2008; Chapter 12, Desai S, Scannapieco FA, Lepore M, Anolik R, Glick M. Diseases of the respiratory tract. pp. 297–322.

8. Ibid, pp. 305–6.

9. Paju S, Scannapieco FA. Oral biofilms, periodontitis, and pulmonary infections. *Oral Dis*. 2007 Nov;13(6):508–12.

10. Heymann. op. cit., p. 644

11. Little JW, Falace DA, Miller CS, Rhodus NL. *Dental management of the medically compromised patient*. 7th ed. St. Louis: Mosby Elsevier; 2008. Chapter 9, Tuberculosis; pp. 115–23.

12. Little, Falace, Miller, Rhodus. op. cit., pp. 97–104.

13. Department of Health and Human Services (US); National Institutes of Health; National Heart, Lung, and Blood Institute. National asthma education and prevention program expert panel report 3: guidelines for the diagnosis and management of asthma-summary report. Bethesda (MD): NHLBI Health Information Center; 2007. 74 p. NIH Publication No.: 08-5846.

14. Desai, Scannapieco, Lepore, Anolik, Glick. op. cit., pp. 314–15.

15. Little, Falace, Miller, Rhodus. op. cit., pp. 92.

16. Gold PM. The 2007 GOLD guidelines: a comprehensive care framework. *Respir Care*. 2009 Aug;54(8):1040–9.

17. Hupp WS. Dental management of patients with obstructive pulmonary diseases. *Dent Clin North Am*. 2006 Oct;50(4):513–27.

18. Wang Z, Zhou X, Zhang J, Zhang L, Song Y, Hu FB, Wang C. Periodontal health, oral health behaviours, and chronic obstructive pulmonary disease. *J Clin Periodontol*. 2009 Sep;36(9):750–5.

19. Desai, Scannapieco, Lepore, Anolik, Glick. op. cit., p. 319.

20. Prince AS. Biofilms, antimicrobial resistance, and airway infection. *N Engl J Med*. 2002 Oct 3; 347(14):1110–11.

21. Desai, Scannapieco, Lepore, Anolik, Glick. op. cit., pp. 318–19.

The Patient With a Cardiovascular Disease

ESTHER M. WILKINS, BS, RDH, DMD

Chapter Outline

Cardiovascular, as the name implies, includes diseases of the heart and blood vessels. Patients with cardiovascular conditions are encountered frequently in a dental office or clinic and may be from any age group, although the highest incidence is among older people. A heart disease may be present for many years before the symptoms are recognized. The patients seen in dental hygiene practice range from those with no obvious symptoms to those nearly disabled.

■ Chronic infections, including chronic advanced periodontitis, are risk factors for coronary vascular disease and stroke.

■ Microorganisms found in subgingival biofilm of periodontal pockets have been identified in atheromatous plaques. The links between periodontal inflammation and cardiovascular disease clearly point to the need for maintenance of healthy oral tissues and prevention of periodontal infections.

- Dental hygienists need to take responsibility to inform patients of the significant relationship between oral and systemic health.
- The major cardiovascular diseases are included in this chapter with their principle symptoms and treatments as well as applications for dental hygiene care.
- Key words and terminology are defined in **Box 66-1**. Prefixes and suffixes to clarify the terminology are listed in Appendix VI on page 1118.

CLASSIFICATION

A. Anatomic Classification

- Diseases of the heart: pericardium, myocardium, endocardium, heart valves
- Diseases of the blood vessels and peripheral circulation

B. Etiologic Classification

- Congenital anomalies

BOX 66-1	**Key Words**

Cardiovascular Diseases

Aneurysm: sac formed by the localized dilatation of the wall of an artery, a vein, or the heart.

Angina: a condition marked by spasmodic suffocative attacks.

Angina pectoris: acute pain in the chest from decreased blood supply to the heart muscle.

Anoxia: absence of oxygen in the tissues; may be accompanied by deep respirations, cyanosis, increased pulse rate, and impairment of coordination.

Anticoagulant: a substance that suppresses, delays, or nullifies coagulation of the blood.

Apnea: temporary cessation of breathing.

Arrhythmia: variation from the normal rhythm, especially with reference to the heart.

Arterial blood: oxygenated blood carried by an artery away from the heart to nourish the body tissues.

Asphyxia: a condition in which there is a deficiency of oxygen in the blood and an increase in carbon dioxide.

Atheroma: lipid (cholesterol) deposit on the intima (lining) of an artery; also called atheromatous plaque.

Bradycardia: slowness of heartbeat with slowing of pulse rate to less than 60 per minute.

Cyanosis: bluish discoloration of the skin and mucous membranes caused by excess concentration of reduced hemoglobin in the blood.

Diaphorosis: profuse perspiration.

Dyspnea: labored or difficult breathing.

Echocardiography: recording of the position and motion of the heart walls and internal structures of the heart and neighboring tissue by the echo obtained from beams of ultrasonic waves directed through the chest wall; used to show valvular and other structural deformities; the record produced is called an echocardiogram.

Edema: abnormal accumulation of fluid in the intercellular spaces of the body.

Electrocardiography: the graphic recording from the body surface of the potential of electric currents generated by the heart as a means of studying the action of the heart muscle; the record produced is called an electrocardiogram (EKG).

Embolism: the sudden blocking of an artery by a clot of foreign material, an embolus, that has been brought to its

site of lodgment by the bloodstream; the embolus may be a blood clot (most frequently) or an air bubble, a clump of bacteria, or a fat globule.

Heparin: anticoagulant; prevents platelet agglutination and thrombus formation.

Hypoxia: diminished availability of oxygen to blood tissues.

Infarct: localized area of ischemic necrosis produced by occlusion of the arterial supply or venous drainage of the part.

Ischemia: deficiency of blood to supply oxygen in part resulting from functional constriction or actual obstruction of a blood vessel.

Lumen: the cavity or channel within a tube or tubular organ, such as a blood vessel or the intestine.

Murmur: irregularity of heartbeat caused by a turbulent flow of blood through a valve that has failed to close.

Myocardium: the middle and thickest layer of the heart wall, composed of cardiac muscle.

Occlusion: blockage; state of being closed.

Prolapse: downward displacement.

Restenosis: recurrent stenosis.

Sclerosis: induration, hardening.

   Arteriosclerosis: group of diseases characterized by thickening and loss of elasticity of the arterial wall.

Shunt: abnormal communication between chambers or blood vessels; *verb,* to bypass, divert.

Stenosis: narrowing or contraction of a body passage or opening.

Tachycardia: abnormally rapid heart rate, usually taken to be over 100 beats per minute.

Tetralogy: a group or series of four.

Tetralogy of Fallot: congenital, cyanotic malformation of the heart that includes pulmonary stenosis, ventricular septal defect, hypertrophy of the right ventricle, and dextroposition of the aorta.

Thrombus: blood clot attached to the intima of a blood vessel; may occlude the lumen; contrast with embolus, which is detached and carried by the bloodstream.

Venous blood: nonoxygenated blood from the tissues; blood pumped from the heart to the lungs for oxygenation.

- Atherosclerosis, hypertension
- Infectious agents, immunologic mechanisms

CONGENITAL HEART DISEASES

I. THE NORMAL HEALTHY HEART

- A diagram of the normal heart is shown in **Figure 66-1** to provide a comparison with the anatomic changes that may appear in a defective heart.
- In the healthy heart, the blood flows in one direction as each chamber contracts, with the valves acting as trap doors that snap shut after each contraction to prevent backflow of blood.
- The right side of the heart contains deoxygenated blood from the body cells on its way to the lungs for re-oxygenation. The left side of the heart contains oxygenated blood from the lungs being pumped out to the aorta on its way to the cells of the body. The septal wall divides the left and right sides of the heart.

II. ANOMALIES

- Anomalies of the anatomic structure of the heart or major blood vessels result following irregularities of development during the first 9 weeks in utero.
- The fetal heart is completely developed by the ninth week.
- Early diagnosis is necessary because one-fourth to half of the infants born with cardiovascular anomalies require treatment during the first year of life.
- Treatment usually involves surgical correction.

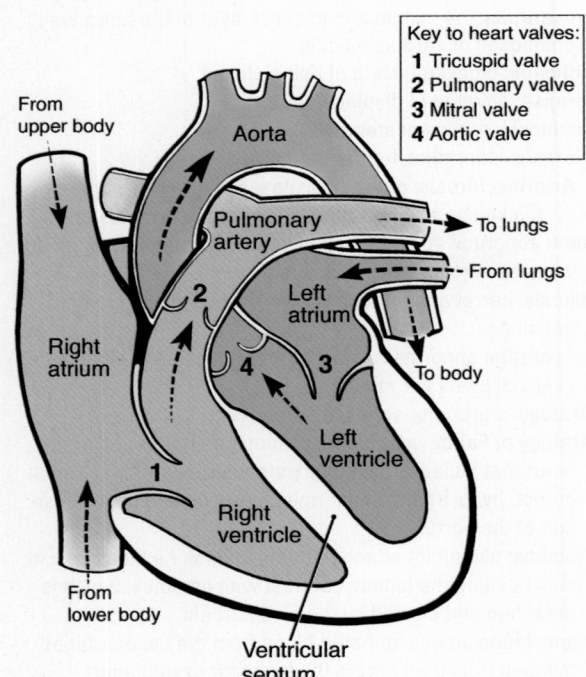

Key to heart valves:
1 Tricuspid valve
2 Pulmonary valve
3 Mitral valve
4 Aortic valve

From upper body
Aorta
Pulmonary artery
To lungs
From lungs
Left atrium
To body
Right atrium
Left ventricle
Right ventricle
From lower body
Ventricular septum

FIGURE 66-1 The Normal Heart. The major vessels and the location of the tricuspid, pulmonary, aortic, and mitral valves are shown.

III. ETIOLOGY

Causes may be genetic, environmental, or a combination of both. Many are unknown.

A. Genetic

- Heredity is apparent in some types of defects.
- An example of a chromosomal defect is Down syndrome, in which congenital heart anomalies occur frequently (described in Chaper 60, page 922).

B. Environmental

- Most congenital anomalies originate between the fifth and eighth weeks of fetal life, when the heart is developing.
- Viral infections from the mother (rubella, cytomegalovirus)
- Drugs (thalidomide)

IV. TYPES OF DEFECTS[1]

- Many types of heart defects exist. Those that occur most frequently are the ventricular septal defect, patent ductus arteriosus, atrial septal defect, and transposition of the great vessels.
- Defects (openings) in the septal wall cause a mixing of oxygenated and deoxygenated blood.
- Atrial and/or ventricular septal defects result in mixing of the blood from the left and right sides of the heart.
- Other defects include a passageway between the great arteries and veins, which also causes mixing of oxygenated and deoxygenated blood. Two of the more common anomalies are described here.

A. Ventricular Septal Defect

- In this type of defect, the left and right ventricles exchange blood through an opening in their dividing wall (septum).
- The oxygenated blood from the lung, which is normally pumped by the left ventricle to the aorta and then to the entire body, can pass across to the right ventricle through the septal defect, as shown in **Figure 66-2**.
- The severity of symptoms is directly related to the specific location and size of the defect. Small defects may close without surgical correction.

B. Patent Ductus Arteriosus

- A patent ductus arteriosus means the passageway (shunt) is open between the two great arteries that arise from the heart, namely, the aorta and the pulmonary artery.
- Normally, the opening closes during the first few weeks after birth.

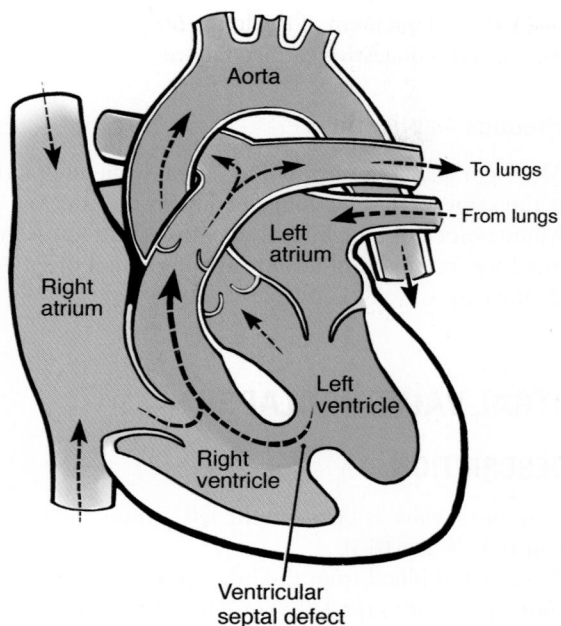

FIGURE 66-2 **Ventricular Septal Defect.** The right and left ventricles are connected by an opening that permits oxygenated blood from the left ventricle to shunt across to the right ventricle and then re-circulate to the lungs. Compare with Figure 66-1, in which the septum separates the ventricles.

- When the opening does not close, blood from the aorta can pass back to the lungs, as shown in **Figure 66-3**.
- The heart compensates in the attempt to provide the body with oxygenated blood and becomes overburdened.

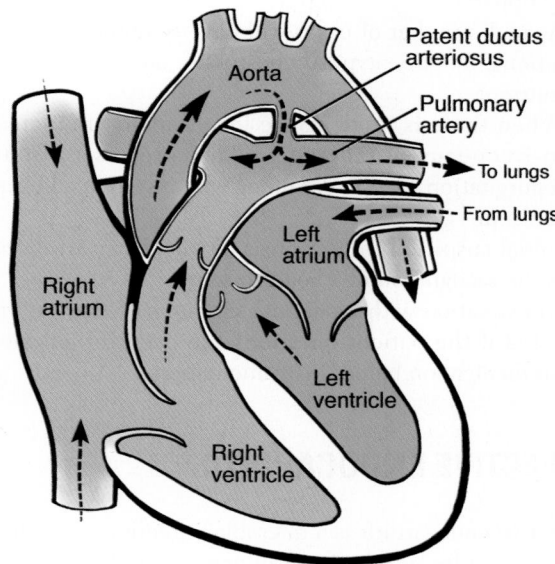

FIGURE 66-3 **Patent Ductus Arteriosus.** An open passageway between the aorta and the pulmonary artery permits oxygenated blood from the aorta to pass back into the lungs. Arrows show directions of flow through the patent ductus. Compare with normal anatomy in Figure 66-1.

V. PREVENTION

- Use of rubella vaccine for childhood immunization.
  - Vaccination confers indefinite immunity.
  - Vaccination for women of childbearing age is highly advised for those not vaccinated in childhood.
  - The vaccine is neither given during pregnancy nor within 3 months of becoming pregnant, because of potential risks to the fetus.
- No medications to be used during pregnancy without prior consultation with the physician.
- Appropriate use of radiologic equipment. A lead apron can be used when oral radiographs are made.
- Control of tobacco, drug, and alcohol addictions.
- Genetic counseling

VI. CLINICAL CONSIDERATIONS

A. Signs and Symptoms of Congenital Heart Disease

General conditions that may be present and that influence patient management are:

- Easy fatigue
- Exertional dyspnea; fainting
- Cyanosis of lips and nail beds
- Poor growth and development
- Chest deformity
- Heart murmurs
- Congestive heart failure

B. Dental Hygiene Concerns

- *Prevention of Infective Endocarditis.* Certain defective heart valves are at risk for endocarditis from bacteremia produced during oral treatments. The American Heart Association Recommendations for premedication are consulted for procedure with this group of patients.[2]
- *Elimination of Oral Disease.* Maintenance of a high level of oral health.

RHEUMATIC HEART DISEASE

Rheumatic heart disease is a complication following rheumatic fever. A rather high percentage of patients with a history of rheumatic fever have permanent heart valve damage. The damaged heart valve, as in congenital heart disease, is susceptible to infective endocarditis.

I. RHEUMATIC FEVER[3,4]

A. Incidence

- Approximately 90% of initial attacks occur between ages 5 and 15 years.
- The patient is left susceptible to future attacks, which may cause additional damage to previously damaged heart valves.
- The tendency to recurrence diminishes with age.

B. Etiology

- The onset of acute rheumatic fever usually appears 2 to 3 weeks after a beta-hemolytic group A streptococcal pharyngeal infection.
- Rheumatic fever and rheumatic heart disease are believed to be immunologic disorders caused by sensitization to antigens of beta-hemolytic group A streptococci.

C. Prevention

- The persistence and severity of the pharyngeal infection are significant factors in determining whether rheumatic fever follows.
- Early diagnosis and treatment of streptococcal throat and pharyngeal infections are necessary.

D. Symptoms of Rheumatic Fever

Over a period of several months of low-grade fever, the joints, heart muscles, central nervous system, skin, and subcutaneous tissues become involved. All the following symptoms disappear with recovery, except the cardiac valve damage.

- *Arthritis.* Migratory polyarthritis is present, which may affect more than one joint at a time. The temporomandibular joint is rarely involved.
- *Carditis.* In a severe case, death may result from heart failure during the acute stage of rheumatic fever, or valvular damage may be sustained with disability. Severity varies, and many patients do not have heart symptoms at the time of the acute illness, some never have, and others may have rheumatic heart disease diagnosed later in life without having had evidence of rheumatic fever.
- The mitral valve is most commonly affected, followed by the aortic valve (**Figure 66-1**). Rheumatic carditis is almost always associated with a significant murmur of insufficiency.

II. THE COURSE OF RHEUMATIC HEART DISEASE

Many factors influence the outlook after rheumatic fever symptoms subside. Usually, no symptoms persist except the effects of the valvular deformity.

A. Symptoms

- Stenosis or incompetence of valves; most commonly, the aortic and mitral valves
- Heart murmur influenced by the amount of scarring of the valves and myocardium
- Cardiac arrhythmias
- Late symptoms include shortness of breath, murmur, angina pectoris, epistaxis, elevation of diastolic blood pressure, enlargement of the left ventricle, and increasing signs of congestive cardiac failure

B. Practice Applications

- The significance in dental and dental hygiene practice is the same as that for congenital heart disease.
- Maintenance of a high level of oral health to prevent a need for treatment of advanced periodontal disease or dental caries.

MITRAL VALVE PROLAPSE

I. DESCRIPTION

- The mitral valve is between the left atrium and the left ventricle (**Figure 66-1**).
- Oxygenated blood from the lungs passes from the pulmonary vein into the left ventricle, where it is pumped through the aortic valve and into the aorta for distribution to the body cells.
- When the mitral valve leaflets are damaged, the closure is imperfect and oxygenated blood can backflow or regurgitate.
- Mitral valve prolapse is the most common disorder of the valve that causes regurgitation.
- The mitral valve is prolapsed into the atrium during systole.

II. SYMPTOMS

- Most patients with mitral valve prolapse are without symptoms.
- A small number of cases will have symptoms of palpitations, fatigue, atypical chest pain, and a late systolic murmur.
- When there is more severe involvement, an increase in frequency of palpitations and progressive mitral regurgitation is apparent along with a systolic click and murmur.
- Initial suspicion for diagnosis of valvular heart disease is the recognition of a heart murmur.
- Consultation with a patient's cardiologist may be indicated if the patient questions the need for antibiotic premedication before instrumentation.

INFECTIVE ENDOCARDITIS[5,6]

Infective endocarditis is a microbial infection of the heart valves or endocardium that is of concern in the dental and dental hygiene care of high-risk patients.

- A bacteremia, or presence of microorganisms in the bloodstream, is necessary for the development of infective endocarditis.

■ A transitory bacteremia can be created during invasive dental and dental hygiene treatment when bleeding occurs.

I. DESCRIPTION

■ Infective endocarditis is a serious disease, the prognosis of which depends on the degree of cardiac damage, the valves involved, the duration of the infection, and the treatment.
■ Patients are prone to develop heart failure leading to death unless the infection is promptly controlled.
■ Infective endocarditis is characterized by the formation of vegetations composed of masses of bacteria and blood clots on the heart valves.
■ The vegetations may arise on normal valves but are most likely to occur on previously damaged valves.
■ When bacteremia occurs, the heart valves may become infected, and infective endocarditis can develop.

II. ETIOLOGY

A. Microorganisms

■ Almost any species of microorganisms may cause infective endocarditis.
■ Streptococci and staphylococci are responsible in most cases, with alpha-hemolytic streptococci being the most prevalent.
■ As yeast, fungi, and viruses have been implicated, the choice of the name "infective" endocarditis is more inclusive than "bacterial" endocarditis.

B. Risk Factors

■ *Preexisting Cardiac Abnormalities.* Bacteria lodge on the endocardial (valvular) surface during bacteremia.
■ *Prosthetic Heart Valves.* There is an increased number of patients who have had valve replacement surgery who are susceptible. Patients who have had prosthetic valve replacements have a risk of developing prosthetic valve endocarditis (PVE).
■ *History of Previous Endocarditis.*
■ *Intravenous Drug Abuse.* Infected material is injected by contaminated needles directly into the bloodstream. Intravenous drug abusers are at high risk for endocarditis, which can initiate on previously normal valves.

C. Precipitating Factors

■ *Self-induced Bacteremia.* In the oral cavity, self-induced bacteremias may result from eating, bruxism, chewing gum, or any activity that can force bacteria through the wall of a diseased sulcus or pocket. Interdental aids for oral hygiene can also cause self-induced bacteremia.
■ *Infection at Portals of Entry.* Infections at sites where microorganisms may enter the circulating blood provide a constant source of potential infectious microorganisms. In the oral cavity, organisms enter the blood by way of periodontal and gingival pockets, where multitudes of many species of microorganisms are harbored. An open area of infection, such as an ulcer caused by an ill-fitting denture, may also provide a site of entry. Patients are exposed daily to bacteremias.
■ *Trauma to Tissues by Instrumentation.* Bacteremias are created during general or oral surgery, endodontic procedures, periodontal therapy, scaling, and, particularly, any therapy that causes bleeding.

III. DISEASE PROCESS

A. Bacteremia Initiated

■ Trauma from instrumentation can rupture blood vessels in the gingival sulcus or pocket.
■ Pressure from trauma forces oral microorganisms into the blood vessels. Ease of entry of organisms directly relates to the severity of trauma and the severity of the gingivitis or periodontitis.

B. Bacterial Implantation

■ Circulating microorganisms attach to a damaged heart valve, prosthetic valve, or other susceptible area. The mitral valve is most often affected.
■ Microorganisms proliferate to form vegetative lesions containing masses of plasma cells, fibrin, and bacteria.
■ Heart valve becomes inflamed; function is diminished.
■ Clumps of microorganisms (emboli) may break off and spread by way of the general circulation; complications result.

C. Clinical Course

■ A small number of patients are symptomatic within 2 days, but usually symptoms appear within 2 weeks.
■ Severe symptoms of fever, loss of appetite and weight loss, weakness, arthralgia, and heart murmurs require hospitalization. Diagnosis is based on symptoms, echocardiography, blood cell count, and positive blood cultures.
■ Complications lead to eventual susceptibility to reinfection with infective endocarditis, congestive heart failure, and cerebrovascular disease.

IV. PREVENTION

The basic areas for attention in dental and dental hygiene care that contribute to the prevention of infective endocarditis are shown in **Box 66-2**.

A. Patient History

■ *Special Content.* Specific questions need to be directed to elicit any history of rheumatic fever and its related

BOX 66-2	Prevention of Infective Endocarditis

- ■ Identification of risk patients
  - ☐ Medical and personal history
- ■ Consultation with physician
- ■ Prophylactic antibiotic coverage during appointments
- ■ Upgrading and maintenance of the patient's oral health
  - ☐ Personal: daily dental biofilm removal
- ■ Professional: supervision, instruction, and motivation

symptoms, congenital heart defects, cardiac transplant, presence of prosthetic valves, acquired valvular defects, or previous episode of infective endocarditis.

- ■ *Consultation with Patient's Physician.* Consultation can be assumed necessary for all patients with a history of rheumatic fever, heart defects, and any other condition suggesting the need for prophylactic antibiotic premedication.
- ■ *Withhold Instrumentation.* The use of a probe or explorer during assessment of the patient is withheld until the medical status is cleared.

B. Prophylactic Antibiotic Premedication

- ■ *Recommended Regimens.* The current recommendations of the American Heart Association are followed.[2]
- ■ Boxes 9-2A and B and Table 9-4 include the specific information in Chapter 9, pages 131 to 133.
- ■ When premedication is indicated, question the patient at the time of the appointment to ascertain that the antibiotic was taken on schedule. In the patient record, document the name of the antibiotic, time, and dosage that was taken by the patient.

C. Dental Hygiene Care

1. *Oral Health.* Maintenance of a high degree of oral health is necessary for each patient susceptible to infective endocarditis.
2. *Instruction.* Instruction in brushing and flossing at initial appointments can be provided while the patient is under antibiotic coverage.
3. *Sequence of Treatment.* Biofilm removal instruction precedes instrumentation for scaling to bring the tissues to as healthy a state as possible. The more severe the gingival or periodontal inflammation, the higher the incidence of bacteremia during and following instrumentation.
4. *Instrumentation.* Reduce the microbial population about the teeth and on the oral mucosa prior to instrumentation by having the patient brush, floss, and rinse thoroughly with an antiseptic mouth rinse.

HYPERTENSION[7]

Hypertension means an abnormal elevation of arterial blood pressure. It has been called the "Silent Killer," as one-third of people who have it do not have symptoms. It is a contributing risk factor in many vascular diseases, or it may be a result or an effect of underlying pathologic changes.

- ■ Detection of blood pressure for dental and dental hygiene patients has become an essential step in patient assessment prior to treatment.
- ■ Early detection, with referral for additional diagnosis and treatment when indicated, can prove to be lifesaving for certain people.
- ■ Knowledge of the health problems of patients is needed for the treatment to be safe and free from threats of emergencies likely to arise.

I. ETIOLOGY

A. Primary or Essential Hypertension

1. *Incidence.* Approximately 95% of all hypertension is primary or essential.
2. *Predisposing or Risk Factors.* Combinations of the factors listed are more significant than any one alone. Risk factors for atherosclerosis are interrelated (page 1041).
   - ■ *Tobacco Use*
   - ■ *Heredity*
   - ■ *Overweight*
   - ■ *Race.* The incidence is higher among African–Americans than among white Americans, the illness is more severe, and the mortality rate is higher at a younger age.
   - ■ *Salt.* Particularly in excess in the diet
   - ■ *Sex.* Men are more affected before age 45 years; women slightly more than men in later years.
   - ■ *Age.* General increase from birth to age 20 years; levels off until 40 years of age; then a slow increase into the older age group.
   - ■ *Environment.* Environmental conditions that increase stress factors.

B. Secondary Hypertension

About 5% of all hypertension is secondary to other underlying medical conditions. In secondary hypertension, usually both systolic and diastolic blood pressures are elevated. Examples of causes are:

1. *Oral Contraceptives*
   - ■ Severe hypertension from contraceptives is uncommon.
   - ■ Increased hypertension over years of using contraceptives has been shown to be a common cause of secondary hypertension in women.

2. *Renal Disease*
   - Renal artery obstruction
   - Pyelonephritis
   - Renal failure
3. *Endocrine Disorders*
   - Hyperthyroidism
   - Diabetes
   - Cushing's syndrome
   - Pheochromocytoma tumor of the adrenal medulla
4. *Medications*
   - Decongestants
   - Steroids

II. BLOOD PRESSURE LEVELS

- The **diastolic** blood pressure is the pressure exerted by the blood within the arteries during the total resting resistance after the contraction of the left ventricle.
- The **systolic** blood pressure is the pressure exerted against the arterial walls during the ventricular contraction. It is altered by the cardiac output, resistance of the capillary bed, and volume and viscosity of the blood. Diseases can have an effect on any of these factors, altering the blood pressure.
- Blood pressure fluctuates, so more than one reading is needed to determine the average level. The baseline blood pressure needs to be measured two or three times and the average reading entered in the patient's record.

A. Normal and High Blood Pressure[8]

Table 66-1 shows the normal readings for blood pressure and the stages of hypertension for adults 18 years and over.

B. Low Blood Pressure

- Many healthy people have a normal systolic pressure under 90 mm Hg, which may be considered "low blood pressure."

TABLE 66-1	CLASSIFICATION OF BLOOD PRESSURE FOR ADULTS AGED 18 YEARS OR OLDER	
BLOOD PRESSURE CATEGORY	**SYSTOLIC (mm Hg)**	**DIASTOLIC (mm Hg)**
Normal	<120	<80
Pre-hypertension	120–139	80–89
Stage 1 hypertension	140–159	90–99
Stage 2 hypertension	≥160	≥100

Data from National High Blood Pressure Education Program. The seventh report of the Joint National Committee on Prevention, Detection, Evaluation, and Treatment of High Blood Pressure. Bethesda (MD): National Heart, Lung, and Blood Institute (US); 2003 Dec. NIH Publication No. 03-5233.

- Such a level is normal for that person, and no clinical problems are evident.
- A marked sudden drop in blood pressure is usually associated with an emergency, such as severe blood loss, shock, myocardial infarction, sepsis, or other medical problem.
- Immediate attention, in the category of a medical emergency, is indicated.
- Referral to specific procedures can be found in Table 69-4 (page 1076).

C. Postural Hypotension

- Postural or orthostatic hypotension is a condition in which there is a sudden drop in the arterial blood pressure when a person sits up quickly from a supine position or stands up quickly from a sitting position.
- Postural hypotension is an adverse effect associated with many medications, mostly antihypertensives and antidepressants.

III. CLINICAL SYMPTOMS OF HYPERTENSION

Essential hypertension is frequently recognized only by blood pressure readings. The condition may go unrecognized because of the lack of clinical symptoms.

A. High Blood Pressure

Those who have early symptoms may describe them as:

- Occipital headaches
- Dizziness
- Visual disturbances
- Weakness
- Ringing in the ears
- Tingling of the hands and feet

B. Long-standing Severe Elevation of Blood Pressure

Hypertensive crisis is a life-threatening disorder. The brain, eyes, heart, or kidney may undergo marked changes in function. In the severe state, if any or all of the following are noted, the patient is referred immediately.

- Any of the symptoms associated with early symptoms.
- Mental confusion leading to stupor, coma, convulsions.
- Blurring of vision; possible loss of sight.
- Severe dyspnea
- Chest pains similar to angina pectoris.

C. Major Sequela

- Hypertensive heart disease; enlarged heart with eventual cardiac failure.
- Cerebral vascular accident (stroke, described in Chapter 58, pages 890 to 892).

- Hypertensive renal disease
- Ischemic heart disease

D. Malignant Hypertension

- Malignant hypertension occurs in approximately 5% of patients who have primary or secondary hypertension.
- The blood pressure rises rapidly to levels greater than 200 mm Hg systolic and 100 mm Hg diastolic.
- **Activate Emergency Medical Service (EMS) immediately.** This is a hypertensive crisis.
- Malignant hypertension presents a risk for a cerebrovascular accident (CVA).

IV. TREATMENT

A. Goals

- *Primary Hypertension*
  A. Achieve and maintain diastolic pressure level below 80 mm Hg.
  B. Lower the risk of serious complications and premature death.
- *Secondary Hypertension*
  A. Surgical or other correction of the cause is needed.

B. Lifestyle Changes (Box 66-3)

1. *Weight and Exercise.* Control weight and exercise daily.
2. *Diet.* Salt restriction and weight loss may be all that are needed for the control of mild elevations of blood pressure.
3. *Tobacco Use.* All forms of tobacco must be eliminated.
4. *Other Risk Factors.* In addition to factors listed in **Box 66-3**, life activity contributions to stress and tension need to be minimized.

BOX 66-3	**Lifestyle Modifications for Hypertension Control and/or Overall Cardiovascular Risk**

- Lose weight if overweight.
- Limit alcohol intake to no more than 1 ounce of ethanol per day (24 ounces of beer, 8 ounces of wine, or 2 ounces of 100-proof whiskey).
- Exercise (aerobic) daily.
- Reduce sodium intake.
- Maintain adequate dietary potassium, calcium, and magnesium intake.
- Stop smoking.
- Reduce dietary saturated fat and cholesterol intake for overall cardiovascular health. Reducing fat intake also helps to reduce caloric intake—important for control of weight and type 2 diabetes.

V. HYPERTENSION IN CHILDREN

- Children 3 years of age and older need to have blood pressure determinations made at least annually.
- When a child between ages 3 and 12 years has a diastolic pressure greater than 90 mm Hg, further investigation is indicated.
- Hypertension has a familial tendency. Determining the pressure levels for children of parents known to have hypertension may reveal important information about the health of the child.

HYPERTENSIVE HEART DISEASE[9]

- Hypertensive heart disease results from the increased load on the heart because of elevated blood pressure.
- When the peripheral arterial resistance to the flow of blood pumped from the heart is increased, the blood pressure rises. The heart attempts to maintain its normal output.
- To cope with the increased workload resulting from the peripheral resistance, muscle fibers are stretched and the heart enlarges.
- The effect of hypertension on the heart is at first a thickening of the left ventricle. In later stages, the entire heart is enlarged. This may be discerned by radiographic and medical examination.
- Cardiac enlargement has no specific symptoms, but the patient may have symptoms of hypertension, such as headaches, weakness, and others listed on previous page.
- When undiagnosed and untreated, the severity increases and left ventricular congestive failure occurs, resulting from the disturbance of cardiac function.

ISCHEMIC HEART DISEASE

Ischemic heart disease is the cardiac disability, acute and chronic, that arises from reduction or arrest of blood supply to the myocardium.

- The heart muscle (myocardium) is supplied through the coronary arteries, which are branches of the descending aorta.
- Because of the relationship to the coronary arteries, the disease is often referred to as coronary heart disease or coronary artery disease.
- Ischemia means oxygen deprivation in a local area from a reduced passage of fluid into the area.
- Ischemic heart disease is the result of an imbalance of the oxygen supply and demand of the myocardium, which, in turn, results from a narrowing or blocking of the lumen of the coronary arteries.

I. ETIOLOGY[10]

Other factors may be involved, but the principal cause of the reduction of blood flow to the heart muscle is **athero-sclerosis** of the vessel walls, which narrows the lumen, thus obstructing the flow of blood.

A. Definition of Atherosclerosis

■ Atherosclerosis is an inflammatory disease of medium and large arteries in which atheromas deposit and thicken the intimal layer of the involved blood vessel.

■ An atheroma is a fibro-fatty deposit or plaque containing several lipids, especially cholesterol.

■ With time, the plaques continue to thicken and, eventually, close the vessel **(Figure 66-4)**.

■ Some plaques calcify, whereas others may develop an overlying thrombus.

B. Risk Factors for Atherosclerosis

■ Inflammation plays a significant role in the formation of atheromas. Low-grade chronic inflammation in other parts of the body, including chronic periodontitis has been shown involved in adverse cardiovascular outcomes.

■ Periodontal pathogenic microorganisms have been associated with the development of atheromas.[11,12,13] The bacteria enter the blood stream at the bottom of periodontal pockets where the epithelial attachment has been broken down by disease, and travel to blood vessels to participate in the formation of atheromas.

■ Many risk factors for periodontal disease are also risk factors for atherosclerosis.

■ Each of the risk factors listed here is significant alone. When these factors occur in combinations, the risk of atherosclerosis, and therefore that of ischemic heart disease, is increased. Prevention depends on educational programs along with early identification of persons at risk.

■ Risk factors include: elevated levels of blood lipids, the result of an increased dietary intake of cholesterol, saturated fat, carbohydrate (especially sucrose), alcohol, and calories.

■ Tobacco use, diabetes, obesity, insufficient physical activity, increased tensions, emotional stress, and family history may all be significant.

■ Genetic inheritance can be one factor along with the perpetuation of familial lifestyle habits such as diet, tobacco habits, tensions, and tendencies toward lack of exercise.

II. MANIFESTATIONS OF ISCHEMIC HEART DISEASE

■ Angina pectoris
■ Myocardial infarction
■ Congestive heart failure

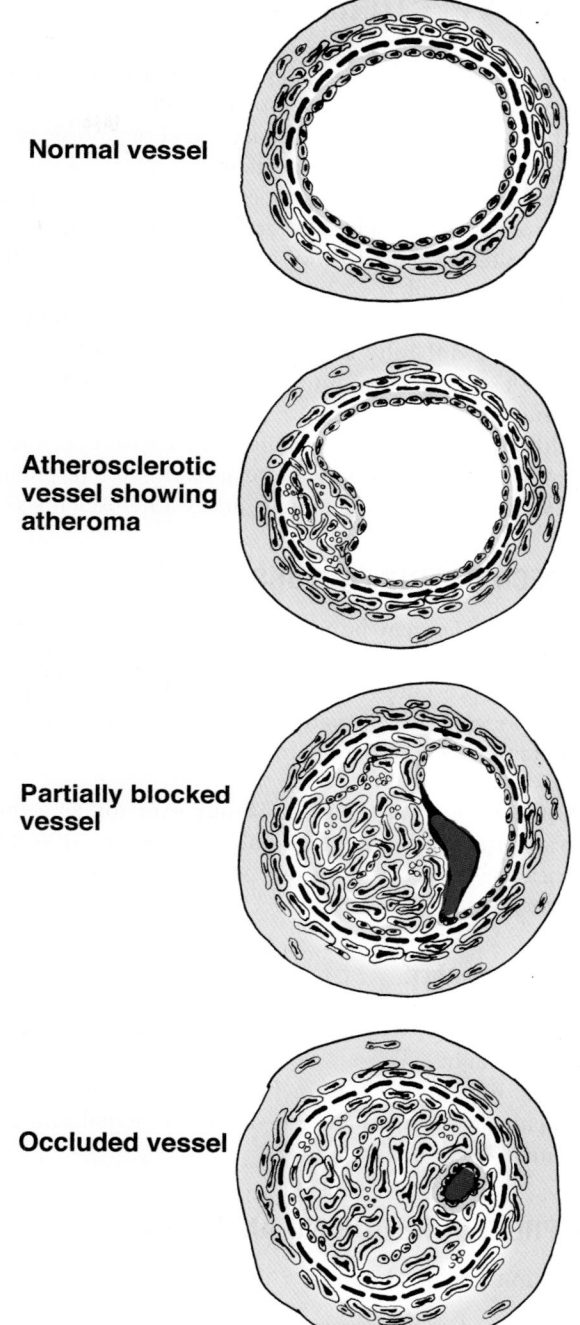

Normal vessel

Atherosclerotic vessel showing atheroma

Partially blocked vessel

Occluded vessel

FIGURE 66-4 **Atherosclerosis.** An atheroma develops within the lining of the normal blood vessel. The atheroma is made of a fatty deposit containing cholesterol. At first, the atheroma is small and no symptoms are apparent, but eventually it enlarges and completely blocks the vessel, thus depriving the area served by the vessel of oxygen. (*Source:* Report of the Working Group on Arteriosclerosis of the National Heart, Lung, and Blood Institute, National Institutes of Health, United States Department of Health and Human Services. [Bethesda, (MD)]: National Institute of Health: 1981 Jun. NIH Publication No. 81–2034.)

ANGINA PECTORIS

- Angina pectoris is chest pain, the most common symptom of coronary atherosclerotic heart disease.
- The pain is described as a heavy, squeezing pressure or tightness in the mid-chest region.
- The pain may radiate to the left or right arm and neck or even the mandible. On rare occasion, the pain may be limited to one of these areas and not occur in the chest area at all.
- The patient may be pale and also experience faintness, sweating, difficulty in breathing, anxiety, or fear. The pain lasts 1 to 5 minutes if precipitating factors are eliminated.
- Although other forms of coronary disease may cause similar pain symptoms, approximately 90% of angina attacks are related to coronary artery atherosclerosis.

I. PRECIPITATING FACTORS

- *Stable angina* may be precipitated by exertion or exercise, emotion, or a heavy meal. In the dental office or clinic, a preventive atmosphere of calmness and quiet can do much to alleviate stress. Stable angina is predictable and consistent in frequency, intensity, and duration.
- *Unstable angina* occurs without exertion or other precipitating factors. The pain may occur while the patient is at rest, and it may vary in intensity at each attack.

II. TREATMENT

- A vasodilator, usually nitroglycerin, is administered sublingually.
- Basic life support that includes supplemental oxygen is part of the treatment provided in a dental office or clinic.

III. PROCEDURE DURING AN ATTACK

A. Terminate Treatment

- Stop the dental or dental hygiene procedure.
- Call for assistance and the emergency kit or cart.

B. Position Patient

- Bring the seat up to a comfortable position.
- Reassure the patient.

C. Administer Vasodilator

- Administer nitroglycerin sublingually.
- Use of the patient's own supply is preferable. Prior to starting procedures of the appointment, the patient's supply should be placed within reach.

- The patient can be asked when the nitroglycerin was purchased because the potency is lost after 6 months out of a sealed storage container.
- Patient with xerostomia may not have sufficient saliva to moisten the nitroglycerin. A few drops of water from the unit syringe can be placed on the tablet under the tongue.

D. Check Patient Response

- Give additional vasodilator. Usually, the first tablet relieves the condition within minutes.
- When it is suspected that the patient's supply may not be fresh and the first tablet has been ineffective, use of a second tablet from the dental office emergency kit may be advisable.

E. Call for Medical Assistance

- When the patient does not respond to the second dose of vasodilator, assume the attack to be a myocardial infarction.
- **Call EMS.**
- **Administer oxygen.**

F. Record Vital Signs

- Use the *Medical Emergency Report,* Figure 69-1 (page 1064).
- Measure blood pressure, check pulse rate, and count respirations, as described in Chapter 10 starting on page 137.

G. Observe Recovery

- For the patient who recovers without additional medical assistance, allow a rest period before dismissal.
- Record vital signs again.

IV. SUBSEQUENT DENTAL AND DENTAL HYGIENE APPOINTMENTS

Keep a copy of the *Medical Emergency Report* in the patient's permanent file for reference when planning future appointments.

MYOCARDIAL INFARCTION

- Myocardial infarction is the most extreme manifestation of ischemic heart disease.
- Other names: heart attack, coronary occlusion, or coronary thrombosis.
- The infarction results from a sudden reduction or arrest of coronary blood flow.
- The most common artery associated with a myocardial infarction is the anterior descending branch of the left

coronary artery. That is also the most common site of advanced atherosclerosis.

I. ETIOLOGY

- Immediate cause: can be a thrombosis that blocks an artery already narrowed by atherosclerosis.
- The blockage creates an area of infarction, which leads to necrosis of the area.
- Necrosis of the area can occur within a few hours.
- A few patients die immediately or within a few hours. Sudden death may be caused by ventricular fibrillation.

II. SYMPTOMS

A. Pain

- *Location.* Pain symptoms may start under the sternum, with feelings of indigestion, or in the middle to upper sternum. Pain may last for extended periods, even hours.
- When the pain is severe, it gives a pressing or crushing heavy sensation and is not relieved by rest or nitroglycerin.
- *Onset.* The pain may have a sudden onset, sometimes during sleep or following exercise. The pain may be radial, similar to angina pectoris, which extends to the left or right arm, neck, and mandible.

B. Other Symptoms

- Cold sweat, weakness and faintness, shortness of breath, nausea, and vomiting may occur.
- Blood pressure falls below baseline.
- Women do not always present with symptoms similar to men; they may be diaphoretic, nauseated, and agitated with a sense of presentiment.

III. MANAGEMENT DURING AN ATTACK

A. Terminate Treatment

- Sit the patient up for comfortable breathing.
- Give nitroglycerin, and reassure the patient.

B. Summon Medical Assistance

- When nitroglycerin does not reduce the angina-like pain within 3 minutes, prepare for basic life support (Table 69-4 page 1078).
- **CALL EMT. Administer oxygen.**
- Use *Medical Emergency Report,* Figure 69-1 (page 1064) and record vital signs.
- Apply basic life support measures (Chapter 69, page 1066), if indicated, while waiting for medical assistance.
- Transport to hospital.

IV. TREATMENT AFTER ACUTE SYMPTOMS

A. Medical Supervision

- Current medical care for heart attack calls for a shortened rest period with increased activity, in keeping with the strength and progress of the patient.
- Most patients experience extreme fatigue during their convalescence.

B. Lifestyle Changes

- Dietary changes and elimination of smoking and stressful activities, as well as control of diseases that exacerbate ischemic heart disease, are essential.
- Periodontal health has particular significance.
- Many patients need considerable education, reassurance, and motivation.

C. Subsequent Appointments

- Elective dental appointments are postponed until the patient's physician has given consent.

CONGESTIVE HEART FAILURE

- Heart failure is a syndrome in which an abnormality of cardiac function is responsible for the inability or failure of the heart to pump blood at a rate necessary to meet the needs of the body tissues.
- Because of the collection of fluids in various body organs and the inability of the heart to empty each chamber with sufficient contractile force, the term congestive heart failure is used.

I. ETIOLOGY

The many causes of heart failure fall into two categories: underlying and precipitating causes.

A. Underlying Causes

Examples of cardiovascular disease that result in heart failure are:

- Heart valve damage (rheumatic heart disease, congenital heart disease).
- Myocardial failure as a result of an abnormality of heart muscle or secondary to ischemia.

B. Precipitating Causes

Examples that place an additional load on a chronically burdened myocardium are:

1. *Acute Hypertensive Crisis.* Severe symptoms of headache, mental confusion, dizziness, shortness of breath, and chest pain may predispose to heart failure.

2. *Massive Pulmonary Embolism.* A thrombus may form in a lower extremity of an inactive person with low cardiac output and circulatory stasis. The thrombus may break loose and, carried by the blood, lodge in the pulmonary artery to cause a pulmonary embolism. Severe dyspnea, cyanosis, congestive failure, and shock result.

3. *Arrhythmia.* After resuscitation of a person with myocardial infarction, ventricular fibrillation, a type of arrhythmia, is the major risk leading to sudden death.

II. CLINICAL MANIFESTATIONS

■ The clinical manifestations coincide with the parts of the heart involved.

■ Signs and symptoms are different, depending, in general, on whether the left or the right side of the heart or both are affected. The general effects are extreme weakness, fatigue, fear, and anxiety.

A. Left Heart Failure

The left side of the heart receives oxygenated blood from the lungs and pumps the blood into the aorta to the rest of the body. A pathologic condition of the left ventricle or the mitral valve alters output, and causes respiratory difficulty because of the backup of serous fluid into the lungs. Clinical symptoms are more prominent at night. The patient rests better in a sitting or semi-sitting position with more than one pillow.

1. *Subjective Symptoms*
   ■ Weakness, fatigue
   ■ Dyspnea, particularly evident on exertion. Shortness of breath when lying supine, relieved when sitting up
   ■ Cough and expectoration
   ■ Nocturia
2. *Objective Symptoms*
   ■ Pallor; sweating, cold skin
   ■ Breathing obviously difficult
   ■ Diastolic blood pressure increased
   ■ Heart rate rapid
   ■ Anxiety, fear

B. Right Heart Failure

The right heart receives the venous blood from the vena cava and pumps it to the lungs for oxygenation. Right heart failure shows evidence of systemic venous congestion with peripheral edema. When left heart failure precedes right heart failure, the heart is already congested. Resistance to receiving the venous blood is an additional factor.

1. *Subjective Symptoms*
   ■ Weakness, fatigue
   ■ Swelling of the feet and/or ankles. The edema progresses to the thighs and abdomen (ascites) in advanced stages of heart failure.
   ■ Cold hands and feet

2. *Objective Symptoms*
   ■ Cyanosis of mucous membranes and nail beds
   ■ Prominent jugular veins
   ■ Congestion with edema in various organs: enlarged spleen and liver; gastrointestinal distress with nausea and vomiting; central nervous system involvement with headache and irritability
   ■ Anxiety, fear

III. TREATMENT DURING CHRONIC STAGES

A patient with an appointment in a dental office or clinic may be receiving a variety of medical treatments. These are revealed by questioning during preparation of histories. Nearly all patients with heart failure complications have the following in their medical treatment plan:

A. Drug Therapy

Physicians may prescribe many different medications for patients with cardiovascular disease.

B. Dietary Control

■ Limited sodium intake to alleviate fluid retention
■ Limited fluid intake
■ Weight reduction

C. Limitation of Activity

■ Activity is limited depending on the severity of the health problem and the advice of the physician.

IV. EMERGENCY CARE FOR HEART FAILURE AND ACUTE PULMONARY EDEMA

A medical emergency that demands urgent attention may occur anywhere. The patient with heart failure or acute pulmonary edema is usually conscious.

■ Position the patient upright for comfortable breathing (Table 69-4, page 1077).
■ **Call EMS. Administer oxygen.**
■ Use the *Medical Emergency Report,* Figure 69-1 (page 1064) and monitor vital signs (blood pressure, respiratory rate, and pulse).
■ Reassure the patient

BASIC NONINVASIVE TREATMENT

1. *Counseling.* With a brief history of angina pain, the patient is counseled to be reassured that lifestyle changes are necessary but that a productive life can be led.

2. *Lifestyle Changes.* Necessary changes in lifestyle (**Box 66-3**) are emphasized, notably diet, exercise, and no tobacco.

3. *Medications.* A variety of medications may be required depending on individual needs.

SURGICAL TREATMENT

I. CORONARY DILATION

A. Percutaneous Transluminal Coronary Angioplasty (PTCA)[14]

■ Widely used procedure to stretch the coronary blood vessel using fluoroscopic guidance allows various tools to be inserted.

■ An inflatable balloon widens the narrowed lumen.

■ An atherectomy may be used to remove atheromatous plaque from the vessel lining.

B. Coronary Stent

■ The stent is placed to maintain the open vessel lumen. Stents are made of metal and become covered with endothelium.

■ The coronary stent provides a semirigid scaffolding within the lumen, which helps prevent restenosis or renarrowing of the lumen.

II. CORONARY BYPASS

A. Coronary Artery Bypass Grafting (CABG)[15]

■ Coronary bypass is primarily for patients with significant obstruction.

■ The purpose is to "jump-pass" over arteries that have been narrowed with atherosclerosis.

■ The beneficial effects are relief from anginal pain, less workload for the heart, and an increase of oxygen and blood supply to the myocardium.

■ **Figure 66-5** shows the use of a vein graft and the internal mammary artery for bypasses.

III. CARDIAC PACEMAKER

■ The natural pacemaker, or center where the normal heartbeat is initiated, is the sinoatrial (S-A) node located in the right atrium.

■ From that node, impulses are sent along the muscle walls to stimulate and regulate the contractions of the ventricles, which pump the blood throughout the body.

■ When the natural pacemaker cells are not able to maintain a reliable rhythm, or when the impulses are interrupted because of heart block, cardiac arrest, various arrhythmias, or other disease conditions, treatment by a cardiologist may include the placement of an artificial pacemaker.

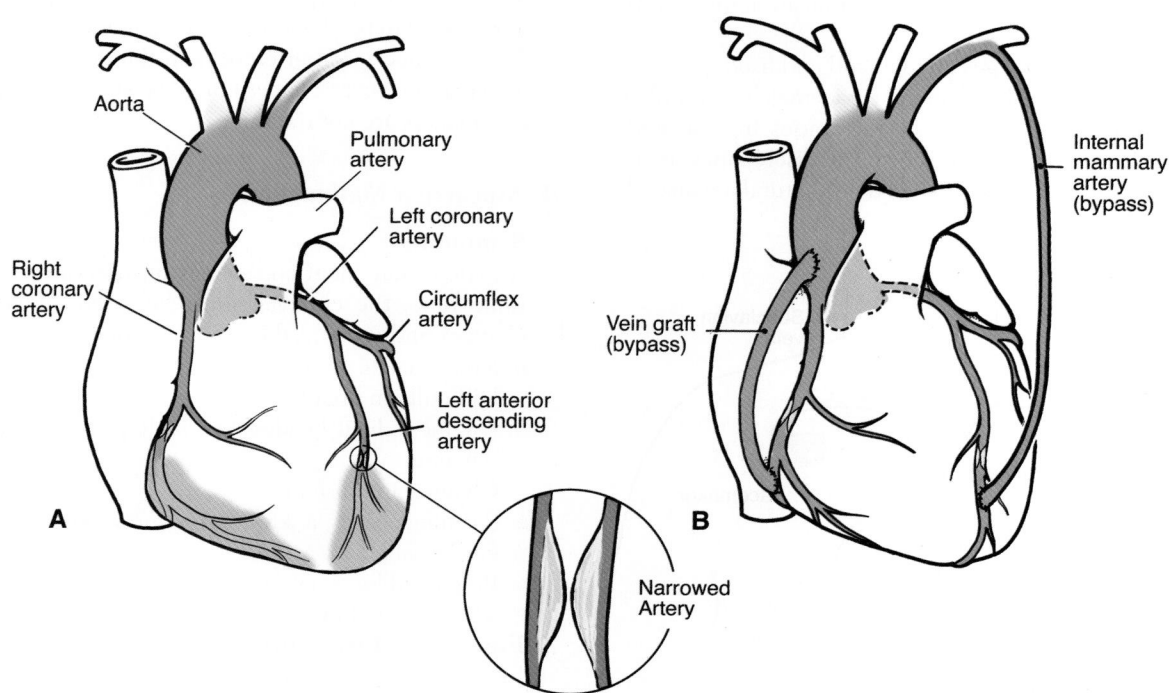

FIGURE 66-5 **Coronary Bypass Surgery. (A)** Heart showing infarcted (shaded) areas created by coronary arteries narrowed by atherosclerosis. **(B)** Vein graft from saphenous vein connected with aorta to bypass narrowed area of right coronary artery, and internal mammary artery used to bypass narrowed left anterior descending artery.

A. Description

1. **Definition**
   - A cardiac pacemaker is an electronic stimulator used to send a specified electrical current to the myocardium to control or maintain a minimum heart rate.
   - It may be single-chambered (to ventricle or atrium) or dual-chambered to sense and pace both heart chambers.

2. **Parts and Power**
   - A permanently implanted pacemaker has electrodes inserted transvenously to the endocardium. Less commonly, the leads may go to the pericardium of the external heart wall.
   - The electrodes are connected to the power source, a plastic- or metal-encased, hermetically sealed pulse generator containing a lithium anode battery.
   - The pulse generator is implanted under the skin in the thorax or upper abdomen. The area selected depends on the individual condition as determined by the cardiologist **(Figure 66-6)**.

B. Types

- Research has provided many advancements in pacemaker technology. Each patient is evaluated for the type of pacemaker that is best for the condition of that individual's heart.
- Current systems involve rate-responsive or physiologic pacing. Sensors may be alert to muscle or physical activity vibrations, body temperature, or respiration rate. The research will have a significant impact on the future of pacing.
- The two general types are demand and fixed rate.
  1. *Demand.* The demand pacemaker stimulates the heart only when the rate varies from a predetermined norm. By sensing a discrepancy in the electrical signals produced by natural means, the pacemaker sends a signal or stimulus, which regulates the heartbeat.
  2. *Fixed Rate.* A preset rate of electrical stimuli is provided independent of the natural heart activity when the natural beat is too slow. The fixed rate is used infrequently.

C. Interferences and Their Effects

- Electromagnetic interferences can stop or alter the function of a pacemaker.
- Models of pacemakers and their sensitivities to interference vary. Newer models are made with a special shielding to protect against interference.
- Historically, ultrasonic scaling units, electrodesensitizing equipment, pulp testers, electric toothbrushes, electrosurgery machines, and certain casting equipment were among the potential sources of interference with a pacemaker in a dental care setting. Dental devices that apply an electric current directly to the patient were considered those most likely to interfere.
- The dental environment has been shown to be a source of moderate electromagnetic interference. All dental equipment needs to be kept in good repair. Electric devices that contact or can contact the patient are checked for leakage because leakage can be a source of interference. Electrical appliances must be earth-grounded.
- The effect of distance has not been sufficiently researched; hence, patients in adjacent dental treatment rooms need to be checked before equipment is used.
- The evidence for interferences in the dental setting is not great; however, concern must be shown because all pacemakers are not the same.

D. Pacemaker Malfunction

1. **Symptoms**
   A patient may mention feelings of discomfort. At the same time, the clinician must be aware of possible changes and signs in the event of stopping or altering of a pacemaker.
   - Difficulty in breathing
   - Dizziness, light-headedness, feelings of faintness, or syncope
   - Changes in pulse rate
   - Swelling of legs, ankles, arms, and wrists
   - Chest pain
   - Prolonged hiccoughing
   - Muscle twitching

2. **Emergency Procedures**
   In the event a pacemaker should be turned off, immediate action is needed.
   - Turn off all suspected sources of interference.
   - Call for medical assistance; a defibrillator may be needed.

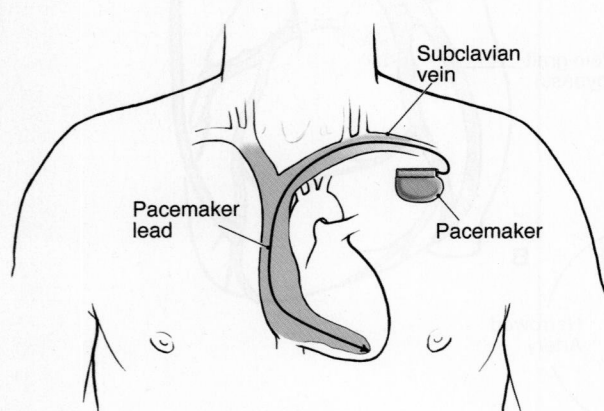

FIGURE 66-6 Cardiac Pacemaker. The pulse generator is implanted under the skin in the thorax or upper abdomen. The lead electrodes may go to the ventricle or to the atrium or both to provide the necessary stimulus for regulation of the heartbeat.

■ Position the patient for cardiopulmonary resuscitation. The procedure is described on page 1066.
■ Observe the patient. When the heart is forced to assume its rhythm again as a result of artificial circulation, the pacemaker is set into action to resume the generation and regulation of the pulse.

E. Appointment Guidelines for the Patient With a Pacemaker

General procedures for all patients with cardiovascular involvement apply to the patient wearing a pacemaker. In addition, certain adaptations are recommended.

1. **Informed Consent**
   ■ The signature of the patient or the patient's parent or guardian on a formal statement is a necessary protection against any legal liability in the event of complications or undesirable effects.
   ■ The patient is provided careful instruction about the anticipated procedures and materials to be used.
   ■ *Implied Consent* allows for provision of emergency lifesaving measures if a patient becomes unconscious/unresponsive and unable to indicate consent for such measures.
   ■ Dental and dental hygiene records need to be accurate and all-inclusive, with a detailed record for each appointment.

2. **Patient Histories**
   ■ The usual health history is supplemented with information about the type of pacemaker, how long it has been in use, where it is located, the underlying disease condition, and other information pertinent to the patient's safety during dental and dental hygiene appointments.
   ■ Consultation with the patient's cardiologist is indicated.

3. **Prophylactic Antibiotic Premedication**
   ■ The underlying cardiovascular disease is the basic determinant for the use of antibiotic prophylaxis.
   ■ Infective endocarditis has occurred in patients with pacemakers.
   ■ Although the patient with a pacemaker appears to be at low risk for endocarditis, the dentist and the cardiologist may choose to use antibiotics to cover dental and dental hygiene procedures.

4. **Patient Preparation**
   ■ *Chair Position*
      ■ Positioning the patient to support breathing and circulation is important.
      ■ If the patient experiences difficulty in breathing when in the supine position, the chair back is elevated to reduce stress.
      ■ The patient may experience some discomfort from wire tension or strain at the implant site if

the chair is positioned too far back. That depends on the location of the pulse generator.
      ■ Care must be taken that no pressure is placed over the site of a pacemaker in the patient's chest.
   ■ *Lead Apron*
      ■ Protection of the pulse generator and the lead wires may be indicated.
      ■ A lead apron can serve to interrupt interferences that may be created by electric devices, including handpieces. A lead apron can be heavy and uncomfortable, however, and therefore may require some consideration.

5. **Instrumentation**
   ■ The use of manual procedures is advisable.
   ■ Ultrasonic instruments can be an annoyance for the patient.

ANTICOAGULANT THERAPY

■ Anticoagulants are used in the treatment of many cardiovascular diseases to prevent embolus and thrombus formation.
■ A prescribed drug may be continued indefinitely by the patient as a preventive measure.
■ Drugs most commonly used to prevent or delay blood coagulation are heparin (hospital-administered intravenous) and coumarin derivatives.
■ Although precautions are needed to prevent hemorrhage, discontinuing the drug may be more hazardous for the patient than performing dental and dental hygiene therapy with precautions. When extensive surgical procedures are required, the patient may need to be hospitalized.

I. CLINICAL PROCEDURES

A. Consultation

■ Information about the patient's prothrombin time is obtained from the physician during an initial consultation.
■ The prothrombin time is a test of the coagulation phase of blood clotting used to monitor therapy with anticoagulants. A therapeutic range of 1½ to 2½ times the normal level is preferred.

B. Treatment Planning[16]

1. Pretest for Prothrombin Time
   ■ Determine the prothrombin time within 24 hours before an appointment. The patient can have the test made on the day of a dental appointment by preplanning with the physician and the laboratory. Most patients have a routine appointment for monitoring of the blood, and dental appointment dates can be planned to coincide.

■ Safe level for dental and dental hygiene procedures is considered to be 1 1/2 times the normal, provided precautions are taken during instrumentation and postoperative care.

2. Quadrant Scaling and Root Planing
   ■ Treat the healthier quadrant first. The least bleeding will occur.
   ■ Teach and emphasize daily dental biofilm control procedures in a series of appointments to prepare the gingival tissue for instrumentation. Healthy, healed tissue does not bleed as readily or as profusely.
   ■ Complete treatment, including removal of all calculus and subgingival biofilm and other irritants, is necessary to contribute to the goal of healthy tissue that does not bleed.

C. Local Hemostatic Measures

■ Instrumentation can be performed for most patients without complication, provided precautions are taken to minimize tissue trauma and control bleeding and not to dismiss the patient until bleeding has stopped.
■ *Pressure.* Pressure with sponges or cotton pellets packed interdentally can aid in control.
■ *Suture.* Sutures may be used to close and adapt the tissue interdentally following deep scaling and root planing.
■ *Periodontal Dressing.* Placement of a dressing is sometimes advisable to provide pressure and protection from trauma that may initiate bleeding. Dressing placement is described in Chapter 42 on page 670.

II. POSTPROCEDURAL INSTRUCTIONS

■ The practice by oral surgeons of closely observing patients for 6 to 8 hours following a surgical procedure has application following certain dental and dental hygiene procedures for selected patients. At the least, a check that post-care instructions are being followed is advisable.
■ The patient is advised to avoid vigorous toothbrushing and rinsing on a treated area for several hours or until the next day.
■ The use of extraoral icepacks may be helpful.
■ General post-care instructions may be found on page 670 for the care of an area with a dressing, see Table 42-2 (pages 671 and 672).
■ The use of a soft diet, cool rather than hot foods, and general moderation of activity may be advisable.
■ Long-term instruction must emphasize the maintenance of gingival health to prevent future bleeding problems.

CARDIAC SURGERY[17]

■ Cardiac surgery has become widely used. Patients in dental offices and clinics who have had or will have surgery are identified and need special procedures.
■ Because the patient with a cardiac prosthesis is at risk for infective endocarditis, all possible dental treatment must be completed before the date of cardiac surgery and preventive measures emphasized.

I. PRESURGICAL

■ Before elective cardiac surgery, the patient is brought to a state of optimum oral health, with all sources of infection removed.
■ All restorations and other dental procedures are completed.
■ Patients requiring cardiac surgery need information and motivation relative to the importance of oral health

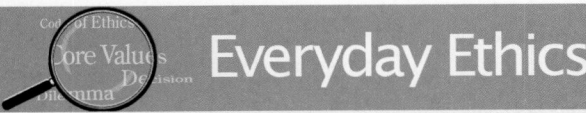

Everyday Ethics

Leo is a 68-year-old, obese, black male with a history of hypertension and hypercholesterolemia. He reminds Kerstin, the dental hygienist, that he has an extreme dislike of dental appointments as he grasps very tightly to the armrests of the dental chair.

   During the medical history review, Leo admitted that he usually remembers to take his blood pressure medications but since he doesn't feel well after the cholesterol-lowering medication, he does not take it regularly. Kerstin takes his right arm blood pressure of 165/90 mm Hg. Leo then starts rubbing his left arm, and Kerstin asks him how he is feeling. Leo says he is having heartburn from a spicy dinner last night and his arm is sore, probably from doing some yard work a couple of days ago.

Questions for Consideration

1. What medical, legal, and ethical questions come to mind to be taken into account when a dental hygienist has a patient like Leo with a complicated medical history that involves medications, patient symptoms, and is a nervous patient about any dental appointments?
2. Which of the dental hygiene core values has application in this scenario? How does each of the core values selected affect the appointment plan?
3. Using the questions in Table V-1 in Section V Introduction, page 362, prepare at least three possible procedure outlines that Kerstin could consider as she decides steps in Leo's treatment that day.

in eliminating a potential source of infective endocarditis.

■ Vigilance in a preventive program that includes biofilm control and self-applied fluorides is essential.

II. POSTSURGICAL

A. Maintenance Appointments

Frequent appointments are necessary for supervision and maintenance.

B. Prophylactic Antibiotic

■ Antibiotic coverage for all dental and dental hygiene procedures for patients with valvular prostheses is essential.[2] Because of the high susceptibility to infections, a special regimen for high-risk patients may be indicated.

■ Patients with implanted vascular *autographs* generally do not need antibiotic premedication before dental and dental hygiene appointments. An example of an implanted vascular autograph is the use of a patient's own blood vessel to provide a coronary bypass **(Figure 66-5)**. The saphenous vein and the internal mammary artery are most commonly used.

C. Immunosuppressive Therapy

■ Principal drugs used for patients with transplants are cyclosporin, azathioprine, and prednisolone to prevent rejection of the transplant.

■ Among the side effects, particularly of cyclosporin, is gingival enlargement.[18] Many patients may receive medication with the nifedipine group, also effective in causing gingival enlargement. Special periodontal care will be needed.

BOX 66-4	Example Progress Note

Patient for 3 months maintenance after initial 4 quads for deep scaling and root planing

Basic extra and intraoral exam: vital signs: blood pressure still stays high, patient says he was on a new drug which he hopes will be easier. Probing in molar areas where pockets had been deeper; a few areas of bleeding on probing; scaled specific areas of the roots again. Mesial #2 to be watched the next time. Patient had slipped back on the biofilm removal so that the program was reviewed; demonstrated use of interdental brush in selected areas. He has had difficulty purchasing his favorite type of floss but hasn't shopped around. Next visit in 3 months again.

Signed: _____, RDH Date: _____

DOCUMENTATION

Documentation for a routine dental hygiene maintenance appointment for a patient with a cardiovascular illness would need to include a minimum of the following items:

■ Note and record the responses to health history review questions about visitations to the cardiologist, and in addition to the patient's report on the state of his health, answers from the MD concerning changes that could influence procedures.

■ Note, record, and compare all findings with previous findings: blood pressure determination, findings in the extraoral and intraoral examination, and the gingival and periodontal clinical examination with complete probing.

■ A sample progress note may be reviewed in **Box 66-4**.

Factors To Teach The Patient

■ Encourage patients who have been diagnosed as hypertensive to continue their prescribed therapy.

Stress Reduction Procedures[19]
■ Select an appointment time that is optimum with respect to that time of the day when the patient is feeling best and may be less fatigued. Most anxious patients prefer a morning appointment.
■ Get adequate sleep and rest, and engage in non-fatiguing activities during the 24 hours before the appointment.
■ Use premedication as prescribed for sleeping the night before. A sedative may be prescribed to be taken 60 minutes before an appointment or at the dental office, if possible. When taken at home 1 hour before, the patient should not drive a car.
■ Allow time to get to the dental office or clinic; bring own reading material, knitting or sewing, or other relaxing activity in the event that waiting is unavoidable.
■ Eat breakfast, lunch, or other usual between-meal food and take usual medications on schedule.
■ When other family members, especially children, have dental or dental hygiene appointments, do not add to their stress by relaying personal negative feelings.

References

1. Schoen FJ. The heart. In: Kumar V, Abbas AK, Fausto N, (eds). Robbins and Cotran's *Pathologic basis of disease.* 7th ed. Philadelphia: WB Saunders; 2005. 564–70 pp.
2. Wilson W, Taubert KA, Gewitz M, Lockhart PB, Baddour LM, Levison M, Bolger A, Cabell CH, Takahashi M, Baltimore RS, Newburger JW, Strom BL, Tani LY, Gerber M, Bonow RO, Pallasch T, Shulman ST, Rowley AH, Burns JC, Ferrieri P, Gardner T, Goff D, Durack DT. Prevention of infective endocarditis: guidelines from the American Heart Association Rheumatic Fever, Endocarditis, and Kawasaki Disease Committee, Council on Cardiovascular Disease

in the Young, and the Council on Clinical Cardiology, Council on Cardiovascular Surgery and Anesthesia, and the Quality of Care and Outcomes Research Interdisciplinary Working Group. *Circulation.* 2007 Oct 9;116(15)1736–54.

3. Schoen. op.cit, pp. 592–4.
4. Little JW, Falace DA, Miller CS, Rhodus NL. *Dental management of the medically compromised patient.* 6th ed. St. Louis: Mosby; 2002. 45–6, 57 p.
5. Little. op.cit, pp. 21–7.
6. Schoen. op.cit, pp. 595–8.
7. Schoen. op.cit, pp. 525–30.
8. National High Blood Pressure Education Program. *The seventh report of the Joint National Committee on Prevention, Detection, Evaluation, and Treatment of High Blood Pressure.* Bethesda (MD): National Heart, Lung, and Blood Institute (US); 2003 Dec. NIH Publication No. 03-5233.
9. Schoen. op.cit, pp. 587–8.
10. Little. op.cit, pp. 79–92.
11. Haraszthy VI, Zambon JJ, Trevisan M, Zeid M, Genco RJ. Identification of periodontal pathogens in atheromatous plaques. *J Periodontol.* 2000 Oct;71(10):1554–60.
12. Renvert S, Pettersson T, Ohlsson O, Persson GR. Bacterial profile and burden of periodontal infection in subjects with a diagnosis of acute coronary syndrome. *J Periodontol.* 2006 Jul;77(7):1110–9.
13. Zaremba M, Górska R, Suwalski P, Kowalski J. Evaluation of the incidence of periodontitis-associated bacteria in the atherosclerotic plaque of coronary blood vessels. *J Periodontol.* 2007 Feb;78(2):322–7.
14. Goldman L, Ausiello D, editors. *Cecil textbook of medicine.* 22nd ed. Philadelphia: Saunders; 2004. 424–27 pp.
15. Goldman. op.cit, pp. 428–9.
16. Little. op.cit, pp. DM 38–41.
17. Little. op.cit, pp. DM 70–1, 504–6.
18. Thomason JM, Seymour RA, Ellis JS, Kelly PJ, Parry G, Dark J, Idle JR. Iatrogenic gingival overgrowth in cardiac transplantation. *J Periodontol.* 1995 Aug;66(8):742–6.
19. Malamed SF. *Handbook of medical emergencies in the dental office.* 5th ed. St. Louis: Mosby; 2000. Chapter 2, Prevention; p. 44–8.

CHAPTER 67

The Patient With a Blood Disorder

BARBARA DAWIDJAN , RDH, MED

Chapter Outline

Oral soft tissue changes, lowered resistance to infection, and bleeding tendencies are major factors to be considered for a patient with a blood disorder. Oral manifestations of blood disorders are generally exaggerated in the presence of dental biofilm and local predisposing factors.

Box 67-1 lists and defines terminology used to describe hematologic conditions. Prefixes, suffixes, and other word derivatives to clarify the terminology are listed in Appnedix VI on page 1118.

ORAL FINDINGS SUGGESTIVE OF BLOOD DISORDERS

- Early signs of systemic conditions frequently appear in the oral soft tissues.
- The patient's medical history may not show the existence of a blood disorder, but clinical examination may reveal tissue characteristics suggestive of disease.
- An important referral for medical examination may lead to diagnosis and treatment of a serious disease.

BOX 67-1	Key Words

Blood Disorders

Anaplasia: loss of structural differentiation with reversion to a more primitive type of cell.

Aplasia: defective development or congenital absence of an organ or tissue.

Chelation therapy: process to remove excess iron acquired from chronic blood transfusions.

Coagulation factor: factor essential to normal blood clotting contained within the blood plasma; designated by Roman numerals I to V and VII to XIII; their absence, diminution, or excess may lead to abnormality of clotting.

Differential cell count: record of number of white blood cells, including the determination of the percentage of each type of cell present; the "differential" is used in the diagnosis of various blood disorders, infections, and other abnormal conditions of the body.

Diffusion hypoxia: lack of adequate amounts of oxygen that can result from the rapid diffusion of nitrous oxide molecules from the bloodstream into the lungs. Occurs if 100% oxygen is not administered at the conclusion of a nitrous oxide sedation procedure.

Ecchymosis: hemorrhagic spot larger than a petechia in the skin or mucous membrane; non-elevated, blue or purplish.

Epistaxis: hemorrhage from the nose.

Erythropoiesis: formation of red blood cells.

Glossitis: inflammation of the tongue.

Glossodynia: pain in the tongue.

Hemarthrosis: blood in a joint cavity.

Hematocrit: volume percentage of erythrocytes (red blood cells) in whole blood.

Hematopoiesis: the formation and development of blood cells, usually in bone marrow.

Hemoglobin: protein in the erythrocyte that transports molecular oxygen to body cells.

Hemolysis: rupture of erythrocytes with the release of hemoglobin into the plasma.

Hemolytic: destruction to blood cells, resulting in liberation of hemoglobin.

Hypoxia: diminished availability of oxygen to body tissues.

Leukocytosis: increase in the total number of leukocytes.

Leukopenia: reduction in total number of leukocytes in the blood; count under 500 per ml.

Lysis: destruction or decomposition, as of a cell, bacterium, or other substance.

Macrocyte: abnormally large red blood cell; contrast with microcyte, abnormally small erythrocyte.

Myelocyte: young cell of the granulocyte series; occurs normally in bone marrow; found in circulating blood in certain diseases.

Neutropenia: diminished number of neutrophils (polymorphonuclear leukocytes or PMNs).

Oxyhemoglobin: oxygenated arterial blood; bright red and about 97% saturated with oxygen; venous blood is a darker color and contains only 20 to 70% oxygen.

Petechia: minute, pinpoint, round, non-raised, purplish-red spot in the skin or mucous membrane, caused by hemorrhage.

Phagocytosis: engulfing of microorganisms and foreign particles by phagocytes, such as macrophages.

Plasma cell: cell in connective tissue converted from B lymphocyte: involved in chronic inflammation and immune response.

Purpura: hemorrhage into the tissues, under the skin, and through the mucous membranes; produces petechiae and ecchymoses.

Thrombocytic purpura: when circulating platelets are decreased.

Vasculopathy: any disease affecting blood vessels.

- In addition, the findings of a laboratory blood examination may provide essential information for safe and effective dental hygiene care.
- Oral soft tissue changes that may occur in patients with blood diseases are not necessarily exclusive to systemic blood disorders.
- The important thing is to recognize change in a previously healthy patient, or an apparently exaggerated response in a patient being examined at an initial appointment.

Findings that may suggest a blood disorder include the following:

- Gingival bleeding, spontaneously or upon gentle probing.
- History of difficulty in controlling bleeding by usual procedures.
- History of bruising easily, with large ecchymoses.
- Numerous petechiae.

- Marked pallor of the mucous membranes.
- Atrophy of the papillae of the tongue.
- Persistent sore or painful tongue (glossodynia).
- Acute or chronic infections, such as candidiasis, that do not respond to usual treatment.
- Severe ulcerations associated with a lack of response to treatment.
- Exaggerated gingival response to local irritants, sometimes with characteristics of necrotizing ulcerative gingivitis (ulceration, necrosis, bleeding, pseudomembrane).

NORMAL BLOOD[1]

I. COMPOSITION

- Blood is composed of 55% plasma fluid and 45% formed elements.

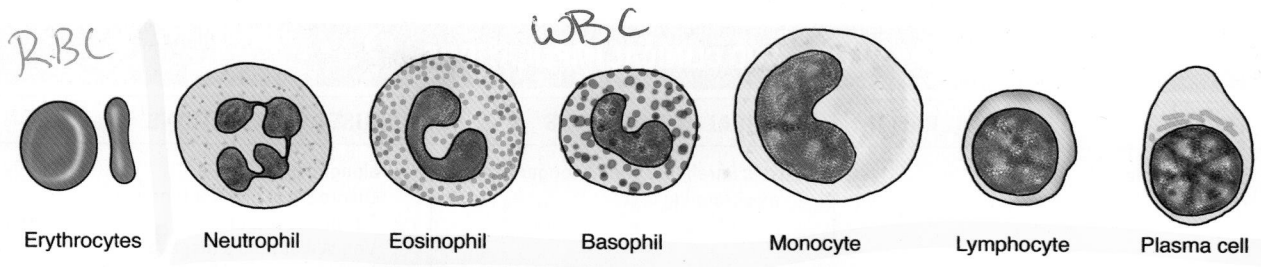

RBC   WBC

| Erythrocytes | Neutrophil | Eosinophil | Basophil | Monocyte | Lymphocyte | Plasma cell |

FIGURE 67-1 **Red and White Blood Cells.** Diagram shows normal cell forms drawn to scale for comparison of cell size. Note the shape of nuclei in each of the white blood cells. The erythrocyte or red blood cell does not have a nucleus; its biconcave disc shape is shown in the lateral view second from the left.

- The 45% formed elements consist of:
  - 44% erythrocytes (red blood cells or corpuscles)
  - 1% leukocytes (white blood cells)
- **Figure 67-1** shows the cell forms and nuclei.
- Hematocrit, a test commonly used in health examinations, shows:
  - A. Percentage packed volume of blood cells
  - B. Normal values are shown in **Table 67-1**.
- Reference values for blood cells are shown in **Table 67-2**, with examples of conditions in which increases and decreases in the normal values occur.

II. ORIGIN OF BLOOD CELLS

- Adult blood cells originate in bone marrow
- Hemocytoblast: the stem cell of origin.
- Erythrocytes and granulocytes leave the bone marrow as mature cells and enter the circulating blood.
- Agranulocytes (lymphocytes and monocytes) leave the bone marrow as immature cells and go to lymphoid tissues for maturing.
- Immature cell forms predominate in certain blood diseases and cancers.

III. PLASMA

- The constituents of the fluid portion of the blood are similar to the fluid constituents of the connective tissue.
- If plasma is allowed to clot, the remaining fluid is called serum.
- The plasma is composed of 90% water and 10% of the following:

A. Plasma Proteins

- Albumin (functions to maintain tissue fluid balance within the vascular system).
- Gamma globulins (are circulating antibodies essential in the immune system).
- Beta globulins (aid in transport of hormones, metallic ions, and lipids).
- Fibrinogen and prothrombin (essential for blood clotting).

B. Inorganic Salts

Sodium, potassium, calcium, bicarbonate, and chloride.

C. Gases

Dissolved oxygen, carbon dioxide, and nitrogen.

D. Substances Being Transported

Hormones, nutrients, waste products, and enzymes.

IV. RED BLOOD CELLS (ERYTHROCYTES)

A. Description

- Although commonly called red blood cells, they are more properly termed corpuscles because they have no nuclei **(Figure 67-1)**.
- Biconcave discs that contain hemoglobin
- Sensitive and flexible; change shape readily as they pass through small capillaries

B. Functions

- Transport hemoglobin.
- Carry oxygen to the body cells in the form of oxyhemoglobin
- Carbon dioxide is transported from the cells.

C. Hemoglobin

- Measured in grams (g) per 100 milliliters (ml).
- Normal values range from 12 to 17.2 g per ml depending on male or female **(Table 67-1)**.
- Values reflect:
  - Anemic state when hemoglobin is lower.
  - Pathologic conditions when hemoglobin increases over normal.

V. WHITE BLOOD CELLS (LEUKOCYTES)

A. Types of Leukocytes

- White blood cells are divided into two general groups, the granulocytes and the agranulocytes.

TABLE 67-1	LABORATORY VALUES AND CLINICAL IMPLICATIONS

TEST	NORMAL RANGE*	CLINICAL IMPLICATIONS	CAUSES OF DEVIATIONS
Bleeding time (BT)	1–6 min	Test is unreliable and no longer used as screening test	Prolonged in: 　Disorders of platelet function 　Thrombocytopenia 　Von Willebrand's disease 　Leukemias 　Aspirin and other drug use
Prothrombin time(PT)	11–15 s	Routine care can be performed when PT is <20 s	Prolonged in: 　Polycythemia vera Prothrombin deficiency 　Anticoagulant therapy 　Vitamin K deficiency 　Liver diseases 　Aspirin use
International normalized ratio (INR)	<2.5	Routine care can be performed when INR 2–3, MD consult when INR > 3.5	Prolonged in: 　Polycythemia vera 　Prothrombin deficiency 　Anticoagulant therapy 　Vitamin K deficiency 　Liver diseases 　Aspirin use
Activated partial thromboplastin time (aPTT)	25–35 s	Routine care when aPTT is <1.5 × normal, MD consult when >57 s	Prolonged in: 　Hemophilia A and B 　von Willebrand's disease 　Anticoagulant therapy
Platelet count	140,000–400,000/mm^3	Routine care 50,000/mm^3	Thrombocytopenia: 　<20,000 mm^3 　<10,000/mm^3 — Potentially life threatening
Hemoglobin (g/dl)	Males: 13.6–17.2 g/ 100 ml Females: 12–15 g/ 100 ml	Delivers O$_2$ through circulation to body tissues and returns CO$_2$ from tissues to lungs	Increased in: 　Polycthemia 　Dehydration Decreased in: 　Anemias 　Hemorrhage 　Leukemias
Hematocrit (volume of packed red cells) (percentage)	Males: 39–49% Females: 33–43%	Indicates relative proportions of plasma and RBCs	Increased in: 　Polycythemia 　Dehydration Decreased in: 　Anemias 　Hemorrhage leukemias

*Ranges vary among health facilities and laboratories. The reference ranges of the facility providing the results are used in interpreting the test result.

- Granulocytes have granules in their cytoplasm, whereas the agranulocytes do not.
- They are further subdivided as shown here:
  - *Granulocytes*: neutrophils, eosinophils, and basophils.
  - *Agranulocytes*: lymphocytes, monocytes.

B. Functions: Amoeboid or Motile

- Phagocytic, immunologic, and other functions related to the inflammatory process in the connective tissue.
- They pass through the walls at the terminal ends of capillaries and into the connective tissue.

- A large number of cells migrate into the area of injury.
- Neutrophils arrive first and are active in the phagocytosis of foreign material and microorganisms.
- The blood functions as a transport medium for the white cells as they pass to areas in the connective tissue where they are needed.
- Numbers and proportions in the blood maintain a constant level in health, as shown in **Table 67-2**.
- Differential cell count of the white blood cells is used in the detection and monitoring of diseased states. Increases and decreases of each cell type can be associated with certain conditions.

TABLE 67-2	BLOOD CELLS REFERENCE VALUES		
CELL TYPE	**NORMAL VALUE**	**CAUSES OF INCREASE**	**CAUSES OF DECREASE**
Red Blood Cells (Erythrocytes)	Males: 4.3–5.9 million per mm^3 Females: 3.5–5.0 million per mm^3	Polycythemia Dehydration	Anemias Leukemias Hemorrhage
Platelets (Thrombocytes) (cell fragments essential for the process of blood clotting)	150,000–400,000 per mm^3 Wintrobe method: 140,000–440,000 per mm^3	Polycythemia vera Chronic myelocytic leukemia Sickle cell anemia Rheumatic fever Hemolytic anemias Bone fractures	Acute severe infections Cirrhosis of the liver Thrombocytopenic purpura Acute leukemias Aplastic anemias Pernicious anemia
White Blood Cells (Leukocytes)	5,000–10,000 per mm^3	Inflammation Overexertion Polycythemia vera Leukemia	Aplastic anemia Granulocytopenia Drug poisoning Thrombocytopenia Radiation Severe infections HIV/AIDS
Differential White Cell Count Granulocytes 1. Neutrophils	60%–70%	Acute infections Myelogenous leukemia Poisoning Erythroblastosis	Aplastic anemia Granulocytopenia
2. Eosinophils	1%–3%	Allergic diseases Dermatitis Hodgkin's disease Scarlet fever	Aplastic anemia Typhoid fever
3. Basophils	1%	Certain chronic infections	Aplastic anemia
Agranulocytes 1. Lymphocytes	20%–35%	Lymphocytic leukemia Chronic infections Viral diseases	Aplastic anemia Myelogenous leukemia Radiation
2. Monocytes	2%–6%	Monocytic leukemias Tuberculosis Infective endocarditis Hodgkin's disease	Aplastic anemia

C. Agranulocytes

- Lymphocytes
  - Small round cells with a round nucleus that nearly fills the cell with a narrow rim of cytoplasm (Figure 67-1)
  - Can move back and forth between the vessels and the extravascular tissues
  - Capable of reverting to blast-like cells of origin and then multiplying as the immunologic need arises
- Monocytes
  - Large cells with a bean-shaped or indented nucleus
  - Actively phagocytic
  - In connective tissue, monocytes differentiate into macrophages, which are important in immunologic processes.

D. Granulocytes

- Neutrophils
  - Also called polymorphonuclear leukocytes "PMNs" or "polys."
  - Most numerous of all the white blood cells.
  - Nucleus has three to five lobes connected by thin chromatin threads.
  - Cells are round in circulation.
  - They are amoeboid in the tissues and function in phagocytosis. Neutrophils are part of the first line of defense of the body.
- Eosinophils
  - Two-lobed nucleus and larger, coarser granules than those of a neutrophil.
  - Microscopically, the cells stain a distinct bright pink; are readily recognized.
  - Few in number; increase markedly during allergic conditions.
- Basophils
  - Nucleus has a "U" or "S" form.
  - Function is to increase vascular permeability during inflammation so that phagocytic cells can pass into the area.

VI. PLATELETS

- Small round or oval formed element without a nucleus
- They are approximately one-fourth the size of a red blood cell.
- Active in the blood clotting mechanism

- Essential in the maintenance of the integrity of blood capillaries by closing them at the time of injury
- Participate in clot dissolution after healing

ANEMIAS

- Anemia, sometimes referred to as "tired blood," is a reduction of the hemoglobin concentration, the hematocrit, or the number of red blood cells to a level below that which is normal for the individual.[2]
- As a result of anemia, oxygen-carrying capacity to the cells is diminished.
- Oxygen is essential in all body tissues for normal maintenance.

I. CLASSIFICATION BY CAUSE

A. Caused by Blood Loss

- Acute: Blood loss from trauma or disease
- Chronic: An internal lesion with constant slow bleeding, usually of gastrointestinal or gynecologic origin, can lead to a chronic loss of blood. An *iron deficiency anemia* can result.

B. Caused by Increased Hemolysis

Hemolysis means the destruction of red blood cells; is also called "hemolytic anemia" because of cell destruction. Causes of hemolytic anemia are listed in **Box 67-2.**

BOX 67-2	Causes of Hemolytic Anemias

Inherited Hemolytic Anemia
- Abnormal hemoglobin
  - ☐ Sickle cell anemia
  - ☐ Thalassemia
- Red blood cell membrane abnormality
- Enzyme deficiencies

Acquired Hemolytic Anemia
- Antibody–related
- Not antibody-related
  - ☐ Liver disease
  - ☐ Uremia
  - ☐ Trauma
  - ☐ Mechanical heart valve
  - ☐ Infection
  - ☐ Toxins
  - ☐ Red blood cell membrane defects

Adapted with permission from Thomas M. Chapter 33: Assessment and management of patients with hematologic disorders. In: Smeltzer S, Bare B, editors. *Medical–surgical nursing.* 10th ed. Philadelphia: Lippincott Williams and Wilkins; 2004. 895 p.

- Hereditary Hemolytic Disorders
  - *Sickle cell disease,* which belongs to the group of hereditary disorders called the hemoglobinopathies
- Acquired Hemolytic Disorders
  - Examples: drugs, infections, and certain physical and chemical agents that may cause red cell destruction
  - In the category of antibody-mediated anemia, *erythroblastosis fetalis* (antibody-mediated anemia) occurs when a mother is Rh-positive; also called hemolytic disease of the newborn.

C. Caused by Diminished Production of Red Blood Cells

A nutritional deficiency or bone marrow failure may be the reason for diminished production.

- Nutritional Deficiency
  - Inadequate dietary choices or inadequate intake.
  - Defective absorption from the gastrointestinal tract.
  - Examples: *pernicious anemia,* which results from a B_{12} vitamin absorption deficiency and celiac sprue, which results from a sensitivity to dietary gluten.
  - Increased demand for nutrients
  - *Iron deficiency anemia,* which may occur during pregnancy or during a growth spurt
- Bone Marrow Failure
  - *Aplastic anemia* (which can be inherited) can occur without apparent cause or can occur when the bone marrow is injured by medications, radiation, chemotherapy, or infection.
  - In aplastic anemia, a combination of anemia, neutropenia, and thrombocytopenia occurs, which leads to a quantitative decrease in all cells formed in the bone marrow.
  - Consult with physician to determine if antibiotic premedication would be indicated.

D. Anemia of Chronic Diseases[3]

- Second most prevalent anemia after iron-deficiency anemia
- Occurs in patients with acute or chronic immune activation
- Patients have a low reticulocyte count, which indicates underproduction of red cells

E. Caused by Genetic Blood Disorders

- *Thalassemia.* Thalassemias are a diverse group of genetic blood disorders characterized by absent or decreased production of normal hemoglobin.[4]
- Thalassemia is an inherited condition that typically affects people of Mediterranean, African, Middle Eastern, and Southeast Asian descent.

- The condition can range in severity from mild to life threatening.
- The most severe form is called Thalassemia major (Cooley's anemia).
- Patient's blood counts to be evaluated and monitored for delayed wound healing.
- Treatment
  - Regular red blood cell transfusions and chelation therapy.
  - Folic acid supplements.
  - Bone marrow transplant is a potential cure if performed during childhood.[5]
  - Hematopoietic stem-cell transplantation is the only available curative approach for Thalassemia.[6]

II. CLINICAL CHARACTERISTICS OF ANEMIA

When a patient's medical history shows the presence of anemia, certain general characteristics may be anticipated for which clinical adaptations may be needed. The general signs and symptoms are:

- Pale thin skin
- Weakness, malaise, easy fatigability
- Dyspnea on slight exertion, faintness
- Headache, vertigo, tinnitus
- Dimness of vision, spots before the eyes
- Brittle nails with loss of convexity

IRON DEFICIENCY ANEMIA

Iron deficiency anemia is a hypochromic microcytic anemia, which means that:

- The hemoglobin is deficient (hypochromic)
- The red blood corpuscles are smaller than normal and deficient in hemoglobin (microcytic)
- Occurs more in younger than older people and more in females than in males
- Plummer-Vinson syndrome can develop as a result of chronic deficiency which includes dysphasia and atrophy of the upper alimentary tract.[7]
- Diagnosis by laboratory test which shows low hemoglobin and a reduced hematocrit value.

I. CAUSES

- Malnutrition or malabsorption
- Chronic infection
- Increased body demand for iron over and above the daily intake. For example, during pregnancy.
- Chronic alchoholism. Blood loss from gastrointestinal tract.[8]
- Chronic blood loss. When iron deficiency anemia occurs in men or in postmenopausal women, it usually indicates internal bleeding, and tests are needed to find the source.

- Causes of internal bleeding
  - Gastrointestinal diseases, such as ulcer and cancer
  - Drugs, notably aspirin
  - Hemorrhoids
- Excessive menstrual flow
- Frequent blood donations

II. SIGNS AND SYMPTOMS

A. General

- General weakness, headache, pallor
- Fatigue on slight exertion

B. Oral

- Pallor of the mucosa and gingiva
- Tongue changes: atrophic glossitis with loss of filiform papillae. In moderate and severe anemia, when the hemoglobin is at 10 g/dl or below, the tongue is smooth and shiny. The patient may have burning, painful sensations (glossodynia).
- Secondary irritations to the thinned, atrophic mucosa may result from smoking, mechanical trauma, or hot, spicy foods.
- Angular cheilitis. Description given on page 818.
- Increased risk of candidiasis

III. THERAPY

- Cause to be investigated.
- Treated with oral ferrous iron tablets with vitamin C for 6 to 12 months. To be taken on empty stomach for best absorption rates. Check Recommended Dietary Allowances (RDA) for correct amounts.
- Folic acid supplements
- Nutritional Counseling. Recommend foods high in iron. Sources given on page 504.
- Liquid preparations, which are sometimes used for children, may stain the teeth. Administering the medicine by way of a straw is advised.

MEGALOBLASTIC ANEMIAS[9]

- Characterized by abnormally large (megalo-) red blood cells, many of which are oval shaped
- A megaloblastic anemia can result from a deficiency of either vitamin B_{12} or folate, or both
- Principal types of megaloblastic anemia:
  - Pernicious anemia
  - Folate deficiency anemia
- Vitamin B_{12} and folate are essential in red blood production in the bone marrow
- Pernicious anemia is caused by a deficiency of vitamin B_{12}
- Folate deficiency anemia is from a deficiency of folate, or folic acid.

■ These two vitamins are essential in red blood cell production in the bone marrow.

I. PERNICIOUS ANEMIA

A. Etiologic Factors

■ Deficiency of vitamin B_{12} can be caused by:
- ■ Decreased intake (inadequate diet or impaired absorption)
- ■ Increased requirement (pregnancy, hyperparathyroidism, disseminated cancer)
- ■ Impaired absorption of B_{12}
■ Due to deficiency of intrinsic factor. Failure of production of *intrinsic factor (IF);* a substance created by the stomach parietal cells that is necessary for the absorption of Vitamin B_{12}.
■ Lack of production of *intrinsic factor* is either chronic atrophic gastritis or surgical removal of partial or all of the stomach.

B. Age Characteristics

■ Pernicious anemia is primarily a disease of people over 40 years of age.
■ Childhood form of the disease: no gastric abnormality exists. Although more research is needed, the cause may either be a hereditary inability to produce intrinsic factor or the ineffective nature of intrinsic factor produced.

C. Clinical Findings

■ General
- ■ Fatigue, weakness, tingling, or numbness of fingers and toes
- ■ Palpitations, weight loss, and syncope
■ Central Nervous System Involvement
- ■ Dizziness, confusion, hypotension
- ■ Severe paresthesia[10]
- ■ Dimmed vision, abdominal pain, weight loss
■ Oral Findings
- ■ Tongue (atrophic glossitis, burning tongue). Painful and inflamed, flabby, red, smooth, and shiny; loss of filiform papillae.
- ■ Sensitivity to hot or spicy foods
- ■ Painful swallowing
- ■ Gingiva and mucosa: pale, atrophic similar to vitamin B deficiency

D. Treatment

■ Vitamin B_{12} administered by injection twice weekly until the condition is controlled, and then monthly, indefinitely.
■ Good dietary sources of vitamin B_{12} are meat, kidney, fish, oyster, clams, milk, cheese, and eggs. Liver is a rich source and was originally used in therapy before the development of synthetic B_{12}.

II. FOLATE DEFICIENCY ANEMIA[11]

Folate deficiency anemia has the same characteristics as pernicious anemia, except clinically, no neurologic changes are evident.

A. Etiologic Factors

■ Decreased Intake
- ■ Inadequate diet
- ■ Impaired absorption
■ Increased Requirement
- ■ Pregnancy
- ■ Disseminated cancer
- ■ Patients who smoke tobacco
- ■ Patients who take a lot of aspirin or antacids
- ■ Certain drugs impair the utilization of folate, for example, cancer chemotherapy drugs and arthritis medications.

B. Dietary Factors: Sources

■ Fresh fruits, green leafy vegetables, and cruciferous vegetables (cauliflower, broccoli, and brussels sprouts)
■ Liver and kidney
■ Dairy products and whole grain cereals
■ Vegetables need to be eaten raw or lightly cooked
■ Only minimal subsistence diets or special diets influenced by such factors as poverty, food faddism, or alcoholism, when the use of alcohol takes precedence over food, are likely to be deficient in folates.
■ Folate deficiency anemia is not uncommon, but it may be more frequently related to malabsorption than inadequate intake.
■ Check RDAs for adults and children.

C. Deficiency

■ Only minimal subsistence
■ Folate deficiency anemia is not uncommon.

D. Fetal Development

■ Folic acid deficiency can cause neural tube defects.
■ Spina bifida: a severe condition affecting the formation of the nerves of the spinal cord, and resulting in infant paralysis. Spina bifida is described in Chapter 58 on pages 900 to 901.

SICKLE CELL DISEASE (SCD)[12]

■ Sickle cell disease is a hereditary form of hemolytic anemia, resulting from a defective hemoglobin molecule.
■ The name is derived from the crescent or "sickle" shape assumed by the erythrocytes when they become deoxygenated.

■ It is described as an autosomal recessive trait disorder having a mild form with no symptoms (sickle cell trait) and affecting about 10% of carriers and a more severe form (sickle cell disease) affecting up to 98% of carriers.[13]

■ Sickle cell anemia is the most common genetic disorder of the blood.[14]

I. DISEASE PROCESS

■ Occurs primarily in the African–American population and in white populations of Mediterranean origin.

■ Testing: A simple blood test, hemoglobin electrophoresis, will detect sickle cell disease or sickle cell trait (parental carrier).

■ Genetic counseling can play an important role in prevention.

■ Detection of the presence of sickle cell disease is possible before birth, so that proper observation and supervision of the infant and young child can be provided.

■ Signs and symptoms start appearing within the first 6 months, with anemia and vasculopathy.[14]

■ Growth and development may be impaired during the early years. Young children are markedly susceptible to communicable diseases and especially to pneumococcal infections. The disease abnormality is in the type and solubility of hemoglobin.

■ The defective hemoglobin loses oxygen, and the red blood cells become distorted into sickle shapes **(Figure 67-2)**.

■ Increases in fluid viscosity result, and blood stasis occurs, which can lead to thrombosis and infarction.

II. CLINICAL COURSE

A. Severe Hemolytic Anemia

■ Adults: chronic hemolytic sickle cell disease can be severe. The hematocrit may range between 18% and 30%.

■ Life span of red blood cells normally is from 90 to 120 days, whereas in hemolytic anemia, such as sickle cell anemia, the red blood cell survival rate is about 10 to 15 days.

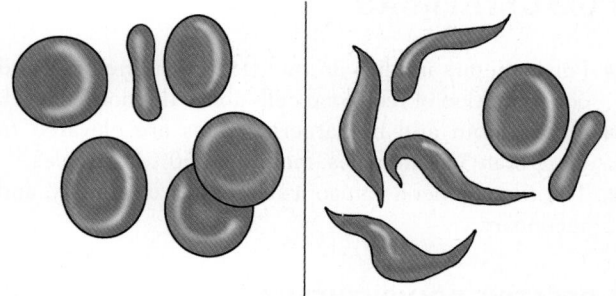

FIGURE 67-2 **Sickle Cell Disease.** *Left, diagrammatic drawing of normal red blood cells.* Right, sickle shapes of red blood cells of a patient with sickle cell disease.

B. Sickle Cell Crisis

Periodic recurrences of clinical exacerbations of the disease with periods of remission characterize childhood and adolescence. The acute form of the disease is called sickle cell crisis.

■ Precipitating Factors
  ■ Crisis may appear at any time with or without stimuli.
  ■ Viral or bacterial infections and other systemic diseases
  ■ Hypoxia, dehydration, sudden changes in temperature
  ■ Physical activity (tissue anoxia), extreme fatigue, acidosis
  ■ Stress/anxiety, additional physical burden (pregnancy), trauma
  ■ Cold causes vasoconstriction which slows the blood flow.

■ Clinical Signs and Symptoms
  ■ A crisis is characterized by self-limited, reversible pain episodes involving the extremities, head, back, chest, and abdomen.
  ■ Swelling, fever, and dehydration
  ■ Infarctions occur in various tissues and organs.
  ■ Symptoms of seizure, stroke, or coma may develop when the nervous system becomes involved.

■ Emergency Procedure
  ■ Stop all clinical procedures.
  ■ Activate emergency medical system for transport to hospital.
  ■ Administer oxygen.

■ Effects and Outcomes of a Crisis
  ■ Effects of crisis may be reversible; severe physical conditions can result.
  ■ Infection or other complications reduce red cell production and there is increased trapping of red cells in the spleen and liver.
  ■ A crisis can be fatal.
  ■ High mortality rate in young children may be the result of the effects of crisis or of severe bacterial infections.
  ■ Children younger than 3 years of age are at great risk for fatal sepsis and meningitis.

C. Systemic Changes That May Occur

■ Chronic changes may occur in any organ system at any age.

■ Major organ affected: kidney

■ Cardiopulmonary system can result in enlargement of the heart, heart murmurs, and coronary insufficiency.

■ Ocular disturbances, even leading to blindness

■ Some patients are susceptible to cerebrovascular accidents with hemiplegia.

■ Lungs, liver, and spleen may be damaged.

■ Changes in bones, including the mandible, result from thrombosis with infarction and from infection.

■ Skin and peripheral vasculature changes with skin ulcers, decreased wound healing, and pain.

D. Preventive Procedures

■ Use folate supplements daily to cope with increased need by the bone marrow.
■ Avoid and/or promptly treat infections; administer pneumococcal polyvalent vaccine to children.
■ Obtain genetic counseling for those with sickle cell trait.
■ Allogeneic stem-cell transplantation may provide a cure for young patients with symptomatic sickle cell disease.[15]
■ Daily penicillin until age 6 years to prevent infection.

E. Treatment and Disease Management

■ Supportive and palliative treatments include those for specific symptoms during crises.
■ Pain relief. Some patients develop problems with substance abuse due to pain medications.[16]
■ Antibiotics for infectious diseases
■ Oxygen therapy and blood transfusions are not used for routine pain episodes but may have limited selective use.
■ Pharmacologic therapy using a chemotherapy agent (Hydroxyurea) to increase hemoglobin F, thereby decreasing the permanent formation of sickle cells.[16]
■ Treatment for sickle cell diseases is evolving,[17] and includes widespread use of penicillin for prophylaxis and new transfusion regimens.

III. ORAL IMPLICATIONS

A. Radiographic Findings[18,19]

■ Decreased radiodensity; increased osteoporosis.
■ Coarse trabecular pattern appearing as horizontal rows between teeth ("step-ladder"), with large marrow spaces.
■ Significant bone loss in children, indicating the presence of periodontitis.
■ Thinning of the border of the mandible.[14]

B. Oral Manifestations

■ Generalized pallor of tissues
■ Jaundiced color from liver disease
■ SCD patients are not prone to an increase in developing periodontal disease; periodontal involvement can lead to a sickle cell crisis.[20]
■ Periodontal evaluation is likely to reveal pockets, infection, and bleeding.
■ Patient requires strict preventive treatment program.
■ Delayed eruption, malocclusion, and dentin hypomineralization.
■ Facial and dental pain.

IV. APPOINTMENT MANAGEMENT[21]

■ The objective during therapy is to provide care without precipitating a sickle cell crisis. During a sickle cell crisis, treatment is limited to emergency relief.
■ A physician consultation to determine disease control including complete blood count
■ Teach and supervise a comprehensive preventive program to minimize oral infection and control etiologic factors.
■ Plan routine care in noncrisis periods; short appointments
■ Stress reduction protocol may be considered in anxious patients. Stress reduction suggestions are described in Chapter 66 with Factors To Teach The Patient on page 1023.
■ Prepare or review the comprehensive medical history. Gather information on the patient's:
  ▪ Related complications specific to organ damage and other problems since birth
  ▪ Characteristics of pain control (frequency, duration, average number, date of last crisis)
  ▪ Past and current medical treatment (surgeries, transfusions, medications, allergies)
  ▪ Presence of venous access catheters and orthopedic prostheses
  ▪ Growth and development issues[14]
■ Some patient's require the use of prophylactic antibiotics. For a patient so highly susceptible to infection, antibiotics can be considered routine, because any form of tissue manipulation can create a bacteremia. Consult physician as this remains a controversial issue.
■ Use local anesthesia with low doses of vasoconstrictors to avoid intravascular occlusion of red blood cells.[22]
■ Use nitrous oxide–oxygen with greater than 50% oxygen, high flow rate, and good ventilation.
■ Avoid long complicated dental appointments by maintaining good personal oral health and arranging frequent appointments with the dental hygienist.
■ Supplemental oxygen during treatment is strongly recommended.[23]
■ If therapy with bisphosphonates is going to be started, all dental treatment is be completed before therapy initiation.[14]

POLYCYTHEMIAS

■ Polycythemia implies an increase in the number and concentration of red blood cells above the normal level.
■ Hemoglobin and hematocrit values are elevated to more than 55% in males, more than 50% in females.[24]
■ The three general categories are relative, primary, and secondary.

I. RELATIVE POLYCYTHEMIA

■ Loss of plasma occurs without a corresponding loss of red blood cells.

- The concentration of cells increases and a relative polycythemia results.
- Causes of fluid loss may be conditions such as dehydration, diarrhea, repeated vomiting, sweating, or loss of fluid from burns.
- Other contributing factors may be smoking, hypertension, becoming mildly overweight, and stress, particularly in middle-aged men.
- The risk of cerebrovascular accidents and myocardial infarction is increased in these patients.[25]

II. POLYCYTHEMIA VERA (PRIMARY POLYCYTHEMIA)[25]

- Results from actual increase in red blood cell count and hemoglobin value.
- White cell and platelet counts are elevated.
- Blood viscosity increases, affecting oxygen transport to tissues.

A. Cause

- Polycythemia vera is a neoplastic condition resulting from a bone disorder in which the primitive red cells or stem cells proliferate.
- The cause is unknown.

B. Oral Signs and Symptoms

- The tongue, mucous membranes, and gingiva are deep purplish–red.
- The gingiva are enlarged, with bleeding on slight provocation.
- Submucosal petechiae, ecchymosis, and hematoma formation.

C. Treatment

- Chemotherapy or radiation
- Phlebotomy, to reduce the total volume, and particularly the red cell volume, of the blood.
- Patient's to avoid iron supplements and aspirin containing medications with a history of bleeding.[24]

D. Dental Hygiene Treatment Considerations

- Frequent maintenance appointments needed to maintain superior health.
- Review medical history, for there is an increased risk of cerebral vascular accident and myocardial infarction.
- Evaluate patient's blood test results, especially hemoglobin and hematocrit.

III. SECONDARY POLYCYTHEMIA

- Secondary polycythemia is also called erythrocytosis, which means an increase in the numbers of red blood cells.

- The increased red cell production can result from hypoxia such as that experienced by residents of high altitudes, chronic obstructive pulmonary disease, cyanotic heart disease, emphysema, and tobacco smoking.
- Can occur from neoplasms (e.g., renal cell carcinoma)[26]
- Bleeding tendencies may be partially controlled with control of gingival irritants.

DISORDERS OF WHITE BLOOD CELLS

- Disorders of the white blood cells may occur because of a decrease (leukopenia) or an increase (leukocytosis) in cell numbers.
- The types of white blood cells are described in **Table 67-2** and illustrated in **Figure 67-1**.

I. LEUKOPENIA[27]

A decrease in the total number of white blood cells results when cell production cannot keep pace with the turnover rate or when an accelerated rate of removal of cells occurs, as in certain disease states.

A. Conditions in Which Leukopenia Occurs

- *Specific Infections.* HIV/AIDS, typhoid fever, influenza, malaria, measles (rubeola), and German measles (rubella) are examples.
- *Disease or Intoxification of the Bone Marrow.* Chronic drug poisoning, ionizing radiation, and autoimmune or drug-induced immune reactions may be implicated.

B. Agranulocytosis (Malignant Neutropenia)

- Rare, serious disease involving the destruction of bone marrow.
- A reduction in circulating neutrophils which has serious consequences.
- The cause of the primary form is unknown and the secondary form is most commonly produced by drugs and other chemicals.[28]
- Causes can relate to toxicity from drugs and chemicals, antipsychotic drugs, and autoimmune reactions.
- Increased susceptibility to infection; oral ulceration and necrosis of tissue.
- Clinical course of sharp drop in white cells, depression of bone marrow, and rapid acute illness leading to death.
- Orally the most characteristic feature is the presence of infection.[28]

II. LEUKOCYTOSIS

■ Increase in the number of circulating white blood cells.

■ Caused by inflammatory and infectious states, trauma, exertion, and other conditions listed in **Table 67-2**.

■ The most extreme abnormal cause of leukocytosis is leukemia.

■ Leukemias are malignant neoplasms of immature white blood cells that multiply uncontrollably and become cancerous.

■ Acute stage progresses very rapidly and can lead to death within weeks to months without aggressive treatment.[28]

■ Characterized by abnormally large numbers of immature leukocytes. There are many types.

■ Cancer cells are located within the circulating blood and in bone marrow; infiltrated into other body tissues and organs like the spleen and lymph nodes.

III. LYMPHOCYTOPENIA

■ Abnormally low number of lymphocytes in the blood

■ Treatment depends on cause, if patient has AIDS and antivirals are taken.

■ Gamma globulin is often administered.

■ Hereditary immunodeficiency requires bone marrow transplantation.

■ If infection occurs, then antibiotic, antifungal, antiviral, or antiparasitic drugs are indicated.[1]

BLEEDING DISORDERS

■ Blood clotting or hemostasis is the body's mechanism for stopping injured blood vessels from forming clots, which can cause serious health problems.[1]

■ The three main processes of blood clotting include constriction of bleeding vessels, activity of platelets, and activity of blood clotting factors.[1]

■ Bleeding disorders have in common the tendencies to spontaneous bleeding and moderate to excessive bleeding following trauma or a surgical procedure.

■ Spontaneous bleeding occurs as small hemorrhages into the skin or mucous membranes and other tissues, and appears as petechiae or purpura.

■ Moderate to excessive bleeding or prolonged bleeding may follow dental hygiene therapy, including nonsurgical instrumentation.

■ A history or suspicion of a bleeding problem requires careful evaluation before treatment can be started.

■ Risk factors for bleeding in patients with hematologic disorders are listed in **Box 67-3**.

I. TYPES OF BLEEDING DISORDERS[29]

The general types are caused by:

BOX 67-3	**Risk Factors for Development of Bleeding in Patients with Hematologic Disorders**

■ Severity of thrombocytopenia
■ Duration of thrombocytopenia
■ Sepsis
■ Liver dysfunction
■ Renal dysfunction
■ Alcohol abuse
■ Medications
■ Increased intracranial pressure

Adapted with permission from Thomas M. Chapter 33: Assessment and management of patients with hematologic disorders. In: Smeltzer S, Bare B, editors. *Medical–surgical nursing*. 10th ed. Philadelphia: Lippincott Williams and Wilkins; 2004. 894 p.

A. Pathology of the Blood Vessel Walls

Vascular fragility is increased; petechial and purpuric hemorrhages appear in the skin or mucous membranes, including the gingiva.

B. Platelet Deficiency or Dysfunction

1. Thrombocytopenia
   ■ A lowered number of platelets may be caused by decreased production in the bone marrow.
   ■ Bone marrow depression may be due to an invasive disease, for example, leukemia; or deficiencies, such as folate or vitamin B_{12} deficiency anemias.
   ■ If severe, a blood transfusion may be necessary.[2]
2. Platelet Dysfunction
   ■ Interference with the blood clotting mechanism leads to a prolonged bleeding time.
   ■ Defects occur as a result of certain hereditary states, uremia, von Willebrand's disease, autoimmune disease, and certain drugs such as aspirin and NSAIDs (nonsteroidal anti-inflammatory drugs).

C. Disorders of Coagulation[30]

1. Acquired Disorders
   ■ Vitamin K deficiency: Vitamin K is essential for prothrombin synthesis and factors VII, IX, and X.
   ■ Good food sources include dark leafy vegetables and liver.
   ■ Liver disease: Nearly all the clotting factors are produced in the liver. When the liver is not functioning properly, the clotting factors may be altered.
   ■ Anticoagulation drugs: Following are the examples of some common medications
      ■ Heparin
      ■ Coumarin
      ■ Aspirin and NSAIDs

2. Hereditary Disorders
   - At least 30 hereditary coagulation disorders exist, each resulting from a deficiency or abnormality of a plasma protein.
   - Clinically, signs and symptoms are similar. The following three are described in this chapter:
     - Hemophilia A (factor VIII abnormality)
     - Hemophilia B (factor IX abnormality)
     - von Willebrand's disease (von Willebrand factor)

HEMOPHILIAS

- The hemophilias are the oldest known hereditary bleeding disorders that are caused by low levels or complete absence of a blood protein essential for clotting.
- Most patients do well with proper medical management involving the administration of drugs to decrease bleeding or the infusion of platelets or plasma containing factors.[31]
- It is advised to avoid (wherever possible) the administration of regional nerve blocks in which the risk of positive aspiration is great.[32]
- The three most common forms of hemophilia are:

I. HEMOPHILIA A (CLASSIC HEMOPHILIA)

- Caused by a reduced amount or reduced activity of factor VIII. 85% of people with hemophilia have this form.

II. HEMOPHILIA B (CHRISTMAS DISEASE)

- Caused by a deficiency of a blood plasma protein called factor IX, that affects the clotting properties of blood.
  - Both hemophilia A and B are X-linked recessive genetic diseases. The defective gene is located on the X chromosome, thus the disorder occurs primarily in males.
  - Severity of the disease can be related directly to the level of the clotting factor in the circulating blood.

III. VON WILLEBRAND'S DISEASE

- Characterized by prolonged bleeding time in the presence of a normal platelet count.
- Most common hereditary disorder of platelet function.
- Patients have a compound defect involving platelet function and the coagulation pathway.
- Rarely is a female affected by hemophilia A or B, but von Willebrand's disease occurs in males and females.
- Extroral signs may include petechiae of skin.

IV. EFFECTS AND LONG-TERM COMPLICATIONS

A. Effects of Minor Trauma

Bleeding and bruising from minor trauma vary depending on the severity of the disease.

B. Hemarthroses

- Bleeding into the soft tissue of joints (knees, ankles, and elbows) begins in the very young with severe hemophilia.
- Much swelling, pain, and incapacitation are created.

C. Joint Deformity and Crippling

Permanent joint damage can result, and the patient may need splints, braces, or orthopedic surgery.

D. Intramuscular Hemorrhage

Hemorrhage into the muscles is accompanied by pain and limitation of motion.

E. Oral Bleeding

- Bleeding from the gingiva is common and more extensive when periodontal infection is more severe.
- Because of the fear of bleeding, patients may neglect toothbrushing and flossing; doing so can lead to increased dental biofilm accumulation and inflammation.
- Small children may injure the oral area when they tumble, and severe bleeding can result.
- Management of Uncontrolled Bleeding:[33] When uncontrolled bleeding is observed, stop dental treatment.
  - If clotting does not occur within a few minutes, apply digital pressure to area with sterile gauze.
  - If needed, local hemostatic agents can be applied, such as absorbable gelatin sponge. Absorbs for 3 to 5 days.
  - Medical attention required if unsuccessful in stopping bleeding.

DENTAL HYGIENE CARE PLAN

- Although prevention and control of bleeding are the main issues when treating a patient with a blood clotting defect, other factors require attention.
- Patients with bleeding disorders have many emotional stresses related to the disease, its treatment, and excessive cost.
- Patients now can take more responsibility for self-care regimens as opposed to previous issues of long

hospitalizations and separations from family, friends, and school.

■ As a result of internal and cerebral hemorrhages, a few patients may become multihandicapped, have mental and physical problems, or may be limited intellectually.

■ Suggestions for appointments from Chapter 56 may be useful for the patient who has had hemarthroses and orthopedic treatment.

I. PATIENT HISTORY

■ Medical history needs to include information regarding the type, severity, treatment, medications, and family history of the blood clotting defect. Blood dyscrasia adverse drug effects are uncommon.

■ Question patient specifically regarding bleeding after clinical and surgical procedures, such as tooth extractions.

■ A careful review of a patient's drug, supplements, and herb use is critical to determine potential oral and physiologic effects. The primary purpose of the drug and potential side effects needs careful review in a current drug reference guide.

■ A variety of drugs and herbs may be factors in increased bleeding. Herbs and supplements associated with increased bleeding are listed in **Box 67-4**.

■ Antithrombotic agents such as aspirin and clopidogrel alter the ability of platelets to stick or clump together and form a clot.[34]

■ Dental history: Discussion with the patient to include previous dental care and perceived treatment needs to be taken into consideration when developing the current care plan.

■ Request reports of current blood tests.

BOX 67-4	Herbs and Supplements Associated With Increased Bleeding

Alfalfa	Cat's claw	Garlic
Allspice	Chamomile	Ginkgo
Angelica	Chrondroitin	Ginger
Anise	Co-enzymen Q10	Gingseng
Billberry	Cranberry	Glucosamine
Blackhaw	Evening Primrose	Guggul
Bogbean	Fenugreek	Horse chestnut
Boldo	Feverfew	Poplar
Bucho	Flax	White willow
Capsicum	Vitamin E	

Adapted from Alberto PL. Alternative medicine for the dental professional. Access. 2009 Jan;23(1):20–4. Available at http://www.thefreelibrary.com/Alternative+medicine+for+the+dental+professio nal-a0193298316.

II. CONSULTATION WITH PHYSICIAN/HEMATOLOGIST

■ Consultation with the physician/hematologist is necessary to obtain complete and accurate information. The American Dental Association has developed a joint policy with the American Heart Association, the American College of Cardiology, the Society for Cardiovascular Angiography and Interventions, and the American College of Surgeons to advise healthcare providers who perform invasive or surgical procedures, such as those associated with oral care, to contact the cardiologist and discuss patient management before discontinuing antiplatelet drugs. The risk for intravascular clot formation is greater than the risk for hemorrhage.[35]

■ Consult physician/hematologist to determine whether premedication is required during dental procedures to prevent infection in joint prostheses and/or indwelling catheter.

■ Many procedures require factor replacement therapy just prior to the dental appointment.

III. PREPARATION FOR CLINICAL APPOINTMENT

■ Certain tests may be needed on the same day as treatment because blood values fluctuate.

For example, the patient taking coagulants is required to have a PT (prothrombin time) within 24 hours of an appointment or report their most recent INR (international normalized ratio) level to the oral health provider.

■ It is critical to assess the patient's prescription and over-the-counter (OTC) medications to provide important information about the patient's current medical status, disease severity, compliance with drug and treatment recommendations, and orientation to health and wellness.[36]

■ Patients taking either coumarin (for prevention of recurrent thrombosis), heparin (for short-term use following a total joint replacement procedure), or medication for long-term anticoagulation (such as aspirin) may need special consultation. The most common side effect of both warfarin and heparin is hemorrhage. Hemorrhages may present as gingival bleeding or submucosal bleeding with hematoma formation.[34]

■ Patient's on cancer chemotherapeutic agents may secondarily induce profound thrombocytopenia (<20,000 mm^3) **(Table 67-2)**. Hemorrhage may occur anywhere in the mouth and may be spontaneous or precipitated by trauma or existing disease.[37]

■ There are many herb–drug interactions, hence it is necessary to refer to a reference book such as Dental Drug Reference by Pickett and Terezhalmy, to help avoid medical emergencies. Common herbs and supplements that are associated with increased bleeding are shown in **(Box 67-3)**. It is recommended to discontinue these herbs and supplements 2 weeks prior to receiving invasive surgical procedures.[36]

- Use of dietary supplements has the potential to:[36]
  - Cause a bleeding condition
  - Exacerbate an existing bleeding condition
  - Alter the effectiveness of other OTC and prescription medications being taken concurrently.

IV. PRIMARY SCREENING TESTS[39]

- Basic tests are listed in **Table 67-1** with their ranges or values
- Indications for screening and pre-appointment tests:
  - When the patient gives a history of a bleeding problem
  - A family member has a history of a bleeding problem
  - Clinical examination reveals signs of a bleeding disorder
  - Patient is being treated with anticoagulation therapy
- Purposes
  - Primary screening tests provide a presumptive diagnosis.
  - They serve to check the current status for the patient.
- The tests are:
  - PT measures the status of extrinsic and common pathways of coagulation. This test reflects the ability of blood lost from vessels in the area of injury to coagulate.
  - INR is a standard method of measuring PT independent of thromboplastin reagent, but is more accurate than the PT test. Used to determine the clotting tendency of blood, in the measure of warfarin dosage, liver damage, and vitamin K status.[37]
  - Activated partial thromboplastin time (aPTT) measures the status of the intrinsic and common pathways of coagulation. This test reflects the ability of the blood still within vessels in the area of injury.
  - Platelet count screens for possible bleeding problems because of thrombocytopenia (number of platelets in the circulating blood).
  - Hemoglobin carries oxygen to cells and is necessary for wound healing.
  - Hematocrit measures the volume of packed red cells in percentage.
  - An examination of a blood smear (or film) may be requested by a physician in response to abnormality in blood counts.

V. CLINICAL IMPLICATIONS FOR PATIENT CARE

- Prevention of gingival infection and dental caries is an essential aspect of care for patients with a bleeding disorder.
- Preliminary tissue conditioning can help prevent severe bleeding during instrumentation. Teach daily personal

biofilm removal at the initial appointment and reinforce at each session.

- Plan scaling in small segments. When care planning local anesthesia injections, try to avoid injections that are at a higher risk for bleeding. For example, a posterior superior alveolar nerve block.
- *Postoperative*: Never use aspirin or nonsteroidal anti-inflammatory drugs for a patient with a bleeding disorder. The bleeding tendency is greatly increased by a drug-induced platelet dysfunction caused by aspirin. Ask the patient to call if bleeding occurs within first 24 to 48 hours.[40]
- *Frequency of Maintenance Care*: Frequent appointments can aid in keeping the oral tissues in an optimum state of health and help to prevent the need for complex or lengthy dental appointments.
- *Radiographic Imaging System*: Films/sensor (infection control barriers) can cut and press on the mucous membranes. Care in placement is to be exercised.
- *Impressions*. Beading the rims of the trays protects the mucosa from pressure and damage from a hard, possibly rough surface, as described in Chapter 13, page 197.
- *Evacuation*: High-vacuum suction tips may be sharp. Caution in the use of suction is necessary to prevent pulling the sublingual or other mucosal tissues into the suction tip and causing hematomas. Hematoma requires no treatment as the lesion will spontaneously resolve.
- *Stress Reduction Protocol*: Prevention or reduction of stress begins before the appointment, is continued throughout the treatment, and followed through into the postoperative period, if necessary.

VI. ORAL HYGIENE PROGRAM

- Encourage each patient to improve and maintain good oral health. Spontaneous oral bleeding problems can be partially controlled by the elimination of oral infections.
- Meticulous dental biofilm removal is practiced and repeated. A soft toothbrush is indicated. If patient indicates using a power brush, proper demonstration of technique is necessary.
- Teach flossing carefully and correctly to prevent cutting the gingiva and inducing proximal bleeding.
- Patients with limited manual dexterity can benefit from special oral hygiene aids in Chapter 56 on pages 864 to 867.
- Select age-appropriate preventive measures including fluoride treatments, remineralizing agents, sealants, biofilm control, and professional dental supervision.
- A nutritional counseling assessment is recommended for caries control and periodontal health but also to stress on choosing foods that provide a well-balanced diet.
- Many vitamins have a role in blood cell formation as listed in Chapter 34, pages 502 to 505.

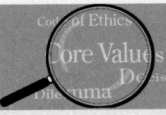

Everyday Ethics

Just as Dena, the dental hygienist, begins to probe for recording the gingival examination for Mr. Bennett, the patient, the receptionist interrupts to give Dena a medical clearance form that has been faxed from the patient's physician. As Dena reviews the information, she understands that the patient has a blood disorder but is unclear as to its extent from the laboratory values in the report. She briefly questions Mr. Bennett about any medical tests and he indicates that he was in the hospital 4 days the previous month.

As Dena continues the probing, she notices considerable bleeding with oozing around the gingival margins.

Questions for Consideration

1. What action, if any, does Dena need to take to ensure she is performing beneficently on behalf of this patient?

2. It appears that Mr. Bennett has not given sufficient information about his medical condition prior to this maintenance appointment. What obligation does a patient have to update the medical history at each appointment? And what obligation does the professional person have to help the patient understand this obligation?

3. While Dena quietly acknowledges to herself that she used to know the information about bleeding conditions, she is currently uncertain of the meaning of the laboratory values in this patient's report. Ethically, how can this realization be assessed? What is the immediate need? What can be done to prevent such a situation from occurring in the future?

DOCUMENTATION

Documentation in the permanent record for each appointment with a blood disorder includes a minimum of the following factors.

- Review or update medical history thoroughly. Document laboratory findings.
- Document extra- and intraoral examinations findings. Use written description and a picture if possible.
- Note treatment planning considerations such as shorter appointments, stress reduction protocols that need to be implemented, and oral hygiene considerations.
- Note consultations with other health professionals involved in the patient's care.
- Reference any difficulties with bleeding control during appointment.

Factors To Teach The Patient

- Meticulous oral hygiene techniques to practice daily: toothbrushing, flossing, and other appropriate oral hygiene aids.
- How to self-evaluate the oral cavity for deviations from normal. Watching for changes in size, shape, color and contacting oral health professional when lesions last longer than 2 weeks.
- Selection of non-cariogenic foods to prevent caries, and knowledge about the diet's relationship to health.
- Avoid use of salicylates (aspirin).
- Importance of informing the dental hygienist of any changes to the medical history, including drugs, herbs, supplements, and hospitalizations and providing recent laboratory values before beginning treatment.

BOX 67-5	Example Progress Notes: Patient With a Blood Disorder

Date— Medical history updated. Patient currently taking Warfarin. Patient states that INR is 2.8. Oral cancer examination is negative. Prophylaxis completed with no incidence of excessive bleeding. Four digital bite-wings exposed and fluoride varnish applied. Reviewed technique of oral hygiene aids and stressed to patient the need for meticulous homecare and recommended 4-month re-care appointment due to moderate plaque and calculus present.

Signed: _____, RDH Date: _____

References

1. Young B, Heath J. *Wheater's functional histology.* 4th ed. London: Churchill & Livingstone; 2000. 46–66 pp.
2. Beebe SN. Blood simple. Dimens. 2008 Sep;6(9):40–3.
3. Weiss G, Goodnough LT. Anemia of chronic disease. *N Engl J Med.* 2005 Mar;352(10):1011–23.
4. Al-Wahadni AM, Taani DQ, Al-Omari MO. Dental diseases in subjects with beta-thalassemia major. *Community Dent Oral Epidemiol.* 2002 Dec;309(6):418–22.
5. Thomas M. Chapter 33: Assessment and management of patients with hematologic disorders. In: Smeltzer S, Bare B, editors. *Medical–surgical nursing.* 10th ed. Philadelphia: Lippincott Williams and Wilkins; 2004. 891 p.
6. Rund D, Rachmilewitz E. Beta-thalassemia. *N Engl J Med.* 2005 Sep;353(11):1135–46.
7. Ibsen OAC, Phelan JA, Vernillo AT. Chapter 9: Oral manifestations of systemic diseases. In: Ibsen OAC, Phelan JA, editors. *Oral pathology for the dental hygienist.* 5th ed. Philadelphia: W.B. Saunders Co.; 2009. 295 p.
8. Smeltzer, Bare.op.cit., p.881.

9. Kumar V, Abbas AK, Fausto N. *Robbins and cotran pathologic basis of disease.* 7th ed. Philadelphia: Elsevier Saunders Co.; 2005. 638–42 pp.

10. Palmer C. *Diet and nutrition in oral health.* 2nd ed. Upper Saddle River: Pearson Prentice Hall; 2007. 177 p.

11. Wardlaw G. *Perspectives in nutrition.* 6th ed. New York: McGraw Hill Co.; 2004. 343–6 pp.

12. Platt A, Eckman JR, Beasley J, Miller G. Treating sickle cell pain: an update from the Georgia comprehensive sickle cell center. *J Emerg Nurs.* 2002 Aug;28(4):297–303.

13. Smeltzer, Bare.op.cit., p. 886.

14. Queis H, daFonsceca M, Casamassimo P. Sickle cell anemia: a review for the pediatric dentist. *J Clin Pediatr Dent.* 2007 Mar/Apr;29(2):159–69.

15. Walters MC, Patience M, Leisenring W, Eckman JR, Scott JP, Mentzer WC, Davies SC, Ohene-Frempong K, Bernaudin F, Matthews DC, Storb R, Sullivan KM. Bone marrow transplantation for sickle cell disease. *N Engl J Med.* 1996 Jun;335(6):369–76.

16. Smeltzer, Bare.op.cit., p.889.[CE: Plz chk this ref]

17. Steinberg MH. Management of sickle cell disease. *N Engl J Med.* 1999 Apr;340(13):1021–30.

18. Taylor LB, Nowak AJ, Giller RH, Casamassimo PS. Sickle cell anemia: a review of the dental concerns and a retrospective study of dental and bony changes. *Spec Care Dentist.* 1995 Jan/Feb;15(1):38–42.

19. Ibsen, Phelan, Vernillo. op.cit.,p.297.

20. Rada RE, Bronny AT, Hasiakos PS. Sickle cell crisis precipitated by periodontal infection: report of two cases. *J Am Dent Assoc.* 1987 Jun;114(6):799–801.

21. Little JW, Falace DA, Miller CS, Rhodus NL. *Dental management of the medically compromised patient.* 7th ed. St. Louis: Mosby; 2002. 367–70 pp.

22. Pickett F, Gurenlian J. *Preventing medical emergencies.* 2nd ed. Philadelphia: Lippincott Williams and Wilkins; 2005. 132 p.

23. Malamed S. *Medical emergencies in the dental office.* 6th ed. St. Louis: Mosby; 2000. 27 p.

24. Smeltzer, Bare.op.cit., p. 894.

25. Ibsen, Phelan, Vernillo.op.cit., p. 298.

26. Smeltzer, Bare.op.cit., p. 895.

27. Little, Falace, Miller, Rhodus. op.cit., p374.

28. Ibsen, Phelan, Vernillo.op.cit.,p.300.[CE:

29. Little, Falace, Miller, Rhodus. op.cit., p. 397.

30. Little, Falace, Miller, Rhodus. op.cit., p. 411.

31. Pickett, Gurelian.op.cit.,p.118.

32. Malamed.op.cit.,p.25.

33. Pickett, Gurelian.op.cit.,p.53.

34. Pickett FA, Sharuga C. Addressing adverse drug effects. Dimens. 2010 Jan;8(1):38–42.

35. Pickett, Gurelian.op.cit.,p.52.

36. Andrews L, Spolarich AE. An examination of the bleeding complications associated with herbal supplements, antiplatelet and anticoagulant medications. *J Dent Educ.* 2007 Summer;81(3):2–14.

37. Picket FA, Terezhalmy G. *Dental drug reference.* 2nd ed. Baltimore: Lippincott Williams and Wilkins; 2010. 34 p.

38. Alberto PL. Alternative medicine for the dental professional. Access. 2009 Jan;23(1):20–4.

39. Little, Falace, Miller, Rhodus. op. cit., pp. 421.

40. Little, Falace, Miller, Rhodus. op. cit., pp. 425.

The Patient With Diabetes Mellitus

KATHRYN RAGALIS DAVIS, RDH, MS, DMD

Chapter Outline

An effective dental hygiene program is vital for the patient with diabetes mellitus. Signs and symptoms of diabetes can be identified by thorough medical history questions. Clinical assessment can reveal oral changes that are indicative of this systemic disease. Dental professionals may be the first to recognize the warnings and refer the patient for early diagnosis. Early diagnosis and treatment can significantly reduce the life-threatening complications of the disease and improve quality of life.

A patient with diabetes may have a lowered resistance to infections, delayed healing, multiple systemic complications, and is prone to life-threatening emergencies. The presence of infection, including periodontitis, may intensify symptoms and make diabetes more difficult to regulate.

The dental clinician has a significant responsibility to:

■ Recognize signs and symptoms of diabetes to promote early diagnosis.

BOX 68-1	Key Words

Diabetes Mellitus

Beta cells: insulin-producing cells of the islets of Langerhans in the pancreas.

Brittle diabetes: term formerly used to describe very unstable type 1 diabetes; characterized by unexplained oscillation between hypoglycemia and diabetic ketoacidosis.

Casual plasma glucose: blood glucose level at any time of day with no regard to time of eating.

Charcot's joints: A joint that is deprived of any pain or position sense due to severe osteoarthritis or as a result of disease such as diabetic neuropathy.

Exocrine: secreting externally via a duct.

Exogenous insulin: insulin from source outside patient.

Gastroparesis: delayed gastric emptying. Occurs when the vagus nerve is damaged or stops functioning normally and movement of food is slowed or stopped.

Gestational diabetes: diabetes that occurs during pregnancy.

Gluconeogenesis: synthesis of glucose from noncarbohydrate sources, such as amino acids and glycerol; can occur in the liver and kidneys when the carbohydrate intake is insufficient to meet the body's needs.

Glycated or glycosylated hemoglobin (HbA1c): the primary assay for assessing long-term glycemic control. Indicates blood glucose levels for the previous 6–8 weeks.

Glycemia: presence of glucose in blood.

Hyperglycemia: very high blood glucose: opposite of hypoglycemia, abnormally low glucose in the blood.

Hyperpnea: abnormal increase in depth and rate of respiration.

Hypogeusia: abnormally diminished acuteness of the sense of taste.

Hypoglycemia: an abnormally low level of glucose in the blood; opposite of hyperglycemia, very high blood glucose.

Insulin: a powerful hormone secreted by the beta cells in the islets of Langerhans of the pancreas; the major fuel-regulating hormone; enters the blood in response to a rise in concentration of blood glucose and is transported immediately to bind with cell surface receptors throughout the body.

Ketoacidosis: diabetic coma; too little insulin; accumulation of ketone bodies in the blood.

Ketone bodies: normal metabolic products of lipid (fat) within the liver; excess production leads to urinary excretion of these acidic chemicals.

Ketonuria: excess concentration of ketone bodies in the urine.

Oral glucose tolerance test: a test of the body's ability to utilize carbohydrates; aid to the diagnosis of diabetes mellitus. After ingestion of a specific amount of glucose solution, the fasting blood glucose rises promptly in a nondiabetic person, then falls to normal within an hour. In diabetes mellitus, the blood glucose rise is greater and the return to normal is prolonged.

Oral hypoglycemic agent: synthetic drug that lowers the blood sugar level; stimulates the synthesis and release of insulin from the beta cells of the islets of Langerhans in the pancreas; used to treat patients with type 2 diabetes mellitus.

Polydipsia: excessive thirst.

Polyphagia: excessive ingestion of food.

Polyuria: excessive excretion of urine.

Postprandial: after a meal.

Prediabetes: IFG and IGT are risk factors for future diabetes and cardiovascular disease.

Pruritus: itching.

Retinopathy: noninflammatory degenerative disease of the retina; called diabetic retinopathy when it occurs with diabetes of long standing.

- Assess the status of diabetes to determine the impact on the oral health of the patient and dental treatment.
- Work with the patient and other healthcare professionals to provide instruction and oral care aimed at maintaining health and preventing infections and emergencies.
- Identify and treat acute emergencies.

Modifications in dental and dental hygiene procedures may be indicated. The status of the diabetes is determined before any treatment can begin. Key words and abbreviations used in this chapter are found in Boxes 68-1 and 68-2, respectively.

DIABETES MELLITUS

I. DEFINITION[1]

- Diabetes mellitus is a group of metabolic diseases characterized by hyperglycemia. The symptoms of hyperglycemia are listed in Box 68-3.

- Hyperglycemia results from an insulin deficiency, resistance to insulin action, or both. There is a relative or absolute lack of insulin or an inadequate function of insulin.
- Chronic hyperglycemia is associated with long-term damage, dysfunction, and failure of numerous organs, especially the eyes, kidneys, nerves, heart, and blood vessels.

II. IMPACT

- Almost 8% of the population in the United States is estimated to have diabetes. Approximately a third that have the disease have not yet been diagnosed.
- As the population ages and with increases in obesity, diabetes becomes more prevalent.
- Due to the prevalence, cost of treatment, and lost productivity, diabetes is one of the most costly health conditions.

Diabetes Mellitus

A1c (A One C): common abbreviation for glycosylated hemoglobin (HbA1c)
EMS: Emergency Medical Service
FPG: fasting plasma glucose
GDM: gestational diabetes mellitus
HbA1c: glycosylated hemoglobin
HDL: high-density lipoprotein
IDDM: insulin-dependent diabetes mellitus
IFG: impaired fasting glucose
IGT: impaired glucose tolerance
LDL: low-density lipoprotein
NIDDM: non-insulin-dependent diabetes mellitus
OGTT: oral glucose tolerance test
PCOS: polycystic ovarian syndrome
PP: postprandial
SMBG: self-monitoring of blood glucose
WHO: World Health Organization

BOX 68-3	Symptoms of Hyperglycemia

- Polyuria
- Polydipsia
- Weight loss
- Polyphagia
- Blurred vision
- Increased susceptibility to infections
- Impaired growth

II. DESCRIPTION

- Food is ingested and converted into glucose.
- Increase in blood glucose level stimulates the pancreas to release insulin into the blood stream.
- Insulin enables glucose transport into cells to use as energy.
- Blood glucose level then decreases.
- **Figure 68-1A** shows the healthy pancreas and the action of insulin as it is taken up by the body cells.

INSULIN

I. DEFINITION

Insulin is a hormone produced by the beta cells in the pancreas. Insulin directly or indirectly affects every organ in the body.

III. FUNCTIONS

The functions of insulin are listed in **Box 68-4**. Without insulin, glucose accumulates in the blood, resulting in hyperglycemia. Normal blood glucose levels in healthy individuals usually range from 60–150 mg/dl. In diabetes, levels range much higher.

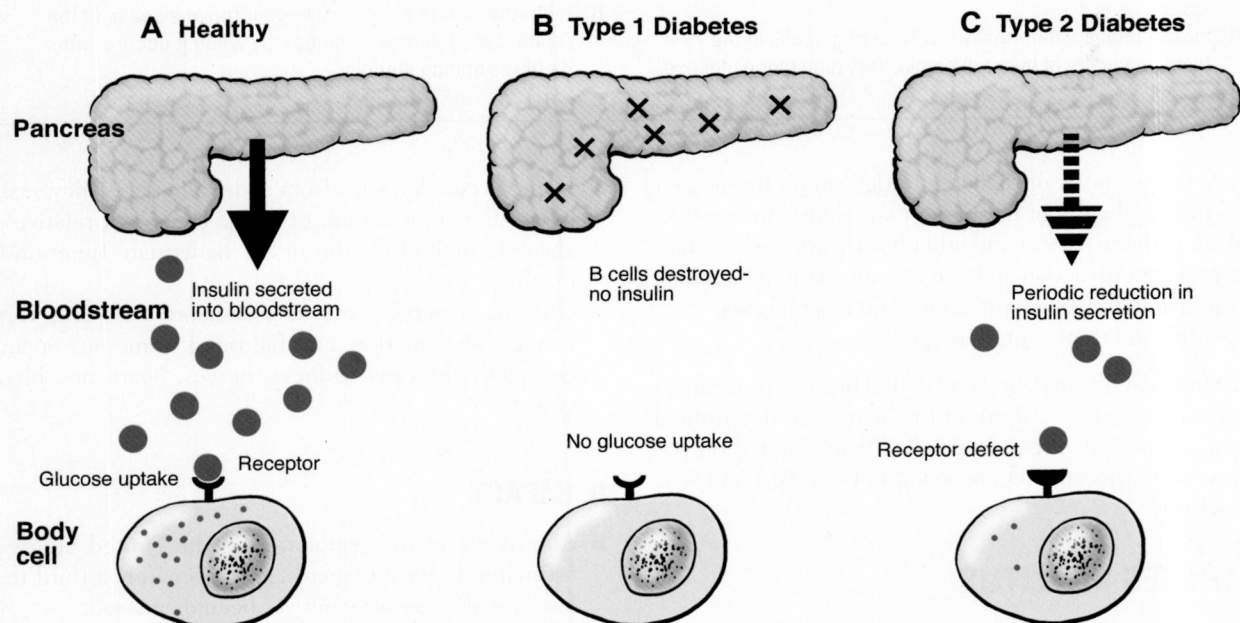

FIGURE 68-1 **Pancreas and Action of Insulin on Body Cell in Health, and Type 1 and 2 Diabetes.** **(A)** Healthy pancreas excretes insulin into bloodstream that enables glucose uptake by body cell. **(B)** Type 1 diabetes shows no insulin produced by pancreas and no glucose uptake by cell. **(C)** Type 2 diabetes shows normal, increased, or decreased insulin production by pancreas and the defective receptor on cell that hampers insulin uptake.

BOX 68-4	Functions of Insulin

1. Facilitates glucose uptake from blood into tissues, which lowers blood glucose level.
2. Speeds the oxidation of glucose within the cells to use for energy.
3. Speeds the conversion of glucose to glycogen to store in the liver and skeletal muscles and to prevent the conversion of glycogen back to glucose.
4. Facilitates conversion of glucose to fat in adipose tissue.

IV. EFFECTS OF DECREASED INSULIN (TYPE 1 DIABETES)

- Less glucose is transmitted through cell walls into the cells.
- Glucose increases in the circulating blood (hyperglycemia) until a threshold is reached and glucose spills over into the urine (glycosuria).
- Increased glycosuria induces osmotic diuresis with excretion of large amounts of urine (polyuria). Water and electrolytes are lost.
- Fluid loss signals excessive thirst to the brain (polydipsia).
- Cells starving for glucose may cause the patient to increase food intake (polyphagia), but weight loss may still occur.
- Without glucose to use for energy, the body metabolizes fat for energy.
  A. End products of fat metabolism are harmful ketones that accumulate in the blood.
  B. Ketones are acidic, and when they accumulate, they are usually neutralized in the blood. When the quantity is large, the neutralizing effect is depleted rapidly and an acidic condition (metabolic acidosis) results.
  C. Metabolic acidosis leads to diabetic coma (ketoacidosis) if not treated promptly.
- **Figure 68-1B** shows changes in pancreas function that occur in type 1 diabetes.

V. EFFECTS OF DECREASED ACTION OF INSULIN (TYPE 2 DIABETES)

- Insulin production and secretion by the pancreas remains at normal levels.
- Cell surface insulin receptors develop defects, and glucose cannot be transmitted into the cell.
- Blood glucose level increases as the insulin resistance of the cells increases. This stimulates more insulin to be released.
- Over time, insulin secretion may also decline and lead to both decrease of insulin in the blood as well as increased insulin resistance of cells.

- **Figure 68-1C** shows the effects of decreased insulin and action of insulin that can occur in type 2 diabetes. Note the defective receptor on the body cell.

VI. INSULIN COMPLICATIONS

- Earlier diagnosis, improved treatment, and better informed patient, family, and friends have reduced the occurrence of emergency insulin complications.
- Constant verbal and visual contact is maintained with a patient to identify early behavioral and physical changes indicative of a developing crisis.

A. Hypoglycemia/Insulin Shock

- Too much insulin (hyperinsulinism), which lowers level of blood glucose (hypoglycemia).
- Hypoglycemia is the emergency more likely to occur in the dental setting.

B. Hyperglycemic Reaction/Diabetic Coma (Ketoacidosis)

- Too little insulin (hypoinsulinism) with increased levels of blood glucose (hyperglycemia).
- **Table 68-1** shows a comparison of the characteristics of hyperglycemic and hypoglycemic reactions, along with the respective treatment procedures.

DIABETES MELLITUS ETIOLOGIC CLASSIFICATION

- In 1997, an international expert committee, organized by the American Diabetes Association, revised the classification of diabetes. The system is based on the etiology of the disease wherever possible.
- The assignment of the type of diabetes is frequently dependent on the circumstances at the time of diagnosis. Many patients do not fit into a single type of diabetes therefore the focus is to understand the pathogenesis of the hyperglycemia and effective treatment.[1]
- A comparison of types 1 and 2 diabetes is found in **Table 68-2**.

I. TYPE 1 DIABETES

A. Description

Figure 68-1B illustrates the changes in type 1 diabetes.

- An absolute insulin deficiency.
- Results from the destruction of the insulin-producing beta cells in the pancreas. The loss of the beta cells is due to either a cell-mediated autoimmune destruction or an unknown etiology and unclear environmental factors.

TABLE 68-1	COMPARISON OF INSULIN REACTION AND DIABETIC COMA	
	HYPOGLYCEMIA/INSULIN SHOCK	**DIABETIC COMA/KETOACIDOSIS**
History/Predisposing Factors	Too much insulin Too little food: omitted or delayed Excessive exercise Stress	Too little insulin: omission of dose or failure to increase dose when requirements increased Too much food Less exercise than planned Infection, illness of any sort Trauma, drugs, alcohol abuse Stress
Occurrence	More common complication than ketoacidosis, especially with less stable type 1 diabetes	Type I diabetes especially if poorly controlled, unstable
Onset	Sudden	Develops slowly over hours/days
Behavioral Changes	Confusion, stupor Drowsy, restless Anxious, irritable, agitated Incoordination, weakness	Any hypoglycemia behavioral change
Physical Findings	Skin: moist, sweaty, perspiration Hunger Headache Tremor, shakiness, weakness Pallor Dilated pupils, blurry vision Dizziness, staggering gait	Skin: flushed, dry Abdominal pain Nausea, vomiting Lack of appetite Dry mouth, thirst Fruity smelling breath Increased urination
Vital Signs Temperature Respiration Pulse Blood Pressure	Normal or below Normal Fast, irregular Normal or slightly elevated	Elevated when infection Hyperpnea, rapid and labored Acetone or fruity smelling breath Rapid, weak Lowered, person may go into shock
If Left Untreated	Possible convulsions, eventual coma and death	Eventual coma and death
Treatment	GIVE SUGAR to raise blood glucose level (apple juice, cake frosting, glucose tablets) Revival is prompt If unconscious/unresponsive: injection of glucagon or intravenous glucose	Immediate professional care Activate EMS, hospitalize Monitor vital signs Keep patient warm Fluids for conscious patient Insulin injection after medical assessment
Prevention	Smooth regulation of blood sugar and frequent blood glucose monitoring	Smooth regulation of blood sugar and frequent blood glucose monitoring

- Patients are dependent on exogenous insulin to sustain life.
- Patients are prone to ketoacidosis.
- Usually arises in childhood or puberty, but may occur at any age.
- Accounts for 5–10% of those with diabetes.

B. Former Names

Type 1 diabetes, insulin-dependent diabetes mellitus (IDDM), juvenile diabetes, juvenile-onset diabetes, ketosis-prone diabetes, brittle diabetes.

II. TYPE 2 DIABETES

A. Description

Figure 68-1C shows changes listed below.

- Pancreatic insulin secretion may be low, normal, or even higher than normal, but the patient exhibits an insulin resistance that impairs the use of insulin.
- Patients have insulin resistance with a relative, not absolute, insulin deficiency.
- Insulin resistance is the inability of the peripheral tissues to respond to insulin.

TABLE 68-2	COMPARISON OF TYPE I AND TYPE 2 DIABETES MELLITUS	
CHARACTERISTIC	**TYPE 1**	**TYPE 2**
Age of Onset	Young, usually before or during puberty, but may appear later	Adult, usually after 30 years, but may occur at younger age
Body Weight	Normal or thin	Most are obese, body fat particularly in abdominal area
Ethnicity	More common in Caucasians	More common in African Americans, Asian Americans, Hispanics, Native Americans, Pacific Islanders
Hereditary	Yes, but less frequent occurrence than type 2	Much more frequent occurrence in families
Lifestyle	Restrictions very difficult for young patients	More frequent in sedentary individuals with high-fat diets
Onset of Symptoms	Rapid, abrupt symptoms of hyperglycemia	Slow, insidious progression over years, frequently goes undiagnosed for years
Symptoms	Weight loss, weakness Polyuria Frequent/recurrent infections Polydipsia slow healing Polyphagia Tingling/numb extremities Blurred vision Fatigue Mimic flu Eye/kidney/cardiovascular problems	Any type 1 symptom
Severity	Severe, life-threatening	Early mild but progressively serious
Complications	Acute hypoglycemic/hyperglycemic emergencies and chronic long-term complications common	Acute complications rare, chronic long-term complications common
Ketoacidosis	Common	Rare
Stability	Unstable, difficult and much effort to control	More stable, easier to manage
Insulin	No insulin production, exogenous insulin required	Insulin levels normal, elevated, or low; exogenous insulin needed by some
Prevention	None, due to multiple genetic predispositions and unclear environmental factors	May be possible to prevent or delay with lifestyle changes, increased activity, and weight loss

- Risk factors for developing this type of diabetes are listed in **Box 68-5**. The risk increases with increased number of risk factors.
- Onset typical after 30 years of age, but may occur at any age. Incidence has increased dramatically in children and adolescents in recent years, possibly due to increases in sedentary lifestyle and obesity in children.
- Most prevalent type of diabetes, accounts for 90–95% of all patients with diabetes.

B. Screening[2]

Type 1 diabetes is usually identified after acute symptoms of hyperglycemia prompt immediate evaluation. Screening is recommended for type 2 diabetes and to assess risk for diabetes due to the slower onset and lack of early symptoms. Screening is done for those who are asymptomatic. Basic criteria for testing in healthcare setting:

- Age 45 and above, repeated every 3 years or more frequently.
- Screening begins earlier and more frequently if the patient is overweight and has other risk factors listed in **Box 68-5**. This includes testing children and adolescents who are overweight and have other risk factors.

C. Former Names

- Type 2 diabetes, non-insulin-dependent diabetes mellitus (NIDDM), adult-onset diabetes, maturity-onset diabetes, ketosis-resistant diabetes.

BOX 68-5	Risk Factors for Type 2 Diabetes[2]

- Overweight adults (BMI 25 kg/m2, which may be lower is some ethnic groups)
- Immediate, first-degree, blood relative (parent/sibling) has diabetes
- Habitual physical inactivity
- High-risk race/ethnicity: African/Asian//Native American, Latino, Pacific Islander
- Had baby weighing more than 9 pounds
- Had gestational diabetes mellitus
- History of polycystic ovary syndrome
- Hypertension ($\geq$140/90 mm Hg)
- Age 45 years or greater
- HDL cholesterol level <35 mg/dl (0.90 mmol/l)
- Triglyceride level >250 mg/dl (2.82 mmol/l)
- Had prior IGT or IFG
- History of c vascular disease
- Have other clinical condition associated with insulin resistance such as severe obesity or acanthosis nigrans.
  - ☐ HbA1C of 5.7–6.4%
  - ☐ Fasting plasma glucose 100–125 mg/dl (5.6–6.9 mmol/l)

III. GESTATIONAL DIABETES MELLITUS (GDM)

- Defined as any degree of glucose intolerance with onset or first recognition during pregnancy.
- Related to genetics, obesity, and hormones causing insulin resistance usually in third trimester.
- Occurs in about 4% of pregnancies in the United States.
- Diagnosis is reclassified 6 or more weeks after pregnancy ends.
- Insulin adjustment, carefully supervised prenatal care, and improved obstetric practices have lessened much of the potential danger for the mother.
- Infants are larger; premature births more frequent; incidence of congenital malformations and perinatal death high; lower rate with improved prenatal care.
- Have tendency to develop type 2 diabetes later in life.

IV. OTHER SPECIFIC TYPES OF DIABETES[1]

Other types of diabetes result from genetic defects, diseases, endocrinopathies, surgery, drugs, malnutrition, infections, and injury.

- Genetic defects of the beta cell.
- Genetic defects in insulin action.
- Diseases of the exocrine pancreas
  A. Diseases that injure or destroy beta cells.
  B. Include pancreatitis, trauma, pancreatectomy, carcinoma, cystic fibrosis.
- Endocrinopathies
  A. Several hormones, such as growth hormone, cortisol, glucagons, epinephrine, antagonize insulin action and cause diabetes.

B. Include acromegaly, Cushing syndrome, hyperthyroidism.
- Drug- or chemical-induced diabetes
  A. Chemicals do not cause diabetes but may impair insulin secretion, impair insulin action, destroy beta cells, and precipitate diabetes.
  B. Includes glucocorticoids, thyroid hormone, dilantin, thiazides.
- Infections
  A. Some viruses can destroy beta cells.
  B. Include congenital rubella, cytomegalovirus, mumps.
- Uncommon forms of immune-mediated diabetes.
- Other genetic syndromes sometimes associated with diabetes include Down syndrome, Huntington's chorea, Prader–Willi syndrome.

DIAGNOSIS OF DIABETES

I. SYMPTOMS SUGGESTIVE OF DIABETES

Questions are asked to obtain the risk factors (Box 68-5) and symptoms (Box 68-3 and **Table 68-2**) of diabetes.

II. DIAGNOSTIC TESTS

- Patients with signs or symptoms suggestive of diabetes are referred to a physician immediately for complete evaluation.
A. Criteria for diagnosis of diabetes
  - A1c greater than or equal to 6.5%.
  - Fasting plasma glucose greater than or equal to 126 mg/dl (7.0 mmol/l). Fasting is defined as no caloric intake for a minimum of 8 hours.
  - A 2-hour plasma glucose greater than or equal to 200mg/dl (11.1 mmol/l) during an Oral Glucose Tolerance Test (OGTT).
  - Patient with classic symptoms of hyperglycemia or hyperglycemic crisis, listed in Box 68-3, plus a random (any time of day) plasma glucose greater than or equal to 200 mg/dl (11.1 mmol/l).
B. Criteria 1–3 are repeated in the absence of unequivocal hyperglycemia to confirm diagnosis of diabetes.

COMPLICATIONS OF DIABETES

Patients with tightly controlled blood glucose levels tend to develop fewer complications and later in life than those whose diabetes is less well controlled.[3–5]

I. INFECTION

- Patients are more susceptible to infections and impaired healing, which can worsen prognosis.

- Presence of infection affects blood glucose levels.
- Infections may involve the urinary tract, skin, lungs (pneumonia or tuberculosis), and the oral cavity (opportunistic infections such as oral candidiasis and chronic infections such as periodontitis).
- Failure to treat an infection intensifies the symptoms and increases severity of diabetes; can progress to life-threatening infections or precipitate diabetic coma.
- Insulin requirements may increase with fever, infection, inflammation, trauma, bleeding, pain, or stress. When the condition is eliminated, prescribed insulin may be reduced.
- Numerous factors are involved including impaired immune response, alterations in metabolism of carbohydrate and protein, vascular changes and impaired circulation, and altered nutritional state.

II. PERIPHERAL NEUROPATHY

- Neuropathy can cause pain, numbness, or tingling of mouth, face, and extremities.
- Lack of feeling can delay patient identification of, for example, foot ulceration and infection.
- Leads to increased incidence of amputations and Charcot's joints.

III. AUTONOMIC NEUROPATHY

- Can cause gastrointestinal tract symptoms, such as gastroparesis.
- Food is delayed in the stomach, leading to delay in absorption and complications in managing blood glucose levels.
- Food may harden into masses that can be an obstruction in the stomach or intestines.
- May lead to overgrowth of bacteria.
- Can lead to cardiovascular symptoms, such as:
  A. Hypertension.
  B. Abnormalities in lipoprotein metabolism.
- Can also lead to genitourinary symptoms and sexual dysfunction.

IV. NEPHROPATHY

- Diabetes is a leading cause of renal disease, and the most common cause of end-stage renal disease (ESRD) in the United States and Europe. Dialysis or kidney transplant is needed.
- Patients diagnosed with diabetes are screened for microalbuminuria.

V. RETINOPATHY

- Diabetes is a leading cause of blindness through the progression of diabetic retinopathy.
- Patients are more likely to have glaucoma and cataracts.

VI. CARDIOVASCULAR DISEASE

- Includes:
  A. Heart disease.
  B. Peripheral vascular disease.
  C. Cerebrovascular disease.
  D. Hypertension.
- May lead to myocardial infarction and stroke.
- Due to the excessive risk of coronary heart disease (CHD), aggressive treatment for dyslipidemia (elevated triglyceride and decreased HDL cholesterol levels) is usually recommended.
- Low-dose aspirin therapy may be recommended for prevention of cardiovascular disease in patients with diabetes with increase risk factors. Daily aspirin intake may increase bleeding time.

VII. AMPUTATION

Diabetes is a major cause of limb amputation (usually foot) from possible complications of neuropathy and vascular disease.

VIII. PREGNANCY COMPLICATIONS

Patients with diabetes are at higher risk for spontaneous miscarriages, having babies with birth defects, and increased weight.

IX. PSYCHOSOCIAL

- Complications of diabetes and daily life of patient as well as those close to patient are significantly affected by diabetes.
- Treatment regimens may be challenging to cope with and lead to emotional and social problems, including depression.
- A suggestion for the patient to discuss psychosocial issues with the physician may improve patient's compliance with treatment and daily oral personal care.

X. SILENT KILLER

- Average life span is reduced.
- Diabetes and its complications are leading causes of death.

MEDICAL TREATMENT AND MODIFICATIONS FOR DIABETES CONTROL

There is no known cure for diabetes. Treatment methods depend on the severity of the disease and on the individual. Consideration is given to individualized needs related to age, activities, vocation, lifestyle, knowledge, attitudes, personality, culture, emotional and psychological needs, as well as the health status and nutritional and weight issues of the patient.

I. GENERAL PROCEDURES

- Early diagnosis.
- Patient education for self-care.
- Attain and maintain the best possible overall personal, physical, and psychological health; practice a healthy lifestyle including diet and exercise.
- Maintain tight glycemic control to reduce the complications of diabetes.
- Receive preventive general physical examinations and specialty examinations on a routine basis to identify effectiveness of treatment and early complications of diabetes.
- Seek immediate treatment to manage acute symptoms.
  A. Aggressive treatment of infections.
  B. Eliminate sources of infection, including oral diseases.
  C. Prevent injuries.

II. INSTRUCTION

A. Health Team

- Initial and ongoing individualized education is provided by the health team.
- Members include physicians, registered nurses, dietitians, pharmacists, mental health professionals, dental professionals, and other specialists, such as endocrinologist, cardiologist, ophthalmologist, and podiatrist.

B. Instructional Materials

- *Books and journals.* A number of excellent books, professional journals, and other printed materials have been prepared for the patient and for health professionals. Review of these materials can provide the dental team members with greater insight into the background and knowledge of the patient in preparation for oral health instruction.
- *Internet.* An extensive resource for information, support groups, and products that can be helpful to the dental team, patient, family, friends, and other health professionals. Note strategies to determine validity of information on Web sites are discussed on page 20 in Chapter 2.

III. EXERCISE

- An essential part of the treatment program.
- Contributes to lowering insulin requirements.
- Lowers the cardiovascular risk factors of obesity, inactivity, and LDL cholesterol level.
- Many cases of type 2 diabetes can be controlled with weight reduction and exercise alone.

IV. DIET

Diet counseling is basic and planned by the physician, dietitian, and patient. Diet planning is ongoing and based on individual needs and treatment goals. There is no specific diabetes diet. Healthy, well-controlled individuals can have a diet very similar to a healthy person without diabetes. No foods are prohibited but eaten in moderation at observed times.

A. Goals of Medical Nutritional Therapy[6]

- Medical nutritional therapy is involved in preventing diabetes and managing and slowing the development of diabetes complications through beneficial nutritional interventions.
- Consideration to personal and cultural preferences and maintenance of the pleasure of eating by limiting food choices only when indicated by scientific evidence.

B. Fundamentals of Diet

- Basic diet selection is based on individual quantitative need; may be identical to an individual without diabetes.
- Proper food selection is stressed so adequate calories are provided to attain and maintain ideal body weight and health. High fiber, low fat, low cholesterol, and low sodium to reduce risk of vascular and heart disease.
- Amount of carbohydrates consumed are monitored and controlled with less regard to source. Foods containing high proportions of sugars are used sparingly.
- The obese patient benefits from a weight-reduction diet that is more successful when combined with exercise and behavior modification.
- Food lost, as in vomiting, may affect glucose balance.
- Consistent, specific times for medication and food intake to control blood glucose levels is needed. Usually three on-time meals and three interval feedings are planned.

V. HABITS

A. Tobacco

- Patient must avoid all types of tobacco.
- Smoking is a major health hazard for everyone and is especially dangerous for those with diabetes. It increases risk of heart disease, stroke, myocardial infarction, limb amputations, periodontal disease, and numerous other health problems.
- Refer patient to appropriate tobacco cessation program as described in Chapter 33 on page 489.

B. Alcohol

- Avoid excessive alcohol; alcohol can raise blood pressure and contribute to other health problems.

MEDICATIONS

I. INSULIN THERAPY

All patients with type 1 diabetes require exogenous insulin for survival. Type 2 patients may need to use insulin for control. Insulin available in the United States is manufactured in a laboratory.

A. Types of Insulin

Insulin is classified as rapid, short, intermediate, or long acting based on the onset, peak, and duration of action. The types of insulin and range of peak action are found in **Table 68-3**.

B. Dosage

Depends on the individual.

- *Objective.* Attain optimum utilization of glucose throughout each 24 hours.
- *Factors affecting the need for insulin.* Food intake, illness, stress, variations in exercise, or infections.
- *"Sick Day Rules."* Insulin dose is adjusted if there are any factors that are affecting the need for insulin.

C. Methods for Insulin Administration

- *Subcutaneous injection with syringe.* A syringe is filled from vial of insulin. Injection sites are rotated usually on abdomen, thighs, or upper arm.
- *Insulin pen.* Prefilled cartridge of single type of insulin injected with attached needle. May be disposable or a reusable type.
- *Continuous subcutaneous insulin infusion with a battery-operated insulin pump.*
  - A. The insulin pump delivers preprogrammed continuous basal rate of insulin and bolus doses when needed.
  - B. Offers greater flexibility, smoother control of glycemia, but may increase the risk of hypoglycemia.

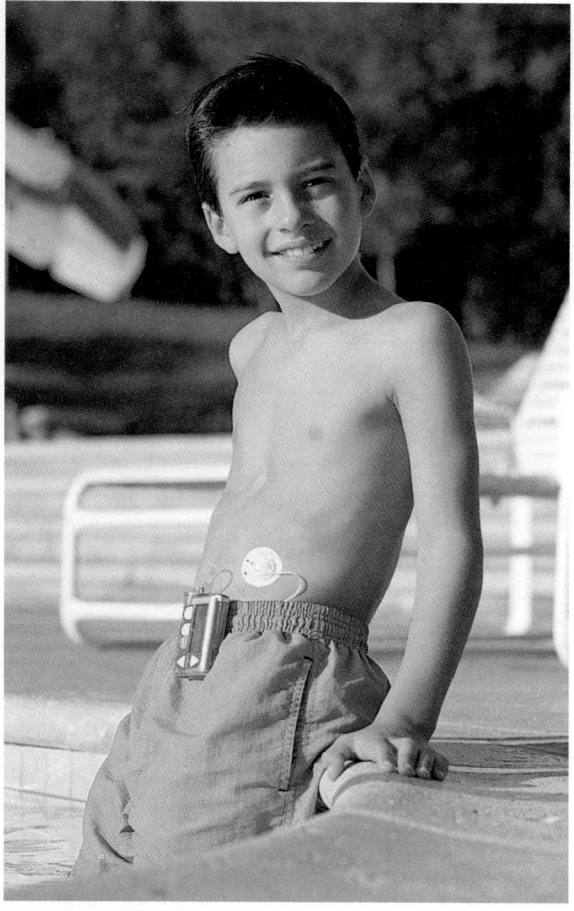

FIGURE 68-2 **Patient Wearing Insulin Pump.** Young boy with active lifestyle wearing an insulin pump. Photo courtesy of Minimed.

  - C. The pager-size pump can be worn in a pocket or on a belt or waistband, as shown in **Figure 68-2**.
- *Inhalable insulin*
  - A. Short-acting, "mealtime" insulin is taken through an inhaler.
  - B. Side effects include lower lung function, cough, dry mouth, or chest discomfort.
  - C. Brand name Exubera™.
- Future modes for insulin administration include an insulin patch, and implantable insulin pumps.

II. ORAL HYPOGLYCEMIC AGENTS

Oral medications are commonly used to treat type 2 diabetes in conjunction with diet, exercise, and possibly the injection of insulin. The medications, listed in **Table 68-4**, may be used individually or in certain combinations.

PANCREAS TRANSPLANTATION

- Pancreas transplantation can be a successful option for treatment of selected patients.
- Successful transplantation has eliminated the need for exogenous insulin in many type 1 patients.

TABLE 68-3	TYPES AND ACTION OF INSULIN	
CLASS OF INSULIN	**TYPE/NAME**	**PEAK ACTION**
Rapid Acting	Lispro, Aspart	30–90 min
Short Acting	Regular	2–3 h
Intermediate Acting	NPH Lente	4–10 h 4–12 h
Long Acting	Ultralente, Glargine	12–16 h
Inhalable	Exubera	30–90 min

TABLE 68-4	ORAL HYPOGLYCEMIC AGENTS USED FOR TREATMENT OF TYPE 2 DIABETES	
AGENT	**EXAMPLE**	**ACTION/FUNCTION**
Sulfonylureas	First generation: chloropamide, tolbutamide, tolazamide, acetohexamide Second generation: glyburide, glipizide, glimepiride	■ Act by stimulating insulin release by the pancreas ■ May cause hypoglycemia
Biguanides	Metformin	■ Prevents liver glycogen breakdown to glucose ■ Increases tissue sensitivity to insulin
Alpha-Glucosidase Inhibitors	Acarbose	■ Slows digestion and glucose uptake into blood
Thiazolidinediones	Rosiglitazone, pioglitazone	■ Increases tissue sensitivity to insulin
Meglitinides	Repaglinide, nateglinide	■ Lowers blood glucose by increasing insulin release by pancreas ■ May cause hypoglycemia
Dipeptidyl Peptidase-4 (DPP-4) Inhibitors	Sitagliptin phosphate	■ Inhibits DPP-IV enzyme, which prolongs active incretin levels. ■ Incretin hormones regulate glucose levels by increasing insulin synthesis and release from pancreatic beta cells and decreasing glucagon secretion from pancreatic alpha cells. ■ Decreased glucagon secretion results in decreased hepatic glucose production.

■ Lifelong immunosuppression therapy is required to prevent rejection and the autoimmune process that may destroy the islet cells again.

■ A complete medical history is confirmed along with any additional recommendations for antibiotic premedication for these patients.

■ Pancreatic islet cell transplantation is experimental at this time and holds hope for the future.

■ Due to the shortage of available human donors, research is underway to develop an implantable artificial pancreas.

■ An artificial pancreas consists of three components: a continuous blood glucose monitor, an insulin pump to deliver the appropriate amount, and a control system to complete a closed feedback loop.

BLOOD GLUCOSE TESTING

■ Blood glucose testing is used to diagnose diabetes and to monitor blood glucose levels.

■ Patients with type 1 diabetes typically do self-monitoring of blood glucose level three or more times per day. Frequency of testing for type 2 patients varies.

■ Blood glucose testing can be accomplished in the dental setting to confirm a safe blood glucose level prior to treatment.

■ Interpretation of routine tests is in **Table 68-5**.

I. SELF-ADMINISTERED TESTS

Self-administered glucose tests also may be sent to a laboratory for analysis and comparison of accuracy of patient's technique.

A. Types of Blood Sugar Level Measurements

■ *Fasting plasma glucose (FPG)*: measurement taken after fasting at least 8 hours.

■ *Postprandial (PP)*: measurement taken after consuming a meal.

■ *Casual plasma glucose*: measurement taken with no regard for time or food ingestion.

B. Tests

■ Blood glucose tests
  A. *Test strip.* Finger prick blood placed on a test strip. Color change of strip is compared to a chart; used at home or in the dental setting.

TABLE 68-5	INDIVIDUAL BLOOD GLUCOSE TEST VALUES RELATED TO CONTROL OF DIABETES		
LEVEL OF DIABETES CONTROL	**FPG**	**PP**	**HbA1c**
Healthy, well controlled	<126 mg/dl	<160 mg/dl	<6%
Moderate control	<160 mg/dl	160–200 mg/dl	6–7%
Uncontrolled	>160 mg/dl	>200 mg/dl	>8%

FPG = fasting plasma glucose; HbA1c = glycosylated hemoglobin; PP = postprandial.

B. *Glucose meter.* Finger prick blood placed on test strip and inserted into the glucose meter; self-monitoring equipment for accurate measurement of blood glucose level; used at home or in the dental setting.

■ Urine ketone test
  A. Objective. To measure ketones; indicates burning of fat instead of glucose.
  B. Use. Used during illness or stress. Performed by patient at home or can be analyzed in a laboratory.

II. LABORATORY TEST

Glycated hemoglobin assay (HbA1c)

■ *Objective.* To measure amount of glucose irreversibly bound to a hemoglobin molecule.
■ *Use.* Value is proportional to blood glucose status over the half-life of the red blood cell; complements daily monitoring and helps predict risk for developing complications by indicating glycemic control over a 2–3 month period so usually performed every 3 months.
■ Along with the FPG, HbA1c has become the measurement of choice for monitoring the treatment of diabetes.
■ Also referred to as glycosylated hemoglobin, glycohemoglobin, A1c test.

ORAL RELATIONSHIPS

The oral cavity of a patient with diabetes may show unusual susceptibility and marked reactions to injury, infections, and all local irritants. Responses are related to lowered resistance and the delayed healing that are especially prevalent in undiagnosed, uncontrolled, and poorly controlled diabetes. Oral findings may be indicative of undiagnosed diabetes and are referred to a physician for evaluation and early detection testing.

I. PERIODONTAL INVOLVEMENT[7,8]

Diabetes increases the risk for periodontal diseases. Periodontal infections may also affect control of blood glucose levels by increasing insulin resistance in a manner similar to obesity. A sudden deterioration of periodontal health may indicate a patient with undiagnosed diabetes or a reduction in the control of a patient's diabetes.

A. Diabetes Effect on Periodontal Disease

■ Marked periodontal disease occurs at young age, and is related to lack of glycemic control. Patients with uncontrolled glucose levels have more severe periodontal disease at younger ages.
■ Diabetes is a conditioning, modifying, and accelerating factor for disease.

■ Inadequate dental biofilm control contributes to more severe tissue response because of decreased resistance.

B. Periodontal Status Effect on Diabetes

■ Poorly controlled periodontal health may alter blood glucose levels. Infection affects insulin requirements and may lead to unstable diabetes.
■ Treatment of periodontal infection and reduction of periodontal inflammation is associated with improved glycemic control through a reduction in level of glycosylated hemoglobin (HbA1c).[9,10]

II. OTHER ORAL FINDINGS

Diabetes does not cause oral disease but may lower resistance and increase susceptibility to the oral findings listed in **Table 68-6**.

TABLE 68-6	ORAL FINDINGS THAT MAY OCCUR WITH DIABETES
LOCATION	**FINDINGS**
Gingiva	Increased gingival inflammation
Periodontium	Periodontitis: more frequent, severe, longer duration Attachment loss: more frequent, more extensive Probing depths: more teeth with deep pockets Alveolar bone loss: more Tooth mobility and migration: increased Healing: delayed, increased infection after surgery
Teeth	Poorly controlled diabetes: increased risk of caries related to decreased saliva, diet, and less successful resolution of endodontic therapy related to decreased resistance to infection Well-controlled diabetes: decreased caries related to low sugar, regular eating habits, dental maintenance appointments
Lips	Dry, cracking, angular cheilitis
Saliva	Decreased flow Glucose in sulcular fluid Xerostomia, contributes to opportunistic infection such as oral candidiasis
Mucosa	Edematous, red Oral candidiasis Burning mouth and/or tongue, burning mouth syndrome Poor tolerance for removable prostheses Delayed healing May have increased prevalence of lichen planus and aphthous stomatitis
Taste	Hypogeusia, diminished taste perception

III. ENDODONTIC INFECTIONS

Patients with diabetes have increased periodontal disease in teeth involved endodontically and have a reduced likelihood of success of endodontic treatment in cases with preoperative periradicular lesions.[11]

IV. DENTAL IMPLANTS[12,13]

- Diabetes that is under metabolic control is not a contraindication for implant placement.
- Patients with diabetes appear to have an impaired bone healing response to implant placement both quantitatively and qualitatively in comparison to the control groups without diabetes.
- Osseointegration can occur in a similar manner for the patient with good metabolic control and the patient without diabetes.

DENTAL HYGIENE CARE PLAN

- The control of oral infections is vital. Infections can progress more quickly and can alter the course and treatment of diabetes.
- Frequent, thorough care, with supervision, is needed and requires the patient's utmost cooperation and motivation.
- The patient with diabetes is prone to life-threatening emergencies.
- Emergency practice drills can help the dental team prevent an emergency, identify early indications of a developing emergency, and act swiftly and appropriately.

I. PATIENT HISTORY

A. Refer for Early Diagnosis

- Questions regarding signs and symptoms of diabetes are basic on any standard medical history

BOX 68-6	Common Medical History Questions to Screen for Diabetes		
■ Have you ever been diagnosed with diabetes?		YES	NO
■ Have any members of your family ever been diagnosed with diabetes?		YES	NO
■ Do you urinate (pass water) more than six times per day?		YES	NO
■ Are you thirsty much of the time?		YES	NO
■ Does your mouth frequently become dry?		YES	NO
■ Have you had any unexplained weight loss?		YES	NO
■ Do you experience excessive hunger?		YES	NO
■ Have you had recent blurred vision?		YES	NO

BOX 68-7	Information to Obtain From Patient With Diabetes

- Adherence to treatments prescribed by health team
- Medications taken on schedule
- Meals and snacks eaten on schedule
- Recent history of glycemic control
- History of hypoglycemia/hyperglycemia and symptoms experienced
- Results of recent blood glucose level testing, including HbA1c
- Symptoms suggestive of the complications of diabetes
- Medical changes, including other recent illnesses
- Current medications, prescribed and over-the-counter, including aspirin
- Other vitamins, homeopathic, or herbal supplements used (check side effects)
- History of exercise, tobacco use, and alcohol use
- Stress such as life, psychological, and social changes
- Date of most recent physical exam and findings

questionnaire. Appropriate questions to ask are listed in **Box 68-6**.
- If an unexplained positive response is present, the patient is referred to a physician for evaluation.

B. Medical History

- Supplement the basic medical history to obtain additional information about diabetes found in **Box 68-7**.
- Update history at each appointment.
- Inquire about recent hypoglycemic reactions: patient who recently had a hypoglycemic reaction may be more likely to have another.
- Identify other health problems or complications of diabetes that may influence dental treatment. Refer to specialist when indicated.
- Ask about exercise and tobacco use; review effect on health.

II. CONSULTATION WITH PHYSICIAN

If unable to obtain complete and accurate information from a patient, or if diabetes is not well controlled, a consultation between dental professional and physician is necessary before treatment.

III. APPOINTMENT PLANNING

Stress, including that created during a dental or dental hygiene appointment, can affect blood sugar levels. Appointment planning centers around many factors, including stress prevention.

A. Antibiotic Premedication

■ *Well-controlled diabetes.* In general, the patient with well-controlled diabetes is treated the same as the patient without diabetes and requires no premedication related to diabetes.

■ *Uncontrolled, unstable diabetes.* Routine dental treatment is deferred until diabetes is stabilized. Only emergency care is given to the uncontrolled patient. Consult patient's physician if question need for antibiotic premedication.

B. Time

■ Treat patient on full stomach.
■ Avoid peak insulin level noted in **Table 68-3**.
■ Ideal time of appointment varies with individual patient's lifestyle and method of insulin intake.
■ Preferred appointment may be morning, soon after the patient's normal breakfast and medication, during the ascending portion of the blood glucose level curve. Note: a patient who eats breakfast at 6 AM does not have a full stomach for a 9 AM appointment.

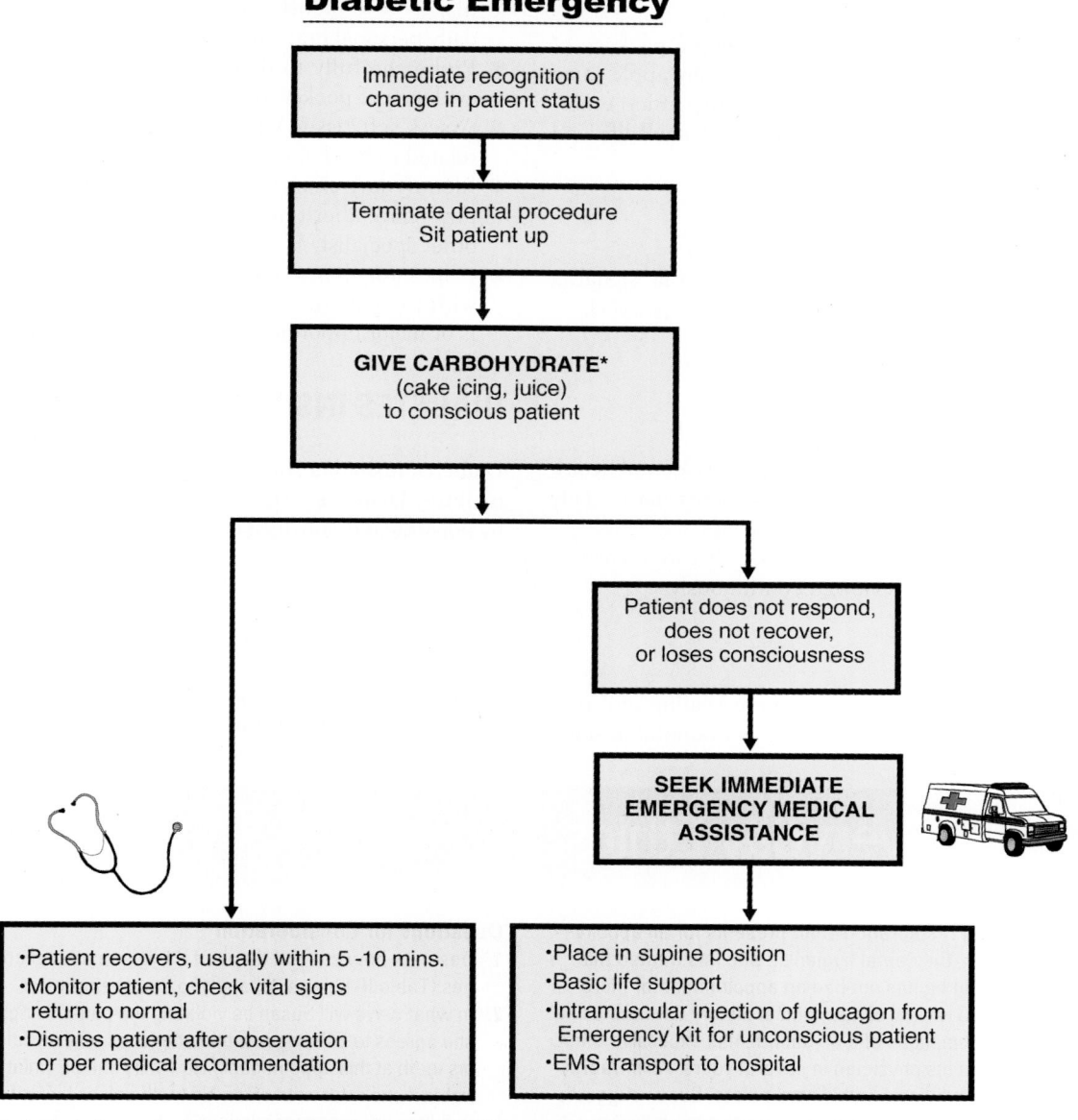

Diabetic Emergency

Immediate recognition of change in patient status

↓

Terminate dental procedure
Sit patient up

↓

GIVE CARBOHYDRATE*
(cake icing, juice)
to conscious patient

↓

Patient does not respond, does not recover, or loses consciousness

↓

SEEK IMMEDIATE EMERGENCY MEDICAL ASSISTANCE

• Patient recovers, usually within 5 -10 mins.
• Monitor patient, check vital signs return to normal
• Dismiss patient after observation or per medical recommendation

• Place in supine position
• Basic life support
• Intramuscular injection of glucagon from Emergency Kit for unconscious patient
• EMS transport to hospital

*Carbohydrate can be given for any diabetic emergency. If hypoglycemia (insulin reaction), patient will have rapid recovery. If hyperglycemia (diabetic coma), there will be no improvement but no worsening of condition. If ketoacidosis or diabetic coma is suspected, seek immediate emergency medical care.

FIGURE 68-3 **Diabetes Emergency Action.** Flow chart to show steps to take when patient exhibits signs of diabetic complications.

■ Alternative appointment time may be after lunch. Always ask if patient has eaten.

C. Precautions: Prevent/Prepare for Emergency

■ Do not keep the patient waiting.
■ Do not interfere with the patient's regular meal and between-meal eating schedule.
■ Avoid long, stressful procedures; dental and dental hygiene care can be divided into short appointments appropriate to the individual's needs.
■ Take additional precautions indicated for the patient with long-term diabetes with complications related to atherosclerosis and other cardiovascular diseases. Needs of the elderly patient may be applied.
■ Prevent and treat all infections promptly.
■ Prepare for diabetic emergencies. Keep a package of glucose gel, cake frosting, or a jar of baby apple juice for the conscious patient as part of the office emergency supplies. These items have a long shelf life and are less likely to be consumed by staff.

D. Emergency

■ Recognize any change in patient behavior that signals a diabetes emergency. Follow flow chart in **Figure 68-3.**

IV. CLINICAL PROCEDURES

A. Dental Biofilm Control Instruction

■ Because of the impact of diabetes on periodontal health and the effect of oral infection on diabetes status, daily meticulous oral personal care is crucial.
■ A biofilm check and individualized self-care measures for biofilm control is reviewed continuously.

B. Instrumentation

■ *Quadrant or area scaling.* Complete scaling and root planing reduces the possibility of periodontal abscess

formation. Allow several short appointments if needed for stress management.
■ *Healing.* Undue trauma to tissues is avoided due to the complications that may be associated with healing

C. Fluoride Application

■ Fluoride treatments, varnishes, and home use of fluoride are encouraged, particularly with xerostomia.
■ Methods for daily self-fluoride application are described in Chapter 35 on page 530.

V. MAINTENANCE PHASE

■ Appointment for supervision and examination on regular 3- to 6-month basis as needed. Effectiveness of daily personal oral care is evaluated.
■ Probe carefully to detect early gingival bleeding and evidence of pocket formation.
■ Assess soft tissue with attention to areas of irritation related to fixed and removable prostheses.
■ Identify any changes that require referral to patient's physician, dietitian, mental health professional, or other specialist.
■ Check for dental biofilm control and review control with the patient at each appointment. Gingival health is of major importance. Keep the patient motivated.

DIABETES INSIPIDUS

Diabetes insipidus should not be confused with diabetes mellitus. Diabetes insipidus is a rare disease characterized by polyuria and polydipsia. It is induced by an antidiuretic hormone defect.

DOCUMENTATION

■ Record status of blood glucose control, including most recent HbA1c and other daily monitoring such

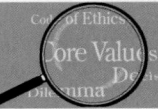
Everyday Ethics

Ed, a 45-year-old restaurant owner, presents for an appointment with Susan, the dental hygienist. She has treated this patient before but he has not had an appointment for more than 2 years. The review of his medical history determines he is overweight, complains of a dry mouth, has excessive thirst, and has not seen his physician in several years. An intraoral exam reveals candidiasis on his hard palate. Susan suggests that he see his physician, but he refuses to even talk about it. He insists that he just wants "clean teeth" for his daughter's upcoming wedding.

Questions for Consideration
1. Describe how each of the dental hygiene ethical core values (Table II-1, page 38) apply to this scenario.
2. In what ways will Susan be violating the patient's rights if she agrees to Ed's request that she focus only on "cleaning" his teeth at this appointment? How may she be violating his rights if she refuses to clean his teeth unless he first agrees to follow her recommendations?
3. Explain choices or alternative actions Susan can consider as she decides how to continue treatment during Ed's appointment unless he first agrees to follow her recommendations.

as fasting, postprandial, or casual blood glucose levels that the patient may have performed.

■ Update current medications and doses.
■ Confirm compliance of medication intake and food consumption.
■ Record patient's status.
■ Record discussion about relationship between oral health status, oral hygiene status, risk factors, and diabetes.
■ **Box 68-8** contains an example progress note for a patient with diabetes.

Factors To Teach The Patient

Factors to Teach Patients With Diabetes
■ Why regular medical examinations are necessary.
■ Why the patient needs to understand status of diabetes, names and doses of medications including over-the-counter medications, and other changes in medical history.
■ How to recognize the early warnings of hypoglycemia and hyperglycemia and know how to treat them.
■ How to control diabetes and blood sugar level through diet, exercise, medications, and glucose monitoring. This may reduce the long-term, life-threatening complications of diabetes.
■ How to prevent and treat the complications of diabetes through regular medical and dental care, eye examinations, blood pressure checks, blood tests for cholesterol, lipids, and kidney readings, and practice self-examination, particularly of feet, for nerve involvement or delayed healing.
■ Why they should seek immediate medical attention for any complications.
■ Factors that affect a healthy lifestyle, including healthy diet, daily exercise, no tobacco products, avoid alcohol, and attain ideal weight.
■ The need to accept assistance for smoking cessation.
■ How to practice meticulous oral hygiene to prevent dental disease and help control blood sugar levels.
■ Ways to reduce stress.

Factors to Teach Patients Not Diagnosed With Diabetes
■ Need for regular medical examinations and screening for diabetes.
■ How to recognize the early warning signs of diabetes and seek medical consult.
■ Factors that affect a healthy lifestyle, including healthy diet, daily exercise, no tobacco products, avoid alcohol, and maintain ideal weight.
■ The need to accept assistance for smoking cessation.
■ How to practice meticulous oral hygiene to prevent dental and periodontal disease.
■ Reduce stress.

BOX 68-8	Example Progress Note: Patient With Diabetes Mellitus

Update on status of diabetes: patient reports the recent daily blood glucose readings indicate moderate control. Most recent HbA1C reading on July 4, = 7.1%. Fasting blood glucose this morning was 111. Patient reports feeling well, took medications and ate breakfast approximately 1 hour ago and is due for snack in 2 hours. Blood pressure 128/80.

Signed: _____, RDH Date: _____.

References

1. American Diabetes Association. Diagnosis and classification of diabetes mellitus. *Diabetes Care*. 2010 Jan;33(Suppl 1):S62–9.
2. American Diabetes Association. Standards of medical care in diabetes—2010. *Diabetes Care*. 2010 Jan;33(Suppl 1):S11–61.
3. Diabetes Control and Complications Trial Research Group. The effect of intensive treatment of diabetes on the development and progression of long-term complications of insulin-dependent diabetes mellitus. *N Engl J Med*. 1993 Sep 30;329(14):977–86.
4. American Diabetes Association. Diabetes control and complications trial research group: hypoglycemia in the diabetes control and complications trial. *Diabetes*. 1997 Feb;46(2):271–86.
5. American Diabetes Association. Implications of the United Kingdom prospective diabetes study. *Diabetes Care*. 2003 Jan;26(Suppl 1): S28–32.
6. American Diabetes Association. Nutrition recommendations and interventions for diabetes. A position statement of the American diabetes association. *Diabetes Care*. 2008 Jan;31(Suppl 1): S61–78.
7. Measley BL, Oates TW. Diabetes mellitus and periodontal diseases. *J Periodontol*. 2006 Aug;77(8):1289–1303.
8. Scannapieco FA. Position paper of The American Academy of Periodontology: periodontal disease as a potential risk factor for systemic diseases. *J Periodontol*. 1998 Jul;69(7):841–50.
9. Teeuw WJ, Gerdes VE, Loos BG. Effect of periodontal treatment on glycemic control of diabetic patients: a systematic review and meta-analysis. *Diabetes Care*. 2010 Feb;33(2):421–7.
10. Faria-Almeida R, Navarro A, Bascones A. Clinical and metabolic changes after conventional treatment of type 2 diabetic patients with chronic periodontitis. *J Periodontol*. 2006 Apr;77(4):591–8.
11. Fouad AF, Burleson J. The effect of diabetes mellitus on endodontic treatment outcome: data from an electronic patient record. *J Am Dent Assoc*. 2003 Jan;134(1):43–51.
12. Kotsovilis S, Karoussis IK, Fourmousis I. A comprehensive and critical review of dental implant placement in diabetic animals and patients. *Clin Oral Implants Res*. 2006 Oct;17:587–99.
13. Javed F, Romanos GE. Impact of diabetes mellitus and glycemic control on the osseointegration of dental implants: a systematic literature review. *J Periodontol*. 2009 Nov;80(11):1719–30.

Emergency Care

LANE WILSON-FOREMAN, CDA, RDH, BS
CYNTHIA BIRON LEISECA, RDH, EMT, MA

Chapter Outline

EMERGENCY PREPAREDNESS

This chapter is designed to help prevent emergencies from escalating into more serious conditions. The more emergency drills practiced the more competent the dental team can become in managing an emergency. Emergencies in the dental office are rare, but the following suggests ways to increase emergency preparedness:

- Public expects competence in emergency situations.
- Periodic review of drills is necessary.
- Equipment is kept in a convenient place.

BOX 69-1	Key Words

Emergencies

Angioneurotic edema: sudden and temporary appearance of large areas of painless swelling in the subcutaneous tissue or submucosa; a symptom related to allergy; also called angioedema.

Arrhythmia: variation from normal rhythm, especially the heartbeat.

Autoinjector: a syringe with a spring-loaded needle that delivers a preloaded dose of medication; often used for self-administration of epinephrine to relieve anaphylaxis.

Basic life support: the phase of emergency cardiac care that supports the ventilation of a victim of respiratory arrest with rescue breathing and supports the ventilation and circulation of a victim of cardiac arrest with cardiopulmonary resuscitation.

Cannula: a tube for insertion into a duct or cavity.

> **Nasal cannula:** a semicircle of plastic tubing with two plastic tips that fit into the patient's nostrils.

Cardiac arrest: sudden and often unexpected stoppage of heart action; circulation ceases and vital organs are deprived of oxygen.

Crepitation: dry crackling sound, such as that produced by the grating of the ends of a fractured bone.

Cricothyrotomy: incision through the skin and the cricothyroid membrane to secure a patent airway for emergency relief of upper airway obstruction.

Defibrillation: termination of atrial or ventricular fibrillation, usually accomplished by electric shock.

Defibrillator: an apparatus used to produce defibrillation by application of brief electric shock to the heart directly or through electrodes placed on the chest wall.

Dyspnea: labored or difficult breathing; indication of inadequate ventilation or of insufficient oxygen in the circulating blood.

Fibrillation: involuntary muscular contraction caused by spontaneous activation of single muscle cells or fibers.

Ventricular fibrillation: a cardiac arrhythmia marked by fibrillary contractions of the ventricular muscle caused by rapid repetitive excitation of myocardial fibers without coordinated ventricular contraction; a frequent cause of cardiac arrest.

Hypoxemia: deficient oxygenation of the blood; insufficient oxygenation of the blood eventually leads to **hypoxia,** which is diminished oxygen to body tissues.

Kussmaul breathing: loud, slow, labored breathing common to patients in diabetic coma.

Orthostatic hypotension: a drop in systolic and diastolic blood pressure due to change in body position, usually from lying back or sitting to a standing position, The resulting reduction in blood flow can cause temporary shortage of oxygen to the brain and a feeling of lightheadedness or syncope.

Parenteral: not through the alimentary canal; administered by subcutaneous, intramuscular, or intravenous injection.

Pruritis: itching

Recovery position: Patient is placed on one side with the top leg bent at the hip and knee to form a right angle. The arm closest to the floor is outstretched above the head so that it will stabilize the upper body, while the bent knee stabilizes the lower body.

Rescue breathing: a rescuer delivers a volume of 800–1200 ml with each ventilation; the exhaled air contains 16–17% oxygen, sufficient for the needs of the victim.

Syncope: temporary loss of consciousness caused by a sudden fall in blood pressure resulting in generalized cerebral ischemia; can have serious consequences, particularly in patients with a cardiovascular disease; commonly referred to as **fainting.**

Trendelenburg's position: the patient is supine with the heart higher than the head on a surface inclined downward about 45°.

Urticaria: vascular reaction of the skin with transient appearance of slightly elevated patches (wheals) that are redder or paler than the surrounding skin; may be accompanied by severe itching; also called hives.

- Quick reference (posted chart) readily available.
- The principal objectives are to include symptoms, equipment needed, and management of common emergencies.
- Key terms and definitions (Box 69-1).

PREVENTION OF EMERGENCIES

I. ATTENTION TO PREVENTION

Prevention of emergencies requires preparedness, alertness, and anticipation. The best way to prevent an emergency is to employ proper patient assessment techniques, including the following:

- Thorough medical history questionnaires.
- Documentation of vital signs at each appointment.
- Documentation of findings on Medical Alert Tags; wrist or ankle bracelet or necklace that provides information on patient's medical condition. Available from Medic Alert Foundation International, Turlock, CA 95380.
- Completion of a physical assessment begins with the first interaction with a patient
  - If by telephone: voice, communication style, attitude.
  - Visual: gait, physical appearance.
  - Handwriting on medical history indicates steadiness, ability to communicate, and education.
  - Extraoral and intraoral examinations.

BOX 69-2 | **Five-Point Plan to Prevent Emergencies**

1. Use careful, routine patient assessment procedures.
2. Document and update accurate, comprehensive patient records.
3. Implement stress reduction protocols.
4. Recognize early signs of emergency distress.
5. Organize team management plan for emergency preparedness.

- Incorporation of proper risk management and stress reduction protocols into the patient care plan.
- Careful review and update of the patient record before each appointment so that preparatory steps can be taken.
- **Box 69-2** suggests a basic five-point plan for emergency prevention.

II. FACTORS CONTRIBUTING TO EMERGENCIES

- Increased number of older patients in society with natural teeth and dental diseases that require invasive procedures.
- Older patients and many other patients are taking medications that interact adversely with drugs used in dentistry.
- More complex dental procedures require longer appointments.
- Increased use of drugs in dentistry.
  - Anesthesia: local, general, conscious sedation.
  - Tranquilizers.
  - Pain medications (CNS depressants).
  - Antibiotics.

PATIENT ASSESSMENT

I. ASSESSMENT FOR ROUTINE TREATMENT

A. First Contact

- Start with the first interaction with the patient.
- Note abnormalities of patient's voice on the telephone during appointment scheduling.
- Assess overall appearance and gait when patient enters the dental office or clinic.
- Document findings in the patient's chart.

B. Parts of the Assessment

- Physical assessment (signs and symptoms).
- Comprehensive medical history.
- Vital signs.
- Extraoral and intraoral examination.
- Comprehensive documentation of findings.

C. Emergency Indicators

Changes in a patient's appearance on the day of an appointment may suggest indicators that encourage preparation for emergencies.

II. THE PATIENT'S MEDICAL HISTORY

A. Update and Document Changes

- Review at each appointment.
- Discuss changes with dental team members who are providing treatment for the patient.
- A comprehensive medical history includes all the items listed in Tables 9-1, 9-2, and 9-3 (pages 123 to 130).

B. Use of Medical Alert Box

- Many dental offices are digital but some are limited to paper records.
- Folders are required for confidentiality and HIPAA.
- Only the patient's name and/or record number may be included on the folder.
- The "Medical Alert Box" includes information that may predispose a patient to a medical emergency before, during or post dental treatment and is located on the first page of the patient chart. Significant items include:
  - physical conditions that may lead to an emergency.
  - diseases the patient has or previously had.
  - medical emergencies the patient experienced previously.
  - medications the patient has taken within the past 2 years.
  - allergies and adverse drug reactions.
  - previous adverse reactions to dental treatments.

III. VITAL SIGNS

- Vital signs are essential to assess a patient's overall health status and to evaluate the severity of a medical emergency.
- A well-prepared dental team takes vital signs routinely, not only during the earliest sign of emergency distress.

A. The Six Vital Signs

Pulse, blood pressure, respirations, temperature, height, weight, and the information from the Medical Alert Tag (bracelet, necklace, anklet) provide essential information for patient care.

B. Baseline Vital Signs

The vital signs taken at a routine appointment are considered baseline. The ranges of vital signs are described in Figure 10-1, page 136.

C. During Emergency

In a medical emergency, the vital signs that are taken are compared to the baseline findings.

- *"Compensating."* In most medical emergencies, patients will experience a "fight or flight" reaction, during which time they are said to be compensating. The vital signs are elevated above the baseline findings.
- *"Decompensating."* The vital signs have fallen below baseline, and the patient could be going into a state of shock.
- *Shock.* A state of lack of perfusion (saturation) of oxygenated blood to all cells of the brain and body. When brain cells are deprived of oxygenated blood, they cease to provide respiratory and circulatory function.

IV. EXTRAORAL AND INTRAORAL EXAMINATIONS

Extraoral and intraoral examinations can provide significant findings that are clues to underlying disease processes that predispose a patient to a medical emergency. Thorough examinations are an integral part of the prevention of medical emergencies.

A. Extraoral

Blood disorders and endocrine disorders may be suspected or discovered from extraoral palpation, skin color changes, abnormalities of the eyes, and asymmetry of the face or neck.

B. Intraoral

Oral manifestations and lesions can be indications of many disease states, such as diabetes, anemia, leukemia, lupus, or HIV/AIDS.

V. RECOGNITION OF INCREASED RISK FACTORS

The carefully prepared and regularly updated medical and personal history, with adequate follow-up consultation with the patient's physician for integration of dental and medical care, can prevent many emergencies by alerting dental personnel to the individual patient's needs and idiosyncrasies. Special needs may include:

- Specific physical conditions that may lead to an emergency, for example, genetic predispositions, seizures, diabetes.
- Diseases for which the patient is (or has been) under the care of a physician and the type of treatment, including medications.
- Allergies or drug reactions or interactions.

STRESS MINIMIZATION

- Stress and anxiety are the basis for many of the common emergencies that occur in a dental office or clinic.

- The clinic atmosphere and the warmth and sincerity of the personnel can help a patient feel accepted and secure.
- The apprehension and anxiety that can be associated with dental treatment compounds the risk factors for medical emergencies.

I. RECOGNIZE THE PATIENT WITH STRESS PROBLEMS

A. Apprehensive about any dental appointment.
B. Elderly patients are prone to medical emergencies, as they may have cardiovascular diseases or other conditions that have or have not been diagnosed.
C. Essential medications: certain prescriptions are required to be taken on schedule or the patient is at risk for an emergency. The medications may cause adverse reactions that can lead to a medical emergency such as orthostatic hypotension.

II. SUGGESTIONS FOR EFFECTIVE COMMUNICATION

Any patient who is apprehensive or medically predisposed to emergencies can be provided with a stress reduction plan. Reduction of stress includes the development of patient rapport through effective communication between the dental team and the patient.

A. Actively Listen to a Patient's Fears

- Develop rapport so the patient senses that the listener is empathetic and interested in alleviating the apprehension.
- Communicate with a patient about fear. A discussion can be very beneficial for emergency prevention.

B. Effects of Fear

Patients who try to repress their fears are more likely to hyperventilate or experience syncopal episodes.

III. REDUCTION OF STRESS

A. Appointment Scheduling[1]

- *New patient.* Initial appointment for a new patient used for consultation and assessment will build rapport and provide opportunity to evaluate the level of anxiety. Stress reduction can be built into treatment appointments.
- *Time of appointment.* Plan in accord with personal health requirements.
- *Waiting time minimized.* First appointment in the morning prevents building of anxiety by waiting all day for the appointment. In addition, anxiety can be decreased by taking the patient into the treatment room immediately and starting treatment promptly.

- *Eating requirements.* Usual mealtime and previous meal checked to prevent hunger anxiety or hypoglycemia.
- *Length of appointment.* Limited to the patient's durability.

B. Medication

- Premedication when indicated and prescribed by the physician or dentist.
- Pain control during treatment.
- Patient's own prescriptions. Patients subject to emergencies are instructed to bring their own prescribed medicines; for example, the patient with asthma or one who is subject to attacks of angina pectoris.

C. Posttreatment Care

- Postcare instructions for prevention and/or relief of discomfort.
- Place a follow-up telephone call to an anxious patient to make certain there were no postoperative complications.

EMERGENCY MATERIALS AND PREPARATION

Organization is a key concept in emergency preparedness. The first steps in preparing for managing emergencies include setting up the emergency equipment and a systematic protocol. Group planning and individual acceptance of responsibility can provide the team with efficiency, composure, and freedom from fear at the time of crisis.

I. COMMUNICATION: TELEPHONE NUMBERS FOR MEDICAL AID

Telephone numbers can be posted near each extension from which outside calls can be made.

- Rescue squads with paramedics (fire, police, flying squad, or 911 in many cities in the United States).
- Ambulance service.
- Nearest hospital emergency department.
- Poison information center: 1-800-222-1222.
- Physicians
  - Patient's physician is listed in the permanent record in a standard, convenient place.
  - Physicians available for emergency calls.

II. EQUIPMENT FOR USE IN AN EMERGENCY

- Every dental office or clinic plans and sets up an emergency kit or cart,[1,2] and everyone in the office becomes familiar with its contents. The kit is kept in order, its contents replenished, and outdated materials replaced as needed.

- The emergency equipment is portable (on wheels), and kept in a place readily accessible to all treatment rooms.
- Materials are plainly marked and kept separate from other office supplies.
- Materials included are selected to accomplish emergency treatment by current methods.
- The items included in the kit imply proper training in their use.
- Members of a team can work out additions to the list in keeping with their training and abilities.
- **Table 69-1**, Emergency Equipment, provides a typical list of essential items.

III. CARE OF DRUGS

- All dental personnel become familiar with the emergency drugs maintained in the particular office or clinic.
- Only specially trained, experienced persons will administer injectable medications.
- The only drugs kept in the dental office are those that the dentist or emergency team is comfortable with and trained to use.[3]

A. Identification

- The purpose and method of administration of each drug is clearly identified on the container.
- Use of a compartmentalized clear plastic cabinet or box can be useful for this purpose because the labels and instructions can be seen from the outside and efficient selection can be made.
- The replacement date appears clearly on each item that has a limited shelf life.
- When narcotics are included in the list of drugs available for emergencies, they are stored in a less accessible place than the emergency kit, and purchased in predosed amounts for specific emergency situations.

B. Record of Drugs

- Label each with information about shelf life and due date for replacement. Example: Nitroglycerin is replaced at 6 months.
- Check weekly to maintain emergency kit in workable order.
- Dispose of an outdated narcotic drug in the presence of a witness to prevent question that the drug may have been stolen. Discard drugs by dumping contents of ampules/vials in a sink drain and place broken drug ampules in a sharps container.
- A complete record of each available drug is kept. The following are recorded:
  - Name of drug
  - Dosage
  - Date purchased

TABLE 69-1	EMERGENCY EQUIPMENT		
EQUIPMENT	**INJECTABLE DRUGS**	**NONINJECTABLE ITEMS**	**SUPPLEMENTARY EQUIPMENT**
Pocket masks for each clinician	Epinephrine	Oxygen	Pen flashlight
Series E portable oxygen tank	Diphenhydramine	Antiplatelet: aspirin	Stopwatch
Low flow oxygen regulator	Cortisone*	Nifedipine*	Scissors
Nasal cannula	Glucagon*	Respiratory stimulant: ammonia vaporoles	Emesis Basin
Simple face mask	Midazolam*	Bronchodilator: albuterol inhaler	Blanket
Nonrebreather mask	Atropine*	Antihypoglycemic for conscious patients: frosting, sugar, glucagon paste	Backboard, 12" × 24", for patients who cannot be moved for CPR
Bag-valve masks adult and pedo		Sterile irrigating solution for eyes	Quick-activated cold packs
Demand valve resuscitator		Vasodilator: nitroglycerine tablets, nitrolingual spray	Medical emergency report form and pen on clipboard
Oropharyngeal airways⁶ sizes: pedo to adult large		Diphenhydramine tablets	Sterile packages of gauze 2" × 2", 4" × 4"
Nasopharyngeal airways⁶ sizes: pedo to adult large			Adhesive bandages
Water-soluble lubricant for insertion of nasopharyngeal airway			Rolled bandage: 1" × 5 yd, 2" × 5 yd
Suction tips (tonsil suction)			Adhesive tape
Sphygomanometer			Inflatable splints
Blood pressure cuffs: child, adult-regular, adult-large			Pillow
Magils forceps			Cotton pliers
Cricothyrotomy equipment*			Thermometer
Syringes: 2–3 ml luer lock tip 21-gauge needles			Betadine wipes
I.V. equipment*			Glucose monitor
Automatic external defibrillator			

*Treatment methods administered only by those who have had advanced medical training.

- Address of source if different from the usual local pharmacy
- Itemized record, signed by the staff member responsible
- Specific entry as each drug is used
- Expiration dates checked at routine intervals

IV. MEDICAL EMERGENCY REPORT FORM

- **Figure 69-1** shows an example of a form that can be used to record the essential information during an emergency.

- Such a form can be filed in the computerized patient record control system to include in patient's permanent record.
- A pad of the forms on noncarbon replication paper (NCR paper) is placed on a clipboard on the emergency cart.
- A copy of the emergency report is given to the EMS personnel to present to those in the emergency room at the hospital or other medical facility when the patient is admitted.

Medical Emergency Report

Patient's Name	*Smith, Joe*	Today's Date	*10/27/20*

Description of incident: *Patient exhibited signs of anaphylaxis after exposure to latex gloves. Urticaria and pruritus were evident on arms, neck and chest. Signs of lip, tongue and laryngeal edema were exhibited with difficulty swallowing and breathing. Quickly explained to patient that he was having an allergic reaction. Patient was immediately given epinephrine (.3mg) via EpiPen autoinjector and EMS was summoned. 50mg of Benadryl and 100mg of Solu-Cortef were also administered IM. Oxygen was delivered by non-rebreather at 15 L/min. Within 5 minutes vital signs and symptoms improved. At 8 minutes vital signs were near baseline. Patient was released to EMS in 15 minutes and transported to the hospital.*

Time of onset		Time EMS summoned		Time EMS arrived		Time patient was released	
Stopwatch	Clock time	Stopwatch	Clock time	Stopwatch	Clock time	Stopwatch	Clock time
0:00 minutes	*10:30 am*	*0:10 minutes*	*10:30 am*	*13:00 minutes*	*10:43 am*	*15:00 minutes*	*10:45 am*

Patient released to: *EMS who transported patient to Tallahassee Memorial Regional Medical Center*

Cessation of breathing: Ø		Cessation of pulse: Ø		CPR initiated: Ø	
Stopwatch	Clock time	Stopwatch	Clock time	Stopwatch	Clock time
N/A	*N/A*	*N/A*	*N/A*	*N/A*	*N/A*

	Initial findings	Stopwatch times	Followup finding	Stopwatch times	Followup finding	Stopwatch times
Blood pressure	*90/60*	*2:15 minutes*	*110/80*	*5:15 minutes*	*120/80*	*8:15 minutes*
Pulse	*50 bpm*	*1:00 minutes*	*68 bpm*	*5:00 minutes*	*72 bpm*	*8:30 minutes*
Respirations	*10*	*1:30 minutes*	*12*	*5:30 minutes*	*16*	*8:00 minutes*
O₂ delivery method	*non-rebreather (15 L/min)*	*1:45 minutes*	*non-rebreather (15 L/min)*	*5:30 minutes*	*non-rebreather (15 L/min)*	*8:30 minutes*

Drugs administered	Route	Dosage	Stopwatch times
Epinephrine via EpiPen ®	*I.M. (Quad)*	*.3 mg*	*0:45*
Benadryl ®	*I.M. (Deltoid)*	*50 mg*	*1:15*
Solu-Cortef ®	*I.M. (Deltoid)*	*100 mg*	*1:30*

FIGURE 69-1 **Sample Medical Emergency Report.** The form is prepared in duplicate. One copy accompanies the patient to the emergency clinic, and the second copy is retained in the patient's dental record file.

A. Purposes

- Organize data collected during the emergency.
- Serve as a time reference during the monitoring of vital signs.
- Prepare a record from which the medical personnel can interpret the patient's condition at the time of transfer from the dental facility.

B. Uses

- Evaluation for planning dental and dental hygiene appointments so that future emergencies for the patient can be avoided.
- Provide a reference in the event legal questions arise. A well-kept record can be vital, and each emergency, however insignificant the incident may seem, is recorded.

V. PRACTICE AND DRILL

A. Staff Instruction

- In an emergency situation, moments count and there is no time for fumbling or discussion.

- Each member of the clinic and office staff is thoroughly familiar with the location, purpose, effect, and application of each item of equipment and its source.
- Each staff member also knows the order of procedures in all types of emergencies, and can assume any role when needed.

B. Assignments

- *Preparation.* The assignment of specific responsibilities during an emergency is the result of planning by the whole team.
- *Substitutions.* Because a staff member may be absent from the scene at the time of an emergency, each person learns and practices the duties for all positions so that substitutions can be made and duties doubled with a minimum of discussion and no confusion.
- **Figure 69-2** shows an example of a possible distribution of duties when three people are available to attend to the patient.
- *Advantages of assignments*
  - Organization efficiently uses personnel.
  - Sharing responsibility relieves pressure.

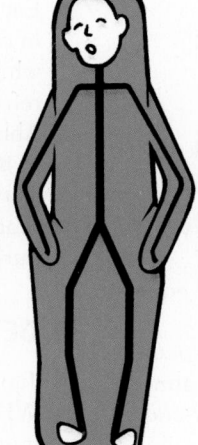

Team Member 2
1. Starts stopwatch
2. Brings cart and oxygen
3. Assists with oxygen
4. Prepares medications
5. Assists Team Leader
6. Assists with CPR

Oxygen

Emergency Kit or Cart

Team Leader 1
1. Provides basic life support
2. Evaluates vital signs
3. Initiates CPR
4. Positions patient
5. Manages airway
6. Directs emergency care
7. Administers oxygen
8. Administers drugs

Team Member 3
1. Calls for medical aid
2. Monitors vital signs
3. Records data
4. Assists Team Leader
5. Suctions
6. Loosens tight clothing
7. Relieves others in CPR

FIGURE 69-2 **Division of Duties for Three-Person Emergency Team.** Suggested distribution of responsibilities to be memorized and practiced by the dental personnel who form the emergency team.

- Duties can be carried out quietly, without excess discussion or attention from others in the clinic.
- Necessary work gets done without duplication and without omissions.

C. Drills

- Regular reviews and rehearsals for each type of emergency are conducted, preferably on a "surprise" basis, at least once a month.
- A specific emergency code call can be used when an intercom or other message system is available. Mentioning "code" in front of a number or phrase may panic the other patients; therefore it is best to use only a number like "17."
- For each type of emergency, practice in the use of procedures, including oxygen administration, resuscitation, and airway maneuvers, as well as specific positioning of a patient for all emergencies, is indicated.
- Equipment and materials can be checked at the time of the drill to ensure their availability and that each is in working order. Outdated supplies can be replaced. One staff member is designated to be in charge of the emergency supplies.
- A record of drills is kept with a diary of dates, procedures practiced, and names of those present.

D. New Staff Member

- Assignment of duties and practice for the new member are a part of the first working day's orientation.
- New members are expected to renew CPR certificates by taking necessary refresher courses within a specified time. Most states require a renewal certificate for annual licensure.
- The American Dental Association Commission on Dental Accreditation (ADA CODA) has established standards that require all clinic personnel to be Healthcare Provider CPR Certified.

E. Procedures Manual

A loose-leaf manual is a valuable study and work reference.

- Reviewed and updated three or four times each year.
- Useful during the orientation of a new member.
- Contains work assignments and checklists for equipment and resources.
- Provides reference information concerning specific emergencies with their symptoms and initial treatment placed in alphabetical order in specially color-coded sections.
- Members of the team keep the manual current by bringing references and notes from readings and courses.

BASIC LIFE SUPPORT

I. PATIENT IN EMERGENCY DISTRESS

The AHA *BLS for Healthcare Providers Manual* is updated regularly to reflect the most current information and BLS procedures to follow when responding to an emergency situation.

This information is based on the 2010 American Heart Association Guidelines for CPR.[4]

- Sudden cessation of effective respiration and circulation are treated immediately.
- Without breathing and heart action, oxygenated blood cannot be carried to the cells and a deficiency occurs quickly.
- The flowchart in **Figure 69-3** shows the steps to take in every emergency.
- *Irreversible brain tissue damage may occur within 4 to 6 minutes in the absence of oxygenated blood perfusion. After 6 minutes, brain damage nearly always occurs.*

A. Assess

- The cause of collapse, respiratory arrest, or cardiac arrest cannot always be determined at the outset.
- Survival rates depend on prompt entry into emergency medical service (EMS) for state-of-the-art medical attention.
- Preliminary assessment of the state of consciousness (response, breathing, and pulse rate) are made immediately, and the EMS activated promptly.

B. Act

- It is necessary to keep calm and act promptly, but not hastily.
- The incorrect procedure may be more harmful than none at all.
- Each member of the dental team participates in courses in emergency procedures and resuscitation techniques while in school and periodically since graduation for refresher, renewal, and updating.
- Abbreviations pertaining to emergency care are listed in **Box 69-3**.
- The steps described are carried out in rapid succession.
- Start a stopwatch **(Figure 69-4)** to assess time accurately during an emergency.

II. DETERMINE STATE OF CONSCIOUSNESS

- Tap and shout "Are you OK?"
- WHEN NO RESPONSE: Have someone call 911 immediately and begin basic life support.[4]
- The acronym CAB (compressions, airway, breathing) identifies the order of actions to take for basic life support.

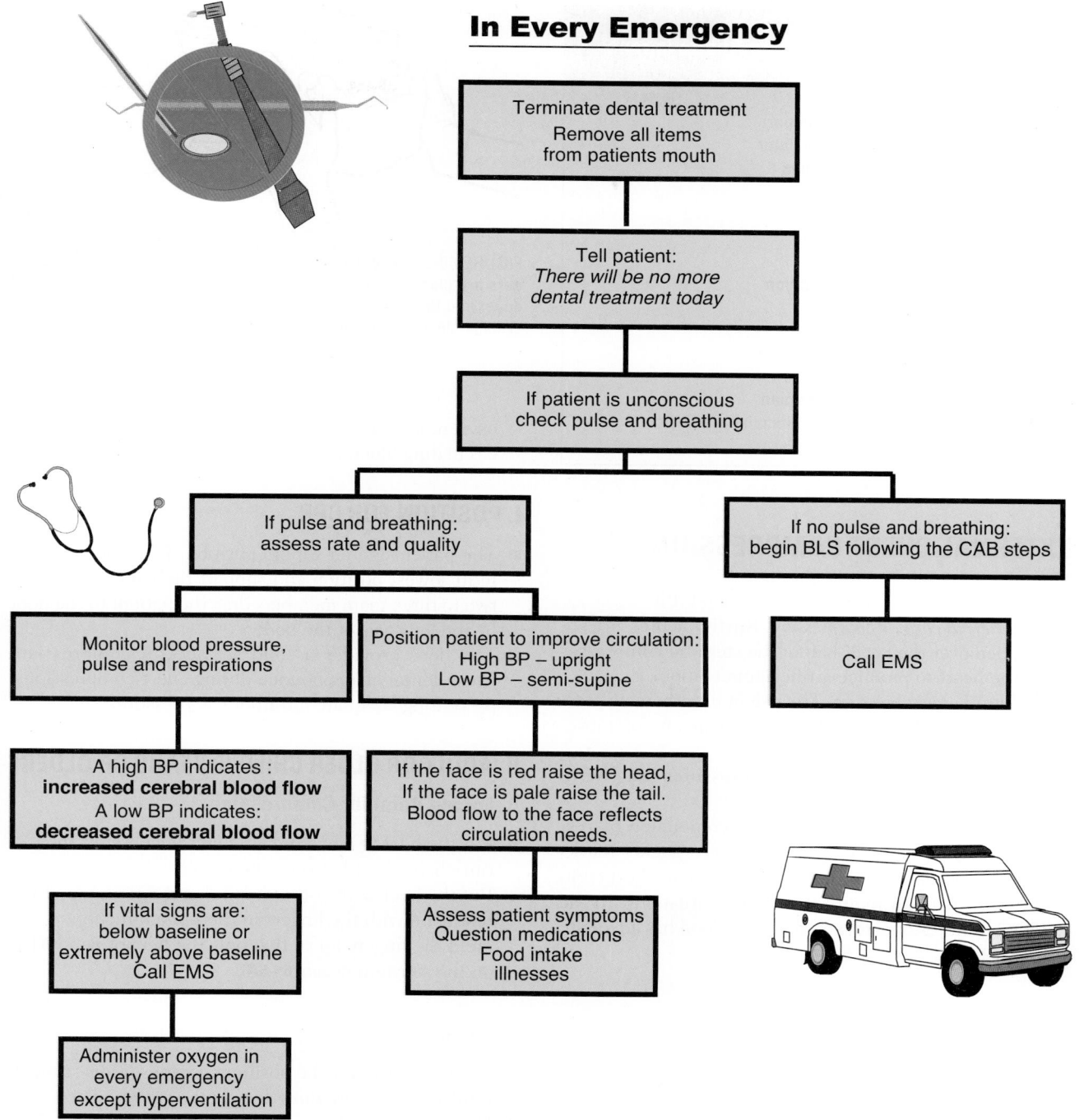

In Every Emergency

Terminate dental treatment
Remove all items
from patients mouth

↓

Tell patient:
*There will be no more
dental treatment today*

↓

If patient is unconscious
check pulse and breathing

If pulse and breathing:
assess rate and quality

If no pulse and breathing:
begin BLS following the CAB steps

Monitor blood pressure,
pulse and respirations

Position patient to improve circulation:
High BP – upright
Low BP – semi-supine

Call EMS

A high BP indicates :
increased cerebral blood flow
A low BP indicates:
decreased cerebral blood flow

If the face is red raise the head,
If the face is pale raise the tail.
Blood flow to the face reflects
circulation needs.

If vital signs are:
below baseline or
extremely above baseline
Call EMS

Assess patient symptoms
Question medications
Food intake
illnesses

Administer oxygen in
every emergency
except hyperventilation

FIGURE 69-3 **Flowchart: In Every Emergency.**

III. CHECK PULSE: BEGIN COMPRESSIONS AND AED

A. Location of Pulse Check

- *Adult.* Carotid pulse in neck (Figure 69-5).
- *Child* (ages 1–8 years). Carotid pulse in neck.
- *Infant* (younger than 1 year). Brachial pulse of the inner upper arm (Figure 10-3).

B. If No Pulse, Begin Compressions and Get the AED Immediately

- 30 chest compressions: 2 breaths until the AED arrives.

PUSH HARD AND FAST (at least 2 inches and 100/minute) AND RELEASE COMPLETELY, MINIMIZE INTERRUPTIONS IN COMPRESSIONS: UNTIL AED ARRIVES.

BOX 69-3	Emergency Care Abbreviations

ACLS: advanced cardiac life support
AED: automated external defibrillator
AHA: American Heart Association
ALS: advanced life support
BLS: basic life support
BCLS: basic cardiac life support
CAD: coronary artery disease
CPR: cardiopulmonary resuscitation
ECC: emergency cardiac care
ECG: electrocardiogram
EMD: emergency medical dispatcher
EMS: emergency medical service
EMT: emergency medical technician
EMT-P: emergency medical technician paramedic

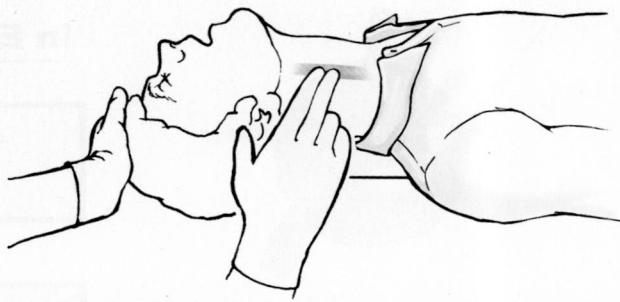

FIGURE 69-5 **Carotid Pulse.** To locate the pulse, two or three fingers are placed on the patient's pharynx. The fingers are then slid down into the groove between the trachea and the neck muscles. With gentle pressure, the pulse can be detected.

EXTERNAL CHEST COMPRESSIONS

- Two mechanisms for blood flow during CPR.
  A. *External cardiac compression.* Rhythmic pressure applied over the lower half of the sternum compresses the heart to produce artificial circulation.
  B. *Intrathoracic pressure.* The rise in intrathoracic pressure provides a significant mechanism for movement of blood to the brain.
- Both cardiac and intrathoracic pressures may be in effect during resuscitation efforts.
- Chest compressions are usually accompanied by rescue breathing, but in situations where pocket masks were not available, rescuers have performed chest compressions without mouth-to-mouth ventilations. In the first 2 minutes of cardiac arrest, the blood has adequate

oxygen, and deep chest compressions are effective at circulating blood to provide perfusion.[5]

I. POSITION FOR CPR

- The patient is in a supine position. Place dental chair in its lowest position and support the patient's head as two to three team members drag the patient to the floor by the long axis of the body.
- The floor provides a solid surface for compression. Most dental chairs bounce during chest compressions, preventing adequate intrathoracic pressure.

II. ADULT OR OLDER CHILD (8 YEARS OR OLDER)

A. Locate Point for Compression

1. Put the heel of one hand (#1) on the center of the victim's bare chest between the nipples.
2. Put the heel of the other hand (hand #2) on top of the first hand with the fingers in the same direction.
3. Hold the fingers up so that only the heel of hand #1 is on the sternum **(Figure 69-6A)**.

B. Compression

1. Lean forward over the positioned hands, arms straight, until shoulders are directly over the sternum.
2. Use a firm, steady, vertical pressure (not a blow). The sternum moves down at least 2 inches **(Figure 69-6B)**.[4]
3. Release pressure but maintain contact and position of the hands with sternum.
4. Compress at a rate of at least 100 times per minute.[4]
   - Make the compressions smooth and uninterrupted, with compression and relaxation of equal duration.
   - Use the natural weight of the upper body to prevent pushing from the shoulders or depending on arm strength.
   - As the heart is compressed between the sternum and the spine, blood is forced out of the heart into the circulation.

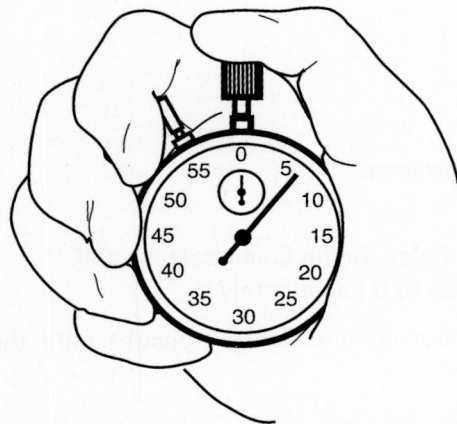

FIGURE 69-4 **Stopwatch.** An essential part of every emergency kit. It is turned on at the onset of an emergency and turned off when the EMS takes the patient to the hospital, or when the medical emergency is over. Time is recorded on the *Medical Emergency Report.*

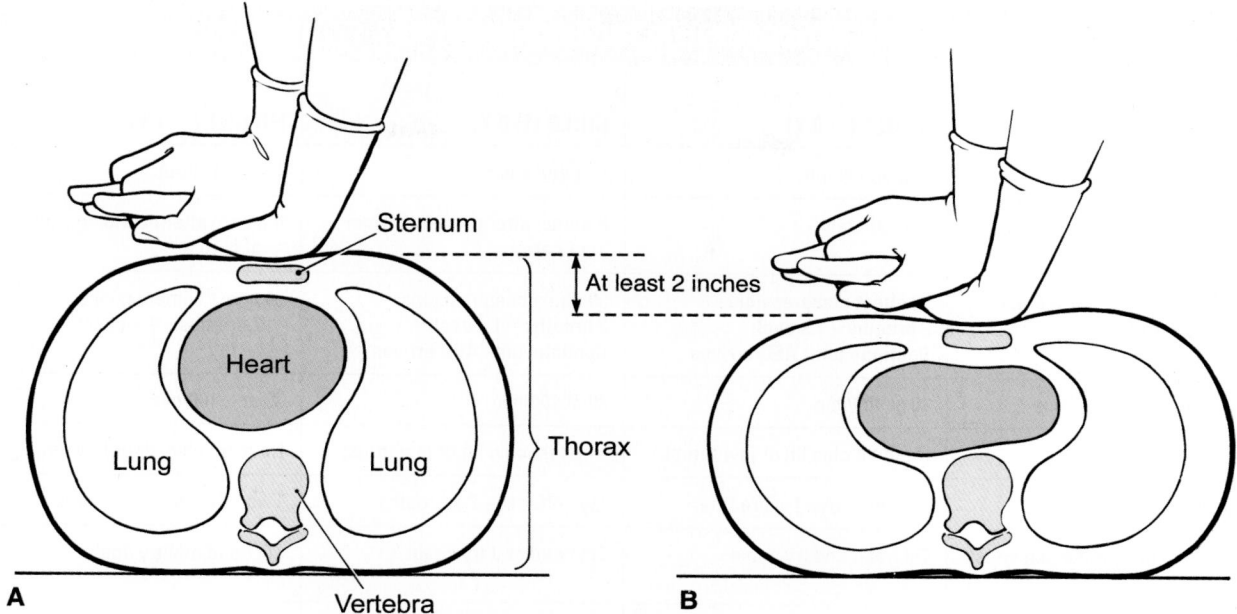

FIGURE 69-6 **External Chest Compression. (A)** Hands in position on the sternum with fingers turned up. **(B)** Application of firm vertical pressure compresses the heart. The sternum is compressed at least 2 inches and then released to allow full recoil. Hands are held in position for the next compression. For all victims, compressions are repeated at a rate of at least 100 per minute.

- Release to allow chest to return to normal level.[4]
- Release of pressure allows blood to flow into the heart.
- Regardless of whether one-rescuer or two-rescuers CPR is being performed, the exact ratio of chest compressions to ventilations is 30:2.
5. When an AED arrives, it is used immediately. See Table 69-2 for a CPR Quick Reference for Healthcare Providers.

III. CHILD (1–8 YEARS OLD)

A. Locate Point for Compression

- Follow the lower edge of the rib cage to the notch where the sternum and ribs meet.
- Place the middle finger in the notch with the index finger beside it.
- Place the heel of the other hand next to the index finger.

B. Compression

- Use the heel of one hand for small child; or two hands, heel of one with second hand on top; compress at least 2 inches.[4]
- Release to allow chest to return to normal level.
- Compress at a rate of at least 100 per minute, using a smooth, even rhythm.[4]
- Keep fingers up, off the chest.

IV. INFANT (UP TO 1 YEAR OLD)

A. Locate Point for Compression

- Place fingers along the sternum, with the index finger just below an imaginary line between the nipples. Lift the index finger. If the fingers are on the xiphoid process, move the fingers closer to the nipples.
- Use the area under the middle and ring fingers.

B. Compression

- One rescuer: compress with two fingers.
- Two rescuers: compress with two thumbs and hands encircling body to a depth of at least 1.5 inches; release to allow chest to return to normal after each compression.
- Compress at a rate of at least 100 per minute, using a smooth rhythm.[4]

V. COORDINATED ACTIVITY FOR CPR

A. Lone Rescuer

- Provide compressions and ventilation.
- *Adult patient*
  - Use ratio of 30 compressions followed by two breaths (1 second each).
  - Compress at the rate of at least 100 per minute (count "1, 2, 3").
  - Continue until AED or EMS arrives.

TABLE 69-2	CPR QUICK REFERENCE FOR HEALTHCARE PROVIDERS		
PROCEDURES FOR HEALTH CARE PROVIDER*	**ADULT (> 8 Y)**	**CHILD (1–8 Y)**	**INFANT (< 1 Y)**
Check responsiveness	Tap and shout	Tap and shout	Tap and shout
If unresponsive: Call EMS and get AED	Immediately	If alone: after providing 2 min of care	If alone: after providing 2 min of care
If no pulse after 10 seconds, begin CPR:	**30 chest compressions: 2 breaths – 1 s each Continue until AED arrives**	30 chest compressions: 2 breaths – 1 s each Continue until AED arrives	30 chest compressions: 2 breaths – 1 s each
C: Chest compressions	30 at 100/min	30 at 100/min	30 at ≥100/min
A: Open airway	Head tilt chin lift or jaw thrust	Head tilt chin lift or jaw thrust	Head tilt chin lift or jaw thrust
B: Rescue breathing	Two effective 1-s breaths	Two effective 1-s breaths	Two effective 1-s breaths
If breath does not make chest rise:	Tilt head and try again	Tilt head and try again	Tilt head and try again
Circulation	Carotid pulse check	Carotid pulse check	Brachial pulse check
Compression landmarks	Center of nipple line	Center of nipple line	One finger width below mammary line
Compression technique	Heel of one hand Interlace fingers of other hand and place on top Push hard and fast	Heel of just one hand or include second hand on top of first Push hard and fast	1 rescuer: 2 fingers 2 rescuers: thumb encircling hands Push hard and fast
Compression depth	At least 2 inches	At least 2 inches	At least 1.5 inches
Compression rate	At least 100/min	At least 100/min	≥100/min
Compression: ventilation ratio	30:2 1 or 2 rescuers Unprotected airway	1 rescuer: 30:2 HCP if 2 rescuers 15:2	1 rescuer: 30:2 HCP if 2 rescuers 15:2
AED	Give 30:2 before AED If shockable rhythm: Give 1 shock then 5 cycles of CPR between each (1) shock	Give 30:2 before AED If shockable rhythm: Give 1 shock then 5 cycles of CPR between each (1) shock	

*The AHA BLS for Healthcare Provider's manual is updated regularly to reflect the most current information and BLS procedures to follow when responding to an emergency situation.

- *Child and infant—single HCP rescuer*
  - Use ratio of 30 compressions followed by two breaths (1 second each).
  - Compress at the rate of at least 100 per minute for a child; minimum of 100 for an infant.
  - Continue until EMS arrives.

B. Two Rescuers

1. *First rescuer* begins compressions, airway and breathing (CAB) treatment as has been described.
2. *Second rescuer* calls for medical assistance and retrieves AED, then promptly takes over compression after first rescuer has completed 2 minutes of compressions.

- Use coordinated rhythm of two breaths after 30 compressions.
- The rescuer at the patient's head maintains the open airway, monitors the carotid pulse, and provides rescue breathing.
- The compressor calls the time for a switch of positions between ventilation and compression.
- Always finish the cycle with a ventilation.
- Start the cycle with compressions.

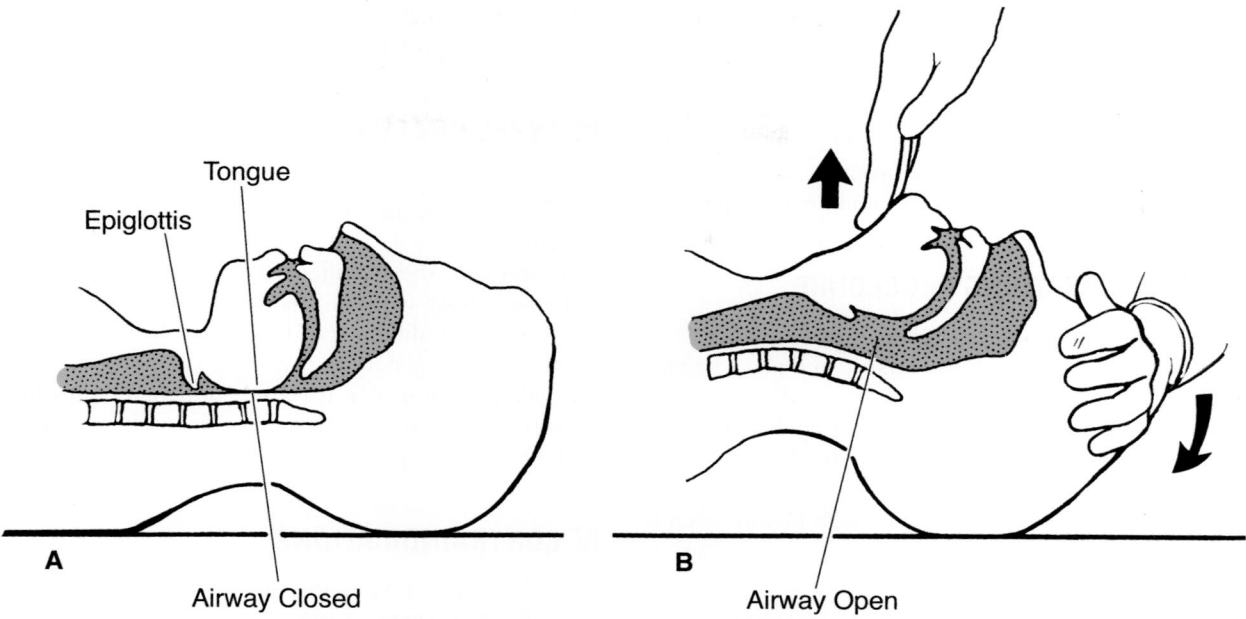

Tongue

Epiglottis

A

Airway Closed

B

Airway Open

FIGURE 69-7 **Chin Lift to Open Airway. (A)** Unconscious person with tongue falling back against posterior wall of pharynx and obstructing the air passage. **(B)** Head is tilted back and chin is lifted by light pressure under the mandible. When neck injury is suspected, a jaw thrust is used. See text for instructions.[6]

VI. LENGTH OF TREATMENT

- *Signs of recovery*: normal skin color returns, patient may gasp or show other sign of breathing, and the body may move or wiggle.
- Do not stop heart compressions while patient is being transported to the hospital.
- *Do not leave patient* when circulation and breathing appear to have returned.
- Watch for need to continue resuscitation in case of relapse. Place the patient in the "Recovery Position."

VII. SEQUELAE

Cardiopulmonary resuscitation is continued until medical assistance arrives or the patient begins to recover. Continue resuscitation while the patient is transported to a hospital.

- For emergencies that do not require hospitalization, the patient can be moved to a couch for rest but is watched carefully.
- Determine the cause of the emergency and need for additional treatment if indicated.
- Send the *Medical Emergency Report* with monitored vital signs with the patient to the medical care facility for reference by the persons assuming responsibility.
- The copy or computer printout is for the patient's permanent record file, and is marked clearly with recommendations for prevention of future emergencies.

RESCUE BREATHING

I. CLEAR THE MOUTH

- Turn the patient's head to the side to clear the mouth of mucus, vomitus, and other foreign material.
- Use suction, gauze, and finger.
- Dentures are left in place to provide support unless the dentures are very loose and could cause throat obstruction if displaced.

II. OPEN AIRWAY

- If breath does not make chest rise, retilt the head and try another breath.
- If the breath still does not make the chest rise, assume the airway is obstructed.
- Give cycles of 30 chest compressions, look for an object in the mouth, remove any visible object, and give 2 breaths.

A. Head Tilt With Chin Lift or Jaw Thrust

- Place palm of hand on the forehead to apply a backward pressure.
- Place fingertips (not thumb) of other hand under the chin with light pressure on the mandible to bring the chin up **(Figure 69-7)**.

B. Modified Jaw Thrust

- Indication. When a neck or spinal injury is suspected, the airway can be opened without extending the neck.

- DO NOT use head tilt/chin lift maneuver when spinal injury is suspected.
- Procedure
  1. From over the top of the head, place thumbs on zygomas and grasp angles of the mandible with fingertips.
  2. Lift fingers upward to open airway.
  3. Never tilt the head when spinal injury is suspected.

III. RESCUE BREATHING PROCEDURE

- Place resuscitation mask on patient.
- Hold with thumbs (on sides of mask) and place fingers on the border of the ramus to obtain a seal.
- Apply modified jaw thrust to open airway if necessary.
- Deliver two breaths (1 second each breath).
  - Avoid giving full, deep breaths.
  - For child or infant, use only enough breath volume for chest to rise.

IV. REPEAT THE BREATHS (VENTILATIONS)

- Provide two breaths following each cycle of 30 chest compressions.
- Rescue breathing is considered effective when the patient's chest rises with each breath.

DEFIBRILLATION WITH THE AUTOMATIC EXTERNAL DEFIBRILLATOR (AED)

I. INDICATIONS

- Patients who are in cardiac arrest have an initial rhythm of ventricular fibrillation (VF), which is an erratic rhythm that is ineffective at producing normal contractile force of the ventricles.
- Purpose: Electrical defibrillation interrupts VF, establishing a normal sinus rhythm.
- Without defibrillation intervention, VF shifts to asystole (no rhythm) in a matter of minutes.
- For every minute that defibrillation is delayed, survival from cardiac arrest declines by as much as 10%. This is why it is crucial to begin using the AED as soon as it arrives.[4]

II. PROCEDURE

- Adhesive electrode pads are placed on the patient.
- AED will advise the rescuer to press the "shock" button to defibrillate the heart, or the AED voice prompt will say "shock not indicated."
- The AED analyzes the ECG signals to determine if the patient's heart is in VF, ventricular tachycardia (VT), or pulseless.
- If the heart has a normal rhythm, the AED will advise the rescuer.

- After each single shock, continue with CPR for 2 minutes before pressing shock button again.

III. TYPES OF AEDS

- Many commercial AEDs are available for dental offices, physician's offices, airlines, and public health centers.
- Training on the specific AED purchased is necessary. Being familiar with the emergency equipment available increases confidence and accuracy in managing any medical emergency.
- A defibrillator may be used only by dental professionals who are trained in a special program on how to use the defibrillation equipment.

IV. CONTRAINDICATIONS

The AED may not be indicated or effective in some situations. Examples are:

- The patient is less than 1 year old.
- The patient is in or near some type of puddle or standing water.
- The patient has an implanted pacemaker or defibrillator.
- The patient has a transdermal patch in the place where the electrode pads are to be placed.
- The patient has hair on the area where the electrode pads are to be placed and the hair interferes with the adhesion of the pads.
- The patient is perspiring so much that the skin is too wet for the electrode pads to properly adhere to the skin.

AIRWAY OBSTRUCTION

A procedure for subdiaphragmatic abdominal thrusts, the Heimlich maneuver, is recommended for removal of a foreign body obstructing an airway in adults and children.

I. PREVENTION

With thought and planning, care can be exercised to prevent aspiration of objects by a patient during a dental or dental hygiene appointment. A few of the procedures that contribute to safety are as follows:

- Place the patient in supine position during examination and treatment. The throat is closed (**Figure 69-7**).
- Use a rubber dam for all appropriate procedures.
- Use a length of floss to tie to small objects, such as a rubber dam clamp or a bite block. Floss hangs out from angle of lips.
- Use a low-speed handpiece to prevent splashing or spinning masses of agents into the throat.

- Have assistant use an aspirator for various procedures that involve large pieces of calculus, copious blood clots, excess saliva, excess water for ultrasonic scaling, restorative materials, and other potentially inhalable items.
- Pay attention to mobile permanent or exfoliating primary teeth that could be inadvertently displaced.

II. RECOGNITION OF AIRWAY OBSTRUCTION

- *Immediate recognition is essential.*
- Differentiation from other emergencies, such as fainting, heart attack, or stroke, in which a sudden respiratory failure may also occur, may be necessary when no object or material was involved that could have been inhaled.
- When no doubt exists that an object has been inhaled, medical aid is obtained.
- A radiograph may be needed to confirm the location of a radiopaque object.

A. Signs and Symptoms of "Mild" Obstruction

- Good air exchange.
- Coughing and irregular breathing.

B. Signs of "Severe" Obstruction

- Poor air exchange.
- Breathing difficulty, or inability to speak or breathe.
- Silent cough.
- Cyanosis.

III. OUTLINE OF TREATMENT

- *An airway established within 4 to 6 minutes prevents possible brain damage from oxygen deficiency.*
- With total obstruction, the patient may become unconscious within a few seconds.
- Treatment begins with the CAB of Basic Life Support, unless inhalation of a specific item was observed.
- When the inspiration is known, the rescuer can proceed directly to attempt to dislodge the obstructing object.

A. Conscious Adult Patient With "Mild" Airway Obstruction

- Good air exchange, let patient cough.
- Object may become dislodged; follow up with medical examination.

B. Conscious Adult Patient With "Severe" Airway Obstruction

- Ask one question, "Are you choking?"

- If the victim nods yes, proceed with airway obstruction management.

IV. FOREIGN BODY AIRWAY OBSTRUCTION (FBAO)

- Manual thrusts are made to the upper abdomen or, in selected cases, the chest. The abdominal thrust is never used during pregnancy.
- The thrusts are given to provide pressure against the diaphragm that compresses the lungs. In turn, the pressure in the lungs is increased, thereby forcing air through the trachea and perhaps forcing out the obstructing object.

A. Patient Standing or Sitting: Conscious

- From behind, wrap the arms around the waist of the patient. Make a fist.
- Hold thumb side of the fist on the patient's upper abdomen above the navel and below the xiphoid. Grab the fist with the other hand.
- Press the fist into the abdomen with quick upward thrusts until the object is dislodged, or the patient may become unconscious.

B. Patient in Supine Position: Unconscious

- Open the airway
- Stand beside and facing the head of the chair when the patient is in the dental chair. On the floor, a more direct thrust can be applied from astride the patient.
- Hold the heel of one hand over the upper abdomen, with the other hand on top.
- Apply 5 quick upward thrusts followed by a finer sweep and several ventilations.
- If no airway: Repeat abdominal thrusts, finger sweeps, and ventilations.

V. CHEST THRUST

The chest thrust is not used routinely but is recommended only when it is not possible to use the abdominal thrust, such as during pregnancy and for very obese individuals.

A. Patient Standing or Sitting With Clinician Behind Patient

- From behind, wrap arms around the chest of the patient at level of armpits.
- Make a fist. Position the thumb side of the fist on the sternum. The thrust is not made on the ribs or on the xiphoid because fracture is possible.
- Grasp the fist with the other hand and apply quick backward thrusts.

B. Patient in Supine Position

- Open the airway.
- Position hands on the lower sternum in the same position as for external cardiac compression (**Figure 69-6**).
- Apply quick downward thrusts.

VI. IN THE EVENT OF UNCONSCIOUSNESS

- If the patient becomes unconscious due to FBAO, CPR is provided without the extra step of abdominal thrusts.
- Chest compressions performed during CPR increase intrathoracic pressure equal to or greater than abdominal thrusts.[6]
- Before ventilations are performed, the oral cavity is checked for the foreign object.[6]
- When object is visible, it is removed with a finger sweep; if it is not visible, CPR is continued.[6]

VII. INFANT

A. Conscious

- If good air exchange, "*mild*" obstruction, encourage coughing.
- If poor air exchange, "*severe*" obstruction, proceed with airway obstruction management.
- Hold the infant face down over the forearm, with the head supported in the hand. Head is lower than the body.
- Apply up to five back blows with the heel of the hand, between the infant's shoulder blades.
- Turn the infant over by placing the free arm over the back and supporting the infant's head with the hand. Place the infant across the thigh with the infant's head lower than its body.
- Apply five chest thrusts. The point of pressure is the same as for external cardiac compression in the infant.
- Repeat back blows and chest thrusts until object is dislodged or infant becomes unconscious.

B. Unconscious

- Begin CPR.
- **Call EMS**.
- Before ventilations look in mouth for object; if visible, use a finger sweep to remove it.
- If object not removed, continue CPR.[5]

OXYGEN ADMINISTRATION

- Oxygen is useful in most emergencies.
- High concentration of oxygen is contraindicated for chronic obstructive lung diseases, especially emphysema.

- Oxygen is also not indicated in the presence of hyperventilation because the patient is receiving increased amounts of oxygen in air inhaled and is in need of carbon dioxide.
- The use of oxygen is beneficial in all other emergencies.
- When the patient is not breathing, positive pressure oxygen (also known as demand valve resuscitator) delivery is needed.

I. EQUIPMENT

Oxygen delivery systems with indications, flow rate, and percentage of oxygen delivered are shown in **Table 69-3**.

A. Parts

Oxygen resuscitation equipment consists of the following:

- An oxygen tank
- A reducing valve
- A flow meter
- Tubing
- Mask
- A positive pressure bag

The *E* cylinder, which can provide oxygen for 30 minutes, is the minimum size recommended. Smaller tanks provide little oxygen for short periods only, and larger tanks are less portable.

B. Directions

Box 69-4 outlines the steps for operation of an oxygen tank. Clear, readable directions are permanently attached to the tank's portable carriage. Practice is a definite part of team drills.

II. PATIENT BREATHING: USE SUPPLEMENTAL OXYGEN

- Apply a full-face clear mask or a nasal cannula.
- Supplemental oxygen is started at 4 to 6 l per minute.
- Monitor breathing; if breathing stops, proceed with positive pressure oxygen.

III. PATIENT NOT BREATHING: USE POSITIVE PRESSURE

For persons not trained in the use of the bag-valve-mask or positive pressure delivery, a mouth-to-mask procedure is used.

- Apply full-face clear mask so that a tight seal is formed. One dental team member may need to apply pressure to the facemask to maintain a complete seal.
- Adjust oxygen flow so that the positive pressure bag remains filled.

TABLE 69-3	OXYGEN DELIVERY SYSTEMS		
DEVICE	**INDICATIONS**	**FLOW RATE**	**OXYGEN DELIVERY**
Cannula	For patient who is breathing and needs low levels of oxygen	2–6 l/min	25–40%
Face Mask	For patient who is breathing and needs moderate levels of oxygen: ■ When cannula is not tolerated ■ When more oxygen is desired ■ Patient is in shock	8–12 l/min	60%
Nonrebreather Mask	For patient who is breathing and needs high levels of oxygen: ■ Patient is in shock ■ When more oxygen is desired	10–15 l/min	60–90%
Bag Mask	When patient has stopped breathing; bag mask is used instead of mouth-to-mouth resuscitation	10–15 l/min	90–100%
Demand Valve Resuscitation	Positive pressure delivery of oxygen on demand	Used by EMTs or others professionally trained	100%

LAMINATE AND AFFIX TO THE OXYGEN TANK.

■ Compress the bag manually, one ventilation every 5–6 seconds to provide 10–12 respirations per minute for an adult. For a child, 1 ventilation every 3 seconds.
■ Watch chest rise. When the chest does not rise, recheck airway for obstruction. Proceed with airway obstruction management.
■ *Call EMS.*

BOX 69-4	Operation of Oxygen Tank

TO TURN ON:
1. Attach oxygen delivery system to tank.
2. Turn **key** on top of tank in *counterclockwise direction* to open flow of oxygen.
3. Read **Low Flow Regulator Knob:**
   To increase O₂ flow: turn the knob in the direction the arrow indicates. (Many regulators are the opposite of sink faucets and open clockwise instead of counter-clockwise.)
4. Attach oxygen delivery system from patient.

TO TURN OFF:
1. Remove oxygen delivery system from patient.
2. Turn **key** on top of tank in *clockwise direction* to shut off flow of oxygen.
3. Turn the **Low Flow Regulator Knob** to open position to bleed oxygen from the system.
4. After bleeding, gently close the **Low Flow Regulator Knob.**

LAMINATE AND AFFIX TO OXYGEN TANK

SPECIFIC EMERGENCIES

Certain systemic disease conditions and physical injuries require specific treatment during an emergency. In **Tables 69-4** and **69-5**, the *Emergency Reference Charts*, several conditions are listed with their symptoms and treatment procedures. Some of the same conditions have been described in detail in Section VIII of this book.

DOCUMENTATION

All details about the patient, the treatments, reactions, healing, and comments by the patient, provide crucial information in a medical emergency or posttreatment complication.

I. COMPREHENSIVE RECORD KEEPING

■ All medical findings and changes.
■ Treatments provided, including types and amounts of local anesthesia, general anesthesia, nitrous oxide, or other types of sedation.
■ Regimens of medications prescribed for patients are crucial information should a medical emergency or a posttreatment complication occur.

II. CONSULTS

In the patient's record, document telephone and written responses of consultations with physicians.

(continued page 1082)

TABLE 69-4	EMERGENCY REFERENCE CHART: MEDICAL EMERGENCIES

EMERGENCY	SIGNS/SYMPTOMS	PROCEDURE

All Cases
Call EMS immediately
  if problem with:
  Breathing
  Unconsciousness
  Anaphylaxis
  Bleeding
  Poisoning
  Chest Pain
		I. Determine consciousness (tap and shout): yell for help.
		If patient is unconscious: Call EMS and get AED
		II. Conduct primary assessment:
		  C. Circulation: Check for pulse for 10 s, if none: Start CPR.
		  A. Airway: open with head tilt-chin lift.
		  B. Breathing: (look, listen, feel) if none: Give 2 (1-s) breaths.
		  D. Defibrillate: 1 shock: then 5 cycles of CPR.
		If patient is breathing and conscious:
		III. Conduct secondary assessment:
		  A. Evaluate level of consciousness.
		    1. Does patient know own name, location, date?
		    2. Use penlight to see if pupils react equally to light.
		    3. If conscious: check for equal hand strength by asking patient to squeeze your hands.
		    4. Position according to signs/symptoms.
		      If face is red, raise the head.
		      If face is pale, raise the tail.
		    5. Evaluate heart rate, blood pressure, respirations.
		  B. Findings in patient record or medical alert bracelet
		    1. Disabilities, diseases, drugs, baseline vital signs:
		    Call EMS.

Respiratory Failure	Labored or weak respirations or cessation breathing Cyanosis or ashen-white with blood loss Pupils dilated Loss of consciousness	Position: semi-supine if not breathing; upright if breathing. Check for and remove foreign material from mouth. Establish airway. Rescue breathing: Adult: initially give 2 breaths of 1 second each followed by 1 breath every 5 s. Infant to child: initially give 2 breaths of 1 second each followed by 1 breath every 3 s. If patient does not spontaneously breathe: **Call EMS.** Monitor vital signs: blood pressure, pulse, respirations. Administer oxygen by nonrebreather mask if patient is already breathing.
Mild Airway **Obstruction**	Good air exchange, coughing, wheezing (patient can speak)	Sit patient up. Loosen tight collar, belt. No treatment; let patient cough.
Severe Airway **Obstruction**	Poor air exchange; noisy breathing; weak, ineffective cough; difficult respirations; gasping. Unable to speak, breathe, cough. Cyanosis, dilated pupils	Reassure patient. Treat for complete obstruction. **Conscious patient** Perform Heimlich maneuver. Patient becomes unconscious: **Begin CPR.** **Unconscious patient** **Call EMS.**
Hyperventilation **Syndrome**	Light-headedness, giddiness Anxiety, confusion Dizziness Overbreathing (25–30 respirations/min) Feelings of suffocation Deep respirations Palpitations (heart pounds) Tingling or numbness in the extremities	Terminate oral procedure. Remove rubber dam and objects from mouth. Position upright. Immediately tell patient: "There will be no more dental treatment today." Loosen tight collar. Reassure patient. Explain overbreathing; request that each breath be held to a count of 10. Ask patient to breathe deeply (7–10 per min) into a paper bag adapted closely over nose and mouth. Never use a bag for a patient with diabetes or patients exhibiting signs of diabetic coma, e.g., fruity breath odor, Kussmaul breathing, lethargy, dry skin.

(*continued*)

TABLE 69-4	EMERGENCY REFERENCE CHART: MEDICAL EMERGENCIES *(Continued)*

EMERGENCY	SIGNS/SYMPTOMS	PROCEDURE
Heart Failure	Difficult or labored breathing Pulmonary congestion with cough and difficulty breathing May cough up pink sputum Rapid, weak pulse Dilated pupils May have chest pain	Place patient in upright position. **Call EMS.** Make patient comfortable: cover with blanket. Administer oxygen by nonrebreather mask. Reassure patient. Basic life support.
Cardiac Arrest	Skin: ashen gray, cold, clammy No pulse No heart sounds No respirations Eyes fixed, with dilated pupils; no constriction with light Unconscious	**Call EMS.** Check oral cavity for debris or vomitus; leave dentures in place for a seal. **Begin CPR.**
Asthma Attack	Difficulty breathing, wheezing, (extreme cases—silence, indicating little to no air exchange) Cyanosis Dilated pupils Confusion due to lack of oxygen Chest pressure Sweating	Position patient upright with arms up and supported forward. Assist with patient's own bronchodilator. Administer supplemental oxygen by nasal cannula. Epinephrine if patient decompensates. Supplemental cortisone to patients who are or have been on corticosteroid therapy. Basic life support—may need demand valve resuscitator if patient experiences respiratory depression. **Call EMS.**
Syncope (Fainting)	Pale gray face, anxiety Dilated pupils Weakness, giddiness, dizziness, faintness, nausea Profuse cold perspiration Rapid pulse at first, followed by slow pulse Shallow breathing Drop in blood pressure Loss of consciousness	Position: Trendelenburg. Open airway. Loosen tight collar, belt. Place cold, damp towel on forehead. Crush ammonia vaporole under patient's nose. Keep warm (blanket). Monitor vital signs: blood pressure, pulse, respirations. Keep airway open. Administer oxygen by nasal cannula. Keep in supine position 10 min after recovery to prevent nausea and dizziness. Reassure patient, especially during recovery.
Shock	Skin: pale, moist, clammy Rapid, shallow breathing Low blood pressure Weakness and/or restlessness Nausea, vomiting Thirst, if shock is from bleeding Eventual unconsciousness if untreated	Position: Trendelenburg Open airway. Keep quiet and warm. Monitor vital signs: blood pressure, respirations, pulse. Keep airway open. Administer oxygen by nonrebreather bag. If patient does not recover fully and/or vital signs not at baseline: **Call EMS.**
Stroke (Cerebrovascular Accident)	*Premonitory* Dizziness, vertigo Transient paresthesia or weakness Transient speech defects Serious Headache (with cerebral hemorrhage) Breathing labored, deep, slow Chills Paralysis one side of body Nausea, vomiting Convulsions Loss of consciousness (slow or sudden onset)	**Conscious patient** **Call EMS.** Turn patient on paralyzed side; semi-upright. Loosen clothing about the throat. Reassure patient; keep calm, quiet. Monitor vital signs: blood pressure, pulse, respirations. Administer oxygen by nasal cannula. Clear airway; suction vomitus because the throat muscles may be paralyzed. **Unconscious patient** Position: supine Basic life support Cardiopulmonary resuscitation if indicated

TABLE 69-4	EMERGENCY REFERENCE CHART: MEDICAL EMERGENCIES *(Continued)*

EMERGENCY	SIGNS/SYMPTOMS	PROCEDURE
Cardiovascular Diseases	Symptoms vary depending on cause	**For all patients** **Call EMS.** Be calm and reassure patient. Keep patient warm and quiet; restrict effort. Always administer oxygen when there is chest pain.
Angina Pectoris	Sudden crushing, paroxysmal pain in sub-sternal area Pain may radiate to shoulder, neck, arms Pallor, faintness Shallow breathing Anxiety, fear	Position: upright, as patient requests, for comfortable breathing. If patient has been diagnosed with angina and has own nitroglycerine: Place nitroglycerin sublingually only when the blood pressure is at or above baseline. Administer oxygen by nasal cannula. Reassure patient. Without prompt relief from nitroglycerin: **Call EMS.** Treat as a myocardial infarction.
Myocardial Infarction (Heart Attack)	Sudden pain similar to angina pectoris, which may radiate, but of longer duration Pallor; cold, clammy skin Cyanosis Nausea Breathing difficulty Marked weakness Anxiety, fear Possible loss of consciousness	**Call EMS** Position: with head up for comfortable breathing. Symptoms are not relieved with nitroglycerin. Administer 162–325 mg of chewable aspririn.[6] Monitor vital signs: blood pressure, pulse, respirations. Administer oxygen by nonrebreather bag. Alleviate anxiety; reassure.
Adrenal Crisis (Cortisol Mental Deficiency)	Anxious, stressed Confusion Pain in abdomen, back, legs Muscle weakness Extreme fatigue Nausea, vomiting Lowered blood pressure Elevated pulse Loss of consciousness Coma	**Conscious patient** Terminate oral procedure. **Call EMS.** Request telephone call for medical assistance. Administer oxygen by nonrebreather mask. Monitor blood pressure and pulse. Place patient on stable side with legs slightly raised. **Unconscious patient** Basic life support. Try ammonia vaporole when cause is undecided. Administer oxygen. **EMS transport to hospital.**
Insulin Reaction (Hyperinsulinism, hypoglycemia)	Sudden onset Skin: moist, cold, pale Confused, nervous, anxious Bounding pulse Salivation Normal to shallow respirations Convulsions (late)	**Conscious patient** Administer oral sugar (cubes, apple juice, candy, or frosting). Observe patient for 1 h before dismissal. Determine time since previous meal, and arrange next appointment following food intake. **Unconscious patient** **Call EMS.** Basic life support. Position: supine. Maintain airway. Administer oxygen by nonrebreather bag. Monitor vital signs. Administer intramuscular glucagon or intravenous glucose.
Diabetic Coma (Ketoacidosis) (Hyperglycemia)	Slow onset Skin: flushed and dry Breath: fruity odor Dry mouth, thirst Low blood pressure Weak, rapid pulse Exaggerated respirations (Kussmaul breathing)	**Conscious patient** **Call EMS.** Keep patient warm. Administer oxygen by nasal cannula. **Unconscious patient** Basic life support. Position: supine.

(continued)

TABLE 69-4	EMERGENCY REFERENCE CHART: MEDICAL EMERGENCIES *(Continued)*	
EMERGENCY	**SIGNS/SYMPTOMS**	**PROCEDURE**
- Seizure 1. Generalized tonic-clonic 2. Generalized absence	Coma Anxiety or depression Pale, may become cyanotic Muscular contractions Loss of consciousness Brief loss of consciousness Fixed posture Rhythmic twitching of eyelids, eyebrows, or head May be pale	**Call EMS.** Position supine: Do not attempt to move from dental chair. Make safe by placing movable equipment out of reach. Do not force anything between the teeth; a soft towel or large sponges may be placed while mouth is open. Open airway; monitor vital signs. Administer oxygen by nasal cannula or face mask. Allow patient to sleep during postconvulsive stage. EMS to determine need for transport to hospital. Take objects from patient's hands to prevent their being dropped.
Allergic Reaction 1. Delayed (anaphylactic shock)	Skin Erythema (rash) Urticaria (wheals, itching) Angioedema (localized swelling of mucous membranes, lips, larynx, pharynx) Respiration Distress, dyspnea Wheezing Extension of angioedema to larynx: may have obstruction from swelling of vocal apparatus	Skin. Administer antihistamine. Respiration. Position: upright. Administer oxygen by nasal cannula. Epinephrine may be needed if breathing difficulty. If airway obstruction: Position: supine. Airway maintenance. Epinephrine (Epi-Pen).
2. Immediate anaphylaxis	Skin Urticaria (wheals, itching) Flushing Nausea, abdominal cramps, vomiting, diarrhea Angioedema Swelling of lips, membranes, eyelids Laryngeal edema with difficulty swallowing Respiration distress Cough, wheezing Dyspnea, airway obstruction Cyanosis Cardiovascular collapse Profound drop in blood pressure Rapid, weak pulse Palpitations Dilation of pupils Loss of consciousness (sudden) Cardiac arrest	Rapid treatment needed. Administer epinephrine via autoinjector. **Call EMS.** Position: supine (except when dyspnea predominates). Administer oxygen by nonrebreather mask. Basic life support. Monitor vital signs. Cardiopulmonary resuscitation if airway obstructed.
Local Anesthesia Reactions 1. Psychogenic 2. Allergic (very rare) 3. Toxic overdose	Reaction to injection, not the anesthetic Syncope Hyperventilation syndrome Anaphylactic shock Allergic skin and mucous membrane reactions Allergic bronchial asthma attack Effects of intravascular injection rather than increased quantity of drug more common Stimulation phase Anxious, restless, apprehensive, confused Rapid pulse and respirations Elevated blood pressure Tremors Convulsions Depressive phase Follows stimulation phase Drowsiness, lethargy Shocklike symptoms: pallor, sweating Rapid, weak pulse and respirations Drop in blood pressure Respiratory depression or respiratory arrest Unconsciousness	Page 1077 (syncope). Page 1077 (hyperventilation). See earlier in this table. Mild reaction. Stop injection. Position: supine. Loosen tight clothing. Reassure patient. Monitor blood pressure, heart rate, respirations. Administer oxygen by nasal cannula. Severe reaction **Call EMS.** Basic life support: maintain airway. Administer oxygen by nonrebreather mask. Continue to monitor vital signs. Cardiopulmonary resuscitation. Administration of anticonvulsant.

TABLE 69-5	EMERGENCY REFERENCE CHART: TRAUMATIC INJURIES	
EMERGENCY	**SIGNS/SYMPTOMS**	**PROCEDURE**
Hemorrhage	Prolonged bleeding Spurting blood: artery Oozing blood: vein	Compression over bleeding area A. Apply gauze pack with direct pressure. B. Bandage pack into place firmly where possible. C. Elevate injury above the heart if possible. Severe bleeding: digital pressure on pressure point of supplying vessel. If shock symptoms: **Call EMS.**
	Bleeding from tooth socket	Pack with folded gauze; do not dab. Have patient bite down firmly. If bleeding does not stop, instruct patient to gently bite down on a damp tea bag and hold in place for 10 min. Do not rinse.
	Bleeding of an extremity	**Call EMS.** Elevate the part: support with pillows. Apply tourniquet only when limb is amputated, mangled, or crushed.
	Nosebleed	Seat patient upright, head elevated. Tell patient to breathe through mouth. Apply cold application to nose. Press nostril on bleeding side for a few minutes. Advise patient not to blow the nose for an hour or more. If bleeding does not stop, wet cotton rolls with water and lubricate with water-soluble lubricant. Pack nostril. Instruct patient to breathe through the mouth. Leave packing in place until patient sees a physician.
Burns 1. First Degree	Skin reddened Swelling Pain	*First- and second-degree burns.* Do not give food or liquids; anticipate nausea. Be alert for signs of shock.
2. Second Degree	Skin reddened, blisters Swelling Wet surface Pain (more than third degree) Heightened sensitivity to touch	Do not apply ointment, grease, or bicarbonate of soda. Immerse in cool water to relieve pain; do not apply ice. Gently clean with a mild antiseptic. Dress lightly with a dry sterile bandage. Elevate burned part. **Call EMS.**
3. Third Degree (full thickness)	Leathery look Insensitive to touch	**Call EMS.** Treat for shock. Basic life support: maintain airway. Check for other injuries. Wrap in clean sheet: EMS transport.
4. Chemical Burn	Reddened, discolored	Immediate: copious irrigation with water for ½ h. Check directions on container from which the chemical came for antidote or other advice. Burn caused by an acid may be rinsed with bicarbonate of soda, burn caused by alkali may be rinsed in weak acid such as acetic (vinegar).

(*continued*)

TABLE 69-5	EMERGENCY REFERENCE CHART: TRAUMATIC INJURIES *(Continued)*

EMERGENCY	SIGNS/SYMPTOMS	PROCEDURE
Internal Poisoning	Signs of corrosive burn around or in oral cavity Evidence of empty container or information from patient Nausea, vomiting, cramps	Call Poison Control Center. 1-800-222-1222. Be calm and supportive. Basic life support: airway maintenance. Artificial ventilation (inhaled poison). Record vital signs. Do NOT give water or milk or Ipecac unless instructed to do so by Poison Control Center. Avoid nonspecific and questionably effective antidotes, stimulants, sedatives, or other agents, which may do more harm. **Call EMS.**
Foreign Body in Eye	Tears Blinking	Wash hands. Ask patient to look down. Bring upper lid down over lower lid for a moment; move it upward. Turn down lower lid and examine: if particle is visible, remove with moistened cotton applicator. Use eye cup: wash out eye with plain water. When unsuccessful, seek medical attention: prevent patient from rubbing eye by placing gauze pack over eye and stabilizing with adhesive tape.
Chemical Solution in Eye	Tears Stinging	Irrigate promptly with copious amounts of water. Turn head so water flows away from inner aspect of the eye; continue for 15–20 min.
Dislocated Jaw	Mouth is open: patient is unable to close	Stand in front of seated patient. Wrap thumbs in towels and place on occlusal surfaces of mandibular posterior teeth. Curve fingers and place under body of the mandible. Press down and back with thumbs, and at the same time pull up and forward with fingers (Figure 69-8). As joint slips into place, quickly move thumbs outward. Place bandage around head to support under chin.
Facial Fracture	Pain, swelling Ecchymoses Deformity, limitation of movement Crepitation on manipulation Zygoma fracture: depression of cheek Mandibular fracture: abnormal occlusion	Place patient on side. Basic life support. Support with bandage around face, under chin, and tied on the top of the head (Barton). **Call EMS.**
Tooth Forcibly Displaced (avulsed tooth)	Swelling, bruises, or other signs of trauma depending on the type of accident	Instruct patient or parent to hold the tooth by the crown, and avoid touching the root(s). If the tooth is dirty, rinse it gently in cool water, but do not scrub it or remove tissue fragments from its root surface. Keep the tooth moist by placing it in milk to transport to dentist. Bring the tooth and the patient to dental office or clinic *immediately*. The longer the time lapse between avulsion and replantation, the poorer the prognosis.

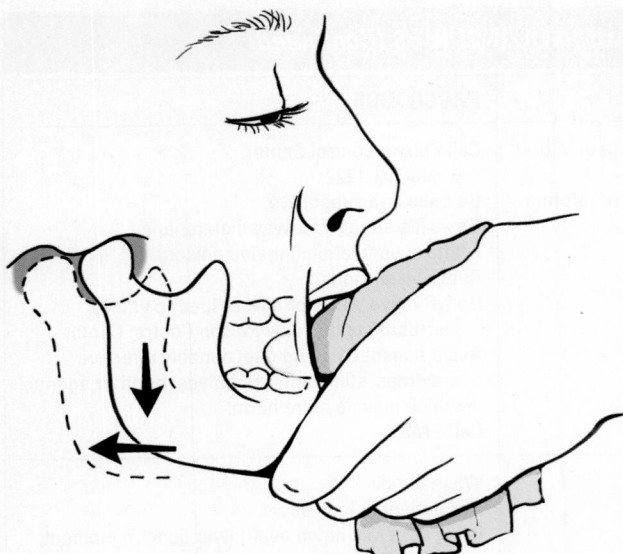

FIGURE 69-8 Treatment for a Dislocated Mandible. With thumbs wrapped in toweling and placed on the buccal cusps of the mandibular teeth, the fingers are curved under the body of the mandible. The jaw is pressed down and back with the thumbs while pulling up and forward with the fingers to permit the condyle to pass over the articular eminence into its normal position in the glenoid fossa. As the jaw slips into place, the thumbs must be moved quickly aside.

(continued page 1075)

III. NEW ENTRIES

- *Response to treatment.* Document a patient's reactions and responses to treatments, whether they are unremarkable or remarkable.
- *Previous appointment review.* Complete a comprehensive review of previous appointment documentation before providing additional treatment at sequential appointments.

BOX 69-5	Example Progress Note: For Emergency During Patient Treatment

Patient presented with blatant signs of anaphylaxis after exposure to latex gloves. Urticaria and pruritus were evident on the arms, neck and chest. Signs of lip, tongue and laryngeal edema were exhibited with difficulty swallowing and breathing. Quickly explained to the patient that he was having an allergic reaction and needed an injection of epinephrine. The dentist immediately gave an injection via EpiPen® and EMS was summoned. 50 mg of Benadryl and 100 mg of Solu-Cortef were also administered IM. Within 5 min, the patient's symptoms seemed to subside and vitals returned closer to baseline. Oxygen was delivered by nonrebreather at 15 l/min. At 8 min, the patients vital signs were near baseline. The patient was released to EMS after 15 min. A Medical Emergency Report Form was completed and given to EMS with one copy included in the patient's chart and the other sent to the patient's physician. See the Medical Emergency Report Form for complete documentation (Figure 69-1). Patient was transported in stable condition by EMS to Tallahassee Memorial Regional Medical Center.

Signed: _____, RDH Date: _____

- *Current information.* Update information about the patient's health status as an integral part of the prevention of medical emergencies.
- *Emergency documentation.* Include a copy of the emergency Medical Emergency Report Form **(Figure 69-1)** that was completed during the emergency in the patient's permanent record.
- *Progress notes.* **Box 69-5** contains an example progress note for an emergency that happens during an appointment.

Everyday Ethics

A 12-year-old patient, Jonathan, had just received local anesthesia in Dr. Spar's treatment room in preparation for a restorative procedure. Suddenly Jonathan started to have a rhythmic twitching of the eyelids and appeared pale. Dr. Spar's assistant, Loraine, called the usual emergency alarm, and Elisa, the dental hygienist joined in the team protocol for medical emergencies

In a few minutes the generalized absence (petit mal) seizure was over and the patient was conscious with no other symptoms evident. Dr. Spar went about the dental procedure as if nothing had happened. Neither Loraine nor Dr. Spar made an entry in the record at the time. Elisa glanced over the patient's record and nothing she could find in the history showed that Jonathan had a susceptibility to seizures. As Elisa went back to her own treatment room, she wondered if she needed to record the emergency or ask Dr. Spar about it.

Questions for Consideration

1. Which of the dental hygiene core values apply in this situation, explain the relationship?
2. Who needs to be informed of the event, and what potential ethical responsibilities are related to the patient?
3. What considerations for future treatment appointments are needed? From an ethical point of view, in what way were the patient's best interests compromised?

Factors To Teach The Patient

■ Stress minimization to prevent emergencies.

■ Take medication prescribed by dentist at times indicated on the prescription.

■ Schedule appointments when there is no waiting, first appointment of the morning or afternoon.

■ Eat breakfast before morning appointment, or lunch before afternoon appointment unless instructed by the patient's physician NOT to eat before the appointment.

■ If patient has prescription medications for emergency episodes, bring those medications to the appointment. Examples: nitroglycerine tablets for angina, asthma inhaler, glucagon for hypoglycemia.

References

1. Meiller TF, Wynn RL, McMullin AM, Biron C, Crossley HL. *Dental office medical emergencies*. 3rd ed. Hudson, Ohio: Lexi-Comp; 2008. 44–5 pp.
2. Hass DA. Emergency drugs. *Dent Clin North Am*. 2002 Oct;46(4): 815–30.
3. Malamed SF. *Medical emergencies in the dental office*. 6th ed. St. Louis: Mosby; 2007. 39, 66, 124–7 pp.
4. Berg RA, Hemphill R, Abella BS, Aufderheide TP, Cave DM, Hazinski MF, Lerner EB, Rea TD, Sayre MR, Swor RA. Adult basic life support: 2010 American Heart Association Guidelines for Cardiopulmonary Resuscitation and Emergency Cardiovascular Care. *Circulation*. 2010;122(Suppl 3):S685–S705.
5. Hallstrom A, Cobb L, Johnson E, Copass M. Cardiopulmonary resuscitation by chest compression alone or mouth-to-mouth ventilation. *N Engl J Med*. 2000 May 25;342(21):1546–53.
6. American Heart Association. American Heart Association Guidelines for Cardiopulmonary Resuscitation and Emergency Cardiovascular Care. International Consensus on Science. *Circulation*. 2005 Dec 13; 112(24 Suppl):IV1–203.

American Dental Hygienists' Association Code of Ethics for Dental Hygienists*

PREAMBLE

As dental hygienists, we are a community of professionals devoted to the prevention of disease and the promotion and improvement of the public's health. We are preventive oral health professionals who provide educational, clinical, and therapeutic services to the public. We strive to live meaningful, productive, satisfying lives that simultaneously serve us, our profession, our society, and the world. Our actions, behaviors, and attitudes are consistent with our commitment to public service. We endorse and incorporate the Code into our daily lives.

PURPOSE

The purpose of a professional code of ethics is to achieve high levels of ethical consciousness, decision making, and practice by the members of the profession. Specific objectives of the Dental Hygiene Code of Ethics are:

■ To increase our professional and ethical consciousness and sense of ethical responsibility.
■ To lead us to recognize ethical issues and choices and to guide us in making more informed ethical decisions.
■ To establish a standard for professional judgment and conduct.

*Reprinted with permission from The American Dental Hygienists' Association. http://www.adha.org

■ To provide a statement of the ethical behavior the public can expect from us.

The Dental Hygiene Code of Ethics is meant to influence us throughout our careers. It stimulates our continuing study of ethical issues and challenges us to explore our ethical responsibilities. The Code establishes concise standards of behavior to guide the public's expectations of our profession and supports existing dental hygiene practice, laws, and regulations. By holding ourselves accountable to meeting the standards stated in the Code, we enhance the public's trust on which our professional privilege and status are founded.

KEY CONCEPTS

Our beliefs, principles, values, and ethics are concepts reflected in the Code. They are the essential elements of our comprehensive and definitive code of ethics and are interrelated and mutually dependent.

BASIC BELIEFS

We recognize the importance of the following beliefs that guide our practice and provide context for our ethics:

■ The services we provide contribute to the health and well-being of society.
■ Our education and licensure qualify us to serve the public by preventing and treating oral disease and helping individuals achieve and maintain optimal health.

- Individuals have intrinsic worth, are responsible for their own health, and are entitled to make choices regarding their health.
- Dental hygiene care is an essential component of overall healthcare, and we function interdependently with other healthcare providers.
- All people should have access to healthcare, including oral healthcare.
- We are individually responsible for our actions and the quality of care we provide.

FUNDAMENTAL PRINCIPLES

These fundamental principles, universal concepts, and general laws of conduct provide the foundation for our ethics.

UNIVERSALITY

The principle of universality assumes that if one individual judges an action to be right or wrong in a given situation, other people considering the same action in the same situation would make the same judgment.

COMPLEMENTARITY

The principle of complementarity assumes the existence of an obligation to justice and basic human rights. It requires us to act toward others in the same way they would act toward us if roles were reversed. In all relationships, it means considering the values and perspectives of others before making decisions or taking actions affecting them.

ETHICS

Ethics are the general standards of right and wrong that guide behavior within society. As generally accepted actions, they can be judged by determining the extent to which they promote good and minimize harm. Ethics compel us to engage in health promotion/disease prevention activities.

COMMUNITY

This principle expresses our concern for the bond between individuals, the community, and society in general. It leads us to preserve natural resources and inspires us to show concern for the global environment.

RESPONSIBILITY

Responsibility is central to our ethics. We recognize that there are guidelines for making ethical choices and accept responsibility for knowing and applying them. We accept the consequences of our actions or the failure to act and are willing to make ethical choices and publicly affirm them.

CORE VALUES

We acknowledge these values as general for our choices and actions.

INDIVIDUAL AUTONOMY AND RESPECT FOR HUMAN BEINGS

People have the right to be treated with respect. They have the right to informed consent prior to treatment, and they have the right to full disclosure of all relevant information so that they can make informed choices about their care.

CONFIDENTIALITY

We respect the confidentiality of client information and relationships as a demonstration of the value we place on individual autonomy. We acknowledge our obligation to justify any violation of a confidence.

SOCIETAL TRUST

We value client trust and understand that public trust in our profession is based on our actions and behavior.

NONMALEFICENCE

We accept our fundamental obligation to provide services in a manner that protects all clients and minimizes harm to them and others involved in their treatment.

BENEFICENCE

We have a primary role in promoting the well-being of individuals and the public by engaging in health promotion/disease prevention activities.

JUSTICE AND FAIRNESS

We value justice and support the fair and equitable distribution of healthcare resources. We believe all people should have access to high-quality, affordable oral healthcare.

VERACITY

We accept the obligation to tell the truth and assume that others will do the same. We value self-knowledge and seek truth and honesty in all relationships.

STANDARDS OF PROFESSIONAL RESPONSIBILITY

We are obligated to practice our profession in a manner that supports our purpose, beliefs, and values in accordance with the fundamental principles that support our ethics. We acknowledge the following responsibilities:

TO OURSELVES AS INDIVIDUALS

- Avoid self-deception, and continually strive for knowledge and personal growth.
- Establish and maintain a lifestyle that supports optimal health.
- Create a safe work environment.
- Assert our own interests in ways that are fair and equitable.
- Seek the advice and counsel of others when challenged with ethical dilemmas.
- Have realistic expectations of ourselves and recognize our limitations.

TO OURSELVES AS PROFESSIONALS

- Enhance professional competencies through continuous learning in order to practice according to high standards of care.
- Support dental hygiene peer-review systems and quality-assurance measures.
- Develop collaborative professional relationships and exchange knowledge to enhance our own lifelong professional development.

TO FAMILY AND FRIENDS

- Support the efforts of others to establish and maintain healthy lifestyles and respect the rights of friends and family.

TO CLIENTS

- Provide oral healthcare utilizing high levels of professional knowledge, judgment, and skill.
- Maintain a work environment that minimizes the risk of harm.
- Serve all clients without discrimination, and avoid action toward any individual or group that may be interpreted as discriminatory.
- Hold professional client relationships confidential.
- Communicate with clients in a respectful manner.
- Promote ethical behavior and high standards of care by all dental hygienists.
- Serve as an advocate for the welfare of clients.
- Provide clients with the information necessary to make informed decisions about their oral health and encourage their full participation in treatment decisions and goals.
- Refer clients to other healthcare providers when their needs are beyond our ability or scope of practice.
- Educate clients about high-quality oral healthcare.

TO COLLEAGUES

- Conduct professional activities and programs, and develop relationships in ways that are honest, responsible, and appropriately open and candid.
- Encourage a work environment that promotes individual professional growth and development.
- Collaborate with others to create a work environment that minimizes risk to the personal health and safety of our colleagues.
- Manage conflicts constructively.
- Support the efforts of other dental hygienists to communicate the dental hygiene philosophy and preventive oral care.
- Inform other healthcare professionals about the relationship between general and oral health.
- Promote human relationships that are mutually beneficial, including those with other healthcare professionals.

TO EMPLOYEES AND EMPLOYERS

- Conduct professional activities and programs and develop relationships in ways that are honest, responsible, open, and candid.
- Manage conflicts constructively.
- Support the right of our employees and employers to work in an environment that promotes wellness.
- Respect the employment rights of our employers and employees.

TO THE DENTAL HYGIENE PROFESSION

- Participate in the development and advancement of our profession.
- Avoid conflicts of interest and declare them when they occur.
- Seek opportunities to increase public awareness and understanding of oral health practices.
- Act in ways that bring credit to our profession while demonstrating appropriate respect for colleagues in other professions.
- Contribute time, talent, and financial resources to support and promote our profession.
- Promote a positive image for our profession.
- Promote a framework for professional education that develops dental hygiene competencies to meet the oral and overall health needs of the public.

TO THE COMMUNITY AND SOCIETY

- Recognize and uphold the laws and regulations governing our profession.
- Document and report inappropriate, inadequate, or substandard care and/or illegal activities by a healthcare provider to the responsible authorities.
- Use peer review as a mechanism for identifying inappropriate, inadequate, or substandard care provided by dental hygienists.
- Comply with local, state, and federal statutes that promote public health and safety.

- Develop support systems and quality-assurance programs in the workplace to assist dental hygienists in providing the appropriate standard of care.
- Promote access to dental hygiene services for all, supporting justice and fairness in the distribution of healthcare resources.
- Act consistently with the ethics of the global scientific community of which our profession is a part.
- Create a healthful workplace ecosystem to support a healthy environment.
- Recognize and uphold our obligation to provide pro bono service.

TO SCIENTIFIC INVESTIGATION

We accept responsibility for conducting research according to the fundamental principles underlying our ethical beliefs in compliance with universal codes, governmental standards, and professional guidelines for the care and management of experimental subjects. We acknowledge our ethical obligations to the scientific community:

- Conduct research that contributes knowledge that is valid and useful to our clients and society.
- Use research methods that meet accepted scientific standards.
- Use research resources appropriately.

- Systematically review and justify research in progress to ensure the most favorable benefit-to-risk ratio to research subjects.
- Submit all proposals involving human subjects to an appropriate human subject review committee.
- Secure appropriate institutional committee approval for the conduct of research involving animals.
- Obtain informed consent from human subjects participating in research that is based on specification published in Title 21 Code of Federal Regulations Part 46.
- Respect the confidentiality and privacy of data.
- Seek opportunities to advance dental hygiene knowledge through research by providing financial, human, and technical resources whenever possible. Report research results in a timely manner.
- Report research findings completely and honestly, drawing only those conclusions that are supported by the data presented.
- Report names of investigators fairly and accurately.
- Interpret the research and the research of others accurately and objectively, drawing conclusions that are supported by the data presented and seeking clarity when uncertain.
- Critically evaluate research methods and results before applying new theory and technology in practice.
- Be knowledgeable concerning currently accepted preventive and therapeutic methods, products, and technology and their application to our practice.

Canadian Dental Hygienists Association Code of Ethics*

PREAMBLE

Dental hygienists believe that oral health is an integral part of a person's overall health, well-being, and quality of life. The profession of dental hygiene is devoted to promoting optimal oral health for all. Dental hygiene has an identified body of knowledge and a distinctive expertise which dental hygienists use to serve the needs of their clients and promote the public good.

The Code of Ethics sets down the ethical principles and ethical practice standards of the dental hygiene profession. The **principles** express the broad ideals to which dental hygienists aspire and which guide them in their practice. The **standards** provide more specific direction for conduct. They are more precise and prescriptive as to what a given principle requires under particular circumstances. Clients, colleagues, and the public in general can reasonably expect dental hygienists to be guided by, and to be accountable under, the principles and standards articulated in this Code.

The purpose of the Code of Ethics is to

■ Elaborate the ethical principles and standards by which dental hygienists are guided and under which they are accountable.
■ Serve as a resource for education, reflection, self-evaluation, and peer review.

■ Educate the public about the ethical principles and standards of the profession.
■ Promote accountability.

The Code of Ethics is a public document that augments and complements the relevant laws and regulations under which dental hygienists practise. By elaborating on the profession's ethical principles and standards, the Code promotes accountability and worthiness of the public's trust.

The Code of Ethics applies to dental hygienists and dental hygiene students in all practice settings, including, but not limited to, private practice, institutions, research, education, administration, community health, and industry.

Interpretation and application of the Code in specific circumstances requires individual judgment. Several aids are appended to the Code to assist in this.

SUMMARY OF THE MAIN PRINCIPLES IN THE CODE

The fundamental principle underlying this Code is that the dental hygienist's primary responsibility is to the client, whether the client is an individual or a community.

PRINCIPLE I: BENEFICENCE

Beneficence involves caring about and acting to promote the good of another. Dental hygienists use their knowledge and skills to assist clients to achieve and maintain optimal oral health and to promote fair and reasonable access to quality oral health services.

*Reprinted with permission from The Canadian Dental Hygienists Association. http://www.cdha.ca

PRINCIPLE II: AUTONOMY

Autonomy pertains to the right to make one's own choices. By communicating relevant information openly and truthfully, dental hygienists assist clients to make informed choices and to participate actively in achieving and maintaining their optimal oral health.

PRINCIPLE III: PRIVACY AND CONFIDENTIALITY

Privacy pertains to the individual's right to decide the conditions under which others will be permitted access to his or her personal life or information. Confidentiality is the duty to hold secret any information acquired in the professional relationship. Dental hygienists respect the privacy of clients and hold in confidence information disclosed to them, subject to certain narrowly defined exceptions.

PRINCIPLE IV: ACCOUNTABILITY

Accountability pertains to the acceptance of responsibility for one's actions and omissions in light of relevant principles, standards, laws, and regulations and the potential to self-evaluate and to be evaluated accordingly. Dental hygienists practise competently in conformity with relevant principles, standards, laws, and regulations and accept responsibility for their behaviour and decisions in the professional context.

PRINCIPLE V: PROFESSIONALISM

Professionalism is the commitment to use and advance professional knowledge and skills to serve the client and the public good. Dental hygienists express their professional commitment individually in their practice and communally through their professional associations and regulatory bodies.

PRINCIPLE I: BENEFICENCE

Beneficence involves caring about and acting to promote the good of another. Dental hygienists use their knowledge and skills to assist clients to achieve and maintain optimal oral health and to promote fair and reasonable access to quality oral health services.

STANDARDS FOR PRINCIPLE I

Dental hygienists:

1a. provide services to their clients in a caring and respectful manner, in recognition of the inherent dignity of human beings;

1b. provide services to their clients with respect for their individual needs and values and life circumstances;

1c. provide services fairly and without discrimination, in recognition of fundamental human rights;

1d. put the needs, values, and interests of their clients first and avoid exploiting their clients for personal gain;

1e. seek to improve the quality of care and advance knowledge in the field of oral health through such activities as quality assurance, research, education, and advocacy in the public arena.

PRINCIPLE II: AUTONOMY

Autonomy pertains to the right to make one's own choices. By communicating relevant information openly and truthfully, dental hygienists assist clients to make informed choices and to participate actively in achieving and maintaining their optimal oral health.

STANDARDS FOR PRINCIPLE II

Dental hygienists:

2a. actively involve clients in their oral health care and promote informed choice by communicating relevant information openly, truthfully, and sensitively in recognition of the client's needs, values, and capacity to understand;

2b. in the case of clients who lack the capacity for informed choice, actively involve and promote informed choice on the part of the client's substitute decision-makers, involving the client to the extent of the client's capacity;

2c. honour the client's informed choices, including refusal of treatment, and regard informed choice as a precondition of treatment;

2d. do not rely upon coercion or manipulative tactics in assisting the client to make informed choices;

2e. recommend or provide only those services they believe are necessary for the client's oral health or as consistent with the client's informed choice.

Note: Critical elements of informed choice include disclosure (i.e., revealing pertinent information, including risks and benefits); willingness (i.e., the choice is not coerced or manipulated); and capacity (i.e., the cognitive capacity to understand and process the relevant information). "Informed choice" encompasses what is sometimes referred to as "informed consent."

PRINCIPLE III: PRIVACY AND CONFIDENTIALITY

Privacy pertains to the individual's right to decide the conditions under which others will be permitted access to his or her personal life or information. Confidentiality is the duty to hold secret any information acquired in the professional relationship. Dental hygienists respect the privacy of clients and hold in confidence information disclosed to them, subject to certain narrowly defined exceptions.

STANDARDS FOR PRINCIPLE III

Dental hygienists:

3a. demonstrate regard for the privacy of their clients;

3b. hold confidential any information acquired in the professional relationship and do not use or disclose it to others without the client's express consent, except:

3b i   as required by law

3b ii   required by the policy of the practice environment (e.g., quality assurance)

3b iii   in an emergency situation

3b iv   in cases where disclosure is necessary to prevent serious harm to others

3b v   to the guardian or substitute decision-maker of a client in these cases, disclose to others only as much information as is necessary to accomplish the purpose for the disclosure;

3c. may infer the client's consent for disclosure to others directly involved in delivering and administering services to the client, provided there is no reason to believe the client would not give express consent if asked;

3d. obtain the client's express consent to use or share information about the client for the purpose of teaching or research;

3e. inform their clients in advance of treatment about how they will use or share their information, in particular about any uses or sharing that may occur without the client's express consent;

3f. promote practices, polices, and information systems that are designed to respect client privacy and confidentiality.

PRINCIPLE IV: ACCOUNTABILITY

Accountability pertains to the acceptance of responsibility for one's actions and omissions in light of relevant principles, standards, laws, and regulations and the potential to self-evaluate and to be evaluated accordingly. Dental hygienists practice competently in conformity with relevant principles, standards, laws and regulations, and accept responsibility for their behavior and decisions in the professional context.

STANDARDS FOR PRINCIPLE IV

Dental hygienists:

4a. accept responsibility for knowing and acting consistently with the principles, standards, laws, and regulations under which they are accountable;

4b. accept responsibility for providing safe, quality, competent care, including, but not limited to, addressing issues in the practice environment within their capacity that may hinder or impede the provision of such care;

4c. take appropriate action to ensure first and foremost the client's safety and quality of care when they suspect unethical or incompetent care;

4d. practice within the bounds of their competence, scope of practice, and personal and/or professional limitations, and refer clients requiring care outside these bounds;

4e. inform the dental hygiene regulatory body when an injury, dependency, infection, condition, or any other serious incapacity has immediately affected, or may affect over time, their continuing ability to practice safely and competently;

4f. promote workplace practices and policies that facilitate professional practice in accordance with the principles, standards, laws, and regulations under which they are accountable.

PRINCIPLE V: PROFESSIONALISM

Professionalism is the commitment to use and advance professional knowledge and skills to serve the client and the public good. Dental hygienists express their professional commitment individually in their practice and communally through their professional associations and regulatory bodies.

STANDARDS FOR PRINCIPLE V

Dental hygienists:

5a. uphold the principles and standards of the professions before clients, colleagues, and others;

5b. maintain and advance their knowledge and skills in dental hygiene through continuing education and the quality of the care they provide through ongoing self-evaluation and quality assurance;

5c. advance general knowledge and skills in the field of oral health by supporting, participating in, or conducting ethically approved research;

5d. participate in professional activities such as meetings, committee work, peer review, and participation in public forums to promote oral health;

5e. participate in mentoring, education, and dissemination of knowledge and skills in oral health care;

5f. support the work of their professional associations and regulatory bodies to promote oral health and professional practice;

5g. inform potential employers about the principles, standards, laws, and regulations to which they are accountable and determine whether employment conditions facilitate professional practice accordingly.

5h. collaborate with colleagues in a cooperative, constructive, and respectful manner toward the primary end of providing safe, competent, fair, quality to clients;

5i. communicate the nature and costs of professional services fairly and accurately.

ETHICAL CHALLENGES/PROBLEMS

No code of ethics can be expected to resolve definitively all ethical challenges or problems that may arise in practice. The analysis below is intended to help dental hygienists understand the nature of ethical challenges or problems and thereby better resolve them.

Ethical challenges or problems faced by practicing dental hygienists tend to fall into the categories of ethical violations, ethical dilemmas, and ethical distress.

Ethical violations: when dental hygienists fail to meet or neglect their specific ethical responsibilities as expressed in the Code's standards. An example would be a dental hygienist who recommends unnecessary treatment in order to achieve personal gain at the expense of the client.

Ethical dilemmas: when one or more ethical principles conflict either with other ethical principle(s) or with self-interest(s) and no apparent course of action will satisfy both sides of the dilemma. An example would be a client with a hip prosthesis who may refuse to be pre-medicated prior to receiving invasive dental treatment. In this case, the principle of autonomy conflicts with the principle of beneficence.

Ethical distress: when dental hygienists experience constraints or limitations in relation to which they are or feel powerless and which compromise their ability to practise in full accordance with their professional principles or standards. An example would be a dental hygienist who is expected by the employer to complete dental hygiene treatment in a length of time insufficient to render quality care or to provide an acceptable level of infection control.

This Code is a useful guide in helping dental hygienists to identify, work through, and put into words ethical issues in light of their responsibilities as articulated in the Code's principles and standards, and to decide on an ethically responsible course of action. It is important to realize that some challenges or problems are perceived to be primarily ethical in nature when, in fact, they arise less from conflicting principles than from poor communication or lack of information. Reflecting on a perceived challenge or problem in light of the Code can help determine to what extent the problem or challenge is truly rooted in conflicting ethical principles, and to what extent it can be resolved by improved communication or by new information.

The Code provides clear direction for avoiding ethical violations. When a course of action is mandated by a standard in the Code or by a principle where there exists no opposing principle, ethical conduct requires that course of action.

In the case of ethical dilemmas and ethical distress, the Code cannot always provide a clear direction. The resolution of dilemmas often depends on the specific circumstances of the case in question. Total satisfaction by all parties involved may not be achieved. Resolution may also depend on which opposing ethical principle is considered to be more important, a matter on which reasonable people may disagree. Ethical distress often arises in situations where the dental hygienist is significantly limited by factors beyond his or her immediate control that may not be resolvable in the specific context.

In all cases, dental hygienists are accountable for how they conduct themselves in professional practice. Even in situations of ethical dilemma or distress where the Code does not prescribe a specific course of action, the hygienist can be expected to give account of his or her chosen action in light of the principles and standards expressed in the Code. Ultimately, dental hygienists must reconcile their actions with their consciences in caring for clients.

REPORTING SUSPECTED INCOMPETENCE OR UNETHICAL CONDUCT

The first consideration of the dental hygienist who suspects incompetence or unethical conduct in colleagues or associates is the welfare of present clients and/or potential harm to future clients. Adherence to the following guidelines could be helpful:

1. First, confirm the facts of the situation.
2. Ensure you are familiar with existing protocols in the practice setting for reporting incidents, incompetence, or unethical care, and follow those protocols.
3. Document and report issues that cannot be resolved within the practice setting and report to the appropriate authority or regulatory body.

The dental hygienist who attempts to protect clients threatened by incompetent or unethical conduct should not be placed in jeopardy (e.g., loss of employment). Colleagues and professional organizations are morally obligated to support dental hygienists who fulfill their ethical obligations under the Code.

DECISION-PROCEDURE

GUIDANCE REGARDING THE PROCESS FOR RESOLVING ETHICAL CHALLENGES

Ethical problems or challenges arise in a variety of contexts and require thoughtful analysis and careful judgment. The following guide may be useful to assist dental hygienists faced with an ethical challenge, recognizing that other stakeholders may need to be involved in resolving the matter. Talking with or getting advice from others at any step on the way to a decision can be very helpful.

1. Identify in a preliminary way the nature of the challenge or problem. What is the issue? What kind of issue is it? What ethical principles are at stake?
2. Become suitably informed and gather information (e.g., talk to others to find out the facts; research relevant policy statements) relevant to the challenge or problem, including:
   a. Factual information about the situation. What has happened? What is the sequence of events?
   b. Applicable policies, laws, or regulations. Does a workplace policy address the issue? What does the Code say? What does law or regulation say?

c. Who are the relevant stakeholders? How do they view the situation?

3. Clarify and elaborate the challenge or problem after getting this information. Now that you are better informed, What is the issue? What ethical principles are at stake? What stakeholders need to be consulted or involved in resolving the challenge or problem?

4. Identify various options for actions, recognizing that the best option may not be obvious at first and realizing it may require creativity or imagination.

5. Assess the various options in light of applicable policy, law, or regulation, being as clear as possible in your mind of the pluses and minuses of each option as assessed in this light.

6. Decide on a course of action, mindful of how you would justify or defend your decision in light of the applicable policy, law, or regulation, if you are called to account.

7. Implement your decision as thoughtfully and sensitively as possible, communicating a willingness to explain or justify the reasons for taking it.

8. Assess the consequences of your decision. Evaluate the process you used to arrive at the decision and the decision itself in light of those consequences. Did things turn out as you thought they would? Would you do the same thing again? What went wrong? Or, what went right?

In all of this, bear in mind that reasonable people can disagree about what is the right thing to do when faced with an ethical challenge or problem. If you cannot be certain whether you have made the right decision, you can at least have some assurance that you came to your decision in a responsible way. The test for this is whether you are able to defend your decision in light of relevant laws, principles, and regulations and to defend the process by which you came to your decision. Reference to the above guidelines will help in this.

In addition, there is a very rich literature on ethics that can be very helpful for thinking through ethical challenges and problems in dental hygiene or for ongoing professional education and development.

Dental hygienists may also find it useful to familiarize themselves with various ethical theories, which tend to guide or orient ethical thinking along different lines. The main ethical theories current today are briefly described below:

- DEONTOLOGY guides ethical thinking in terms of duties and rights, which the philosopher Immanuel Kant grounds in the fundamental imperative to act in relation to others according to principles that apply universally to all people, and that one would also wish for others to apply in their actions in relation to oneself.

- UTILITARIANISM guides ethical thinking in terms of harms and benefits, which the philosopher J.S. Mill grounds in the fundamental imperative to promote the greatest good for the greatest number.

- THE ETHIC OF CARE guides ethical thinking in terms of preserving and enhancing relationships and service to others. This theory derives from the work of Carol Gilligan, who found in her research that this style of ethical thinking tends to be more associated with females than with males.

- VIRTUE ETHICS guides ethical thinking in terms of habits of acting and assesses actions in terms of virtues and vices of character. This theory derives from the work of the philosopher Aristotle, who emphasized that ethics cannot be reduced to rules or formulas and held that the person of good character (the "good man") is the ultimate standard of right and wrong and should be emulated by others as a role model.

- FEMINIST ETHICS guides ethical thinking in terms of sensitivity to the power or political dimension of human interaction. The philosopher Susan Sherwin grounds feminist ethics in the allegiance to those who are oppressed, vulnerable, or disadvantaged and the imperative to improve their situation.

This is by no means a complete listing of ethical theories, nor is the richness of these theories captured in the condensed descriptions given. Moreover, considerable controversy exists not only among these theories but also among adherents of each theory.

References

American Dental Hygienists Association. Code of ethics for dental hygienists. Chicago: ADHA; 1995.

Canadian Dental Hygienists Association. "Dental hygiene: client's bill of rights." Ottawa: CDHA; October 2001.

Canadian Dental Hygienists Association. Code of ethics. Ottawa: CDHA; July 1997.

College of Dental Hygienists of Ontario. Code of ethics. Toronto: CDHO; 1996.

College of Dental Hygienists of British Columbia. Code of ethics. Victoria: CDHBC; March 1, 1995.

Canadian Dental Association. Code of ethics. Ottawa: CDA; August 1991.

Canadian Dental Assistants Association. CDAA code of ethics. Ottawa: CDAA; 2000.

Canadian Medical Association. Code of ethics of the Canadian Medical Association. Ottawa: CMA; 1997.

Canadian Nurses Association. Code of ethics for registered nurses. Ottawa: CNA; March 1997.

International Federation of Dental Hygienists Code of Ethics*

INTRODUCTION

The fundamental responsibility of dental hygienists is to promote and restore oral health.

Dental hygienists promote oral health by providing clinical, therapeutic remedies, and health education.

Dental hygienists serve the public as oral health professionals and thus contribute to the public's general health and well-being.

The need for dental hygiene services is universal and unrestricted by race, colour, age, sex, language, religion, political or other opinion, national or social origin, property, birth or other status.

Dental hygienists are called upon to deliver care to the individual, the family and the community.

In a business relationship in which a dental hygienist is an employee the dental hygienist exhibits competence, loyalty and fair return of work for compensation. However, employee status does not minimize a dental hygienist's ethical responsibility to account for a patient's well-being. Nor does it lessen the dental hygienist's right to act competently, accountably and knowledgably on behalf of the patient.

Dental hygiene care is provided with integrity and respect and in collaboration with other health care professionals.

VALUES EMBEDDED IN THE CODE OF ETHICS

Dental Hygienists value integrity and respect.

*Reprinted with permission from The International Federation of Dental Hygienists. http://ifdh.org

1. **Integrity:** moral soundness; uprightness; sincerity; freedom from corrupting influence or motive
   a. Dental hygienists value personal integrity and are honest, truthful, and respectful when interacting with other human beings.
   b. Dental hygienists value professional integrity and practice according to the profession's standards and values.
   c. Ethical practice requires both personal integrity and professional integrity.
2. **Respect:** to regard with special attention, to care for, to avoid violation of, or interference with. Dental hygienists value respect for *persons and personal dignity as human beings are unique, in their abilities, strengths, weaknesses and needs.*
   a. *Dental hygienists value respect for* truthfulness. Truthfulness is essential when assisting the patient to obtain relevant information about dental hygiene services, diagnosis, treatment and probable outcomes. Truthfulness builds trust.
   b. Dental hygienists value respect for *individual choice. Patients have choices and can decide which services to accept or decline.*
   c. *Dental hygienists value respect for* patient confidentiality. Confidentiality is preserved unless such confidentiality could pose substantial risk or serious harm and where that risk or harm is greater than the harm of breaking the confidentiality.
   d. Dental hygienists respect the natural *environment.*

These **values** are embedded in the four principle elements of the Code.

CODE OF ETHICS

The code of ethics has four principal elements that outline the standards of ethical conduct. This establishes the standards of behavior of dental hygienists and embodies integrity and respect.

1. Dental Hygienists and People/Society
2. Dental Hygienists and Practice
3. Dental Hygienists and Co-workers
4. Dental Hygienists and the Profession

DENTAL HYGIENISTS AND PEOPLE/SOCIETY

- The dental hygienist strives to promote an environment in which the human rights, values, customs, and spiritual beliefs of the individual, family and community are respected.
- The dental hygienist endeavors to ensure that the individual receives sufficient and appropriate information on which to base consent for care and related dental hygiene treatment.
- The dental hygienist provides services consistent with the patient's needs and requests.
- The dental hygienist holds personal information confidential and uses professional reasoned judgment in sharing this information.
- The dental hygienist protects the environment by responsible disposal of all wastes in the dental hygiene practice.
- The dental hygienist's own personal interests, if in conflict with her/his professional obligation should be declared and resolved for the well-being of the client.

DENTAL HYGIENISTS AND PRACTICE

- The dental hygienist has the qualifications, knowledge, training, skills, judgment and attitudes to practice safely.
- The dental hygienist has a thorough knowledge of the profession and its related laws.

- The dental hygienist at all times practices with integrity and adheres to the standards of practice and personal conduct of her/his legislative jurisdiction.
- The dental hygienist is personally responsible for remaining competent and current in her/his professional knowledge by continual education and training.
- The dental hygienist provides a choice of services within a range of safe affordable options consistent with the patient's needs.
- The dental hygienist provides timely competent care and charges reasonable fees for professional services.
- The dental hygienist, in providing care, ensures that use of technology and scientific advances are compatible with the safety, dignity and rights of people.

DENTAL HYGIENIST AND CO-WORKERS

- The dental hygienist sustains a co-operative and collaborative relationship with co-workers in oral health and other fields.
- A dental hygienist recognizes particular skills and expertise of health care personnel working collaboratively in the patient's care.
- A dental hygienist advocates for the patient when another oral health provider is giving inappropriate or incompetent care, inconsistent with the patient's well-being.

DENTAL HYGIENISTS AND THE PROFESSION

- The dental hygienist adheres to and may exceed the standards of dental hygiene practice within the jurisdiction of the country of practice.
- The dental hygienist is active in developing and publishing a core of research based on the ongoing pursuit of professional knowledge.
- The dental hygienist, acting through the professional organization, participates in creating and maintaining equitable social and economic working conditions in oral health.
- The dental hygienist promotes respect for human beings ensuring the profession protects their right to health.

Guidelines for Infection Control in Dental Health-Care Settings—2003*

RECOMMENDATIONS

Each recommendation is categorized on the basis of existing scientific data, theoretical rationale, and applicability. Rankings are based on the system used by the Centers for Disease Control and Prevention (CDC) and the Healthcare Infection Control Practices Advisory Committee (HICPAC) to categorize recommendations:

Category IA. Strongly recommended for implementation and strongly supported by well-designed experimental, clinical, or epidemiologic studies.
Category IB. Strongly recommended for implementation and supported by experimental, clinical, or epidemiologic studies and a strong theoretical rationale.
Category IC. Required for implementation as mandated by federal or state regulation or standard. When IC is used, a second rating can be included to provide the basis of existing scientific data, theoretical rationale, and applicability. Because of state differences, the reader should not assume that the absence of an IC implies the absence of state regulations.
Category II. Suggested for implementation and supported by suggestive clinical or epidemiologic studies or a theoretical rationale.

Unresolved issue. No recommendation. Insufficient evidence or no consensus regarding efficacy exists.

I. PERSONNEL HEALTH ELEMENTS OF AN INFECTION-CONTROL PROGRAM

A. General Recommendations

1. Develop a written health program for dental health-care personnel (DHCP) that includes policies, procedures, and guidelines for education and training; immunizations; exposure prevention and postexposure management; medical conditions, work-related illness, and associated work restrictions; contact dermatitis and latex hypersensitivity; and maintenance of records, data management, and confidentiality (IB).[5,16–18,22]

2. Establish referral arrangements with qualified healthcare professionals to ensure prompt and appropriate provision of preventive services, occupationally related medical services, and postexposure management with medical follow-up (IB, IC).[5,13,19,22]

B. Education and Training

1. Provide DHCP 1) on initial employment, 2) when new tasks or procedures affect the employee's occupational exposure, and 3) at a minimum, annually, with education and training regarding occupational exposure to potentially infectious agents and infection-control procedures/protocols appropriate for and specific to their assigned duties (IB, IC).[5,11,13,14,16,19,22]

---

*Excerpted from: Centers for Disease Control and Prevention. Control in Dental Health-Care Settings—2003. *MMWR*. Dec 2003;52(RR-17):1–61. Additional resource materials available from: http://www.cdc.gov/oralhealth/infectioncontrol/guidelines.

2. Provide educational information appropriate in content and vocabulary to the educational level, literacy and language of DHCP (IB, IC).[5,13]

C. Immunization Programs

1. Develop a written comprehensive policy regarding immunizing DHCP, including a list of all required and recommended immunizations (IB).[5,17,18]
2. Refer DHCP to a prearranged qualified healthcare professional or to their own health-care professional to receive all appropriate immunizations based on the latest recommendations as well as their medical history and risk for occupational exposure (IB).[5,17]

D. Exposure Prevention and Postexposure Management

1. Develop a comprehensive postexposure management and medical follow-up program (IB, IC).[5,13,14,19]
   A. Include policies and procedures for prompt reporting, evaluation, counseling, treatment, and medical follow-up of occupational exposures.
   B. Establish mechanisms for referral to a qualified healthcare professional for medical evaluation and follow-up.
   C. Conduct a baseline tuberculin skin test (TST), preferably by using a two-step test, for all DHCP who might have contact with persons with suspected or confirmed infectious TB, regardless of the risk classification of the setting (IB).[20]

E. Medical Conditions, Work-Related Illness, and Work Restrictions

1. Develop and have readily available to all DHCP comprehensive written policies regarding work restriction and exclusion that include a statement of authority defining who can implement such policies (IB).[5,22]
2. Develop policies for work restriction and exclusion that encourage DHCP to seek appropriate preventive and curative care and report their illnesses, medical conditions, or treatments that can render them more susceptible to opportunistic infection or exposures; do not penalize DHCP with loss of wages, benefits, or job status (IB).[5,22]
3. Develop policies and procedures for evaluation, diagnosis, and management of DHCP with suspected or known occupational contact dermatitis (IB).[32]
4. Seek definitive diagnosis by a qualified healthcare professional for any DHCP with suspected latex allergy to carefully determine its specific etiology and appropriate treatment as well as work restrictions and accommodations (IB).[32]

F. Records Maintenance, Data Management, and Confidentiality

1. Establish and maintain confidential medical records (e.g., immunization records and documentation of tests received as a result of occupational exposure) for all DHCP (IB, IC).[5,13]
2. Ensure that the practice complies with all applicable federal, state, and local laws regarding medical record-keeping and confidentiality (IC).[13,34]

II. PREVENTING TRANSMISSION OF BLOODBORNE PATHOGENS

A. HBV Vaccination

1. Offer the hepatitis B virus (HBV) vaccination series to all DHCP with potential occupational exposure to blood or other potentially infectious material (IA, IC).[2,13,14,19]
2. Always follow U.S. Public Health Service/CDC recommendations for hepatitis B vaccination, serologic testing, follow-up, and booster dosing (IA, IC).[13,14,19]
3. Test DHCP for hepatitis B surface antibody (anti-HBs) 1–2 months after completion of the 3-dose vaccination series (IA, IC).[14,19]
4. DHCP should complete a second 3-dose vaccine series or be evaluated to determine if they are hepatitis B surface antigen (HBsAg)-positive if no antibody response occurs to the primary vaccine series (IA, IC).[14,19]
5. Retest for anti-HBs at the completion of the second vaccine series. If no response to the second 3-dose series occurs, nonresponders should be tested for HBsAg (IC).[14,19]
6. Counsel nonresponders to vaccination who are HBsAg-negative regarding their susceptibility to HBV infection and precautions to take (IA, IC).[14,19]
7. Provide employees appropriate education regarding the risks of HBV transmission and the availability of the vaccine. Employees who decline the vaccination should sign a declination form to be kept on file with the employer (IC).[13]

B. Preventing Exposures to Blood and OPIM (Other Potentially Infectious Materials)

- General recommendations
  A. Use standard precautions (Occupational Safety and Health Administration's [OSHA's]) blood-borne pathogen standard retains the term universal precautions) for all patient encounters (IA, IC).[11,13,19,53]
  B. Consider sharp items (e.g., needles, scalers, burs, lab knives, and wires) that are contaminated with patient blood and saliva as potentially infective and establish engineering controls and work practices to prevent injuries (IB, IC).[6,13,113]
  C. Implement a written, comprehensive program designed to minimize and manage DHCP exposures to blood and body fluids (IB, IC).[13,14,19,97]
- Engineering and work-practice controls
  A. Identify, evaluate, and select devices with engineered safety features at least annually and

as they become available on the market (e.g., safer anesthetic syringes, blunt suture needle, retractable scalpel, or needleless IV systems) (IC).[13,97,110–112]

B. Place used disposable syringes and needles, scalpel blades, and other sharp items in appropriate puncture-resistant containers located as close as feasible to the area in which the items are used (IA, IC).[2,7,13,19,113,115]

C. Do not recap used needles by using both hands or any other technique that involves directing the point of a needle toward any part of the body. Do not bend, break, or remove needles before disposal (IA, IC).[2,7,8,13,97,113]

D. Use either a one-handed scoop technique or a mechanical device designed for holding the needle cap when recapping needles (e.g., between multiple injections and before removing from a nondisposable aspirating syringe) (IA, IC).[2,7,8,13,14,113]

■ Postexposure management and prophylaxis

A. Follow CDC recommendations after percutaneous, mucous membrane, or nonintact skin exposure to blood or other potentially infectious material (IA, IC).[13,14,19]

III. HAND HYGIENE

A. General Considerations

■ Perform hand hygiene with either a nonantimicrobial or antimicrobial soap and water when hands are visibly dirty or contaminated with blood or other potentially infectious material. If hands are not visibly soiled, an alcohol-based hand rub can also be used. Follow the manufacturer's instructions (IA).[123]

■ Indications for hand hygiene include

A. when hands are visibly soiled (IA, IC);

B. after bare-handed touching of inanimate objects likely to be contaminated by blood, saliva, or respiratory secretions (IA, IC);

C. before and after treating each patient (IB);

D. before donning gloves (IB); and

E. immediately after removing gloves (IB, IC).[7–9, 11,13,113,120–123,125,126,138]

■ For oral surgical procedures, perform surgical hand antisepsis before donning sterile surgeon's gloves. Follow the manufacturer's instructions by using either an antimicrobial soap and water, or soap and water followed by drying hands and application of an alcohol-based surgical hand-scrub product with persistent activity (IB).[121–123,127–133,144,145]

■ Store liquid hand-care products in either disposable closed containers or closed containers that can be washed and dried before refilling. Do not add soap or lotion to (i.e., top off) a partially empty dispenser (IA).[9,120,122,149,150]

B. Special Considerations for Hand Hygiene and Glove Use

1. Use hand lotions to prevent skin dryness associated with handwashing (IA).[153,154]

2. Consider the compatibility of lotion and antiseptic products and the effect of petroleum or other oil emollients on the integrity of gloves during product selection and glove use (IB).[2,14,122,155]

3. Keep fingernails short with smooth, filed edges to allow thorough cleaning and prevent glove tears (II).[122,123,156]

4. Do not wear artificial fingernails or extenders when having direct contact with patients at high risk (e.g., those in intensive care units or operating rooms) (IA).[123,157–160]

5. Use of artificial fingernails is usually not recommended (II).[157–160]

6. Do not wear hand or nail jewelry if it makes donning gloves more difficult or compromises the fit and integrity of the glove (II).[123,142,143]

IV. PPE (PERSONAL PROTECTIVE EQUIPMENT)

A. Masks, Protective Eyewear, and Face Shields

1. Wear a surgical mask and eye protection with solid side shields or a face shield to protect mucous membranes of the eyes, nose, and mouth during procedures likely to generate splashing or spattering of blood or other body fluids (IB, IC).[1,2,7,8,11,13,137]

2. Change masks between patients or during patient treatment if the mask becomes wet (IB).[2]

3. Clean with soap and water, or if visibly soiled, clean and disinfect reusable facial protective equipment (e.g., clinician and patient protective eyewear or face shields) between patients (II).[2]

B. Protective Clothing

1. Wear protective clothing (e.g., reusable or disposable gown, laboratory coat, or uniform) that covers personal clothing and skin (e.g., forearms) likely to be soiled with blood, saliva, or OPIM (IB, IC).[7,8,11,13,137]

2. Change protective clothing if visibly soiled[134]; change immediately or as soon as feasible if penetrated by blood or other potentially infectious fluids (IB, IC).[13]

3. Remove barrier protection, including gloves, mask, eyewear, and gown before departing work area (e.g., dental patient care, instrument processing, or laboratory areas) (IC).[13]

C. Gloves

1. Wear medical gloves when a potential exists for contacting blood, saliva, OPIM, or mucous membranes (IB, IC).[1,2,7,8,13]

2. Wear a new pair of medical gloves for each patient, remove them promptly after use, and wash hands

immediately to avoid transfer of microorganisms to other patients or environments (IB).[1,7,8,123]

3. Remove gloves that are torn, cut, or punctured as soon as feasible and wash hands before regloving (IB, IC).[13,210,211]

4. Do not wash surgeon's or patient examination gloves before use or wash, disinfect, or sterilize gloves for reuse (IB, IC).[13,138,177,212,213]

5. Ensure that appropriate gloves in the correct size are readily accessible (IC).[13]

6. Use appropriate gloves (e.g., puncture- and chemical-resistant utility gloves) when cleaning instruments and performing housekeeping tasks involving contact with blood or OPIM (IB, IC).[7,13,15]

7. Consult with glove manufacturers regarding the chemical compatibility of glove material and dental materials used (II).

D. Sterile Surgeon's Gloves and Double Gloving During Oral Surgical Procedures

1. Wear sterile surgeon's gloves when performing oral surgical procedures (IB).[2,8,137]

2. No recommendation is offered regarding the effectiveness of wearing two pairs of gloves to prevent disease transmission during oral surgical procedures. The majority of studies among health-care personnel (HCP) and DHCP have demonstrated a lower frequency of inner glove perforation and visible blood on the surgeon's hands when double gloves are worn; however, the effectiveness of wearing two pairs of gloves in preventing disease transmission has not been demonstrated (Unresolved issue).

V. CONTACT DERMATITIS AND LATEX HYPERSENSITIVITY

A. General Recommendations

1. Educate DHCP regarding the signs, symptoms, and diagnoses of skin reactions associated with frequent hand hygiene and glove use (IB).[5,31,32]

2. Screen all patients for latex allergy (e.g., take health history and refer for medical consultation when latex allergy is suspected) (IB).[32]

3. Ensure a latex-safe environment for patients and DHCP with latex allergy (IB).[32]

4. Have emergency treatment kits with latex-free products available at all times (II).[32]

VI. STERILIZATION AND DISINFECTION OF PATIENT-CARE ITEMS

A. General Recommendations

1. Use only Food and Drug Administration (FDA)-cleared medical devices for sterilization and follow the manufacturer's instructions for correct use (IB).[248]

2. Clean and heat-sterilize critical dental instruments before each use (IA).[2,137,243,244,246,249,407]

3. Clean and heat-sterilize semicritical items before each use (IB).[2,249,260,407]

4. Allow packages to dry in the sterilizer before they are handled to avoid contamination (IB).[247]

5. Use of heat-stable semicritical alternatives is encouraged (IB).[2]

6. Reprocess heat-sensitive critical and semicritical instruments by using FDA-cleared sterilant/high-level disinfectants or an FDA-cleared low-temperature sterilization method (e.g., ethylene oxide). Follow manufacturer's instructions for use of chemical sterilants/high-level disinfectants (IB).[243]

7. Single-use disposable instruments are acceptable alternatives if they are used only once and disposed of correctly (IB, IC).[243,383]

8. Do not use liquid chemical sterilants/high-level disinfectants for environmental surface disinfection or as holding solutions (IB, IC).[243,245]

9. Ensure that noncritical patient-care items are barrier-protected or cleaned, or if visibly soiled, cleaned and disinfected after each use with a U.S. Environmental Protection Agency (EPA)-registered hospital disinfectant. If visibly contaminated with blood, use an EPA-registered hospital disinfectant with a tuberculocidal claim (i.e., intermediate level) (IB).[2,243,244]

10. Inform DHCP of all OSHA guidelines for exposure to chemical agents used for disinfection and sterilization. Using this report, identify areas and tasks that have potential for exposure (IC).[15]

B. Instrument Processing Area

1. Designate a central processing area. Divide the instrument processing area, physically or, at a minimum, spatially into distinct areas for 1) receiving, cleaning, and decontamination; 2) preparation and packaging; 3) sterilization; and 4) storage. Do not store instruments in an area where contaminated instruments are held or cleaned (II).[173,247,248]

2. Train DHCP to employ work practices that prevent contamination of clean areas (II).

C. Receiving, Cleaning, and Decontamination Work Area

1. Minimize handling of loose contaminated instruments during transport to the instrument processing area. Use work-practice controls (e.g., carry instruments in a covered container) to minimize exposure potential (II). Clean all visible blood and other contamination from dental instruments and devices before sterilization or disinfection procedures (IA).[243,249–252]

2. Use automated cleaning equipment (e.g., ultrasonic cleaner or washer-disinfector) to remove debris to improve cleaning effectiveness and decrease worker exposure to blood (IB).[2,253]

3. Use work-practice controls that minimize contact with sharp instruments if manual cleaning is necessary (e.g., long-handled brush) (IC).[14]

4. Wear puncture- and chemical-resistant/heavy-duty utility gloves for instrument cleaning and decontamination procedures (IB).[7]

5. Wear appropriate PPE (e.g., mask, protective eyewear, and gown) when splashing or spraying is anticipated during cleaning (IC).[13]

D. Preparation and Packaging

1. Use an internal chemical indicator in each package. If the internal indicator cannot be seen from outside the package, also use an external indicator (II).[243,254,257]

2. Use a container system or wrapping compatible with the type of sterilization process used and that has received FDA clearance (IB).[243,247,256]

3. Before sterilization of critical and semicritical instruments, inspect instruments for cleanliness, then wrap or place them in containers designed to maintain sterility during storage (e.g., cassettes and organizing trays) (IA).[2,247,255,256]

E. Sterilization of Unwrapped Instruments

1. Clean and dry instruments before the unwrapped sterilization cycle (IB).[248]

2. Use mechanical and chemical indicators for each unwrapped sterilization cycle (i.e., place an internal chemical indicator among the instruments or items to be sterilized) (IB).[243,258]

3. Allow unwrapped instruments to dry and cool in the sterilizer before they are handled to avoid contamination and thermal injury (II).[260]

4. Semicritical instruments that will be used immediately or within a short time can be sterilized unwrapped on a tray or in a container system, provided that the instruments are handled aseptically during removal from the sterilizer and transport to the point of use (II).

5. Critical instruments intended for immediate reuse can be sterilized unwrapped if the instruments are maintained sterile during removal from the sterilizer and transport to the point of use (e.g., transported in a sterile covered container) (IB).[258]

6. Do not sterilize implantable devices unwrapped (IB).[243,247]

7. Do not store critical instruments unwrapped (IB).[248]

F. Sterilization Monitoring

- Use mechanical, chemical, and biological monitors according to the manufacturer's instructions to ensure the effectiveness of the sterilization process (IB).[248,278,279]

- Monitor each load with mechanical (e.g., time, temperature, and pressure) and chemical indicators (II).[243,248]

- Place a chemical indicator on the inside of each package. If the internal indicator is not visible from the outside, also place an exterior chemical indicator on the package (II).[243,254,257]

- Place items/packages correctly and loosely into the sterilizer so as not to impede penetration of the sterilant (IB).[243]

- Do not use instrument packs if mechanical or chemical indicators indicate inadequate processing (IB).[243,247,248]

- Monitor sterilizers at least weekly by using a biological indicator with a matching control (i.e., biological indicator and control from same lot number) (IB).[2,9,243,247,278,279]

- Use a biological indicator for every sterilizer load that contains an implantable device. Verify results before using the implantable device, whenever possible (IB).[243,248]

- The following are recommended in the case of a positive spore test:
  A. Remove the sterilizer from service and review sterilization procedures (e.g., work practices and use of mechanical and chemical indicators) to determine whether operator error could be responsible (II).[8]
  B. Retest the sterilizer by using biological, mechanical, and chemical indicators after correcting any identified procedural problems (II).
  C. If the repeat spore test is negative, and mechanical and chemical indicators are within normal limits, put the sterilizer back in service (II).[9,243]

- The following are recommended if the repeat spore test is positive:
  A. Do not use the sterilizer until it has been inspected or repaired or the exact reason for the positive test has been determined (II).[9,243]
  B. Recall, to the extent possible, and reprocess all items processed since the last negative spore test (II).[9,243,283]
  C. Before placing the sterilizer back in service, rechallenge the sterilizer with biological indicator tests in three consecutive empty chamber sterilization cycles after the cause of the sterilizer failure has been determined and corrected (II).[9,243,283]

- Maintain sterilization records (i.e., mechanical, chemical, and biological) in compliance with state and local regulations (IB).[243]

G. Storage Area for Sterilized Items and Clean Dental Supplies

1. Implement practices on the basis of date- or event-related shelf-life for storage of wrapped, sterilized instruments and devices (IB).[243,284]

2. Even for event-related packaging, at a minimum, place the date of sterilization, and if multiple sterilizers are used in the facility, the sterilizer used, on the outside of the packaging material to facilitate the retrieval of processed items in the event of a sterilization failure (IB).[243,247]

3. Examine wrapped packages of sterilized instruments before opening them to ensure the barrier wrap has not been compromised during storage (II).[243,284]

4. Reclean, repack, and resterilize any instrument package that has been compromised (II).

5. Store sterile items and dental supplies in covered or closed cabinets, if possible (II).[285]

VII. ENVIRONMENTAL INFECTION CONTROL

A. General Recommendations

1. Follow the manufacturers' instructions for correct use of cleaning and EPA-registered hospital disinfecting products (IB, IC).[243–245]

2. Do not use liquid chemical sterilants/high-level disinfectants for disinfection of environmental surfaces (clinical contact or housekeeping) (IB, IC).[243–245]

3. Use PPE, as appropriate, when cleaning and disinfecting environmental surfaces. Such equipment might include gloves (e.g., puncture- and chemical-resistant utility), protective clothing (e.g., gown, jacket, or lab coat), and protective eyewear/face shield, and mask (IC).[13,15]

B. Clinical Contact Surfaces

1. Use surface barriers to protect clinical contact surfaces, particularly those that are difficult to clean (e.g., switches on dental chairs) and change surface barriers between patients (II).[1,2,260,288]

2. Clean and disinfect clinical contact surfaces that are not barrier-protected, by using an EPA-registered hospital disinfectant with a low- (i.e., human immunodeficiency virus [HIV] and HBV label claims) to intermediate-level (i.e., tuberculocidal claim) activity after each patient. Use an intermediate-level disinfectant if visibly contaminated with blood (IB).[2,243,244]

C. Housekeeping Surfaces

1. Clean housekeeping surfaces (e.g., floors, walls, and sinks) with a detergent and water or an EPA-registered hospital disinfectant/detergent on a routine basis, depending on the nature of the surface and type and degree of contamination, and as appropriate, based on the location in the facility, and when visibly soiled (IB).[243,244]

2. Clean mops and cloths after use and allow to dry before reuse; or use single-use, disposable mop heads or cloths (II).[243,244]

3. Prepare fresh cleaning or EPA-registered disinfecting solutions daily and as instructed by the manufacturer (II).[243,244]

4. Clean walls, blinds, and window curtains in patient-care areas when they are visibly dusty or soiled (II).[9,244]

D. Spills of Blood and Body Substances

1. Clean spills of blood or OPIM and decontaminate surface with an EPA-registered hospital disinfectant with low-level (i.e., HBV and HIV label claims) to intermediate-level (i.e., tuberculocidal claim) activity, depending on size of spill and surface porosity (IB, IC).[13,113]

E. Carpet and Cloth Furnishings

1. Avoid using carpeting and cloth-upholstered furnishings in dental operatories, laboratories, and instrument processing areas (II).[9,293–295]

F. Regulated Medical Waste

■ General Recommendations

A. Develop a medical waste management program. Disposal of regulated medical waste must follow federal, state, and local regulations (IC).[13,301]

B. Ensure that DHCP who handle and dispose of regulated medical waste are trained in appropriate handling and disposal methods and are informed of the possible health and safety hazards (IC).[13]

■ Management of Regulated Medical Waste in Dental Health-Care Facilities

A. Use a color-coded or labeled container that prevents leakage (e.g., biohazard bag) to contain non-sharp regulated medical waste (IC).[13]

B. Place sharp items (e.g., needles, scalpel blades, orthodontic bands, broken metal instruments, and burs) in an appropriate sharps container (e.g., puncture resistant, color-coded, and leakproof). Close container immediately before removal or replacement to prevent spillage or protrusion of contents during handling, storage, transport, or shipping (IC).[2,8,13,113,115]

C. Pour blood, suctioned fluids, or other liquid waste carefully into a drain connected to a sanitary sewer system, if local sewage discharge requirements are met and the state has declared this an acceptable method of disposal. Wear appropriate PPE while performing this task (IC).[7,9,13]

VIII. DENTAL UNIT WATERLINES, BIOFILM, AND WATER QUALITY

A. General Recommendations

1. Use water that meets EPA regulatory standards for drinking water (i.e., ≤500 CFU/mL of heterotrophic water bacteria) for routine dental treatment output water (IB, IC).[341,342]

2. Consult with the dental unit manufacturer for appropriate methods and equipment to maintain the recommended quality of dental water (II).[339]

3. Follow recommendations for monitoring water quality provided by the manufacturer of the unit or waterline treatment product (II).

4. Discharge water and air for a minimum of 20–30 seconds after each patient, from any device connected to the dental water system that enters the patient's mouth (e.g., handpieces, ultrasonic scalers, and air/water syringes) (II).[2,311,344]

5. Consult with the dental unit manufacturer on the need for periodic maintenance of antiretraction mechanisms (IB).[2,311]

B. Boil-Water Advisories

■ The following apply while a boil-water advisory is in effect:
A. Do not deliver water from the public water system to the patient through the dental operative unit, ultrasonic scaler, or other dental equipment that uses the public water system (IB, IC).[341,342,346,349,350]
B. Do not use water from the public water system for dental treatment, patient rinsing, or handwashing (IB, IC).[341,342,346,349,350]
C. For handwashing, use antimicrobial-containing products that do not require water for use (e.g., alcohol-based hand rubs). If hands are visibly contaminated, use bottled water, if available, and soap for handwashing or an antiseptic towelette (IB, IC).[13,122]

■ The following apply when the boil-water advisory is cancelled:
A. Follow guidance given by the local water utility regarding adequate flushing of waterlines. If no guidance is provided, flush dental waterlines and faucets for 1–5 minutes before using for patient care (IC).[244,346,351,352]
B. Disinfect dental waterlines as recommended by the dental unit manufacturer (II).

IX. SPECIAL CONSIDERATIONS

A. Dental Handpieces and Other Devices Attached to Air and Waterlines

1. Clean and heat-sterilize handpieces and other intraoral instruments that can be removed from the air and waterlines of dental units between patients (IB, IC).[2,246,275,356,357,360,407]

2. Follow the manufacturer's instructions for cleaning, lubrication, and sterilization of handpieces and other intraoral instruments that can be removed from the air and waterlines of dental units (IB).[361–363]

3. Do not surface-disinfect, use liquid chemical sterilants, or ethylene oxide on handpieces and other intraoral instruments that can be removed from the air and waterlines of dental units (IC).[2,246,250,275]

4. Do not advise patients to close their lips tightly around the tip of the saliva ejector to evacuate oral fluids (II).[364–366]

B. Dental Radiology

■ Wear gloves when exposing radiographs and handling contaminated film packets. Use other PPE (e.g., protective eyewear, mask, and gown) as appropriate if spattering of blood or other body fluids is likely (IA, IC).[11,13]

■ Use heat-tolerant or disposable intraoral devices whenever possible (e.g., film-holding and positioning devices). Clean and heat-sterilize heat-tolerant devices between patients. At a minimum, high-level disinfect semicritical heat-sensitive devices, according to manufacturer's instructions (IB).[243]

■ Transport and handle exposed radiographs in an aseptic manner to prevent contamination of developing equipment (II).

■ The following apply for digital radiography sensors:
A. Use FDA-cleared barriers (IB).[243]
B. Clean and heat-sterilize, or high-level disinfect, between patients, barrier-protected semicritical items. If the item cannot tolerate these procedures, then, at a minimum, protect with an FDA-cleared barrier and clean and disinfect with an EPA-registered hospital disinfectant with intermediate-level (i.e., tuberculocidal claim) activity, between patients. Consult with the manufacturer for methods of disinfection and sterilization of digital radiology sensors and for protection of associated computer hardware (IB).[243]

C. Aseptic Technique for Parenteral Medications

■ Do not administer medication from a syringe to multiple patients, even if the needle on the syringe is changed (IA).[378]

■ Use single-dose vials for parenteral medications when possible (II).[376,377]

■ Do not combine the leftover contents of single use vials for later use (IA).[376,377]

■ The following apply if multidose vials are used:
A. Cleanse the access diaphragm with 70% alcohol before inserting a device into the vial (IA).[380,381]
B. Use a sterile device to access a multiple-dose vial and avoid touching the access diaphragm. Both the needle and syringe used to access the multidose vial should be sterile. Do not reuse a syringe even if the needle is changed (IA).[380,381]
C. Keep multidose vials away from the immediate patient treatment area to prevent inadvertent contamination by spray or spatter (II).
D. Discard the multidose vial if sterility is compromised (IA).[380,381]

■ Use fluid infusion and administration sets (i.e., IV bags, tubings, and connections) for one patient only and dispose of appropriately (IB).[378]

D. Single-Use (Disposable) Devices

1. Use single-use devices for one patient only and dispose of them appropriately (IC).[383]

E. Preprocedural Mouthrinses

1. No recommendation is offered regarding use of preprocedural antimicrobial mouthrinses to prevent clinical infections among DHCP or patients. Although studies have demonstrated that a preprocedural antimicrobial rinse (e.g., chlorhexidine gluconate, essential oils, or povidoneiodine) can reduce the level of oral microorganisms in aerosols and spatter generated during routine dental procedures and can decrease the number of microorganisms introduced in the patient's bloodstream during invasive dental procedures,[391–399] the scientific evidence is inconclusive that using these rinses prevents clinical infections among DHCP or patients (see discussion, Preprocedural Mouthrinses) (Unresolved issue).

F. Oral Surgical Procedures

- The following apply when performing oral surgical procedures:
  A. Perform surgical hand antisepsis by using an antimicrobial product (e.g., antimicrobial soap and water, or soap and water followed by alcohol-based hand scrub with persistent activity) before donning sterile surgeon's gloves (IB).[127–132,137]
  B. Use sterile surgeon's gloves (IB).[2,7,121,123,137]
  C. Use sterile saline or sterile water as a coolant/irritant when performing oral surgical procedures.
  D. Use devices specifically designed for delivering sterile irrigating fluids (e.g., bulb syringe, single-use disposable products, and sterilizable tubing) (IB).[2,121]

G. Handling of Biopsy Specimens

1. During transport, place biopsy specimens in a sturdy, leakproof container labeled with the biohazard symbol (IC).[2,13,14]
2. If a biopsy specimen container is visibly contaminated, clean and disinfect the outside of a container or place it in an impervious bag labeled with the biohazard symbol, (IC).[2,13]

H. Handling of Extracted Teeth

1. Dispose of extracted teeth as regulated medical waste unless returned to the patient (IC).[13,14]
2. Do not dispose of extracted teeth containing amalgam in regulated medical waste intended for incineration (II).
3. Clean and place extracted teeth in a leakproof container, labeled with a biohazard symbol, and maintain hydration for transport to educational institutions or a dental laboratory (IC).[13,14]
4. Heat-sterilize teeth that do not contain amalgam before they are used for educational purposes (IB).[403,405,406]

I. Dental Laboratory

1. Use PPE when handling items received in the laboratory until they have been decontaminated (IA, IC).[2,7,11,13,113]
2. Before they are handled in the laboratory, clean, disinfect, and rinse all dental prostheses and prosthodontic materials (e.g., impressions, bite registrations, occlusal rims, and extracted teeth) by using an EPA-registered hospital disinfectant having at least an intermediate-level (i.e., tuberculocidal claim) activity (IB).[2,249,252,407]
3. Consult with manufacturers regarding the stability of specific materials (e.g., impression materials) relative to disinfection procedures (II).
4. Include specific information regarding disinfection techniques used (e.g., solution used and duration), when laboratory cases are sent off-site and on their return (II).[2,407,409]
5. Clean and heat-sterilize heat-tolerant items used in the mouth (e.g., metal impression trays and face-bow forks) (IB).[2,407]
6. Follow manufacturers' instructions for cleaning and sterilizing or disinfecting items that become contaminated but do not normally contact the patient (e.g., burs, polishing points, rag wheels, articulators, case pans, and lathes). If manufacturer instructions are unavailable, clean and heat-sterilize heat-tolerant items or clean and disinfect with an EPA-registered hospital disinfectant with low-level (HIV, HBV effectiveness claim) to intermediate-level (tuberculocidal claim) activity, depending on the degree of contamination (II).

J. Laser/Electrosurgery Plumes/ Surgical Smoke

1. No recommendation is offered regarding practices to reduce DHCP exposure to laser plumes/surgical smoke when using lasers in dental practice. Practices to reduce HCP exposure to laser plumes/surgical smoke have been suggested, including use of a) standard precautions (e.g., high-filtration surgical masks and possibly full face shields)[437]; b) central room suction units with in-line filters to collect particulate matter from minimal plumes; and c) dedicated mechanical smoke exhaust systems with a high-efficiency filter to remove substantial amounts of laser-plume particles. The effect of the exposure (e.g., disease transmission or adverse respiratory effects) on DHCP from dental applications of lasers has not been adequately evaluated (see previous discussion, Laser/Electrosurgery Plumes or Surgical Smoke) (Unresolved issue).

K. Mycobacterium Tuberculosis

- General Recommendations
  A. Educate all DHCP regarding the recognition of signs, symptoms, and transmission of tuberculosis (TB) (IB).[20,21]

B. Conduct a baseline TST, preferably by using a two-step test, for all DHCP who might have contact with persons with suspected or confirmed active TB, regardless of the risk classification of the setting (IB).[20]

C. Assess each patient for a history of TB as well as symptoms indicative of TB and document on the medical history form (IB).[20,21]

D. Follow CDC recommendations for 1) developing, maintaining, and implementing a written TB infection-control plan; 2) managing a patient with suspected or active TB; 3) completing a community risk-assessment to guide employee TSTs and follow-up; and 4) managing DHCP with TB disease (IB).[2,21]

■ The following apply for patients known or suspected to have active *TB*:

A. Evaluate the patient away from other patients and DHCP. When not being evaluated, the patient should wear a surgical mask or be instructed to cover mouth and nose when coughing or sneezing (IB).[20,21]

B. Defer elective dental treatment until the patient is noninfectious (IB).[20,21]

C. Refer patients requiring urgent dental treatment to a previously identified facility with TB engineering controls and a respiratory protection program (IB).[20,21]

L. Creutzfeldt-Jakob Disease (CJD) and Other Prion Diseases

1. No recommendation is offered regarding use of special precautions in addition to standard precautions when treating known CJD or vCJD patients. Potential infectivity of oral tissues in CJD or vCJD patients is an unresolved issue. Scientific data indicate the risk, if any, of sporadic CJD transmission during dental and oral surgical procedures is low to nil. Until additional information exists regarding the transmissibility of CJD or vCJD during dental procedures, special precautions in addition to standard precautions might be indicated when treating known CJD or vCJD patients; a list of such precautions is provided for consideration without recommendation (see Creutzfeldt Jakob Disease and Other Prion Diseases) (Unresolved issue).

M. Program Evaluation

1. Establish routine evaluation of the infection-control program, including evaluation of performance indicators, at an established frequency (II).[470,471]

ACKNOWLEDGMENT

The Division of Oral Health thanks the working group as well as CDC and other federal and external reviewers for their efforts in developing and reviewing drafts of this report and acknowledges that all opinions of the reviewers might not be reflected in all of the recommendations.

Reference

A comprehensive list of references can be found in the original article: Centers for Disease Control and Prevention. Guidelines for Infection Control in Dental Health-Care Settings—2003. *MMWR*. Dec 2003;52(RR-17):1–61. Additional resources are available from: http://www.cdc.gov/oralhealth/infectioncontrol/guidelines [accessed Oct 2011].

Average Measurements of Human Teeth

TABLE A-1	AVERAGE MEASUREMENTS OF THE PRIMARY TEETH (IN MILLIMETERS)				
		OVERALL LENGTH	**LENGTH OF CROWN**	**LENGTH OF ROOT**	**WIDTH OF CROWN (MESIALDISTAL AT WIDEST POINT)**
Maxillary	Central Incisor	16.0	6.0	10.0	6.5
	Lateral Incisor	15.8	5.6	11.4	5.1
	Canine	19.0	6.5	13.5	7.0
	First Molar	15.2	5.1	10.0	7.3
	Second Molar	17.5	5.7	11.7	8.2
Mandibular	Central Incisor	14.0	5.0	9.0	4.2
	Lateral Incisor	15.0	5.2	10.0	4.1
	Canine	17.5	6.0	11.5	5.0
	First Molar	15.8	6.0	9.8	7.7
	Second Molar	18.8	5.5	11.3	9.9

(Reprinted with permission from Black, G.V. *Descriptive Anatomy of the Human Teeth*, 4th ed. Philadelphia, The S.S. White Dental Manufacturing Company, 1897, according to Ash, M.M.: *Wheeler's Dental Anatomy, Physiology, and Occlusion*, 7th ed. Philadelphia, W.B. Saunders, Co., 1993, p. 58.)

TABLE A-2	AVERAGE MEASUREMENTS OF THE PERMANENT TEETH (IN MILLIMETERS)

		OVERALL LENGTH	LENGTH OF CROWN	LENGTH OF ROOT	WIDTH OF CROWN (MESIALDISTAL AT WIDEST POINT)
Maxillary	Central Incisor	23.5	10.5	13.0	8.5
	Lateral Incisor	22.0	9.9	13.0	6.5
	Canine	27.0	10.0	17.0	7.5
	First Premolar	22.5	8.5	14.0	7.0
	Second Premolar	22.5	8.5	14.0	7.0
	First Molar	B* L 19.5 20.5	7.5	B L 12 13	10.0
	Second Molar	B L 17.0 19.0	7.0	B L 11 12	9.0
	Third Molar	17.5	6.5	11.0	8.5
Mandibular	Central Incisor	21.5	9.0	12.5	5.0
	Lateral Incisor	23.5	9.5	14.0	5.5
	Canine	27.0	11.0	16.0	7.0
	First Premolar	22.5	8.5	14.0	7.0
	Second Premolar	22.5	8.0	14.5	7.0
	First Molar	21.5	7.5	14.0	11.0
	Second Molar	20.0	7.0	13.0	10.5
	Third Molar	18.0	7.0	11.0	10.0

* = Buccal measurement; L = Lingual measurement.
(Reprinted with permission from Ash, M.M.: Wheeler's Dental Anatomy, Physiology, and Occulsion, 7th ed. Philadelphia, W.B. Saunders, Co., 1993, p. 15.)

Prefixes, Suffixes, and Combining Forms

A

a-, an- absence, lack, without, e.g., *a*morphous
ab- from, away, e.g., *ab*normal
ad- (change d to c, f, g, p, s, or t before words beginning with those consonants) to, toward, e.g., *ad*hesion, *ac*cretion
adeno- gland, e.g., *adeno*fibroma
-algia pain, e.g., neur*algia*
ambi- all (both) sides, round, e.g., *ambi*dexterity
amelo- enamel, e.g., *amelo*genesis
amphi-, ampho- on both sides, double, e.g., *ampho*diplopia
ana- up, excessive, again, e.g., *ana*bolism
andro- masculine, male, e.g., *andro*gen
angio- vessel, e.g., *angio*ma
ante- before, e.g., *ante*febrile
anti- against, e.g., *anti*dote
aqu-, aqua- water, e.g., *aqu*eous
arthro-, arth- joints, e.g., *arth*ritis
-ase denotes an enzyme, e.g., dextrin*ase*
-asthenia weakness, e.g., my*asthenia* gravis
auto-, aut- self, e.g., *auto*transplant

B

bi- two, twice, double, e.g., *bi*furcation
bio-, bi- life, living, e.g., *bio*psy
-blast formative cell, e.g., osteo*blast*
-brachy- short, e.g., *brachy*dactylic
brady- slow, e.g., *brady*cardia
bucc- cheek, e.g., *bucc*inator

C

calc- stone, calcium, lime, e.g., *calc*ification
cardio-, cardi- heart, e.g., *cardio*vascular
cata- down, against, e.g., *cata*bolism
-cele swelling, protrusion, hernia, e.g., meningo*cele*
cephalo-, cephal- head, e.g., *cephalo*metry
cerebro-, cerebr- brain, e.g., *cerebr*al palsy
cheilo-, cheil- lip, e.g., *cheil*itis
chloro-, chlor- pale green, e.g., *chloro*phyll
chromo-, chromat- color, pigmentation, e.g., *chromo*genic
-cidal killing, e.g., bacter*icidal*
-clast break up, divide into parts, e.g., osteo*clast*
-clus- shut, e.g., oc*clus*ion
co-, com-, con-, cor- with, together, e.g., *con*genital
coll- glue, e.g., *coll*oid
contra- opposite, e.g., *contra*lateral
cryo, cry- cold, freezing, e.g., *cry*otherapy
cuti- skin, e.g., *cuti*cle
cyan- blue, e.g., *cyan*otic
-cyto-, -cyt- cell, e.g., leuko*cyte*

D

-dactyl, dactylo- fingers, e.g., *dactyl*edema
de- down, away from, separation, e.g., *de*calcification
denti-, dent- tooth, e.g., *dent*ition
-derm-, derma- skin, e.g., hypo*derm*ic
dextr-, dextro- right, toward right, e.g., *dextro*cardia
di- twice, two, e.g., *di*plopia
dis- separation, opposite, taking apart, e.g., *dis*infect
disto-, dist- posterior, distant from center, e.g., *disto*buccal

-drome course, e.g., syn*drome*
dur- hard, e.g., in*dur*ation
dys- bad, ill, difficult, e.g., *dys*trophy

E

ecto-, ect- without, outer side, e.g., *ecto*derm
-ectomy surgical removal, e.g., gingi*vectomy*
-emia (-aemia) blood condition, e.g., bacter*emia*
en- in, on, into, e.g., *en*demic
encephal-, encephalo- brain, e.g., *encephalo*meningitis
endo- inside, e.g., *endo*dontics
entero-, enter- intestine, e.g., *entero*toxin
epi- upon, after, in addition, e.g., *epi*dermis
erythro-, eryth- red, e.g., *eryth*ema
esthesio-, esthesia (-aesthesia) sensation, perception, e.g., an*esthesia*
ex- beyond, from, out of, e.g., *ex*udate
extra- outside of, beyond the scope of, e.g., *extra*cellular

F

faci- face, e.g., *faci*al
-facient causes or brings about, e.g., rube*facient*
-ferent carry, bear, e.g., af*ferent*
fibro-, fibr- fibers, fibrous tissue, e.g., *fibro*blast
fract- break, e.g., *fract*ional

G

galacto-, galact- milk, e.g., *galact*ose
gastro-, gastr- stomach, e.g., *gastr*itis
-gen- produced, e.g., glyco*gen*
genio- chin, lower jaw, e.g., *genio*plasty
germ- bud, early growth, e.g., *germ*inal
gero- old age, e.g., *gero*dontics
glosso-, gloss- tongue, e.g., *gloss*itis
gluco-, glue- glucose, e.g., *gluco*neogenesis
glyco-, glyc- sweet, e.g., *glyc*erin
gnatho-, gnath- jaw, e.g., *gnatho*dynamometer
-gnosis knowledge, e.g., pro*gnosis*
-gram, -graph write, draw, e.g., radio*graphic*
gran- grain, particle, e.g., *gran*uloma
gyn-, gyne-, gynec- woman, e.g., *gyne*cology

H

hemi- half, e.g., *hemi*section
hemo- (haemo-) blood, e.g., *hemo*rrhage
hepato-, hepat- liver, e.g., *hepat*itis
hetero-, heter- other, different, e.g., *hetero*geneous
histo-, hist- tissue, e.g., *hist*ology
homo-, homeo- like, similar, e.g., *homeo*stasis
hydro-, hydr- water, e.g., *hydro*cephalic
hygro-, hygr- moisture, e.g., *hygro*phobia
hyper- abnormal, excessive, e.g., *hyper*trophy
hypno-, hypn- sleep, e.g., *hypn*otic

hypo-, hyp- deficiency, lack, below, e.g., *hypo*tonic
hystero-, hyster- uterus or hysteria, e.g., *hyster*ectomy

I

-ia state or condition, e.g., glycosur*ia*
iatro- relation to medicine, a physician, dentist, or other health professional, e.g., *iatro*genic
-ic of, pertaining to, e.g., gastr*ic*
idio- one's own, separate, distinct, e.g., *idio*pathic
in- not, without, e.g., *in*activate
infra- beneath, below, e.g., *infra*orbital
inter- between, among, e.g., *inter*cellular
intra- within, into, e.g., *intra*oral
ischo-, isch- suppression, stoppage, e.g., *isch*emia
iso- equality, similarity, e.g., *iso*tonic
-ist one who practices, holds certain principles, e.g., hygien*ist*
-itis inflammation, e.g., dermat*itis*

J

-ject- throw, e.g., in*ject*ion
juxta- next to, near, e.g., *juxta*position

K

karyo-, kary- nucleus of a cell, e.g., *kary*olysis
kerato-, kerat- horny, keratinized tissue, e.g., *kerat*inization
kin- move, e.g., *kin*etic

L

labio- lip, e.g., *labio*version
lacto-, lact- milk, e.g., *lact*ation
laryngo-, laryn- larynx, e.g., *laryn*gitis
later- side, e.g., *later*oversion
leuko-, leuk- white, e.g., *leuko*plakia
linguo-, lingu- tongue, e.g., *lingu*al
lipo-, lip- fat, fatty, e.g., *lip*oma
-logy doctrine, science, e.g., periodonto*logy*
lympho-, lymph- lymph, e.g., *lymph*angioma
-lysin, -lysis, -lytic dissolving, destructive, e.g., hemo*lysis*

M

macro-, macr- enlargement, elongated part, e.g., *macro*dontia
mal- bad, ill, e.g., *mal*nutrition
mast-, mastro- breast, e.g., *mast*ectomy
-megalo-, -megal- large, great, e.g., *megalo*blast
melano- dark-colored, relating to melanin, e.g., *melano*genesis
meningo-, mening- meninges, e.g., *mening*itis
meno- month, e.g., *meno*pause

mes-, medi, mesio- middle, intermediate, e.g., *mes*oderm

meta-, met- over, beyond, transformation, e.g., *meta*bolism

metro-, metra- uterus, e.g., *metro*fibroma

-metry measure, e.g., cephalo*metry*

micro-, micr- small, e.g., *micr*oorganism

mono- one, single, e.g., *mono*saccharide

morpho-, morph- form, shape, e.g., *morph*ology

muco-, muc- relating to mucous membrane, e.g., *muco*gingival

myel-, myelo- bone marrow, spinal cord, e.g., *myelo*blast

mylo- molar teeth or posterior portion of mandible, e.g., *mylo*hyoid

myo-, my- muscle, e.g., *my*ocardium

N

naso- nose, e.g., *naso*palatine

necr- death, e.g., *necr*otic

neo-, ne- new, recent, e.g., *neo*plasm

nephro-, nephr- kidneys, e.g., *nephr*itis

neuro-, neuri-, neur- pertaining to nerves, e.g., *neur*asthenia

nucleo-, nucle- pertaining to nucleus, e.g., *nucleo*protein

O

ob- (change b to c before words beginning with c) against, toward, e.g., *oc*clusion

odonto-, odont- tooth, e.g., *odont*algia

-oid like, resembling, e.g., ame*boid*

-olig-, oligo- a few, a little, e.g., *oligo*dontia

-oma swelling, tumor, e.g., lip*oma*

-opia, -opy sight, eye defect, e.g., my*opia*

oro- mouth, oral, e.g., *oro*nasal

ortho-, orth- straight, normal, e.g., *ortho*dontics

-osis condition, state, e.g., cyan*osis*

osteo-, oste- bone, e.g., *osteo*porosis

oto-, ot- ear, e.g., *oto*plasty

-ous full of, having, e.g., aque*ous*

ovi-, ovo-, ovu- egg, e.g., *ovu*lation

P

pan- all, every, general, e.g., *pan*acea

para- beyond, beside, near, e.g., *para*site

patho-, path- disease, e.g., *patho*gnomonic

pedia-, pedo- (paedo-) child, e.g., *pedo*dontics

-penia deficiency, e.g., leuko*penia*

per- throughout, completely, e.g., *per*cussion

peri- around, near, e.g., *peri*apical

phago- to eat, e.g., *phago*cytic

-phile, -phil- loving, e.g., hemo*philia*

phlebo-, phleb- vein, e.g., *phleb*itis

-phobe, -phobia fear, dread, e.g., photo*phobia*

pilo- hair, e.g., *pilo*erection

-plas- mold, shape, e.g., gingivo*plasty*

plasmo-, plasm form, e.g., cyto*plasm*

-plegia, -plexy paralysis, stroke, e.g., hemi*plegia*

pleo- more, e.g., *pleo*morphism

-pnea (-pnoea) breathing, e.g., dys*pnea*

pneumo- air, lung, e.g., *pneumo*thorax

-poiesis, -poietic production, e.g., erythro*poietic*

poly- many, much, e.g., *poly*saccharide

pont- bridge, e.g., *pont*ic

poro-, -por- opening, pore, duct, e.g., *por*ous

post- behind, after, e.g., *post*natal

pre- before, in front of, e.g., *pre*maxilla

pro- before, in front of, e.g., *pro*gnathic

proprio- one's own, e.g., *proprio*ceptive

proto- first, e.g., *proto*plasm

pseudo- false, deceptive, e.g., *pseudo*membrane

psycho-, psych- mind, mental processes, e.g., *psycho*somatic

pulmo- lung, e.g., *pulmo*nary

pur- pus, e.g., *pur*ulent

pyo- pus, e.g., *pyo*rrhea

pyro- fever, heat, e.g., *pyro*genic

R

re- back, again, e.g., *re*gurgitate

-renal kidney, e.g., ad*renal*

retro- back, backward, behind, e.g., *retro*molar

-rhage breaking, bursting forth, profuse flow, e.g., hemor*rhage*

-rhea (-rhoea) flow, discharge, e.g., pyor*rhea*

rhino-, rhin- nose, e.g., *rhin*itis

rube- red, e.g., *rube*facient

S

sarco- flesh, muscle, e.g., *sarco*ma

sclero- hard, e.g., *sclero*derma

-scopy examination, inspection, e.g., micro*scopy*

semi- half, partly, e.g., *semi*permeable

sero- serum, serous, e.g., *sero*purulent

sial-, sialo- saliva, e.g., *sialo*graphy

somat-, somato-, -some body, e.g., chromo*some*

-squam- scale, e.g., de*squam*ative

stomat- mouth, e.g., *stomat*itis

sub- beneath, under, deficient, e.g., *sub*acute

super- above, upon, excessive, e.g., *super*numerary tooth

syn- with, together, e.g., *syn*drome

T

tachy- swift, e.g., *tachy*cardia

tact- touch, e.g., *tact*ile

tera-, terato- monster, malformed fetus, e.g., *terato*genic

thermo- heat, e.g., *thermo*phile

thrombo-, thromb- clot, coagulation, e.g., *thromb*in

-thym-, thymo- mind, soul, emotions, e.g., dys*thym*ia

trans- beyond, through, across, e.g., *trans*plantation
tropho-, trophic nutrition, nourishment, e.g.,
  hyper*trophic*
-tropic turning toward, changing, e.g., hydro*tropic*

U

-ule diminutive, small, e.g., tub*ule*
-uria urine, e.g., glucos*uria*

V

vaso- blood vessels, e.g., *vaso*dilation
vita- life, e.g., *vita*min

X

xero- dry, e.g., *xero*stomia

Charting Symbols and Standardized Abbreviations Useful for Documenting Dental Hygiene Care*

SELECTED SYMBOLS COMMONLY USED IN DENTAL CHARTING	
SYMBOL	MEANING
"X" or " = "	Missing tooth or pontic
≠	Fracture
||	Open contact
↑	Increase
↓	Decrease
→ midline ←	Drifted mesially
← midline →	Drifted distally
↻	Rotated clockwise
↺	Rotated counterclockwise
C/	Complete upper denture
/C	Complete lower denture

STANDARDIZED ABBREVIATIONS	
ABBREVIATION	TERM
abn	abnormal
BOP	bleeding on probing
bp	blood pressure
brux	bruxism or bruxer
bw, bwx, or bwxr; pa or pax; pan or pano	bite wing radiograph; periapical radiograph; panoramic radiograph
CAL	clinical attachment level
Calc	calculus
CC	chief complaint
CEJ	cementoenamel junction
chk	check, observe
cm	centimeter
cons	consultation
debrd	debridement
decid	deciduous, primary
demo	demonstrate
dent hx	dental history
dup	duplicate

*Selected from the complete list available in: American Dental Association. Dental abbreviations, symbols, and acronyms. 2nd ed. Chicago; American Dental Association; 2008. 5–20 pp. Used with permission.

ABBREVIATION	TERM
emerg	emergency
esp	especially
eval	evaluate, evaluation
Ex, exam	examination
exf	exfoliate
ext	extraction
f/u	follow-up
F, fl, Ftx APF NaF	fluoride, fluoride treatment; acidulated phosphate fluoride; sodium fluoride;
fgm	free gingival margin
food imp	food impaction
fur, furc	furcation
ging	gingival, gingival
H, hx, hist, h/o	history, history of
HH, med hx	health history, medical history
htn	hypertension
hyg	dental hygiene
IC	informed consent
INS	Insurance
LA; lido xylo; vaso	local anesthesia, Lidocaine; Xylocaine; vasoconstrictor
mand; max	mandibular; maxillary
mdl	midline
meds	medications
n/a; n/c; n/d	not applicable; no change; not determined
NKA; NKDA	no known allergies; no known drug allergies
nv	next visit

ABBREVIATION	TERM
occ, occl	occlusal or occlusion
OHI	oral hygiene instructions
OTC	over the counter
pk, pkt	Pocket
POI	post operative instructions
pol	Polish
pre op; post op	preoperative, postoperative
prev	prevention, preventive
prog, Px	prognosis
pt	patient
quad; LRQ; URQ	quadrant; lower right quadrant; upper right quadrant
reapp, reappt	reappoint(ment)
re-eval	re-evaluation
rp/sc, RPS, S&RP, SRP	scaling and root planing
Rx	prescription
S&Sx, S/S	signs and symptoms
S/D BP	systolic/diastolic blood pressure
stat	immediately
sut	suture
sub, subggv, subgin	subgingival
Supra ggv	supragingival
tb	toothbrush
Tx	treatment
unk	unknown
var	varnish
wnl	within normal limits